Discover Sherpath®

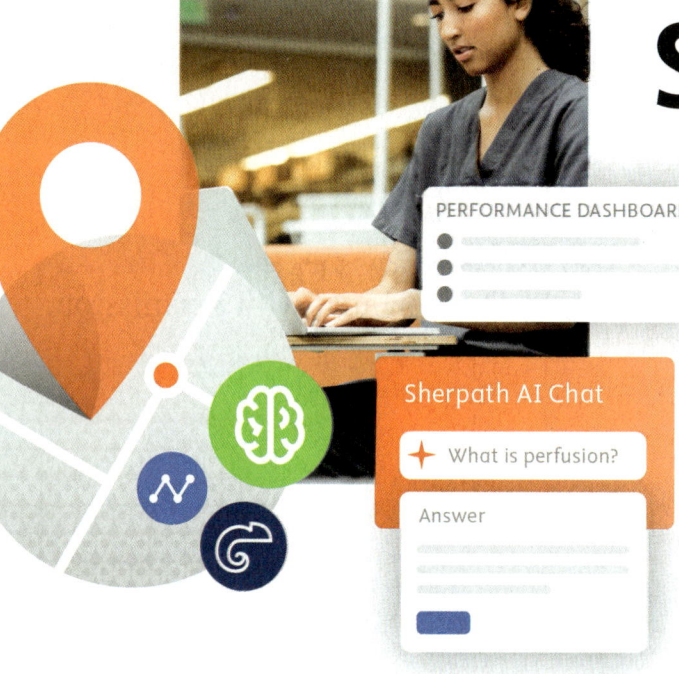

The digital teaching and learning technology built specifically for healthcare education.

Sherpath's all-in-one course delivery solution powers your textbook with innovative resources, including the following:

Digital lessons aligned with learning objectives create an interactive experience with multimedia, adaptive remediation, assignment assessments, and more.*

eBook and resources are seamlessly accessible within Sherpath for quick access to relevant course materials, activities, and reading recommendations.

Elsevier Adaptive Quizzing customizes quizzes based on performance and allows you to choose relevant quiz topics.

Performance dashboard offers a holistic view of course progress and areas of strength and weakness.

Sherpath AI is a conversational AI tool that generates personalized answers to questions, sourced solely from Elsevier's vast library of trusted, evidence-based content.

Osmosis® bite-sized, illustrated health education videos simplify complex concepts and promote active learning. A curated collection of Osmosis videos are seamlessly integrated into your Sherpath course.*

*Only available for select collections.

And more!

STUDENTS — Ask your instructor about enhancing your course experience with Sherpath!

INSTRUCTORS — Scan code or visit myevolve.us/spnu to learn more!

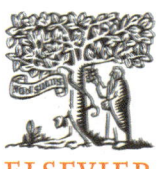

24-0481 TM/AF

ELSEVIER

ABOUT THE COVER
Cover image by Prof. Kenneth Morgan, PhD. Reprinted with permission.

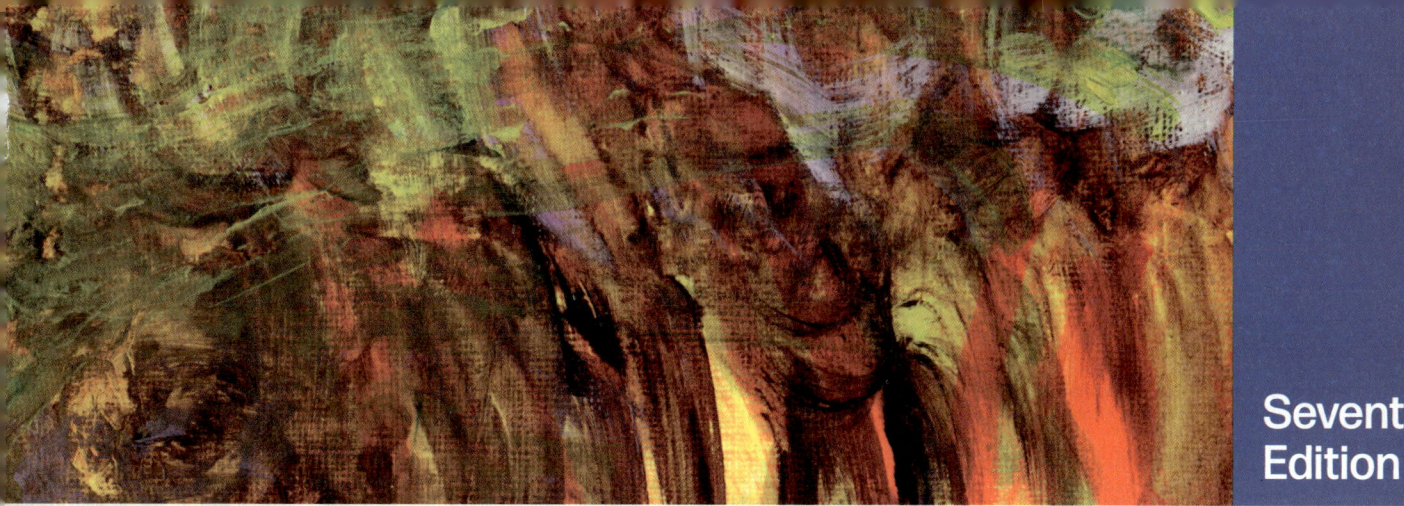

Seventh Edition

GERONTOLOGIC NURSING

Jennifer J. Yeager
PhD, MSN, RN
Associate Professor of Nursing
Tarleton State University
Stephenville, Texas

Mary B. Winton
PhD, MSN, RN
Associate Professor of Nursing
Tarleton State University
Stephenville, Texas

Sue E. Meiner
EdD, APRN, BC-GNP
President
Consultant on Health Issues, Inc.
McKinney, Texas

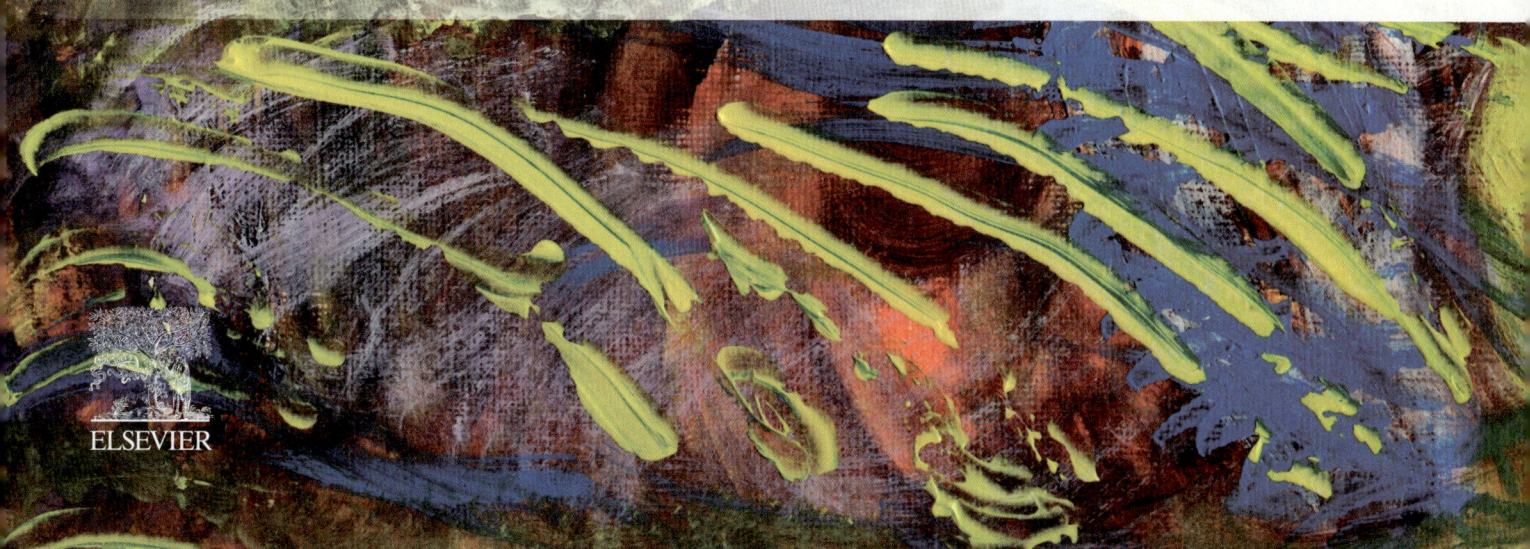

ELSEVIER

Elsevier
3251 Riverport Lane
St. Louis, Missouri 63043

GERONTOLOGIC NURSING, SEVENTH EDITION   ISBN: 978-0-323-87520-2

Copyright © 2025 by Elsevier Inc. All rights are reserved, including those for text and data mining, AI training, and similar technologies.

Publisher's note: Elsevier takes a neutral position with respect to territorial disputes or jurisdictional claims in its published content, including in maps and institutional affiliations.

No part of this publication may be reproduced or transmitted in any form or by any means, electronic or mechanical, including photocopying, recording, or any information storage and retrieval system, without permission in writing from the publisher. Details on how to seek permission, further information about the Publisher's permissions policies and our arrangements with organizations such as the Copyright Clearance Center and the Copyright Licensing Agency, can be found at our website: www.elsevier.com/permissions.

This book and the individual contributions contained in it are protected under copyright by the Publisher (other than as may be noted herein).

Notice

Practitioners and researchers must always rely on their own experience and knowledge in evaluating and using any information, methods, compounds or experiments described herein. Because of rapid advances in the medical sciences, in particular, independent verification of diagnoses and drug dosages should be made. To the fullest extent of the law, no responsibility is assumed by Elsevier, authors, editors or contributors for any injury and/or damage to persons or property as a matter of products liability, negligence or otherwise, or from any use or operation of any methods, products, instructions, or ideas contained in the material herein.

Previous editions copyrighted 2019, 2015, 2011, 2006, 2000, and 1996.

Senior Content Strategist: Sandra Clark
Senior Content Development Specialist: Rae Robertson
Content Development Manager: Danielle Frazier
Publishing Services Manager: Deepthi Unni
Project Manager: Nayagi Anandan
Design Direction: Amy Buxton

Printed in India

Last digit is the print number: 9 8 7 6 5 4 3 2 1

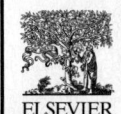 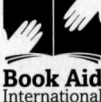

Working together to grow libraries in developing countries

www.elsevier.com • www.bookaid.org

I am dedicating this edition to my dad, Leopold J. Gauvin.
April 21, 1935, to June 4, 2021

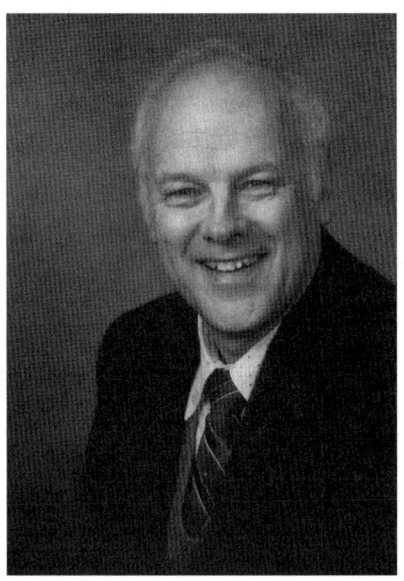

Thank you, Dad, for being you. I'll never forget your patience in teaching me to tie fly fishing flies, do leatherwork, use a compound bow, and so many other things. You always made time for us kids. Our hiking, weekends out fishing, backpacking and camping trips, and trips to many National Parks over the years will always be fond memories.

Jennifer J. Yeager

ABOUT THE AUTHORS

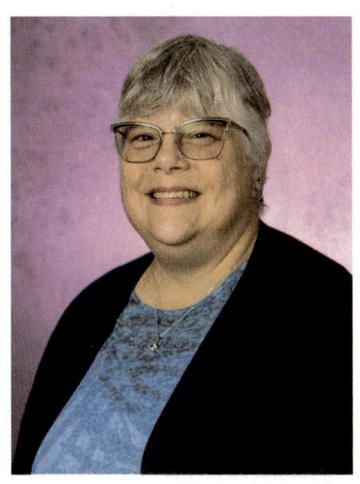

Jennifer J. Yeager, PhD, MSN, RN: I was called to be a nurse during my senior year in high school. I simply woke up one morning knowing that I was supposed to be a nurse; up till the day before, I had planned on becoming an English teacher. I am the only nurse in a large family of teachers and engineers.

I attended the University of Portland in Oregon on an Air Force ROTC nursing scholarship. After graduation, I moved to Texas to be an Air Force nurse at Wilford Hall Medical Center in San Antonio. After six years of service, and earning the rank of Captain, I separated from the Air Force. I stayed in Texas, as I enjoy living in the state..

While I was in school in Portland, I looked at my instructors and knew I was supposed to fill their shoes one day. In the back of my mind, I set the goal to earn my doctoral degree before I turned 50 and become a nursing professor. In 1998, I earned my MSN as an Adult/Gerontological Nurse Practitioner with Educator Role from The University of Texas at Arlington; in 2013 I earned my PhD in Nursing at The University of Texas at Tyler. I met my goal through determination and hard work.

I have taught at Tarleton State University since 2007; I am retiring this year. Teaching students the art and science of nursing is the most wonderful opportunity imaginable. Although my background has been working with the elderly, I have taught a variety of courses at all levels (undergraduate and graduate). I earned the O.A. Grant Excellence in Teaching Award in 2023; the Certificate in Effective College Instruction through the Association of College and University Educators and the American Council on Education in 2020; and in 2018 I earned the Faculty Excellence in Scholarship Award at Tarleton State University, College of Health Science and Human Services. In 2011 I was selected to participate in the Sigma Theta Tau International Nurse Faculty Leadership Academy.

Reaching my goal meant sacrifice for both my family and me, but it has been worth it. Setting goals and reaching them through hard work, dedication, learning through mistakes and never quitting makes reaching the goal all the sweeter.

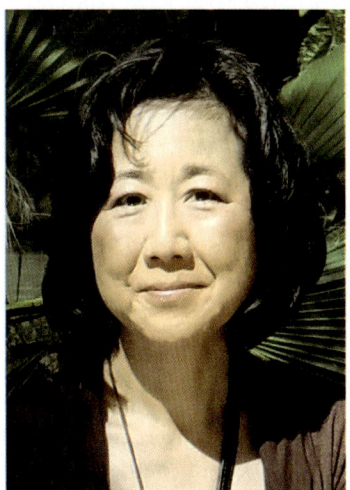

Dr. Mary B. Winton, PhD, MSN, RN, started her nursing career after receiving her Associate Degree in Nursing from Tarleton State University in Stephenville, Texas, a member of the Texas A&M University System. Since then, she obtained her Bachelor and Master of Science in Nursing from the University of Texas at Arlington, and her PhD in Nursing from The University of Texas at Tyler.

Mary has many years of hospital nursing experience in areas including critical care, emergency, and medical-surgical nursing as both a nurse and as a nursing supervisor. Additionally, she was employed with a hospitalist group as a board-certified Acute Care Nurse Practitioner. She is currently an Associate Professor in the College of Health Sciences, School of Nursing, at Tarleton State University. Mary has experience in teaching graduate-level pharmacology, pathophysiology, and nursing informatics, and she has vast experience teaching at all levels of the undergraduate nursing courses, including nursing pathophysiology, pharmacology, medical-surgical nursing, nursing care of older adults, and health assessment. Mary served as faculty advisor for the Student Nurses Association at Tarleton many years. She has been a member of several organizations, including Sigma Theta Tau International Honor Society in Nursing, Tau Chi chapter; American Nurses Association/Texas Nurses Association; Critical Care Nursing Education; and Rural Nurse Organization. She is actively involved in various university, college, school, and departmental committees.

During her career as a nurse educator, Mary was the recipient of the Texas A&M Student Evaluation Teaching Excellence Award and the O.A. Grant Excellence in Teaching Award. She was also the recipient of the AACN 2020-2021 Scholarship of Teaching and Learning Excellence Award. She also taught English as a Second Language at her church of membership.

Mary's research interests include health disparity among minorities, especially among Korean immigrants; student learning outcomes; and the use of technology in classrooms. She has presented at several conferences and has published on the health care of Korean immigrants.

During her spare time, Mary enjoys spending time with her husband, daughters, and grandchildren. She also enjoys traveling, reading, crocheting, and cooking.

ABOUT THE AUTHORS

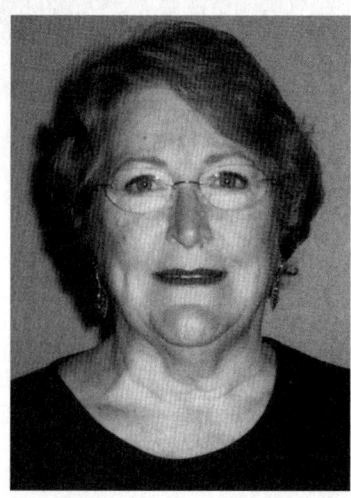

Sue E. Meiner, EdD, APRN, GNP-BC, began her nursing career in 1962 in St. Louis, Missouri. She began as a Licensed Practical Nurse (LPN) prior to the availability of Associate Degree Nursing programs in the Midwest. She graduated from the second class of the Associate in Applied Science degree (ADN) program from St. Louis Community College (Meramec campus). Continuing her education in nursing, she completed a Bachelor of Science in Nursing (BSN) and a Master of Science in Nursing (MSN) from St. Louis University. Later she received her Doctor of Education (EdD) from Southern Illinois University at Edwardsville, and a Certificate as a Gerontological Nurse Practitioner from the Barnes-Jewish Hospital College of Nursing in St. Louis. Dr. Meiner held certifications as both a Gerontological Clinical Nurse Specialist and a Gerontological Nurse Practitioner from the American Nurses Credentialing Center (ANCC) of the American Nurses Association (ANA). She took additional courses toward counseling at Lindenwood College, St. Charles, Missouri. She has received numerous awards and has been asked to speak at local, regional, and national conferences and workshops. Dr. Meiner worked as a staff nurse in hospitals in the St. Louis area as well as home health nursing. Over time she worked as a hospital nursing supervisor and interim director of nursing. While her main clinical interest was in medical-surgical nursing, she began to focus on the special care needs of the older adult. She has practiced nursing for over 50 years; however, the last 30 years have been heavily focused on geriatric nursing. She has taught nursing at the LPN, ADN, BSN, and MSN levels of education. She has been the Director of Nursing Programs at the LPN and ADN levels. Before returning to full-time clinical practice in Las Vegas as a Nurse Practitioner, she taught the final course of clinical nursing at the master's level at the University of Nevada, Las Vegas, School of Nursing. Her clinical practice was directed at chronic and tertiary pain management, with a focus on the needs of the older adult. Dr. Meiner has engaged in the support of nursing through advocacy of both nurses and patients and their families by serving part time as a Forensic Nurse. She has been active in legal nurse consulting since 1988 and incorporated her company in the early 2000s. Throughout those 25 years, she provided case reviews and expert witness testimony at depositions and trials across the United States. She authored and edited **Nursing Documentation: Legal Focus across Practice Setting** in 2000, as well as authored, coauthored, or edited multiple textbooks, and has written multiple professional articles on nursing care and issues. During 5 years in the 1980s, she was elected to serve her community of Creve Coeur, Missouri, as a Director of the Fire Protection District. In her free time, Dr. Meiner enjoys national and international travel and spending time with her family.

CONTRIBUTORS AND REVIEWERS

CONTRIBUTORS

Renae Authement, DNP, MSN, RN
Assistant Professor
School of Nursing
Tarleton State University
Waco, Texas

Linda Bub, MSN, RN, GCNS-BC, NPD-BC
Regional Manager
Nursing Education and Professional Development
Advocate Health
Milwaukee, Wisconsin

Jerilyn W. Bumpas, DNP, MSN
Assistant Professor
School of Nursing
Tarleton State University
Stephenville, Texas

Chiquesha Davis, DNP, MSN, CMSRN
Academic Chair, RN-BSN Program
School of Nursing
Dallas College
Dallas, Texas

Donna L. Hamby, DNP, RN, APRN, ACNP-BC
Clinical Associate Professor
Graduate Nursing
College of Nursing and Health Innovation
University of Texas Arlington
Arlington, Texas

Jennifer Mundine, EdD, MSN, RN, CNE, CHSE
Associate Dean, Faculty
Department of Nursing
Chamberlain University
Irving, Texas

Patti A. Parker, PhD, RN, ACNS, ANP, GNP, BC, GS-C
Assistant Professor
Graduate Nursing
University of Texas at Arlington College of Nursing
Arlington, Texas

Martha Smith, DNP, APRN, FNP-BC
Assistant Professor
Post Licensure Department, School of Nursing
Tarleton State University
Lipan, Texas

REVIEWERS

Dawna Martich, RN, MSN
Wild Iris Medical Education
Compche, California

Emmanuel D. Paragas, Jr., DNS, APRN, FNP-BC, CRRN
Associate Professor of Nursing, Clinical Nursing Coordinator
Department of Nursing, College of Sciences
West Liberty University
West Liberty, West Virginia

Cherie Carnes Rebar, PhD, MBA, RN, CNE, CNEcl, COI, CLNC, FAADN
Professor of Nursing
Galen College of Nursing
Louisville, Kentucky;
Nursing Education Consultant
RH Nursing Education Consultant
Beavercreek, Ohio

Christy Swinson, DNP, FNP-C, CMSRN
Assistant Professor of Nursing
School of Nursing
Fayetteville State University
Fayetteville, North Carolina

Karen A. Thornton, PhD, RN
Associate Professor
Rasmussen University
Odessa, Florida

PREFACE

The field of gerontologic nursing has blossomed over the past decades as the population of Baby Boomers entered retirement age. The provision of quality health care for older adults is an ever-growing challenge. Issues related to health and illness across the care continuum must be addressed within a cost-effective and resource-limited environment. The largest group of patients in hospitals (outside of obstetric and pediatric units) is older adults. Residents of long-term care and rehabilitation facilities are predominantly older adults. The specialty of gerontologic nursing is in greater demand more than ever before.

Gerontologic Nursing, seventh edition, has been revised to provide today's students with a solid foundation to meet the future challenges of gerontologic nursing practice. This textbook provides comprehensive, theoretical, and practical information concerning concepts and issues relevant to the care of older adults across the care continuum. The extensive coverage of material provides the student with the information necessary to make sound clinical judgments while emphasizing the concepts, skills, and techniques of gerontologic nursing practice. Psychologic and sociocultural issues and aspects of older adult care are integrated throughout the textbook, reflecting the reality of practice with this unique population.

Intended for use by nursing students in all levels of professional nursing programs, *Gerontologic Nursing* was developed for use in either gerontologic nursing or medical-surgical courses, or within programs that integrate gerontologic content throughout the educational program.

ORGANIZATION

The 27 chapters in *Gerontologic Nursing* are divided into six parts, with theoretical frameworks to guide gerontologic nursing practice woven throughout:

Part 1, Introduction to Gerontologic Nursing, includes three chapters that serve as the foundation for the remainder of the textbook. These chapters provide a historical overview of gerontologic nursing, and demographics related to aging; practice standards and legal and ethical issues related to care of the older adult across the care continuum; and assessment of the older adult, with a focus on cognition and functional status.

Part 2, Influences on Health and Illness, includes chapters on cultural, family, and socioeconomic and environmental influences. Health promotion and illness/disability prevention are also included.

Part 3, Influences on Quality of Life, details the needs and nursing care of older adults in the areas of nutrition, sleep and activity, safety, issues related to sexuality, pain management, and infection and inflammation.

Part 4, Diagnostic Studies and Pharmacologic Management, focuses on the nurse's role in effectively managing the nursing care of older adults related to drugs and aging, as well as laboratory and diagnostic testing in older adults.

Part 5, Nursing Care of Physiologic and Psychological Disorders, contains chapters detailing nursing management of older adults with diseases or conditions affecting the function of body systems: integumentary, sensory, cardiovascular, respiratory, gastrointestinal, urinary, musculoskeletal, cognitive and neurologic, and endocrine.

Part 6, Health Care Transitions, contains chapters that detail nursing management of older adults as they transition across the care continuum, from wellness, to illness, to end-of-life care.

In organizing the textbook, every attempt was made to ensure a logical sequence by grouping related topics. However, it is not necessary to read the text in sequence. A detailed table of contents and an extensive index is included. It is hoped that this approach provides easy access to information of interest.

FORMAT

The seventh edition has been revised and reflects the growth and change of gerontologic nursing practice and the learning needs of today's students. The presentation of content has been designed for ease of use and reference. The textbook's visual appeal has been carefully planned to make it both aesthetically pleasing and easy to read and follow. Clinical examples depict nurses practicing in many different roles in a wide variety of practice settings, reflecting current practice patterns.

All body system chapters include an overview of age-related changes in structure and function. Common problems and conditions within each of the chapters are presented in a format that includes the definition, etiology, pathophysiology, and typical clinical presentation for each. The Nursing Care Guidelines section of the condition is central to each of these chapters and follows the clinical judgment (nursing process) format of Recognize Cues (Assessment), Analyze Cues and Prioritize Hypotheses (Patient Problems), Generate Solutions (Planning), Take Actions (Nursing Interventions), and Evaluate Outcomes (Evaluation). Nursing Care Plan boxes for selected problems and conditions begin with a realistic clinical situation and emphasize patient problems pertinent to the situation, expected outcomes, and nursing interventions, all within an easy-to-reference, two-column format.

FEATURES

Each chapter begins with Learning Objectives to help the student focus on important subject matter, followed by *What Would You Do?* scenarios to stimulate thinking. Patient/Family Teaching boxes are included where appropriate, providing key information on what to teach patients and families to enhance their knowledge and promote active participation in their care. Health Promotion/Illness Prevention boxes are included in the text, which identify activities and interventions that promote a healthy lifestyle and prevent disease and illness. Nutritional Considerations boxes are found throughout the text to stress the importance of nutrition in the care of older adults. Evidence-Based Practice boxes are presented in each chapter to emphasize the application of relevant research findings to current nursing practice and allow students to reflect on how to integrate evidence-based practice into everyday nursing practice. Cultural Awareness boxes are included where applicable to develop the student's cultural sensitivity and promote the delivery of culturally competent care. Home Care boxes are presented at the end of appropriate chapters to provide pragmatic suggestions for care of the homebound patient and family. Finally, each chapter concludes with a brief summary, followed by Key Points that highlight important principles discussed in the chapter. Clinical Judgment Exercises at the end of every chapter stimulate students to carefully consider the material learned and apply their knowledge to the situation presented. New Next-Generation NCLEX® Examination-Style Case Studies sprinkled throughout the text provide readers with opportunities to develop analytical skills. Answers to these Case Studies can be found on the accompanying Evolve site.

EVOLVE ANCILLARIES

Instructor Resources
- TEACH for Nurses lesson plans
- PowerPoints
- Test Bank
- Clinical Judgment-Style Practice Questions

Student Resources
- Review Questions
- Case Studies
- Answers to Next-Generation NCLEX® Style Case Studies in the text

As the scope of gerontologic nursing practice continues to expand, so must the knowledge guiding that practice reflect the most current standards and guidelines. Every effort has been made to incorporate the most current standards and guidelines from appropriate agencies into the seventh edition of this text.

Jennifer J. Yeager
Mary B. Winton
Sue E. Meiner

ACKNOWLEDGMENTS

Heartfelt thanks must be given to Sue Meiner for placing her trust in me to continue her work on this text, and to Mary Winton for joining me as co-editor on this edition. The development of this seventh edition would not have been possible without the combined efforts of many talented professionals who supported me throughout the entire process. Without the tireless work of the contributing authors, who have dedicated their careers to caring for older adults, this edition would not be possible.

A special recognition goes to the editorial and production team at Elsevier. This team of professionals worked extremely hard to assist me in meeting the deadlines. I want to call special attention to Rae Robertson, who kept me on track down to the last second. Her patience is greatly appreciated!

Jennifer J. Yeager

CONTENTS

About the Authors, vii
Contributors and Reviewers, ix
Preface, xi
Acknowledgments, xiii

PART I Introduction to Gerontologic Nursing

1 Overview of Gerontologic Nursing, 2
Jennifer J. Yeager, PhD, MSN, RN
  Foundations of the Specialty of
    Gerontologic Nursing, 2
    Professional Origins, 2
    Standards of Practice, 3
    Roles, 3
    Terminology, 5
  Demographic Profile of the Older Population, 5
    The Older Population, 6
    Highlights of the Profile of Older Americans, 6
    Sex and Marital Status, 6
    Race and Ethnicity, 7
    Living Arrangements, 7
    Geographic Distribution, 7
    Education, 8
    Income and Poverty, 8
    Employment, 8
  Health Status of Older Adults, 8
    Self-Assessed Health and Chronic Disease, 9
    Functional Status, 9
    Healthcare Expenditure and Use, 9
    Implications for Healthcare Delivery, 9
    Acute Care Setting, 9
    Nursing Facilities, 10
    Home Care, 10
    Continuum of Care, 10
  Effect of an Aging Population on Gerontologic
    Nursing, 11
    Ageism, 11
    Nursing Education, 11
    Nursing Practice, 14
    Nursing Research, 15

2 Healthcare Policy that Affects Older Adults, 18
Donna Leake Hamby, DNP, RN, APRN, ACNP-BC
  Scope of Practice and Professional Standards: Legal
    Significance, 18
  Overview of Relevant Healthcare Policies, 19
    Sources of Law, 19
    *Health Insurance Portability and Accountability Act
      (HIPAA) of 1996, 19*
  Elder Abuse and Protective Services, 20
    Medicare and Medicaid, 21
  Nursing Facility Reform, 21
    OBRA's Three Major Parts, 22
    Affordable Care Act, 25
    The Patient Self-Determination Act, 25
  Autonomy and Self-Determination, 25
    Do Not Resuscitate Orders, 26
    Legal Tools, 26
    *Communication Between Patient's Directives and
      Family Desires, 30*
  Nurses' Ethical Code and Practice Decisions, 30
    Ethical Dilemmas and Considerations, 30
    Experimentation and Research, 31
    Organ Donation, 31
    Ethics Committees, 31
    Social Media, 32

3 Assessment of the Older Adult, 36
Jennifer J. Yeager, PhD, RN
  Special Considerations Affecting Assessment, 37
    *Interrelationship Between Physical and Psychosocial
      Aspects of Aging, 37*
    *Nature of Disease and Disability and Their Effects
      on Functional Status, 38*
    *Tailoring the Nursing Assessment to the Older
      Person, 42*
  The Health History, 42
    The Interviewer, 43
    The Patient, 44
    Electronic Health Records, 44
    The Health History Format, 44
    Approach to Physical Assessment, 47
    Equipment and Skills, 48
  Additional Assessment Measures, 48
    Functional Status Assessment, 48
    Cognitive and Affective Assessment, 51
    Social Assessment, 54
  Laboratory Data, 54

PART II Influences on Health and Illness

4 Family Influences, 60
Jennifer J. Yeager, PhD, MSN, RN
  Role and Function of Families, 60
    Planning in Advance of Need, 61
  Common Late-life Family Issues and Decisions, 61
    The Issue of Driving, 61
    Financial and Legal Concerns, 62
    End-of-Life Healthcare Decisions, 62
    Family Caregiving, 63
  Caregiver Education, 65
    Respite Programs, 65
    Support Groups, 66
  Assessing the Family, 66
    Past Relationships, 66
    Family Dynamics, 66

     Roles, 66
     Dependence and Independence, 67
    Changes in Living Arrangements, 67
     Deciding About a Care Facility, 67
5 **Socioeconomic and Environmental Influences, 70**
    Jennifer J. Yeager, PhD, MSN, RN
    Socioeconomic Factors, 70
     Generational Differences, 70
     Income, 71
     Education, 73
     Health Status and Healthcare Coverage, 74
    Environmental Influences, 75
     Geographic Location of Residence, 76
     Housing, 77
     Transportation, 77
    Advocacy, 77
6 **Health Promotion and Illness/Disability Prevention, 81**
    Jennifer J. Yeager PhD, MSN, RN
    Essentials of Health Promotion for Aging Adults, 81
     Terminology, 82
    Barriers to Health Promotion and Disease Prevention, 82
    Models of Health Promotion, 82
     Transtheoretical Model, 82
     Health Belief Model, 83
     Health Promotion Model, 83
    Disease Prevention, 83
     Primary Preventive Measures, 83
     Secondary Preventive Measures, 85
     Tertiary Preventive Measures, 85
    Nursing Role in Prevention, 85
     Nursing Care Guidelines for Health Promotion and Disease Prevention, 85
     Supporting the Empowerment of Older Adults, 90

PART III Influences on Quality of Life

7 **Nutrition, 94**
    Martha Smith, DNP, APRN, FNP-BC
    Malnutrition, 94
     Factors Influencing Nutritional Risk in Older Adults, 95
     Drug–Nutrient Interactions, 95
     Dehydration, 95
     Micronutrient Deficiency, 97
     Indicators of Malnutrition, 97
     Oral Health, 97
    Nutritional Screening and Assessment, 98
     Nutritional Screening, 98
     Nutritional Assessment, 98
    Patient Problems Associated with Nutritional Problems, 99
    Evidence-based Strategies to Improve Nutrition, 99
     Components of a Healthy Diet, 100
     Dysphagia, 101
     Specialized Nutritional Support, 103

8 **Sleep and Activity, 108**
    Chiquesha Davis, DNP, MSN, CMSRN, RN-BC
    Sleep and Older Adults, 108
     Biologic Brain Functions Responsible for Sleep, 108
     Stages of Sleep, 108
     Sleep and Circadian Rhythm, 109
     Insomnia, 109
     Age-Related Changes in Sleep, 109
     Factors Affecting Sleep, 110
     Sleep Disorders and Conditions, 112
     Components of the Sleep History, 114
     Further Assessment of Sleep, 115
     Getting a Good Night's Sleep, 116
    Activity and Older Adults, 117
     Activities of Daily Living, 117
     Physical Exercise, 118
     Activity as Affected by Lifestyle Changes, 118
     Activity Affected by Alzheimer Disease and Other Dementias, 120
9 **Safety, 124**
    Jerilyn W. Bumpas, DNP, MSN, RN and
    Jennifer J. Yeager, PhD, MSN, RN
    Falls, 125
     Overview and Magnitude of the Problem, 125
     Definition of Falling, 125
     Meaning of Falling, 126
     Normal Age-Related Changes Contributing to Falling, 126
     Fall Risk, 127
     Fall Antecedents and Fall Classification, 130
     Fall Consequences, 131
     History, 132
     Physical Examination, 132
     Special Testing, 132
     Management, 136
    Safety and the Home Environment, 138
     Burn Injuries in the Home, 138
     Other Injuries in the Home, 139
     Foodborne Illnesses, 141
    Seasonal Safety Issues, 141
     Hypothermia and Hyperthermia in Older Adults, 141
    Disasters, 143
    Storage of Medications and Health Care Supplies in the Home, 143
    Crime Prevention, 144
    Automobile Safety, 144
    Abuse and Neglect, 145
    Firearms, 145
10 **Sexuality and Aging, 150**
    Linda A. Bub, MSN, RN, GCNS-BC, NPD-BC
    Older Adult Needs for Sexuality and Intimacy, 150
    The Importance of Intimacy Among Older Adults, 150
    Nursing's Reluctance to Manage the Sexuality of Older Adults, 152

Normal Changes of the Aging Sexual Response, 152
   Physiologic Changes, 152
   Genitourinary Syndrome of Menopause, 153
Pathologic Conditions Affecting Older Adults' Sexual Responses, 153
   Illness, Surgery, and Medication, 153
   Human Immunodeficiency Virus, 153
   Malignancies, 155
   Dementia, 155
Environmental and Psychosocial Barriers to Sexual Practice, 155
Lesbian, Gay, Bisexual, and Transgender Older Adults, 156
Nursing Care Guidelines for Sexuality and Aging, 156
   Recognize Cues (Assessment), 156
   Analyze Cues and Prioritize Hypotheses (Patient Problems), 158
   Generate Solutions (Planning), 158
   Take Actions (Nursing Interventions), 159
   Evaluate Outcomes (Evaluation), 161

11 Pain, 164
Jennifer Mundine, EdD, MSN, RN, CNE
Understanding Pain, 165
   Definition, 165
   Scope of the Problem of Pain, 165
   Consequences of Unrelieved Pain, 165
Pathophysiology of Pain in Older Adults, 167
   Perception of Pain in Older Adults, 167
Barriers to Effective Pain Management in Older Adults, 167
Pain Assessment, 169
   Pain Assessment and Culture, 169
   Pain Assessment Tools, 171
Nursing Care Guidelines for Older Adults with Pain, 173
   Pharmacologic Treatment, 173
   Planning Pain Relief, 178

12 Infection and Inflammation, 182
Mary B. Winton, PhD, MSN, RN
Immunologic Theory, 182
Age-Related Changes in the Immune System, 183
Factors Affecting Immunocompetence, 183
   Nutritional Factors, 183
   Psychosocial Factors, 184
   Drugs, 184
   Complementary and Alternative Medications, 184
   Infections, 184
The Chain of Infection, 184
Common Problems and Conditions, 185
   COVID-19, Influenza, and Pneumonia, 185
   Cancer, 185
   Autoimmunity, 185
HIV Infection in Older Adults, 186
Significant Healthcare-Associated Pathogens, 186
   Clostridium difficile, *186*
   Vancomycin-Resistant Enterococcus, 186
   Methicillin-Resistant Staphylococcus aureus, *187*
   Extended Spectrum β-Lactamase-Positive Escherichia coli, *187*
Nursing Care Guidelines for Infection, 187
   Recognize Cues (Assessment), 187
   Analyze Cues and Prioritize Hypotheses (Patient Problems), 188
   Generate Solutions (Planning), 188
   Take Actions (Nursing Interventions), 188
   Evaluate Outcomes (Evaluation), 189

PART IV Diagnostic Studies and Pharmacologic Management

13 Laboratory and Diagnostic Tests, 196
Donna Leake Hamby, DNP, RN, APRN, ACNP-BC
Hematologic Testing, 198
   Red Blood Cells, 198
   White Blood Cells, 198
   Folic Acid, 198
   Vitamin B_{12}, 199
   Total Iron-Binding Capacity, 199
   Iron, 199
   Uric Acid, 199
   Prothrombin Time, 199
   Partial Thromboplastin Time, 200
   D-dimer Test, 200
   Erythrocyte Sedimentation Rate, 200
   C-Reactive Protein, 200
   Platelets, 200
Components of Blood Chemistry Testing, 200
   Electrolytes, 200
   Amylase, 203
   Total Protein, 204
   Albumin and Prealbumin, 204
   Blood Urea Nitrogen, 204
   Creatinine, 204
   Creatinine Clearance, 204
   Triglycerides, 204
   Total Cholesterol, 204
   High-Density Lipoprotein, 204
   Low-Density Lipoprotein, 204
   Brain Natriuretic Peptide, 205
   Alkaline Phosphatase, 205
   Aspartate Aminotransferase, 205
   Creatine Kinase, 205
   Lactate Dehydrogenase, 205
   Troponin, 205
   Thyroid Function Tests, 205
   Prostate-Specific Antigen, 206
Urinalysis, 206
   Protein, 206
   Glucose, 206
   Bacteria, 206
   Ketones, 207
   pH, 207
   Blood, 207

Components of Arterial Blood Gas Testing, 207
  Partial Pressure of Oxygen, 207
  pH of the Blood, 207
  Bicarbonate, 207
  Oxygen Saturation, 208
Therapeutic Drug Monitoring, 208

14 Drugs and Aging, 211
Patti A. Parker, PhD, RN, ACNS, ANP, GNP, BC, GS-C

Overview of Drug Use and Problems, 211
  Demographics of Drug Use, 211
  Changes in Drug Response With Aging, 211
  Pharmacodynamic Changes: What the Drug Does to the Body, 213
  Drugs and Quality of Life, 214
  Pharmacologic Contributors to Risk, 214
Commonly Used Drugs, 218
  Antipsychotics, 218
  Anxiolytics and Hypnotics, 218
  Antidepressants, 218
  Cardiovascular Drugs, 219
  Antimicrobials, 220
  Opioid Analgesics, 220
  Nonprescription Agents, 220
  Dietary Supplements, 221
Drug Adherence, 221
  Assessing for Risk Factors, 222
  Strategies for Improving Adherence, 222
  Reviewing the Drug List for Problems, 222
Substance Use Disorders, 223
  Definitions and Common Usage, 223
  Difficulty in Identification of SUD, 223
  Physiologic Changes, 223
  Psychological Changes, 224
  Sociologic Changes, 224
Nursing Care Guidelines for SUDs, 224
  Recognize Cues (Assessment), 224
  Analyze Cues and Prioritize Hypotheses (Patient Problems), 225
  Take Actions (Nursing Interventions), 225
  Evaluate Outcomes (Evaluation), 225
Commonly Misused Substances in Older Adults, 225
  Alcohol, 225
  Prescription Drugs, 227
  Nicotine, 228
  Cannabis, 228
Future Trends, 229

PART V Nursing Care of Physiologic and Psychological Disorders

15 Integumentary Function, 236
Patti A. Parker, PhD, RN, ACNS, ANP, GNP, BC, GS-C

Age-Related Changes in Skin Structure and Function, 237
  Epidermis, 237
  Dermis, 237
  Subcutaneous Fat, 237
  Dermal Appendages, 237
  Dermatoporosis, 237
Common Problems and Conditions, 238
  Benign Skin Growths, 238
  Inflammatory Dermatoses, 239
  Psoriasis, 240
  Pruritus, 241
  Candidiasis, 242
  Herpes Zoster (Shingles), 243
  Premalignant Skin Growths: Actinic Keratosis, 244
Malignant Skin Growths, 246
  Basal Cell Carcinoma, 246
  Squamous Cell Carcinoma, 246
  Melanoma, 246
  Nursing Care Guidelines for Malignant Skin Growths, 247
Lower Extremity Ulcers, 248
  Arterial Ulcers, 248
  Venous Ulcers, 249
  Diabetic Foot Lesions, 249
  Nursing Care Guidelines for Lower Extremity Ulcers, 250
Pressure Injuries, 250
  Epidemiology of Pressure Injuries, 251
  Etiology of Pressure Injuries, 251
  Risk Assessment Tools, 253
  Preventive Strategies, 254
  Pressure Injury Management, 257

16 Sensory Function, 270
Mary B. Winton, PhD, MSN, RN

Vision, 270
  Age-Related Changes in Structure and Function, 271
  Common Complaints, 271
  Common Problems and Conditions, 272
Hearing and Balance, 280
  Age-Related Changes in Structure and Function, 281
  Common Problems and Conditions, 281
Taste and Smell, 286
  Age-Related Changes in Structure and Function, 286
  Common Problems and Conditions, 286
Touch, 287

17 Cardiovascular Function, 290
Mary B. Winton, PhD, MSN, RN

Age-Related Changes in Structure and Function, 290
  Conduction System, 290
  Vessels, 290
  Response to Stress and Exercise, 291
Common Cardiovascular Problems, 291
  Hypertension, 291
  Risk Factors for Heart Disease, 296
  Coronary Artery Disease, 298
  Arrhythmia, 303
  Orthostatic Hypotension, 305
  Syncope with Cardiac Causes, 306
  Valvular Heart Disease (VHD), 307
  CHF, 309

Peripheral Artery Disease, 315
Chronic Venous Insufficiency, 316
Anemia, 318

18 Respiratory Function, 325
Jennifer Mundine, EdD, MSN, RN, CNE

Age-Related Changes in Structure and Function, 325
Factors Affecting Lung Function, 328
    Exercise and Immobility, 328
    Smoking, 328
    Obesity, 329
    Anesthesia and Surgery, 329
Respiratory Findings Common in Older Patients, 329
Respiratory Alterations in Older Patients, 330
Obstructive Pulmonary Disease, 330
    Asthma, 330
    Chronic Bronchitis, 334
    Emphysema, 334
    Chronic Obstructive Pulmonary Disease, 334
Restrictive Pulmonary Disease, 341
    Lung Cancer, 341
    Tuberculosis, 342
    Pneumonia, 344
Other Respiratory Alterations, 348
    Cardiogenic and Noncardiogenic Pulmonary Edema, 348
    Pulmonary Emboli, 350
    Obstructive Sleep Apnea, 352

19 Gastrointestinal Function, 357
Renae Authement, DNP, MSN, RN

Age-Related Changes in Structure and Function, 357
    Oral Cavity and Pharynx, 357
    Esophagus, 359
    Stomach, 359
    Small Intestine, 359
    Large Intestine, 359
    Gallbladder, 359
    Pancreas, 359
    Liver, 360
Prevention, 360
Common GI Symptoms, 360
    Nausea and Vomiting, 360
    Anorexia, 361
    Abdominal Pain, 361
    Gas, 362
    Diarrhea, 362
    Constipation, 362
    Fecal Incontinence, 363
Common Diseases of the GI Tract, 364
    Gingivitis and Periodontitis, 364
    Dysphagia, 365
    Gastroesophageal Reflux and Esophagitis, 366
    Vitamin B_{12} Deficiency, 367
    Gastritis, 367
    Peptic Ulcer Disease, 368
    Enteritis, 369
    Intestinal Obstruction, 370
    Diverticula, 373
    Colon Polyps, 373
    Hemorrhoids, 374
Disorders of the Accessory Organs, 374
    Cholelithiasis and Cholecystitis, 374
    Pancreatitis, 375
    Hepatitis, 376
    Cirrhosis Secondary to Alcohol Use Disorder, 378
    Drug-Induced Hepatitis, 380
GI Cancers, 381
    Esophageal Cancer, 381
    Gastric Cancer, 382
    Colorectal Carcinoma, 383
    Pancreatic Cancer, 384
    Liver Cancer, 385

20 Urinary Function, 388
Linda Bub, MSN, RN, GCNS-BC, NPD-BC

Age-Related Changes in Structure and Function, 388
Prevalence of UI, 389
Common Incontinence Problems and Conditions, 389
    Transient Incontinence, 389
    Established Incontinence, 389
Nursing Care Guidelines for Incontinence, 391
    Recognize Cues (Assessment), 391
    Analyze Cues and Prioritize Hypotheses (Patient Problems), 392
    Generate Solutions (Planning), 394
    Take Actions (Nursing Interventions), 394
    Evaluate Outcomes (Evaluation), 397
Age-Related Renal Changes, 398
Common Renal Problems and Conditions, 398
    Acute Kidney Injury, 398
    Chronic Kidney Disease, 399
    Urinary Tract Infection, 403
    Bladder Cancer, 408
    Benign Prostatic Hyperplasia, 408
    Prostate Cancer, 410

21 Musculoskeletal Function, 414
Mary B. Winton, PhD, MSN, RN

Age-Related Changes in Structure and Function, 414
Common Problems and Conditions of the Musculoskeletal System, 415
    Hip Fracture, 416
    Colles Fracture, 419
    Clavicular Fracture, 419
    Casts and Cast Care, 419
    Osteoarthritis, 420
    Spinal Stenosis, 423
    Rheumatoid Arthritis, 424
    Gouty Arthritis, 426
    Osteoporosis, 428
    Paget's Disease, 433
    Osteomyelitis, 434
    Amputation, 435
    Polymyalgia Rheumatica, 437
    Foot Problems, 438
    Muscle Cramps, 440

22 Cognitive and Neurologic Function, 444
Jennifer J. Yeager, PhD, MSN, RN

- The Central Nervous System, 444
  - The Brain, 445
  - Spinal Cord, 445
  - Evaluation of Cognitive Function, 446
  - Cognitive Function in Typical Aging, 447
- Cognitive Disorders Associated with Altered Thought Processes, 448
  - Depression, 448
  - Delirium, 450
  - Dementia, 451
  - Resources, 459
- Other Common Problems and Conditions, 460
  - Suicide, 460
  - Parkinson Disease, 462
  - Cerebrovascular Accident, 469
  - Anxiety, 473
  - Schizophrenia, 474
- Mental Health Resources, 475
  - E4 Center, 476

23 Endocrine Function, 481
Mary B. Winton, PhD, MSN, RN

- Endocrine Physiology in Older Adults, 481
  - Andropause and Menopause, 482
  - Adrenopause, 483
  - Somatopause, 483
- Common Endocrine Pathophysiology in Older Adults, 485
  - Metabolic Syndrome–Diabetes Continuum, 485
  - Type 2 Diabetes Mellitus, 486
  - Hyperthyroidism, 497
  - Hypothyroidism, 497
  - Primary Osteoporosis, 498
  - Sexual Dysfunction, 499

PART VI Health Care Transitions

24 Health Care Delivery Settings and Older Adults, 506
Martha Smith, DNP, APRN, FNP-BC

- Characteristics of Older Adults in Acute Care, 506
- Characteristics of the Acute Care Environment, 507
  - Philosophy of Care, 507
  - Risks of Hospitalization, 507
  - Safety Features, 509
- Nursing in the Acute Care Setting, 509
  - Nursing-Specific Competency and Expertise, 510
  - Critical Care and Trauma Care, 510
- Continuity of Care, 511
  - Benefits of Home Care, 511
  - Role of Home Care Agency, 513
- Implementing the Plan of Treatment, 513
  - The Nurse's Role, 513
  - Role of the Home-Health Aide, 513
- Oasis, 514
- Community-Based Providers, 514
- Factors Affecting the Health Care Needs of Older Adults, 514
  - Functional Status, 514
  - Cognitive Function, 515
  - Housing Options for Older Adults, 515
  - Profile of Community- and Home-Based Services, 515
- Home Health Care, 517
  - Home Health Agency, 518
  - Proprietary Agencies, 518
  - Facility-Based Agencies, 518
  - Visiting Nurse Associations, 518
- Overview of Long-Term Care, 519
  - Definition, 519
  - Factors Associated with Institutionalization, 519
  - Medical and Psychosocial Models of Care, 519
- Clinical Aspects of the Nursing Facility, 520
  - Resident Rights, 520
  - Resident Assessment, 521
  - Skin Care, 521
  - Incontinence, 522
  - Nutrition, 522
  - Drug Administration, 523
  - Rehabilitation, 523
  - Infection Control, 524
  - Mental Health, 525
  - End-of-Life Care, 525
- Management Aspects of the Nursing Facility, 525
  - The Nursing Department, 525
  - Nursing Care Delivery Systems, 525
- Specialty Care Settings, 526
  - Assisted-Living Programs, 526
  - Special Care Units, 526
  - Subacute Care, 526
- Innovations in the Nursing Facility, 527
  - Creativity in "Everyday" Nursing Facilities, 527
  - Nurse Practitioners in the Nursing Facility, 527
- The Future of the Nursing Facility, 528
- Hospice, 528
  - Hospice Philosophy, 528

25 Chronic Illness and Rehabilitation, 534
Martha Smith, DNP, APRN, FNP-BC

- Chronicity, 534
  - Prevalence of Chronic Illness, 535
  - Cultural Competency, 536
  - Quality of Life and Health-Related Quality of Life, 537
  - Adherence in Chronic Illness, 537
  - Patient-Centered Approach, 537
  - Psychosocial Needs of Older Adults With Chronic Illness, 538
  - Physiologic Needs of Chronically Ill Older Adults, 540
  - Effect of Chronic Illness on Family and Caregivers, 541
  - Nursing Implications of Caregiver Stress, 541

Rehabilitation, 541
   Care Environments, 542
   Reimbursement Issues, 542
   Public Policy and Legislation, 542
   Enhancement of Fitness and Function, 543
   Functional Assessment, 543
   The Impact Act of 2014, 543
   Keys for Completing a Functional Assessment, 543
   Health Promotion, 544
   Management of Disabling Disorders, 545
   Life Issues, 545
   Nursing Strategies, 545

26 Cancer, 549
Mary B. Winton, PhD, MSN, RN

Incidence, 549
Racial and Ethnic Patterns, 550
Aging and Its Relationship to Cancer, 551
   Aging and Cancer Prevention, 553
Common Malignancies in Older Adults, 553
   Lung Cancer, 553
   Breast Cancer, 554
   Prostate Cancer, 555
   Colorectal Cancer, 556
Screening and Early Detection: Issues for Older Adults, 556
Major Treatment Modalities, 557
   Surgery, 558
   Radiation Therapy, 558
   Chemotherapy, 559
   Targeted Therapy, 559
   Immunotherapy, 561
   Hormone Therapy, 561
   Bone Marrow/Stem Transplant, 561
Common Physiologic Complications, 561
   Bone Marrow Suppression, 562
   Nausea and Vomiting, 562
   Chemotherapy-Induced Oral Mucositis, 563
   Anorexia and Cachexia, 564
   Diarrhea, 564
   Alopecia, 564
Older Adults' Experience of Cancer, 564
   Quality of Life, 564
   Depression, 566
   Grief and Loss, 566
   Social Isolation and Loneliness, 567
   Resources and Support, 567

27 Loss and End-of-Life Issues, 572
Jerilyn Bumpas, DNP, MSN, RN and Jennifer J Yeager, PhD, MSN, RN

Definitions, 572
   Losses, 572
   Bereavement, 572
   Grief, 573
   Mourning, 575
Approaching Death, 577
   Comfort Theory, 577
   General Health-Care Needs, 577
   Effects of Age-Related Changes, 577
   Nursing Care Guidelines for the Older Adult Who is Dying, 578
Hospice, 584
Palliative Care, 584
Legislative Initiatives, 584

Appendix A: Resources and Advocacy Groups for Older Adults, 588
Index, 591

Answers to Next Generation NCLEX® Examination-style Case Studies can be found on Evolve

PART I

Introduction to Gerontologic Nursing

1

Overview of Gerontologic Nursing

Jennifer J. Yeager, PhD, MSN, RN

http://evolve.elsevier.com/Yeager/gerontologic/

LEARNING OBJECTIVES

On completion of this chapter, the reader will be able to:
1. Trace the historic development of gerontologic nursing as a specialty.
2. Identify the educational preparation, practice roles, and certification requirements of the gerontologic nurse generalist, acute or primary care nurse practitioner, and adult-gerontologic clinical nurse specialist.
3. Discuss the major demographic trends in the United States in relation to the older adult population.
4. Describe the effects of each of the following factors on the health, well-being, and life expectancy of older adults:
   - Sex
   - Marital status
   - Race or ethnicity
   - Living situation
   - Educational status
   - Economic status
   - Functional status
5. Discuss how the aging of society will affect the future of healthcare delivery.
6. Explore the concept of ageism as it relates to the care of older adults in various settings.
7. Identify the issues influencing gerontologic nursing education.
8. Analyze the issues affecting gerontologic nursing research.

WHAT WOULD YOU DO?

What would you do if you were faced with the following situations?
- You have been a nurse for 6 years; many of your patients are over the age of 65. Your supervisor requests you become certified as a gerontology nurse; upon reflection, you realize this is a wonderful idea. What steps would you take to achieve this goal?
- You discover your 78-year-old patient has been cutting their pills in half. Because of this, your patient's hypertension is uncontrolled. What factors might play into this decision? How can you intervene?

Previous author: Sue E. Meiner, EdD, APRN, BC, GNP

FOUNDATIONS OF THE SPECIALTY OF GERONTOLOGIC NURSING

One in six Americans is over the age of 65; by 2030, this number is projected to be one in five (Federal Interagency Forum on Aging-Related Statistics, 2020). Between 2009 and 2019, there was a 36% growth in the number of adults over 65 years of age. The number of older adults has grown steadily since 1900, and they continue to be the fastest growing segment of the population (Administration for Community Living [ACL], 2022). The specialty of gerontologic nursing has grown in recognition since the Baby Boomers began to turn 65 years old in 2011. However, this has not always been the case, and the struggle for recognition can be traced back to the beginning of the 20th century.

Professional Origins

In 1966, the American Nurses Association (ANA) established the Division of Geriatric Nursing Practice and defined geriatric nursing as "concerned with the assessment of the nursing needs of older people; planning and implementing nursing care to meet those needs; and evaluating the effectiveness of such care." In 1976, the name *The Division of Geriatric Nursing Practice* was changed to *The Division of Gerontologic Nursing Practice* to reflect the nursing role of providing care to healthy, ill, and frail older persons. The division came to be called the *Council of Gerontologic Nursing* in 1984 to encompass issues beyond clinical practice. Certification for the Gerontologic Clinical Nurse Specialist (GCNS) was established through the ANA in 1989. In 2013, the differences in acute care and primary care for gerontologic nurse practitioners (GNPs) were identified, and separate certification examinations were established by the American

Nurses Credentialing Center (American Nurses Credentialing Center [ANCC], n.d.).

Standards of Practice

The years 1960 to 1970 were characterized by many "firsts," as the specialty devoted to the care of older adults began its exciting development. Journals, textbooks, workshops and seminars, formal education programs, professional certification, and research with a focus on gerontologic nursing have since evolved. However, the singular event that truly legitimized the specialty occurred in 1969, when a committee appointed by the ANA Division of Geriatric Nursing Practice completed the first *Standards of Practice for Geriatric Nursing*. These standards were widely circulated during the next several years; in 1976, they were revised, and the title was changed to *Standards of Gerontological Nursing Practice*. In 1981, *A Statement on the Scope of Gerontological Nursing Practice* was published. The revised *Scope and Standards of Gerontological Nursing Practice* was published in 1987, 1995, and 2010. The changes to this document reflect the comprehensive concepts and dimensions of practice for the nurse working with older adults. In 2010, the revised *Scope and Standards of Gerontological Nursing Practice* not only reflected the nature and scope of current gerontologic nursing practice but also incorporated the concepts of health promotion, health maintenance, disease prevention, and self-care. The second edition of *Gerontological Nursing: Scope and Standards of Practice* was published by the ANA in 2019. This edition adds information on core role accountabilities, qualifications, and ethics, as well as issues, trends, and opportunities impacting gerontologic nursing practice (ANA, 2019).

In addition to the ANA, the Canadian Gerontological Nursing Association (CGNA) has played a large role in the development of specialized nursing practice. First published in 1989, the fourth edition of the *Gerontological Nursing Standards of Practice and Competencies* was published in 2020. The purpose of these standards is to:

- Define the scope and depth of gerontological nursing practice
- Establish criteria and expectations for high-quality nursing practice and safe, ethical care
- Provide criteria for measuring actual and desired performance
- Support the ongoing development of gerontological nursing
- Promote gerontological nursing as a specialty, providing the foundation for certification of gerontological nursing by the Canadian Nurses Association
- Promote components of gerontological nursing knowledge as entry-to-practice competencies, setting a benchmark for new graduates
- Inspire excellence in, commitment to, and accountability for gerontological nursing practice (CGNA, 2020, p. 12).

The *Nursing Scope and Standards of Practice* (4th ed.) was updated in 2021. This update included a revised definition of nursing.

"Nursing integrates the art and science of caring and focuses on the protection, promotion, and optimization of health and human functioning; prevention of illness and injury; facilitation of healing; and alleviation of suffering through compassionate presence. Nursing is the diagnosis and treatment of human responses and advocacy in the care of individuals, families, groups, communities, and populations in recognition of the connection of all humanity" (ANA, 2021, p. 12).

Additionally, the ANA reaffirmed that nursing takes place within the nursing process, stating, "the nursing process is conceptualized as a cyclic, iterative, and dynamic process, including assessment, diagnosis, outcomes identification, planning, implementation and evaluation" (ANA, 2021, p. 20).

Roles

In 1973, the first gerontologic nurses were certified through the ANA. Certification is an additional credential granted by the ANCC (a subsidiary of the ANA), providing a means of recognizing specialized knowledge and clinical competence (ANCC, n.d.). Certification is usually voluntary. From the initial certification offering as a generalist in gerontologic nursing to the first GNP examination offering in 1979 to the GCNS examination first administered in 1989, the gerontologic nursing specialty has continued to grow and attract a high level of interest. The first combined certification for either the acute care Adult-Gerontologic Nurse Specialist (AGCNS) or primary care AGCNS examination took place in 2014. Eligibility criteria for the application process to take any one of the four certification examinations can be found in Box 1.1. Because changes are fluid, contact the ANCC for up-to-date requirements. Additional information can be retrieved from https://www.nursingworld.org/our-certifications/. Information about certification as a gerontology nurse in Canada can be found at https://cna-aiic.ca/en/certification/about-certification.

The Generalist Nurse

The growth of the nursing profession, increasing educational opportunities, demographic changes, and changes in healthcare delivery systems have all influenced the development of the generalist nurse's role in adult and gerontologic nursing and the advanced practice roles. The generalist in gerontologic nursing has completed a basic entry-level educational program and is licensed as a registered nurse (RN). A generalist nurse may practice in a wide variety of settings, including home and the community, long-term care, and acute care. The gerontologic nurse provides care and support for older adults and their families. The challenge of the gerontologic nurse generalist is to identify older adults' strengths and assist them in maximizing their independence, promoting healthy aging, supporting the mental health of the older adult, providing health promotion and disease prevention, and implementing dementia-friendly initiatives (Smith, J. et al., 2022). Older adults should participate as much as possible in decision-making about their care. The generalist nurse consults with the advanced practice nurse and other interdisciplinary healthcare professionals to meet the complex care needs of older adults.

The Clinical Nurse Specialist

The AGCNS requires at least a master's degree in nursing and must be licensed as an RN. The first clinical nurse specialist program was launched in 1966 at Duke University.

> **BOX 1.1 American Nurses Credentialing Center Eligibility Requirements for Certification in Gerontologic Nursing**
>
> **Gerontological Nurse (Registered Nurse—Board Certified (GERO-BC)**
> The nurse must meet all the following requirements before applying for an examination:
> 1. Currently hold an active RN license in the United States or its territories or the professional, legally recognized equivalent in another country.
> 2. Have practiced the equivalent of 2 years, full-time, as an RN.
> 3. Have completed clinical practice of at least 2000 hours in gerontologic nursing within the past 3 years.
> 4. Have had 30 contact hours of continuing education applicable to gerontologic nursing within the past 3 years.
>
> **Adult-Gerontology Acute Care Nurse Practitioner (AGACNP-BC)**
> The nurse must meet all the following requirements:
> 1. Currently hold an active RN license in the United States or its territories or the professional, legally recognized equivalent in another country.
> 2. Hold a master's, postgraduate, or doctorate degree from an acute care AGCP program accredited by the Commission on Collegiate Nursing Education (CCNE) or the Accreditation Commission for Education in Nursing (ACEN).
> 3. A minimum of 500 faculty-supervised clinical hours must be included in the acute care AGNP role and population.
> 4. Three separate, comprehensive graduate-level courses in the following:
>   a. Advanced physiology/pathophysiology, including general principles that apply across the life span.
>   b. Advanced health assessment, which includes assessment of all human systems and advanced assessment techniques, concepts, and approaches.
>   c. Advanced pharmacology, which includes pharmacodynamics (PD), pharmacokinetics, PK and pharmacotherapeutics (PT) of all broad categories of agents.
> 5. Content in:
>   a. Health promotion and/or maintenance.
>   b. Differential diagnosis and disease management, including the use and prescription of pharmacologic and nonpharmacologic interventions.
>
> **Adult-Gerontology Primary Care Nurse Practitioner (AGPCNP-BC)**
> The nurse must meet all the following requirements:
> 1. Currently hold an active RN license in the United States or its territories or the professional, legally recognized equivalent in another country.
> 2. Hold a master's, postgraduate, or doctorate degree from an AGPCNP program accredited by the CCNE or the ACEN.
> 3. A minimum of 500 faculty-supervised clinical hours must be included in the AGPCNP role and population.
> 4. Three separate, comprehensive graduate-level courses in the following:
>   a. Advanced physiology/pathophysiology, including general principles that apply across the life span.
>   b. Advanced health assessment, which includes assessment of all human systems and advanced assessment techniques, concepts, and approaches.
>   c. Advanced pharmacology, which includes PD, PK, and PT.
> 5. Content in:
>   a. Health promotion and/or maintenance.
>   b. Differential diagnosis and disease management, including the use and prescription of pharmacologic and nonpharmacologic interventions.
>
> **Adult-Gerontology Clinical Nurse Specialist (AGCNS-BC)**
> The nurse must meet all the following requirements:
> 1. Currently hold an active RN license in the United States or its territories or the professional, legally recognized equivalent in another country.
> 2. Hold a master's, postgraduate, or doctorate degree from an AGCNS program accredited by the CCNE or the ACEN.
> 3. A minimum of 500 faculty-supervised clinical hours must be included in the AGCNS role and population. The AGCNS program must include content across the health continuum, from wellness through acute care.
> 4. Three separate, comprehensive graduate-level courses in the following:
>   a. Advanced physiology/pathophysiology, including general principles that apply across the life span.
>   b. Advanced health assessment, which includes assessment of all human systems and advanced assessment techniques, concepts, and approaches.
>   c. Advanced pharmacology, which includes PD, PK, and PT of all broad categories of agents.
> 5. Content in:
>   a. Health promotion and/or maintenance.
>   b. Differential diagnosis and disease management, including the use and prescription of pharmacologic and nonpharmacologic interventions.
>
> More details on these certifications can be found online at https://www.nursingworld.org/our-certifications/.

Modified from ANCC Certification Center. (n.d.). Retrieved from https://www.nursingworld.org/our-certifications/.
To keep abreast of the changing scope, standards, and education requirements, the eligibility criteria are reviewed annually and are subject to change. When applying to take a certification examination, request a current catalog from ANCC; compliance with the current eligibility criteria is required. Applications can be downloaded from the Internet.

The gerontologic master's program typically focuses on the advanced knowledge and skills required to care for younger and older adults in a wide variety of settings, and the graduate is prepared to assume a leadership role in the delivery of that care. AGCNSs have an expert understanding of the dynamics, pathophysiology, and psychosocial aspects of aging. They use advanced diagnostic and assessment skills and nursing interventions to manage and improve patient care (ANCC, n.d.). The AGCNS functions as a clinician, educator, consultant, administrator, or researcher to plan care or improve the quality of nursing care for adults and their families. Specialists provide comprehensive care based on theory and research. Today, AGCNSs may be found practicing in acute care hospitals, long-term care or home care settings, or independent practices.

The Nurse Practitioner

The Adult Gerontologic Acute Care Nurse Practitioner or Primary Care Nurse Practitioner (AGACNP/AGPCNP) may be educationally prepared in various ways but must hold a license as an RN. In the early 1970s, the first AGNPs were prepared primarily through continuing education programs.

Another early group of AGNPs received their training and clinical supervision from physicians. Only since the late 1980s has a master's-level education with a focus on primary care been available. In 2004, the American Association of Critical-Care Nurses (AACN) endorsed the position statement that the Doctor of Nursing Practice (DNP) degree was the most appropriate entry-to-practice degree for advanced practice RNs (APRNs). However, only 14% of APRNs hold their DNP. Cost, practicum experience hours, and a failure of professional nursing associations to agree upon entry-to-practice requirements have derailed the enactment of national standards requiring a DNP for APRNs (McCauley et al., 2020).

As a primary care provider and a case manager, the AGNP conducts health assessments, identifies nursing diagnoses, and plans, implements, and evaluates nursing care for adult and older patients. The AGNP has the knowledge and skills to detect and manage limited acute and chronic stable conditions; coordination and collaboration with other healthcare providers is a related essential function. The AGACNP or AGPCNP activities include health promotion, maintenance, and restoration interventions. AGNPs provide acute or primary ambulatory care in independent practice or in a collaborative practice with a physician; they also practice in settings across the continuum of care, including the acute care hospital, subacute care center, ambulatory care setting, and long-term care setting. In most states in the United States, AGNPs hold prescriptive authority for most drugs. Each state has determined the type and extent of prescriptive authority permitted.

Terminology

Any discussion of older adult nursing is complicated by the wide variety of terms used interchangeably to describe the specialty. Some terms are used because of personal preference or because they suggest a certain perspective. Still others are avoided because of the negative inferences they evoke. As described in the preceding overview of the evolution of the specialty, the terminology has changed over the years. The following are the most commonly used terms and definitions:

- *Geriatrics*—derived from the Greek word *geras*, meaning "old age"—is the branch of medicine that deals with the diseases and problems of old age. Viewed by many nurses as having limited application to nursing because of its medical and disease orientation, the term *geriatrics* is generally not used when describing the nursing care of older adults.
- *Gerontology*—derived from the Greek word *geron*, meaning "old man"—is the scientific study of the process of aging and the problems of older adults; it includes biologic, sociologic, psychological, and economic aspects.
- *Gerontologic nursing*—this specialty of nursing involves assessing the health and functional status of older adults, planning and implementing healthcare and services to meet identified needs, and evaluating the effectiveness of such care. *Gerontologic nursing* is the term most often used by nurses specializing in this field.
- *Gerontic nursing*—this term was developed by Gunter and Estes in 1979 and is meant to be more inclusive than *geriatric* or *gerontologic nursing* because it is not limited to diseases or scientific principles. Gerontic nursing connotes the nursing of older persons—the art and practice of nurturing, caring, and comforting. This term has not gained wide acceptance, but some view it as a more appropriate description of the specialty.

These terms and their usage spark a great deal of interest and controversy among nurses practicing with older adults. As the specialty continues to grow and develop, it is likely that the terminology will too.

DEMOGRAPHIC PROFILE OF THE OLDER POPULATION

Nursing care for older adults has come a long way from its beginning in almshouses and nursing homes. Nurses today find themselves caring for older adults in a wide variety of settings, including, but not limited to, emergency departments (EDs), medical-surgical, and critical-care units in hospitals, outpatient clinics and surgical centers, home care agencies, hospices, and rehabilitation and long-term care centers. Nurses in any of these settings need to only count the number of adults 65 or older to understand firsthand what demographers have termed the *graying of America*. Although this trend has already attracted the attention of the healthcare marketplace, it promises to become an even greater influence on healthcare organizations. It is clearly a trend that promises to shape the future practice of nursing in profound and dramatic ways.

Demography is the science dealing with the distribution, density, and vital statistics of human populations. What follows is a review of basic demographic facts about older adults. Keep in mind while reading that the rates and intensity of aging are highly variable and individual. Aging occurs gradually and in no predictable sequence.

Before examining the statistics surrounding aging in America, it is important to understand that President Franklin D. Roosevelt signed the Social Security Act in 1935, setting the retirement age at 65. Although considered arbitrary, the program designers looked at the payments distributed to Civil War veterans and their survivors, as well as the social insurance program adopted by Germany's Chancellor Otto von Bismark, and the International Labour Organization (ILO) which established international social security standards. The government wanted the age set at 70, but the citizens, coping with unemployment from the Great Depression, were asking for age 60. The government considered age 60 too expensive to maintain the program, and age 65 was adopted to appease the citizens and encourage older adults to leave the labor force (Ovaska-Few, 2018).

When the American Social Security program was established in 1935, it was believed that age 65 would be a reasonable age for allocating benefits and services. In 1983, Congress passed legislation slowly raising the retirement age. The current age is 66 years and 2 months for those born in 1955. The age will gradually increase to 67 for those born in 1960 or later, but the earliest a person can receive Social Security will remain at 62 (Social Security Administration [SSA], 2022). However, demographic information and other forms of data are still reported using age 65 as the defining standard for *old*. Considering the heterogeneity of older adults, they are often classified as young-old (65 to 74 years), middle-old (75 to 84 years), or old-old (≥85 years) (Lee et al., 2018). The older adult population has become increasingly older. In 2020, the 65–74 age group (32.5 million) was more than 14 times larger than in 1900 (2.2 million); the 75–84 age group (16.5 million) was 21 times larger (771,369), and the 85+ age group (6.7 million) was more than 54 times larger (122,362) (ACL, 2022, p. 4).

Although grouping older adults is useful in some circumstances, nurses are cautioned against thinking all persons older than 65 years as similar. In fact, older persons are far from a homogeneous group. Landmarks for human growth and development are well established for infancy through middle age, but few landmarks have been discretely defined for older adulthood. In fact, most developmental landmarks described for later life categorize all older persons in the older-than-65 group. One could argue, from a developmental perspective, that great differences exist among 65-, 75-, 85-, and 95-year-olds as they do among 2-, 3-, 4-, and 5-year-olds; yet no definitive landmarks for older adult development have been established. Consequently, nurses are urged to view each older patient as one would any patient—a being with a richly diverse and unique array of internal and external variables that ultimately influence how the person thinks and acts. Understanding how the variables interact with and affect older adults enables the nurse to provide individualized care. Additionally, nurses are encouraged to use each patient as their own standard, comparing the patient's current pattern of health and function with their past status.

The Older Population

The federal government maintains aging statistics available to the public. These publications include an annual chart book with the name of the year. Information can be found at https://www.acl.gov/aging-and-disability-in-america/data-and-research/profile-older-americans. This is now part of the public census and reporting data.

The rapid growth of the older adult population segment is not just an American issue. According to the World Health Organization (WHO), it is expected that between 2015 and 2050, the proportion of the world's population over 60 years will nearly double from 12% to 22% (WHO, 2022). Between 2000 and 2019, life expectancy increased from 66.8 years to 73.4 years worldwide (Global Health Observatory (GHO), n.d.). However, in the United States, life expectancy is at its lowest point in two decades. Life expectancy declined by 1.8 years in 2020 to 76.4 years. The decline in life expectancy is influenced by several factors, including COVID-19, which accounted for 60% of the decline (Noguchi, 2022; ACL, 2022), and the mental health crisis, where 106,000 deaths in the last year were caused by drug overdose (Noguchi, 2022). Other contributing factors include suicide and alcohol-related liver disease (Noguchi, 2022), which have also shortened the life span of Americans, as well as unintentional injuries, homicide (ACL, 2022), heart disease, and diabetes (ACL, 2022; Noguchi, 2022).

Highlights of the Profile of Older Americans

Adults 65 and older account for 55.7 million in America, which is an increase of 38% since 2010. One in every six Americans is an older adult. This accounts for 17% of the population of the United States (ACL, 2022). There were 104,819 persons age 100 and older in 2020—more than triple the 1980 figure of 32,194 (ACL, 2022, p. 4). See Fig. 1.1 for population trends for persons 65 years of age or older.

Sex and Marital Status

Despite the overall decline in longevity in America, females continue to live longer than males. In fact, females live longer than males throughout the world. High-income countries have a greater difference in longevity than low-income countries. However, as gender equity has been achieved, the difference in longevity in high-income countries has narrowed. But narrowing the difference in longevity is not as clear-cut as it seems; class, country of birth, race, socioeconomic status, rurality, and other inequities all play a role in the difference in longevity between males and females (Baum et al., 2021).

Older males are much more likely to be married than older females—69% of males versus 47% of females. In 2021, 30% of females older than 65 were widows. Well over a third (43%) of older females over the age of 75 live alone (ACL, 2022).

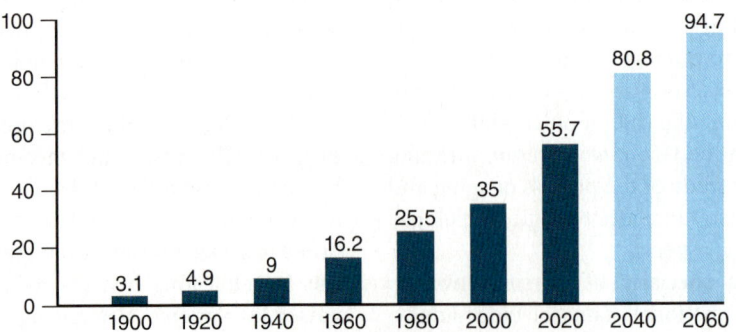

Note: Lighter bars (2040 and 2060) indicate projections.
Source: U.S. Census Bureau, Population Estimates and Projections

Fig. 1.1 Population estimates and projections of persons 65 and older: 1900 to 2060 (numbers in millions). (From Administration for Community Living. [2022]. *2021 profile of older Americans*. Washington, DC: Administration on Aging, U.S. Department of Health and Human Services. Retrieved from https://acl.gov/aging-and-disability-in-america/data-and-research/profile-older-americans.)

Marital status is an important determinant of health and well-being because it influences income, mobility, housing, intimacy, and social interaction.

This demographic fact has important healthcare and policy implications because most older females are likely to be poor, live alone, and have a greater degree of functional impairment and chronic disease. Because of these considerations, many gerontologists view aging as a significant female problem. The nursing profession and gerontologic nurses must assume a prominent role in the political arena and advocate for an agenda that addresses this important issue.

Race and Ethnicity

Statistics from 2020 indicate that 24% of persons 65 or older were minorities: 9% were African Americans (not Hispanic), 5% were Asian Americans (not Hispanic), and fewer than 1% were American Indian, Alaska Native, or Native Hawaiian/Pacific Islander (not Hispanic). In addition, 0.8% of persons older than 65 identified themselves as being of two or more races. Persons of Hispanic origin (of any race) were 8% of the older population (ACL, 2022).

The 2020 census report continues to show the increasing diversity of the American population. Latino or Hispanic and Asian Americans are the fastest growing ethnic groups in America; Latino or Hispanic residents make up 18.7% of the population, African American residents are 12.1%, and Asian Americans are 6.1% (Frey, 2021). The nursing profession must consider the effect of such changing demographic characteristics, as the health status of diverse populations presents unique nursing care challenges.

Living Arrangements

Living arrangements differ according to the needs and preferences of each person. Most older adults prefer to live in their own homes and communities (referred to as *aging in place*). The arrangements might include living alone, with family members, or with an unrelated individual. For those living independently, additional in-home care may be required; assisted-living communities, continuing care retirement communities, group homes, and the controlled environments of long-term care are also options. A person's overall degree of health and well-being greatly influences the selection of housing as they age. Ideally, housing should be selected to promote functional independence, but the need for safety and social interaction must also be considered.

Statistics show that approximately 11% of all adults older than 65 are institutionalized in long-term care facilities or nursing homes. About 27% of community-dwelling older adults, or 15.2 million persons, live alone. Females make up most of this group, numbering 10.1 million compared with 5.2 million males. Of females older than 75, 43% live alone (ACL, 2022) (Fig. 1.2).

As people age, they are more vulnerable to multiple losses and frailty. Frail older adults need more intensive care across all healthcare settings. Despite the growth of life-extending therapies and the continuous development of highly sophisticated treatment measures, the current healthcare delivery system is still not equipped to effectively manage the needs of this segment of the population (Kojima et al., 2019).

Older adults have unique responses to the factors that influence their health status. Advancing age is associated with more physical frailty because of the increased incidence of chronic disease, greater vulnerability to illness and injury, diminished physical functioning, and the increased likelihood of developing cognitive impairment. Additionally, psychological, social, environmental, and financial factors play a significant role in the level of frailty (Kojima et al., 2019). Nevertheless, not *all* older adults are frail. The expectation of wellness, even in the presence of chronic illness and significant impairment, must be incorporated into the consciousness *and* practice of nurses who interact with this population.

In 2019, the median value of homes owned by older persons was $200,000; the median year of construction for these homes was 1972. However, much of an older adult's income went to housing costs: 36% for homeowners and 786% for renters (ACL, 2022).

Geographic Distribution

Older adults, as a group, are less likely to change residences compared with other age groups. This has been an important factor in the growth of the population 65 or older living in metropolitan and nonmetropolitan areas. However, various factors may influence the decision to move. Functional and

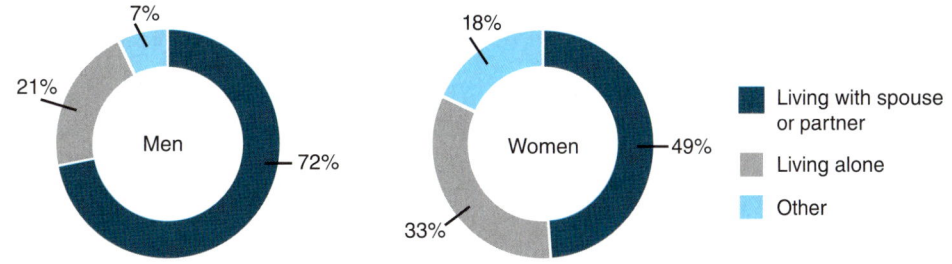

Source: U.S. Census Bureau, Current Population Survey, Annual Social and Economic Supplement 1967 to present

Fig. 1.2 Living arrangements for persons 65 and older: 2021. (Redrawn from Administration for Community Living. [2022]. *2021 profile of older Americans*. Washington, DC: Administration on Aging, U.S. Department of Health and Human Services. Retrieved from https://acl.gov/aging-and-disability-in-america/data-and-research/profile-older-americans.)

health status may require older persons to move to be near caregivers. Dwindling financial resources may necessitate a move to a more economical location; conversely, economic stability or affluence may afford the opportunity to move to a retirement community or a location with a temperate climate and recreational offerings.

Education

The educational level of the older adult population has been steadily increasing. Between 1970 and 2021, the percentage of older adults who had completed high school increased from 28% to 89%. In 2021, about 33% had earned their bachelor's degree or higher (ACL, 2022).

Educational levels are significantly different between Whites and non-Whites. In 2021, 93% of Whites had completed high school, whereas only 83% of Asians, 83% of African Americans, and 62% of Hispanics had achieved the same level of education (ACL, 2022).

Low levels of education may impair an older adult's ability to live a healthy lifestyle, access service and benefit programs, recognize health problems, seek appropriate care, and follow recommendations for care. The literacy level of older adult patients also affects patient educational processes; thus, it is an important consideration in discharge planning, health promotion, and illness/disability prevention (Smith, G. et al., 2022).

Income and Poverty

The median income of older adults in 2020 was $35,808 for older males and $21,245 for older females. For all older persons reporting income in 2020, 12% reported less than $10,000, and 52% reported $25,000 or more (Fig. 1.3). In 2020, the median income of households headed by older adults (adjusting for inflation) decreased by 3.3%. Family households headed by persons 65 or older had a median income of $68.067 in 2020. Non-Whites continued to have substantially lower incomes than their White counterparts. Asian American older adults reported a median income of $67,378, African Americans $54,909, and Hispanics $46,183, whereas non-Hispanic Whites had a median income of $72,855. About 5% of all family households headed by an older adult had annual median incomes of less than $15,000.

More than 5 million older adults were living below the poverty line in 2020. Another 2.6 million older persons were classified as near-poor, with incomes between the poverty level and 125% of the level (ACL, 2022). Sex and race are significant indicators of poverty. Older females had a poverty rate higher than older males in 2020 (10.1% versus 7.6%). Only 6.8% of older non-Hispanic White adults were poor in 2020, compared with 17.2% of older African Americans, 11.5% of Asians, and 16.6% of older Hispanics (ACL, 2022) (Fig. 1.4).

The most important factor in the relationship between income and health is the lifestyle changes imposed by reduced or dwindling financial resources. People unable to meet their basic needs typically reduce the amount spent on healthcare or avoid spending any health-related dollars.

Employment

About 10.6 million older adults (18.9%) were classified as labor force participants (employed or actively seeking employment) in 2021, of which 23%–24% were male and 15.2% were female. (ACL, 2022). The number of older adults in the workforce is roughly 96% of its pre–COVID-19 level. The pandemic hurt older adult workers; while those under 55 were able to work remotely, older adults were unable to work due to vulnerability to the virus, including hospitalization and death. Additionally, older adult workers were more likely to be laid off (22% of those over 55 versus 14% of those under 55). Although the number of older adults in the workforce has decreased, their number is still expected to increase and is expected to be over 25% by 2030 (SeniorLiving.org Team, 2022).

HEALTH STATUS OF OLDER ADULTS

Old age is not synonymous with disease. Although selected portions of this text address disease and disability in old age by emphasizing the provision of age-appropriate nursing care for persons with various conditions, the implication is not that disease is a normal, expected outcome of aging. Clearly, the

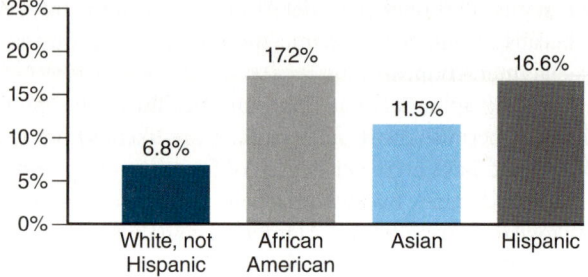

Source: U.S. Census Bureau, Current Population Survey, Annual Social and Economic Supplement

Fig. 1.4 Persons age 65 and over living below the poverty level by race and Hispanic origin, 2020. (From Administration for Community Living. [2022]. *2021 profile of older Americans*. Washington, DC: Administration on Aging, U.S. Department of Health and Human Services. Retrieved July 27, 2023 from https://acl.gov/aging-and-disability-in-america/data-and-research/profile-older-americans.)

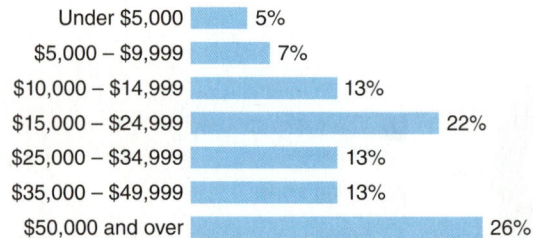

Source: U.S. Census Bureau, Current Population Survey, Annual Social and Economic Supplement

Fig. 1.3 Percentage distribution by income for individuals 65 and older, 2020. (From Administration for Community Living. [2022]. *2021 profile of older Americans*. Washington, DC: Administration on Aging, U.S. Department of Health and Human Services. Retrieved from https://acl.gov/aging-and-disability-in-america/data-and-research/profile-older-americans.)

risks of health problems and disability increase with age, but older adults are not necessarily incapacitated by these problems. They may have multiple, complex health problems resulting in sickness and institutionalization, but nurses should not consider this the norm for older adults.

Because of the high concentration of morbidity and frequent use of health services by certain high-risk groups of older adults, delivery systems are now forced to manage resources more effectively. Strategies to maximize health and prevent disease in older adults are incorporated into health insurance plans. Incentives have prompted the development of innovative programs and service lines that improve outcomes and lower costs for healthy and chronically ill older adults. These proactive developments hold promise for the future care of older adults and provide opportunities to redefine gerontologic nursing practice. The notion of incorporating an expectation of wellness, even when treating those who have chronic disease and functional impairment, is one that is reshaping the care of older adults. Nurses must remember that older adults with disease, disability, or both can be considered healthy and well to some degree on the health–illness continuum. In fact, older adults already tend to view their personal health positively despite the presence of chronic illness, disease, and impairment.

Self-Assessed Health and Chronic Disease

Noninstitutionalized older adults over 75 routinely assessed their health as fair to poor (20%). Most older adults have one or more chronic conditions. In 2021, the most common conditions for community-dwelling older adults were arthritis (47%) and coronary heart disease (14%). In 2021, 75% of those over the age of 65 received their influenza vaccine, 68% reported receiving the pneumococcal vaccine, and 95% reported they had at least one dose of the COVID-19 vaccine. About 30% of adults over the age of 65 were obese, 9% reported that they were current smokers, and 12% reported some form of psychological distress (ACL, 2022). The leading causes of death among older adults are heart disease, cancer, COVID-19, stroke, chronic lower respiratory diseases, Alzheimer disease, and diabetes (National Council on Aging [NCA], 2023).

Functional Status

The degree of functional ability is of greater concern to older adults and nurses than the incidence and prevalence of chronic disease. *Functional ability* is defined as the capacity to carry out the basic self-care activities that ensure overall health and well-being. Functional ability is classified in many measurement tools by activities of daily living (ADLs), such as bathing, dressing, eating, transferring, and toileting (Katz et al., 1963), and instrumental ADLs, which include home-management activities such as shopping, cooking, housekeeping, laundry, and handling money (Lawton & Brody, 1969). These measurement tools were identified more than 45 years ago, but they remain the most used and effective measurement tools available.

The use of such measurement tools or scales to determine the effect of chronic disease and normal aging on physical, psychological, and social functions provides objective information about a person's overall degree of health. Assessment of the effect of chronic disease and age-related decreases in functional status enables nurses to determine needs, plan interventions, and evaluate outcomes.

Chronic disease and disability may impair physical and emotional health, self-care ability, and independence. Interventions to improve the health and functional status of older adults and prevent complications of chronic disease and disability may avert the onset of physical frailty and cognitive impairment, two conditions that increase the likelihood of institutionalization.

Healthcare Expenditure and Use

Through Medicare, the federal government funds most of the healthcare in the United States for persons aged 65 or older. The Medicare insurance program is for people aged 65 or older, younger than 65 with certain disabilities, and any age with end-stage renal disease (ESRD: permanent kidney failure requiring dialysis or a kidney transplantation). The different parts of Medicare include Part A (hospital insurance), Part B (medical insurance), Part C (Medicare Advantage plans such as Health Maintenance Organizations [HMOs] or preferred provider organizations [PPOs]), and Part D (Medicare prescription drug coverage) (Centers for Medicare and Medicaid Services [CMS], 2023). Some basics of these types of coverage include Part A services such as blood transfusions, home health services, hospice care, hospital stays as an inpatient, and residency in a skilled nursing facility (CMS, 2023). For more information on the many benefits or services, go to https://www.medicare.gov or call 800-633-4227.

Implications for Healthcare Delivery

Although the future direction of healthcare is uncertain, based on the demographic profile, it can be confidently surmised that nurses in a wide variety of settings and roles will be challenged to provide care to an increasingly divergent, complex group of older persons. An urgent need exists for gerontologic nurses to (1) create roles that meet the needs of older adults across the continuum of care, (2) develop models of care delivery directed at all levels of prevention, with special emphasis on primary prevention and health promotion services in community-based settings, and (3) assume positions of leadership and influence not only in institutions and settings where care is currently provided to older adults but also in the political arena. The overriding fact to remember is that most of the problems experienced by older adults fall within the scope of *nursing* practice.

The following descriptions of select settings of care are given as an overview and are not intended to be inclusive. Rather, they represent the settings where much of the care is provided to older adults.

Acute Care Setting

The time when the hospital was the hub of the healthcare delivery system has passed. The political climate, market forces, technological advances, and economics are a few of the major external forces that have brought about the significant changes seen in recent years in this traditional care setting. Although the shift is away from the acute care setting toward a wide array of community-based alternatives, a segment of the older adult population will continue to need care in a hospital setting. Acute conditions such as stroke, hip fracture, congestive heart failure (CHF), and infections are common in older adults and are still treated in the hospital, as are critical health problems requiring medical and surgical treatments. However, few acute care hospitals adequately manage the care of their older adult patients in terms of preventing functional decline and promoting independence, which is why the hospital setting continues to be one of the most dangerous for older persons.

Subacute care units are aimed at the high-risk hospitalized older population. Such units typically provide intensive physical and functional interventions to bridge the gap between the hospital and home. These units may be in freestanding facilities, hospital-based, or part of a traditional nursing or rehabilitation facility that has upgraded the physical unit and the staff providing the care. The units provide treatments such as chemotherapy, wound care, intravenous (IV) therapy, and ventilator care.

Because they may be caring for frail, high-risk older adults, nurses in the acute care workforce of today need to recognize that they should quickly acquire the necessary knowledge and skills for delivering timely, age-appropriate care. Knowledge should include (1) an understanding of normal aging and abnormal aging; (2) strong assessment skills to detect subtle changes that indicate impending, serious problems; (3) excellent communication skills when interacting with not only healthy older adults but also those with delirium, dementia, and depression; (4) a keen understanding of rehabilitation principles as they apply to the maintenance and promotion of functional ability in older adults; and (5) sensitivity and patience so that older adults are treated with dignity and respect. It is imperative for acute care nurses to incorporate this knowledge and these skills into their daily practice with older adult patients because hospitalized older adults in the future will likely be even frailer than they are today.

Nursing Facilities

As discussed, the emphasis on reducing costs in the hospital setting through more rapid discharge has led to shifting more acutely ill residents to nursing facilities, which are traditionally referred to as *nursing homes* or *long-term care facilities*. Unfortunately, some of these facilities do not have an adequate number of qualified, professional nursing staff to provide the complex care these residents require. In addition, the nursing staff mix may not be sufficient to meet the needs of this more acutely ill population. Finally, the physical environment and systems for delivering care in the traditional nursing facility may not be the most appropriate for meeting the needs of this acutely ill, more unstable population.

The population of adults older than 85, numbered at 6.7 million in 2020, is expected to double by 2040 (ACL, 2022). Their care needs, coupled with those of the more acutely ill residents who are increasingly being placed in nursing facilities, have already placed great demands on many of these institutions. Economics, particularly as driven by healthcare reform, will determine the future of these institutions.

As the role of the advanced practice nurse continues to progress, opportunities for implementing various models of service delivery for nursing facility residents are growing. For example, AGACNPs are serving as case managers and coordinators of care in this setting. AGPCNPs are providing primary care services to nursing facility residents, demonstrating the delivery of high-quality healthcare. AGCNSs are providing staff education and training and serve as consultants to the nursing staff in assessing and planning nursing care for residents with complex health conditions. Significant gains have been made in the quality of nursing facility resident care because of economic and legislative reforms that have allowed nurses to practice in these innovative ways. Although the momentum is growing, advanced practice nurses are challenged to continue to serve as leaders in promoting continued reform and advocating higher standards of care.

Home Care

The desire and preference of older persons to stay in their own homes for as long as possible is a major driving force influencing the need for increased home care services. Additional factors are the recent economic, governmental, and technological developments that have led to sicker patients being discharged from the hospital after shorter stays, with needs for high-tech care and complex equipment (Mah et al., 2021).

Older home care patients have multiple complex problems. In addition to possessing the knowledge and skills previously noted, home care nurses must be self-directed and capable of functioning with a multidisciplinary team widely dispersed throughout the community. Keen clinical judgment is essential because the home care nurse is often called on to make decisions about whether patients should be referred to a healthcare provider. In addition to physical and psychosocial assessments, the home care nurse is responsible for determining the older adults' functional status. The home care nurse is responsible for assessing home safety and family dynamics, knowledge and use of community resources, knowledge of the older adult's acute and chronic conditions, and lifestyle implications. Excellent coordination and collaboration skills are necessary because the home care nurse is the primary resource for older patients; home care nurses call in other resources as warranted. Finally, a genuine respect for the older adult's wishes, preferences, and rights to live at home is vital.

Nurses caring for homebound older adults need to become involved in conducting community assessments that focus specifically on the aged population. The data obtained from this type of assessment may be used to plan age-specific programs and services aimed at all levels of prevention (i.e., refinement of health screening, health promotion, and health maintenance activities). Linking these activities to existing community-based programs and organizations already used by older persons is a logical place to begin.

Continuum of Care

The shift from acute care and hospital-based organizations to fully integrated health systems has resulted in a highly competitive healthcare market. Managed care organizations (MCOs), patient-centered medical homes (PCMHs), accountable care organizations (ACOs), concierge practices, and pay-as-you-go clinics are types of healthcare organizations and practices in the United States (Arias, 2021). They emphasize health promotion and disease prevention so that maximum health and independence can be achieved. Gerontologic nurses must advocate for *all* older persons along the continuum of care, promoting interventions that result in their highest level of wellness, functionality, and independence.

Continuing efforts to restructure the healthcare system for the older adult population must consider the wide range of care needed by this group. Any healthcare system that evolves for this population must integrate programs of care that allow for ease of movement along the continuum. The future of healthcare for older adults remains in flux. Older adults and their caregivers are anxiously awaiting the new choices that will be presented in hopes of more effectively meeting the needs of a growing and demographically changing population.

EFFECT OF AN AGING POPULATION ON GERONTOLOGIC NURSING

Given the demographic projections presented previously in this chapter and the development of gerontologic nursing as a specialty, the current challenge is to participate in the development of an appropriate healthcare delivery framework for older adults that considers their unique needs. Now is the time for all gerontologic nurses to create a new vision for education, practice, and research.

Ageism

Ageism "refers to the stereotypes (how we think), prejudice (how we feel) and discrimination (how we act) towards others or oneself based on age" (WHO, 2021). Ageism can be seen around us every day: birthday cards that poke fun at aging, sitcoms where jokes are made about the forgetfulness of the older adult characters, and when older adults refer to misplacing their keys as "senior moments" (D'Arrigo, 2022). Allen et al. (2022) concluded that the ageism seen around us every day may be harmful to the health of older adults. Kang & Kim (2022) added that these harmful effects include mental health issues, including anxiety and depression. They determined that interventions aimed at improving self-image and decreasing negative self-talk and emotions can decrease the effects of ageism and improve the psychological well-being of older adults.

Nursing Education

The need for adequately prepared nurses to care for the growing population of older adults continues to intensify. Gerontologic nursing content must be an intricate component throughout the nursing curricula in all nursing educational programs.

The second edition of the *National Gerontological Nursing Association Core Curriculum for Gerontological Nursing* (Luggen & Meiner, 2002) set the tone for the guidelines for essentials in gerontologic education. These texts were developed in conjunction with the now disbanded National Gerontological Nursing Association (NGNA) and were originally conceived as a tool to prepare candidates for the ANCC Certification Examination for the Gerontologic Nurse.

In 2008, the AACN published *The Essentials of Baccalaureate Education for Professional Nursing Practice*. It addressed the inclusion of geriatric nursing content and clinical experience. This document was updated in 2010, with additional information from the Hartford Institute for Geriatric Nursing (HIGN), as *Recommended Baccalaureate Competencies and Curricular Guidelines for the Nursing Care of Older Adults*. The development of the competencies and guidelines came from the need to prepare nurses to care for the burgeoning population of older adults (Box 1.2). Nurses need to graduate with the skills

---

BOX 1.2 Gerontological Nursing Competency Statements

1. Incorporate professional attitudes, values, and expectations about physical and mental aging in the provision of patient-centered care for older adults and their families.
2. Assess barriers for older adults in receiving, understanding, and giving information.
3. Use valid and reliable assessment tools to guide nursing practice for older adults.
4. Assess the living environment as it relates to the functional, physical, cognitive, psychological, and social needs of older adults.
5. Intervene to assist older adults and their support network to achieve personal goals, based on the analysis of the living environment and the availability of community resources.
6. Identify actual or potential mistreatment (physical, mental, or financial abuse, and/or self-neglect) in older adults and refer appropriately.
7. Implement strategies and use online guidelines to prevent and/or identify and manage geriatric syndromes.
8. Recognize and respect the variations in care, the increased complexity, and the increased use of healthcare resources inherent in caring for older adults.
9. Recognize the complex interaction of acute and chronic co-morbid physical and mental conditions and associated treatments common to older adults.
10. Compare models of care that promote safe and quality physical and mental healthcare for older adults, such as Program of All-Inclusive Care for the Elderly (PACE), Nurses Improving Care for Health System Elders (NICHE), Guided Care, Culture Change, and Transitional Care Models.
11. Facilitate ethical, non-coercive decision-making by older adults and/or families/caregivers for maintaining everyday living, receiving treatment, initiating advance directives, and implementing end-of-life care.
12. Promote adherence to the evidence-based practice of providing restraint-free care (both physical and chemical restraints).
13. Integrate leadership and communication techniques that foster discussion and reflection on the extent to which diversity (among nurses, nurse assistive personnel, therapists, healthcare providers, and patients) has the potential to impact the care of older adults.
14. Facilitate safe and effective transitions across levels of care, including acute, community-based, and long-term care (e.g., home, assisted living, hospice, and nursing homes) for older adults and their families.
15. Plan patient-centered care with consideration for the mental and physical health and well-being of informal and formal caregivers of older adults.
16. Advocate for timely and appropriate palliative and hospice care for older adults with physical and cognitive impairments.
17. Implement and monitor strategies to prevent risk and promote quality and safety (e.g., falls, medication mismanagement, and pressure injuries) in the nursing care of older adults with physical and cognitive needs.
18. Utilize resources/programs to promote functional, physical, and mental wellness in older adults.
19. Integrate relevant theories and concepts included in a liberal education into the delivery of patient-centered care for older adults.

Modified from the American Association of Colleges of Nursing and the Hartford Institute for Geriatric Nursing, New York University College of Nursing. (2010). *Recommended baccalaureate competencies and curricular guidelines for the nursing care of older adults*. American Association of Colleges of Nursing. Retrieved from https://www.aacnnursing.org/Portals/0/PDFs/CCNE/AACN-Gero-Competencies-2010.pdf.

to provide quality care across the healthcare continuum to older adults with multiple needs. These works have encouraged nursing educational programs at all levels to add geriatric nursing content with clinical experiences to enhance nurses' responsibilities, knowledge, and skills in the practice of nursing.

However, competencies for nursing students are not the only necessary competencies. Faculty designing and teaching gerontologic nursing content must be competent in gerontologic knowledge and:

> act as role models not only [to] address the complex care needs of older adults, but also to counteract the deep-seated ageism present in nursing as well as society. Needed are nurse educators with crucial gerontological knowledge and instructional skills to facilitate students not only recognizing that older adults will constitute a large part of their care population across most settings, but also having positive attitudes toward their care. (Wyman et al., 2019, p. 454)

The development of the *Core Competencies for Gerontological Nurse Educators* began in 2015. Through an iterative process over the course of two years, a panel of experts developed core competencies addressing the knowledge, skills, and attitudes required to competently teach gerontologic nursing (Wyman et al., 2019) (Box 1.3).

BOX 1.3 Core Competencies for Gerontological Nurse Educators

Competency 1:
Maintains knowledge and skills in the care of older adults.
The Gerontological Nurse Educator possesses the requisite knowledge and skills to prepare students to deliver high-quality nursing care to diverse older adult populations. This includes gerontological, geriatric, and geropsychiatric knowledge and skills that can be obtained through postbaccalaureate formal education or other professional development programs/activities. Experience working with older adults is crucial.
Exemplars that **may** demonstrate competency include:
1.1. Incorporates comprehensive geriatric assessment and evidence-based interventions for older adults and families into their teaching.
1.2. Educates students about normal aging and the complex factors that influence the health, function, and independence of older adults, such as socioeconomic and environmental issues, multiple chronic conditions, geriatric syndromes, atypical illness presentation, and gero-pharmacology.
1.3. Integrates theories and the science of aging into didactic and clinical teaching.
1.4. Maintains national certification(s) in the care of older adults.

Competency 2:
Serves as an advocate and positive role model for quality care for older adults.
2.1. Applies principles of effective teaching, knowledge of the science of learning, national standards of nursing practice, and/or research evidence to inspire and motivate students in the care of older adults, their families, and caregivers within the context of varied healthcare settings.
2.2. Develops collegial working relationships with students, faculty members, interprofessional team members, and community members/partners to promote positive learning environments and commitment in the care of older adults.
2.3. Serves as a consultant or resource for evidence-based practice, theoretical development, and/or teaching in gerontological nursing.
2.4. Provides leadership related to the care of older adults at local/organizational, regional, national, and/or international levels.
2.5. Advocates for policies that promote the health and quality of care for older adults.

Competency 3:
Implements innovative teaching strategies for engaging students in learning about healthy aging and the care of older adults.
Exemplars that may demonstrate this competency include:
3.1. Incorporates conceptual frameworks about aging into teaching.
3.2. Uses evidence-based teaching and learning strategies that generate student value for and interest in the care of older adults.
3.3. Integrates effective learning activities associated with reflection on the aging process and individual experiences.
3.4. Engages students in activities that increase awareness of their own attitudes, values, and expectations about aging and how these influence the care of diverse older adults, families, and communities.
3.5. Develops innovative learning opportunities for students to interact with older adults and their families across the wellness–illness continuum and a variety of settings.

Competency 4:
Facilitates interprofessional learning opportunities for students related to healthy aging and the care of older adults.
The Gerontological Nurse Educator builds strong collaborative relationships with other disciplines to develop meaningful interprofessional education (IPE) and practice opportunities for students to learn about healthy aging and the care of older adults. IPE learning opportunities occur in diverse practice settings, ranging from the hospital to postacute environments and communities.
Exemplars that may demonstrate this competency include:
4.1. Uses nationally recognized competencies for IPE in designing learning opportunities for building team skills and collaborative practice (e.g., Core Competencies for Interprofessional Education and Collaborative Practice [IPECP]).
4.2. Implements learning opportunities that promote positive attitudes towards collaborative practice in the care of older adults and their families/caregivers and prepares students to deliver person- and family-centered care in interprofessional teams.
4.3. Uses case studies, simulation scenarios, and other active learning activities to foster interprofessional practice.
4.4. Creates, implements, or actively participates in practice models that exemplify collaborative practice in diverse settings to foster healthy aging and quality care for older adults and their families/caregivers.

Competency 5:
Facilitates the integration of concepts of healthy aging and care for older adults in academic and/or professional curricula.
The Gerontological Nurse Educator serves as an expert in knowledge of healthy aging and the care of older adults. Using this expertise, the Gerontological Nurse Educator periodically reviews academic and/or professional curricula to ensure that current knowledge and care competencies are integrated throughout courses and education programs.
Exemplars that may demonstrate this competency include:
5.1. Advocates for the integration of concepts of healthy aging and quality care of older adults in academic and/or professional curricula.
5.2. Ensures that didactic and practice learning opportunities in the care of older adults and their families are incorporated into the academic and/or professional curricula.

BOX 1.3 Core Competencies for Gerontological Nurse Educators—cont'd

5.3. Advocates for the periodic review of academic and/or professional curricula to ensure that concepts of healthy aging and care for older adults are well integrated.

5.4. Provides faculty members with current, evidence-based resources to enhance teaching and learning about the care of older adults in a variety of settings.

Competency 6:
Collaborates in the evaluation of learning about healthy aging and the care of older adults in academic and/or professional curricula.

The Gerontological Nurse Educator clearly describes expected learning outcomes for students in prelicensure, graduate, and professional development programs based on nationally recognized gerontological/geriatric nursing competencies and other related competencies (e.g., AACN Competencies to Improve Care for Older Adults, Core Competencies for Interprofessional Collaborative Practice (IPCP), Gerontological Advanced Practice Nurses Association [GAPNA] Consensus Statement on Proficiencies for the APRN Gerontological Specialist, and AACN/HIGN Geropsychiatric Nursing Competency Enhancements). Learning outcomes are evaluated by the Gerontological Nurse Educator in online, classroom, laboratory, simulation, clinical, and community settings using specific criteria for evaluation related to the care of older adults.

Exemplars that may demonstrate this competency include:

6.1. Describes learning outcomes specific to the curriculum expected of students that indicate integration of content and experiences in healthy aging and care of older adults.

6.2. Incorporates reliable, valid criteria, standards, and assessment methods into the evaluation of student learning related to healthy aging and the care of older adults.

6.3. Provides faculty members with development opportunities related to the evaluation of competency-based learning in the care of older adults.

Competency 7:
Demonstrates scholarship and leadership that advances gerontological nursing education and practice and fosters others' professional development.

The Gerontological Nurse Educator demonstrates scholarly leadership in gerontological nursing by disseminating scholarly work in the following areas: teaching, mentorship, and learning related to the care of older adults in academic and professional development programs; discovery that advances new knowledge about healthy aging and care of older adults; integration of gerontology/geriatrics across disciplines and professions; application by engaging in evidence-based practice and policy advocacy and/or leadership related to the care of older adults; or application of new knowledge to improve the care of older adults.

Exemplars that may demonstrate this competency include:

7.1. Presents on gerontological nursing research, education, practice, or policy at local, state, regional, national, or international conferences.

7.2. Provides testimony on aging issues to policymakers.

7.3. Publishes information about research, education, and/or practice projects related to healthy aging and the care of older adults.

7.4. Mentors students, faculty members, and/or clinicians interested in gerontological nursing or interprofessional geriatric practice.

7.5. Demonstrates leadership at the local, state, regional, national, and/or international level that influences the care of older adults.

From the National Hartford Center of Gerontological Nursing Excellence. (n.d.). *Core competencies for gerontological nurse educators*. Retrieved from https://www.nhcgne.org/core-competencies-for-gerontological-nursing-excellence.

EVIDENCE-BASED PRACTICE
The Development of a Deprescribing Competency Framework in Geriatric Nursing Education

Background
On average, older adults take between two and nine medications daily; however, up to 62.5% of these medications have been deemed inappropriate, harmful, or redundant and result in adverse drug reactions. Reducing polypharmacy and adverse drug reactions can be accomplished through deprescribing.

Sample/Setting
Incorporated 24 peer-reviewed qualitative and quantitative manuscripts published between 2005 and 2019.

Methods
The seven steps of the Comprehensive Literature Review Process Model were used to examine the facilitators and barriers faced by nurses regarding the process of deprescribing for older adults and the development of deprescribing competency in geriatric nursing education.

Findings
Analysis revealed three major facilitating factors: (1) effective education and training in deprescribing, (2) the need for continuing education and professional development in medication optimization, and (3) the benefits of multidisciplinary involvement in medication management.

Implications
"The successful development of a nursing deprescribing competency framework [Fig. 1.5] in geriatric care should include effective education and training, continuing education and professional development, and multidisciplinary collaboration. ... The role of the nurse in the deprescribing process includes active participation in a patient's medication management which means a nurse should be able to not only effectively administer and optimize medications, but also recognize medication effects, drug sensitivities, incompatibilities, contraindications, prescribing errors, and polypharmacy impacts. The nurse's role in the deprescribing could also consist of undertaking medication reviews and encouraging discussions with patients about their medications" (p. 1048).

Data from Sun, W., Grabkowski, M., Zou, P., & Ashtarieh, B. (2021). The development of a deprescribing competency framework in geriatric nursing education. *Western Journal of Nursing Research, 43*(11), 1043–1050.

In terms of program evaluation and outcomes, these documents assist in meeting the challenges set forth by evolutions in healthcare, nursing curricula, instructional strategies, and clinical practice models that respond to major trends in healthcare. Nurse educators must develop clinical practice sites for students outside the comfort of the institutional setting that reflect the emerging trends of community-based care, focusing on health promotion, disease prevention, and the preservation of

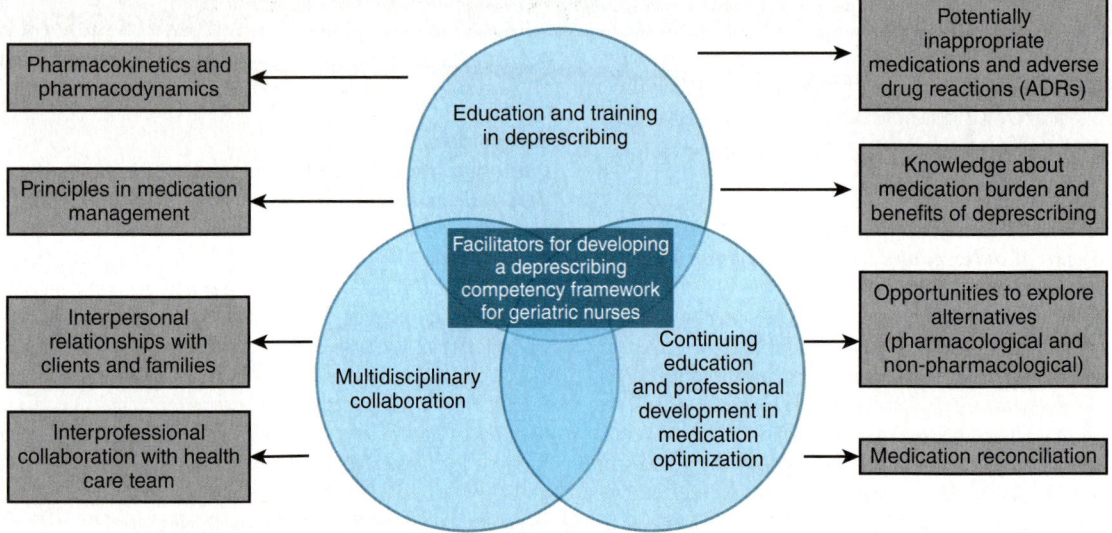

Source: U.S. Census Bureau, Current Population Survey, Annual Social and Economic Supplement

Fig. 1.5 Facilitators for developing a deprescribing competency framework for geriatric nurses. (Redrawn from Sun, W., Grabkowski, M., Zou, P., & Ashtarieh, B. [2021]. The development of a deprescribing competency framework in geriatric nursing education. *Western Journal of Nursing Research, 43*[11], 1043–1050.)

functional abilities. Nurse faculty members with formal preparation in gerontologic nursing are imperative if students are to be adequately prepared to meet the needs of the older adult population.

Assuring nursing students that they will be sufficiently prepared to practice in the future—a future that will increasingly include the care of older adults in a wide variety of settings—necessitates answering many questions concerning nursing education. The primary issue is not whether to include gerontologic nursing content but the extent of its inclusion. Until adequate numbers of nursing faculty are prepared in the specialty, this question will remain unanswered, and students will continue to be inadequately prepared for the future of nursing.

Nursing Practice

Today's older adult healthcare consumers are more knowledgeable and discerning and thus better informed as they become active decision-makers about their health and well-being. Because they have greater financial resources (ACL, 2022) and are more technologically savvy than they were in the past (Faverio, 2022), older adult consumers can exercise more options in all aspects of their daily lives.

As care continues to shift from hospitals to ambulatory or community-based sites, despite older adults having multiple chronic conditions and complex care needs (Roberts et al., 2018, p. 86), older adults are demanding timely care, effective communication and coordination of care, shared decision-making, information about community resources (i.e., transportation), comprehensive discharge planning, and follow-up (Roberts et al., 2018). Gerontologic nurses play an integral role in effecting these changes. As healthcare systems adjust to meet the needs of the growing population of older adults, so will the opportunities for gerontologic nursing practice.

Advanced practice gerontologic nurses practice independently in some states; others work with a collaborating physician in primary care, urgent care, and long-term care facilities. Gerontologic nurses must continue to educate older persons about their care options and lobby for legislation at the state and federal levels to expand reimbursement opportunities for advanced practice nurses who care for older adults.

Considering the increasing number of older adults requiring functional assistance to remain at home, in semi-independent living settings, or in other alternative settings, gerontologic nurses often delegate to unlicensed assistive personnel (UAP, also referred to as nursing assistive personnel [NAP]). UAPs are vital in the delivery of care and in taking on basic nursing tasks. They are trained to assist the nurse in patient care situations. Their typical tasks include (Ohio University, 2022):

- taking vital signs
- providing minor first aid
- assisting with rehabilitative services
- assisting with provision of ADLs.

However, nurses must understand the evolving roles and responsibilities of the various licensed care providers and UAP and delegate them appropriately. In 2019, the National Council of State Boards of Nursing (NCSBN) and the ANA developed *National Guidelines for Nursing Delegation* (Box 1.4) to standardize nurse-UAP delegation.

Gerontologic nurses must consider the effect of many intervening factors on the health status of older adults. Psychological, social, environmental, and economic needs must be given equal consideration as physical needs. The ability to

> **BOX 1.4 Five Rights of Delegation**
>
> **Right Task**
> - The activity falls within the delegatee's job description or is included as part of the established written policies and procedures of the nursing practice setting. The facility needs to ensure the policies and procedures describe the expectations and limits of the activity and provide any necessary competency training.
>
> **Right Circumstance**
> - The health condition of the patient must be stable. If the patient's condition changes, the delegatee must communicate this to the licensed nurse, and the licensed nurse must reassess the situation and the appropriateness of the delegation.
>
> **Right Person**
> - The licensed nurse, along with the employer and the delegatee, is responsible for ensuring that the delegatee possesses the appropriate skills and knowledge to perform the activity.
>
> **Right Directions and Communication**
> - Each delegation situation should be specific to the patient, the licensed nurse, and the delegatee.
> - The licensed nurse is expected to communicate specific instructions for the delegated activity to the delegatee; the delegatee, as part of two-way communication, should ask any clarifying questions. This communication includes any data that need to be collected, the method for collecting the data, the time frame for reporting the results to the licensed nurse, and additional information pertinent to the situation.
> - The delegatee must understand the terms of the delegation and agree to accept the delegated activity.
> - The licensed nurse should ensure that the delegatee understands that they cannot make any decisions or modifications in carrying out the activity without first consulting the licensed nurse.
>
> **Right Supervision and Evaluation**
> - The licensed nurse is responsible for monitoring the delegated activity, following up with the delegatee at the completion of the activity, and evaluating patient outcomes. The delegatee is responsible for communicating patient information to the licensed nurse during the delegation situation. The licensed nurse should be ready and available to intervene as necessary.
> - The licensed nurse should ensure appropriate documentation of the activity is completed.

From the National Council of State Boards of Nursing. (2016). National guidelines for nursing delegation. *Journal of Nursing Regulation, 7*(1), 5–14.

comprehensively assess these areas requires the nurse to possess excellent assessment skills. This is increasingly important as nurses take on more responsibility for caring and treating older adults across all settings. Equally important is the development of coordination and collaboration skills, communication and human relations skills, and the ability to influence others; these skills reflect a true team approach to older adult care.

Nursing Research

Since the early 1980s, nurse researchers have studied the well-being and problems experienced by older adults, designed to improve clinical decision-making and patient outcomes (Bowers, 2020). The results of these and more recent studies can be seen in the publications and organizations that regularly review and disseminate evidence-based practice findings.
- *Journal of Gerontological Nursing*
- *Geriatric Nursing*
- *International Journal of Older People Nursing*
- *Research in Gerontological Nursing*
- *Nursing Older People*
- *Journal of Korean Gerontological Nursing*
- *International Journal of Geriatric Nursing*
- *Perspectives Journal of the Canadian Gerontological Nursing Association*
- *RFP Journal of Gerontology and Geriatric Nursing*
- *Journal of Geriatric Nursing and Health Sciences*

Knowledge built through research is imperative to guide clinical practice and promote quality care and quality of life (QoL) for older adults. Nursing research and evidence-based practice are integral to meeting the *Future of Nursing recommendations*. Additionally, the evidence produced by gerontologic nursing research has informed legislative changes at both the state and national levels (Bowers, 2020). Information concerning federal funding for specific research areas can be found at the National Institute on Aging [NIA] website (https://www.nia.nih.gov/research), the Health Resources and Services Administration (HRSA) website (https://www.hrsa.gov/grants/find-funding), https://www.grants.gov, and the John A. Hartford Foundation website (https://www.johnahartford.org/grants-strategy/). Smaller research grants are available through nursing organizations such as Sigma Theta Tau International, the American Nurses Foundation (ANF), and the Gerontological Advanced Practice Nurses Association (GAPNA).

SUMMARY

Nursing care for older adults is a recognized nursing specialty. The important groundwork that has been laid serves as the basis for guiding future gerontologic nurses. Gerontologic nurses at all levels of educational preparation and in all settings of care should venture into that future with creativity, pride, and determination as they meet their professional responsibility to provide quality care to older adults everywhere. Now is the time to seize the opportunity to advance gerontologic nursing education, practice, and research for the benefit of the older adult population—a population that continues to grow worldwide.

KEY POINTS

- The growth of the nursing profession, increasing educational opportunities, demographic changes, and changes in healthcare delivery systems have all influenced the development of gerontologic nursing roles.
- *Age 65 or older* is widely accepted and used for reporting demographic statistics about older persons; however, turning 65 does not automatically mean a person is "old."
- Nurses are cautioned against thinking of all older adults as alike, even though most demographic data places all adults over 65 into a single reporting group.
- Adults 65 or older currently represent about 17% of the total population of the United States.
- The most rapid and dramatic growth for the older adult population in the United States to date is occurring now as the Baby Boomers reach 65 years old.
- *About* 11% of persons older than 65 live in long-term care facilities, but the percentage increases dramatically with advancing age.
- Sex and race are significant indicators of poverty; older females have a poverty rate significantly higher than older men, and a higher percentage of aging African Americans and Hispanics are poor compared with the percentage of Whites.
- Estimates indicate that most adults over 65 have one or more chronic health conditions.
- Three leading causes of death among older adults are cardiovascular diseases, cancer, and COPD.
- *Ageism* is prejudice against the old just because they are old; it involves how we think, feel, and act towards others based on age.
- Nurses in a variety of settings and roles provide age-appropriate and age-specific care based on a comprehensive and scientific knowledge base.
- Gerontologic nursing content should be included in all nursing education programs.
- Knowledge built through research is imperative to guide clinical practice and promote quality care and QoL for older adults.

CLINICAL JUDGMENT EXERCISES

1. Care for the older person today is considerably more different from what it was in 1960. Cite examples of how and why the care of older adults is different today than it was in the past.
2. When caring for multiple older adults, is it safe to assume that their care will be similar because they are older adults? Why or why not? How can their care be enhanced or compromised if they are treated similarly?
3. At what point in your education do you feel information related to the care of an older adult should be included? In early classes, later in the program, or throughout your nursing program? Support your position.

REFERENCES

Administration for Community Living (ACL). (2022). *2021 profile of older Americans*. Washington, DC: Administration on Aging, U.S. Department of Health and Human Services (HHS). Retrieved from https://acl.gov/aging-and-disability-in-america/data-and-research/profile-older-americans. Accessed July 27, 2023.

Allen, J. O., Solway, E., Kirch, M., Singer, D., Kullgren, J. T., Moïse, V., et al. (2022). Experiences of everyday ageism and the health of older US adults. *JAMA Network Open, 5*(6), e2217240. doi:10.1001/jamanetworkopen.2022.17240.

American Nurses Association (ANA). (2021). *Nursing: Scope and standards of practice* (4th ed.). Silver Spring, MD: ANA.

American Nurses Association (ANA). (2019). *Gerontological nursing: Scope and standards of practice* (2nd ed.). Silver Spring, MD: ANA.

American Nurses Credentialing Center (ANCC). (n.d.). *Our certifications*. NursingWorld.org [website]. Retrieved from https://www.nursingworld.org/our-certifications/. Accessed July 27, 2023.

Arias, A. (2021). *5 Types of healthcare organizations and their medical billing practices*. NCG Medical [website]. Retrieved from https://education.ncgmedical.com/blog/types-of-medical-organizations. Accessed July 27, 2023.

Baum, F., Musolino, C., Gesesew, H. A., & Popay, J. (2021). New perspective on why women live longer than men: An exploration of power, gender, social determinants, and capitals. *International Journal of Environmental Research and Public Health, 18*(2), 661. doi:10.3390/ijerph18020661.

Bowers, B. (2020). Improving practice and informing policy development: The impact of gerontological nursing research. *Geriatric Nursing, 41*(1), 32–37. doi:10.1016/j.gerinurse.2020.01.010.

Canadian Gerontological Nursing Association (CGNA). (2020). *Gerontological nursing standards of practice and competencies 2020* (4th ed.). Toronto, Canada: CGNA.

Centers for Medicare and Medicaid Services (CMS). (2023). *Medicare & you: The official U.S. government medicare handbook*. Washington, DC: CMS. Retrieved from https://www.medicare.gov/publications/10050-Medicare-and-You.pdf. Accessed July 27, 2023.

D'Arrigo, T. (2022). *Ageism takes a toll on physical, mental health*. Psychiatric News [website]. American Psychiatric Association Publishing. doi:10.1176/appi.pn.2022.09.9.5. Retrieved from https://psychnews.psychiatryonline.org/doi/10.1176/appi.pn.2022.09.9.5. Accessed July 27, 2023.

Faverio, M. (2022). *Share of those 65 and older who are tech users has grown in the past decade*. Pew Research Center [website]. Retrieved from https://www.pewresearch.org/fact-tank/2022/01/13/share-of-those-65-and-older-who-are-tech-users-has-grown-in-the-past-decade/. Accessed July 27, 2023.

Federal Interagency Forum on Aging-Related Statistics. (2020). *Older Americans 2020: Key indicators of well-being*. Washington, DC: U.S. Government Printing Office. Retrieved from https://agingstats.gov/docs/LatestReport/OA20_508_10142020.pdf. Accessed July 27, 2023.

Frey, W. H. (2021). *Mapping America's diversity with the 2020 census.* The Brookings Institution [website]. Retrieved from https://www.brookings.edu/research/mapping-americas-diversity-with-the-2020-census/. Accessed July 27, 2023.

Global Health Observatory. (n.d.). *GHE: Life expectancy and healthy life expectancy.* World Health Organization [website]. Retrieved from https://www.who.int/data/gho/data/themes/mortality-and-global-health-estimates/ghe-life-expectancy-and-healthy-life-expectancy. Accessed July 27, 2023.

Gunter, L., & Estes, C. (1979). *Education for gerontic nursing.* New York, NY: Springer.

Kang, H., & Kim, H. (2022). Ageism and psychological well-being among older adults: A systematic review. *Gerontology & Geriatric Medicine, 8,* 23337214221087023. doi:10.1177/23337214221087023.

Katz, S., Ford, A. B., Moskowitz, R. W., Jackson, B. A., & Jaffe, M. W. (1963). Studies of illness in the aged. The index of ADL: A standardized measure of biological and psychosocial function. *JAMA, 185,* 914–919. doi:10.1001/jama.1963.03060120024016.

Kojima, G., Liljas, A. E. M., & Iliffe, S. (2019). Frailty syndrome: Implications and challenges for health care policy. *Risk Management and Healthcare Policy, 12,* 23–30. doi:10.2147/RMHP.S168750.

Lawton, M. P., & Brody, E. M. (1969). Assessment of older people: Self-maintaining and instrumental activities of daily living. *Gerontologist, 9*(3), 179–186. Frailty syndrome: Implications and challenges for health care policy.

Lee, S. B., Oh, J. H., Park, J. H., Choi, S. P., & Wee, J. H. (2018). Differences in youngest-old, middle-old, and oldest-old patients who visit the emergency department. *Clinical and Experimental Emergency Medicine, 5*(4), 249–255. doi:10.15441/ceem.17.261.

Luggen, A. S., & Meiner, S. E. (2002). *NGNA core curriculum for gerontological nursing* (2nd ed.). St. Louis: Mosby.

Mah, J. C., Stevens, S. J., Keefe, J. M., Rockwood, K., & Andrew, M. K. (2021). Social factors influencing utilization of home care in community-dwelling older adults: A scoping review. *BMC Geriatrics, 21*(1), 145. doi:10.1186/s12877-021-02069-1.

McCauley, L. A., Broome, M. E., Frazier, L., Hayes, R., Kurth, A., Musil, C. M., et al. (2020). Doctor of nursing practice (DNP) degree in the United States: Reflecting, readjusting, and getting back on track. *Nursing Outlook, 68*(4), 494–503. doi:10.1016/j.outlook.2020.03.008.

National Council on Aging. (2023). *Get the facts on healthy aging.* NCOA [website]. Retrieved from https://www.ncoa.org/article/get-the-facts-on-healthy-aging. Accessed July 27, 2023.

Noguchi, Y. (2022). *American life expectancy is now at its lowest in nearly two decades.* NPR.org [website]. Retrieved from https://www.npr.org/sections/health-shots/2022/12/22/1144864971/american-life-expectancy-is-now-at-its-lowest-in-nearly-two-decades. Accessed July 27, 2023.

Ohio University. (2022, June 10). *Unlicensed assistive personnel vs. nurses: What are the differences?* Ohio University [website]. Retrieved from https://wp3.onlinemasters.ohio.cds-store.com/blog/unlicensed-assistive-personnel/. Accessed July 27, 2023.

Ovaska-Few, S. (2018). *How 65 became the default retirement age.* Journal of Accountancy [website]. Retrieved from https://www.journalofaccountancy.com/issues/2018/mar/how-65-became-default-retirement-age.html. Accessed July 27, 2023.

Roberts, H., Abonyi, S., & Kryzanowski, J. (2018). What older adults want from their health care providers. *Patient Experience Journal, 5*(3), 81–90. doi:10.35680/2372-0247.1307.

SeniorLiving.org Team. (2022). *Older adult employment: 2021 annual report.* SeniorLiving.org [website]. Retrieved from https://www.seniorliving.org/finance/senior-employment-annual-report/. Accessed July 27, 2023.

Smith, G. D., Ho, K. H. M., Poon, S., & Chan, S. W. C. (2022). Beyond the tip of the iceberg: Health literacy in older people. *Journal of Clinical Nursing, 31*(5-6), E3–E5. doi:10.1111/jocn.16109.

Smith, J., Sawhney, M., Duhn, L., & Woo, K. (2022). The association between new nurses' gerontological education, personal attitudes toward older adults, and intentions to work in gerontological care settings in Ontario, Canada. *The Canadian Journal of Nursing Research, 54*(2), 190–198. doi:10.1177/08445621211063702.

Social Security Administration. (2022). *Fast facts & figures about social security, 2023.* SSA.gov [website]. Retrieved from https://www.ssa.gov/policy/docs/chartbooks/fast_facts/index.html. Accessed July 27, 2023.

World Health Organization. (2022). *Ageing and health.* WHO.int [website]. Retrieved from https://www.who.int/news-room/fact-sheets/detail/ageing-and-health. Accessed July 27, 2023.

World Health Organization. (2021). *Ageing: Ageism.* WHO.int [website]. Retrieved from https://www.who.int/news-room/questions-and-answers/item/ageing-ageism. Accessed July 27, 2023.

Wyman, J. F., Abdallah, L., Baker, N., Bell, C., Cartwright, J., Greenberg, S. A., et al. (2019). Development of core competencies and a recognition program for gerontological nursing educators. *Journal of Professional Nursing, 35*(6), 452–460. doi:10.1016/j.profnurs.2019.04.003.

2

Healthcare Policy that Affects Older Adults

Donna Leake Hamby, DNP, RN, APRN, ACNP-BC

http://evolve.elsevier.com/Yeager/gerontologic/

LEARNING OBJECTIVES

On completion of this chapter, the reader will be able to:
1. Discuss how the Standards of Practice for Registered Nurses guide their legal duties in providing nursing care to older adults.
2. State the sources and definitions of laws such as statutes, regulations, and case law, as well as the levels at which the laws were made, such as federal, state, and local laws.
3. Explore why older adults are considered a vulnerable population, why this is legally significant, and the legal implications of such a designation.
4. Discuss the reasons behind the sweeping nursing facility reform legislation known as the Omnibus Budget Reconciliation Act (OBRA) of 1987 and understand its continuing significance and effect for residents and caregivers in nursing facilities.
5. Identify the OBRA's three major parts and describe the key areas addressed in each part.
6. State the rationale behind the Affordable Care Act and cite who the Act was developed to benefit.
7. Discuss the legal history of the doctrine of autonomy and self-determination and cite major laws that have influenced contemporary thought and practice.
8. Identify the three broad categories of elder abuse, define seven types of abuse, and discuss the responsibility of the nurse in responding to suspected abuse of older adults.
9. Name and state the purpose of tools known as "advance directives" and Physician Orders for Life-Sustaining Treatment (POLST).
10. Explain the purpose of the Patient Self-Determination Act (PSDA) and the nurse's responsibility with respect to advance directives.
11. Discuss ethical challenges for healthcare professionals in preparing patients for end-of-life decisions.

WHAT WOULD YOU DO?

What would you do if you were faced with the following situations?
- You are viewing your social media post received from a coworker who is complaining about a patient's daughter. "She is not happy with any care that her mother is receiving." How will you handle this posting on your social media?
- An elderly patient arrives in the emergency department with their caregiver present. On assessment, you note multiple stages of ecchymosis on their upper arms. The patient is vague about the nature of their injury and states, "Oh, I fell and hurt my arms." The caregiver interjects that the patient is "clumsy and does not follow directions." You suspect there is more to the patient's story and would like to investigate this further. What will you do?
- A patient and their family ask you what the difference is between a living will (advance directive) and a Physician Orders for Life-Sustaining Treatment (POLST) form. How will you explain this to them?

Previous author: Carol Ann Amann, PhD, RN-BC, CDP, FNGNA

Providing nursing care for older adults requires knowledge and understanding of the Registered Nurse's (RN's) scope of practice, as well as the regulatory policies and ethical considerations. Older adults have varied care needs based on their individual physical and mental health status. As such, the RN must be aware of and understand these differences, including promoting and providing quality care so that the individual patient may achieve their highest level of function. This chapter will focus on the RN's professional standards, health policy, and ethical concerns related to the older adult patient.

SCOPE OF PRACTICE AND PROFESSIONAL STANDARDS: LEGAL SIGNIFICANCE

Healthcare providers have an obligation to live up to accepted, prudent, or customary standards of care, which may be determined on a regional or national basis. Nurses are responsible for providing care to their level of education, inclusive of the degree, skill, and diligence measured and recognized by applicable standards of care as established by the RN's state board of nursing.

The duty of care and nurse advocacy roles increase as patients' physical and mental conditions and ability to self-care decline.

Nursing standards of practice are measured according to the expected level of professional practice of those in similar roles and clinical fields. For example, the standards of practice of a gerontological RN practicing at the generalist level would be measured against the practice of other RN generalists practicing in gerontology. The advanced practice gerontological nurse, who holds a minimum of a master's degree in an applicable field, would be expected to conform to standards established for similarly situated advanced practice nurses.

A standard of care is a guideline for nursing practice and establishes an expectation for the nurse to provide safe, effective, and appropriate care. It is used to evaluate whether care administered to patients meets the appropriate level of skill and diligence that can reasonably be expected, given the nurse's level of skill, education, and experience. Standards may originate from many sources. Both state and federal statutes may help establish standards, although conformity with a state's minimum standards does not necessarily prove that due care was provided. Conformity with local, state, and federal standards or comparison with similar facilities (benchmarking) may be considered evidence of proper care (Agency for Healthcare Research and Quality [AHRQ], 2018). Some jurisdictions in the United States call this the *community standard of care.* Note that the community standard of care can be more restrictive within organizations but cannot be lower or hold fewer expectations than the federal standard.

The published standards of professional organizations, representing the opinion of experts in the field, are important in establishing the proper standard of care. The *Gerontological Nursing, Scope and Standards of Practice,* 3rd edition, published in 2010 by the American Nurses Association (ANA), is one example (ANA, 2010). Nurses who care for older patients should be familiar with these standards as well as the newest *Nursing: Scope and Standards of Practice,* released in 2021 by ANA, with the new definition of nursing and the 18 standards (ANA, 2021) (refer to https://www.nursingworld.org).

Most healthcare facilities, at some point, seek accreditation status. This means that they voluntarily undergo a detailed survey by an organization with the skill and expertise to evaluate their services. A major accreditation organization for facilities is The Joint Commission (TJC). The standards established and used by the TJC to review healthcare facilities are often referred to in court cases to ascertain the appropriate standard of care. The standards set by TJC are designed and developed and have proven reasonable and achievable to provide quality and safety for healthcare outcomes (TJC, n.d.).

Federal and state statutes require nursing facilities to have written healthcare and safety policies, and these have been used successfully to establish a standard of care in court cases. Bylaws and internal rules and policies also help establish the standard of care in an organization, although, depending on the circumstances, their importance may vary. In any event, it is important for nurses to be aware of their organization's policies; failure to follow "your own rules" clearly poses a liability risk—both to the nurse and the organization.

OVERVIEW OF RELEVANT HEALTHCARE POLICIES

Sources of Law

Healthcare policy is the law created in the legislative, executive, or judicial branches of the state or federal government. Regulations are rules of action and conduct developed to explain and interpret statutes and to prescribe methods for carrying out statutory mandates. Regulations are also promulgated at the federal and state levels (Mason et al, 2021).

Health Insurance Portability and Accountability Act (HIPAA) of 1996

Recent changes in federal law provide additional protection to individuals and their family members when they need to buy, change, or continue their health insurance. These important laws affect the health benefits of millions of working Americans and their families. It is important that nurses understand these regulations, as well as the laws in their respective states, to help them make more informed choices for themselves or to inform their patients of the options available. HIPAA may:

1. Increase a person's ability to get healthcare coverage when the person begins a new job.
2. Lower the chance of losing existing health coverage, whether the coverage is through a job or through individual health insurance.
3. Help maintain continuous health coverage when a change of job occurs.
4. Help purchase health insurance coverage individually if the coverage is lost under an employer's group health plan and no other health coverage is available (U.S. Department of Health and Human Services [DHHS], 2022a).

Among the specific protections of HIPAA are the following:

1. Limits the use of preexisting condition exclusions.
2. Prohibits group health plans from discriminating by denying coverage or charging extra for coverage based on the person's or a family member's past or present poor health.
3. Guarantees certain small employers and individuals who lost job-related coverage the right to purchase health insurance.
4. Guarantees, in most cases, that employers or individuals who purchase health insurance can renew the coverage regardless of any health conditions of the individuals covered under the insurance policy.
5. Additionally, patients have a right to:
   a. Privacy with third parties
   b. Privacy with the use of electronic health records
   c. Privacy to designate what is shared with family and/or friends
   d. Right to associated fees and timing (DHHS, 2022a)

Several misunderstandings exist about what HIPAA provides. Note the following:

1. HIPAA does *not* require employers to offer or pay for health coverage for employees or family coverage for spouses and dependents.
2. HIPAA does *not* guarantee health coverage for all workers.

3. HIPAA does *not* control the amount an insurer may charge for coverage.
4. HIPAA does *not* require group health plans to offer specific benefits.
5. HIPAA does *not* permit people to keep the same health coverage they had at their old job when they move to a new job.
6. HIPAA does *not* eliminate the use of preexisting condition exclusions.
7. HIPAA does *not* replace the state as the primary regulator of health insurance (DHHS, 2022a).

ELDER ABUSE AND PROTECTIVE SERVICES

As people age, their cognitive decline is often followed by a functional decline. This leads to the inability to perform independent activities of daily living and live independently (McGrath et al, 2020). These changes affect not only older adults but also often their families and others who must see to their care and living needs. Without enacting appropriate interventions and resources, this can lead to the neglect, deliberate abuse, or exploitation of older adults.

In addition, as older adults' abilities to manage their personal affairs are compromised, the necessity of turning the management of certain activities over to others may also open the door to mistreatment. The legal recognition of this vulnerability is reflected in laws enacted specifically to protect older adults. Unfortunately, mistreatment is not defined in the same manner across each state. However, it is known that it occurs recurrently, episodically, and not usually as an isolated incident (Rosen et al, 2018).

The need to protect older adults from abuse is a subject of growing public policy interest. Elder abuse, including neglect and exploitation, is reported to be experienced by one out of every 10 people ages 60 and older (Centers for Disease Control and Prevention [CDC], 2021). However, given the potential for hiding incidents of elder abuse in domestic settings as a "family secret" or out of fear, the incidents of elder abuse are probably underreported. Cultural differences have also led to poor identification of the reaction to abuse.

Elder abuse is defined by state laws, which vary from state to state. However, the following three basic categories of elder abuse exist: (1) domestic elder abuse, (2) institutional elder abuse, and (3) self-neglect or self-abuse (Administration for Community Living [ACL], 2019). Domestic elder abuse refers to forms of maltreatment by someone who has a special relationship with the older adult, for example, a family member or caregiver. Institutional abuse refers to abuse that occurs in residential institutions such as nursing facilities, usually committed by someone who is a paid caregiver, such as a nursing facility staff member. Self-neglect is usually related to a diminished physical or mental decline. It is identified by a failure or refusal to provide oneself with adequate shelter, food, water, hygiene, safety, clothing, or healthcare. Within the three broad categories noted, there are several recognized types of elder abuse.

Definitions of elder abuse are the following:

1. Physical abuse—use of physical force that may result in bodily injury, physical pain, or impairment.
2. Sexual abuse—nonconsensual sexual contact of any kind with an older adult
3. Emotional abuse—infliction of anguish, pain, or distress through verbal or nonverbal acts
4. Financial and material exploitation—illegal or improper use of an older adult's funds, property, or assets
5. Neglect—the refusal or failure of a person to fulfill any part of his or her obligations or duties to an older adult
6. Abandonment—the desertion of an older adult by an individual who has physical custody of the older adult or by a person who has assumed responsibility for providing care to the older adult
7. Self-neglect—behaviors of an older adult that threaten the older adult's health or safety (ACL, 2019.; World Health Organization [WHO], 2022)

Elder abuse generally occurs as the result of many complex factors. Abuse or the potential for abuse may be a result of caregiver stress. The physical and emotional demands of caring for a physically or mentally impaired person can be great, and the lack of supportive resources and financial strain may progress to an abusive relationship (Nguyen et al, 2021; Pickering et al, 2020). Additionally, caregivers with less social support and poor coping mechanisms are at a higher risk of experiencing depression and anxiety disorders, which can lead to burnout and abuse in some situations. Caregivers who have a history of mental illness and drug and alcohol abuse are vulnerable to being abusers if under stress. It is important that nurses are aware of the signs and symptoms of abuse, as well as caregiver stress, when they assess patients (Table 2.1). As the number of older persons requiring care increases, it is paramount that ongoing education

TABLE 2.1 Signs and Symptoms of Elder Abuse

Physical	• Bruises not caused by medications • Wounds that are not treated • Fractures unexplained (spiral)
Sexual	• Bruising in the genital area • Vaginal bleeding or discharge
Emotional or psychological	• Behavioral changes • Depression • Socially withdrawn
Neglect, abandonment, or self-neglect	• Unclean, wearing dirty clothes, or having foul-smelling body odor • Unsanitary environment • Chronic illness not managed • Not taking drugs as prescribed • Increased visits to the Emergency Department • Hungry, malnourished, and/or dehydrated
Financial exploitation	• Diversion of money from the care of a person • Utilities not paid • Medications not purchased (worsening chronic conditions)

Data from ClevelandClinic.org. (2019). *Elder abuse*. Retrieved from https://my.clevelandclinic.org/health/articles/15583-elder-abuse. Accessed July 27, 2023.

inclusive of stress management, abuse identification, and abuse prevention be included as required elements for gerontological nurses.

The term adult protective services refers to the range of laws and regulations enacted to deal with abusive situations. Laws and regulations are administered by a designated agency within each state, which may also work collaboratively with law enforcement. Specific responses to safeguard abused or at-risk older adults may include protective orders and legal involvement to shield older adults from abusive persons; elder abuse statutes that outlaw harmful acts victimizing older adults; and interventions to protect older residents of nursing facilities from abuse, inclusive of the psychological, physical, and social needs of abused older adults (Texas Department of Family and Protective Services, n.d.).

Elder abuse laws levy criminal penalties against those who commit harmful acts against older adults. Many states' laws enhance the penalties for criminal offenses against older persons for example, some violent or property-related offenses outlaw any acts that victimize older adults (e.g., see Texas Administrative Code §705.1001). States may also levy penalties for acts of elder abuse committed by those responsible for the care of older adults in nursing facilities or other institutions. These laws are in addition to those already in effect to protect the rights of patients in facilities governed by federal regulation. Most states have mandatory reporting requirements for nurses, other healthcare workers, and facility employees who have a reasonable suspicion of elder abuse.

States may designate certain professionals, such as nurses or other caregivers, as "mandated reporters." This means that the mandated reporter is required by law to report suspected cases of abuse, neglect, or exploitation. Failure to report as required under this law may result in the imposition of civil penalties, criminal penalties, or both. Tennessee is a mandatory state to report elder abuse (Tennessee Commission on Aging and Disability, n.d.).

Nurses must be aware of their responsibility to respect and preserve the autonomy and individual rights of older adults. All people, including older adults, have the right to healthcare decisions and the right to exercise maximum control over their personal environments and living conditions. The nurse's responsibility in this regard emanates from both legal and professional standards.

Medicare and Medicaid

The federal government, under the Social Security Act, has the primary responsibility for providing medical services to certain older adults, those with disabilities, or certain other classified American citizens. The government fulfills this obligation through the Medicare and Medicaid programs. These programs were enacted as part of the Social Security Amendments of 1965 (P.L. No. 89–97, July 30, 1965 [42 U.S.C. §3001]). Several amendments have been added over the years, and the continuation or proposed modifications of amendments are ongoing.

The U.S. Department of Health and Human Services (DHHS) promulgated regulations for the Medicare and Medicaid programs until July 1, 2001. At that time, the Health Care Financing Administration (HCFA) became the Centers for Medicare and Medicaid Services (CMS).

The Centers for Medicare and Medicaid Services are focused on health equity, expanding services, and improving health outcomes (CMS, 2020). In 2022, CMS has identified six areas for a strategic plan:

1. Advance equity to address the disparities in the current health system
2. Expand access by building on the Affordable Care Act
3. Engage partners in communities with policy and implementation in healthcare services
4. Drive innovation to create solutions for the challenges currently in the healthcare system
5. Protect programs with sustainability and wise spending
6. Foster excellence within CMS and in improving healthcare outcomes (Fig. 2.1)

Programs provided by Medicare for persons 65 years of age or older are for healthcare coverage and treatments. Coverage is limited to services and items that are considered reasonable and necessary to diagnose and/or treat illness (CMS, n.d.[a]).

Medicare Part A covers hospitalization, skilled nursing facilities (limited length of stay), hospice, and select home health services. Part A services are paid through payroll taxes during the beneficiary's employed time and do not have a cost at retirement age 65 years and older. Part B covers physician services and outpatient care. Additional services of physical therapy, occupational therapy, and home health services not covered under Part A are included under Part B. Part D is prescription drug coverage and is available only with a Medicare-eligible plan. Both Parts B and D have a monthly premium based on the beneficiary's income. Income Related Monthly Adjustment (IRMA) is a calculator that is based on last year's reportable salary but may be adjusted for income changes for the current year (CMS, n.d.[a]).

Medicare Part C was effective in January 1999 as the *Medicare +Choice*. Public and private companies were authorized to offer optional health plan coverages to Medicare beneficiaries (i.e., Health Maintenance Organizations [HMO] or Preferred Provider Organizations [PPO]). In December 2003, Part C was amended to include Part D and called *Medicare Advantage* (CMS, n.d.[a]).

NURSING FACILITY REFORM

The Omnibus Budget Reconciliation Act (OBRA) of 1987 focused on the safety and quality of skilled and nursing home patients. Patient abuse, neglect, and monetary misappropriation had been identified as a wide-spread issue nationwide (DHHS, 2022a). The focus was to improve safety and care for the residents in skilled nursing and long-term care (Table 2.2). It is important to note that while Medicare Part A covers skilled nursing, it does not cover long-term care services. OBRA regulations cover both skilled nursing and long-term care services.

In April 2022, the National Academies of Sciences, Engineering, and Medicine (2022) issued a report on quality

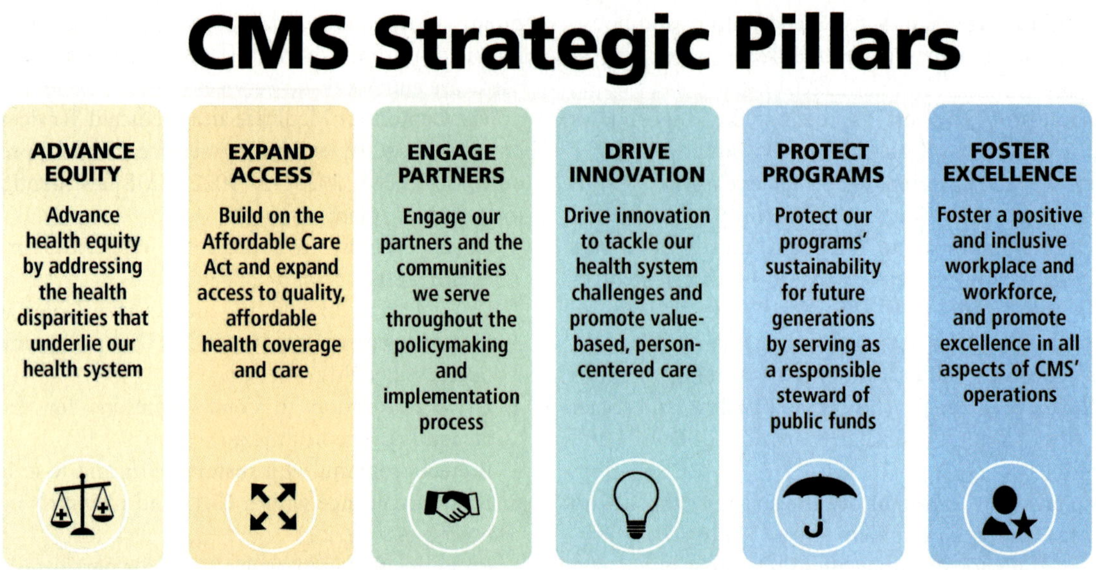

CMS Strategic Pillars

ADVANCE EQUITY — Advance health equity by addressing the health disparities that underlie our health system

EXPAND ACCESS — Build on the Affordable Care Act and expand access to quality, affordable health coverage and care

ENGAGE PARTNERS — Engage our partners and the communities we serve throughout the policymaking and implementation process

DRIVE INNOVATION — Drive innovation to tackle our health system challenges and promote value-based, person-centered care

PROTECT PROGRAMS — Protect our programs' sustainability for future generations by serving as a responsible steward of public funds

FOSTER EXCELLENCE — Foster a positive and inclusive workplace and workforce, and promote excellence in all aspects of CMS' operations

Fig. 2.1 Centers for Medicare and Medicaid Services strategic areas. (From the U.S. Centers for Medicare and Medicaid Services. [2022]. *CMS strategic plan*. Retrieved from https://www.cms.gov/cms-strategic-plan.)

TABLE 2.2 Nursing Care Requirements for the Omnibus Budget Reconciliation Act

42 CFR § 483.15	• Provide services for resident's quality of life • Maintain resident's dignity
42 CFR § 483.20	• Develop a comprehensive plan based on a comprehensive assessment of resident's health at admission
42 CFR § 483.25	• Prevention plan for declining activities of daily living • Prevent pressure sores • Provide treatment to promote healing of pressure sores • Provide care for urinary incontinence and prevent adverse effects • Avoid unnecessary urinary catheters • Prevent weight loss with sufficient nutritional intake • Prevent falls • Prevent dehydration with sufficient fluid intake • Prevent medication errors
42 CFR § 483.30	• Provide sufficient nursing staff
42 CFR § 483.40	• Ensure resident's rights to select activities and schedules • Ensure resident's right to maintain healthcare
42 CFR § 483.60	• Provide a medication service to meet the physical and psychological needs of each resident
42 CFR § 483.75	• Maintain accurate and complete medical records for each resident

Data from the Centers for Medicare and Medicaid Services. (2022). *Nursing homes*. Retrieved from https://www.cms.gov/medicare/provider-enrollment-and-certification/guidanceforlawsandregulations/nursing-homes. Accessed July 27, 2023.

BOX 2.1 Recommendations Established for Improving Nursing Home Quality

1. Deliver comprehensive, person-centered, equitable care that ensures residents' health, quality of life, and safety; promotes autonomy; and manages risks.
2. Ensure a well-prepared, empowered, and appropriately compensated workforce.
3. Increase transparency and accountability in finances, operations, and ownership.
4. Design a more effective and responsive system of quality assurance.
5. Expand and enhance quality measurement and continuous quality improvement.
6. Adopt health information technology in all nursing homes.

Data from the National Academies of Sciences, Engineering, and Medicine & the Committee on the Quality of Care in Nursing Homes. (2022). *The national imperative to improve nursing home quality: Honoring our commitment to residents, families, and staff.* Washington, DC: The National Academies Press.

OBRA's Three Major Parts

The OBRA provisions are divided into three parts: (1) provision of service requirements for nursing facilities, (2) survey and certification processes, and (3) enforcement mechanisms and sanctions.

The provision of service requirements for nursing facilities includes resident assessments, preadmission and annual screening of residents, maintenance and public posting of minimal nurse staffing levels, required and approved nurse aide training programs and competency levels, and professional social worker services in facilities with 120 or more beds. The important focus is on specifying and ensuring resident rights (CMS, 2022a).

The survey and certification processes are conducted annually. Complaints received at a nursing facility are also investigated and may result in a full survey, pending the investigation's findings. Enforcement with fines and sanctions ensures the correction of a problem affecting the health and safety of the residents (CMS, 2022a).

in nursing facilities. As a result of the findings and goals established, changes in regulations and care will be implemented that are not available at the time of this book's printing (Box 2.1).

Provision of Service Requirements

Quality of care. Nurses are the primary healthcare providers for nursing home facilities. They care for the residents 24 hours a day, 7 days a week. Additional providers such as a social worker, physical therapist, and occupational therapist are supportive, but the total care of the resident is dependent on the nurses and nurse aides. Important skills for the nurses are to assess and analyze (recognize and analyze cues, hypothesized needs) for changes in the resident's health, then plan (generate solutions) for care needs, implement (take action), and then evaluate the outcomes.

In Medicare- and Medicaid-certified long-term care facilities, physicians and advanced practice providers evaluate residents at the time of admission, and then reassessment must be completed by a healthcare provider at 30 days and 90 days, with any change in condition, and at 1-year intervals. A state-specified instrument must be used to conduct the initial or intake assessment, which is based on a uniform data set, referred to as the Minimum Data Set (MDS), established by the CMS (2017).

A similar uniform approach to the assessment of adult home care patients, known as the Outcome and Assessment Information Set (OASIS-C), is used across the country. The goal of this tool is to provide a set of essential data items necessary for measuring patient outcomes that have utility for such purposes as outcome monitoring, clinical assessment, and care planning. As of January 1, 2015, the CMS (2012) issued new rules relating to home health agencies that include the required collection of OASIS-C data.

The advent of the OBRA and nursing facility reform has ushered in increased professional accountability. It has increased the demands on nursing time and performance, forced nursing facilities to change the structure of their operation, and resulted in a different image of what nursing facilities are and how they care for their residents.

Nursing assistants must be trained according to regulatory specifications and pass state-approved competency evaluations. They must receive classroom training before any contact with residents and training in areas such as interpersonal skills, infection control, safety procedures, and resident rights. Regulations specific to curriculum and training requirements are developed at the individual state level to govern the profession. Many but not all states require ongoing continuing education in topics such as elder care or working with cognitively impaired residents, for example (NursingLicensure.org, n.d.).

Resident rights. A primary thrust of the OBRA's nursing facility reform provision is to protect and promote the rights of residents to enhance their quality of life. Thus, the legislation contains numerous requirements to ensure the preservation of a resident's rights (OBRA '87 at § 4211[a]). Disclosure obligations on nursing facilities to apprise residents of their rights have been required by the OBRA; residents are to be notified, both orally and in writing, of their rights and responsibilities and of all rules governing resident conduct. Notification and disclosure must take place before or up to the time of admission and must be updated and reviewed during the residents' stay. Box 2.2 provides an example of statements from the OBRA's resident bill of rights, as adapted from the Code of Federal Regulations (CFR). Most facilities have developed a contract for new residents (or a family member or other responsible person) to sign at the time of admission. This is usually called the admission agreement. This agreement sets forth the rights, obligations, and expectations of each party. It is an effective way to inform residents of a facility's rules, regulations, and philosophy of care. This is a practical way to meet the OBRA's notification and disclosure requirements.

Transfer or discharge of residents is permissible by the facility as per the OBRA regulations in the following situations: (1) if the facility cannot meet the residents' needs, (2) if their stay is no longer required for their medical condition, (3) if they fail to pay for their care as agreed to, or (4) if the facility ceases to operate. These provisions provide a 30-day notice and are designed to establish the basic right of a resident to remain in a facility and not be transferred involuntarily unless one of these conditions exists; they also ensure that a resident has been given proper notice with the opportunity to appeal the decision. This was, in part, a response to situations in which older residents of nursing facilities were "ousted" without notice and perhaps without regard to the detrimental effects (both physical and emotional) of being uprooted from familiar surroundings (CMS, 2022b).

OBRA strengthened and enhanced the importance of these requirements by enforcing them as part of the facility survey process. Although the specific contents of resident's rights laws vary considerably from state to state, both the state and federal contents have some similarities. Both are concerned with physician selection, medical decision-making, privacy, dignity, the ability to pursue grievances, discharge and transfer rights, and access to visitors and services (Medicare.gov, n.d.).

Unnecessary drug use and chemical and physical restraints. The OBRA regulations require nursing facility residents to be free of unnecessary drugs; chemical restraints, commonly thought of as psychotropic drugs; and physical restraints. Chemical restraints are inclusive of drugs used to limit or inhibit specific behaviors or

---

BOX 2.2 Resident Bill of Rights

A facility must protect and promote the exercise of rights for all residents. The following are some of those rights:
1. The right to select a personal attending physician and to receive complete information about one's care and treatment, including access to all records pertaining to the resident.
2. Freedom from physical or mental abuse, corporal punishment, involuntary seclusion, and any unwarranted physical or chemical restraints.
3. Privacy regarding accommodations, medical treatment, mail and telephone communication, visits, and meetings of family and resident groups.
4. Confidentiality regarding personal and clinical records.
5. Residing in a facility and receiving services with reasonable accommodation for individual needs and preferences.
6. Protesting one's treatment or care without discrimination or reprisal, including the refusal to participate in experimental research.
7. Participation in resident and family groups.
8. Participation in social, religious, and community activities.
9. The right to examine the federal or state authorities' surveys of a nursing facility.

Note: Modified from 42 CFR § 483.10.

movements, such as antipsychotics, benzodiazepines, other anxiolytic and sedative drugs, and hypnotics. The drug use guidelines are based on the principle that certain issues can be handled with nonpharmacologic methods, and interventions should be utilized and underlying medical concerns ruled out before drug therapy is initiated. Furthermore, when used, drugs must either maintain or demonstrate improvement in a resident's functional status (CMS, 2022b; DHHS, 2024).

Surveyors review the duration of drug therapy regimens and look for documentation of indications for the use of the drug therapy. Nurses should also carefully document the observed effects of drug therapy. This is an area in which the nurse should exercise their skill, knowledge, critical thinking, and leadership by working with others on the resident's care team to ensure that the resident is not unnecessarily medicated. For example, the nurse may work with the interdisciplinary care team to plan and generate solutions for nondrug interventions.

The nurse, as an advocate for the resident, is in a position to inform the healthcare provider about the OBRA's guidelines regarding drug use. This may not only be new information for the provider but also provide a sound explanation that can be used when speaking with a resident's family, who may request drug interventions. In fact, the nurse is in the best position to work with residents and their families to provide information, give instruction on alternative nonpharmacological interventions, and reinforce best practices about this important approach to care.

Reasons for the use of antipsychotic drugs must be documented in the physician's orders and in the resident care plan. They should not be used for unusual behaviors, such as restlessness, insomnia, yelling or screaming, and wandering, or because of the staff's inability to manage the resident.

The OBRA mandates a 25% reduction in dose trials, unless the drug has been tried previously and has resulted in decompensation for the resident or if the resident has one of the following conditions:

1. Schizophrenia
2. Schizoid-affective disorder
3. Delusional disorder
4. Acute psychosis
5. Mania with a psychotic mood
6. Brief reactive psychosis
7. Atypical psychosis
8. Tourette syndrome
9. Huntington chorea
10. Short-term symptomatic treatment of nausea, vomiting, hiccups, or itching
11. Dementia associated with psychotic or violent features that represent a danger to the patient or others (CMS, 2022b)

Physical restraints are appliances that inhibit free physical movement, for example, limb restraints, vests, jackets, and waist belts. Wheelchairs, geriatric chairs, and side rails may, in some circumstances, be considered forms of physical restraint. This type of restraint may be used only when specific medical indications exist and when a provider has written a specific order for their use. The order must include the type of restraint, the condition or specific behavior for which it is to be applied, and a specified time or duration for its use. Orders for a restraint must be reevaluated and, if use is to be continued, periodically reassessed (Texas Health and Safety Law §576.024).

Reductions in the use of physical restraints and almost universal use of CMS's resident assessment system are indications that nursing facility reform is working. Nurses have been successful in employing interventions directed toward avoiding the use of chemical or physical restraints. Some of these interventions are as follows: companionship; increased patient supervision; meeting physical needs such as toileting, exercise, or hunger; staff training; 1:1 safety sitters; and distraction and other psychosocial approaches. Nurses are in a unique position to positively affect the quality of life of institutionalized older adults. Nurses should continue to educate others about behavior management techniques to decrease the incidence of chemical and physical restraint usage.

A facility or nurse is not absolved from regulatory liability by the mere presence of a provider's written order for restraints of any kind. Nurses have a legal duty to know the legal obligations and protections in the state in which they practice (Schroeter, 2021). The American Nurses' Association (ANA, 2015) has published a booklet discussing ethical practice with models for decision-making. Nurses should participate in the development of problem-solving procedures established to provide constructive and effective ways to resolve disputes involving patient care issues.

Urinary incontinence. Urinary incontinence is commonly noted in skilled nursing facilities (SNFs). In fact, more than half of nursing facility residents are incontinent. Left untreated, this condition may lead to other physical problems such as infections and skin breakdown. Urinary incontinence in a nursing home resident is associated with a higher risk of mortality (Huang et al, 2021). Because this is a prevalent condition and one that has implications for the quality and enjoyment of life, it may be expected to remain a major area of regulatory scrutiny. Under OBRA, nursing facilities are required to include incontinence in the comprehensive assessment of a resident's functions and to provide the necessary treatment, including bladder retraining, prompted voiding, pelvic floor exercises, etc. (CMS, 2022b). Furthermore, a designated state agency's surveyors focus on this problem by evaluating its occurrence in the nursing facilities they survey and assessing the extent to which residents have interventions such as incontinence therapy and wound prevention. It is important for the nurse to understand the different types of incontinence and work with the interprofessional team to develop and implement (generate solutions and take action) a plan of care (Kane et al, 2018a).

Facility Survey and Certification

The CMS (2022b) is determined to see that every nursing facility implements and complies with the letter and spirit of the OBRA's requirements. This determination is enforced through a process of surveying facilities that certifies a facility's compliance with OBRA's laws and regulations. The enactment of the OBRA created a new survey process. In general, the standard survey is conducted to review the quality of care by evaluating criteria such as medical, nursing, and rehabilitative care, dietary services, infection control, and the physical environment.

Written care plans and resident assessments are evaluated for their adequacy and accuracy, and the surveyors look for compliance with residents' rights. OBRA's long-term care survey processes place a renewed emphasis on the outcome of resident care rather than mere documented compliance with regulatory requirements.

By contractual arrangement with the DHHS, state survey agencies are authorized to certify facilities' compliance. States are also required to educate facility staff regarding the survey process and are further authorized to investigate complaints of all types. Based on reports of persistent problems in nursing facilities that spearheaded government involvement, CMS (2022b) strives to strengthen federal oversight of nursing facility quality and safety standards. These steps include increasing the frequency of inspections for repeat offenders or facilities with serious violations.

Surveys are conducted by a multidisciplinary survey team of professionals, including at least one RN. Survey participants include facility personnel, residents and their families, and the state's long-term care public advocate who investigates complaints, known as an ombudsman. Surveyors interview residents and ask them about facility policies and procedures. They observe staff in the performance of their duties, and staff may be asked to complete forms required by the survey team.

Enforcement Mechanisms and Sanctions

The DHHS and the states may apply sanctions or penalties against a facility for failure to meet requirements and standards. Such sanctions include civil monetary penalties, the appointment of a temporary manager to run a facility while deficiencies are remedied, or even the closure of a facility or the transfer of residents to another facility (or both). In addition, CMS (n.d.[b]) and some State Department of Health offices publish individual nursing facility survey results and violation records on their nursing home comparison website to increase accountability and flag repeated offenders for families and the public.

The nurse needs to understand that officials, authorized by the state or federal agencies that oversee the operation of nursing facilities (or any licensed healthcare institution or setting), may enter and review activities within an organization at any time. They are not required to announce their visit in advance; OBRA's regulations specifically prohibit this for the annual standard survey, and nurses must respond to their questions and requests for information and records once proper identification is shown.

The nurse should be aware that a surveyor may find information suggesting that the practice of a licensed nurse may have been improper or may not have met the proper standard of care. For example, a nurse may have a high incidence of medication errors or may not have taken proper action when a patient or resident experienced a change in condition. In such cases, the surveyor has the option to forward this finding to the State Board of Nursing. This again underscores the need for nurses to be diligent, current, conscientious, and accountable in their professional practice.

Affordable Care Act

The Affordable Care Act (ACA) was passed by Congress on March 21, 2010, and signed into law on March 23, 2010, by former President Barack Obama. The ACA represents the largest change in the United States Health Care System since 1965, when Medicare and Medicaid were enacted and initiated. The main goal of the ACA is to reduce the number of Americans who do not have health insurance and to further reduce the overall costs of healthcare in the United States (DHHS, 2022b).

Legislative changes to the ACA in 2017 repealed the individual mandate, eliminated cost-sharing reductions, increased state Medicaid waivers, and expanded Association Health Plans (AHPs) (Beaton, 2018). The overall impact of these changes on the ACA is yet to be determined.

All Americans will be able to obtain health insurance regardless of their community rating, preexisting medical conditions, or age. Everyone within the same age group and location must be charged the same premium. Failure to secure coverage may lead to penalties assessed by a health insurance tax.

The Patient Self-Determination Act

The PSDA came into effect in 1990 as an amendment to Titles XVIII and XIX of the Social Security Act. The law's intent is to ensure that patients are informed about the extent to which their rights are protected under state law. The PSDA requires hospitals, nursing facilities, and other healthcare providers who receive federal funds, such as Medicare or Medicaid, to give patients written information explaining their legal options for refusing or accepting treatment should they become incapacitated (Teoli & Ghassemzadeh, 2022).

This law is significant because it empowers patients to make decisions about their healthcare and express their desired Advanced Medical Directives (AMDs). All healthcare professionals have a duty to ensure that patients know and understand their healthcare-related rights (Teoli and Ghassemzadeh, 2022).

AUTONOMY AND SELF-DETERMINATION

The right to self-determination has its basis in the doctrine of informed consent. Informed consent is the process by which competent individuals are provided with information that enables them to make a reasonable decision about any treatment or intervention to be performed on them. It is generally accepted that for consent to be valid and legally sufficient, a standard of disclosure must be met that includes the diagnosis, the nature and purpose of the treatment, the risks of the treatment, the probability of success of the treatment, available treatment alternatives, and the consequences of not receiving the treatment.

To ensure decisions, various documents can be used, such as a living will or medical power of attorney. It is important for the nurse to understand that a lack of documents does not mean a decision has not been made. There are alternative methods for individuals to use rather than the documents. Nurses must remember that the right to decide what shall be done for and to themselves is a fundamental right. Legal tools should be used to assist, not detract, from that basic human right. The nurse's role as advocate has a high degree of importance in this regard.

The right to self-determination covers all decisions about one's care and treatment, including the removal of life support or life-sustaining treatments and life-prolonging or life-saving measures. These issues are particularly relevant to older adults. Although individuals of all ages are concerned with these matters and young persons do die, incapacity and infirmity are more common in old age. Therefore, more frequent discussion of the need to preserve the right to self-determination occurs among older adults.

The doctrine and standards of informed consent are intended to apply to the decision-making capability of one who makes such a decision. There is a distinct difference between decision-making capacity and competency. *Competence* is a legal term that presumes a person is competent unless found not to be by the court system. Competency may be related to one specific area or could be for all major decisions. A person may not be competent to manage finances, but they can be competent in other areas of their life. Decision-making capability is provided by the medical provider, with substantial documentation to support this fact (Amaral et al, 2022). Nurses must remember that all persons have the right to decide what treatments they want or do not want. Even if a person has been evaluated by the medical provider to not have decision-making capability, the nurse must be aware that this is related to consent to medical treatment. For example, a resident in the nursing home has the right to choose their clothing to wear for a particular day.

Do Not Resuscitate Orders

A DNR order is a specific order from a healthcare provider, entered on the patient/resident's order sheet or by using computerized physician order entry (CPOE) systems. Code status or DNR orders have been used for many years. The order instructs healthcare providers not to use or order specific methods of life-saving therapy, referred to as *cardiopulmonary resuscitation* (CPR). This generally includes measures and therapies used to restore cardiac function or to support ventilation in the event of a cardiac or respiratory arrest (McKinney's consolidated laws of New York annotated, Public Health Law § 2961[4]) and to handle emergencies caused by sudden loss of oxygen supply to the brain because of lung or cardiac failure. In some states, consent to CPR is presumed unless a DNR order has been issued (McKinney's consolidated laws of New York annotated, Public Health Law § 2962[1], 1993). The DNR order is written based on the individual's choice of no treatment, partial treatment, or maximum treatment without resuscitation.

For a person to choose to accept or reject medical care, it is assumed that they have decision-making capacity (Amaral et al, 2022). The capacity to make decisions is applicable only to the decision being made at the time. Even if a person has appointed an agent to manage their affairs, this does not necessarily mean that the person does not have decision-making capability. For example, a person may have difficulty seeing and may need assistance from a child, sibling, or other trusted individual to help with financial responsibilities. This does not mean that they do not have the capacity to make decisions.

A challenge for older adults is issues concerning the right to self-determination, and in such matters, patients' statements and other indications of their wishes, as well as their state of mind, are critical. Nurses should keep these points in mind when they are responsible for the care of older adults, and they should make certain that records and notations, assessments, and other ongoing observations are carefully, objectively, and accurately documented. If a time comes when a nurse needs to refer to records to testify in a court proceeding, the information provided will be used to help determine how an individual's basic rights are being addressed. A nurse can be secure in knowing that everything morally, ethically, and legally has been performed to ensure that the resident's rights are respected.

Guidelines for DNR Policies in Nursing Facilities

DNR orders are used in hospitals. In many states, an Out of Hospital form signed by a clinician is used in nursing facilities (Texas Administrative Code § 157.25). Nurses are responsible for knowing the policies for the nursing facility as well as state regulations. Because the nurse may be the only healthcare professional present in the nursing facility at any given time, it is imperative for the nurse to request that the facility have a detailed and specific policy to provide the necessary guidance.

Legal Tools

There are several tools available for individuals that assist with decision-making if they become incapable of expressing their wishes. These documents vary from state to state; however, the most commonly used are:
- AMDs.
- Living wills (LWs) or designation of healthcare agents.
- Physician orders for life-sustaining treatment.
- Durable power of attorney.

Advanced Medical Directives

AMDs are documents that permit people to express in writing their wishes and preferences regarding healthcare. These legal documents are used to indicate the patient/resident's healthcare decisions if the time comes when they are unable to speak for themselves. Some AMDs also permit people to designate someone to convey their wishes in the event they are rendered unable to do so. The AMD is helpful to professionals because it provides information and guidance based on the person's wishes for their treatment decisions. (Mayo Clinic, 2022). An AMD is not a living will. Both are directives for a person's treatment wishes; however, the AMD may or may not have a designated person to convey their wishes. Most often, the AMD has more specific information than the living will.

Living Wills or Designation of Healthcare Agents

LWs are intended to provide written expressions of a patient's wishes regarding the use of medical treatments in the event of a terminal illness or condition. Healthcare agent designations entail appointing a trusted person to express the patient's wishes regarding the withholding or withdrawal of life support when the patient is cognitively stable and aware of their decisions (Boxes 2.3 and 2.4).

Allowing for variations among states, LWs are generally not effective until (1) the attending physician has the document and

CHAPTER 2 Healthcare Policy that Affects Older Adults

BOX 2.3 Living Will Example

Connecticut General Statutes § 19A-575. Form of Document

Any person 18 years of age or older may execute a document that contains directions as to specific life support systems that such person chooses to have administered. Such document shall be signed and dated by the maker with at least two witnesses and may be substantially in the following form:

Document Concerning Withholding or Withdrawal of Life Support Systems

If the time comes when I am incapacitated to the point where I can no longer actively take part in decisions for my own life and am unable to direct my physician as to my own medical care, I wish this statement to stand as a testament to my wishes.

I .... (NAME) request that, if my condition is deemed terminal or if it is determined that I will be permanently unconscious, I be allowed to die and not be kept alive through life support systems. By terminal condition, I mean that I have an incurable or irreversible medical condition that, without the administration of life support systems, will, in the opinion of my attending physician, result in death within a relatively short time. By permanently unconscious, I mean that I am in a permanent coma or persistent vegetative state, which is an irreversible condition in which I am at no time aware of myself or the environment and show no behavioral response to the environment. The life support systems that I do not want included, but are not limited to:

Artificial respiration
Cardiopulmonary resuscitation
Artificial means of providing nutrition and hydration (cross out any initial life support systems you want to be administered.)

I do not intend any direct taking of my life, but only that my dying not be unreasonably prolonged.

Other specific requests:

This request is made after careful reflection while I am of sound mind.

.... (Signature)
.... (Date)

This document was signed in our presence by the above-named

.... (NAME) who appeared to be 18 years of age or older, of sound mind, and able to understand the nature and consequences of healthcare decisions at the time the document was signed.

.... (Witness)
.... (Address)
.... (Witness)
.... (Address)

BOX 2.4 Healthcare Agent Example

Connecticut Healthcare Agent (C.G.S. § 19A-577)

(a) Any person 18 years of age or older may execute a document that may, but need not, be substantially in the following form:

Document Concerning the Appointment of a Healthcare Agent

I appoint .... (NAME) to be my healthcare agent. If my attending physician determines that I am unable to understand and appreciate the nature and consequences of healthcare decisions and to reach and communicate an informed decision regarding treatment, my healthcare agent is authorized to:
1) convey to my physician my wishes concerning the withholding or removal of life support systems.
2) take whatever actions are necessary to ensure that my wishes are given effect.

If this person is unwilling or unable to serve as my healthcare agent, I appoint .... (NAME) to be my alternative healthcare agent.

This request is made after careful reflection while I am of sound mind.

.... (Signature)
.... (Date)

This document was signed in our presence by the above-named

.... (NAME) who appeared to be 18 years of age or older, of sound mind, and able to understand the nature and consequences of healthcare decisions at the time the document was signed.

.... (Witness)
.... (Address)
.... (Witness)
.... (Address)

the patient has been determined to lack decision-making capacity, (2) the physician has determined the patient has a terminal condition or a condition such that any therapy provided would only prolong dying, and (3) the physician has written the appropriate orders in the medical record (Mayo Clinic, 2022).

Most statutes require that the patient's signature be witnessed. The witness usually does not have to attest to the patient's mental competence; however, many forms require that the witness indicate that the principal "appeared" to be of sound mind. In general, it is also prohibited for an owner or employee of a facility where a person is a resident or patient to serve as a witness to a signature (Mayo Clinic, 2022). It is important for the nurse to know that a resident or patient has the right to revoke or change their LW or AMD at any time if they remain cognizant and aware of the changes and possible repercussions.

Physician Orders for Life-Sustaining Treatment

Physician Orders for Life-Sustaining Treatment (POLST) is a process of communicating healthcare wishes during a medical crisis or decline in health (National POLST Collaborative, 2022). This tool is seeing more frequent use and allows the patient to communicate with their physician to set forth medical orders to be followed. The POLST form does not replace traditional end-of-life care communication tools such as advance directives, "no code," or DNR statuses. Rather, it augments these tools to provide a comprehensive set of patient preferences for care, more so than simply a DNR.

The POLST is an ongoing order that reflects the patient's wishes for care when severely ill (National POLST Collaborative, 2019) (Fig. 2.2). Importantly, although POLST forms may vary slightly from state to state, they all include sections where patients can identify their wishes related to resuscitation (Section A), intubation (Section B), instructions related to other medical interventions such as blood transfusions and dialysis (Section C), and artificial nutrition (Section D). The second page of the form identifies emergency contacts and a section

HIPAA PERMITS DISCLOSURE OF POLST ORDERS TO HEALTH CARE PROVIDERS AS NECESSARY FOR TREATMENT WHENEVER TRANSFERRED OR DISCHARGED

National POLST Model Form: A Portable Medical Order   Copyright © 2019 by NPC. All rights reserved*

Health care providers should complete this form only after a conversation with their patient or the patient's representative. The POLST decision-making process is for patients who are at risk for a life-threatening clinical event because they have a serious life-limiting medical condition, which may include advanced frailty (www.polst.org/guidance-appropriate-patients-pdf).

Patient Information.	Having a POLST form is always voluntary.
This is a medical order, not an advance directive. For information about POLST and to understand this document, visit: www.polst.org/form	Patient First Name: _____ Middle Name/Initial: _____ Preferred name: _____ Last Name: _____ Suffix (Jr, Sr, etc): _____ DOB (mm/dd/yyyy): __/__/____ State where form was completed: _____ Gender: ☐ M ☐ F ☐ X Social Security Number's last 4 digits (optional): xxx-xx-__ __ __ __

A. Cardiopulmonary Resuscitation Orders. Follow these orders if patient has no pulse and is not breathing.

Pick 1
- ☐ YES CPR: Attempt Resuscitation, including mechanical ventilation, defibrillation and cardioversion. (Requires choosing Full Treatments in Section B)
- ☐ NO CPR: Do Not Attempt Resuscitation. (May choose any option in Section B)

B. Initial Treatment Orders. Follow these orders if patient has a pulse and/or is breathing.

Reassess and discuss interventions with patient or patient representative regularly to ensure treatments are meeting patient's care goals. Consider a time-trial of interventions based on goals and specific outcomes.

Pick 1
- ☐ **Full Treatments (required if choose CPR in Section A).** Goal: Attempt to sustain life by all medically effective means. Provide appropriate medical and surgical treatments as indicated to attempt to prolong life, including intensive care.
- ☐ **Selective Treatments.** Goal: Attempt to restore function while avoiding intensive care and resuscitation efforts (ventilator, defibrillation and cardioversion). May use non-invasive positive airway pressure, antibiotics and IV fluids as indicated. Avoid intensive care. Transfer to hospital if treatment needs cannot be met in current location.
- ☐ **Comfort-focused Treatments.** Goal: Maximize comfort through symptom management; allow natural death. Use oxygen, suction and manual treatment of airway obstruction as needed for comfort. Avoid treatments listed in full or select treatments unless consistent with comfort goal. Transfer to hospital **only** if comfort cannot be achieved in current setting.

C. Additional Orders or Instructions. These orders are in addition to those above (e.g., blood products, dialysis).
[EMS protocols may limit emergency responder ability to act on orders in this section.]

D. Medically Assisted Nutrition (Offer food by mouth if desired by patient, safe and tolerated)

Pick 1
- ☐ Provide feeding through new or existing surgically-placed tubes
- ☐ No artificial means of nutrition desired
- ☐ Trial period for artificial nutrition but no surgically-placed tubes
- ☐ Not discussed or no decision made (provide standard of care)

E. SIGNATURE: Patient or Patient Representative (eSigned documents are valid)

I understand this form is voluntary. I have discussed my treatment options and goals of care with my provider. If signing as the patient's representative, the treatments are consistent with the patient's known wishes and in their best interest.

✘ (required) _____

If other than patient, print full name:	Authority:	The most recently completed valid POLST form supersedes all previously completed POLST forms.

F. SIGNATURE: Health Care Provider (eSigned documents are valid)   Verbal orders are acceptable with follow up signature.

I have discussed this order with the patient or his/her representative. The orders reflect the patient's known wishes, to the best of my knowledge. [Note: Only licensed health care providers authorized by law to sign POLST form in state where completed may sign this order]

✘ (required) _____   Date (mm/dd/yyyy): Required __/__/____   Phone #: ( )

Printed Full Name: _____   License/Cert. #: _____

Supervising physician signature: ☐ N/A   License #: _____

A copied, faxed or electronic version of this form is a legal and valid medical order. This form does not expire.   2019

Fig. 2.2 Components of a POLST form. Section A designates orders related to CPR. Option A - Full Treatments must be selected in Section B (which concerns intubation) if CPR is desired. Any option in Section B may be selected when a person does NOT desire CPR. Section C addresses additional orders such as blood transfusions or dialysis. Section D concerns artificial nutrition (and, in some states, artificial hydration) for when the patient cannot eat. The second page of the form identifies emergency contacts and a section where the healthcare provider verifies they have reviewed the document. (From National POLST Collaborative. [2019]. *National POLST model form: A portable medical order.* https://polst.org/national-form/.)

CHAPTER 2 Healthcare Policy that Affects Older Adults

National POLST Model Form – Page 2　*****ATTACH TO PAGE 1*******　Copyright © February 2019 by NPC. All rights reserved*

Patient Full Name:

Contact Information (Optional but helpful)

Patient's Emergency Contact. (Note: Listing a person here does **not** grant them authority to be a legal representative. Only an advance directive or state law can grant that authority.)

Full Name:	☐ Legal Representative ☐ Other emergency contact	Phone #: Day: (　) Night: (　)
Primary Care Provider Name:		Phone: (　)
☐ Patient is enrolled in hospice	Name of Agency: Agency Phone: (　)	

Form Completion Information (Optional but helpful)

Reviewed patient's advance directive to confirm no conflict with POLST orders: (A POLST form does not replace an advance directive or living will)	☐ Yes; date of the document reviewed:_____ ☐ Conflict exists, notified patient (if patient lacks capacity, noted in chart) ☐ Advance directive not available ☐ No advance directive exists
Check everyone who participated in discussion:	☐ Patient with decision-making capacity　☐ Court Appointed Guardian　☐ Parent of Minor ☐ Legal Surrogate / Health Care Agent　☐ Other: _____

Professional Assisting Health Care Provider w/ Form Completion (if applicable): Full Name:	Date (mm/dd/yyyy): 　/　/	Phone #: (　)

This individual is the patient's:　☐ Social Worker　☐ Nurse　☐ Clergy　☐ Other:

Form Information & Instructions

- **Completing a POLST form:**
  - Provider should document basis for this form in the patient's medical record notes.
  - Patient representative is determined by applicable state law and, in accordance with state law, may be able execute or void this POLST form only if the patient lacks decision-making capacity.
  - Only licensed health care providers authorized to sign POLST forms in their state or D.C. can sign this form. See www.polst.org/state-signature-requirements-pdf for who is authorized in each state and D.C.
  - Original (if available) is given to patient; provider keeps a copy in medical record.
  - Last 4 digits of SSN are optional but can help identify / match a patient to their form.
  - If a translated POLST form is used during conversation, attach the translation to the signed English form.
- **Using a POLST form:**
  - Any incomplete section of POLST creates no presumption about patient's preferences for treatment. Provide standard of care.
  - No defibrillator (including automated external defibrillators) or chest compressions should be used if "No CPR" is chosen.
  - For all options, use medication by any appropriate route, positioning, wound care and other measures to relieve pain and suffering.
- **Reviewing a POLST form:** This form does not expire but should be reviewed whenever the patient:
  - (1) is transferred from one care setting or level to another;
  - (2) has a substantial change in health status;
  - (3) changes primary provider; or
  - (4) changes his/her treatment preferences or goals of care.
- **Modifying a POLST form:** This form cannot be modified. If changes are needed, void form and complete a new POLST form.
- **Voiding a POLST form:**
  - **If a patient or patient representative (for patients lacking capacity) wants to void the form**: destroy paper form and contact patient's health care provider to void orders in patient's medical record (and POLST registry, if applicable). State law may limit patient representative authority to void.
  - **For health care providers**: destroy patient copy (if possible), note in patient record form is voided and notify registries (if applicable).
- **Additional Forms.** Can be obtained by going to www.polst.org/form
- As permitted by law, this form may be added to a secure electronic registry so health care providers can find it.

State Specific Info	For Barcodes / ID Sticker/Medical Record #

*No part of this publication may be reproduced, stored in or introduced into a retrieval system, or transmitted in any form or by any means (electronic, mechanical, photocopying, recording, or otherwise), without written permission of the National POLST Collaborative (NPC). Requests for permission may be directed to natlpolstcollaborative@gmail.com. This publication may be reproduced and distributed for personal use or for instructional purposes only by academic or professional organizations

For more information, visit www.polst.org　　　Copied, faxed or electronic versions of this form are legal and valid.　2019

Fig. 2.2, cont'd

where the healthcare provider verifies they have reviewed the document. POLST is also known as MOLST (Medical Orders for Life-Sustaining Treatment) or MOST (Medical Orders for Sustaining Treatment) in varying states (Tark et al, 2019).

Durable or General Power of Attorney: Differences and Indications

The durable power of attorney for healthcare (DPAHC) is a legal instrument by which a person may designate someone else to make healthcare decisions at a time in the future when they may be rendered incapable of decision-making for medical care. The role of the designated surrogate in this situation is to make the decisions that most closely align with the patient's wishes, desires, and values (Mayo Clinic, 2022).

The DPAHC has an advantage over the LW in that the designated agent may assess the current situation, ask questions, and gather information to assist in determining the probable wishes of the patient. The LW, however, speaks for the patient who cannot speak for themself.

All states now have laws providing for different types of LW documents, DPAHCs, or both. Because the specifics of the laws vary from state to state, it is important for the nurse to be knowledgeable of the laws in the state in which they practice. Depending on a nurse's work environment, resources for this information may be the facility administration, risk management staff, legal counsel, social worker, or another appropriate source.

Communication Between Patient's Directives and Family Desires

It is not uncommon for the nurse to encounter families that may disagree with an individual's advanced directives. Although the law consistently upholds the expressed desires of patients and residents, families often continue to exert influence over medical decisions, even when they support decisions known to be contrary to the patient's wishes. This can put healthcare providers and nurses in a challenging situation. Designated healthcare agents, whether court-appointed or selected by the individual, may also find themselves in conflict with family members who question the control of the agent and may not understand why the agent has been given this control. Yet, it is the nurse's duty to uphold the patient or court decision. Communication early in the illness with the family and interprofessional team decreases the potential for conflict (Calton & Russell, 2022).

NURSES' ETHICAL CODE AND PRACTICE DECISIONS

Ethics relate to the moral actions, behavior, and character of an individual. Nurses occupy one of the most trusted positions in society, and conforming to a code of ethics gives evidence of acceptance of that responsibility and trust. A code of ethical conduct offers general principles to guide and evaluate nursing actions. The role of the healthcare professional is to advocate, promote, and improve patient autonomy, maintain or improve health status, and do no harm (Winland-Brown, 2020).

The nurse–patient relationship is built on trust, and nurses' understanding of the key ethical principles is the basis of a trusting relationship. The key ethical principles should serve as a framework for nursing decision-making and the application of professional judgment. These key ethical principles are autonomy or self-determination, beneficence (doing good), nonmaleficence (avoiding evil), justice (allocation of resources), and veracity (truthfulness) (ANA, 2015). Issues related to ageism, ethnicity, sexual orientation, sex, gender, physical or mental disability, and race are critical areas of difference that may affect the nurse–patient relationship (Block et al, 2022). These factors must be acknowledged and addressed if the moral and ethical principles of the provider-patient relationship are to be respected. More importantly, the ethical code serves to regulate professional practice from within the profession and ensure ethical conduct in the professional setting. Ethical directives guide and direct the nurse caring for dying patients. Care for the terminally ill and dying should be performed with professional and ethical deliberation.

Ethical Dilemmas and Considerations

Euthanasia, Suicide, and Assisted Suicide

The issue of physician-assisted suicide is a major ethical debate. Calls to legalize physician-assisted suicide have increased, and public support and interest in the subject have grown in recent years (Sulmasy & Mueller, 2017). Personal and professional views on this issue are at best controversial. However, grass roots efforts to change and shape public policy on this issue will continue. The American Medical Association (AMA) and the American College of Physicians (ACP) have maintained their opposition to physician-assisted suicide, stating, "The ACP does not support the legalization of physician-assisted suicide, the practice of which raises ethical, clinical, and other concerns" (Sulmasy & Mueller, 2017, para 14).

Currently, Oregon, Washington, Vermont, and California have laws to allow physician-assisted suicide. Montana allows this by court case ruling (Kane et al, 2018b).

Additionally, the *Code of Ethics for Nurses* prohibits nurses from participating in assisted suicide. The ANA's position statement holds that "The nursing profession's opposition to nurse participation in euthanasia does not negate the obligation of the nurse to provide compassionate, ethically justified end-of-life care which includes the promotion of comfort and the alleviation of suffering, adequate pain control, and at times, foregoing life-sustaining treatments" (ANA, 2015).

> ### EVIDENCE-BASED PRACTICE
> #### Depression and Spousal Self-Euthanasia
>
> **Background**
> This article provides the first qualitative account of spousal self-euthanasia in older people, a previously unexplored phenomenon. The researchers investigate the lived experience of a Dutch elderly couple who strongly wished—and chose—to die together at a self-directed moment, despite not suffering from a life-threatening disease or severe depression. The anticipatory fear of further deterioration, further losing control, and not being able to control the time and manner of death in the future compelled the couple to make this ultimate decision.

CHAPTER 2 Healthcare Policy that Affects Older Adults

> **EVIDENCE-BASED PRACTICE—cont'd**
>
> **Sample/Setting**
> This research focused on the experience of one elderly couple (aged over 70 years) by presenting two personal accounts from an insider perspective. Interviews inclusive of personal accounts from an insider perspective regarding an elderly couple aged over 70 years were conducted.
>
> **Methods**
> A case study through family interviews was completed regarding two married older adults who committed simultaneous suicide through a "lived experience." A thematic existential phenomenological method was utilized to report the data.
>
> **Findings**
> After self-directed spousal self-euthanasia, the respondent confirmed that both (husband and wife) feared separation, dependency, and physical decline more than death. "They wanted to abandon life in all serenity."
>
> **Implications**
> The article outlines practical implications that nurses and healthcare providers working in gerontology should be aware of regarding the consequences of the effects of depression and the relationship between self-euthanasia and depression in elderly people. The authors felt that encouraging people to discuss the emotional tensions about the different concerns and sense of time was the most appropriate intervention to understand the desire to end one's life.

Data from van Wijngaarden, E., Leget, C., & Goossensen, A. (2016). Till death do us part: The lived experience of an elderly couple who chose to end their lives by spousal self-euthanasia. *The Gerontologist, 56*(6), 1062–1071.

Experimentation and Research

As previously discussed, nursing facility residents are accorded specific rights with respect to their treatments. The patient's or resident's bill of rights entitles them to choose a primary physician and terminate their relationship if so desired. Furthermore, they have the right to be informed about their medical conditions and proposed treatment plans. Nursing facility residents, or any patient in a healthcare facility, may refuse to participate in experimental research. For example, see Annotated Code of Maryland, 1957, § 19-344(f); and Vermont Statutes Annotated, Title 18 § 1852(a)(10) and Title 33 § 3781(3), as redesignated by Act 219, L. 1990, effective July 1, 1990.

Residents may refuse to be examined, observed, or treated by students or other staff without jeopardizing their access to care (see 1990 edition, General Laws of Massachusetts, supplemented by the 1991 Supplement, Chapter 111: 70E9h).

The goals of research are different from the goals of care. Research seeks to acquire knowledge that may or may not benefit the subjects because much clinical research is conducted to determine effective treatments or the potential benefits of new drugs and medical devices. Key points to consider in this research are as follows: 1) the goals and value of the research, 2) conflicts between institutional interests and researchers, and 3) the medical interests of the individual that do no harm (Resnik, 2020). The federal policy for the protection of human subjects was published in 1991 (DHHS, 2021). An appropriate institutional review board (IRB) should examine all research involving humans prior to implementation (U.S. Food & Drug Administration, 2019). All aspects of the proposed study must be evaluated to ensure that the research is justified and of benefit and that the individual rights of all persons, including those of volunteer participants, are not sacrificed. Nurses, as a professional group closely involved with the clinical aspects of human research, should be represented on the review board.

Organ Donation

Technological and medical advances have facilitated the successful transplantation of vital organs, and such procedures have become routine at many medical centers. However, this success has exacerbated the ethical questions involving the allocation of scarce donor organs. Recognizing that the number of recipients waiting is greater than the number of available donors, the federal government has taken steps to promote organ donation. Hospitals in the United States are now required to report *all* deaths to the local organ procurement organization (OPO) or Organ Procurement and Transplantation Network (OPTN). This would permit the nation's OPOs, which collect organs and coordinate donations daily, to determine whether a person is a suitable donor while following specific guidelines set forth based on the organ and potential recipient (OPTN, n.d.) The DHHS believes that this measure, which is now a condition for participating in the Medicare program, will save lives by substantially increasing organ donations in the United States. Standards of informed consent must be adhered to with respect to both donors and recipients (Center for Organ Recovery and Education, 2018). In dealing with the ethical issues faced in these situations, the answers are not clear-cut and may depend on individual values. However, when it is necessary to sort out conflicts or report anything believed to be illegal or unethical, the nurse should consider obtaining guidance from an institutional ethics committee or other ethical resource.

Ethics Committees

Institutional biomedical ethics committees play a pivotal role in dealing with sensitive conflicts about treatment decisions. Ethics committees act as the primary organizational mechanism for studying, educating about, and providing advice on value conflicts and dilemmas faced in healthcare (Hummel et al, 2021). Ethics committees serve in a voluntary capacity in a consultative role and do not act as a decision-making body. Their primary objective is to carefully evaluate differing positions to achieve a consensus that is ethically and legally acceptable to all parties. Ethics committees do not have any legal authority. Their main purpose is to create a forum where patients, patient representatives, and providers can express and consider different points of view.

Two-thirds of general hospitals with more than 200 beds have ethics committees. Their presence in nursing facilities is not as common. Membership on ethics committees should be diverse to help maintain a balanced view among professionals, laypersons, and special interest groups. If constructed in this manner, the committee will offer a variety of perspectives to those seeking guidance. The nurse's role as a member of an ethics committee is crucial. Representation should include administrative and staff nurses, as well as nurses practicing in specialty areas.

Ethics committees' primary purposes are to (1) provide education and help guide policy making regarding ethical issues,

BOX 2.5 ANA's Principles for Social Networking

1. Nurses must not transmit or place individually identifiable patient information online.
2. Nurses must observe ethically prescribed professional patient–nurse boundaries.
3. Nurses should understand that patients, colleagues, institutions, and employers may view postings.
4. Nurses should take advantage of privacy settings and seek to separate personal and professional information online.
5. Nurses should bring content that could harm a patient's privacy, rights, or welfare to the attention of appropriate authorities.
6. Nurses should participate in developing institutional policies governing online conduct.

Tips for Social Media

1. Remember that standards of professionalism are the same online as in any other circumstance.
2. Do not share or post information or photos gained through the nurse–patient relationship.
3. Maintain professional boundaries in the use of electronic media. Online contact with patients blurs this boundary.
4. Do not make disparaging remarks about patients, employers, or coworkers, even if they are not identified.
5. Do not take photos or videos of patients on personal devices, including cell phones.
6. Promptly report a breach of confidentiality or privacy.

Modified from American Nurses Association. (n.d.). *Social media.* Retrieved from https://www.nursingworld.org/social/. Accessed September 19, 2022.

(2) facilitate the resolution of ethical dilemmas, and (3) take an activist role in involving all interested parties in promoting the best care for patients (Hummel et al, 2021).

Issues and topics that might be discussed by an ethics committee include but are not limited to euthanasia; patient competency and decision-making capacities; guardianship issues; DNR orders and policies; patient refusal of treatment; starting, continuing, or stopping treatment; informed consent; use of feeding tubes; use of restraints; and so on. Basically, anything that composes an ethical dilemma can be brought before the committee.

Social Media

Social media has taken the world by storm and will continue to do so. Rarely can we go anywhere without connectivity to the world around us. This type of media has raised ethical issues within the healthcare environment. Social media can benefit all healthcare professionals; however, there are risks to using social media, including poor quality of information and misinformation, the posting of unprofessional content that can damage the professional image of nursing, and breaches of patient privacy, whether intentional or accidental. The National Council of State Boards of Nursing and seven other nursing organizations released a policy statement (NCSBN, 2021) that nurses disseminating misinformation regarding COVID-19 vaccines jeopardizes the health of the public and may affect their license and career. Nurses are expected to meet the ethical standards of practice. The ANA added "Social Networking Principles" and "Social Media Tips" to their website to set forth the expectations of professional nurses in this digital age (ANA, n.d.) (Box 2.5). Nurses are a well-respected profession, and they must remember not to promote personal health biases or non–evidence-based treatments/recommendations on media sites.

HOME CARE

- Remember that home care agencies' standards are based on *Gerontological Nursing: Scope and Standards of Practice*, originally published by the American Nurses Association (1995) and revised in 2010.
- Assess for older adult abuse and notify the proper authorities (e.g., local older adult protective services or ombudsman programs).
- On the initial assessment, inform homebound older adults and their caregivers of home care patient rights. Have them sign a copy of the documents stating that they have been informed of their rights.
- Inform caregivers and homebound older adults of their right to self-determination. Document that homebound older adults, caregivers, or both have been informed by obtaining signatures. AMDs must be part of a clinical assessment.
- Obtain a copy of homebound older adults' AMDs and keep them on file in their charts. Send copies to the physicians to file.
- Remember that the physician must sign a DNR order within 48 hours, as specified by Medicare regulations.
- To help caregivers and homebound older adults make decisions about treatment used to prolong life, consider using a values history. The values history is an instrument that asks questions related to quality versus length of life and the values that persons see as important to maintain during terminal care.

SUMMARY

Legal and ethical issues associated with the nursing care of older adults involve federal regulation since Medicare is the primary source of healthcare insurance for persons 65 years of age and older. Professional standards of practice are the legal measure against which nursing practice is judged, and it is a professional responsibility for nurses to understand their legal duties in the care of older adults. It is important for the nurse to be aware of all laws and regulations affecting the care of older adults in the facilities where he or she practices. Nurses need to be knowledgeable about the legal documents for patients to ensure their healthcare-related rights as well as understand the patient's decision-making rights. The Nurses' Code of Ethics should guide ethical considerations and issues that nurses encounter (ANA, 2015).

Nurses have a significant role in assisting the older adult to meet their healthcare needs. The unique characteristics, vulnerabilities, and needs of older adults present great and varied challenges. The older individual's quality of life is affected to a great extent by the quality of nursing care received.

KEY POINTS

- The nurse's duty to patients is to provide care according to a measurable standard. When patients' physical and mental conditions and their ability to care for themselves decline, the duty of care increases.
- Older adults, particularly frail older adults, are considered a vulnerable population; therefore, their treatment in licensed healthcare institutions and other settings (including the home) is carefully regulated.
- Evidence provided to the US Congress in 1983 suggested widespread abuse of residents in nursing facilities and resulted in the enactment of the OBRA, the most sweeping reform affecting Medicare and Medicaid nursing facilities since those programs began. Concern for quality in nursing facilities has led to closer regulation and more stringent enforcement.
- OBRA focuses on the quality of life of residents in nursing facilities and assurances of the preservation of their human rights and due process interests. The regulations address virtually every element of life in a nursing facility. OBRA's regulations are enforced through a survey process that focuses on the outcomes of residential care and includes sanctions designed to force compliance, analyzed according to the scope and severity of violations.
- A strong judicial deference toward individual autonomy ensures that every human has the right to determine what shall be done with his or her own body. These rights are guaranteed in the US Constitution and have been additionally interpreted in case law and state laws.
- Legal tools and instruments such as AMDs, DNR, POLST, designation of healthcare agents, and durable powers of attorney help people plan for future decision-making so that their wishes can be carried out even when they are no longer able to speak for themselves. The presence of these instruments may add to the information available about an individual's wishes, but care should be taken to avoid equating the instruments themselves with the existence of these fundamental human rights.
- The right to self-determination was given even more emphasis with the passage of the PSDA in 1990. This law requires healthcare providers to inform and educate patients about their rights as they exist under the laws of each state.
- Physician-assisted suicide and issues surrounding the care of terminally ill older persons are subjects of national interest and debate, as well as judicial and legislative interest, and the role and obligation of the nurse in such matters must be carefully monitored.
- The technological and medical advancements that help people live longer also contribute to the complicated ethical dilemmas that exist in the care of older adults. Ethics committees help in these matters by responding to the need for education and communication between caregivers and patients.
- It is preferable to resolve patient care dilemmas at the bedside rather than in the courtroom. The courts prefer that patients, their families, and healthcare professionals handle such matters. With careful guidance and discussion, this can often be achieved.

CLINICAL JUDGMENT EXERCISES

1. An 85-year-old male has been able to care for himself with minimum assistance until recently. Should he and his family decide that it is time for him to move to a long-term care facility? How will his rights as an individual be protected because he will be giving up his independence? Explain.
2. A 95-year-old male resides in a long-term care facility. He has signed an AMD in case he becomes seriously ill. A 73-year-old female is being treated in the hospital for a recent cerebral vascular accident that has left her severely incapacitated. Her family has requested a DNR order. How do these two instruments differ? In what ways do they protect each person's rights?
3. You are the nurse in charge of a wing of a nursing facility. During rounds one evening, an older, sometimes confused resident tells you that a nurse aide "pushed her around" during dinner that evening. What issues are presented, and what actions should you take?

REFERENCES

Administration for Community Living (ACL). (2019). *What is elder abuse?* Retrieved from https://acl.gov/programs/elder-justice/what-elder-abuse. Accessed July 27, 2023.

Agency for Healthcare Research and Quality (AHRQ). (2018). *AHRQuality indicators™*. Retrieved from https://www.ahrq.gov/cpi/about/otherwebsites/qualityindicators.ahrq.gov/qualityindicators.html. Accessed July 27, 2023.

Amaral, A. S., Afonso, R. M., Simões, M. R., & Freitas, S. (2022). Decision-making capacity in healthcare: Instruments review and reflections about its assessment in the elderly with cognitive impairment and dementia. *The Psychiatric Quarterly*, 93(1), 35–53. doi:10.1007/s11126-020-09867-7.

American Nurses Association (ANA). (2021). *Nursing: Scope and standards of practice* (4th ed.). Silver Spring, MD: ANA.

American Nurses Association (ANA). (2015). *Code of ethics for nurses with interpretive statements.* Silver Spring, MD: American Nurses Association.

American Nurses Association (ANA). (2010). *Gerontological nursing: Scope and standards of practice* (3rd ed.). Silver Spring, MD: ANA.

American Nurses Association (ANA). (n.d.). *Social media*. Retrieved from https://nursingworld.org/social. Accessed July 27, 2023.

Beaton, T. (2018). *Affordable Care Act changes may bring a rocky 2018 for payers*. HealthPayerIntelligence.com. Retrieved from https://healthpayerintelligence.com/news/affordable-care-act-changes-may-bring-a-rocky-2018-for-payers. Accessed July 27, 2023.

Block, L., Powell, W. R., Gilmore-Bykovskyi, A., & Kind, A. J. H. (2022). Social determinants of health, health disparities, and health equity. In J. B. Halter, J. G. Ouslander, S. Studenski, K. P. High, S. Asthana, M. A. Supiano, et al. (Eds.), *Hazzard's geriatric medicine and gerontology* (8th ed., pp. 95–106). New York: McGraw Hill.

Calton, B., & Russell, M. L. (2022). Effective communication strategies for patients with serious illness. In J. B. Halter, J. G. Ouslander, S. Studenski, K. P. High, S. Asthana, M. A. Supiano, et al. (Eds.). *Hazzard's geriatric medicine and gerontology* (8th ed., pp. 1089–1096). New York: McGraw-Hill.

Center for Organ Recovery and Education (CORE). (2018). *Donation process*. Retrieved from https://www.core.org/understanding-donation/donation-process/. Accessed July 27, 2023.

Centers for Disease Control and Prevention (CDC). (2021). *Elder abuse*. Retrieved https://www.cdc.gov/violenceprevention/elderabuse. Accessed July 27, 2023.

Centers for Medicare and Medicaid Services (CMS). (2022a). *Nursing homes*. Retrieved from https://www.cms.gov/medicare/provider-enrollment-and-certification/certificationandcomplianc/nhs. Accessed July 27, 2023.

Centers for Medicare and Medicaid Services (CMS). (2022b). *Nursing homes: Medicare and Medicaid programs; reform of requirements for long-term care facilities*. Retrieved from https://www.cms.gov/medicare/provider-enrollment-and-certification/guidanceforlawsandregulations/nursing-homes. Accessed July 27, 2023.

Centers for Medicare and Medicaid Services (CMS). (2020). *Quality, safety, & oversight – general information – CMS national background check program*. Retrieved from https://www.hhs.gov/guidance/document/quality-safety-oversight-general-information-cms-national-background-check-program. Accessed July 27, 2023.

Centers for Medicare and Medicaid Services (CMS). (2017). *2017 RAI user's manual provider updates*. Retrieved from https://downloads.cms.gov/files/MDS-RAI-Users-Manual-Provider-Updates.pdf. Accessed July 27, 2023.

Centers for Medicare and Medicaid Services (CMS). (2012). *OASIS-C PBQI/Process measures*. Retrieved from https://edit.cms.gov/Medicare/Quality-Initiatives-Patient-Assessment-Instruments/HomeHealthQualityInits/Downloads/HHQI-OASIS-PBQI.pdf. Accessed July 27, 2023.

Centers for Medicare and Medicaid Services (CMS). (n.d.[a]). *Get started with medicare*. Retrieved from https://medicare.gov/basics/get-started-with-medicare. Accessed July 27, 2023.

Centers for Medicare and Medicaid Services (CMS). (n.d.[b]). *Find & compare providers near you*. Retrieved from https://www.medicare.gov/care-compare. Accessed July 27, 2023.

Huang, P., Luo, K., Wang, C., Guo, D., Wang, S., Jiang, Y., et al. (2021). Urinary incontinence is associated with increased all-cause mortality in older nursing home residents: A meta-analysis. *Journal of Nursing Scholarship*, 53(5), 561–567. doi:10.1111/jnu.12671.

Hummel, P., Adam, T., Reis, A., & Littler, K. (2021). Taking stock of the availability and functions of National Ethics Committees worldwide. *BMC Medical Ethics*, 22(1), 56. doi:10.1186/s12910-021-00614-6.

Joint Commission. (n.d.). *Standards*. Retrieved from https://www.jointcommission.org/standards/about-our-standards/. Accessed July 27, 2023.

Kane, R. L., Ouslander, J. G., Resnick, B., & Malone, M. L. (Eds.). (2018a). Incontinence. In *Essentials of clinical geriatrics* (8th ed., pp. 201–242). New York: McGraw-Hill.

Kane, R. L., Ouslander, J. G., Resnick, B., & Malone, M. L. (Eds.). (2018b). Ethical issues in the care of older persons. In *Essentials of clinical geriatrics* (8th ed., pp. 499–522). New York: McGraw-Hill.

Mason, D. J., Dickson, E., McLemore, M. R., & Perez, G. A. (2021). Frameworks for action in policy and politics. In D. Mason, E. Dickson, M. McLemore, & G. Perez (Eds.), *Policy & politics in nursing and healthcare* (8th ed., pp. 1–16). St. Louis: Elsevier.

Mayo Clinic. (2022). *Living wills and advance directives for medical decisions*. Retrieved from http://www.mayoclinic.org/healthy-lifestyle/consumer-health/in-depth/living-wills/art-20046303. Accessed July 27, 2023.

McGrath, R., Vincent, B. M., Hackney, K. J., Sohan, A. S., Graham, J., Thomas, L., et al. (2020). Weakness and cognitive impairment are independently and jointly associated with functional decline in aging Americans. *Aging Clinical and Experimental Research*, 32(9), 1723–1730. doi:10.1007/s40520-019-01351-y.

Medicare.gov. (n.d.). *Rights & protections in a nursing home*. Retrieved from https://www.medicare.gov/what-medicare-covers/what-part-a-covers/rights-protections-in-a-nursing-home. Accessed July 27, 2023.

National Academies of Sciences, Engineering, and Medicine. (2022). *The national imperative to improve nursing home quality: Honoring our commitment to residents, families, and staff*. Washington, DC: The National Academies Press. http://doi.org/10.17226/26526.

National Council of State Boards of Nursing (NCSBN). (2021). *Policy statement: Dissemination of non-scientific and misleading COVID-19 information by nurses*. Retrieved from https://www.ncsbn.org/PolicyBriefDisseminationofCOVID19Info.pdf. Accessed July 27, 2023.

National POLST Collaborative. (2022). *POLST & advance directives*. Retrieved from https://polst.org/polst-and-advance-directives/. Accessed July 27, 2023.

National POLST Collaborative. (2019). *National POLST form: Portable medical order*. Retrieved from https://polst.org/national-form/. Accessed July 27, 2023.

Nguyen, A. L., Mosqueday, L., Windisch, N., Axelrod, J., & Han, S. D. (2021). Perceived types, causes, consequence of financial exploitation: Narratives from older adults. *Journal of Gerontology Social Sciences*, 76(5), 996–1004. doi:10.1093/geronb/gbab010.

NursingLicensure.org. (n.d.). *Certified nursing assistant requirements*. Retrieved from https://www.nursinglicensure.org/cna. Accessed July 27, 2023.

Organ Procurement and Transplantation Network (OPTN). (n.d.). *How organ allocation works*. Retrieved from https://optn.transplant.hrsa.gov/learn/about-transplantation/how-organ-allocation-works/. Accessed July 27, 2023.

Pickering, C. E. Z., Yefimova, M., Maxwell, C., Puga, F., & Sullivan, T. (2020). Daily context for abusive and neglectful behavior in family caregiving for dementia. *The Gerontologist*, 60(3), 483–493. doi:10.1093/geront/gnz110.

Resnik, D. B. (2020). *What is ethics in research & why is it important?* National Institute of Environmental Health Sciences [website]. Retrieved from https://www.niehs.nih.gov/research/resources/bioethics/whatis/. Accessed July 27, 2023.

Rosen, T., Stern, M. E., Elman, A., & Mulcare, M. R. (2018). Identifying and initiating intervention for elder abuse and neglect in the emergency department. *Clinical Geriatric Medicine*, 34(3), 435–451. doi:10.1016/j.cger.2018.04.007.

Schroeter, K. (2021). Is the Code of Ethics for Nurses a legal document? *American Nurse*, 16(5), 48.

Sulmasy, L. S., & Mueller, P. S. (2017). Ethics and the legalization of physician-assisted suicide: An American College of Physicians position paper. *Annals of Internal Medicine*, 167(8), 576–578. Retrieved from https://www.acpjournals.org/doi/10.7326/m17-0938. Accessed July 27, 2023.

Tark, A., Agarwal, M., Dick, A. W., & Stone, P. W. (2019). Variations in physician orders for life-sustaining treatment program across the nation: Environmental scan. *Journal of Palliative Medicine*, 22(9), 1032–1038. doi:10.1089/jpm.2018.0626.

Tennessee Commission on Aging and Disability. (n.d.). *Reporting elder abuse and neglect*. Retrieved from https://www.tn.gov/aging/resources/community-resource-guide/reporting-elder-abuse. Accessed July 27, 2023.

Teoli, D., & Ghassemzadeh, S. (2022). Patient Self-Determination Act. In *StatPearls*. Retrieved from https://www.ncbi.nlm.nih.gov/books/NBK538297/. Accessed July 27, 2023.

Texas Department of Family and Protective Services. (n.d.). Retrieved from http://www.dfps.state.tx.us/. Accessed July 27, 2023.

U.S. Department of Health and Human Services (DHHS). (2024). *CMS/CDRH letter regarding physical restraint definition*. Retrieved from https://www.accessdata.fda.gov/scripts/cdrh/cfdocs/cfcfr/CFRSearch.cfm?fr=880.6760. Accessed September 24, 2024.

U.S. Department of Health and Human Services (DHHS). (2022a). *Health information privacy*. Retrieved from https://www.hhs.gov/hipaa/. Accessed July 27, 2023.

U.S. Department of Health and Human Services (DHHS). (2022b). *About the affordable care act*. Retrieved from https://www.hhs.gov/healthcare/about-the-aca/index.html. Accessed July 27, 2023.

U.S. Department of Health and Human Services (DHHS). (2021). *Federal policy for the protection of human subjects ('common rule')*. Retrieved from https://www.hhs.gov/ohrp/regulations-and-policy/regulations/common-rule/index.html. Accessed July 27, 2023.

U.S. Food and Drug Administration. (2019). *Institutional review boards (IRBs) and protection of human subjects in clinical trials*. Retrieved from https://www.fda.gov/about-fda/center-drug-evaluation-and-research-cder/institutional-review-boards-irbs-and-protection-human-subjects-clinical-trials. Accessed July 27, 2023.

Winland-Brown, J. E. (2020). Staying alert to ethical challenges. *Journal of the American Association of Nurse Practitioners*, 32(10), 642–644. doi:10.1097/JXX.0000000000000512.

World Health Organization (WHO). (2022). *Abuse of older people*. Retrieved from https://www.who.int/news-room/fact-sheets/detail/abuse-of-older-people. Accessed July 27, 2023.

3
Assessment of the Older Adult

Jennifer J. Yeager, PhD, RN

http://evolve.elsevier.com/Yeager/gerontologic/

LEARNING OBJECTIVES

On completion of this chapter, the reader will be able to:
1. Explain the interrelationship between the physical and psychosocial aspects of aging as it affects the assessment process.
2. Describe how the atypical presentation of illness in older adults affects the assessment process.
3. Compare the clinical presentation of delirium and dementia.
4. Describe the assessment modifications that may be necessary when assessing older adults.
5. Describe strategies to ensure collection of relevant and comprehensive health histories for older adults.
6. Identify the basic components of a health history for older adults.
7. List the principles to observe when conducting physical examinations of older adults.
8. Explain the rationale for assessing functional status in older adults.
9. Describe the elements of a functional assessment.
10. Describe the basic components of cognitive assessment.
11. Explain the rationale for assessing social function in older adults.
12. Conduct a comprehensive health assessment on an older adult patient.

WHAT WOULD YOU DO?

What would you do if you were faced with the following situations?
- Your older adult patient is recovering from open reduction and internal fixation of the right femur. The femur was fractured during a fall at home. Since surgery yesterday morning, your patient has been oriented to person only. When you bring their breakfast into the room this morning, the patient pushes the tray away, holds out their hand, and with a big smile says, "Look, look, he finally proposed. Clint Eastwood asked me to marry him." What is going on with your patient? How would you determine this?
- Your older adult patient has been diagnosed with leukemia and is undergoing chemotherapy. During the home health intake at 3 p.m., you note the patient is frail and sitting on the sofa with their head on their chest. The patient is unshaven and wearing pajamas. Their feet are bare on the carpeted floor. What additional assessments should you complete to ensure optimal outcomes from your nursing intervention?

Previous author: Sue E. Meiner, EdD, APRN, BC, GNP

The nursing process is a problem-solving process that provides the organizational framework for providing nursing care. Assessment, the crucial foundation on which the remaining steps of the process are built, includes the collection and analysis of data and results in a nursing diagnosis. A nursing-focused assessment is crucial in determining patient problems amenable to nursing interventions. Unless the approach to assessment maintains a *nursing* focus, the sequential steps of the nursing process—diagnosis, planning, implementation, and evaluation—cannot be carried out.

A nursing focus evolves from an awareness and understanding of the definition of nursing. This is defined by the American Nurses Association (ANA, 2015):

> *Nursing is the protection, promotion, and optimization of health and abilities, prevention of illness and injury, facilitation of healing, alleviation of suffering through the diagnosis and treatment of human response, and advocacy in the care of individuals, families, groups, communities, and populations. (p. 1)*

Furthermore, the ANA (2015) identifies tenets that characterize the practice of nursing across all settings:
1. Caring and health are central to the practice of the registered nurse.
2. Nursing practice is individualized.

3. Registered nurses use the nursing process to plan and provide individualized care for health-care consumers.
4. Nurses coordinate care by establishing partnerships.
5. A strong link exists between the professional work environment and the registered nurse's ability to provide quality health care and achieve optimal outcomes (pp. 8–9).

Tenet number 3 establishes the nursing process as the foundation of nursing care. As stated previously, assessment provides the basis for all components of the nursing process. During assessment, the nurse collects subjective and objective data about the patient and their environment that assist the nurse in determining a response to health and illness. A comprehensive, *nursing-focused* assessment of these responses establishes a database about a patient's ability to meet the full range of "physical, functional, psychosocial, emotional, cognitive, sexual, cultural, age-related, environmental, spiritual/transpersonal, and economic needs" (ANA, 2015, p. 53). Patient responses that reveal an inability to meet these needs satisfactorily indicate a need for nursing care.

Nursing-focused assessment of older adults occurs across all settings: hospitals, homes, long-term care facilities, senior centers, congregate living units, hospice facilities, and independent or group nursing practices. The setting dictates how data collection and analysis should be managed to serve patients best. Although the setting may vary, the purpose of nursing-focused assessment of older adults remains to determine the older person's ability to meet any health- and illness-related needs. Specifically, the purpose of older adult assessment is to identify patient strengths and limitations so that effective and appropriate interventions can be delivered to support, promote, and restore optimal function, and prevent disability and dependence.

Gerontological nurses recognize that assessing the older adult involves applying a broad range of skills and abilities and considering many complex and varied issues. Nursing-focused assessment based on a sound, scientific gerontological knowledge base, coupled with repeated practice to acquire the *art* of assessment, is essential for the nurse to recognize responses that reflect unmet needs. Many frameworks and tools are available to guide the nurse in assessing older adults. Regardless of the framework or tool used, the nurse should collect the data while observing the following key principles: (1) the use of an individual, person-centered approach; (2) a view of patients as participants in health monitoring and treatment; and (3) an emphasis on patients' functional ability.

SPECIAL CONSIDERATIONS AFFECTING ASSESSMENT

Nursing assessment of older adults is a complex and challenging process that must consider the following points to ensure a patient-centered approach. The first is the interrelationship between physical and psychosocial aspects of aging. Next is assessing the nature of disease and disability and their effects on functional status. The third is to tailor the nursing assessment to the individual older adult.

Interrelationship Between Physical and Psychosocial Aspects of Aging

Although many theories pose mechanisms for the aging process (Table 3.1), the health of people of all ages is subject to multiple extrinsic factors (i.e., environmental, sociologic, spiritual, and psychologic factors). The balance (homeostasis) achieved within the factors greatly influences a person's health status. Factors such as reduced ability to respond to stress, increased frequency and multiplicity of loss, and physical changes associated with normal aging may place older adults at high risk for loss of functional ability. Consider the following case, which illustrates how the interaction of select physical and psychosocial factors may seriously compromise function.

Mrs. M, age 83, arrived in the emergency room after a neighbor found her in her home. The neighbor had become concerned because he noticed Mrs. M had not picked up her newspapers for the past 3 days. She was found in her bed, weak and lethargic. She stated that she had the flu for the past week, so she was unable to eat or drink much because of the associated nausea and vomiting. Except for her mild hypertension (HTN), which is medically managed with an antihypertensive agent, she had enjoyed relatively good health before this acute illness. She was admitted to the hospital with pneumonia. Because of the emergent nature of the admission, Mrs. M has no personal belongings, including her hearing aid, glasses, and dentures. She develops congestive heart failure (CHF) after treatment of her dehydration with intravenous (IV) fluids. She becomes confused and agitated, and haloperidol is administered. Her impaired mobility, resulting from the chemical

TABLE 3.1 Theories of Aging

Theory of Aging	Mechanism
Telomere shortening	Each time a cell divides, a proportion of the protective sheath at the end of the telomere is lost, eventually leading to errors in deoxyribonucleic acid (DNA) replication
Damage accumulation	Aging is the result of the accumulation of damage at a molecular and cellular level due to a reduction in maintenance and repair mechanisms
Free radical	Free radicals due to oxidation reactions accumulate over time, causing damage to the cell and triggering cellular senescence
Disposable soma	An evolutionary theory that organisms preferentially use resources for reproduction rather than repair and longevity
Mutation accumulation	The accumulation of DNA mutations over time; mutations that occur after reproductive age wcannot be passed on to future generations
Antagonistic pleiotropy	Genes that are beneficial to survival in earlier life become detrimental in later life

From Preston, J., & Biddell, B. (2021). The physiology of ageing and how these changes affect older people. *Medicine, 49*(1), 1–5.

restraint, has caused urinary and fecal incontinence, and she has developed a stage 2 pressure injury on her coccyx. She needs to be fed because of confusion and eats very little. She sleeps at intervals throughout the day and night, and when awake, she usually cries.

Undue emphasis should not be placed on individual weaknesses; the gerontological nurse should identify the patient's strengths and abilities and build the plan of care on this foundation. In older adults, the cause of one problem is often best understood in light of associated problems. Careful consideration must be given to the interrelationships among physical, psychosocial, and environmental aspects of every patient situation.

Nature of Disease and Disability and Their Effects on Functional Status

Aging does not necessarily result in disease and disability. Although the prevalence of chronic disease increases with age, older adults remain functionally independent. However, what cannot be ignored is that chronic disease increases older adults' vulnerability to functional decline. Comprehensive assessment of physical and psychosocial function and environmental issues is important because it can provide valuable clues to a disease's effect on functional status. Self-reported vague signs and symptoms such as lethargy, incontinence, decreased appetite, and weight loss may be indicators of functional impairment. Ignoring older adults' vague symptomatology exposes them to an increased risk for physical frailty. Physical frailty, or impairment of physical abilities needed to live independently, is a major contributor to the need for long-term care. Therefore, it is essential to thoroughly investigate reports of nonspecific signs and symptoms to determine whether underlying conditions may contribute to the older person's frailty.

Declining organ and system function and diminishing physiologic reserve with advancing age are well documented in literature. Such normal aging changes may make the body more susceptible to disease and disability, the risk of which increases with advancing age. It may be difficult for the nurse to differentiate normal age-related findings from indicators of disease or disability. It is common for nurses and older adults to mistakenly attribute vague signs and symptoms to normal aging changes or just "growing old." However, it is essential for the nurse to determine what is "normal" versus what may indicate disease or disability so that treatable conditions are not disregarded.

Age-Related Changes

Declining physiologic function and increased prevalence of disease result from a reduction in the body's ability to respond to stress in all forms. Typical physiologic changes include decreased renal and hepatic blood flow and mass, decreased lean body mass and muscle mass, along with decreased total body water and increased adipose tissue, all leading to a potential for altered pharmacokinetic (PK) and pharmacodynamic (PD) responses to drugs. With age, the immune system has a decreased ability to respond to invading microorganisms secondary to decreased T- and B-cell function. Additionally, as individuals age, they are more susceptible to cancer due to an increase in damage to cellular DNA and a decreased ability to repair this damage.

Baroreceptors have a reduced response to physiologic changes, increasing the risk for syncope in older adults. Secondary to increased insulin resistance and glucose intolerance, the incidence of diabetes increases.

The important point is that older adults are less able than younger adults to manage issues such as acute illness, blood loss, the high-technology environment of the hospital, or other issues. It is important for nurses to assess older adults for the presence of physical, psychosocial, and environmental stressors and their physical and cognitive manifestations.

Atypical Presentation of Illness

Determining older adults' physical and psychosocial health status is not easy, and is secondary to altered presentation of illness. Vague signs and symptoms of illness, coupled with altered parameters for laboratory values and drug dosages, make diagnosis and treatment difficult in older adults. The body does not respond as vigorously to illness or disease with advanced age because of diminished physiologic reserve. The diminished reserve poses no particular problems for older people as they carry out their daily routines; however, in times of physical and emotional stress, older people will not always exhibit the expected or classic signs and symptoms. The characteristic presentation of illness in older adults is more commonly one of blunted or atypical signs and symptoms (Jung et al, 2017).

The signs and symptoms exhibited by older adults often differ from the "classic" examples provided in pathophysiology textbooks. For example, in the case of pneumonia, older adults may exhibit a dry cough instead of the classic productive cough. Also, the presenting signs and symptoms may be unrelated to the actual problem, for example, the confusion accompanying a urinary tract infection (UTI). Finally, the expected signs and symptoms may not be present at all, as in the case of a myocardial infarction (MI) that occurs without chest pain (Table 3.2). All these atypical presentations challenge the nurse to conduct careful and thorough assessments and analyses of symptoms to ensure appropriate treatment.

The nurse should assume heterogeneity rather than homogeneity when caring for older people. It is crucial to respect the uniqueness of each person's life experiences, strengths, cultural practices, values, and beliefs, and to preserve the individuality created by those experiences. The older person's experiences represent a rich and vast background that the nurse can use to develop an individualized plan of care. The nurse can compare the older adult's own previous patterns of physical and psychosocial health and function with the current status, using the individual as the standard.

TABLE 3.2 Atypical Presentation of Illness in Older Adults

Problem	Classic Presentation in Young Patients	Presentation in Older Adult Patients
Urinary tract infection (UTI)	Dysuria, frequency, urgency, nocturia	Dysuria, frequency, and urgency often *absent*; nocturia *sometimes* present Incontinence, delirium, falls, dizziness, confusion, fatigue, weakness, and anorexia are other signs
Myocardial infarction (MI)	Severe substernal chest pain, diaphoresis, nausea, dyspnea	Sometimes *no* chest pain; or atypical pain location such as in jaw, neck, shoulder, epigastric area Dyspnea may or may not be present Other signs are tachypnea, arrhythmia, hypotension, restlessness, syncope, confusion, and fatigue/weakness A fall may be a prodrome
Pneumonia	Cough productive of purulent sputum, chills and fever, pleuritic chest pain, elevated white blood cell (WBC) count	Cough may be mild and nonproductive, or absent; chills and fever and/or elevated white blood cells (WBCs) also may be absent Tachypnea, slight cyanosis, delirium, anorexia, nausea and vomiting, confusion, malaise, and tachycardia may be present
Congestive heart failure (CHF)	Increased dyspnea (orthopnea, paroxysmal nocturnal dyspnea [PND]), fatigue, weight gain, pedal edema, nocturia, bibasilar crackles	Anorexia, confusion, agitation, weakness, restlessness, delirium, cyanosis, and falls may be present Cough, may not report dyspnea
Hyperthyroidism	Heat intolerance, fast pace, exophthalmos, increased pulse, hyperreflexia, tremor	Subtle symptoms, lethargy, weakness, depression, atrial fibrillation (AFib), tachycardia, weight loss, fatigue, palpitations, tremor, and HF
Hypothyroidism	Weakness, fatigue, cold intolerance, lethargy, skin dryness and scaling, constipation	Often presents without overt symptoms; cognitive dysfunction, fatigue, anorexia, and arthralgias may be present Delirium, dementia, depression/lethargy, constipation, weight loss, and muscle weakness/unsteady gait are common
Depression	Dysphoric mood and thoughts, withdrawal, crying, weight loss, constipation, insomnia	Any of classic symptoms *may or may not* be present Memory and concentration problems, cognitive and behavioral changes, increased dependency, anxiety, and increased sleep Muscle aches, abdominal pain or tightness, flatulence, nausea and vomiting, dry mouth, and headaches Be alert for CHF, diabetes, cancer, infectious diseases, and anemia Cardiovascular (CV) agents, anxiolytics, amphetamines, narcotics, and hormones may also play a role

Data from Vonnes, C., & El-Rady, R. (2021). When you hear hoof beats, look for the zebras: Atypical presentation of illness in the older adult. *The Journal for Nurse Practitioners*, *17*(4), 458–461; and Flaherty, E., & Zwicker D. (2020). *Atypical presentation*. Hartford Institute for Geriatric Nursing. Retrieved from https://hign.org/consultgeri/resources/protocols/atypical-presentation.

EVIDENCE-BASED PRACTICE
Recognition of Atypical Presentation of Illness in Older Adults

Background
Prompt recognition of acute myocardial infarction (AMI) symptoms and initiation of lifesaving measures in the emergency department (ED) is necessary to save lives. Symptom recognition is challenging in older adults who arrive at the ED with atypical symptoms.

Sample and Setting
Cardiac units at three regional hospitals in Hong Kong participated in this study. Consecutive samples were recruited, consisting of patients over 18 years of age with confirmed diagnosis of AMI. The developmental cohort consisted of 300 participants; the validation cohort consisted of 97 participants.

Methods
This was a risk-prediction model development study, designed to develop and validate a risk scoring system to predict atypical symptom presentation among AMI patients.

Findings
The development cohort consisted of 24.3% of the patients whereas the validation cohort included 24.7% of those who presented with atypical symptoms. Five (5) predictors made statistically significant contribution to atypical AMI presentation: age ≥75; female; diagnosis of diabetes; previous AMI; and no history of hyperlipidemia.

Implications
Timely recognition of AMI and initiation of lifesaving treatment is crucial to decreasing morbidity and mortality. Identification of predictors of atypical presentation has the potential to improve recognition of atypical presentation of AMI for triage nurses in the ED.

Data from Li, P. W. C., & Yu, D. S. F. (2017). Recognition of atypical symptoms of acute myocardial infarction: Development and validation of a risk scoring system. *Journal of Cardiovascular Nursing*, *32*(2), 99–106.

Cognitive Assessment

As can be seen in Box 3.1, delirium is one of the most common, atypical presentations of illness in older adults, representing a wide variety of potential problems. As an advocate for older adults, the nurse may need to remind other team members that a sudden change in cognitive function is often the result of illness, not aging. Knowing older adults' baseline mental status is essential to avoid overlooking a serious illness manifesting itself with delirium. Box 3.1 outlines the multivariate causes of delirium that the nurse must consider during the assessment. The Confusion Assessment Method (CAM) is an evidence-based tool to assist health-care providers in the identification of delirium, both quickly and accurately. The CAM evaluates 4 features related to delirium. Delirium is diagnosed if features 1 and 2, and either 3 or 4 are present (Box 3.2):

One of the more challenging aspects of the assessment of an older adult is distinguishing reversible delirium from irreversible cognitive changes such as those seen in dementia and

---

BOX 3.1 Causes of Delirium

Reversible causes of delirium are outlined by the following acronym (DELIRIUM):

- **D**rugs, including any new medications, increased dosages, drug interactions, over-the-counter drugs, alcohol, etc
- **E**lectrolyte disturbances, especially dehydration and thyroid problems
- **L**ack of drugs, such as when long-term sedatives (including alcohol and sleeping pills) are stopped, or when pain drugs are not being given adequately
- **I**nfection, commonly urinary or respiratory tract infection (UTI / RTI)
- **R**educed sensory input, which happens when vision or hearing are poor
- **I**ntracranial (referring to processes within the skull) such as a brain infection, hemorrhage, stroke, or tumor (rare)
- **U**rinary problems or intestinal problems, such as constipation or inability to urinate
- **M**yocardial (heart) and lungs, such as heart attack, problems with heart rhythm (arrhythmia), worsening of heart failure, or chronic obstructive pulmonary disease (COPD)

Delirium can result from an imbalance in brain chemicals (neurotransmitters), which are crucial molecules that relay signals between nerves. A particularly important neurotransmitter is acetylcholine. One reason that people with dementia (such as Alzheimer disease) are at high risk of delirium is that the brain damage found in dementia kills the brain cells that produce acetylcholine. If oxygen or glucose levels in the brain decrease, even a little, the amount of acetylcholine drops even more dramatically. In such cases, the brain functions abnormally, producing delirium.

Other brain chemicals, such as dopamine, also contribute to delirium, because they regulate the amount of acetylcholine in the brain.

- **Medications.** Side effects of familiar medications or sudden withdrawal from drugs are the most common and most treatable causes of delirium. Because many older people take multiple medications which may interact in harmful ways, it is important that health-care professionals are told about every prescription and nonprescription medication being taken.
- **Alcohol.** Alcohol abuse is frequently overlooked as a cause of delirium in older adults. Either excessive use (intoxication) or a sudden withdrawal from alcohol can cause delirium. Delirium caused by withdrawal of alcohol appears to be as common in older adults with alcoholism as in their younger counterparts, although the death rate after withdrawal is higher in older alcoholics.
- **Medical conditions.** Virtually any physical illness or condition can bring on delirium, especially when more than one illness is present. Sometimes, delirium is also the first sign of a serious, life-threatening illness such as a heart attack. In a hospital, the most common causes are sudden blood loss, dehydration, low blood pressure, fluid retention, infections, low levels of oxygen (hypoxia), kidney or liver failure, high blood sugar (hyperglycemia) or low blood sugar (hypoglycemia), intestinal blockage (impaction), sleep deprivation, or inability to urinate. Delirium caused by a sudden change in the nervous system, such as a stroke, brain tumor, or brain infection, is less common. Immobility, sleep deprivation or fragmented sleep, and pain can all contribute to bringing on delirium.
- **Environmental conditions.** Delirium can also result from too little stimulation of the senses, especially in people who already have some degree of mental impairment, or who are confined to a featureless room in a hospital or nursing home. In one study, delirium after an operation occurred twice as often in patients in intensive care units (ICUs) without windows as in patients in similar units with windows. In addition, a form of delirium that occurs **in the evening** (known as "sundowning") may be partly due to sensory deprivation. Vision and hearing loss may also make it more difficult for the person to perceive reality and increases the likelihood of delusions or hallucinations.
- **Delirium after surgery.** Delirium may be the most common complication after surgery in older adults, and leads to longer hospital stays, a higher death rate, and a greater need for nursing home care afterward. It may also signal that there will be complications after surgery.

The chance that a patient will become delirious after an operation increases if a patient is an older adult already has dementia or a physical disability, drinks excessive alcohol, or has very abnormal blood tests. Also, certain types of operations are more frequently associated with delirium. For example, delirium is much more common after hip surgery and heart surgery.

From the American Geriatric Society (AGS) Health in Aging Foundation. (2020). *Delirium.* HealthInAging.org [website]. Retrieved from https://www.healthinaging.org/a-z-topic/delirium/causes.

BOX 3.2 The Confusion Assessment Method (CAM) Diagnostic Algorithm

- **Feature 1: Acute Onset or Fluctuating Course.** This feature is usually obtained from a family member or nurse and is shown by positive responses to the following questions: Is there evidence of an acute change in mental status from the patient's baseline? Did the (abnormal) behavior fluctuate during the day, that is, tend to come and go, or increase and decrease in severity?
- **Feature 2: Inattention.** This feature is shown by a positive response to the following question: Did the patient have difficulty focusing attention, for example, being easily distractible, or having difficulty keeping track of what was being said?
- **Feature 3: Disorganized thinking.** This feature is shown by a positive response to the following question: Was the patient's thinking disorganized or incoherent, such as rambling or irrelevant conversation, unclear or illogical flow of ideas, or unpredictable switching from subject to subject?
- **Feature 4: Altered level of consciousness.** This feature is shown by any answer other than "alert" to the following question: Overall, how would you rate this patient's level of consciousness? (alert [normal]), vigilant [hyperalert], lethargic [drowsy, easily aroused], stupor [difficult to arouse], or coma [unarousable])?

From Inouye, S., van Dyck, C., Alessi, C., Balkin, S., Siegal, A., & Horwitz, R. (1990). Clarifying confusion: The confusion assessment method. *Annals of Internal Medicine, 113*(12), 941–948. © 2003 Sharon K. Inouye MD, MPH.

related disorders. In contrast to the characteristics of delirium noted previously, dementia is a global, sustained deterioration of cognitive function in an alert patient. Other diagnostic features of dementia include significant cognitive decline over time and deficits in learning and memory, language, executive function, attention, perceptual and motor skills, and social interactions (UpToDate, 2018). Table 3.3 depicts the distinguishing features of delirium, dementia, and depression. Keep in mind that delirium predominantly affects attention and is typically reversible; dementia predominantly affects memory and is irreversible.

TABLE 3.3 Characteristics Comparison between Dementia, Delirium, and Depression

Characteristic	Dementia	Delirium	Depression
Onset/duration	Slow, progressive onset; deterioration over time	Abrupt onset	Changes in mood persisting for at least 2 weeks
Progression	Irreversible; symptoms progress over time; trajectory dependent on underlying disease process	Acute with symptoms fluctuating throughout day; reversible with treatment of the underlying cause	Relapsing, chronic; responds to treatment
Psychomotor activity (motor actions that result directly from environmental stimulus)	BPSD (agitation, irritability, apathy, disinhibition / inappropriate behavior, paranoia, repetitive movements, and vocalizations)	Hyperactive delirium: agitation, restlessness, hallucinations Hypoactive delirium: somnolence, speech may be garbled, nonsensical Mixed: fluctuates between above	Usually withdrawn Apathy Psychomotor agitation or retardation
Sleep-wake cycle	Impaired; day / night reversal	Impaired; frequent changes	Hypersomnia or abnormal patterns
Alertness (appropriate response to stimulus; sensory awareness)	Alert during the day	Fluctuates	Normal
Focus (ability to focus on a particular aspect of a stimulus)	Normal	Impaired or fluctuates, distractable	Decreased concentration and ability to think
Affect (internal feelings)	Emotional changes Depression accompanied by appetite changes	Fluctuating emotions	Lack of interest or pleasure in usual activities Appetite changes resulting in increase or decrease in weight
Thinking (reasoning)	Impaired judgment Amnesia, aphasia, apraxia, agnosia	Disorganized, distorted, incoherent	Hopelessness, sadness, emptiness Feelings of worthlessness Thoughts of death or suicide
Perception (interpreting the senses)	Delusions and hallucinations may be present	Distorted – illusions, hallucinations, delusions; difficulty distinguishing between reality and misperceptions	Usually intact (hallucinations and delusions only present in severe cases)
Screening	MoCA MMSE Mini-Cog	CAM CAM-ICU	GDS
Management	Multi-disciplinary approach with pharmacological and non-pharmacological therapies Address polypharmacy Cholinesterase inhibitors, NMDA SSRIs may delay progression of MCI and treat agitation and delusions Patient-centered care with family / caregiver involvement	Treat underlying cause Symptom management Antipsychotics (quetiapine or risperidone) if safety is a concern Patient-centered care with family / caregiver involvement	Pharmacological treatment combined with cognitive therapies Patient-centered care with family / caregiver involvement

MCI, Mild cognitive impairment; *BPSD*, Behavioral and psychological symptoms of dementia; *SSRIs*, selective serotonin reuptake inhibitors; *SNRIs*, selective serotonin and norepinephrine reuptake inhibitors; *NDRIs*, norepinephrine and dopamine reuptake inhibitors; *NaSSA*, noradrenergic and specific serotonergic; *NMDA*, N-methyl-D-aspartate receptor antagonist; *GDS*, Geriatric Depression Scale; *MoCA*, Montreal Cognitive Assessment; *MMSE*, Mini-Mental State Exam; *Mini-Cog*, Mini-Cog Cognitive Impairment Screening; *CAM*, Confusion Assessment Method; *CAM-ICU*, Confusion Assessment Method Intensive Care Unit.

Data from: Burton, R. D. (2019). 3D pharmacology: Management of depression, delirium, and dementia in older adults. *GeriNotes*, 26(1), 28–31; Dening, K. H., & Aldridge, Z. (2021). The three Ds: dementia, delirium and depression. *Journal of Community Nursing*, 35(6), 59–64; Harris, M. (2017). Decline, delirium, depression, dementia. *Nursing Clinics of North America*, 52, 363–374; Holle, C. H., Turnquist, M. A, & Rudolph, J. L. (2019). Safeguarding older adults with dementia, depression, and delirium in a temporary disaster shelter. *Nursing Forum*, 54, 157–164; Laske, R. A., & Stephens, B. A. (2018). Confusion states: Sorting out delirium, dementia, and depression. *Nursing Made Incredibly Easy! 16*(6), 13–16; Mack, L., Zonsius, M. C., Newman, M., & Emery-Tiburcio, E. E. (2022). Recognizing and acting on mentation concerns. *American Journal of Nursing*, 122(5), 50–55; Victoria State Government, Department of Health. (2015). *Differential diagnosis – depression, delirium and dementia*. State of Victoria. Retrieved from https://www.health.vic.gov.au/patient-care/differential-diagnosis-depression-delirium-and-dementia. Accessed May 6, 2024.

Assessment may be complex because of the multiple associated characteristics of delirium and dementia. It is not uncommon for delirium to be superimposed on dementia. In this case, the symptoms of a new illness may be accentuated or masked, thus confounding assessment. Therefore, the nurse must have a clear understanding of the differences between delirium and dementia and must recognize that only subtle evidence may be present to indicate the existence of a problem. Also, completing the total assessment during the first encounter with the patient may not be possible or desirable. In conducting the initial assessment of the course of the presenting symptoms, the nurse should remember that families and friends of the patient may be valuable sources of data regarding the onset, duration, and associated symptoms.

CULTURAL AWARENESS

Cultural Assessment

Culturally sensitive assessment is necessary to achieve quality care outcomes. At a minimum, the following questions should be included as part of every geriatric assessment:
- What is your ethnicity?
- What is your preferred language?
- Do you know that interpreter services are available free of charge? Do you want to choose one of the available interpreter services (online, telephone, in person)?
- How much education did you complete (none, <7th grade, ≥7th grade)?

From American Geriatrics Society (AGS) Ethnogeriatrics Committee. (2016). Achieving high-quality multicultural geriatric care. *Journal of the American Geriatrics Society, 64*(2), 255–260.

Tailoring the Nursing Assessment to the Older Person

The health assessment may be collected in various physical settings, including the hospital, home, office, daycare center, and long-term care facility. Any of these settings may be adapted to be conducive to the free exchange of information between the nurse and an older adult. The overall atmosphere established by the nurse should be one that conveys trust, caring, and confidentiality. The following general suggestions are related to preparing the environment and considering individual patient needs to foster the collection of meaningful data.

Environmental modifications made during the assessment should consider sensory and musculoskeletal changes in the older adult. The following points should be considered in preparing the environment:
- Provide adequate space, particularly if the patient uses a mobility aid
- Minimize noise and distractions like those generated by television, radio, intercom, or other nearby activity
- Set a comfortable, sufficiently warm temperature and ensure no drafts are present
- Use diffuse lighting with increased illumination; avoid directional or localized light
- Avoid glossy or highly polished surfaces, including floors, walls, ceilings, and furnishings
- Place the patient in a comfortable seating position that facilitates information exchange
- Ensure the older adult's proximity to a bathroom
- Keep water or other preferred fluids available
- Provide a place to hang or store garments and belongings
- Maintain absolute privacy
- Plan the assessment, considering the older adult's energy level, pace, and adaptability; more than 1 session may be necessary to complete the assessment
- Be patient, relaxed, and unhurried
- Allow the patient plenty of time to respond to questions and directions
- Maximize the use of silence to allow the patient time to collect thoughts before responding
- Be alert to signs of increasing fatigue such as sighing, grimacing, irritability, leaning against objects for support, dropping the head and shoulders, and progressive slowing
- Conduct the assessment during the patient's peak energy time

Regardless of the degree of disability and decline an older adult patient may exhibit, they have assets and capabilities that allow functioning within the limitations imposed by chronic disease. During the assessment, the nurse must provide an environment that allows the older adult to demonstrate those abilities. Failure to do so could result in inaccurate conclusions about the older adult's functional ability, which may lead to inappropriate care and treatment:
- Assess more than once and at different times of the day
- Measure performance under the most favorable of conditions
- Take advantage of natural opportunities that elicit assets and capabilities; collect data during bathing, grooming, and mealtime
- Ensure that assistive sensory devices (glasses, hearing aid) and mobility devices (walker, cane, prosthesis) are in place and functioning correctly
- Interview family, friends, and significant others involved in the patient's care to validate assessment data
- Use body language, touch, eye contact, and speech to promote the patient's maximum degree of participation
- Be aware of the patient's emotional state and concerns; fear, anxiety, and boredom may lead to inaccurate assessment conclusions regarding functional ability

THE HEALTH HISTORY

The nursing health history—the first phase of a comprehensive, nursing-focused health assessment—provides a subjective account of the older adult's current and past health status. The interview forms the basis of a therapeutic nurse–patient relationship in which the patient's well-being is a mutual concern. Establishing this relationship with the older adult is essential for gathering useful, significant data. The data obtained from the health history alerts the nurse to focus on key areas of the physical examination that require further investigation. By talking with the nurse about health concerns, the older adult increases their awareness of health, and topics for health teaching can be identified. Finally, recounting a patient's history in a purposeful, systematic way may have the therapeutic effect of serving as a life review.

Although many formats exist for the nursing health history, all have similar basic components. The nursing health history for the older adult should include an assessment of functional, cognitive, affective, and social well-being. Specific tools for collecting these data are addressed later in this chapter.

The physical, psychosocial, cultural, and functional aspects of the older adult patient require adaptations in interviewing styles and techniques. Making adaptations that reflect a genuine sensitivity toward the older adult and a sound, theoretic knowledge base of aging enhances the interview process.

The Interviewer

The interviewer's ability to elicit meaningful data from the patient depends on the interviewer's attitudes and stereotypes about aging and older people. The nurse must be aware of these factors because they affect nurse–patient communication during the assessment (see Cultural Awareness box).

CULTURAL AWARENESS
Cultural Considerations and the Interviewer

Healthcare personnel must be mindful of the different approaches to health care each culture prefers. Research indicates that persons who consider themselves without prejudice tend to express overt prejudice. Self-awareness can help overcome this issue and facilitate compassionate, culturally appropriate care (American Geriatrics Society [AGS] Ethnogeriatrics Committee, 2016).

- Be respectful of, interested in, and understanding of other cultures without being judgmental
- Avoid stereotyping by race, gender, age, ethnicity, religion, sexual orientation, socioeconomic status, and other social categories
- Know the traditional health-related beliefs and practices prevalent among members of a patient's cultural group and encourage patients to discuss their cultural beliefs and practices
- Learn about the traditional or folk illnesses and folk remedies common to patients' cultural groups
- Try to understand patient perceptions of appropriate wellness and illness behaviors and expectations of health-care providers in times of health and illness
- Study the cultural expressions and manifestations of caring and noncaring behaviors expected by patients
- Avoid stereotypical associations with violence, poverty, crime, low-level education, nonadherent behaviors, and nonadherence to time-regimented schedules, and avoid any other stereotypes that may adversely affect nurse–patient relationships
- Be aware that patients who have lived in the United States for many years may have become increasingly westernized and have fewer remaining practices of their birth culture
- Learn to value the richness of cultural diversity as an asset rather than a hindrance to communication and effective intervention

Attitude is a feeling, value, or belief about something that determines behavior. If the nurse has an attitude that characterizes older adults as less healthy, alert, and more dependent, then the interview structure will reflect this attitude. For example, if the nurse believes that dependence in self-care normally accompanies advanced age, the patient will not be questioned about strengths and abilities. The resulting inaccurate functional assessment will do little to promote patient independence. Myths and stereotypes about older adults also may affect the nurse's questioning. For example, believing that older adults do not participate in sexual relationships may result in the nurse's failure to interview the patient about sexual health matters. The nurse's own anxiety and fear of personal aging, as well as a lack of knowledge about older people, contribute to commonly held negative attitudes, myths, and stereotypes about older people. Gerontological nurses have a responsibility to themselves and their older adult patients to improve their understanding of the aging process and aging people.

To ensure a successful interview, the nurse should explain the reason for the interview to the patient and give a brief overview of the format to be followed. This alleviates anxiety and uncertainty, and the patient can focus on telling the story. Another strategy that can be employed in some settings is to give the patient selected portions of the interview form to complete *before* meeting with the nurse. This allows patients sufficient time to recall their life histories, thus facilitating the collection of important health-related data.

Older people have lengthy and often complicated histories. A goal-directed interviewing process helps the patient share pertinent information, but the tendency to reminisce may make it difficult for the patient to stay focused. *Guided reminiscence,* however, can elicit valuable data and promote a supportive therapeutic relationship. Using such a technique helps the nurse balance the need to collect the required information with the patient's need to relate what is personally important. For example, the patient may relate a story about a social outing that seems irrelevant but may reveal important information about available resources and support systems. The interplay of the previously noted factors may necessitate more than one encounter with the patient to complete the data collection. Setting a time limit in advance helps the patient focus on the interview and aids with the problem of diminished time perception. Keeping an easy-to-read clock within view of the patient may be helpful.

To promote patient comfort and data sharing, the nurse should work with the patient to establish the organization of the interview. The patient should feel that the nurse is a caring person who treats others with respect. Self-esteem is enhanced if the patient feels included in the decision-making process.

At the beginning of the interview, the nurse and patient must determine the most effective and comfortable distance and position for the session. The ability to see and hear is critical to the communication process with an older adult, and adaptations to account for any disability must consider personal space requirements.

The appropriate use of touch during the interview may reduce the anxiety associated with the initial encounter. The importance and comfort of touch is highly individual, but older persons need and appreciate it. Touch should always convey respect, caring, and sensitivity.

Finally, the nurse does not have to obtain the entire history in the traditional manner of a seated, face-to-face interview.

Depending on the situation, this technique may be inappropriate with an older adult. The nurse should not overlook the natural opportunities available in the setting for gathering information. Interviewing the patient at mealtime or even while participating in a game, hobby, or other social activity often provides more meaningful data about a variety of areas.

The Patient

Several factors influence the patient's ability to participate meaningfully in the interview. The nurse must be aware of these factors because they affect the older adult's ability to communicate all the information necessary for determining appropriate, comprehensive interventions. Sensory–perceptual deficits, anxiety, reduced energy level, pain, multiple and interrelated health problems, and the tendency to reminisce are the major patient factors requiring special consideration as the nurse elicits the health history. Table 3.4 contains recommendations for managing these factors.

Electronic Health Records

With the advent of electronic health records (EHRs), patients and providers have voiced concerns that their connection with each other has been undermined and has become impersonal. To alleviate some issues related to their use, keep the keyboard or monitor in a position that lets you face the patient. Patients have noted that eye contact with their health-care provider is an important component of communication. Input as much data into the EHR before talking to the patient, then alternate talking and inputting data to maintain eye contact and personal connection with the older adult. On a positive note, patients like the use of the EHR as it reduces the repetition of information; additionally, when health-care providers shared the information in the EHR with the patient, they felt it facilitated communication and made them feel a part of the health-care planning process (Rose et al, 2014).

The Health History Format

Table 3.5 provides a brief overview of the components of the health history. When possible, refer to old records to obtain information that will lessen the time required of the patient and the interviewer.

Patient Profile or Biographic Data

This profile is basic, factual data about the older adult. In this section, it is often useful to comment on the reliability of the information source. For example, if the patient's cognitive ability prevents giving accurate information, secondary sources such as family or other medical records should be consulted. Knowledge of the data source alerts the reader or user to the context within which they must consider the information. Take time to clarify advance directives such as the existence of a living will, powers of attorney for health care and finances, and code status.

Family Profile

This information about immediate family members gives a quick overview of who may be living in the patient's home or who may represent important support systems for the patient. These data also establish a basis for a later description of family health history.

Occupational Profile

Information about work history and experiences may alert the nurse to possible health risks or exposures, lifestyle or social

TABLE 3.4 History-Taking Recommendations for the Older Adult

Factor	Recommendations
Sensory deficits	Dentures, eyeglasses, or hearing aids, if normally worn, should be worn to facilitate communication during the interview; adequate lighting and elimination of visual or auditory distraction also help
Underreporting of symptoms	Older patients may not report symptoms that they may incorrectly consider part of normal aging (e.g., dyspnea, hearing or vision deficits, memory problems, incontinence, gait disturbance, constipation, dizziness, falls); however, no symptom should be attributed to normal aging unless a thorough evaluation is done and other possible causes have been eliminated
Unusual manifestations of a disorder	In older adults, typical manifestations of a disorder may be absent; instead, older patients may present with nonspecific symptoms (e.g., fatigue, confusion, weight loss)
Functional decline as the only manifestation	Disorders may manifest solely as functional decline; in such cases, standard questions may not apply; for example, when asked about joint symptoms, patients with severe arthritis may not report pain, swelling, or stiffness, but if asked about changes in activities, they may, for example, report that they no longer take walks or volunteer at the hospital; questions about duration of functional decline (e.g., "How long have you been unable to do your own shopping?") can elicit useful information; identifying people when they have just started to have difficulty doing basic activities of daily living (ADLs) or instrumental ADLs may provide more opportunities for interventions to restore function or to prevent further decline and thus maintain independence
Difficulty recalling	Patients may not accurately remember past illnesses, hospitalizations, operations, and drug use; clinicians may have to obtain these data elsewhere (e.g., from family members, a home-health aide, or medical records)
Fear	Older adults may be reluctant to report symptoms because they fear hospitalization, which they may associate with dying
Age-related disorders and problems	Depression (common among older adults who are vulnerable and sick), the cumulative losses of old age, and discomfort due to a disorder may make older adults less apt to provide health-related information to clinicians; patients with impaired cognition may have difficulty describing problems, impeding the physician's evaluation

From the MSD Manual Professional Version, edited by Sandy Falk. Copyright © 2024 Merck & Co., Inc., Rahway, NJ, USA and its affiliates. All rights reserved. Available at https://www.msdmanuals.com/professional. Accessed May 2024.

TABLE 3.5 Basic Components of a Health History

Domain	Suggested Items for Assessment
Physical health and medical conditions	Comorbid conditions and disease severity Medical review Nutritional status Polypharmacy Urinary continence Sexual function Vision / Hearing Dentition
Mental health and psychologic status	Cognition Mood and anxiety Fears Goals of care Advance care preferences Spirituality
Functioning	Functional capacity: core functions such as mobility and balance, fall risk Activities of daily living (ADIs) Life roles that are important to the patient
Social circumstances	Social support and networks Informal support available from family Wider network of friends and contacts Statutory care Financial concerns and poverty
Environment	Living situation: housing, comfort, facilities, and safety Use or potential use of "telehealth" technology Transport facilities Accessibility to local resources

From Spirgiene, L., & Brent, L. (2018). Comprehensive geriatric assessment from a nursing perspective. In: K. Hertz & J. Santy-Tomplinson (Eds.). *Fragility fracture nursing: holistic care and management of the orthogeriatric patient.* New York: Springer, pp 41-52.

use of health-care and related services, perceptions of such resources, and attitudes about the importance of health maintenance and promotion. The importance of religion in all its dimensions, including participation in church-related activities, is an important area to assess. Frequently, the church "family" is a significant source of support for the older adult.

CULTURAL AWARENESS
Health Literacy

Health literacy is "the degree to which individuals have the capacity to obtain, process, and understand basic health information and services needed to make appropriate health decisions" (AGS Ethnogeriatrics Committee, 2016, p. 257). Nearly 60% of older adults have limited health literacy; this number rises when the older adult has less than a high school education and is a minority. Limited health literacy has been associated with an increased risk for mortality, poor understanding of prescribed drugs on discharge, and failure to use preventive health services. Universal adoption of the "teach-back" technique and keeping printed and oral education at the sixth-grade reading level or lower (in the preferred language of the older adult) has been shown to compensate for limited health literacy (AGS Ethnogeriatrics Committee, 2016).

Description of a Typical Day
Identifying the activities of a patient during a full 24-hour period provides data about practices that either support or hinder healthy living. Analysis of the usual activities carried out by the patient may explain symptoms described later in the Review of Systems section. Clues about the patient's relationships, lifestyle practices, and spiritual dimensions may also be uncovered.

Present Health Status
The patient's perception of health in the past year and in the past 5 years, coupled with information about health habits, reveals much about their physical integrity. Based on how the patient responds, the nurse may be able to ascertain whether the patient needs health maintenance, promotion, or restoration.

The chief complaint, stated in the patient's own words, enables the nurse to identify why the patient is seeking health care specifically. It is best to ask about this using a term other than *chief complaint* because patients may take offense at that choice of words. If a symptom is the reason, usually its duration is also included. A complete and careful symptom analysis may be carried out for the chief complaint by collecting information on the factors identified in Table 3.6. When the patient does not display specific symptomatology but has broader health concerns, the nurse should identify those concerns to establish potential nursing interventions.

Information about the patient's knowledge and understanding of their current health state, including treatments and management strategies, helps the nurse focus on possible areas of health teaching and reinforcement, identify a patient's access to and use of resources, discover coping styles and strategies, and determine health behavior patterns. Data about the patient's perception of functional ability regarding perceived health problems and medical diagnoses provide valuable insight into the individual's overall sense of physical, social, emotional, and cognitive well-being.

patterns, activity level, and intellectual performance. Retirement concerns may also be identified. Obtaining the patient's perception of the adequacy of income for meeting daily living needs may have implications for designing nursing interventions. Financial resources and health have an interdependent relationship.

Living Environment Profile
Any nursing interventions for the patient must be planned considering the living environment. A patient's living environment affects the degree of function, safety and security, and feelings of well-being.

Recreation or Leisure Profile
Identifying what the patient does to relax and have fun and how the patient uses free time may provide clues to some of their social and emotional dimensions.

Resources or Support Systems Used
Obtaining information about the various health-care providers and agencies the patient uses may alert the nurse to patterns of

TABLE 3.6 The Provocation, Quality, Region / Radiation, Severity, and Time (PQRSTU) Assessment

The mnemonic is often used to assess pain but can also be used to assess many signs and symptoms related to the client's main health needs and other signs and symptoms that are discussed during the complete subjective health assessment. This lists examples of prompting questions using this mnemonic.

PQRSTU	Questions Related to Pain	Questions Related to Other Symptoms
Provocative	• What makes your pain worse?	• What makes your breathing worse?
Palliative	• What makes your pain feel better?	• What makes your nausea better?
Quality	• What does the pain feel like? **Note**: If the client struggles to answer this question, you can provide suggestions such as "aching," "stabbing," "burning."	• What does the itching feel like?
Quantity	• How bad is your pain?	• How bad is the itching?
Region	• Where do you feel the pain? • Point to where you feel the pain.	• Where exactly do you feel the nausea?
Radiation	• Does the pain move around? • Do you feel the pain elsewhere?	• Do you feel the nausea elsewhere?
Severity (severity scale)	• How would you rate your pain on a scale of 0 to 10, with 0 being *no pain* and 10 being the *worst pain you've ever experienced*? **Note**: The severity scale is an important assessment of pain and when used can provide evaluation of a treatment's effectiveness. After eliciting a baseline, you may provide some sort of pain control intervention and then reassess the pain to see if it was effective.	• How would you rate your breathing issues on a scale of 0 to 10, with 0 being *no problems* and 10 being the *worst breathing issues you've ever experienced*?
Timing	• When did the pain start? • What were you doing when the pain started? • Where were you when the pain started? • Is the pain constant or does it come and go? • If the pain is intermittent, when did it last occur? • How long does the pain last?	• When did your breathing issues begin? • What were you doing when the itching first started? • Where were you when the itching first started? • Is the nausea constant or does it come and go? • If the nausea is intermittent, when did it last occur? • How long did the nausea last?
Treatment	• Have you taken anything to help relieve the pain? • Have you tried any treatments at home for the pain?	• Have you taken anything to relieve the itching better? • Have you tried any treatments at home for the itching?
Understanding	• What do you think is causing the pain?	• What do you think is causing the rash?

From Lapum, J., St-Amant, O., Hughes, M., Petrie, P., Morrell, S., & Mistry, S. (2019). *The complete subjective health assessment* (pp. 35–40). Creative Commons Attribution-ShareAlike (4.0 International [CC BY-SA] license: https://creativecommons.org/licenses/by-sa/4.0/). Retrieved from https://ecampusontario.pressbooks.pub/healthassessment/chapter/the-pqrstu-assessment/.

Drugs

Assessment of the older adult's current drugs is usually accomplished by having the patient bring in *all* prescription and over-the-counter drugs, as well as regularly and occasionally used home remedies. The nurse should also inquire about the patient's use of supplements, herbal and other related products, and ask how each drug is taken—orally, topically, inhalation, or other route. Obtaining the drugs in this manner allows the nurse to examine drug labels, which may show the use of multiple physicians and pharmacies. Also, this helps the nurse determine the patient's pattern of drug taking (including adherence), their knowledge of drugs, the expiration dates of drugs, and the potential risk for drug interactions.

Immunization and Health Screening Status

The older adult's immunization status for specific diseases and illnesses is essential because of the degree of risk for this age group. More attention is increasingly paid to the immunization status of the older adult population, primarily because of the underuse of vaccines in the past, especially the influenza and pneumococcal vaccines. Tetanus, diphtheria, and pertussis (Tdap) or tetanus and diphtheria toxoids (Td) boosters are recommended at 10-year intervals for those who have been previously immunized as adults or children (Centers for Disease Control and Prevention [CDC], 2022). Adults over the age of 60 years should receive herpes zoster immunization even if they do not remember having chickenpox. Additionally, older adults should receive an updated COVID-19 vaccine based on CDC recommendations. As of 2023, the CDC also recommends adults over age 60 receive a single dose of the respiratory syncytial virus (RSV) vaccine (CDC, 2023).

Older adults should still participate in health screenings for the most recent recommendations. Tuberculosis, a disease that was once well-controlled, is now resurfacing in this country. Older adults who may have had a tubercular lesion at a young age may experience a reactivation because of age-related immune system changes, chronic illness, and poor nutrition. Frail and institutionalized older adults are particularly vulnerable and should be screened for exposure or active disease through an annual purified protein derivative (PPD) test.

Allergies

Determining the older adult's drug, food, and other contact and environmental allergies is essential for planning nursing interventions. It is important to note the patient's reaction to the allergen and the usual treatment.

Nutrition

A 24-hour diet recall is a useful screening tool that provides information about the intake of daily requirements, including the intake of "empty" calories, adherence to prescribed dietary therapies, and the practice of unusual or "fad" diets. The nurse should also assess the time meals and snacks are eaten. If a 24-hour recall cannot be obtained or the information gleaned raises more questions, having the patient keep a food diary for a select time (5 to 7 days) may be indicated. The diets of older adults may be nutritionally inadequate because of advanced age, multiple chronic illnesses, lack of financial resources, mobility impairments, dental health problems, and loneliness. The diet recall and diary provide nutritional assessment data reflecting the patient's health and well-being.

CULTURAL AWARENESS
Cultural Assessment of Nutritional Needs

- What is the meaning of food and eating to the patient?
- What does the patient eat during:
  - a typical day
  - special events such as secular or religious holidays? (e.g., Muslims fast during the month of Ramadan; Catholics may not eat meat on Fridays during Lent)
- How does the patient define food? (for some, food may mean survival; for others, food is a reflection of status; food can be pleasure or mean community)
- What is the timing and sequencing of meals?
- With whom does the patient usually eat? (e.g., alone, with others of the same gender, with spouse)
- What does the patient believe constitutes a "healthy" versus "unhealthy" diet?
- From what sources (e.g., ethnic grocery store, home garden, restaurant) does the patient obtain food items? Who usually does the grocery shopping?
- How are foods prepared? (e.g., type of preparation; cooking oil used; length of time food is cooked; amount and type of seasoning added before, during, and after preparation)
- Has the patient chosen a nutritional practice such as vegetarianism or abstinence from alcoholic beverages?
- Do religious beliefs and practices influence the patient's diet or eating habits (e.g., amount, type, preparations, or designation of acceptable food items or combinations)? Ask the patient to explain the religious calendar and guidelines that govern these dietary practices, including exemptions for older adults and the sick.

Previous Health Status

Because a person's present health status may depend on past health conditions, gathering data about common childhood illnesses, serious or chronic illnesses, trauma, hospitalizations, operations, and obstetric history is essential. The patient's history of measles, mumps, rubella, chickenpox, diphtheria, pertussis, tetanus, rheumatic fever, and poliomyelitis should be obtained to identify potential risk factors for future health problems.

An older adult patient may not know what diseases are considered serious or may not fully appreciate why it is important to ask about the history of certain diseases. In such cases, the nurse should ask the patient specifically about the history of certain diseases. It is also important to note the dates of onset or occurrence and the treatment measures prescribed for each disease.

For the older adult, the history of traumatic injuries should be completely described, and the date, time, place, circumstances surrounding the incidents, and effect of the incidents on the patient's overall function should be noted. Additional data may be needed to gain a complete picture of the older adult's health status based on the information gathered about previous hospitalizations, operations, and obstetric history. The patient may need to be guided through this process because of forgetfulness or a lengthy, complicated personal history.

Family History

Collecting a family health history provides valuable information about inherited diseases and familial tendencies, whether environmental or genetic, to identify risks and determine the need for preventive services. In surveying the health of blood relatives, the nurse should note the degree of overall health, the presence of disease or illness, and age (if deceased, the cause of death). By collecting these data, the nurse may also be able to identify the existence and degree of family support systems. Data are usually recorded in a family tree format.

Review of Systems

The review is generally a head-to-toe screening to ascertain the presence or absence of key symptoms within each of the body's systems. It is important to question the patient in lay terminology and, if a positive response is elicited, conduct a complete symptom analysis to clarify the course of the symptomatology (see Table 3.6). To reduce confusion and ensure accurate data collection, the nurse should ask the patient for only one piece of information at a time. Information obtained here alerts the nurse about what to focus on during the physical examination.

Approach to Physical Assessment

The objective information acquired in the physical assessment adds to the subjective database already gathered. Together, these components serve as the basis for establishing nursing diagnoses and planning, developing interventions, and evaluating nursing care.

Physical assessment is typically performed after the health history. The approach should be a systematic and deliberate one that allows the nurse to (1) determine patient strengths and capabilities, as well as disabilities and limitations; (2) verify and gain objective support for subjective findings; and (3) gather objective data not previously known.

No single right way exists to assemble the physical assessment, but a head-to-toe approach is generally the most efficient. The sequence used to conduct the physical assessment within this approach is highly individual, depending on the older adult patient. In all cases, however, a side-to-side comparison of findings is made using the patient as the control. To increase mastery in conducting an integrated and comprehensive physical assessment, the nurse should develop a method of organization and use it consistently.

Ultimately, the practice setting and patient condition determine the type and method of examination. For example, an older adult admitted to an acute care hospital with a medical diagnosis of CHF initially requires respiratory and cardiovascular system assessments to plan appropriate interventions for improving activity tolerance. In the home-care setting, assessing the patient's musculoskeletal system is a priority for determining the potential for fall-related injuries and the ability to perform basic self-care tasks. In a long-term care setting, the frail, immobile patient requires an initial skin assessment to determine the risk for pressure injury development and the required preventive measures. Regular examination of the skin thereafter is necessary to assess the effectiveness of the preventive measures instituted.

In all situations, complete physical assessments are important and should eventually be carried out with the patient and setting dictating priorities. Consider the subjective patient data already obtained regarding the urgency of the situation, the acute or chronic nature of the problem, the extent of the problem in terms of body systems affected, and the interrelatedness of physical and psychosocial factors in determining where to begin.

SPICES is an efficient acronym to help gather information necessary to identify patient problems in 6 common areas identified as increasing mortality risk, leading to increased cost and longer hospitalizations in older adults. Positive findings in these areas guide the nurse to implement preventive and therapeutic interventions. The acronym SPICES stands for:

Sleep disorders: Ask the patient how well they usually sleep.
Problems with eating or feeding: Ask the patient why they do not feel like eating.
Incontinence (of bowel or bladder): Ask the patient if they usually make it to the bathroom on time.
Confusion: Assessed through observation and use of appropriate assessment tools.
Evidence of falls: Ask the patient how often they have fallen. Obtain additional data from secondary sources (e.g., family, caregivers, or long-term care facility).
Skin breakdown: Assess for risk factors using appropriate assessment tools.

When using this tool, alterations in any area should lead to additional assessment in the area indicated (Fulmer, 2019).

General Guidelines

Regardless of the approach and sequence used, the following principles should be considered during the physical assessment of an older adult:
- Recognize that the older adult may have no previous experience with a nurse conducting a physical assessment. Each step should be explained, and the patient should be reassured. The examiner should project warmth, sincerity, and interest to allay anxiety or fear.
- Be alert to the older patient's energy level. If the situation warrants it, complete the most important parts of the assessment first and the other parts at a later time. Generally, the head-to-toe assessment should take approximately 30 to 45 minutes.
- Respect the patient's modesty. Allow privacy for changing into a gown; if assistance is needed, assist in a way that does not expose the patient's body or cause embarrassment.
- Keep the patient comfortably draped. Do not unnecessarily expose a body part; expose only the part to be examined.
- Sequence the assessment to minimize position changes. Patients with limited range of motion and strength may require assistance. Be prepared to use alternative positions if the patient is unable to assume the usual position for assessing a body part.
- Develop an efficient sequence for assessment that minimizes nurse and patient movement. Variations that may be necessary will not be disruptive if the sequence is consistently followed. Working from one side of the patient; generally the right side, promotes efficiency.
- Make sure the patient is comfortable. Offer a blanket for added warmth or a pillow or alternative position for comfort.
- Explain each step in simple terms. Give clear, concise directions and instructions for performing required movements.
- Warn of any discomfort that might occur. Be gentle.
- Probe painful areas last.
- For reassurance, share findings with the patient when possible. Encourage the patient to ask questions.
- Take advantage of "teachable moments" that may occur while conducting the assessment (e.g., breast self-examination).
- Develop a standard format on which to note selected findings. Not all data need to be recorded, but the goal is to reduce the potential for forgetting certain data, particularly measurements.

Equipment and Skills

Because the older adult patient may become easily fatigued during the physical assessment, the nurse should ensure proper function and equipment readiness before the assessment begins to avoid unnecessary delays. Place the equipment within easy reach and in the order in which it will be used. The traditional inspection techniques, palpation, percussion, and auscultation are used with older adults, with age-specific variations for some areas.

ADDITIONAL ASSESSMENT MEASURES

Standardized tools and measures of functional status are important adjuncts to traditional assessment, as they enable health-care providers to objectively determine the older person's ability to function independently despite disease, altered cognition, and other disability. These assessments include determining the patient's ability to perform ADLs and instrumental ADLs (IADSs) and the patient's cognitive, affective, and social levels of function. Obtaining these additional data provides a more comprehensive view of the interrelated variables' effect on the older adult's total functioning.

Functional Status Assessment

Functional status is a significant component of an older adult's quality of life (QoL). Assessing functional status has long been viewed as an essential piece of the overall clinical evaluation of an older person. Functional status assessment measures the older adult's ability to perform basic self-care tasks, or ADLs, and tasks requiring more complex independent living activities, or IADLs. Determination of the degree of functional independence in these areas helps identify a patient's abilities and limitations, leading to appropriate interventions (Factora, 2023).

The patient's situation determines the location and time when any of the scales or tools should be administered and the number of times the patient may need to be tested to ensure accurate results. Many tools are available, but the nurse should use only those tools that are valid, reliable, and relevant to the practice setting. The following sections describe the appropriate tools for older adults in most settings.

The Katz Index of ADLs (Fig. 3.1) is a tool widely used to determine the results of treatment and prognosis in older and chronically ill people. The index ranks adequacy of performance in 6 functions: bathing, dressing, toileting, transferring, continence, and feeding. A dichotomous rating of independence or dependence is made for each function. One point is given for each dependent item. Only people who can perform the function without help are rated as independent. The Katz Index is a useful tool for the nurse because it describes the patient's functional level at a specific point in time and objectively measures the effects of the treatment intended to restore function. The tool takes only about 5 minutes to administer and may be used in most settings (McCabe, 2019).

Older adults in most health-care settings benefit from functional status assessment. However, those in acute care settings are particularly in need of such an assessment because of their advanced age, level of acuity, comorbidity, and risk for iatrogenic conditions such as urinary incontinence, falls, delirium, and polypharmacy. The hospitalization experience for older adults may cause loss of function and self-care ability because of the many extrinsic risk factors associated with this setting, including aggressive treatment interventions, bed rest, lack of exercise, insufficient nutritional intake, and iatrogenic infection (Palleschi et al, 2018). Box 3.3 provides a clinical practice protocol to guide acute care nurses in the functional assessment process for older adults. Nurses in this setting are in a key position to assess the older adult's function and implement interventions to prevent decline. Specialized care units known as *acute care for elders* (ACE) units have been developed in

Katz Index of Independence in Activities of Daily Living

ACTIVITIES POINTS (1 OR 0)	INDEPENDENCE: (1 POINT) NO supervision, direction or personal assistance	DEPENDENCE: (0 POINTS) WITH supervision, direction, personal assistance or total care
BATHING POINTS:_____	**(1 POINT)** Bathes self completely or needs help in bathing only a single part of the body such as the back, genital area or disabled extremity.	**(0 POINTS)** Needs help with bathing more than one part of the body, getting in or out of the tub or shower. Requires total bathing.
DRESSING POINTS:_____	**(1 POINT)** Gets clothes from closets and drawers and puts on clothes and outer garments complete with fasteners. May have help tying shoes.	**(0 POINTS)** Needs help with dressing self or needs to be completely dressed.
TOILETING POINTS:_____	**(1 POINT)** Goes to toilet, gets on and off, arranges clothes, cleans genital area without help.	**(0 POINTS)** Needs help transferring to the toilet, cleaning self or uses bedpan or commode.
TRANSFERRING POINTS:_____	**(1 POINT)** Moves in and out of bed or chair unassisted. Mechanical transferring aides are acceptable.	**(0 POINTS)** Needs help in moving from bed to chair or requires a complete transfer.
CONTINENCE POINTS:_____	**(1 POINT)** Exercises complete self control over urination and defecation.	**(0 POINTS)** Is partially or totally incontinent of bowel or bladder.
FEEDING POINTS:_____	**(1 POINT)** Gets food from plate into mouth without help. Preparation of food may be done by another person.	**(0 POINTS)** Needs partial or total help with feeding or requires parenteral feeding.

TOTAL POINTS = _____ 6 = High (*patient independent*) 0 = Low (*patient very dependent*)

Fig. 3.1 Katz Index of Independence in Activities of Daily Living. (Adapted from Katz, S., Down, T. D., Cash, H. R., & Grotz, R. C. [1970]. Progress in the development of the index of ADL. *The Gerontologist, 10*[1], 20–30. Copyright © The Gerontological Society of America.)

BOX 3.3 Nursing Standard of Practice Protocol: Assessment of Function in Acute Care

The following nursing care protocol has been designed to assist bedside nurses in monitoring function in older patients, preventing decline, and maintaining the function of older adults during acute hospitalization.

Objective: The goal of nursing care is to maximize the physical functioning and prevent or minimize declines in ADL function.

I. Background
A. The functional status of individuals describes the capacity to safely perform ADLs. Functional status is a sensitive indicator of health or illness in older adults and therefore a critical nursing assessment.
B. Some functional decline may be prevented or ameliorated with prompt and aggressive nursing intervention (e.g., ambulation, enhanced communication, adaptive equipment).
C. Some functional decline may occur progressively and is not reversible. This decline often accompanies chronic and terminal disease states such as Parkinson disease and dementia.
D. Functional status is influenced by physiologic aging changes, acute and chronic illness, and adaptation. Functional decline is often the initial symptom of acute illness such as infections (pneumonia, UTI). These declines are usually reversible.
E. Functional status is contingent on cognition and sensory capacity, including vision and hearing.
F. Risk factors for functional decline include injuries, acute illness, drug side effects, depression, malnutrition, and decreased mobility (including the use of physical restraints).
G. Additional complications of functional decline include loss of independence, loss of socialization, and increased risk for long-term institutionalization and depression.
H. Recovery of function can also be a measure of return to health such as in those individuals recovering from exacerbations of cardiovascular disease.

II. Assessment Parameters
A. A comprehensive functional assessment of older adults includes independent performance of basic ADLs, social activities, or IADLs; the assistance needed to *accomplish* these tasks; and the sensory ability, cognition, and capacity to ambulate.
   1. Basic ADLs
      a. Bathing
      b. Dressing
      c. Grooming
      d. Eating
      e. Continence
      f. Transferring
   2. IADLs
      a. Meal preparation
      b. Shopping
      c. Drug administration
      d. Housework
      e. Transportation
      f. Accounting
B. Older adult patients view their health in terms of how well they can function rather than in terms of disease alone.
C. The clinician should document functional status and recent or progressive declines in function.
D. Function should be assessed over time to validate capacity, decline, or progress.
E. Standard instruments selected to assess function should be efficient to administer and easy to interpret and provide useful, practical information for clinicians.
F. Multidisciplinary team conferences should be scheduled.

III. Care Strategies
A. Strategies to maximize function:
   1. Maintain individual's daily routine; help the patient to maintain physical, cognitive, and social functions through physical activity and socialization: encourage ambulation; allow flexible visitation, including pets; and encourage reading the newspaper
   2. Educate older adults and caregivers on the value of independent functioning and the consequences of functional decline:
      a. physiologic and psychologic value of independent functioning
      b. reversible functional decline associated with acute illness
      c. strategies to prevent functional decline—exercise, nutrition, and socialization
      d. sources of assistance to manage decline
   3. Encourage activity, including routine exercise, range-of-motion exercises, and ambulation to maintain activity, flexibility, and function
   4. Minimize bed rest
   5. Explore alternatives to physical restraint use
   6. Judiciously use psychoactive drugs in geriatric dosages
   7. Design environments with handrails, wide doorways, raised toilet seats, shower seats, enhanced lighting, low beds, and chairs
   8. Help individuals regain baseline function after acute illnesses by the use of exercise, physical therapy consultation, and increasing nutrition
   9. Obtain assessment for physical and occupational therapies needed to help regain function
B. Strategies to help individuals cope with functional decline:
   1. Help older adults and family determine realistic functional capacity with interdisciplinary consultation
   2. Provide caregiver education and support for families of individuals when decline cannot be ameliorated in spite of nursing and rehabilitative efforts
   3. Carefully document all intervention strategies and patient responses
   4. Provide information to caregivers on causes of functional decline related to the patient's disorder
   5. Provide education to address safety care needs for falls, injuries, and common complications; alternative care settings may be required to ensure safety
   6. Provide sufficient protein and calories to ensure adequate intake and prevent further decline
   7. Provide caregiver support and community services such as home care, nursing, and physical and occupational therapy services to manage functional decline

IV. Expected Outcomes
A. Patients can:
   1. Maintain a safe level of ADLs and ambulation
   2. Make necessary adaptations to maintain safety and independence, including assistive devices and environmental adaptations
B. Provider can demonstrate:
   1. Increased assessment, identification, and management of patients susceptible to or experiencing functional decline
   2. Ongoing documentation of capacity, interventions, goals, and outcomes
   3. Competence in preventive and restorative strategies for function
C. Institution can demonstrate:
   1. Decrease in incidence and prevalence of functional decline in all care settings
   2. Decrease in morbidity and mortality rates associated with functional decline
   3. Decreased use of physical restraints
   4. Decreased incidence of delirium
   5. Increase in prevalence of patients who leave hospital with baseline functional status
   6. Decreased readmission rate
   7. Increased use of rehabilitative services (occupational and physical therapy)
   8. Support of institutional policies and programs that promote function:
      a. caregiver educational efforts
      b. walking programs
      c. continence programs
      d. self-feeding initiatives
      e. elder group activities

ADL, Activities of daily living; *IADL,* instrumental activities of daily living.
Modified from Kresevic, D. M., & Mezey, M. (1997). Assessment of function: Critically important to acute care of elders. *Geriatric Nursing, 18*(5), 216–222.

hospitals nationwide to address these issues better. Research has demonstrated this age-specific, comprehensive approach reduces morbidity and mortality associated with hospitalizing older adults (Palmer, 2018).

Nurses practicing in all settings should begin incorporating valid and reliable tools into routine assessments to determine a patient's baseline functional ability. However, the nurse should remember the following points:
- Environment in which the tool is administered will affect scores
- Patient's affective and cognitive state will affect performance
- Result represents but one piece of the total assessment

Cognitive and Affective Assessment

The purpose of a mental status assessment in the older adult is to determine the patient's level of cognitive function (which implies all those processes associated with mentation or intellectual function). This assessment is usually integrated into the interview and physical examination, and testing is conducted in a natural, nonthreatening manner with consideration of ethnicity. Table 3.7 identifies typical areas assessed in a mental status assessment.

The multiple physiologic, psychologic, and environmental causes of cognitive impairment in older adults, coupled with the view that mental impairment is a normal, age-related process, often lead to incomplete assessment of this problem. Standardized examinations test a variety of cognitive functions, aiding the identification of deficits that affect overall functional ability. Formal, systematic mental status testing helps the nurse determine which behaviors are impaired and warrant intervention.

The Montreal Cognitive Assessment (MoCA) (Fig. 3.2) was developed as a quick screening tool for MCI and Alzheimer

TABLE 3.7 Examination of Mental Status

The mental status examination is an assessment of current mental capacity through evaluation of general appearance, behavior, any unusual or bizarre beliefs and perceptions (e.g., delusions, hallucinations), mood, and all aspects of cognition (e.g., attention, orientation, memory).
Examination of mental status is done in anyone with an altered mental status or evolving impairment of cognition whether acute or chronic. Many screening tools are available; the following are particularly useful:
- Montreal Cognitive Assessment (MOCA) for general screening because it covers a broad array of cognitive functions (e.g., attention, concentration, executive functions, memory, language, visuospatial skills, abstraction, calculation, orientation)
- Mini-Mental State Examination when evaluating patients for Alzheimer disease because it focuses on testing memory

Baseline results are recorded, and the examination is repeated yearly and whenever a change in mental status is suspected.
Patients should be told that recording of mental status is routine and that they should not be embarrassed by its being done.
The examination is done in a quiet room, and the examiner should make sure that patients can hear the questions clearly. Patients who do not speak English as their primary language should be questioned in the language they speak fluently.
Mental status examination evaluates different areas of cognitive function. The examiner must first establish that patients are attentive—e.g., by assessing their level of attention while the history is taken or by asking them to immediately repeat 3 words. Testing an inattentive patient further is not useful.
The parameters of cognitive function to be tested and examples of how to test them include the following:

Orientation	Test 3 parameters of orientation: • Person (What is your name?) • Time (What is today's date?) • Place (What is the name of this place?)
Short-term memory	Ask the patient to recall 3 objects after about 2 to 5 minutes
Long-term memory	Ask the patient a question about the past, such as "What was the color of the suit you wore at your wedding?" or "What was the make of your first car?"
Math	Use any simple mathematical test. Serial 7s are common: The patient is asked to start with 100 and to subtract 7, then 7 from 93, etc. Alternatively, ask how many nickels are in $1.35.
Word finding	Ask the patient to name as many objects in a single category, such as articles of clothing or animals, as possible in 1 minute.
Attention and concentration	Ask the patient to spell a 5-letter word forward and backward. "World" is commonly used.
Naming objects	Present an object, such as a pen, book, or ruler, and ask the patient to name the object and a part of it.
Following commands	Start with a 1-step command, such as "Touch your nose with your right hand." Then test a 3-step command, such as "Take this piece of paper in your right hand. Fold it in half. Put the paper on the floor."
Writing	Ask the patient to write a sentence. The sentence should contain a subject and an object and should make sense. Spelling errors should be ignored.
Spatial orientation	Ask the patient to draw a house or a clock and mark the clock with a specific time. Or ask the patient to draw 2 intersecting pentagons.
Abstract reasoning	Ask the patient to identify a unifying theme between 3 or 4 objects (e.g., all are fruit, all are vehicles of transportation, all are musical instruments). Ask the patient to interpret a moderately challenging proverb, such as "People who live in glass houses should not throw stones."
Judgment	Ask the patient about a hypothetical situation requiring good judgment, such as "What would you do if you found a stamped letter on the sidewalk?" Placing it in the mailbox is the correct answer; opening the letter suggests a personality disorder.

From the MSD Manual Professional Version, edited by Sandy Falk. Copyright © 2024 Merck & Co., Inc., Rahway, NJ, USA and its affiliates. All rights reserved. Available at https://www.msdmanuals.com/professional. Accessed May 2024.

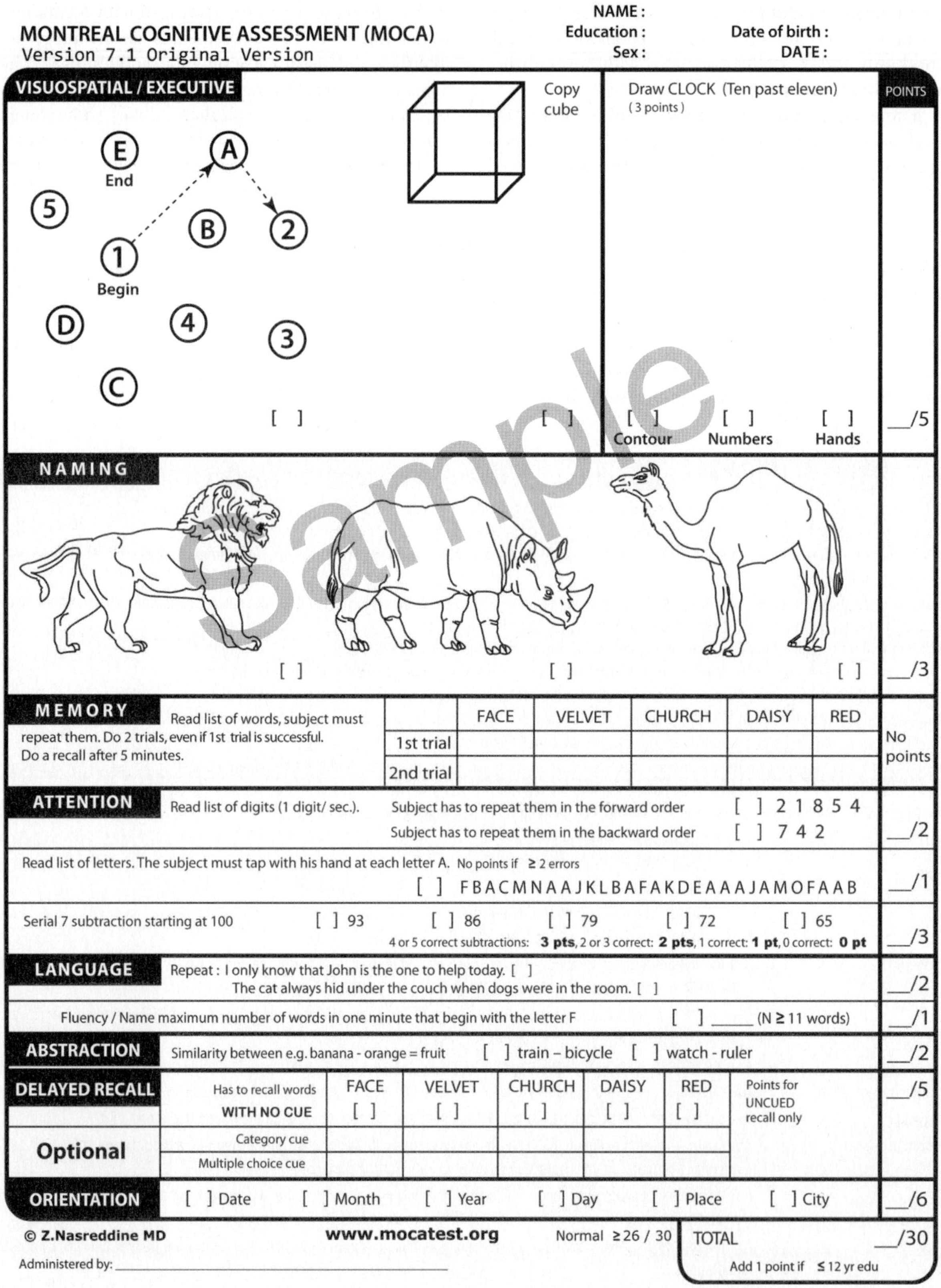

MONTREAL COGNITIVE ASSESSMENT (MOCA)
Version 7.1 Original Version

NAME :
Education : Date of birth :
Sex : DATE :

VISUOSPATIAL / EXECUTIVE		POINTS
(E) End, (A), (5), (B), (2), (1) Begin, (D), (4), (3), (C) [ ]	Copy cube [ ]	
Draw CLOCK (Ten past eleven) (3 points)	[ ] Contour [ ] Numbers [ ] Hands	__/5

NAMING [ ] [ ] [ ] __/3

MEMORY		FACE	VELVET	CHURCH	DAISY	RED	
Read list of words, subject must repeat them. Do 2 trials, even if 1st trial is successful. Do a recall after 5 minutes.	1st trial						No points
	2nd trial						

ATTENTION Read list of digits (1 digit/ sec.). Subject has to repeat them in the forward order [ ] 2 1 8 5 4
Subject has to repeat them in the backward order [ ] 7 4 2 __/2

Read list of letters. The subject must tap with his hand at each letter A. No points if ≥ 2 errors
[ ] FBACMNAAJKLBAFAKDEAAAJAMOFAAB __/1

Serial 7 subtraction starting at 100 [ ] 93 [ ] 86 [ ] 79 [ ] 72 [ ] 65
4 or 5 correct subtractions: **3 pts,** 2 or 3 correct: **2 pts,** 1 correct: **1 pt,** 0 correct: **0 pt** __/3

LANGUAGE Repeat : I only know that John is the one to help today. [ ]
The cat always hid under the couch when dogs were in the room. [ ] __/2

Fluency / Name maximum number of words in one minute that begin with the letter F [ ] ____ (N ≥ 11 words) __/1

ABSTRACTION Similarity between e.g. banana - orange = fruit [ ] train – bicycle [ ] watch - ruler __/2

DELAYED RECALL	Has to recall words WITH NO CUE	FACE [ ]	VELVET [ ]	CHURCH [ ]	DAISY [ ]	RED [ ]	Points for UNCUED recall only	__/5
Optional	Category cue							
	Multiple choice cue							

ORIENTATION [ ] Date [ ] Month [ ] Year [ ] Day [ ] Place [ ] City __/6

© Z.Nasreddine MD www.mocatest.org Normal ≥26 / 30 TOTAL __/30
Add 1 point if ≤ 12 yr edu

Administered by: ____________________

Fig. 3.2 Montreal Cognitive Assessment. (Copyright © Z. Nasreddine, MD. Reproduced with permission. It is mandatory to follow the online MoCA© Training and Certification Program to administer and score the MoCA©. Copies are available at www.mocacognition.com.)

dementia. It assesses attention, concentration, executive functions, memory, language, visuoconstructional skills, conceptual thinking, calculations, and orientation. The tool has extensive testing in multiple languages in older adults over 85 years of age, covering a wide range of disorders affecting cognition. The total possible score is 30 points, with a score of 26 or higher considered normal. To compensate for a limited educational background, older adults with only 4 to 9 years of education should have 2 points added to the total score; for those with only 10 to 12 years of education, 1 point should be added to the total score. A modified version of the tool is available for use in older adults with visual impairment (MoCA Cognition, n.d.).

The Mini-Cog is an instrument that combines a simple memory test with a clock drawing test. It was created by researchers at the University of Washington led by Soo Borson (Borson et al. 2003). The Mini-Cog is quick and easy to use and is as effective as longer, more time-consuming instruments in accurately identifying cognitive impairment (Doerflinger, 2019). It is relatively uninfluenced by education level or language.

Affective status measurement tools are used to differentiate serious depression that affects many domains of function from the low mood common to many people. Depression is common in older adults and is often associated with confusion and disorientation, so older people with depression are often mistakenly labeled as having dementia. It is important to note here that depressed people usually respond to items on mental status examinations by saying, "I don't know," which leads to poor performance. Because mental status examinations are not able to distinguish between dementia and depression, a response of "I don't know" should be interpreted as a sign that further affective assessment is warranted (Mukku et al, 2021).

The Geriatric Depression Scale: Short-Form (GDS; Fig. 3.3), a valid and reliable tool, is derived from the original 30-question scale. It is a convenient instrument explicitly designed for use with older people to screen for depression. Of the 15 items on the short-form GDS, 10 indicates depression when answered positively; the remaining 5 (questions 1, 5, 7, 11, and 13) indicate depression when answered negatively. A score of 0 to 4 is considered normal; a score ≥ 5 indicates depression (Greenberg, 2023).

The instruments described here for assessing cognitive and affective status are valuable screening tools that the nurse may use to supplement other assessments and monitor a patient's condition over time. The results of any mental or affective status

---

Geriatric Depression Scale: Short Form

Choose the best answer for how you have felt over the past week:

1. Are you basically satisfied with your life? YES / **NO**

2. Have you dropped many of your activities and interests? **YES** / NO

3. Do you feel that your life is empty? **YES** / NO

4. Do you often get bored? **YES** / NO

5. Are you in good spirits most of the time? YES / **NO**

6. Are you afraid that something bad is going to happen to you? **YES** / NO

7. Do you feel happy most of the time? YES / **NO**

8. Do you often feel helpless? **YES** / NO

9. Do you prefer to stay at home, rather than going out and doing new things? **YES** / NO

10. Do you feel you have more problems with memory than most? **YES** / NO

11. Do you think it is wonderful to be alive now? YES / **NO**

12. Do you feel pretty worthless the way you are now? **YES** / NO

13. Do you feel full of energy? YES / **NO**

14. Do you feel that your situation is hopeless? **YES** / NO

15. Do you think that most people are better off than you are? **YES** / NO

Answers in **bold** indicate depression. Score 1 point for each bolded answer.

A score >5 points is suggestive of depression.
A score ≥10 points is almost always indicative of depression.
A score >5 points should warrant a follow-up comprehensive assessment.

Fig. 3.3 Geriatric Depression Scale: Short Form. (Adapted from Aging Clinical Research Center. [n.d.] *Geriatric depression scale*. Retrieved from https://web.stanford.edu/~yesavage/GDS.html.)

examination should never be accepted as conclusive; they are subject to change based on further workup or after treatment interventions have been implemented.

Social Assessment

First, social function is correlated with physical and mental function. Alterations in activity patterns may negatively affect physical and mental health and vice versa. Second, an individual's social well-being may positively affect their ability to cope with physical impairments and remain independent (Ward and Reuben, 2023). Third, a satisfactory level of social function is a significant outcome in and of itself. The QoL an older person experiences is closely linked to social function dimensions such as self-esteem, life satisfaction, socioeconomic status, and physical health and functional status.

The relationship the older adult has with family plays a central role in the overall level of health and well-being. Assessing this aspect of the patient's social system may yield vital information about an important part of the total support network. Contrary to popular belief, families provide substantial help to their older members. Consequently, the level of family involvement and support cannot be disregarded when collecting data.

Support for people outside the family plays an increasingly significant role in the lives of many older persons today. Faith-based community support, especially in the form of the parish nurse program, is evolving as a meaningful source of help for older persons who have no family or who have family in distant geographic locations. The nurse must regard these "nontraditional" sources of social support as legitimate when assessing the older adult's social system.

One of the components of the Older Adults Resources and Services (OARS) Multidimensional Functional Assessment Questionnaire (OMFAQ), developed at Duke University, is the Social Resource Scale (Fig. 3.4). The questions extract data about family structure, patterns of friendship and visiting, availability of a confidant, satisfaction with the degree of social interaction, and availability of a helper in the event of illness or disability. Different questions (noted in italics in Fig. 3.4) are used for patients residing in institutions. The interviewer rates the patient using a 6-point scale ranging from "excellent social resources" to "totally socially impaired" based on the responses to the questions (Duke University Center for the Study of Aging and Human Development OARS Program, 1975).

For all the additional assessment measures discussed previously, the nurse should remember that they are meant to augment the traditional health assessment, not replace it. Care needs to be taken to ensure the tools are used appropriately regarding purpose, setting, timing, and safety. Doing so leads to a more accurate appraisal on which to base nursing diagnostic statements and to plan suitable and effective interventions.

LABORATORY DATA

The last component of a comprehensive assessment is the evaluation of laboratory tests. The results of laboratory tests validate history and physical examination findings and identify potential health problems not pointed out by the patient or the nurse. Data are considered in relation to established norms based on age and gender.

SUMMARY

This chapter presented the components of a comprehensive nursing-focused assessment for an older adult, including special considerations to ensure an age-specific approach and pragmatic modifications for conducting the assessment with this unique age group. Components of the health history and physical assessment were discussed, and consideration was given to additional functional status assessment measures that can be used with older adults. Compiling an accurate and thorough assessment of an older adult patient, which serves as the foundation for the remaining steps of the nursing process, involves blending many skills and is an art not easily mastered.

KEY POINTS

- The less vigorous response to illness and disease in older adults because of the diminished physiologic reserve, coupled with the diminished stress response, causes an atypical presentation of and response to illness and disease.
- Cognitive change is one of the most common manifestations of illness in old age.
- Delirium in older adults requires a complete workup to identify the cause so that appropriate interventions can be developed to reverse it.
- Conducting a health assessment with an older adult requires modifying the environment, considering the patient's energy level and adaptability, and observing the opportunity for demonstrating assets and capabilities.
- Sensory-perceptual deficits, anxiety, reduced energy level, pain, multiple and interrelated health problems, and the tendency to reminisce are the major factors requiring special consideration by the nurse while conducting the health history with the older adult.
- An older adult's physical health alone does not provide a reliable measure of functional ability; physical, cognitive, affective, and social assessment provides a comprehensive view of the older adult's total degree of function.
- The purpose of a nursing-focused assessment of the older adult is to identify patient strengths and limitations so that effective and appropriate interventions can be delivered to promote optimum function and prevent disability and dependence.

Now I'd like to ask you some questions about your family and friends.

Are you single, married, widowed, divorced, or separated?

1 Single   3 Widowed   5 Separated

2 Married   4 Divorced   ____ Not answered

If "2" ask following:

Does your spouse live here also?*

1 yes   0 no

____ Not answered

Who lives with you?

(Check "Yes" or "No" for each of the following.)

Yes	No	
___	___	No one
___	___	Husband or wife
___	___	Children
___	___	Grandchildren
___	___	Parents
___	___	Grandparents
___	___	Brothers and sisters
___	___	Other relatives (does not include in-laws covered in the above categories)
___	___	Friends
___	___	Nonrelated paid help (includes free room)
___	___	Others (specify) _____

In the past year about how often did you leave here to visit your family and/or friends for weekends or holidays or to go on shopping trips or outings?*

  1 Once a week or more
  2 One to three times a month
  3 Less than once a month or only on holidays
  4 Never
  ____ Not answered

How many people do you know well enough to visit with in their homes?

  3 Five or more
  2 Three to four
  1 One to two
  0 None
  ____ Not answered

About how many times did you talk to someone—friends, relatives, or others—on the telephone in the past week (either you called them or they called you)? (If subject has no phone, question still applies.)

  3 Once a day or more
  2 Twice
  1 Once
  0 Not at all
  ____ Not answered

How many times during the past week did you spend some time with someone who does not live with you, that is, you went to see them, or they came to visit you, or you went out to do things together?

  3 Once a day or more
  2 Two to six
  1 Once
  0 Not at all
  ____ Not answered

How many times in the past week did you visit with someone, either with people who live here or people who visited you here?*

  3 Once a day or more
  2 Two to six
  1 Once
  0 Not at all
  ____ Not answered

Do you have someone you can trust and confide in?

  1 Yes
  0 No
  ____ Not answered

Do you find yourself feeling lonely quite often, sometimes, or almost never?

  0 Quite often
  1 Sometimes
  2 Almost never
  ____ Not answered

Do you see your relatives and friends as often as you want to, or not?

  1 As often as wants to
  0 Not as often as wants to
  ____ Not answered

Is there someone (outside this place) who would give you any help at all if you were sick or disabled (e.g., your husband/wife, a member of your family, or a friend)?

  1 Yes
  0 No one willing and able to help
  ____ Not answered

If "yes," ask A and B.

A. Is there someone (outside this place) who would take care of you as long as needed, or only for a short time, or only someone who would help you now and then (e.g., taking you to the doctor, or fixing lunch occasionally)?

  3 Someone who would take care of subject indefinitely (as long as needed)
  2 Someone who would take care of subject for a short time (a few weeks to six months)
  1 Someone who would help subject now and then (taking him to the doctor or fixing lunch, etc.)
  ____ Not answered

B. Who is this person?

Name _____

Relationship _____

RATING SCALE

Rate the current social resources of the person being evaluated along the 6-point scale presented below. Circle the one number

Fig. 3.4 OARS Social Resources Scale, modified for community and institutional use. *Indicates questions that are intended for residents of institutions. (Reprinted from the OARS Multidimensional Functional Assessment Questionnaire. [1988]. With permission of the Center for the Study of Aging and Human Development, Duke University Medical Center, Durham, NC.)

that best describes the person's present circumstances.
1. *Excellent Social Resources:* Social relationships are very satisfying and extensive; at least one person would take care of him (her) indefinitely.
2. *Good Social Resources:* Social relationships are fairly satisfying and adequate and at least one person would take care of him (her) indefinitely, or social relationships are very satisfying and extensive, and only short-term help is available.
3. *Mildly Socially Impaired:* Social relationships are unsatisfactory, of poor quality, few; but at least one person would take care of him (her) indefinitely, or social relationships are fairly satisfactory and adequate, and only short-term help is available.
4. *Moderately Socially Impaired:* Social relationships are unsatisfactory, of poor quality, few; and only short-term care is available, or social relationships are at least adequate or satisfactory, but help would only be available now and then.
5. *Severely Socially Impaired:* Social relationships are unsatisfactory, of poor quality, few; and help would be available only now and then, or social relationships are at least satisfactory or adequate, but help is not available even now and then.
6. *Totally Socially Impaired:* Social relationships are unsatisfactory, of poor quality, few; and help is not available even now and then.

Fig. 3.4.—cont'd

- An older adult's reduced ability to respond to stress and the physical changes associated with normal aging combine to place the older adult at high risk for losing functional ability.
- A comprehensive assessment of an older adult's report of nonspecific signs and symptoms is essential for determining underlying conditions that may lead to a functional decline.
- To compensate for the lack of definitive standards for what constitutes "normal" in older adults, the nurse may compare the older patient's own previous patterns of physical and psychosocial health and function with the patient's status.

CLINICAL JUDGMENT EXERCISES

1. You are interviewing an older adult just admitted to the hospital. They state that they are hard of hearing; you note that the patient is restless and apprehensive. How would you revise your history-taking interview based on these initial observations?

2. Three (3) individuals, 65, 81, and 95 years of age, have blood pressure readings of 152/88, 168/90, and 170/92 mm Hg, respectively. The nurse infers that all older people are hypertensive. Analyze the nurse's conclusion. Is faulty logic being used in this situation? What assumption(s) did the nurse make regarding older people in general?

REFERENCES

American Geriatrics Society (AGS) Ethnogeriatrics Committee. (2016). Achieving high-quality multicultural geriatric care. *Journal of the American Geriatrics Society, 64*(2), 255–260. doi:10.1111/jgs.13924.

American Nurses Association (ANA). (2015). *Nursing: Scope and standards of practice* (3rd ed.). Silver Spring, MD: ANA.

Borson, S., Scanlan, J. M., Chen, P., & Ganguli, M. (2003). The Mini-Cog as a screen for dementia: Validation in a population-based sample. *Journal of the American Geriatrics Society, 51*(10), 1451–1454.

Centers for Disease Control and Prevention (CDC). (2023). *Respiratory syncytial virus (RSV) vaccine VIS.* U.S. Department of Health and Human Services. Retrieved from https://www.cdc.gov/vaccines/hcp/vis/vis-statements/rsv.html. Accessed November 9, 2023.

Centers for Disease Control and Prevention (CDC). (2022). *Diphtheria, tetanus, and whooping cough vaccination.* U.S. Department of Health and Human Services. Retrieved from https://www.cdc.gov/vaccines/vpd/dtap-tdap-td/public/index.html. Accessed November 9, 2023.

Doerflinger, D. M. C. (2019). *Mental status assessment of older adults: The Mini-Cog™.* Try This Series, Issue No. 3. The Hartford Institute for Geriatric Nursing, New York University, Rory Meyers College of Nursing. Retrieved from https://hign.org/sites/default/files/2020-06/Try_This_General_Assessment_3.pdf. Accessed November 9, 2023.

Duke University Center for the Study of aging and human development Older Adults Resources & Services (OARS) program. (1975). Retrieve from https://osf.io/94qv5/.

Factora, R. (2023). Optimizing functional status in the elderly. *BMJ Best Practice.* Retrieved from https://bestpractice.bmj.com/topics/en-us/887. Accessed November 9, 2023.

Fulmer, T. (2019). *Fulmer SPICES: An overall assessment tool for older adults.* Try This Series, Issue No. 1. The Hartford Institute for Geriatric Nursing, New York University, Rory Meyers College of Nursing. Retrieved from https://hign.org/sites/default/files/2020-06/Try_This_General_Assessment_1.pdf. Accessed November 9, 2023.

Greenberg, S. A. (2023). *The Geriatric Depression Scale (GDS).* Try This Series. Issue No. 4. The Hartford Institute for Geriatric Nursing,

New York University, Rory Meyers College of Nursing. Retrieved from https://hign.org/sites/default/files/2022-11/GDS%20General%20Assessment.pdf. Accessed November 9, 2023.

Jung, Y. J., Yoon J. L., Kim, H. S., Lee, A. Y., Kim, J. Y., & Cho, J. J. (2017). Atypical clinical presentation of geriatric syndrome in elderly patients with pneumonia or coronary artery disease. *Annals of Geriatric Medicine and Research*, *21*(4), 158–163. doi:10.4235/agmr.2017.21.4.158.

McCabe, D. (2019). *Katz Index of Independence in Activities of Daily Living (ADL)*. Try This Series, Issue No. 2. The Hartford Institute for Geriatric Nursing, New York University, Rory Meyers College of Nursing. Retrieved from https://hign.org/sites/default/files/2020-06/Try_This_General_Assessment_2.pdf. Accessed November 9, 2023.

MoCA Cognition. (n.d.). *Montreal cognitive assessment (MoCA) full*. Retrieved from https://mocacognition.com/paper/. Accessed November 9, 2023.

Mukku, S. S. R., Dahale, A. B., Muniswamy, N. R., Muliyala, K. P., Sivakumar, P. T., & Varghese, M. (2021). Geriatric depression and cognitive impairment—An update. *Indian Journal of Psychological Medicine*, *43*(4), 286–293. doi:10.1177/0253717620981556.

Palleschi, L., Galdi, F., & Pedone, C. (2018). Acute medical illness and disability in the elderly. *Geriatric Care*, *4*(3). doi:10.4081/gc.2018.7561.

Palmer, R. M. (2018). The Acute Care for Elders Unit model of care. *Geriatrics*, *3*(3), 59. doi:10.3390/geriatrics3030059.

Rose, D., Richter, L. T., & Kapustin, J. (2014). Patient experiences with electronic medical records: Lessons learned. *Journal of the American Association of Nurse Practitioners*, *26*(12), 674–680. doi:10.1002/2327-6924.12170.

UpToDate. (2018). *DSM-IV and DSM-5 criteria for dementia*. Wolters Kluwer. Retrieved from https://doctorabad.com/UpToDate/d/image.htm?imageKey=NEURO/91276. Accessed November 22, 2023.

Ward, K. T., & Reuben, D. B. (2023). Comprehensive geriatric assessment. In K. E. Schmader & J. Givens (Eds.), *UpToDate*. Waltham, MA: UpToDate, Inc. Retrieved from https://www.uptodate.com/contents/comprehensive-geriatric-assessment. Accessed November 9, 2023.

WEBSITES

Try This:® Series, a clinical website of The Hartford Institute for Geriatric Nursing. https://hign.org/consultgeri-resources/try-this-series.

Montreal Cognitive Assessment (MoCA). http://www.mocatest.org/splash/.

The Registered Nurses' Association of Ontario (RNAO). http://rnao.ca/.

PART II

Influences on Health and Illness

4

Family Influences

Jennifer J. Yeager, PhD, MSN, RN

http://evolve.elsevier.com/Yeager/gerontologic/

LEARNING OBJECTIVES

On completion of this chapter, the reader will be able to:
1. Gain an understanding of the role of families in the lives of older adults.
2. Identify demographic and social trends that affect families of older adults.
3. Understand the common dilemmas and decisions older adults and their families face.
4. Develop collaborative plans of care to solve aging-related concerns.
5. Identify common stresses that family caregivers experience.
6. Identify interventions to support families.
7. Plan strategies for working more effectively one-on-one with families of older adult patients.

WHAT WOULD YOU DO?

What would you do if you were faced with the following situations?
- Following 45 years of marriage, your partner has a severe stroke and cannot communicate. They managed the family finances and made all the family decisions. You do not know anything about your financial affairs. What would you do?
- Your parents, in their late 70s, are mentally competent, but their physical condition means they cannot manage alone in their home. They require all kinds of help and reject any other living situation or paying outsiders for services. What do you do?
- Your parent is dying. You promised that no heroic measures would be taken to prolong their life; they did not want to die "with tubes hooked up to my body." Your sibling demands the physician use all possible measures to keep your parent alive. What do you do?
- Your parent's reactions and eyesight are poor. You do not want your children with them when they are driving. Your parent always takes the grandchildren to get ice cream and will be hurt if you say the children cannot ride with them. How do you approach this situation?

ROLE AND FUNCTION OF FAMILIES

Each year, millions of older adults receive long-term services and supports (LTSS) from unpaid caregivers. Most often, these services include assistance with daily functioning and personal activities, which are provided by family members and friends, and enable older adults to age in place instead of moving to long-term care (Favreault et al., 2023). Demographic and social trends affect families' abilities to provide support as follows:

- **The aging population.** The number of older adults has increased by 15.2 million since 2010, compared to a 2% increase in those under 65. The older adult population is expected to be 22% of the population by 2040 (Administration for Community Living [ACL], 2022a). "The older population itself became increasingly older. In 2020, the 65–74 age group (32.5 million) was more than 14 times larger than in 1900 (2.2 million); the 75–84 group (16.5 million) was 21 times larger (771,369), and the 85+ group (6.7 million) was more than 54 times larger (122,362)" (ACL, 2022a, p. 4).
- **Living arrangements.** Sixty percent of community-dwelling older adults lived with a spouse or partner in 2021, while 27% lived alone. Females (33%) are more likely than males (21%) to live alone (ACL, 2022a). Roughly 6% of older adults have never married or had any children (Spillman et al., 2020).
- **Functioning.** "In 2020, 18% of adults age 65 and older reported they could not function at all or had a lot of difficulty with at least one of six functioning domains. Specifically, 21% had trouble seeing (even if wearing glasses), 29% had difficulty hearing (even if wearing hearing aids), 39% had trouble with mobility (walking or climbing stairs), 8% had difficulty with communication (understanding or being understood by others), 28% had trouble with cognition (remembering or concentrating), and 8% had difficulty with self-care (such as washing all over or dressing)" (ACL, 2022a, pp. 18–19).

Previous author: Elizabeth C. Mueth, MLS, AHIP

- **Employment.** In 2021, nearly 20% of older adults were either working or actively seeking employment (ACL, 2022a).
- **Family caregivers.** Nearly 66% of caregivers are under the age of 45, caring for their baby boomer parents experiencing chronic disease and disability (Lee, 2023). Family caregivers between 55 and 64 years old account for 24% of nonpaid caregivers, followed by those aged 45 to 54 (21%), and those aged 65 and older (18%). Fifteen percent of caregivers cared for someone they lived with; 83% cared for someone they did not live with. Of those living with the person they cared for, 35% also had children in the home under the age of six, and 65% had children in the home between 6 and 17 years old. On average, family caregivers spend 3 hours a day providing care (ACL, 2022b). Over half of caregivers report increased stress due to caregiving, and caregivers under the age of 35 experience high levels of anxiety. Nearly 40% of caregivers state they never feel relaxed (Horovitz, 2023). They also experience financial strain, a lack of "reciprocated support," and fatigue from the multiple demands placed on them (Lee, 2023).

Planning in Advance of Need

Making plans to age in place should begin before the need for assistance arises. Personal preferences concerning the support services required for the older adult to stay at home and remain as independent as possible should be discussed with family and planned in advance. These services include personal care, household chores, meals, financial management, healthcare (i.e., drug administration and wound care), transportation, and home safety (National Institute on Aging [NIA], 2023a).

Planning requires anticipating all situations—dependency, disability, incapacity, and death—and exploring actions to be taken. Discussing these subjects may be uncomfortable for family members. For some people, talking about their potential incapacity and inability to manage finances is more difficult than talking about death.

Waiting to make plans until a family member shows signs of a degenerative disease such as Alzheimer reduces the options. Although prior planning does not prevent all complications, it does prepare families to act more effectively should a crisis occur. Planning may also:
- Prevent decision-making during a crisis
- Reduce emotional and financial upheaval
- Ensure that the older person's lifestyle, personal philosophies, and choices are known in advance
- Decrease the possibility that the family will have to take more intrusive, restrictive actions, such as petitioning the court for guardianship or conservatorship if their older family member becomes incapacitated
- Reduce disagreements and misunderstandings among family members

Prior planning should begin with a family meeting to discuss current and future needs. It should allow everyone to have a voice, give space for varied perspectives and feelings, and formulate a plan where all family members work together to care for the older adult family member. Vock (n.d.) provides the following guiding principles:
- Inclusivity: everyone has the opportunity to have a voice.
- Respect for each family member's feelings, opinions, and perspectives. How is respect conveyed?
- All feelings and perspectives are acknowledged.
- No one is made wrong.
- Use "I" statements rather than "you" statements in order to speak from your own experience and preferences.
- The goal from which everything else needs to pivot is providing the best care possible for the older adult.

COMMON LATE-LIFE FAMILY ISSUES AND DECISIONS

When changes occur in an older adult's functioning, family members are often involved in making decisions about the person's living situation and arranging for social services, healthcare, and caregiving. Some of the most common issues and difficult decisions families face include issues with driving, financial and legal concerns, end-of-life healthcare decisions, family caregiving issues, including educational needs and managing resistance to care, and nursing facility placement.

The Issue of Driving

In 2020, there were 48 million licensed drivers over 65. Driving helps to maintain freedom, independence, and social interaction. However, each day, 20 older adults are killed, and almost 540 are injured in motor vehicle accidents; death rates among older drivers are higher than those of middle-aged drivers, most likely due to increased vulnerability to injury. Often, older adults limit driving at night, avoid challenging situations, and reduce the hours they drive in advance of need. Age-related changes in vision, hearing, and physical functioning; the ability to reason and remember; and chronic disease and medical treatments impact older adults' driving ability (Centers for Disease Control and Prevention, 2022).

Visual changes include difficulty seeing at night. Glaucoma, cataracts, and macular degeneration can result in altered visual fields, making seeing cars and other objects difficult. Changes in hearing may make it harder to notice horns, sirens, and other noises that warn a driver to move out of the way or pull over. Physical changes that affect driving include joint stiffness due to arthritis. Arthritic changes may limit range of motion and make the movements required to steer, press the brake pedal, or turn the head painful. Slower reaction times and reflexes make it difficult to react quickly; loss of feeling or altered sensation, like that caused by diabetic neuropathy, may make it difficult to use the brakes. Chronic diseases such as Parkinson's may make driving unsafe due to uncontrollable movements and loss of coordination and balance; a stroke may slow reaction time, cause muscle weakness, and reduce coordination, making driving unsafe (Barco and Carr, 2022; NIA, 2022a).

Older adults should talk to their healthcare providers about any health concerns that may impact safety while driving. Additionally, older adults must remain active to improve

BOX 4.1 Key Steps to Staying Safe on the Roads

- Always wear a seat belt as a driver or passenger.
- Drive when conditions are the safest.
- Do not drink and drive.
- Follow a regular activity program to increase strength and flexibility.
- Ask your doctor or pharmacist to review prescription and over-the-counter medicines to reduce side effects and interactions.
- Have your eyes checked by an eye doctor at least once a year. Wear glasses and corrective lenses as required.
- Plan your route before you drive.
- Find the safest route with well-lit streets, intersections with left-turn signals, and easy parking.
- Leave a large following distance between your car and the car in front of you.
- Avoid distractions in your car, such as listening to a loud radio, talking or texting on your phone, and eating.
- Consider potential alternatives to driving, such as riding with a friend, using ride sharing services, or taking public transit.

Modified from the Centers for Disease Control and Prevention. (2022). *Older adult drivers.* Retrieved from https://www.cdc.gov/older-adult-drivers/about/?CDC_AAref_Val=https://www.cdc.gov/transportationsafety/older_adult_drivers/index.html

strength and flexibility and maintain annual auditory and ophthalmic evaluations to ensure conditions affecting driving are found early (NIA, 2022a; see Box 4.1 for further safety tips).

Families face a difficult time when an older family member shows signs of unsafe driving, including frequent close calls, increased citations, problems with memory, and changes in the way they drive, such as drifting into other lanes and braking or accelerating suddenly without reason. Family members may be both worried about safety and reluctant to raise concerns or take action with their older adult family members. The issue is even more complicated when the older adult is cognitively impaired and does not perceive their deterioration and potential driving risk.

The following tips are provided for talking to a family about driving (Segal et al., 2023):

- Be respectful. Driving is often an integral part of independence. At the same time, do not be intimidated or back down if you have a true concern.
- Give specific examples. Instead of generalizations like "You can't drive safely anymore," outline specific concerns you have noticed. For example: "You have a harder time turning your head than you used to," or "You braked suddenly at stop signs three times the last time we drove."
- Find strength in numbers. If more than one family member or close friend has noticed, it is less likely to be taken as nagging. A loved one may also listen to a more impartial party, such as a doctor or driving specialist.
- Help find alternatives. People may be so used to driving that they have never considered alternatives. You can offer concrete help by researching transportation options or offering rides when possible.
- Understand the difficulty of the transition. Your loved one may experience a profound sense of loss after giving up the keys, and not being able to drive can lead to isolation and depression. Try to help with the transition as much as possible. If it is safe, try slowly transitioning the senior out of driving to give them time to adjust. For example, your loved one may begin the transition by no longer driving at night or on the freeways, or by using a shuttle service to specific appointments, such as the doctor's.

Financial and Legal Concerns

Major financial issues families face include paying for long-term care, helping an older adult who has problems managing money, knowing about and accessing resources for the older adult family member whose income is insufficient, and planning for and talking about potential incapacity.

One of the most important things a nurse can do is become knowledgeable about the community resources that can help families faced with financial and legal concerns, eligibility requirements for programs, program access issues, and options for older persons who need assistance in managing their finances. If a family and their older relative have not already discussed potential financial concerns, encourage them to do so.

Many families do not discuss finances before a crisis, and then it is often too late. Sometimes adult children hesitate to discuss financial concerns for fear of appearing overly interested in their inheritance. Children should convey that they do not want to know how much their parents have—or might leave in their will; rather, they want to ensure that a current and complete plan exists. When a person has been diagnosed with Alzheimer disease or a related disorder, the family must make financial and legal plans while the older adult can participate. At this point, it would also be appropriate to execute a general durable power of attorney, which appoints someone to act as an agent for legal and financial purposes when the person can no longer do so (NIA, 2023b). Once the person becomes incapacitated, if plans have not been made, the options are fewer, more complex, and more intrusive. A family may need to seek a conservatorship, which requires court action.

Older persons with limited mobility, diminished vision, or loss of hand dexterity may need only minimum assistance with finances (e.g., help with reading fine print, balancing a checkbook, preparing checks for signature, or dealing with Medicare or other benefit programs). Others who are homebound because of poor health but can still direct their finances may need someone to implement their directives. In such situations, a family's objective should be to assist, not to take away control. The goal is to choose the least intrusive intervention to enable the older person to remain as independent as possible.

End-of-Life Healthcare Decisions

The end of life is different for everyone, often determined by the person's preferences, needs, and choices. The main interests of patients nearing the end of life are physical comfort, mental and emotional needs, spiritual needs, and practical tasks (NIA, 2022b).

"End-of-life care planning refers to an ongoing care planning process for terminal conditions. It includes formal documents and verbal discussions. Advance care planning is 'a process that supports adults at any age or stage of health in understanding and sharing their values, life goals, and preferences regarding future medical care'" (Rahemi et al., 2023, p. 320; Fig. 4.1). Planning for the end of life in advance (e.g., living wills, durable power of attorney for healthcare, and holding informal discussions with family members) can protect older adults from unwanted medical treatments should they become unable to express their preferences (Population Reference Bureau, 2012) (Table 4.1).

Family Caregiving

Family caregiving is primarily provided by the adult children of the older individual. Often, the varying levels of participation among siblings may cause stress within the family. Providing care to frail, dependent older adults is becoming increasingly common because of the rapidly aging population. "In 2019, at least 53 million people were providing informal, usually unpaid, care and support to aging family members and people of all ages with disabilities (including mental health conditions). … When family caregivers do not have training, support, and opportunities for rest and self-care, their own health, well-being, and quality of life suffer" (ACL, 2022b). Although 88% of family caregivers feel the experience is rewarding, many family caregivers experience significant stress and depression. Caregiving syndrome, also referred to as caregiver burnout and stress, is characterized by physical, mental, and emotional exhaustion. Often a result of neglecting oneself, other symptoms of caregiving syndrome include anger, irritability, anxiety, lack of energy, trouble sleeping or sleeping too much, loss of interest

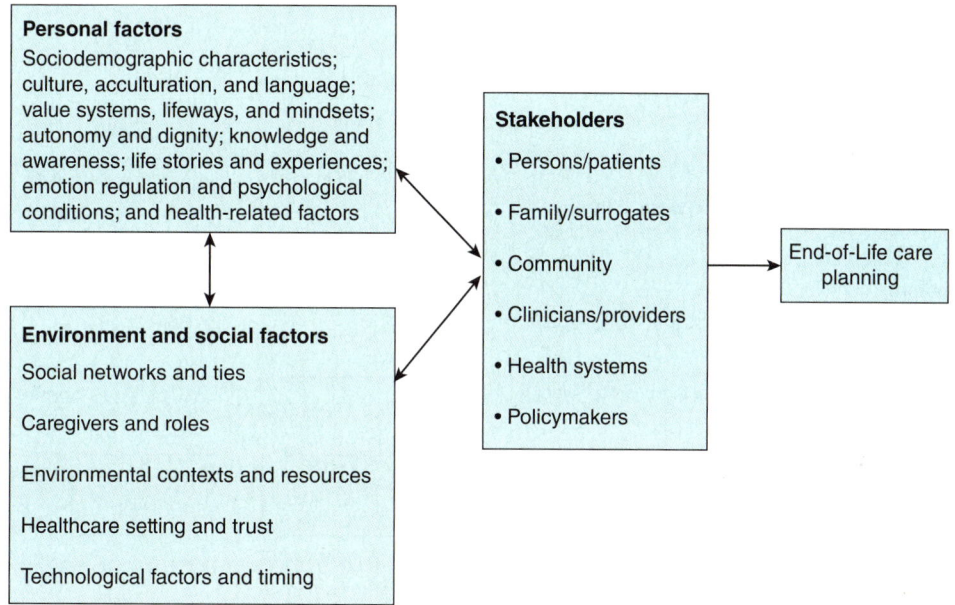

Fig. 4.1 End-of-life care planning model. (From Rahemi, Z., Malatyali, A., Wiese, L. A. K., & Dye, C. J. [2023]. End-of-life care planning in diverse individuals across age groups: A proposed conceptual model of nursing. *Journal of Nursing Care Quality, 38*[4], 319–326.)

TABLE 4.1 Common End-of-Life Documents

Type of Document	Definition	Signature
Do-not-resuscitate (DNR) order	Executed by a competent person, indicating that if heartbeat and breathing cease, no attempts to restore them should be made.	Physician, nurse practitioner, or patient (state law dependent)
Out of hospital DNR or physician orders for life-sustaining treatment (POLST)	This gives the EMS providers permission not to perform CPR. Without an out-of-hospital DNR order or POLST, emergency crews must perform CPR.	Patient signature and signature of physician and two witnesses (state law dependent)
Healthcare proxy or medical power of attorney	Designates a surrogate decisionmaker for healthcare matters that takes effect on one's incompetency. Decisions must be made following the person's relevant instructions or in their best interests.	Patient or witnesses (state law dependent)
Living will	Directs that extraordinary measures not be used to artificially prolong life if recovery cannot reasonably be expected. These measures may be specified.	Patient or witnesses (state law dependent)
Advance health directive	Explains a person's wishes about treatment in the case of incompetency or inability to communicate. Often used in conjunction with a healthcare proxy or power of attorney.	Patient or witnesses (state law dependent)

in previously enjoyed activities, and reduced resistance to illness (Brandon and Williams, 2023).

The Modified Caregiver Strain Index (MCSI) is a 13-item tool that can be used to quickly screen for caregiver stress (Fig. 4.2). In addition to identifying actual stressors—which may or may not be a direct result of caregiving—the nurse must assess their significance to the caregiver. Other useful areas to assess are a caregiver's style of coping, the caregiver's support system, the caregiver's evaluation of the adequacy of their support system, the care needs of the older person, including behavioral and emotional problems, and the caregiver's perception of those care needs; and financial resources.

Modified Caregiver Strain Index

Directions: Here is a list of things that other caregivers have found to be difficult. Please put a checkmark in the columns that apply to you. We have included some examples that are common caregiver experiences to help you think about each item. Your situation may be slightly different, but the item could still apply.

	Yes, On a Regular Basis = 2	Yes, Sometimes = 1	No = 0
My sleep is disturbed (For example: the person I care for is in and out of bed or wanders around at night)	_____	_____	_____
Caregiving is inconvenient (For example: helping takes so much time or it's a long drive over to help)	_____	_____	_____
Caregiving is a physical strain (For example: lifting in or out of a chair; effort or concentration is required)	_____	_____	_____
Caregiving is confining (For example: helping restricts free time or I cannot go visiting)	_____	_____	_____
There have been family adjustments (For example: helping has disrupted my routine; there is no privacy)	_____	_____	_____
There have been changes in personal plans (For example: I had to turn down a job; I could not go on vacation)	_____	_____	_____
There have been other demands on my time (For example: other family members need me)	_____	_____	_____
There have been emotional adjustments (For example: severe arguments about caregiving)	_____	_____	_____
Some behavior is upsetting (For example: incontinence; the person cared for has trouble remembering things; or the person I care for accuses people of taking things)	_____	_____	_____
It is upsetting to find the person I care for has changed so much from his/her former self (For example: he/she is a different person than he/she used to be)	_____	_____	_____
There have been work adjustments (For example: I have to take time off for caregiving duties)	_____	_____	_____
Caregiving is a financial strain	_____	_____	_____
I feel completely overwhelmed (For example: I worry about the person I care for; I have concerns about how I will manage)	_____	_____	_____

(Sum responses for "Yes, on a regular basis" [2 pts each] and "yes, sometimes" [1 pt each])

Total Score =

Fig. 4.2 Modified Caregiver Strain Index. (From Thornton, M., & Travis, S. S. [2003]. Analysis of the reliability of the Modified Caregiver Strain Index. *The Journals of Gerontology, Series B, Psychological Sciences and Social Sciences, 58*[2], S129. Copyright The Gerontological Society of America.)

However, the best thing is to prevent caregiving syndrome in the first place. The following measures may help prevent caregiving syndrome (Brandon and Williams, 2023):
- Do not be afraid to ask for help. Sometimes it may seem easier or quicker to do tasks yourself, but asking family, friends, or others for help is OK.
- Build a support network. Find people you can talk to about your feelings, whatever they may be, or seek professional help if needed. Sometimes, spiritual or inspirational avenues help. In other words, talk to your higher power or creator. You can also consult with other caregivers who understand what you are experiencing and who may offer help.
- Take regular breaks or even a vacation. Getting away for a few days helps clear your head and obtain some much-needed rest.
- Eat healthy meals and exercise to relieve stress.
- Get enough sleep.
- See your doctor regularly. Do not skip appointments, and share what you are experiencing as a caregiver. Doctors can also help make your role as a caregiver easier by ordering special equipment or other services.
- Do not neglect your social life. For example, take time to see a movie, go to a concert, or visit your place of worship.

CAREGIVER EDUCATION

Respite Programs

Respite programs are one of the few services designed specifically to benefit caregivers. The programs allow caregivers to plan time away from their caregiving role. Researchers agree that respite care could potentially improve the well-being of the caregiver and possibly delay the institutionalization of the older person in their care. The two basic premises of respite care are (1) shared responsibility for caregiving and (2) caregiver support (NIA, 2023c).

The nurse can help the caregiver understand that it is normal to need a break and that seeking respite care will not label them as

---

EVIDENCE-BASED PRACTICE

Latino Family Caregivers

Background
Family caregivers of persons with dementia spend an average of $8,978 per year on out-of-pocket expenses. Many expenses, such as home modifications, are not covered by Medicare or other insurance. Additionally, many caregivers experience loss of income due to reduced work hours or leaving the workforce due to caregiving responsibilities. Caregivers, on average, spend 26% of their annual household income on caregiving. However, Latino caregivers spend 47% of their average annual income (about $11,293 per year) on caregiving expenses. The researchers sought to understand why Latino caregivers spend more money proportionate to their income on care-related costs and how these out-of-pocket expenses affect Latino caregivers and their families.

Sample
A purposeful sample of 14 Latino caregivers living in California (n = 7) and Texas (n = 7) was recruited through community organization newsletters, social media, educational events, and email invitations. Eligibility criteria included Latino/Latina/Latinx ethnicity, English- or Spanish-speaking, and currently providing unpaid care to a person living with dementia for at least 4 hours per week. Additionally, they needed to assist with at least one activity of daily living or two instrumental activities of daily living.

Methods
The researchers conducted a one-time, semi-structured, and in-depth qualitative interview with Latino caregivers. The study design was guided by a conceptual model of financial hardship, which comprises material, psychosocial, and behavioral components.

Findings
The average age of the caregivers was 60 years old, with 71% being female. The caregivers were either children, children-in-law, or spouses. Of the participants, only two were employed, with the others being unemployed or retired.
Three themes were revealed:
1. Making ends meet—despite the cumulative costs of day-to-day expenditures, most caregivers expressed reluctance to be reimbursed by the care recipients. Expenses were often incurred to support the older adults' desire to age in place rather than in a nursing home, where these costs would be covered by Medicaid. Caregivers saw these costs as worthwhile and wanted to show respect for their parents. Caregivers often make sacrifices to cover caregiving, including spending their savings and incurring interest on financing the costs of care. Sacrifices also included reduced work hours and deciding to leave the workforce.
2. The psychological impact of caregiving costs—caregivers described the costs of caregiving on their mental and physical health, often due to worrying about finances. Caregivers were also worried about their own financial future and their ability to retire and cover the costs of their own needs and those of their family. Often, caregivers expressed the pressure they felt due to social expectations—females felt obligated to provide direct care. In contrast, males felt worried about being able to pay the rent, provide food and clothes, and pay other expenses.
3. Frustration with accessing resources—caregivers expressed frustration with trying to access community-based support resources, including lengthy administrative processes, and being offered services that did not meet their needs or that they did not qualify for. Additionally, it was noted that when family members do not ask the care recipient for reimbursement, the recipient does not "spend down" their assets and is therefore not eligible for need-based services. Other participants stated they did not know how to access resources. Finally, frustration was voiced that other family members did not help or contribute.

Implications
Latino caregivers would likely benefit from financial support to help manage the material and psychosocial effects of financial hardship, and current policy-level responses may not meet the needs of Latino family caregivers. This study's use of the material-psychosocial-behavioral model offers a helpful framework that can be replicated in future studies. The model offers a promising framework to guide intervention content. Additionally, interventions that help caregivers navigate community and healthcare resources to help displace some out-of-pocket caregiving costs should be developed and implemented.

Data from Mage, S., Benton, D., Gonzales, A., Zaragoza, G., Wilber, K., Tucker-Seeley, R., et al. (2024). "I lay awake at night": Latino family caregivers' experiences covering out-of-pocket costs when caring for someone living with dementia. *The Gerontologist, 64*, 1-11.

a failure. According to the Alzheimer's Association, respite services also benefit the patient. Caregivers need time to spend with family and friends, run errands, get a haircut, or see a doctor while still having the comfort of knowing that their loved one is well cared for. Benefits to the patient may include interactions with others in a similar situation, a safe, supportive environment, and activities that will match their needs and abilities (NIA, 2023c).

Respite services may be provided at home or out-of-home and for a few hours a day, overnight, a weekend, or longer. In-home respite care can include companion sitter programs or the temporary use of homemakers or home health services. Out-of-home respite services include adult day programs or short stays in adult foster care homes, long-term care facilities, or hospitals (NIA, 2023c).

Support Groups

In many communities, caregiver support groups have developed. Some support groups are oriented toward specific diseases such as cancer, Parkinson disease, lung disease, stroke, or Alzheimer disease and related dementia. Others are for family caregivers in general.

A support group may be where caregivers get advice, gain knowledge about their older relatives' medical conditions and problems, share experiences and feelings, develop new coping strategies, and learn about community resources and care alternatives. A support group may help normalize a caregiver's experience. Discovering that they are not alone may provide much-needed emotional relief to some caregivers. For the isolated caregiver, deprived of intimacy and support from the care receiver, a support group may also provide an acceptable outlet for socializing. More information on support groups and finding the right support group is available at https://www.caregiveraction.org/.

ASSESSING THE FAMILY

No easy answers exist when an older person's life situation or physical or mental status changes. What may be the best answer for one older person and their family may be inappropriate for another family whose situation seems the same.

Each older person and family system is different. It may be just as important to understand the family's history, current life circumstances, and needs as it is to know about an older person's needs and level of functioning. For example, a family's willingness to provide care says nothing about their ability to do so. Sometimes, the care an older person needs exceeds what an individual or family can provide, and the caregiver becomes the "hidden patient." As one adult daughter stated, "My father was the person with Alzheimer disease, but his illness also killed my mother." Failing to evaluate the ability of family members to provide caregiving is a disservice to older patients.

Information from a family assessment may result in more effective older adult care planning and decision-making. Another benefit of assessing how well a caregiver is doing is that it validates a person's caregiving efforts and sends a message that the nurse is concerned about the caregiver's well-being and the older adult's health.

Depending on the family, the older adult, and the decisions to be made, the following may be among the important factors to consider in conducting a family assessment:

Past Relationships

Lifetime relationships may influence the family's ability to plan, to make decisions together, and to provide support. Remember, every adult child has a different history with an aging parent, even if they share the same family events. Families with a history of alcoholism, poor relationships, or abusive behavior cannot always be expected to provide the assistance an older person needs.

Consider the degree of emotional intensity—the closeness, affection, and openness—in the relationships among family members. Parental or spousal disability sometimes threatens a person's identity or the level of emotional relationship that has been established. For example, some married couples, parents, and children have been emotionally distant for many years. Some spouses have shared the same household but have lived separate lives. Some adult children have maintained an emotional distance from a parent by living and working at a geographic distance. People in these situations may be reluctant to enter the care system or have more difficulty with caregiving. It may be unrealistic to expect such family members to meet the emotional needs of the older person; they may feel more comfortable meeting a person's instrumental needs, that is, doing tasks.

Family Dynamics

Family dynamics are the ways family members interact with one another, including their communication patterns, family alliances, and symbiotic relationships. What are family members' views about how decisions should be made? How do they view the older adult's role in decisions about their life? To what degree are family members paternalistic, that is, to what degree do they expect the older person to submit to their decisions or a healthcare professional's recommendation?

Roles

It is useful to know whether individual family members have distinctive roles. If so, what role or roles does each person have? What expectations are held by the person fulfilling the role and by other family members? Do any of the roles generate conflict for the people who bear them? For example, family members may have always assumed that if a parent needed care, a particular daughter would provide the care because she is the oldest, lives the closest, is a nurse, or has always taken care of everyone who needed help. The daughter may also have viewed caregiving as her role. However, this "assigned" role may or may not be realistic given the daughter's current life situation or the parent's needs. Sometimes, an older adult or a family member may not make a decision until the "decision-maker" in the family is consulted. The importance of considering who plays which roles is exemplified by this daughter's comments:

> I lived in the same town as my Dad, so when he needed help, I was the one who provided it daily. Dad expected me to help because I was his daughter. But when it came to making decisions, my opinions never counted with him. His son's opinions, however, mattered, and he would listen to them. I think his basic view throughout his life was "women are there to serve men" and "men are, by far, more knowledgeable than women." It didn't matter that I had a college education, and my brother didn't.

Knowing who does what for the older adult makes for more effective planning. Old family roles may also come to the foreground when siblings are brought together to address a parent's care needs. One daughter stated:

I lived in the same community as my parents, so when they became ill, I did everything that needed to be done and arranged for support services. Both of my sisters lived hundreds of miles away. Although I am a competent businesswoman, it seemed that when both of my older sisters came home, I immediately became the "baby of the family" again.

It may be helpful to identify how family roles, especially those of the older adult, are affected by the older adult's increased frailty. What are family members' perceptions regarding the role of the older adult? Do any adult children perceive that their role is now to "parent their parents"?

Sometimes, people talk about "role reversal." Although a family member may take on parent-like responsibilities, in the emotional sense, a parent is still a parent, and a spouse is still a spouse, no matter how dependent a person has become. Decades of adult experiences cannot be repressed. If family members think of an older family member as a child, they are more likely to treat that person as they would treat a child and, in return, get childish behavior.

Consider the older adult's view of their role with respect to the rest of the family. For example, does the older adult believe they are still a contributing family member, or do they feel a loss of role? Does the person think they are entitled to care from family members, for example, "just because I am your parent?" Paulette tells her story:

I could see Dad deteriorating. When Dad could no longer live alone at home, he refused to consider anyone but "his daughter helping him." When the time came that Dad had to move from his home, he said to me adamantly, "Your mother took care of her mother and my father until they died," implying that I also should do the same with him. To Dad, "taking care of" meant he would live in our home. He felt that this is "what daughters are supposed to do."

Dependence and Independence

Some families accept and adjust more easily than other families to the increased dependence of a family member. Answers to the following questions can help determine how well family members are dealing with or will deal with increased frailty in an older family member:

- What are the attitudes and expectations of family members, including the older person, about dependency?
- Has the family experienced a shift in who is dependent? If so, what is the response of individual family members to this shift?
- Are any family members threatened by the increased dependence of the older person?
- Is the older person giving family members mixed messages about how independent or dependent they are?
- Do family members perceive the dependency needs of the person realistically? Is anyone denying, minimizing, or exaggerating the dependence? Is anyone overprotecting or forcing dependency?

Providing caregiving to a family member may be more difficult if the caregiver is the dependent person in the relationship. The care receiver may also resent the caregiver exercising more control.

CHANGES IN LIVING ARRANGEMENTS

Family members are often emotionally torn between allowing someone to be as independent as possible and creating a more secure environment. They may wonder how hard they should push for change, particularly if they believe the person's decisions are not in their best interest. The family may be focused on the advantages of a group living situation (e.g., good nutrition, socialization, and security). However, an older adult may view a move as a loss of independence or control.

The nurse plays an important role in:
- Providing an objective assessment of an older adult's functional ability
- Exploring ways to maintain an older relative in their home and the advantages and disadvantages of other living arrangement options
- Helping families understand the older adult's perspective on the meaning of home and the significance of accepting help or moving to a new environment

Deciding About a Care Facility

Until about 25 years ago, only two options were available to older adults who could no longer live alone: move in with their children or move into a long-term care facility. In the mid-1980s, a new option was born: assisted living. Many older people needed help with things such as housekeeping, meals, laundry, or transportation, but otherwise they could function independently. Baby boomers latched onto this concept, and the industry has grown exponentially. Perhaps the fastest-growing care facility option is the continuing-care retirement community (CCRC), also known as Life Plan Communities (LPCs). Amenities may include chapels/sanctuaries, restaurants, pools, fitness centers, and spas. The attraction of CCRCs is healthcare for life. This type of community typically allows residents to live independently as long as they can and gives them access to increased care (e.g., skilled nursing, assisted living, and memory care), in the same location when they need it. Today, more than 1900 CCRCs exist nationwide. The biggest drawback to CCRCs is their cost. Entrance fees (buy-in fee) range from $100,000 to $1 million, with monthly rent ranging from $3000 to $5000 (Bretschneider, 2023).

Moving an older family member into any care facility is difficult for most families. It is often a decision filled with guilt, sadness, anxiety, doubt, and anger—even when the older person makes the decision. Dealing with the family's feelings about placement is as important as stressing the need for long-term care. Many families view facilities negatively because of what they have seen in the media concerning neglect, abuse, and abandonment. Cultural considerations may also affect feelings about placement.

It may be helpful to talk with family members about the potential benefits of a care facility. For many people, walking into a care facility for the first time is not easy. It is helpful to prepare families about what to expect and to give guidelines for evaluating facilities, moving an older family member into a care facility, and helping an older family member adjust to the changes.

Further information on moving a family member to a care facility can be found on the AgingCare website (https://www.agingcare.com/articles/moving-into-a-nursing-home-a-CHECKLIST-209625.htm). Additionally, invaluable information about individual facilities can be found on the Centers for Medicare and Medicaid Services Nursing Home Care Compare website (https://www.medicare.gov/care-compare/), which provides information on staffing, quality measures, inspections, and penalties.

SUMMARY

Providing high-quality care to older adults requires recognizing the family's role and assessing and responding to the needs of family members, particularly the caregivers. Family members should be considered a part of the care team, not outsiders. The nurse should invite families to share the knowledge they have gained through caregiving, particularly when placing an older adult family member in a care setting.

It is also important to be nonjudgmental and remember that each family has its history and values. Nurses need to be aware of their own values regarding what constitutes a family and their feelings about family behavior and relationships. It is important that nurses not allow personal values to prevent them from working effectively with families whose values or relationships with each other may be different. Nurses should not label such families as "dysfunctional." It is necessary to identify each family's strengths and build on those strengths while recognizing the family's limitations in providing support and caregiving.

KEY POINTS

- Families are significant in the lives of older persons and provide most of the support for older adults.
- Common dilemmas and decisions families face in later life involve changes in living arrangements, nursing facility placement, financial and legal issues, end-of-life medical treatments, the safety of an older family member's driving, and caregiving.
- Moving an older family member to a nursing facility is a difficult decision for most families.
- When working with older adults, it is as important to address the family's needs as to focus on the older person's needs. If only the older person's needs are considered, a care plan is less likely to be successful, particularly if the family is responsible for implementing it.
- Caregiving tends to be more stressful if the care receiver has a degenerative condition, behavioral problem, or emotional disturbance than if the care receiver is only physically disabled.
- The meaning a caregiver ascribes to a stressor is a stronger predictor of its effect than the actual stressor.
- Family caregivers often experience restrictions on personal activities and social life, emotional strain, competing demands, role conflict, and financial stress. They may need to adjust their expectations regarding their ill family member, themselves as caregivers, and their stage of life.
- Respite is most effective when a caregiver use it early to prevent physical and emotional exhaustion rather than later to treat it.
- The family meeting is one strategy for a family to decide how to share caregiving responsibilities and reach a consensus about problems, needs, and decisions.
- Factors to consider in conducting a family assessment include a history of relationships, family dynamics, the effect of increased dependence on an older adult on all family members, the family's ability to provide the needed care, and the nature and degree of caregiver stress.

CLINICAL JUDGMENT EXERCISES

1. Think about your own family relationships. What individual and family values might influence your care of an older adult family member? How might your current perceptions change over the next decade?
2. An older adult is recovering from pneumonia. They have Alzheimer disease and have become increasingly unmanageable in the home setting. The adult child caregiver feels guilty about the idea of placing their parent in a long-term care facility but feels they are not able to care for them. What is the role of the nurse in this situation?

REFERENCES

Administration for Community Living (ACL). (2022a). *2021 Profile of older Americans*. Retrieved from https://acl.gov/aging-and-disability-in-america/data-and-research/profile-older-americans. Accessed February 5, 2024.

Administration for Community Living (ACL). (2022b). *2022 National strategy to support family caregivers*. Retrieved from https://acl.gov/sites/default/files/RAISE_SGRG/NatlStrategyToSupportFamilyCaregivers-2.pdf. Accessed February 5, 2024.

Barco, P. P., & Carr, D. B. (2022). The older driver. In *Merck manual consumer version*. Merck & Co., Inc. Retrieved from https://www.merckmanuals.com/home/older-people%E2%80%99s-health-issues/the-older-driver/the-older-driver. Accessed February 5, 2024.

Brandon, D., & Williams, W. (2023). *The role of a family caregiver*. Extension [website]. Alabama Cooperative Extension System. Retrieved from https://www.aces.edu/blog/topics/home-family-urban/the-role-of-a-family-caregiver/. Accessed February 5, 2024.

Bretschneider, A. (2023). *Continuing care retirement communities: Your 2024 guide*. Seniorly [website]. Retrieved from https://www.seniorly.com/continuing-care-retirement-community. Accessed February 5, 2024.

Centers for Disease Control and Prevention. (2022). *Older adult drivers*. Retrieved from https://www.cdc.gov/transportationsafety/older_adult_drivers/index.html. Accessed February 5, 2024.

Favreault, M. M., Johnson, R., Dey, J., Anderson, L., Lamont, H., & Marton, W. (2023). *The economic value of unpaid care provided to older adults with needs for long-term services and supports (Issue Brief)*. Washington, DC: Office of the Assistant Secretary for Planning and Evaluation, U.S. Department of Health and Human Services. Retrieved from https://aspe.hhs.gov/sites/default/files/documents/03e41402bed72b426b68246b06b2cfe2/economic-value-unpaid-ltss-care.pdf. Accessed February 4, 2024.

Horovitz, B. (2023). *More than 60% say caregiving increased their level of stress and worry, new AARP report finds*. AARP.org [website]. Retrieved from https://www.aarp.org/caregiving/health/info-2023/report-caregiver-mental-health.html. Accessed February 12, 2024.

Lee, J. (2023, March 28). The agony of putting your life on hold to care for your parents. *The New York Times*.

National Institute on Aging (NIA). (2022a). *Safe driving for older adults*. National Institutes of Health. Retrieved from https://www.nia.nih.gov/health/safety/safe-driving-older-adults. Accessed February 5, 2024.

National Institute on Aging (NIA). (2022b). *Providing care and comfort at the end of life*. National Institutes of Health. Retrieved from https://www.nia.nih.gov/health/end-life/providing-care-and-comfort-end-life. Accessed February 5, 2024.

National Institute on Aging (NIA). (2023a). *Aging in place: Growing older at home*. National Institutes of Health. Retrieved from https://www.nia.nih.gov/health/aging-place/aging-place-growing-older-home. Accessed February 5, 2024.

National Institute on Aging (NIA). (2023b). *Getting your affairs in order checklist: Documents to prepare for the future*. National Institutes of Health. Retrieved from https://www.nia.nih.gov/health/advance-care-planning/getting-your-affairs-order-checklist-documents-prepare-future. Accessed February 5, 2024.

National Institute on Aging (NIA). (2023c). *What is respite care?* National Institutes of Health. Retrieved from https://www.nia.nih.gov/health/caregiving/what-respite-care. Accessed February 5, 2024.

Population Reference Bureau. (2012). Planning for retirement and end-of-life care. *Today's research on aging*, No. 24. Retrieved from https://www.prb.org/wp-content/uploads/2020/11/TRA24-2012-Reitrement-end-of-life-aging.pdf. Accessed February 5, 2024.

Rahemi, Z., Malatyali, A., Wiese, L. A. K., & Dye, C. J. (2023). End-of-life care planning in diverse individuals across age groups: a proposed conceptual model of nursing. *Journal of Nursing Care Quality*, 38(4), 319–326. doi:10.1097/NCQ.0000000000000705.

Segal, R., White, M., & Robinson, L. (2023). *Age and driving*. HelpGuid.org [website]. Retrieved from https://www.helpguide.org/articles/alzheimers-dementia-aging/how-aging-affects-driving.htm. Accessed February 5, 2024.

Spillman, B. C., Favreault, M. M., & Allen, E. H. (2020). *Family structures and support strategies in the older population: Implications for Baby Boomers*. Urban Institute. Retrieved from https://www.urban.org/research/publication/family-structures-and-support-strategies-older-population. Accessed February 5, 2024.

Vock, J. (n.d.). *Guide on how to hold a family meeting*. Elizz [website]. Retrieved from https://www.elizz.com/family/guide-on-how-to-hold-a-family-meeting/. Accessed February 5, 2024.

5

Socioeconomic and Environmental Influences

Jennifer J. Yeager, PhD, MSN, RN

http://evolve.elsevier.com/Yeager/gerontologic/

LEARNING OBJECTIVES

On completion of this chapter, the reader will be able to:
1. Identify the major socioeconomic and environmental factors that influence the health of older adults.
2. Explain the importance of age cohorts in understanding older adults.
3. Describe the economic factors that influence the lives of older persons.
4. Identify components of the Medicare health insurance programs.
5. Discuss the influences of income, education, and health status on quality of life (QoL).
6. Discuss environmental factors that affect the safety and security of older adults.
7. Compare and contrast the housing options available for older adults.
8. Assess the ability of older adults to advocate for their own well-being, including avoiding fraud.

WHAT WOULD YOU DO?

What would you do if you were faced with the following situations?
- You are the medical-surgical nurse on an inpatient unit. An older adult is 2 days postsurgery and set to be discharged. You determine that your patient was homeless before their admission through the emergency department (ED) and has no place to go. What options for discharge will your patient have? What can you, as a nurse, do to help your patient after discharge?
- You are a nurse at an internal medicine clinic. You are working with a patient who is 85 years old and lives alone. They have a diagnosis of coronary heart disease (CHD) and hypertension (HTN) and are interested in making some health changes. Based on where they fall in an age cohort, what interventions and suggestions would you have for them to make health changes?

Each person is a unique product of genetic inheritance, life experiences, education, and environment. In addition to the typical risk factors of tobacco use, alcohol use, and inactivity, the leading predictors of morbidity and mortality in older adults are economic, social, and psychological factors (Puterman et al, 2020). The environment also influences safety and well-being. Therefore, it is imperative that healthcare professionals understand the socioeconomic and environmental status of older adults.

The United States spends more per capita on healthcare than any other country, and the rate at which spending is increasing. Much of this spending is on healthcare that controls or reduces the effects of chronic disease. Data from 2021 indicates older adults spend five times as much on healthcare ($22,356) than that of a child ($4217), and double the expenses of adults under the age of 65 ($9,154) (USAFacts Team, 2024).

SOCIOECONOMIC FACTORS

Generational Differences
Each generation has different expectations from their healthcare experience. While emerging adults (ages 18–29; Generation Z) prefer telemedicine, remote monitoring applications, and other technological advances as part of their healthcare experience, older adults (the Silent Generation and Baby Boomers) focus on health outcomes and high-quality service (Clark, 2020).

The Silent Generation (also named The Greatest Generation)
Persons in the Silent Generation were born between 1928 and 1945. This generation was expected to make advances in life through a strong work ethic. Males and females had traditional roles, with females staying home to raise the children. Males worked the same job their whole lives. Divorce and having children outside of marriage were taboo. Defining events for this generation included the Great Depression, World War II, the Korean War, landing on the moon, and the Cold War. The Silent

---
Previous author: Colleen Steinhauser, MSN, RN-BC, FNGNA

Generation has respect for authority. They are family focused and believe in giving back to society (Clark, 2020).

Although they make up 6% of the population, the Silent Generation accounts for most hospital stays. The Silent Generation trusts their healthcare provider and their opinion. They want guidance from their provider, and they tend to not ask questions and follow orders. When working with people from this generation, it is important not to appear rushed, or they will not ask questions. The teach-back technique is effective in determining if students understand instructions. This generation wants respect and good service. Good service means friendly staff, and being addressed as Mr. or Mrs. They often bring their children with them to appointments (Carroll, 2021). Television, radio, and direct mail are the best means of reaching this population (Gopal, n.d.).

Baby Boomers

Persons in the Baby Boomer generation were born between 1946 and 1964. The name for this generation is derived from the high birth rate following World War II and is the only officially named generation (by the Census Bureau). Baby Boomers have experienced significant social and cultural change. Females of this generation often worked outside the home, although many stayed home to raise the children. Premarital sex and divorce became more common. Defining events for the Baby Boomers include the Vietnam War and the associated protests, Woodstock and the Summer of Love, and the assassinations of John F. Kennedy, Martin Luther King, Jr., and Robert Kennedy. Television became mainstream. Baby Boomers believe in equal rights and equal opportunity. They question authority. They believe in personal growth and want to make a difference in the world. While they traditionally found self-worth in their job, they also believe in a work-life balance (Clark, 2020).

Baby Boomers often understand technology more than caregivers realize. Many competently use smartphones and computers. They are willing to use patient portals. Baby Boomers question and research symptoms, diagnoses, and treatments prior to their appointments. They want their healthcare providers to take the time to discuss their diagnosis and treatments, including the advantages and disadvantages. They want healthcare providers with a good reputation and will change providers if they do not receive high-quality care (Carroll, 2021). Although this generation is technologically savvy, they still prefer in-person visits with the provider rather than telemedicine. Baby Boomers are often caregivers for their aging parents. This population can be reached via television and radio, but also through social media and digital advertising, as nearly 80% of this population is online daily (Gopal, n.d.).

Generation X

Persons in Generation X, born between 1965 and 1980, are the next cohort to become older adults. They are motivated to learn. They are the first generation where females have more education than males. Generation Xers also carry a lot of debt; they are the first generation who are not as well off financially as their parents and the generation to have their children in day care so both parents can work. They make up a third of the workforce. Many parents of Generation Xers are divorced, and persons in Generation X tend to marry later and divorce sooner than previous generations. This generation is defined by the fall of the Berlin Wall, the end of the Cold War, the AIDS crisis, and MTV. They are independent, want a work-life balance, are resourceful, and value diversity, responsibility, and challenge. However, they are also known for their distrust of institutional authority (Clark, 2020). Generation X is also known as the "sandwich generation" as they manage the healthcare needs of their parents and their own children, as well as themselves.

This generation created many of the advances in technology, including video games, artificial intelligence (AI), and others. They are multitaskers. Generation Xers value healthcare quality and convenience in healthcare and the scheduling of appointments, including evening and weekend appointments. They are willing to use healthcare portals for communication, accessing diagnostic reports, and refilling prescriptions. This generation wants their healthcare provider to use technology to improve the patient experience. Persons in this generation are willing to change providers to improve healthcare outcomes. They investigate before making any health-related decisions; they want healthcare options to be provided but do not want to be told what to do. Generation Xers become impatient with long wait times. Affordable healthcare is also a concern for this generation (Carroll, 2021). This population can be reached through television and in-office messages. They actively seek ratings and reviews on the internet (Gopal, n.d.).

Income

Older adults report income from five sources: (1) Social Security, (2) assets, (3) retirement funds, (4) government pensions, and (5) wages. The median income in 2020 was $35,808 for males and $21,245 for females (Fig. 5.1) (Administration for Community Living [ACL] and Administration on Aging [AoA], 2022).

Social Security is derived from payroll taxes, and benefits are earned by accumulating credits based on annual income. There are four types of Social Security benefits:

- Retirement Benefits: A monthly check that replaces part of your income when you stop working. Eligibility is based on work. Most older adults have had Social Security taxes taken out of their paychecks throughout their work lives so they can get the monthly benefit in retirement.

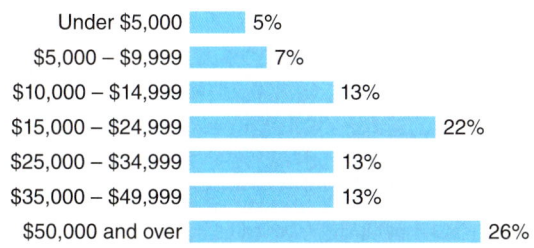

Fig. 5.1 Distribution by income of persons aged 65 and older reporting income, 2020. (Redrawn from Administration for Community Living, Administration on Aging. [2022]. *2021 Profile of older Americans.* U.S. Department of Health and Human Services. Available at: https://acl.gov/aging-and-disability-in-america/data-and-research/profile-older-americans. Accessed March 6, 2024.)

- Social Security Disability Insurance (SSDI): Provides monthly payments to persons with a disability that prevents or limits them from working. Persons must have worked for at least 5 of the past 10 years with quality. For persons who continue to work a limited amount, there are income limits.
- Supplemental Security Income (SSI): Provides monthly payments to people with disabilities and older adults who have little or no income (less than $1,971 a month for an individual) and few resources (assets amounting to less than $2,000 for an individual).
- Survivor Benefits: Paid to widows, widowers, and dependents of eligible persons who have worked long enough to qualify for benefits.

These are brief summaries; specifics can be found at https://www.usa.gov/what-is-social-security.

In 2020, 9% of those age 65 or older were classified as poor, with income at or below the poverty level (in 2024, this level is $15,060 for a family of one; $20,440 for a family of two [Department of HHS, 2024]). Another 4.6% are considered near poor, or at 125% of the poverty level. Over 17% of African Americans over 65 are poor, compared with 6.8% of older Whites, 16.6% of older Hispanics, and 11.5% of older Asians (Fig. 5.2). The poverty rate for older females is 10.1%. In contrast, the rate for older males is 7.6%. Older adults who live alone have a higher incidence of poverty (15.7%), compared to those who live with family (5.6%). Hispanic females over the age of 65 who live alone have the highest rate of poverty (35.6%) (ACL & AoA, 2022). Adults over 80 have the highest poverty rates, at 12.9% (Li & Dalaker, 2022).

Living in poverty increases vulnerability, functional limitations, chronic illnesses, hospital admissions, morbidity, and mortality. Difficulty meeting basic needs, food insecurity, substandard housing, a lack of resources, and limited access to resources often result in depression and anxiety (Dobarrio-Sanz et al, 2023). Facilitating access to services such as food banks, the Supplemental Nutrition Assistance Program (SNAP) (Box 5.1), Meals on Wheels, transportation, community health centers (CHCs) (Box 5.2), and federal housing assistance programs (Box 5.3) can ensure older adults meet the basic needs of food, shelter, and healthcare, which are vital to achieving healthy aging and quality of life (QoL)

(Kean and Lang, 2018). It is important for the nurse caring for older adults to be aware of services and programs available in their state and local area to ensure their patients achieve maximal QoL.

> **BOX 5.1 What is SNAP?**
>
> Created in 1939, the Supplemental Nutrition Assistance Program (SNAP) is a federally funded program to help those with limited income supplement their household food budget. In addition to helping individuals and families afford healthier food, it allows them to spend more of their income on other needs, such as transportation and housing. Eligible food items include meat, poultry, fish, fruits, vegetables, dairy products, bread, cereals, snack foods, and nonalcoholic beverages (MANNA FoodBank, 2023).
>
> SNAP also provides training programs to help individuals gain skills and obtain employment; it also provides educational programs to teach individuals how to cook healthy meals and stay physically active (MANNA FoodBank, 2023).
>
> SNAP was designed so that no one goes hungry; however, its work requirements reflect the importance of work and responsibility (USDA Food and Nutrition Service, 2023). See https://www.fns.usda.gov/snap/work-requirements for SNAP work requirements. Requirements may vary by state.

> **BOX 5.2 What are Community Health Centers?**
>
> Community health centers (CHCs) started to open in 1965 to provide culturally competent, comprehensive primary care that is accessible to all patients, regardless of their ability to pay. They charge for services on a sliding fee scale. CHCs increase health equity by reducing barriers like cost, lack of insurance, distance, and language.
>
> - **Health centers improve the health and well-being of underserved communities** while empowering people to become actively involved in solving issues unique to their needs and communities.
> - **Health centers are innovators, healers, and problem solvers** that reach beyond the walls of the conventional health care delivery system to prevent illness and address the social drivers that may cause poor health—diet, nutrition, mental illness, or homelessness.
> - **The health center mission to promote health equity** has become increasingly important in the fight against COVID-19 and other preventable diseases.
> - **Health centers have been vital in protecting marginalized communities from COVID-19**—including racial and ethnic minorities, migrant and seasonal workers, people experiencing homelessness, those in public housing, and people with limited English proficiency (multilingual interpreter services are available).
> - **Health centers work in partnership** with healthcare payers, entire healthcare systems, the private sector, and the government on all levels to address and respond to the critical public health crises of our time, including the following:
>   - Pandemics
>   - Natural disasters and extreme weather events
>   - National opioid crisis
>   - Maternal mortality and more
> - By mission and by law, health centers offer enabling services to assist patients with specific barriers to care, including the following:
>   - Transportation
>   - Translation
>   - Food security
>   - Accessing other social services
>
> Modified from the National Association of Community Health Centers (NACHC). (n.d.). *What is a community health center?* Retrieved from https://www.nachc.org/community-health-centers/what-is-a-health-center/. Accessed March 6, 2024.

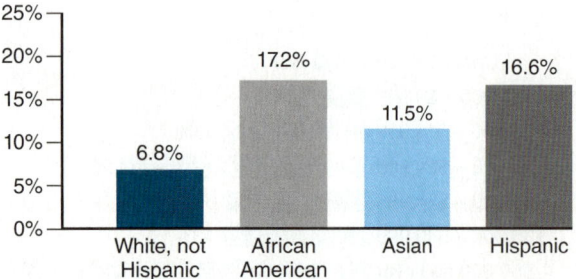

Fig. 5.2 Persons age 65 and over living below the poverty level by race and Hispanic origin, 2020. (Redrawn from Administration for Community Living [ACL], Administration on Aging [AoA]. [2022]. *2021 Profile of older Americans*. U.S. Department of Health and Human Services. Retrieved from https://acl.gov/aging-and-disability-in-america/data-and-research/profile-older-americans. Accessed March 6, 2024.)

BOX 5.3 What are Federal Housing Assistance Programs?

Most federal housing assistance programs are aimed at making housing affordable for low-income families. Affordability—defined as housing that costs no more than 30% of a family's income—is considered to be the largest housing problem today. Rental assistance programs, which are the largest source of direct housing assistance for low-income families, all allow families to pay affordable, income-based rents; however, different forms of assistance target different types of households, including the elderly, persons with disabilities, and families with children (McCarty et al, 2019).

Housing assistance for lower-income households has been available, in some form, since the 1930s, following the Great Depression. Three categories of assistance are monitored by the Department of Housing and Urban Development (HUD): rental housing assistance, assistance to state and local governments, and assistance to homeowners. Within these three categories are multiple forms of housing assistance, including (McCarty et al, 2019; see https://crsreports.congress.gov/product/pdf/RL/RL34591 for full descriptions and eligibility requirements for each of these programs):

- Section 8 vouchers
- Project-based rental assistance
- Public housing
- Housing for the elderly
- Housing for persons with disabilities
- Rural rental assistance
- Community development block grants
- HOME investment partnership block grants
- Low-income housing tax credits
- Homeless assistance programs
- Federal housing authority
- Department of Veterans Affairs mortgage assistance
- Mortgage interest tax deductions

Education

The educational level of older adults continues to increase. The number of older adults who have completed high school has increased from 28% in 1970 to 89% in 2021. Additionally, 33% of older adults had a bachelor's degree or higher in 2021 (Fig. 5.3). The highest level of education achieved is noted to be a strong predictor of hospitalization among older adults in the United States (Yue et al, 2021), and adults with higher educational attainment have increased health and life expectancy compared to those with less education (Raghupathi and Raghupathi, 2020). Older adults with a General Education Development (GED) certificate, compared to those with a high school diploma, have increased odds of cognitive impairment, vision impairment, hearing impairment, limitations in activities of daily living (ACLs), and ambulation limitations; additionally, high-school dropouts have worse outcomes than those with a GED (Fuller-Thomson et al, 2023). Nurses should encourage all older adults, particularly those with low educational attainment or low levels of health literacy, to implement the Ask Me 3® educational program, developed by the Institute for Healthcare Improvement (n.d.). In this program, patients are encouraged to ask three questions to help them manage their health issues:

1. What is my main problem?
2. What do I need to do?
3. Why is it important for me to do this?

Providing older adults with the education necessary to self-manage their chronic health issues can seem overwhelming to the nurse caring for them. See the Patient/Family Teaching box for teaching strategies to use with older adults.

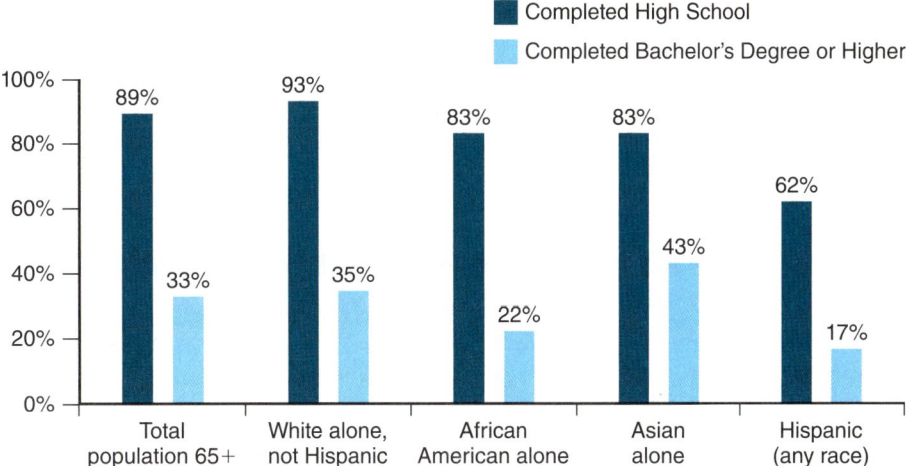

Note: The race categories white, African American, and Asian refer to people who reported only one race category and did not report being Hispanic.

Source: U.S. Census Bureau, Current Population Survey, 2021 Annual Social and Economic Supplement

Fig. 5.3 Percentage of persons age 65 and older who completed high school or a bachelor's degree or higher by race and Hispanic origin, 2021. (Redrawn from Administration for Community Living [ACL], and Administration on Aging [AoA]. [2022]. *2021 Profile of older Americans.* U.S. Department of Health and Human Services [HHS]. Retrieved from https://acl.gov/aging-and-disability-in-america/data-and-research/profile-older-americans. Accessed March 6, 2024.)

PATIENT/FAMILY TEACHING

Patient Teaching Strategies

Older adults often have physical, sensory, or cognitive impairments that affect communication and teaching strategies. To improve comprehension and adherence, consider the following suggestions:

- Speak to them as an adult and speak plainly.
- Avoid "elder speak" and use formal language as a default (such as Mr. or Mrs.) and avoid familiar terms, such as "dear," which could be perceived as disrespectful.
- Ensure they are comfortable.
- Speak slowly and provide time to process information; avoid appearing rushed.
- Use common language and ask if clarification is needed.
- Speak face to face; do not talk with your back turned or while typing.
- Compensate for hearing or visual deficits.
- Write or print takeaway points in the older adult's preferred language.
- Use professional translation services.
- Be sensitive to cultural differences.
- Include family and caregivers as desired by the older adult.
- Check back later to assess understanding.

Data from the National Institute on Aging. (2023). *Talking with your older patients.* National Institutes of Health. Available at: https://www.nia.nih.gov/health/health-care-professionals-information/talking-your-older-patients.

BOX 5.4 Health Status of Older Adults

In 2021 (January–June), among people aged 65 and older:
- 58% reported having diagnosed hypertension during the past 12 months.
- 75% reported that they received an influenza vaccination during the past 12 months.
- 68% reported that they had ever received a pneumococcal vaccination.
- 95% reported that they had at least one dose of the COVID-19 vaccine.

In 2020:
- 9% of persons aged 65 and older reported that they were current smokers.
- 30% were obese.
- 12% of people aged 65 and older reported taking prescription medicine for feelings of worry, nervousness, or anxiety.
- 11% reported taking prescription medicine for depression.
- 97% of persons aged 65 and older reported that they had a usual place to go for medical care.
- 22% had a hospital emergency department (ED) visit in the past year.
- 2% said that they failed to obtain needed medical care during the previous 12 months due to cost.

From Administration for Community Living (ACL), and Administration on Aging (AoA). (2022). *2021 Profile of older Americans.* U.S. Department of Health and Human Services (HHS). Retrieved from https://acl.gov/aging-and-disability-in-america/data-and-research/profile-older-amerians. Accessed March 6, 2024.

Health Status and Healthcare Coverage

Most older adults have at least one chronic disease, and some have more. The leading chronic diseases among older adults in 2020 included the following (ACL and AoA, 2022, p. 17):

- Arthritis (47%)
- Coronary heart disease (CHD) (14%)
- Myocardial infarction (MI) (9%)
- Angina (4%)
- Any cancer (26%)
- Chronic obstructive pulmonary disease (COPD), emphysema, or chronic bronchitis (11%)
- Diagnosed diabetes (21%)

Additional health status information can be found in Box 5.4.

Most older adults have Medicare (94%). Medicare covers most acute care services, with beneficiaries paying out-of-pocket (OOP) the amount Medicare does not cover. Coverage varies based on the services received. OOP healthcare expenses have increased by 38% since 2010; on average, older adults spend $6668 per year. In addition to Medicare, half of older adults had insurance from other sources (6% had military-based health insurance, and 6% were covered by Medicaid), and 1% had no coverage (Fig. 5.4) (ACL and AoA, 2022).

Medicare

Medicare is the federal health insurance program for adults over the age of 65. It also covers persons who are younger if they are disabled, and it covers persons with end-stage renal disease (ESRD) on dialysis or who have had a transplant. There are

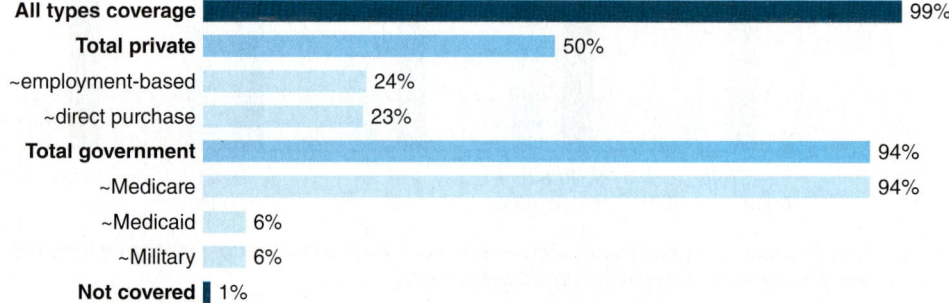

Notes: 1) CPS/ASEC 2021 asks about insurance for 2020. 2) Military includes VA/CHAMPVA/TRICARE
Source: U.S. Census Bureau, Current Population Survey, Annual Social and Economic Supplement

Fig. 5.4 Health insurance coverage, 2020. (Redrawn from Administration for Community Living [ACL], and Administration on Aging [AoA]. [2022]. *2021 Profile of older Americans.* U.S. Department of Health and Human Services [HHS]. Retrieved from https://acl.gov/aging-and-disability-in-america/data-and-research/profile-older-americans. Accessed March 6, 2024.)

several different parts to Medicare (Table 5.1) (Centers for Medicare and Medicaid Services [CMS], n.d.; National Council on Aging [NCA], 2023).

Medicare part A (hospital insurance). Part A covers inpatient hospital stays, care in a skilled nursing facility, hospice care, and some home healthcare. Medicare premiums come from Social Security taxes while working. If Social Security taxes are not paid, Part A can be purchased.

Medicare part B (medical insurance). Part B covers certain doctors' services, outpatient care, medical supplies, and preventive services. Older adults pay for Part B coverage. In 2024, the premium is $174.70 a month, plus an income-related monthly adjustment amount. Part B coinsurance—the portion the patient is expected to pay after reaching their deductible—is 20% of the cost for each Medicare-approved service or item. This can make up a significant portion of OOP costs.

Medicare advantage (part C). Medicare Advantage is a Medicare-approved plan from a private company that offers an alternative to original Medicare for health and drug coverage. These "bundled" plans include Part A, Part B, and usually Part D. Plans may offer some extra benefits that original Medicare does not cover—like vision, hearing, and dental services. Medicare Advantage Plans have yearly contracts with Medicare and must follow Medicare's coverage rules. The plan must notify you about any changes before the start of the next enrollment year (Centers for Medicare and Medicaid Services [CMS], n.d.).

Medicare part D (prescription drug coverage). Medicare Part D helps cover the cost of prescription drugs (including many recommended shots or vaccines). Plans vary in cost, and each has a different formula. To help cover OOP expenses, those with original Medicare coverage can purchase a Medicare Supplement Insurance (Medigap) policy.

ENVIRONMENTAL INFLUENCES

The physical environment affects the QoL of older adults. Environmental factors such as adequate shelter, safety, and comfort contribute to a person's ability to function well. In 2020, nearly 20% of older adults reported they had lost function or had difficulty in one or more of six domains, 21% had trouble seeing (even if wearing glasses), 29% had difficulty hearing (even if wearing hearing aids), 39% had trouble with mobility (walking or climbing stairs), 8% had difficulty with communication (understanding or being understood by others), 28% had trouble with cognition (remembering or concentrating), and 8% had difficulty with self-care (such as washing all over or dressing) (ACL and AoA, 2022, pp. 18-19). The interaction between functional losses and the environment

TABLE 5.1	What You'll Pay in Out-of-Pocket Medicare Costs in 2024
Medicare Plan	**2024 Out-of-Pocket Costs**
Part A (Hospital insurance)	**Premium:** $0 for most people; otherwise, $278 or $505/mo **Deductible:** $1,632 for each inpatient hospital benefit period **Coinsurance:** Varies with location and length of stay **For a hospital stay:** Days 1–60: **$0** Days 61–90: **$408 per day** Days 91–150[a]: **$816 per day** **OOP maximum:** None
Part B (Medical insurance)	**Premium:** $174.70/mo or higher, depending on income **Deductible:** $240 annually **Coinsurance:** 20% of service costs; deductible must be met first **OOP maximum:** None **Preventative benefits:** There are some preventive services under Part B that Medicare covers at 100%
Part C (Medicare Advantage)	**Premium:** Varies by plan, includes Part B premium **Deductible:** Varies by plan; may include Part D deductible **Coinsurance:** Varies by plan and service(s) received **OOP maximum:** $8,850, but some Part C plans set lower limits
Part D (Prescription drug coverage)	**Premium:** Varies by plan; the average basic monthly premium for standard Part D is estimated to be about $55.50/mo in 2024 **Deductible:** Varies by plan, but no more than $545 per year **Coinsurance:** Varies by plan **OOP maximum:** None, but catastrophic coverage kicks in after you hit $8,000 in OOP costs for covered drugs
Medigap (Supplemental insurance)	**Premium:** Varies by plan **Deductible:** $2,800 for Plans F, G, and J **Coinsurance:** Varies by plan **OOP maximum:** OOP maximums for Medigap Plans K and L are $7,060 and $3,530, respectively

[a]These are called "lifetime reserve days" because Medicare will only pay for these extra days once in your lifetime
© National Council on Aging (NCA). Used with permission. All rights reserved.

> **EVIDENCE-BASED PRACTICE**
>
> *Support for Older Adults Living in Low-Income Housing*
>
> **Background**
> Older adults living in low-income housing on a limited fixed income experience difficult choices between necessities, such as toilet paper and food, and healthcare basics, such as medications. The "Living-in-Place" pilot project sought to increase access to care, provide interdisciplinary services, and improve care coordination to promote independent living and improve QoL.
>
> **Sample/Setting**
> The study was conducted in two primary care clinics embedded within low-income older adult apartment complexes. The participants self-selected their participation, and enrollment required a transfer of care from their previous primary care provider. Exclusion from the study included those younger than 55 and not living in either apartment complex.
>
> **Method**
> Measures used in this pilot study included the Patient Health Questionnaire 9-item Scale (PHQ-9), Generalized Anxiety Disorder 7-item Scale (GAD-7), Social Connection and Isolation Panel, Timed Up and Go (TUG) test, BRIEF Health Literacy Scale, and Morse Fall Risk Scale (MSRS). Additionally, quantitative data concerning health characteristics and healthcare utilization throughout the first year of clinic operations were collected through a medical record audit.
>
> **Findings**
> Thirty (30) patients participated in the study. The mean age was 69, and 50% were male. Half of the patients were White, 23.3% were African American, and 3.3% identified their race as other. One patient self-identified as Hispanic/Latino. Seven participants declined to self-identify their race.
> Nineteen (19) patients were insured by Medicaid. Patients in this sample had an average of 6.97 chronic health conditions and took an average of 7.47 prescriptions. Common chronic conditions included hypertension (HTN), diabetes, and mental health conditions. The body mass index (BMI) of 74% of the participants was >25 kg/m^2, and 51.81% had a BMI >30 kg/m^2. Barriers to good nutrition included shopping for fresh foods due to lack of transportation, access to stores with fresh produce, and cost. Of the participants, 36% were current smokers. No patients were interested in smoking cessation. Forty percent (40%) of the participants reported transportation as a barrier to receiving primary care. Participants in the study also reported significant loneliness and isolation.
> While health literacy was assessed, it did not correlate with patient experience. Some patients did show a lack of understanding about their chronic disease, while other patients reported emotional fatigue from chronic care management, which, in turn, affected their desire and ability to participate in prescribed treatments. Other barriers to care included cost, transportation issues, and access to specialty care appointments.
>
> **Implications**
> This pilot study has a small sample size, which limits generalizability. It was determined that some residents were hesitant to switch from their established primary care provider, and others were prescribed controlled substances, which the embedded clinics could not provide. The COVID-19 pandemic also interfered with enrollment.
> Despite the small enrollment, the findings can be used to direct future care, which includes the integration of behavioral health services in the on-site clinics to better support mental health. The researchers also plan to include qualitative data collection to more fully investigate why older adults living in the apartment complexes chose to participate, or not participate, in the healthcare services.

Data from Hughes-Carter, D. L., Faubert, S. J., & Henschel, E. (2021). A novel partnership with low-income housing to support healthy aging. *The Journal for Nurse Practitioners,* 17(1), 718–722.

(home, neighborhood, sidewalks, streets, traffic density, parks, crime, and safety) influences independence (Gobbens and van Assen, 2018).

Geographic Location of Residence

The older adult population is increasing in rural areas (17.5% of the rural population) compared to urban areas (13.8% of the urban population). Healthy aging in rural areas presents unique challenges. Rural populations are considered a health disparity group due to increased chronic disease and mental health issues. Overall health outcomes are worse for older adults in rural areas. They have increased incidences of obesity, diabetes, CHD, cancer, COVID-19, and overall mortality (Cohen and Greaney, 2023). Higher rates of poverty, limited job opportunities, limited access to healthcare services, increased numbers of uninsured, and a lack of transportation contribute to health disparities (Carter and Dean, 2021). Older adults in rural areas also experience poorly maintained roads, low-quality housing, and limited technological infrastructure (internet and cell phone service) (Rhubart et al, 2020), all impacting QoL. Older adults living in rural areas are more likely to forgo medical care due to costs than their urban counterparts (Carter and Dean, 2021). The Centers for Disease Control and Prevention (CDC, 2023) has identified the following measures to improve the health of rural Americans:

- High blood pressure screening and quality management
- Prevention, early detection, and treatment of cancer
- Promotion of physical activity and healthy eating to reduce obesity
- Smoking cessation
- Support for those with mental, behavioral, and developmental disorders
- Motor vehicle safety
- Safe prescribing of opioids

Federal policies have been implemented to assist aging populations, both rural and urban. The One Policy, the Older Americans Act (OAA), provides services and protections for older adults. It includes funding to assist older adults with the greatest economic and social needs to live as independently as they can. Title III grants can help older adults access home and community-based services. Limited access to home and community-based services results in increased nursing home placement (Rhubart et al, 2020). Therefore, nurses must help their older adult patients navigate access to these services.

Housing

Many older adults in America find it difficult to access affordable, safe housing that meets their needs as their health status changes (installation of grab bars, ramps, and stairlifts) while living on a fixed income. Nearly a third of older adults pay 30% of their income for housing, and half of this group pays more than 50%. The number of older adults who qualify for federal housing subsidies is growing (Ludden, 2023), but housing subsidies only reached 36.5% of the older adults who needed them (Holder, 2023).

Older adults comprise nearly half of the homeless population. Older adults with homelessness experience more health-related concerns, have a significantly shorter life expectancy, have an increased incidence of geriatric syndromes (falls, functional impairment, and cognitive impairment), and have higher rates of mental health and substance use disorders (Couch, 2023) (Box 5.3).

Housing options are available in some areas for those who need a little assistance, and options are also available for those who require total assistance. Age-restricted communities are communities where at least 80% of the homes must have at least one resident over 55. Many offer swimming pools, tennis courts, and other amenities. Senior apartments are rental units for those over 55 and often have limited stairs and grab bars in the bathroom. Meal packages may be offered. Some senior apartments are subsidized housing for older adults who qualify for reduced rent. Continuing care retirement communities (CCRCs) offer a continuum of care from independent living to nursing home care. Assisted living offers residents their own room or suite, with around-the-clock care, meals, and medication management. Some assistance can be provided with bathing and dressing. Assisted living facilities (ALFs) are typically private. Group homes are state-licensed homes owned by an individual or company, offer a range of services, and may have shared or private rooms. Memory care is specialized care for older adults living with dementia. They have programs designed to stimulate cognition. Memory care units are often part of a CCRS. Nursing homes provide 24-hour-a-day care and assistance with all needs (Schoch, 2022). The Eldercare Locator can assist with finding a home environment that meets the needs of the individual (https://eldercare.acl.gov/public/Resources/LearnMoreAbout/Housing.aspx).

Transportation

For many older adults, an automobile is a symbol of independence. In 2021, 32 million adults over the age of 70 still had driver's licenses (Insurance Institute for Highway Safety [IIHS], n.d.). In some areas, an automobile is necessary for transportation to shopping areas, medical facilities, and social centers. An older adult's self-assessment, care partner, and clinician involvement may determine when an older adult should stop driving. Driving is a form of independence, and it is hard to "give up." Normal physical aging changes and the effects of chronic health conditions may require adaptations (decreased miles driven, avoidance of driving at night, and avoiding challenging situations). Resources are available from the CDC at https://www.cdc.gov/transportationsafety/older_adult_drivers/index.html to help start the conversation on when to stop driving (National Highway Traffic Safety Administration [NHTSA], n.d.). One challenge for older adults who do not drive is the availability of public transportation. Gimie et al. (2022) reported that 40% of older adults report access to public transportation impedes its use, as one out of five transit stations are not Americans with Disabilities Act (ADA)-compliant and make it difficult for people with visual or hearing impairments to use the resource. Low-cost transportation is an objective of the OOA and is the responsibility of the AoA. Each Area Agencies on Aging (AAA) is charged with ensuring that transportation is available in its area (ACL, 2023). Obstacles preventing public transportation use include cost, scheduling, distance from home, availability in rural areas, lack of awareness of the service, and the reluctance of some older adults to use public transportation (Fig. 5.5) (Fraade-Blanar et al, 2022).

ADVOCACY

Older adults as a group are advocates for their own special needs and interests. They write to legislators, consumer protection groups, government agencies, and other groups that control issues affecting older adults. By advocating for themselves, older adults are taking charge of their environment, resources, mental and physical health, and the future of all older adults. Older adults know from experience that they can make a difference.

However, persons with disabilities, those with less than a high school education, people from some racial and ethnic groups, those with limited English proficiency, and older adults whose incomes are below the federal poverty threshold all need assistance to take advantage of services and programs that may benefit them.

Advocacy is an ongoing process as opposed to a single, isolated event. As a moral concept, advocacy requires the nurse to speak up for the patient's rights and choices, to help the patient clarify their decision, and to protect the patient's privacy and autonomy in decision-making (Potter et al, 2023). The nurse is often the best person to initiate and provide that assistance. The nurse is trained to listen and assess, is aware of aging physiology and psychology, is familiar with community resources, and is motivated to serve older adults. The nurse may be the one member of the formal support group with the most complete information about older adults.

Many organizations in the United States advocate for older adults. Local and regional organizations, including state departments, also advocate for older adults and the local AAA (https://acl.gov/).

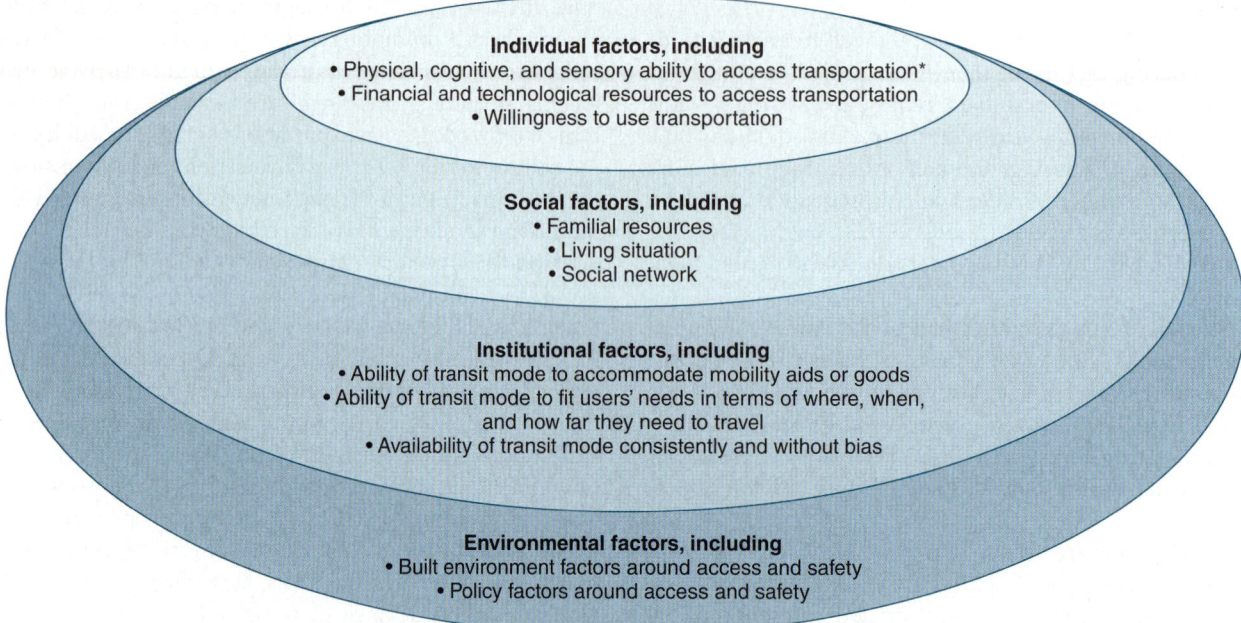

*Access refers to the ability to summon transportation (if using a rideshare model), travel to the transportation mode (e.g., where it is parked), enter the mode, spend the ride safe and informed of the trip's status, exit the mode when the ride is complete, and reach the intended destination. This usage is based on the concept of *complete trips* (Department of Transportation [DoT], undated).

Fig. 5.5 Barriers to transportation. (Redrawn from Fraade-Blanar, L., Best, R., and Shih, R. A. [2022]. *Transportation equity for older adults*. Rand Corporation. Retrieved from https://www.rand.org/content/dam/rand/pubs/perspectives/PEA1600/PEA1615-1/RAND_PEA1615-1.pdf. Accessed March 11, 2024.)

SUMMARY

Older adults' perceptions of the healthcare system in its entirety are influenced by experience. The nurse needs knowledge about the major historical events that have influenced the perceptions of today's older adults to understand their response to healthcare issues.

Socioeconomic issues, including income sources, prosperity or poverty, educational level, health status, and formal and informal support systems, affect the ability of older adults to comprehend and comply with healthcare regimens.

Older adults and their families may need to be made aware of community resources. The nurse should be aware of the housing options, nutrition programs, transportation opportunities, respite programs, and legal assistance programs available in the community.

By understanding the eligibility requirements for benefits and entitlements, the nurse can assist older adults in receiving optimum services. By understanding the necessity for and availability of conservatorship or guardianship, the nurse can help older adults and their families cope with diminishing abilities.

The sensitive nurse understands the concerns of older adults and supports and reassures them. The nurse can also encourage the older adults' informal support systems of friends and family. Often, the nurse can coordinate the formal and informal support systems for the maximum positive effect on the health and well-being of older adults.

Advocates for older persons, whether the older adults themselves or professionals in the field of aging, can help make socioeconomic and environmental factors a positive influence on older adults.

To provide maximum benefits to aging healthcare consumers, the nurse must understand the factors influencing health perception. To successfully work with older adults, the nurse must understand where they are and where they have been.

KEY POINTS

- Socioeconomic factors such as income level, income sources, insurance coverage, benefits and entitlements, and educational level influence older adults' perceptions of their health and approach to healthcare.
- Environmental factors, such as geographic location, housing, transportation, and perception of safety, influence the availability of services and older adults' knowledge and use of those services.
- Experience strongly influences shaping value systems, coping skills, and perceptions. Understanding each generation is important to understand their values and perceptions.

- Education has a strong positive influence on economic well-being and health status. Education prepares persons to make positive decisions that contribute to a higher perceived QoL.
- Medicare is a federal program that provides health insurance for older adults. It consists of two parts: Part A is hospital insurance that helps pay for inpatient care and some follow-up care, and Part B is medical insurance that helps pay for physician and outpatient services.
- Medicaid is a state-administered program that uses federal funds to cover some medical expenses not covered by Medicare. Each state has different coverage and requirements. Medicaid is designed for persons with very low incomes and minimal assets.
- Various housing options are available to meet the needs of older adults, including senior apartments, retirement communities, ALFs, and nursing facilities. Each option provides a different level of service to help older adults maintain maximum independence. However, many older adults are homeless.
- Through advocacy, nurses can protect the dignity of older adults and improve their QoL.

CLINICAL JUDGMENT EXERCISES

1. A 69-year-old chronically ill older adult with few financial resources and no formal education only has one child who can assist them. Their adult child is married, has four children, and has a job that barely manages to support them and their family. Speculate how the person's situation may affect their perception of healthcare. In what ways can the nurse intervene?

REFERENCES

Administration for Community Living (ACL). (2023). *Older Americans Act (OAA)*. Retrieved from https://acl.gov/about-acl/authorizing-statutes/older-americans-act. Accessed March 11, 2024.

Administration for Community Living (ACL), & Administration on Aging (AoA). (2022). *2021 Profile of older Americans*. U.S. Department of Health and Human Services (HHS). Retrieved from https://acl.gov/aging-and-disability-in-america/data-and-research/profile-older-americans. Accessed March 6, 2024.

Carroll, J. (2021). *Understanding generational differences with patients*. Advantage Healthcare Consulting (AHC) [website]. Retrieved from https://www.advadm.com/understanding-generational-differences-with-patients/. Accessed March 7, 2024.

Carter, E., & Dean, O. (2021). *Rural-urban health disparities among US adults ages 50 and older*. AARP.org [website]. Retrieved from https://www.aarp.org/pri/topics/health/prevention-wellness/rural-urban-health-disparities-among-us-adults-ages-50-and-older.html. Accessed March 7, 2024.

Centers for Disease Control and Prevention (CDC). (2023). *About rural health*. Retrieved from https://www.cdc.gov/ruralhealth/about.html. Accessed March 7, 2024.

Centers for Medicare and Medicaid Services (CMS). (n.d.). *What's Medicare?* Medicare.gov [website]. Retrieved from https://www.medicare.gov/what-medicare-covers/your-medicare-coverage-choices/whats-medicare. Accessed March 7, 2024.

Clark, M. (2020). *What different generations want in healthcare* [Blog]. Etactics [website]. Retrieved from https://etactics.com/blog/generations-in-healthcare. Accessed March 7, 2024.

Cohen, S. A., & Greaney, M. L. (2023). Aging in rural communities. *Current Epidemiology Reports*, 10(1), 1–16. doi:10.1007/s40471-022-00313-9.

Couch, L. (2023). *HHS: Older adults fastest growing homelessness group*. LeadingAge.org [website]. Retrieved from https://leadingage.org/hhs-older-adults-fastest-growing-homelessness-group/. Accessed March 7, 2024.

Department of Health and Human Services (HHS). (2024). Annual update of the HHS poverty guidelines [89 FR 2961]. *Federal Register*. Retrieved from https://www.federalregister.gov/documents/2024/01/17/2024-00796/annual-update-of-the-hhs-poverty-guidelines. Accessed March 7, 2024.

Dobarrio-Sanz, I., Chica-Pérez, A., Martínez-Linares, J. M., López-Entrambasaguas, O. M., Fernández-Sola, C., & Hernández-Padilla, J. M. (2023). Experiences of poverty amongst low-income older adults living in a high-income country: A qualitative study. *Journal of Advanced Nursing*, 79(11), 4304–4317. doi:10.1111/jan.15750.

Fraade-Blanar, L., Best, R., & Shih, R. A. (2022). *Transportation equity for older adults*. Rand Corporation. Retrieved from https://www.rand.org/content/dam/rand/pubs/perspectives/PEA1600/PEA1615-1/RAND_PEA1615-1.pdf. Accessed March 11, 2024.

Fuller-Thomson, E., Grossman, R., & MacNeil, A. (2023). Is the health of older Americans with a GED equivalent to their peers with a high school diploma? *International journal of aging and human development*. http://doi.org/10.1177/00914150231208685.

Gimie, A. M., Castillo, A. I. M., Mullins, C. D., & Falvey, J. R. (2022). Epidemiology of public transportation use among older adults in the United States. *Journal of the American Geriatrics Society*, 70(12), 3549–3559. doi:10.1111/jgs.18055.

Gobbens, R. J. J., & van Assen, M. A. L. M. (2018). Associations of environmental factors with quality of life in older adults. *The Gerontologist*, 58(1), 101–110. doi:10.1093/geront/gnx051.

Gopal, S. (n.d.). *Health care decisions by generation: How do patients differ?* Rendia.com [website]. Retrieved from https://rendia.com/resources/insights/health-care-decisions-generation-patients-differ/. Accessed March 7, 2024.

Holder, S. (2023). *America is aging into a housing crisis for older adults*. Bloomberg.com [website]. Retrieved from https://www.bloomberg.com/news/articles/2023-12-07/high-costs-for-housing-and-care-cloud-retirement-for-us-older-adults. Accessed March 7, 2024.

Institute for Healthcare Improvement (IHI). (n.d.). *Ask me 3: Good questions for your good health*. Retrieved from https://www.ihi.org/resources/tools/ask-me-3-good-questions-your-good-health. Accessed March 11, 2024.

Insurance Institute for Highway Safety (IIHS). (n.d.). *Older drivers*. IIHS/HLDI. Retrieved from https://www.iihs.org/topics/older-drivers#:~:text=Based%20on%20data%20reported%20by,2021%20(FHWA%2C%202023).

Kean, N., & Lang, K. (2018). *Supporting older Americans' basic needs: Health care, income, housing and food* [Issue Brief]. Justiceinaging.

org [website]. Retrieved from https://justiceinaging.org/supporting-older-americans-basic-needs-health-care-income-housing-food/. Accessed March 7, 2024.

Li, Z., & Dalaker, J. (2022). *Poverty among the population aged 65 and older* [R45791]. Congressional Research Service. Retrieved from https://sgp.fas.org/crs/misc/R45791.pdf. Accessed March 7, 2024.

Ludden, J. (2023). *Millions of seniors struggle to afford housing—and it's about to get a lot worse*. NPR.org [website]. Retrieved from https://www.npr.org/2023/11/30/1215460460/housing-seniors-affordable-harvard-report-baby-boomers. Accessed March 7, 2024.

MANNA FoodBank. (2023). *Understanding SNAP: A comprehensive guide to food assistance*. MANNAFoodBank.org [website]. Retrieved from https://www.mannafoodbank.org/snap-guide/. Accessed March 7, 2024.

McCarty, M., Perl, L., & Jones, J. (2019). *Overview of federal housing assistance programs and policy* [RL34591]. Congressional Research Service. Retrieved from https://crsreports.congress.gov/product/pdf/RL/RL34591. Accessed March 7, 2024.

National Council on Aging (NCA). (2023). *What you'll pay in out-of-pocket Medicare costs in 2024*. ncoa.org [website]. Retrieved from https://www.ncoa.org/article/what-you-will-pay-in-out-of-pocket-medicare-costs-in-2024. Accessed March 7, 2024.

Potter, P. A., Perry, A. G., Stockert, P. A., & Hall, A. M. (2023). *Fundamentals of nursing* (11th ed.). St. Louis: Elsevier.

Puterman, E., Weiss, J., Hives, B. A., Gemmill, A., Karasek, D., Mendes, W. B., et al. (2020). Predicting mortality from 57 economic, behavioral, social, and psychological factors. *Proceedings of the National Academy of Sciences of the United States of America, 117*(28), 16273–16282. doi:10.1073/pnas.1918455117.

Raghupathi, V., & Raghupathi, W. (2020). The influence of education on health: an empirical assessment of OECD countries for the period 1995–2015. *Archives of Public Health, 78*, 20. doi:10.1186/s13690-020-00402-5.

Rhubart, D. C., Monnat, S. M., Jensen, L., & Pendergrast, C. (2020). The unique impacts of U.S. social and health policies on rural population health and aging. *The Public Policy & Aging Report, 31*(1), 24–29. doi:10.1093/ppar/praa034.

Schoch, D. (2022). *11 housing options for older adults who need a little—or more—help*. AARP.org [website]. Retrieved from https://www.aarp.org/caregiving/basics/info-2022/housing-options.html. Accessed March 7, 2024.

USAFacts Team. (2024). *How much is spent on personal healthcare in the US?* USAFacts.org [website]. Retrieved from https://usafacts.org/articles/how-much-is-spent-on-personal-healthcare/. Accessed March 7, 2024.

USDA Food and Nutrition Service. (2023). *SNAP eligibility*. U.S. Department of Agriculture. Retrieved from https://www.fns.usda.gov/snap/recipient/eligibility. Accessed March 7, 2024.

Yue, D., Ponce, N. A., Needleman, J., & Ettner, S. L. (2021). The relationship between educational attainment and hospitalizations among middle-aged and older adults in the United States. *SSM-Population Health, 15*, 100918. doi:10.1016/j.ssmph.2021.100918.

Health Promotion and Illness/Disability Prevention

Jennifer J. Yeager PhD, MSN, RN

http://evolve.elsevier.com/Yeager/gerontologic/

LEARNING OBJECTIVES

On completion of this chapter, the reader will be able to:
1. Define health promotion, health protection, and disease prevention.
2. Identify models of health promotion and wellness.
3. Describe health-care provider barriers to health promotion activities.
4. Describe patient barriers to health promotion activities.
5. Describe primary, secondary, and tertiary prevention.
6. Plan strategies for nursing's role in health promotion and public policy.
7. Develop approaches to support the empowerment of older adults.

WHAT WOULD YOU DO?

What would you do if you were faced with the following scenarios?

- You are caring for an older adult in the telemetry unit with a history of hypertension (HTN), chronic heart failure (CHF), chronic obstructive pulmonary disease (COPD), and a smoker of 30 packs per year who was admitted for shortness of breath and unstable HTN. While performing a medication review, you realize that the patient is on multiple medications to control blood pressure, including metoprolol, lisinopril, and clonidine. When you ask about medication adherence at home, the patient states, "Sometimes I skip doses of my medication because I have trouble affording them all." What interventions can you do to help your patient?

- You are caring for an older adult in the medical / surgical unit the day she received the news that there is a possibility her breast cancer, which has been in remission for 15 years, could be present again. The internist explained to her that they would like to order a computed tomography (CT) scan, magnetic resonance imaging (MRI), and multiple laboratory tests. Your patient refuses the tests, stating, "I have lived a long and happy life. Even if the cancer is back, I don't plan on wasting my time and energy on treatments. I would rather live each day to the fullest." The internist is adamant that your patient should follow through with the testing because the diagnosis has not yet been confirmed, thus a prognosis cannot be formed. What would you do?

ESSENTIALS OF HEALTH PROMOTION FOR AGING ADULTS

Older adults remain the fastest growing segment of the US population. The number of older adults has increased by 38% since 2010. It is expected that the number of older adults will reach 80 million by 2040 (National Council on Aging (NCA), 2024). According to the Centers for Disease Control and Prevention (CDC), the life expectancy of males is 73.2 years, whereas the life expectancy of females is 79.1 years (CDC, 2022a). This is a decline in life expectancy for the second year in a row; life expectancy is at its lowest level since 1996. The decline in life expectancy is primarily a result of the COVID-19 pandemic (74% of the decline). However, accidents and unintentional injuries also account for this decline (14%); 50% of unintentional injuries are drug overdoses. Heart disease (4.1%), chronic liver disease / cirrhosis (3%), and suicide (2.1%) also play a role in the overall decline in life expectancy.

Health-care spending continues to rise. Per-capita expenses increased by 4.1% in 2022, to $13,493 (American Medical Association [AMA], 2024). The only way to offset the rising costs of health care is to utilize health promotion and disease prevention services so that older adults can minimize or limit the effects of disease. Educating older adults regarding these services is key to decreasing premature mortality and functional disability, increasing quality of life (QoL), and reducing hospital visits and health-care spending.

Healthy People 2030 (Office of Disease Prevention and Health Promotion (OASH), n.d.) has identified 20 objectives for older adults, as they are at increased risk for developing chronic health conditions, experiencing falls, and are more likely to be hospitalized with infectious diseases than the general population. Objective categories cover dementia, foodborne illness, infectious disease, injury prevention, oral conditions, osteoporosis, respiratory disease, and sensory or communication disorders. Visit the Healthy People 2030 website for detailed information about these objectives (https://health.gov/healthypeople).

Previous authors: Ashley N. Davis, MSN, RN, PCCN, Sue E. Meiner, EdD, APRN, BC, GNP, and Dr. Jean Benzel-Lindley, PhD, RN.

> **BOX 6.1 Areas of Health Promotion Most Relevant to Older Adults**
>
> - Increasing physical activity
> - Smoking reduction / cessation
> - Reduction of alcohol consumption
> - Medication safety
> - Spiritual health
> - Cardiac health: heart-healthy diet, exercise, and preventive medication use
> - Psychological / emotional / mental health
> - Environmental health
> - Nutrition
> - Social health
> - Weight maintenance
> - Driving safety
> - Avoiding risky sexual behavior

Terminology

Health promotion is the science and art of helping people change their lifestyle to move toward optimal health, with *optimal health* being a complete and holistic type of health or health that focuses on mind, body, and spirit. The promotion of health provides the pathway or process to achieve this balance. Box 6.1 lists areas of health promotion that are the most relevant to older adults. A distinction should be made between health promotion and disease prevention. Health promotion addresses individual responsibility, whereas preventive services are promoted by health-care providers. Disease prevention focuses on protecting as many people as possible from the harmful consequences of a threat to health.

Primary prevention is the act of seeking out services and education to prevent disease. Primary prevention measures include activities that help prevent a specific condition. Examples include immunization against diseases, receiving health-protecting education and counseling, promoting the use of automobile passenger restraints, home safety, and fall-prevention programs. Because successful primary prevention helps avoid the distress, cost, and burden associated with injury or disease, it is typically considered the most cost-effective form of health care.

Secondary prevention is the act of detecting early disease and seeking care before the disease progresses or symptoms become apparent. Examples of secondary prevention activities include screening tests for cancer and findings of other diseases. If disease is detected early, interventions can be implemented to maintain functional ability and increase the chance of survival and wellness.

Tertiary prevention is defined as activities involving chronic disease care; attempts are made to maintain the person at their highest function, minimize the negative effects of disease, and prevent disease-related complications.

BARRIERS TO HEALTH PROMOTION AND DISEASE PREVENTION

The barriers to health promotion and disease prevention in the United States are not specific to older adults. The issue is systemic inequity within the health-care system. Often, individuals cannot afford to "go to the doctor." Others live in areas with no nearby health-care facilities (e.g., rural areas). Five (5) factors have been identified as barriers with no nearby health-care facilities (i.e., those in rural areas). Five (5) factors have been identified as barriers that must be addressed to help overcome health-care disparities (Wolters Kluwer, 2022).

The first issue is a lack of insurance. While older adults may have Medicare coverage due to fixed incomes, they may not have the resources to meet copays and cover the costs of medications. Often, they skip other basic needs to pay for health care, such as proper nutrition, dental and vision care, and recommended health screenings (Wolters Kluwer, 2022).

Another factor is staffing shortages. There are shortages of physicians, nurses, and technicians, particularly in rural areas (Wolters Kluwer, 2022).

Bias and stigma towards various groups persist in the health-care sector. Discrimination based on age, race and ethnicity, immigration status, sex and gender, and sexual orientation hampers access to care and negatively impacts the individual's willingness to seek out specialized care (e.g., mental health services). Often, the bias is unintentional due to a failure to adhere to current, evidence-based guidelines (Wolters Kluwer, 2022).

Transportation and work-related barriers negatively impact an individual's ability to seek timely health-care and preventive services. Access to transportation, specifically in rural areas, and the inability to take time off from work negatively impact access. Telemedicine has made large strides toward overcoming this barrier and providing after-hours access to care (Wolters Kluwer, 2022).

Language barriers are a growing concern in health care, as 1 in 5 households speaks a language other than English (Wolters Kluwer, 2022). According to Allen et al. (2020), in 2015, the US Census Bureau reported that more than 350 languages were spoken in homes across the United States, including more than 150 Native American languages. Language barriers negatively impact the quality of care. Using family members can risk mistranslation of medical terminology and miscommunication. Interpretation services can better support patients (Wolters Kluwer, 2022).

Healthy People 2030 has identified tools for action to help individuals, organizations, and communities overcome barriers to health equity. Please visit https://health.gov/healthypeople/tools-action for more information.

MODELS OF HEALTH PROMOTION

Models of behavior change address interventions designed to positively influence a person's behavior, decrease health risks, and "facilitate effective adaptation to and coping with illness" (Institute of Medicine, 2001, Introduction).

Transtheoretical Model

The transtheoretical model (TTM) of health promotion focuses on an individual progressing through 6 stages of behavioral changes as follows:
- *Precontemplation:* people do not see that their behavior produces negative consequences. They are not ready to take action within the next 6 months.
- *Contemplation:* People intend to start healthy behavior. They recognize their behavior produces negative consequences

and are pondering the pros and cons of taking action. There is ambivalence about change. These individuals are getting ready to take action within 6 months.
- *Preparation (determination):* Individuals are ready to take action in the next 30 days. They believe taking action will reduce or reverse the negative consequences of their behavior, and they can lead healthier lives.
- *Action:* People have changed their behavior and plan to maintain the changes leading, to healthier lives.
- *Maintenance:* People have sustained their behaviors for 6 months or more. They work hard to prevent relapse.
- *Termination:* There is no desire to return to previous unhealthy behavior. This stage is rarely reached. Most people stay at the maintenance stage.

The amount of time an individual takes to complete each stage is variable and requires different interventions to facilitate moving the person to the next state of change (LaMorte, 2022a).

Health Belief Model

The second model is the health belief model (HBM). This model was developed to identify behaviors that inhibited participation in disease prevention measures. This model is based on the idea that a person's perception of the value of attaining a health goal or service determines how likely they are to take specific actions to attain that goal (LaMorte, 2022b). Key elements include (Boskey, 2024):
- *Perceived severity:* People make behavioral changes based on the perceived severity of the consequences of inaction.
- *Perceived susceptibility:* People will not change their behavior unless they believe they are at risk.
- *Perceived benefits:* People will only change their behavior if there are benefits to their actions.
- *Perceived barriers:* People will not change their behavior if they think the barriers (e.g., amount of effort, discomfort, expense, and inconvenience) are too hard to overcome.
- *Cues to action:* External factors (e.g., a high blood pressure reading) that prompt the person to make the change.
- *Self-efficacy:* Individual belief in the ability to make changes.

This model can be used to develop interventions and educational opportunities designed to prevent health problems, encourage behavior change, and support behavior change.

Health Promotion Model

The health promotion model (HPM) describes health as a dynamic state and provides a framework to explain and predict health-related behavior. There are 4 major concepts in the model (Business Bliss Consultants, 2018):
- *Person:* Individual characteristics and life experiences directly impact their health-related behaviors.
- *Environment:* The environment includes the physical, social, and economic circumstances of the individual. A healthy environment promotes healthy living.
- *Health:* The individual's definition of health directly impacts their actions relative to health promotion and disease prevention.
- *Nursing:* Taking into account the person, environment, and the individual's perception of health, the nurse can develop interventions that facilitate health-promoting behaviors.

This model is person-centered. All interventions are tailored to the individual and designed to meet their needs to promote behavior change.

DISEASE PREVENTION

Primary Preventive Measures

Primary preventive measures refer to specific actions taken to optimize the health of individuals by helping them become more resistant to disease or ensuring an individual's health by helping them become more resistant to disease or ensuring their environment is less harmful. Overall guidelines for Medicare coverage of primary prevention are reviewed in Tables 6.1 and 6.2. Providing ongoing education to the older adult population about the importance of these measures and Medicare coverage may increase the likelihood of service utilization.

Yearly well-visits with a primary care provider are recommended for older adults, as are screening and counseling opportunities. Not only are well-visits important to the overall health of the older adult, so too are routine dental visits. Too often, dental visits are not prioritized due to a lack of access to care, the cost, and the discomfort associated with examinations. However, poor dental hygiene can lead to dental caries, pain, infection, gum disease, tooth loss, a decrease in nutritional intake, cardiovascular disease, and cancer. Due to barriers that prevent older adults from seeking dental care, a culture change is needed to educate and train primary care providers to perform basic oral examinations, provide education, use dental sealants and fluoride varnish, and make dental referrals when needed (Bussenius et al, 2017).

Immunizations are strongly recommended for older adults, especially for those who are considered high-risk due to multiple comorbidities and suppressed immune systems and who are institutionalized. Recommended immunizations include (CDC, 2023):
- COVID-19 vaccines: 2- and 3-dose primary series and booster
- Influenza vaccine: annually
- Respiratory syncytial virus (RSV): 1 dose should provide protection for 2 winters
- Pneumococcal vaccination (PCV): "1 dose of PCV15 or PCV20 should be given if patient has never received a PCV; if PCV15 is administered, it should be followed by a dose of pneumococcal polysaccharide vaccine (PPSV23) >1 year after PCV15 dose; PCV20 vaccination does not require a subsequent dose of PPSV23; in patients with a prior history of only a PPSV23 vaccination, 1 dose of PCV15 or PCV20 should be administered. A minimum 1-year interval between PPSV23 dose and PCV dose is recommended" (Papke & Cochran, 2023, PCV20 section).
- Tetanus, diphtheria, and pertussis vaccines (Tdap): every 10 years
- Zoster vaccine (Shingles): 2 doses

Smoking cessation increases life expectancy, reduces the risk of developing or further complicating heart and lung diseases, reduces the risk of cerebrovascular accidents and erectile dysfunction, reduces respiratory symptoms, and reduces the risk of cancer. These benefits can significantly increase the QoL for older adults. Immediate benefits of quitting smoking

TABLE 6.1 Secondary Prevention: Medicare Reimbursement

Screening / Preventive Procedure	Medicare Guidelines for Reimbursement
Pneumococcal infection vaccination	The initial vaccine and the second vaccine are given 1 year later, and then every 5 years
Influenza vaccination	For all older adults annually
Hepatitis B virus (HBV) vaccination	Older adults at a medium or high risk of contracting HBV: once per lifetime
Mammography	Females older than 40 years are covered for 1 screening every 12 months
Papanicolaou test and pelvic examination	Pap test and screening pelvic examination (including clinical breast examination) are covered at 2-year intervals; annual examinations are covered for females identified as high-risk
Colorectal screening	Annual fecal occult blood test for those older than 50 years
	Flexible sigmoidoscopy every 4 years for those older than 50 who are at higher risk; for those not at high risk, every 10 years
	Colonoscopy every 2 years for those at high risk for those not at high risk, every 10 years
	Screening barium enemas every 2 years for those older than 50 years and are high risk; for those not at high risk, every 4 years
Osteoporosis	Bone density scans every 2 years for those who meet one or more criteria
Diabetes screening	Up to twice a year for those at high risk
Glaucoma screening	Annually for those at high risk (20% and copayment required)
Smoking cessation counseling	Up to 8 face-to-face visits per year
Physical examination	Within first 12 months of joining Medicare, then every 12 months

Data from the Centers for Medicare and Medicaid Services. (n.d.). *Preventive and screening services.* Medicare.gov [website]. Retrieved from https://www.medicare.gov/coverage/preventive-and-screening-services.html. Accessed November 10, 2023.

TABLE 6.2 United States Preventive Services Task Force (USPSTF) Guidelines for Primary and Secondary Health Promotion Activities for Older Adults

Health Promotion Activity	Recommendation	Supportive Evidence
Mammography	Annually starting at age 50 and continue every 2 years until age 74	Based on randomized trials supportive evidence does not correlate with the recommendation as higher-stage tumors are reduced with annual screening
Cervical smear test	Screening is not recommended after age 65; if not high-risk, and previous 3 consecutive screenings were negative within last 10 years, with most recent being within last 5 years	Based on randomized trials and evidence, harm outweighs benefit
Colorectal cancer screening	Screening is recommended from ages 50–75; after age 75, screening should be based on individual and prior screening history; fecal occult screening is recommended yearly, whereas a colonoscopy is recommended every 10 years	Based on randomized trials; supportive evidence does not correlate with recommendation as evidence supports fecal occult screening every 2 years; colonoscopy benefits appear to outweigh the risks
Prostate examination	Evidence is insufficient to support screening with prostate-specific antigen (PSA) testing in males older than 70 years of age; males 55–69 years of age should be evaluated on an individual basis	Based on insufficient evidence to support benefits of screening; risks appear to outweigh benefits
Osteoporosis screening	Screening is recommended for females aged 65 and older; evidence is insufficient for evaluating males for osteoporosis	No current evidence evaluates risks versus benefits

Data from U.S. Preventive Services Task Force. (2018). *USPSTF A and B Recommendations.* Retrieved May 2, 2018 from https://www.uspreventiveservicestaskforce.org/Page/Name/uspstf-a-and-b-recommendations/.

include a reduction in heart rate and blood pressure and decreased carbon monoxide levels in the blood (World Health Organization (WHO), 2020).

Research concerning the health benefits and risks of alcohol consumption yields variable and conflicting results. Additionally, individual health behaviors and genetics confound results further. Current evidence indicates that consumption of 1 drink per day (i.e., 12 ounces 5% alcohol by volume [ABV] beer; 8 ounces 7% ABV malt liquor; 5 ounces 12% ABV wine, or 1.5 ounces 40% ABV [80 proof] distilled spirits [e.g., gin, rum, vodka, whiskey]) or less can increase the risk for some types of cancer and cardiovascular disease (CDC, 2022b).

Polypharmacy occurs when an older adult is prescribed or takes multiple medications concurrently that have the possibility of interacting with one another or when the older adult is taking medications that are prescribed to treat the side effects of other drugs or are not necessary for their conditions. This occurs when care is sought from multiple providers who do not collaborate. Polypharmacy can result in increased hospitalizations and health-care spending due to adverse drug events (ADEs), drug interactions, nonadherence to medications due to a lack of financial resources or misunderstandings, a decline in functional ability, including incontinence and subsequent falls, decreased nutritional intake, and cognitive impairment. As patient advocates, nurses are responsible for assessing the older adult's medication during transitions in care and institutionalizations. Medication reconciliation needs to focus on all medications, including prescribed, over-the-counter, herbals and supplements, and illicit drugs. The list of medications should be reviewed for necessity, interactions, contraindications, and overmedication or overdosing.

The American Geriatrics Society (AGS) Beers Criteria for Potentially Inappropriate Medication (PIM) Use in Older Adults (2023) has been updated to include new criteria, modifications to existing criteria, and changes to make the list easier to use. This list should be considered during all medication reviews in acute, ambulatory, and institutional settings, except for hospice and palliative care settings. To reduce the risk of polypharmacy, the nurse should educate the older adult to keep a complete list of all medications and include the dose, route, frequency, and reason for taking the medication. The older adult's medication list should also have their pharmacy information located on it. The older adult should also keep a list of all health-care providers and their contact information. A copy of these lists should be kept in a wallet or purse for accessibility.

All older adults, especially females, are more susceptible to osteoporosis and fractures. Disease prevention strategies should also focus on bone health. Over 18% of females and over 4% of males age 50+ have osteoporosis and are at risk for fractures. Screening guidelines for females 65 and over include a detailed history, a physical exam, and using an osteoporosis clinical risk assessment tool, such as the Fracture Risk Assessment (FRAX), or other tools to determine risk. Based on risk, bone mineral density (BMD) measurement should be considered. Consideration should be given to the benefit of further investigation versus the risk of treatment and patient wishes (Elam et al, 2024).

Secondary Preventive Measures

Secondary prevention focuses on screening or detection of early disease. In addition, secondary prevention incorporates primary prevention techniques to delay disease progression. For example, encourage people who have had a heart attack to stop smoking and start exercising. Annual screening recommendations for older adults should be made on an individual basis with the use of the guidelines and evidence-based recommendations from the USPSTF (https://www.uspreventiveservicestaskforce.org/uspstf/). Screening for those in good health should continue through age 75. Those older than 75 should talk to their health-care provider to determine if screening should continue. Table 6.3 outlines the advantages and disadvantages of common screenings.

Tertiary Preventive Measures

Tertiary prevention aims to prevent or reduce the long-term effects of a disease by helping patients manage their conditions and chronic symptoms. Many older adults receive tertiary care through specialists who manage complex conditions, such as cardiologists or pulmonologists. Other examples include rehabilitation after stroke, support groups, pain management programs, and follow-up examinations to identify cancer recurrence or metastatic disease.

NURSING ROLE IN PREVENTION

The American Nurses Association (ANA) (1995) position statement, which was developed in 1995 and remains unchanged, supports nurses in their role as advocates of health promotion and disease prevention:

- Increase nurses' knowledge and skills in provision of preventive services
- Encourage partnerships with consumers and other disciplines to identify needs, set priorities, develop strategies, and evaluate progress in promoting health
- Support health-care legislation that holds health insurance plans accountable for preventive care
- Become involved in research to evaluate the extent to which specific preventive interventions at individual, family, group, and community levels can (a) improve health, (b) affect access, use, cost, and desired outcomes, and (c) prevent disease, injury, or disability
- Encourage use of multidisciplinary efforts to call consumers' attention to health-promoting behaviors and environments and development of community-focused primary prevention models for care
- Influence local and national economic and political options toward reconceptualizing health care in preventive and health-promoting models
- Continue to advance nursing's concern that prevention and health promotion be central to reformed health care
- Educate the public to promote health of population through a broader definition of health and its relationship to behavior

Nursing Care Guidelines for Health Promotion and Disease Prevention
Recognize Cues (Assessment)

When assessing older adults, the nurse must look at potential health hazards to identify risk factors for illness or injury. Risk factors include habits and lifestyle choices, personal and family medical histories, and environmental conditions. Environmental risk factors include the lack of access to opportunities to engage in enjoyable social and physical activities and the presence of clutter, poor lighting, and poor footwear, which put the older adult at risk of falling.

Gordon's functional health patterns. Assessment for health promotion and disease prevention begins with collecting data about the older adult. The assessment must be developed in a comprehensive manner. Subjective data are obtained through the health history. Objective data are obtained through a complete

TABLE 6.3 Advantages and Disadvantages of Health Promotion Activities

Activity	Advantages	Disadvantages
Alcohol use	Social benefit Increases high-density lipoprotein (HDL) cholesterol Decreased mortality after a heart attack Decreased risk of congestive heart failure (CHF) Associated with lower C-reactive protein levels and decreased frailty Associated with better memory	Health complications such as gastrointestinal, cardiac, dermatologic, cognitive, and neurologic and impairment of nutritional state Risk of depression Risk of falls Drug interactions
Cervical smear test	An increased risk of cervical cancer occurs with age and may result in unpleasant symptoms if untreated Older females may not have had regular cervical smear tests performed and may want this early screening Only pursue, USPSTF guidelines, if the female is willing to undergo treatment if disease is identified	Life expectancy after diagnosis is small in females over age of 70 Less risk if the patient is not sexually active Testing is difficult and uncomfortable for older females, particularly those who are no longer (or never were) sexually active
Mammography	An increased risk of breast cancer occurs with age If detected, these tumors are generally estrogen-receptor positive and treatable Only pursue if the female is willing to undergo treatment if a disease is identified	False-positive results can place the older adult at risk for additional harmful tests and procedures Tumors in older females tend to be slow growing Discomfort and pain associated with mammography Stress and anxiety over investigations Multiple complications of treatment (e.g., lumpectomy, radiation, or hormone treatment)
Prostate cancer screening	Increased risk for prostate cancer occurs with age Only pursue if male is at increased risk and is willing to undergo treatment if disease is identified	With diagnosis, only a small-to-no reduction in mortality was found
Fecal occult blood test (FOBT)	Early detection of a growth that could cause older adult discomfort and affect QoL if left untreated Easily performed at home with no discomfort and no preparation FOBT has better predictive value in older adults than in young adult population	False-positive results may cause additional testing and anxiety for patient
Colonoscopy	Screening is infrequent Diagnostics and treatments can be performed immediately Lower colorectal cancer (CRC) mortality rate Past age of 75 should only be screened if older adult is at increased risk and willing to undergo treatment if disease is identified	Bowel preparation can cause complications (such as dehydration and electrolyte imbalances), discomfort, and pain Risk of perforation and bleeding Risk of complications from sedation
Diet monitoring	Decreasing cholesterol with dieting reduces morbidity and mortality from cardiovascular disease	Restriction in diet may affect QoL
	Focus should be on eating a healthy diet low in fat and high in fruits, vegetables, and grains, which can facilitate maintenance of an ideal weight while decreasing risk of cancer and other diseases	Restricted diets can result in unneeded weight loss and failure to thrive
Reducing / quitting smoking	Smoking is associated with an increased risk of sudden cardiac death and myocardial infarction (MI) Financial incentive May decrease peripheral vascular problems and may prevent further lung disease and COPD	Nicotine replacement therapy can cause major cardiovascular adverse events (AEs) Electronic cigarettes (vaping) have not been extensively studied
Exercise	Positive physical health benefits Positive mental health benefits Decreased fatigue Decreased pain Maintain weight Maintain physical function	None

physical examination and observation. To obtain a complete, nursing-focused assessment, the nurse must understand the functional health patterns of aging. Eleven (11) of the basic functional health patterns of older adults that are important to assess are as follows (Bitencourt et al, 2023):

1. Self-perception or self-concept pattern
2. Role or relationship pattern
3. Health perception or health management pattern
4. Nutritional or metabolic pattern
5. Coping or stress-tolerance pattern
6. Cognitive or perceptual pattern
7. Value or belief pattern
8. Activity or exercise pattern
9. Rest or sleep pattern
10. Sexuality or reproductive pattern
11. Elimination pattern

The following discussion expands on these identified functional health patterns based on Gordon's typology of 11 functional health patterns. Each pattern presented includes a description and subjective and objective assessments. Within each of these patterns, the nurse needs to identify the older adult's knowledge of health promotion, ability to manage health-promoting activities, and value given to health promotion activities (Bitencourt et al, 2023).

Self-perception or self-concept pattern

Description: This pattern encompasses a sense of personal identity, body image, attitudes toward self, and view of self in cognitive, physical, and affective realms, as well as expressions of sense of worth and self-esteem. Perceptions of self should be explored with direct questions asked with sensitivity. Emotional patterns may be identified during this exploration of perceptual patterns.

Subjective: Determine the older adult's feelings about their competencies and limitations, particularly regarding preventive health behaviors and behavior change, withdrawal from previous activities, self-destructive actions, excessive grieving, and increased dependency on others. Assess changes in eating, sleeping, and physical activity patterns. Explore the person's perception of their identity, self-worth, self-perception, body image, abilities, successes, and failures.

Objective: Identify verbal and nonverbal cues related to these subjective data. Verbal cues elicit feelings about oneself (strengths and limitations), and nonverbal cues include a change in personal appearance. Using tools for assessing anxiety and depression is helpful.

Roles or relationships pattern

Description: This pattern encompasses the achievement of expected developmental tasks. Basic needs for communication and interactions with others, as well as meaningful communication and satisfaction in relationships with others, are examined.

Subjective: Determine family structure, history of relationships, and social interactions with friends and acquaintances. Focus on health behaviors, beliefs, and activities among their social network. Assess the perceived reasons for unsatisfactory relationships and identify attempts to change patterns and outcomes.

Objective: Examine the family or friend dynamics of interdependent, dependent, and independent practices among members.

Health perception or health management pattern

Description: This pattern encompasses the perceived level of health and the current management of any health problems. Determine health maintenance behaviors and the importance the older adult places on these behaviors.

Subjective: Determine the level of understanding of any treatments or therapy required for management of health deficits or activities, including the possible sources of reimbursement and concerns about costs, and include an assessment of the performance of activities of daily living (ADLs), instrumental activities of daily living (IADLs), or both.

Objective: Observe cues that indicate effective management of deficits, including the physical environment in which the patient resides. Assessment should include information about prior health promotion activities (e.g., mammography and vaccinations) and management during sickness and wellness. A home safety checklist should be utilized. Focus specifically on barriers to engaging in these behaviors and what has prevented them from participating in the past.

Nutritional or metabolic pattern

Description: This pattern encompasses the evaluation of dietary and other nutrition-related indicators.

Subjective: Determine the older adult's description, patterns, and perception of food and fluid intake, as well as adequacy for maintaining a healthy body mass index (BMI). It may not be realistic to obtain an accurate 24-hour food and fluid recall; however, the nurse could possibly obtain information on how meals are prepared, who prepares them, and approximately how much is eaten during a typical day. Identify any recent weight loss or gain, and identify food intolerances, fluid intake, and gastrointestinal (GI) symptoms. Consider access to grocery stores and restaurants and opportunities for obtaining appropriate, heart-healthy food sources.

Objective: Observe general appearance and various body system indicators of nutritional status. Note the height, weight, and fit of clothes. If possible, observe the older adult eating a meal. A nutritional examination tool may also be used.

Coping or stress-tolerance pattern

Description: This pattern encompasses the patient's reserve and capacity to resist challenges to self-integrity and their ability to manage difficult situations. The ability to successfully tolerate stress through personal coping behaviors is important to incorporate into any health promotion plan. Of equal importance is the identification of the older adult's support systems.

Subjective: Assess ways to handle big and little problems that occur in everyday life. Determine the past and current amount of stress present in the older adult's life. Discuss recent losses and the methods used to deal with those situations. Identify any stress-reducing activities that are practiced and the usual results obtained.

Objective: Observe coping skills and stress-reducing techniques and note their effectiveness. Consider evidence of health-promoting options for stress reduction (e.g., exercise).

Cognitive or perceptual pattern

Description: This pattern encompasses self-management of pain, communication difficulties, and deficits in sensory function. Modes include vision, hearing, taste, smell, touch, and compensatory assistive devices used when a deficit exists. Pain should be assessed, and also how the older adult treats it.

Subjective: Inquire about sensory function and communication difficulties and assess for any cognitive changes or pain.

Objective: Assess the usual patterns of communication and note the patient's ability to comprehend. Also, note the ability to read, hear the spoken word, smell, and distinguish tactile sensations and tastes. Simple screening may be performed using cognitive assessments.

Value or belief pattern

Description: This pattern encompasses elements of values, beliefs, and spiritual well-being that the older adult perceives as important for a satisfactory daily living experience and the philosophic system that helps them function within society.

Subjective: Identify the older adult's values and beliefs about health and health promotion activities. Explore spirituality and note any special emphasis on how this influences health promotion behaviors (e.g., "God will take care of health promotion and disease prevention").

Objective: Determine what is important to the older adult's life regarding overall goals (e.g., long life versus QoL) and support coping strategies. Note any references made to spirituality or religious affiliation and practices, as well as choices and decisions that are determined by values, beliefs, and spiritual practices.

Activity or exercise pattern

Description: This pattern encompasses information related to HP that encourages the older adult to achieve the recommended 30 minutes of physical activity daily on most days of the week.

Subjective: Screen for safety related to exercise and physical activity using screening measures such as the Exercise Assessment and Screening for You (EASY) (Chodzko-Zajko et al, 2012). The EASY determines whether it is safe for an individual to immediately start an exercise program and, depending on comorbid conditions matches the individual with a recommended exercise program that can be printed out from online resources, thus providing them with a hard copy to use. In addition, assess daily routines and activities, including patterns of exercise, leisure habits, recreation, and hobbies, and inquire about any limitations or changes in these patterns. Identify IADLs that are practiced with or without difficulty. Inquire about the older adult's typical day. Assess for pain, fatigue, and fear of falling and fall potential, and conduct a fall history.

Objective: Obtain vital signs and conduct cardiopulmonary and musculoskeletal system assessments. Assess self-care ability by observing and asking the patient about self-care activities such as bathing, dressing, toileting, and feeding, if possible. Note the use of adaptive tools or equipment. Complete the EASY with the older individual and provide appropriate exercise resources.

Rest or sleep pattern

Description: This pattern encompasses the sleep and rest patterns over a 24-hour period and their effect on function. Assess the rest and sleep patterns of the older adult for the usual pacing of activities with consistent energy reserves that do not require immediate rest.

Subjective: Assess usual sleep patterns, including bedtime and arousal time, quality of sleep, sleep environment, and distribution of sleep hours within a 24-hour period. Inquire about episodes of insomnia and deterrents to sleep such as pain; anxiety; depression; use of pharmacologic agents such as caffeine, over-the-counter agents that may cause arousal, alcohol, and prescribed medications such as some treatments for depression; lack of exercise; and inappropriate sleep hygiene. Identify the time and circumstances for regular rest periods. Record any activities associated with a rest period.

Objective: Have the patient keep a sleep diary that includes nap and rest periods. If possible, observe daily activities and note the effects of sleep disturbances on functional ability.

> ### EVIDENCE-BASED PRACTICE
>
> **Nurses' Health Perception Influences on Health Promotion Activities**
>
> **Background**
> Nurses are responsible for the provision of health promotion (HP) activities that improve QoL and reduce health inequalities. This study was conducted to determine the influence of HP knowledge and perceptions on nurses' HP practice.
>
> **Methods**
> A self-administered questionnaire comprised of 22 closed-ended questions was administered to 184 nurses randomly sampled from a tertiary hospital. Questions were asked about the respondents' demographics, knowledge, perception, and practice of HP.
>
> **Results**
> Male nurses made up 7.6% of the respondents. Most were over 40 years old, and just over 35% had been nurses for 10 years or less. "Of the participating 184 nurses, 56.0% (n = 103) agreed to having adequate knowledge regarding the conditions patients present within their units and their ability to provide HP services. A total of 63.6% (n = 117) of respondents strongly held the perception that health education and counseling from nurses could enhance patients' health, while 51.6% (n = 95) encouraged their patients to observe fitness assessments and health screening."
>
> **Conclusion**
> "Data showed that nurses' knowledge regarding HP had a strong influence on their perception of HP. Their perception of HP, in turn, strongly influenced their practice of the same. Therefore, rigorous efforts must be made by governmental agencies and organizations involved in health-care worker training and nursing accreditation to ensure the HP curriculum is well incorporated in nursing undergraduate training and sustained in service."

Data from Melariri, H., Osoba, T.A., Williams, M., & Melariri, P. (2022). An assessment of nurses' participation in Health Promotion: a knowledge, perception, and practice perspective. *Journal of Preventive Medicine and Hygiene, 63*(1), E27–E34.

Sexuality or reproductive pattern

Description: This pattern encompasses the older adult's behavioral expressions of sexual identity.

Subjective: Assess the patient's satisfaction or dissatisfaction with current circumstances related to sexual function and intimacy, including perceived satisfaction or dissatisfaction with sexuality or sexual experiences.

Objective: Discuss any current sexual relationship. When none is present, elicit the meaning this has for the patient's overall emotional and physical well-being.

Elimination pattern

Description: This pattern encompasses bowel and bladder excretory functions.

Subjective: Assess lifelong elimination habits and excretory self-care routines. Inquire about the patient's perception of normal bowel and bladder functions and explore specifically for recent changes in usual bowel and bladder functions. Assess the effect of elimination patterns and the ability to control elimination on QoL and participation in HP activities such as exercise.

Objective: Perform abdominal and rectal examinations; external genitalia and pelvic examinations may be indicated. Note the daily intake of food, particularly the amount of dietary fiber, and assess total fluid intake over a 24-hour period.

A nurse's approach to completing thorough functional health assessments of older adults must be positive and reassuring. Many of the necessary assessment tools needed to complete a thorough examination of the older adult can be found on the Hartford Institute for Geriatric Nursing (HIGN) *Try This*: Series website: https://hign.org/consultgeri-resources/try-this-series. Permitting older adults to be active participants in this process is important to the success of gaining insight into their needs.

Generate Solutions (Planning)

The nurse's role in promoting health among older adults relies on organized planning. The planning may begin by exploring older adults' personal ideas and beliefs concerning health needs. Reading current literature provided by the US Department of Health and Human Services (HHS), the National Institutes of Health (NIH), the National Institute on Aging (NIA), or the CDC will help the nurse keep abreast of the latest specific HP recommendations. Internet addresses for these and other information centers are provided at the end of this chapter.

Being well-versed in current health policy information will safeguard patient rights. The nurse can then inform older adults of significant policy changes as soon as they are made at the highest (federal) level. Often, the dissemination of health policy is slow, and news reaches the recipient long after the fact. When policies are retroactive or are to be enforced on a certain date, passing the information on to older adults may be crucial to their health and well-being. Moreover, it will help establish and maintain a trusting relationship.

Planning involves understanding behavior change and behavior change theories such as the theory of self-efficacy. The theory of self-efficacy states that the stronger the individual's belief that they can perform a behavior and the stronger their belief in the positive benefit of performing the behavior, the more likely they are to engage in the given activity. Recommendations to facilitate behavior change are shown in Table 6.4.

Take Actions (Nursing Interventions)

Implementation may begin by adopting a proactive stance toward an action plan for the HP of older adults. Seeking activities, locations, and means for disseminating HP information to a group of older adults is an example of implementing a proactive stance. The benefits of proactive activities include an early approach to a problem that has not been acted on previously. Annual HP screenings may be incorporated into programs that provide vaccinations for older adults and may include screenings for cancer, diabetes, osteoporosis, and age-related macular degeneration (AMD), as appropriate. Likewise, monthly health talks provided in senior centers, senior

TABLE 6.4 Interventions to Motivate Individuals to Change Behavior Using a Social-Ecologic Model

Component	Description	Examples of Interventions
Intrapersonal	Demographics (age and gender) Physical health and function Psychosocial factors (e.g., mood, resilience), cognitive status, pain, fatigue, and fear	Encouraging self-efficacy and empowerment through education in disease management and injury prevention
Interpersonal	Social support	Social support through groups of like-minded people or family and friends
	Verbal encouragement	Use of verbal encouragement to strengthen self-efficacy and outcome expectations
	Goal-setting and motivation	Goal identification (e.g., losing weight, being able to walk the dog) and recognizing motivators for completing goals
	Rewards	Identifying personal rewards for completing goals
	Role models	Exposure to others engaging in similar behaviors
Environment	Physical environment	Wide range of social and physical activities and safe walking areas Accessible healthy food choices or restaurants
Policy	Disease prevention guidelines Institutional policies and procedures Laws	Use of guidelines in educational interventions to encourage adherence

housing sites, or continuing-care retirement communities may be a useful way to repeatedly advocate and educate about HP activities such as exercise, prevention of falls, or safe medication use. Area Agencies on Aging (AAA) can provide information on activities and resources specific to older adults in a specific area. This information can aid the nurse in planning HP and disease-prevention activities.

Evaluate Outcomes (Evaluation)

Evaluation involves determining the effectiveness of the care plan. Was the older adult able to achieve the mutually established goals? The nurse should consider why these goals were or were not achieved and coordinate with the older adult to establish appropriate and realistic revised goals and realistic steps to achieve them.

Supporting the Empowerment of Older Adults

Nurses can provide a bridge between the theory of HP and the implementation of HP, protection, and preventive services. The active participation of nurses in encouraging older adults to set HP goals aimed at maintaining the best possible health, function, and QoL throughout the rest of their life span is essential. Nurses can collaborate with other health-care professionals and organizations, such as the AGS and the National Hartford Center for Gerontological Nursing Excellence (NHCGE), to establish guidelines, write papers, and influence policy.

Learning about community resources and local, state, and federal programs that can provide information or services to older adults and then disseminating the information to older adults in various settings are legitimate nursing roles. HP programs and activities may be provided to individuals, small groups, and larger groups where older adults congregate. Many retirement centers, assisted living facilities, church groups and organizations, Salvation Army centers, and senior citizen centers look for speakers on a variety of health subjects. In most cases, the managers of these facilities welcome nursing students or registered nurse (RN) volunteers to present HP or disease prevention programs on a regular basis. Empowering older adults requires initiative, organization, and knowledge of the major areas of HP relevant to this population and governmental policies.

Nurses should ideally use an individualized approach to health promotion when working with older individuals. This approach focuses on providing appropriate education both formally in HP classes and informally during health-care visits. Education should provide current recommendations for HP activities, such as receiving vaccinations and screenings, and helping older patients decide what health behaviors they want to engage in. This type of individualized approach has the advantage of being cost-effective in that screening is not performed if the individual does not intend to act on the results. In addition, individualized HP increases adherence to positive health behaviors such as smoking cessation and exercise.

SUMMARY

As the older adult population in the United States continues to increase, emphasis must be placed on the practices of HP, health protection, and disease prevention in order to increase functional mobility, increase QoL, reduce health-care spending, and decrease premature mortality. Three (3) models of HP activities were presented. The TTM provides insight into behavioral changes in stages. The HBM helps to determine behaviors that prevent participation in preventive measures. Nola Pender's HPM presumes a collaborative effort by the participant and the health-care professionals involved.

Definitions and examples of primary, secondary, and tertiary measures of disease prevention were provided. Primary prevention includes immunizations and counseling programs. Prevention counseling is aimed at healthy living, such as smoking cessation. Other areas of concern include home and medication safety. Secondary prevention (screening) focuses on the detection and early treatment of disease. Tertiary prevention involves eliminating or slowing the progression of symptoms.

The nurse's role in HP and protection or prevention of disease may be based on a framework of functional health patterns. Data about these health patterns are best obtained when the nurse completes a comprehensive nursing assessment of each of the areas of function using positive and reassuring communication.

The best results are achieved when the nursing process is used to assess, plan action, set goals, and implement a plan for HP, behavior change related to health-care activities, or disease prevention, followed by evaluation. Suggested HP activities that offer several levels of commitment are available to nurses who wish to become involved in social policy or political action. Involvement in a proactive movement to increase HP is possible at local, regional, and national levels. The use of an individualized approach and the empowerment of older adults to make their own health-care decisions will help them achieve their optimal level of health, function, and QoL.

CHAPTER 6 Health Promotion and Illness/Disability Prevention

KEY POINTS

- HP, health protection, and disease prevention will continue to be national goals with the *Healthy People 2030* initiative.
- HPMs are available to guide the change process in establishing a local, regional, or national effort.
- HP barriers include lack of insurance, staffing shortages, bias and stigma, transportation and work issues, and language barriers.
- Health protection targets 5 areas: (1) unintentional injuries, (2) occupational health and safety, (3) environmental issues, (4) food and drug safety, and (5) oral health.
- Primary prevention focuses on immunizations and health screening activities.
- Secondary prevention focuses on the detection of occult diseases.
- Tertiary prevention focuses on preventing the progression of symptoms while facilitating rehabilitation.
- The nurse's role in HP begins with a complete health assessment using the functional health patterns framework; this should incorporate an individualized approach for each patient.
- Using the nursing process in HP activities provides a sound foundation for success.
- Involvement in HP activities may be at the local, regional, and national levels.
- Using an individualized approach and empowering older adults to determine their level of HP and primary, secondary, tertiary, and quaternary prevention activities will help them achieve their optimal QoL.

CLINICAL JUDGMENT EXERCISES

1. Several nurses have volunteered to give influenza vaccines to older adults at a senior center. When the line to receive the injections slows down, 1 nurse notices a table of 4 older adults playing cards. None of the older adults have approached the vaccine registration table. What actions, if any, are appropriate for the volunteer nurses in this situation? Does the fact that the nurses are volunteers change any potential course of action?

2. You are caring for an older adult in the acute care setting. Their adult child has been staying with them throughout the admission. You notice the adult child appears to be disheveled and tearful. They state they have not been sleeping due to the stress of managing their mother's care at home and the present illness. What actions would you suggest the nurse take regarding the adult child? If an action is taken, when is it the appropriate time to do so?

REFERENCES

2023 American Geriatrics Society (AGS) Beers Criteria® Update Expert Panel. (2023). American Geriatrics Society 2023 updated AGS Beers Criteria® for potentially inappropriate medication use in older adults. *Journal of American Geriatrics Society*, 71(7), 2052–2081. doi:10.1111/jgs.18372.

Allen, M. P., Johnson, R. E., McClave, E. Z., & Alvarado-Little, W. (2020). Language, interpretation, and translation: A clarification and reference checklist in service of health literacy and cultural respect. *NAM Perspectives*, 2020, 10.31478/202002c. doi:10.31478/202002c.

American Nurses Association (ANA). (1995). *Position statement background information: Promotion and disease prevention.* Nursing World. Retrieved from https://www.nursingworld.org/practice-policy/nursing-excellence/official-position-statements/id/promotion-and-disease-prevention/. Accessed August 12, 2024.

American Medical Association (ANA). (2024). *Trends in health care spending.* Retrieved from https://www.ama-assn.org/about/research/trends-health-care-spending. Accessed August 12, 2024.

Bitencourt, G. R., de Souza, P. A., de Melo Ferreira, A. F., Fernandes, L. L., da Silva, C. S., & dos Santos Fonseca Correa, D. B. (2023). Functional patterns of health nursing theory in the hospital context: Evaluation according to Meleis. *Global Academic Nursing Journal*, 4(1), e336. doi:10.5935/2675-5602.20200336.

Boskey, E. (2024). *How the health belief model influences your behaviors.* Verywell Mind [website]. Retrieved from https://www.verywellmind.com/health-belief-model-3132721. Accessed August 12, 2024.

Business Bliss Consultants FZE. (2018). *Pender's health promotion model.* NursingAnswers.net [website]. Retrieved from https://nursinganswers.net/reflective-guides/penders-model.php?vref=1. Accessed August 12, 2024.

Bussenius, H., Reznik, D., & Moore, C. (2017). Building a culture of oral health care. *The Journal for Nurse Practitioners*, 13(9), 623–627. doi:10.1016/j.nurpra.2017.07.019.

Centers for Disease Control and Prevention (CDC). (2023). *What vaccines are recommended for you.* Retrieved from https://www.cdc.gov/vaccines/adults/rec-vac/index.html. Accessed August 12, 2024.

Centers for Disease Control and Prevention (CDC). (2022a). *Life expectancy in the U.S. dropped for the second year in a row in 2021.* Retrieved from https://www.cdc.gov/nchs/pressroom/nchs_press_releases/2022/20220831.htm. Accessed August 12, 2024.

Centers for Disease Control and Prevention (CDC). (2022b). *Dietary guidelines for alcohol.* Retrieved from https://www.cdc.gov/alcohol/fact-sheets/moderate-drinking.htm. Accessed November 10, 2023.

Chodzko-Zajko, W. J., Resnick, B., & Ory, M. G. (2012). Beyond screening: Tailoring physical activity options with the EASY tool. *Translational Behavioral Medicine*, 2(2), 244–248. doi:10.1007/s13142-012-0134-7.

Elam, R. E. W., Jackson, N. N., Machua, W., & Carbone, L. D. (2024). *Osteoporosis guidelines.* Medscape [website]. Retrieved from https://emedicine.medscape.com/article/330598-guidelines. Accessed August 12, 2024.

Institute of Medicine (US) Committee on Health and Behavior: Research, Practice, and Policy. (2001). *Health and behavior: The* interplay of biological, behavioral, and societal influences. Washington, DC: National Academies Press.

LaMorte, W. W. (2022a). *The Transtheoretical model (stages of change)*. Boston University School of Public Health. Retrieved from https://sphweb.bumc.bu.edu/otlt/mph-modules/sb/behavioralchangetheories/behavioralchangetheories6.html. Accessed August 12, 2024.

LaMorte, W. W. (2022b). *The health belief model*. Boston University School of Public Health. Retrieved from https://sphweb.bumc.bu.edu/otlt/mph-modules/sb/behavioralchangetheories/behavioralchangetheories2.html. Accessed August 12, 2024.

National Council on Aging. (2024). *Get the facts on older Americans*. Retrieved from https://www.ncoa.org/article/get-the-facts-on-older-americans. Accessed August 12, 2024.

Office of Disease Prevention and Health Promotion. (n.d.). *Older adults*. Healthy People 2030. Retrieved from https://health.gov/healthypeople/objectives-and-data/browse-objectives/older-adults. Accessed August 12, 2024.

Papke, J., & Cochran, M. (2023). Pneumococcal vaccines update for 2023. *U.S. Pharmacist*, 48(7), 17–25. Retrieved from https://www.uspharmacist.com/article/pneumococcal-vaccines-update-for-2023. Accessed August 12, 2024.

Wolters Kluwer. (2022). *Five key barriers to healthcare access in the United States*. Retrieved from https://www.wolterskluwer.com/en/expert-insights/five-key-barriers-to-healthcare-access-in-the-united-states. Accessed August 12, 2024.

World Health Organization (WHO). (2020). *Tobacco: Health benefits of smoking cessation*. Retrieved from http://www.who.int/tobacco/quitting/benefits/en/. Accessed August 12, 2024.

WEBSITES

American Association of Retired Persons (AARP). http://www.aarp.org.
Area Agency on Aging. https://areaagencyonaging.org/.
US Aging. https://www.usaging.org/.
International Counsel on Active Aging (ICAA). http://www.icaa.cc.
Administration on Aging (ACL). https://acl.gov/about-acl/administration-aging.
Alliance for Aging Research. http://www.agingresearch.org.
American Geriatrics Society (AGS). http://www.americangeriatrics.org.
American Society on Aging (ASA). http://www.asaging.org.
BenefitsCheckUp. http://www.benefitscheckup.org.
Centers for Disease Control and Prevention (CDC). http://www.cdc.gov.
Healthy People 2030 documents online. http://www.healthypeople.gov.
Information on Wellness Activities (State of Texas). http://www.dshs.texas.gov/Wellness/Activities/.
Medicare. http://www.medicare.gov.
National Council on Aging (NCA). http://www.ncoa.org.
National Hartford Center of Gerontological Nursing Excellence (NHCGNE). https://www.nhcgne.org/resources.
National Health Information Center (NHIC). http://www.health.gov/nhic/.
National Institute on Aging (NIA). http://www.nia.nih.gov.
National Institutes of Health (NIH). http://www.nih.gov.
U.S. Department of Health and Human Services (HHS). http://www.hhs.gov.
U.S. Preventive Services Task Force (USPSTF). http://www.uspreventiveservicestaskforce.org.

PART III

Influences on Quality of Life

7

Nutrition

Martha Smith, DNP, APRN, FNP-BC

http://evolve.elsevier.com/Yeager/gerontologic/

LEARNING OBJECTIVES

On completion of this chapter, the reader will be able to:
1. Differentiate between the factors influencing nutritional risk in older adults.
2. Differentiate between a nutritional screen and a nutritional assessment.
3. Identify the steps and core data collection elements of a nutritional assessment.
4. Describe the changes in nutritional requirements for older adults.
5. Describe the role of nutritional support in nutritional therapies.
6. Identify major dietary guidelines and recommendations for older adults.

WHAT WOULD YOU DO?

What would you do if you were faced with the following situations?
- You are caring for an 85-year-old adult in a long-term care unit. The older adult begins coughing while eating lunch. The older adult has a recent history of stoke. What actions do you take?
- You are making the first home health-care visit to evaluate a 92-year-old who lives alone. You notice that they are very thin (weighs 88 pounds), so you check the refrigerator for food options. The refrigerator has very little food in it and most of what is in there is outdated. How can you provide nutritional support to your patient?

Aging means an ongoing, physiologic, although not linear, decline in physical and mental function loosely associated with a person's age in years (World Health Organization, 2022). The diversity of how people age is not random. Some variations are genetic, but physical and social environments, gender, ethnicity, and socioeconomic status play a larger role. These factors impact opportunities and health behaviors.

Many changes in the body's cells, tissues, and organs are associated with aging (Rolf et al, 2022). These changes affect the digestive and musculoskeletal systems, which can affect food intake, digestion, and absorption of nutrients. This, combined with the poor nutritional value of meals, can lead to malnutrition. Additionally, certain drugs prescribed to older adults potentiate this phenomenon. Studies have shown 25% to more than 60% of older adults are affected by malnutrition or the risk for malnutrition (Greene et al, 2018). Malnutrition can be linked to generalized weakness, a weakened immune system, a higher risk for infection, bone loss, and muscle weakness, followed by an increased risk for falls, hospitalization, and death (Bakhtiari et al, 2020).

Older adults may suffer from loneliness and depression, which can lead to weight gain or loss and, ultimately, malnutrition. Food is an important aspect of life; eating too much or too little can negatively affect an older adult's quality of life (QoL) and overall health. This chapter will review those nutrition topics important to older adults and their overall health.

MALNUTRITION

Malnutrition in older adults is often unrecognized, and its prevalence increases with age. The term *malnutrition* is used to describe a nutritional deficiency that has adverse effects on the body and its normal functions. Poor nutritional status is a negative prognostic indicator in older adults, and unintentional weight loss in those over 60 years of age significantly increases the risk for dying (De Stefani et al. 2018). Although the actual percentages of malnutrition prevalence differ among meta-analyses, the main conclusions are comparable. Older adults in the community setting have the lowest percentage of malnourishment, and the highest percentage is in acute and subacute care settings. As expected, prevalence rises with age, and females are at greater risk (Norman et al, 2021).

Previous author: Neva L. Crogan, PhD, ARNP, GNP-BC, ACHPN, FAAN

Factors Influencing Nutritional Risk in Older Adults

Many factors influence nutritional risk in older adults. These factors can be classified into three major groups: social, psychologic, and biologic (Rashid et al, 2020). Social factors include isolation, loneliness, poverty, and dependency (Burris et al, 2021), but of those, poverty is the most significant cause of weight loss and malnutrition in older adults. Other social factors include lack of caregivers and transportation, culturally determined food habits, and widowhood and bereavement. A systematic review found those at high risk for malnutrition include individuals with a low income level, who live alone, are single, widowed, or divorced, and have a low educational level (Besora-Moreno et al, 2020). An older adult's inability to shop, cook, or feed themselves can lead to weight loss and malnutrition. Psychologic factors that influence nutritional risk in older adults include depression, anxiety, bereavement, and dementia (Rashid et al, 2020). Treating depression can reverse weight loss in nursing home residents (Morley, 2011a).

The prevalence of dementia is increasing in older adults and is often associated with weight loss. Older adults with dementia often forget or refuse to eat. Eight years after diagnosis, 50% of patients with Alzheimer disease have lost the ability to feed themselves (Volicer et al, 1987). Encouraging an older adult with advanced dementia to eat can become a time-consuming process. Often, older adults with advanced dementia wander excessively rather than consume food. They may express paranoid ideation, thereby refusing food because of a fear of being poisoned. Many older adults with dementia are prescribed psychotropic drugs that can cause anorexia. Finally, some older adults with dementia may develop apraxia of swallowing and must be reminded to swallow after each mouthful of food (Rashid et al, 2020).

Many biologic factors influence nutritional risk in older adults. Many medical conditions can cause weight loss and malnutrition by one or more of the following mechanisms: hypermetabolism, anorexia, swallowing difficulty, or malabsorption (Rashid et al, 2020). Specific diseases affecting an older adult's ability to eat or prepare food include stroke, tremors, or arthritis. Swallowing disorders (dysphagia) are associated with an increased risk for aspiration and may result in poor food intake. Infections are another cause of weight loss in older adults. Infections can lead to confusion, anorexia, and negative nitrogen balance.

Another disease that contributes to poor food intake is chronic obstructive pulmonary disease (COPD). Malnutrition occurs in nearly 60% of people with COPD. Older adults with COPD experience malnutrition due to the increased energy spent to do the work of breathing and physical activity, shortness of breath interfering with eating, early satiety, and cachexia related to the disease itself (Shalit et al, 2016). Individuals with Parkinson disease (PD) often experience weight loss in the later stages of the disease; this is presumed to be due to muscle hypertonia and dyskinesias. Persons with PD may need calorie-rich supplements to counteract weight loss (Barichella et al, 2017).

Drug–Nutrient Interactions

Seventy percent of older adults have two or more chronic conditions (National Council on Aging [NCA], 2023). Drugs are typically prescribed to manage these conditions. Adverse effects of these drugs may include unintentional weight loss due to either an altered sense of taste and smell or anorexia. Drugs that alter taste or smell include allopurinol, angiotensin-converting enzyme inhibitors, certain antibiotics, anticholinergics, antihistamines, calcium channel blockers, levodopa, propranolol, selegiline, and spironolactone. Drugs associated with anorexia include amantadine, certain antibiotics, anticonvulsants, antipsychotics, benzodiazepines, digoxin, levodopa, metformin, neuroleptics, opiates, selective serotonin reuptake inhibitors, and theophylline (Gaddey and Holder, 2021).

The interactions between drugs and nutrients may affect drug metabolism, absorption, digestion, or excretion. Table 7.1 lists selected interactions between drugs and nutrients commonly taken by older adults. Many older adults take a variety of vitamins and herbal supplements. The nurse needs to obtain an accurate assessment of all the over-the-counter therapies and drugs the patient may be taking. As the patient's drug profile changes, the nurse must continue to screen for drug–drug or drug–nutrient interactions and consult with a pharmacist or a dietitian, as needed.

Dehydration

Older adults are at a greater risk for dehydration due to several factors, including an age-related decrease in sensitivity to thirst, a decrease in total body water (TBW) resulting in an increased risk for dehydration with small changes in fluid intake, diminished kidney function which causes the kidneys to be less effective at conserving body water, exposure to prescription drugs which affect body water, and mobility problems which affect the ability to obtain fluids. Additionally, situational and psychologic factors, such as confusion, dementia, or depression, may limit access to water and other beverages. Finally, fear of incontinence may affect the volume of fluids consumed (Edmonds et al, 2021).

The human body is comprised of up to 60% water, and proper body water balance is essential for survival (Lacey et al, 2019). The extracellular space contains one-third of body water, distributed in a ratio of approximately 4:1 between extracellular interstitial and vascular compartments. Plasma is almost 60% of circulatory blood volume (Seifter and Chang, 2017).

TBW is regulated by offsetting water gains from drinking, eating, and metabolic water production, with sensible water loss (urine production, loss in feces) and insensible water loss (evaporation from lungs during breathing and perspiration).

Sodium is the major osmotically active ion in the extracellular fluid (ECF), and total body sodium regulates ECF volume (Docherty et al, 2021). Dehydration takes three main forms: *Isotonic dehydration* results from losing sodium and water, such as during a gastrointestinal (GI) illness. *Hypertonic dehydration* results when water losses exceed sodium losses. This type of dehydration is the most common and may occur from fever or limited fluid intake. *Hypotonic dehydration* may occur with diuretic use when sodium loss exceeds water loss (Docherty et al,

TABLE 7.1 Select Drug–Nutrient Interactions

Drug	Class of Drug	Nutrient	Interaction
Acetaminophen/Hydrocodone (Vicodin, Norco)	Narcotic, anti-inflammatory	Caffeine	Increases analgesic effects Increases absorption Increases elimination of drug
		Alcohol	Increases risk for hepatotoxicity Induces CYP2E1
Albuterol (Ventolin, Proventil)	Bronchodilator	None	No significant interactions confirmed
Amlodipine (Norvasc)	Calcium channel blocker	Grapefruit juice	Inhibits CYP3A4; slightly increases plasma concentration of drug
Atorvastatin (Lipitor)	Statin	Grapefruit juice	Increases serum atorvastatin Induces CYP3A4; increases plasma concentration of atorvastatin acid and atorvastatin lactone
		St. John's wort	Increases LDL and total cholesterol
Gabapentin (Neurontin, Neuraptine)	Anticonvulsant	Alcohol	Safe to use in treatment of alcohol dependency; reduces symptoms of alcohol withdrawal
		Cannabis	Reduces symptoms of cannabis withdrawal
Insulin glargine injection (Lantus Solostar)	Insulin analogue	Berberine	Potential significant theoretical interaction
Levothyroxine (Levothroid, Synthroid)	Synthetic thyroxine	Calcium	Decreases absorption of drug; increases TSH
		Vitamin C	Increases absorption of drug; decreases in TSH
		Coffee	Decreases absorption of drug
		Grapefruit juice	Inhibits OATP1A2; slightly decreases absorption of drug
Lisinopril (Prinivil, Zestril)	ACE inhibitor	None	No significant interactions confirmed
Metformin (Glucophage XL, Gluformin)	Biguanide	Berberine (300 mg)	Improves insulin sensitivity; decreases HOMA-IR, total cholesterol, LDL
		Alcohol (>7 drinks per week)	Increases effects of drug; increases lactic acidosis and lactate production
Metoprolol (Lopressor, Toprol-XL)	Beta blocker	None	No significant interactions confirmed
Omeprazole (Prilosec, Zegerid)	Proton pump inhibitor	St. John's wort	Induces CYP2C19 and CYP3A4; decreases effectiveness of drug
		Grapefruit juice	Inhibits CYP3A4; inhibits metabolism of drug
Rosuvastatin (Crestor)	Statin	Grapefruit juice	Inhibits OATP2B1; reduces bioavailability of drug
		EGCG	Significantly reduces systemic exposure of drug

Note: The information provided in this chart is based on a review of literature available at the time of publication. While the content is considered to be accurate at the time of publication, new or updated research released after the publication date may impact the accuracy of the information.
ACE, angiotensin-converting enzyme; *CYP*, cytochrome 450; *EGCG*, epigallocatechin-3-gallate; *HOMA-IR*, Homeostatic Model Assessment for Insulin Resistance; *LDL*, low-density lipoprotein; *TSH*, thyroid-stimulating hormone.
Modified from Fullscript. (2019). *Addressing pharmaceutical interactions in clinical practice*. Fullscript™. Retrieved from https://fs-marketing-files.s3.amazonaws.com/guides/pharmaceutical-interactions.pdf. Accessed July 31, 2023.

2021). Therefore, volume depletion may be a sequela to dehydration (most commonly in isotonic dehydration) but is not synonymous with it.

Dehydration can lead to electrolyte imbalances in older adults. Hypernatremia and hyponatremia are the most common electrolyte imbalances in older adults. (These are discussed more in-depth in Chapter 13, Laboratory and Diagnostic Tests.)

Prevalence estimates of dehydration in older adults vary widely. The prevalence ranges from more than one-third of older adults admitted to the hospital as emergencies to 20% to 88% of older adults in care homes to 60% of community-dwelling older adults (Edmonds et al, 2021). This relates to the inconsistency of methods to measure dehydration. Risk factors include advanced age (>80 years of age), female gender, residing in a nursing home, infection, and a diagnosis of dementia (Schlanger et al, 2010).

Nurses can help prevent dehydration in older adults by (Mentes, 2006):

- Providing fluids that older adults like and enjoy drinking
- Educating older adults to drink fluids even when they are not thirsty
- Identifying at-risk older adults
- Identifying and treating reversible dehydration causes, such as diarrhea and vomiting
- Measuring fluid intake and urinary output
- Providing appropriately-sized cups and glasses for older adults to handle, and straws if necessary
- Educating caregivers to offer small amounts of fluid each time they enter the room

- Educating caregivers to encourage the older adult to drink 8 ounces of fluids between and at each meal
- Providing positive feedback to caregivers who provide fluid

Micronutrient Deficiency

Micronutrients, such as vitamin D, calcium, and B_{12}, are commonly deficient in older adults. Even though the best way to ingest micronutrients is to eat a well-balanced diet, this may not always be possible. A vitamin or mineral supplement may be necessary for those older adults found to be deficient in any micronutrient (Norman et al, 2021).

In older adults, vitamins D and B_{12} may be difficult to gain in adequate supply. Approximately one-third of vitamin D requirements are obtained through diet. The rest is synthesized in the skin via sunlight. This could be problematic for homebound older adults with limited sunlight exposure secondary to decreased mobility or those who reside in a nursing home or assisted-living facility. Also, as one ages, the skin's ability to synthesize vitamin D declines (Chalcraft et al, 2020). Vitamin D deficiency has been linked to cancer progression, bone health (vitamin D is needed to absorb calcium), osteoporosis, and fractures. Vitamin B_{12} deficiency has been linked to pernicious anemia, bone health, and cognitive decline in older adults. Deficiencies of either vitamin can be treated with diet and supplementation (Davies, 2011).

Indicators of Malnutrition

Despite the availability of many validated nutritional screening tools, malnutrition often remains undiagnosed. It can lead to prolonged hospital stays, frequent re-admissions, and an increase in morbidity and mortality (Morley, 2011b). Therefore, it is important for nurses to recognize the causes, signs, and symptoms of malnutrition.

Two major markers of malnutrition are sarcopenia and cachexia. *Sarcopenia* is defined as "the decline in skeletal muscle mass that can result from physical inactivity, disuse of muscles, reduced levels of growth hormone and testosterone, neuromuscular changes, insufficient dietary protein, and impaired protein metabolism" (Brownie, 2013, p.141). Older adults can become sarcopenic after a lengthy hospitalization or illness. On the other hand, *cachexia* is characterized by a loss of fat and muscle mass accompanied by anorexia. It is a complex metabolic process often associated with an underlying terminal illness such as end-stage renal disease or cancer (Morley, 2011a). Older adults with cachexia also will have sarcopenia, but those with sarcopenia may not have cachexia (Crogan, 2017). Older adults with sarcopenia are at increased risk for falls with injuries (see the Evidence-Based Practice box).

Oral Health

Oral health is fast becoming a strong predictor or measure of the QoL for older adults (Spanemberg et al, 2019). Poor oral health in older adults is linked to protracted states of suffering and pain, and functional, nutritional, aesthetic, and psychologic issues. Thus, oral health preventative efforts are paramount to enhancing the QoL in our aging population.

> **EVIDENCE-BASED PRACTICE**
>
> *Patient-Specific Risk Factors for Adverse Outcomes After Geriatric Proximal Femur Fractures*
>
> **Background**
> Proximal femur fractures (PFFs) occur frequently among geriatric patients due to diverse risk factors, such as a lower bone-mineral density and the increased risk for falls.
>
> **Methods**
> In this review, we focus on recent literature of patient-specific risk factors and their impact on common complications and outcome parameters in patients with PFF.
>
> **Results**
> Patient- and treatment-related factors have a significant impact on outcome and are associated with an increased risk for mortality, impairments in functional rehabilitation, and complicative courses.
>
> **Conclusion**
> Geriatric patients at high risk for complications are nursing home inhabitants with severe osteoporosis, dementia, and sarcopenia. The early and ongoing assessment of these individual risk factors is crucial. Strategies including interdisciplinary approaches, addressing comorbidities, and facilitating an optimal risk-factor evaluation result in a beneficial outcome. The ongoing ambulant assessment and therapy of complicating factors (e.g., malnutrition, sarcopenia, frailty, or osteoporosis) must be improved.

Data from Becker, N., Hafner, T., Pishnamaz, M., Hildebrand, F., & Kobbe, P. (2022). Patient-specific risk factors for adverse outcomes following geriatric proximal femur fractures. *European Journal of Trauma and Emergency Surgery, 48*(2), 753–761.

Xerostomia, or dry mouth, is among the most common causes of poor food intake in older adults. Individuals with xerostomia have difficulty forming a bolus, chewing, and then swallowing. They will have a reduced ability to taste food and may have cracked lips or a fissured tongue, resulting in poor food intake. Additionally, xerostomia can lead to mucositis and dental caries (Khoury et al, 2022). Xerostomia in older adults is most likely drug-induced, and the risk increases with greater numbers of drugs taken (Storbeck et al, 2022).

Older adults are at increased risk for dental caries secondary to xerostomia and gingivitis. Almost 50% of older adults have dental caries affecting at least one tooth. Prevention includes the adoption of good oral hygiene and a well-balanced diet. Good oral hygiene includes the use of rotating toothbrushes, topical fluoride, daily mouth rinses, high-fluoride toothpaste, and regular dental checkups that include a fluoride varnish application (Coll et al, 2020).

Older adults with cognitive impairment (CI) are at increased risk for dental caries, oral infections, and periodontal disease (Coll et al, 2020). Older adults with dentures should be encouraged to remove them daily, inspect for damage, clean them before bed, and then return them to the mouth in the morning. Cognitively-impaired older adults may need help or support completing this task. Educating caregivers is important in preventing dental caries in cognitively-impaired older adults.

As the older adult's functional abilities decline with advancing age or disease processes (arthritis), providing modified equipment such as toothbrushes with built-up handles or Velcro grips may help enhance the elder functional ability and sense of well-being (Mac Giolla Phadraig et al, 2020). Other options include using electric toothbrushes, specialized floss holders, or nosey cups for rinsing the mouth. Finally, frequent dental cleanings and examinations can help promote optimal oral health in at-risk older adults.

NUTRITIONAL SCREENING AND ASSESSMENT

Nutritional Screening

Nutritional screening is an abbreviated assessment of nutritional risk factors that identifies patients needing a more comprehensive assessment and nutritional interventions. A variety of tools have been developed to conduct nutritional screening. The Mini Nutritional Assessment (MNA) is the most widely used tool to assess malnutrition or the risk of malnutrition in older adults (Isautier et al, 2019). The MNA is a simple and reliable 18-item questionnaire that examines food intake, weight loss, body mass index (BMI), psychologic stress, neuropsychologic problems, and mobility. The MNA-short form (SF), which reduces screening time to less than 5 minutes, is presently the tool of choice in most clinical practice. Additionally, the MNA-SF is more applicable to older adults with CI because the six items do not contain subjective questions. Go to https://www.mna-elderly.com/sites/default/files/2021-10/mna-guide-english-sf.pdf to view the MNA-SF with instructions for use.

Another tool in use is the Subjective Global Assessment (SGA). This tool incorporates medical history and physical examination findings to classify patients as well-nourished, moderate, or suspected of being malnourished or severely malnourished. Its use is limited in that it does not consider subtle changes in nutritional status or laboratory values. Go to https://nutritioncareincanada.ca/resources-and-tools/hospital-care-inpac/assessment-sga for further information on the SGA.

Nutritional Assessment

A nutritional assessment is a comprehensive evaluation of a patient's nutritional status. It typically includes data collection in the following areas: demographic and psychosocial data, medical history, dietary history, anthropometrics, drugs and laboratory values, and a physical assessment. Nutritional assessment may be performed because of an identified risk on a nutritional screening or when the risk status is obvious without a preliminary screening. The American Society for Parenteral and Enteral Nutrition (ASPEN) published standards that identify nutritionally-at-risk patients (Mueller et al, 2011) (Box 7.1). ASPEN also identified the goals of a nutritional assessment as follows:

- Establishing baseline subjective and objective nutrition parameters
- Identifying specific nutritional deficits
- Determining nutritional risk factors
- Establishing nutritional needs
- Identifying medical and psychosocial factors that may influence the prescription and administration of nutritional support

> **BOX 7.1 Nutritionally-at-Risk Adults**
>
> - Involuntary loss of ≥10% usual body weight within 6 months, or involuntary loss of ≥ 5% or more of usual body weight in 1 month
> - Involuntary loss or gain of 10 pounds within 6 months
> - BMI <18.5 kg/m^2
> - Increased metabolic requirements
> - Altered diets or diet schedules
> - Inadequate nutrition intake, including not receiving food or nutrition products for >7 days

Sources: Blackburn, G. L., Bistrian, B. R., Maini, B. S., Schlamm, H. T., & Smith, M. F. (1977). Nutritional and metabolic assessment of the hospitalized patient. *JPEN. Journal of Parenteral and Enteral Nutrition, 1,* 11–22.; White, J. V., Dwyer, J. T., Posner, B. M., Ham, R. J., Lipschitz, D. A., & Wellman, N. S. (1992). Nutrition screening initiative: development and implementation of the public awareness checklist and screening tools. *Journal of the American Dietetic Association, 92,* 163–167; World Health Organization. BMI classification. Retrieved from http://apps.who.int/bmi/index.jsp?introPage=intro_3.html. Accessed April 11, 2015; Braunschweig, C. L., Levy, P., Sheehan, P. M., & Wang, X. (2001). Enteral compared with parenteral nutrition: A meta-analysis. *American Journal of Clinical Nutrition, 74,* 534–542; In: Robinson, D., Walker R., Adams, S. C., Allen, K., Arnold, M. A., Bechtold, M., et al. (2018). American Society for Parenteral and Enteral Nutrition (ASPEN) Definition of terms, style, and conventions used in ASPEN board of directors–approved documents. Silver Spring, MD: ASPEN.

- Setting goals for nutritional deficits; if applicable, set goals in areas of medical and psychologic factors to be worked on with an interdisciplinary team

Diet History

In addition to a complete history and physical assessment, patients at nutritional risk require a more specific evaluation of their dietary intake patterns. Information that is typically part of a diet history includes the number of meals and snacks per day; chewing or swallowing difficulties; GI problems or symptoms that affect eating; oral health and denture use; history of diseases or surgery; activity level; use of drugs; appetite; need for assistance with meals and meal preparation; and food preferences, allergies, and aversions.

A diet history may also include a *food recall*. For accuracy and relevancy, the food recall must include specific information about the type of food ingested, the preparation method, and an accurate estimate of the amount. The patient should be asked to select days for recording his or her typical intake patterns. It is generally best to select two weekdays and one weekend day to record the best information on intake patterns. Patients should be instructed about how to estimate portion sizes and given samples from which to estimate their intake (e.g., 3 ounces [oz] of meat is the size of a pack of cards; a serving of vegetables is usually half a cup). Using food models or large, specific, and detailed pictures of food category serving sizes may be very helpful as the typical consumer is unfamiliar with standard serving portions. The purpose of the food recall is to estimate the average number of calories and amount of protein ingested daily and to detect any deleterious food intake patterns such as overusing fried foods or lack of vegetables or fruit. Some patients may need assistance from another person to complete the food recall.

For a more detailed picture of a patient's diet and food patterns, a 3- to 7-day food intake diary is obtained. Patients are asked to keep a detailed record of everything they eat, the time they eat, and the amount of each food item consumed. In addition to recording eating habits, patients are also asked to record activities and feelings, allowing the health-care professional to determine whether some emotional issues or activities may interfere with or enhance eating pleasure. Seven-day diet histories may help detect many behavioral issues in patients; however, many individuals have difficulty recording their food intake continuously.

Another way to assess dietary patterns is to look at food frequency. Food frequency questionnaires (FFQs) allow a health-care professional to assess a particular nutrient category, such as calcium, or the adequacy of an individual's entire diet. An FFQ is completed by a medical assistant or the patient during their wait in a health professional's office. FFQs are recommended for new patients because they allow the practitioner to collect reasonable dietary data without compromising the patient's privacy about food intake and diet.

Anthropometrics

Height and weight are the mainstays of anthropometric measurements. Ideally, the patient is weighed in the morning while wearing light clothing. Height is measured, if possible. For patients who are unable to stand without assistance, height may be estimated by measuring the distance from the heel to the top of the knee (knee height) with a broad-bladed caliper. Additional information and instructions on using a broad-bladed caliper and then estimating height using the following formula can be found at https://www.rxkinetics.com/height_estimate.html.

Females
Height in cm = $84.88 - (0.24 \times age) + (1.83 \times knee\ height)$

Males
Height in cm = $64.19 - (0.04 \times age) + (2.02 \times knee\ height)$

Measuring body surface area may help detect those who are overweight or underweight for their height. BMI can be used to determine body fat (BF) levels, with a BMI <18.5 kg/m² indicating underweight and an increased risk for mortality (Klatsky et al, 2017). However, in older adults, BMI may not be accurate in that height measurement may not be accurate secondary to physical changes related to aging.

Other anthropometric measurements include triceps skinfold (TSF) and mid-upper arm muscle circumference (MUAC). These measurements are of limited value when measured only one time. The MUAC is measured using a tape measure placed snugly against the skin at the midpoint of the distance between the tip of the acromial process of the scapula and the olecranon process of the ulna. MUAC was found to be a predictor of mortality in nursing-home residents.

TSF is measured at the midpoint between the acromion process and the olecranon process of the upper arm using a skinfold caliper. An average of at least three measurements is used to ensure accuracy. Nutritional depletion is defined as a skinfold measure of <11.3 mm in females and <4.3 mm in males (Burr and Phillips, 1984).

Another fast, noninvasive, and highly accurate method for assessing lean tissue and bone mass is dual-energy x-ray absorptiometry (DXA). These scanning devices allow the practitioner to evaluate not only bone density at several sites but also evaluate BF in a minimum amount of time (generally less than 20 minutes) with minimum radiation exposure (rem; less than 5 millirem [mrem]) (DXA, Hologic, Inc., Bedford, MA). The advantage of a DXA scan is that the patient can obtain a more reliable picture of his or her body composition (BF versus lean body mass) compared with anthropometric measurement. The disadvantage of DXA scanning is that the patient must be mobile; however, newer models that allow portability into homes and senior centers are now on the market.

Laboratory Values

No single laboratory test is diagnostic of malnutrition. Several tests that reflect protein synthesis may also reflect nutritional status. Serum albumin is the serum protein most frequently cited about malnutrition; it reflects the liver's ability to synthesize plasma protein. Albumin has a half-life of about 21 days, so it does not always reflect current nutritional status. Albumin values may also be affected by immune status and hydration. Given these limitations, albumin levels below 3.5 grams per deciliter (g/dL) may indicate some degree of malnutrition.

Transferrin is a carrier protein for iron and has a shorter half-life of 8 to 10 days. It is a more rapid predictor of protein depletion. Levels below 200 milligrams per deciliter (mg/dL) may indicate mild to moderate depletion, respectively. Levels below 100 mg/dL may indicate severe depletion.

Prealbumin (PAB) is a retinol-binding protein carrier protein with a half-life of 2 to 3 days. It is sensitive to sudden demands on protein synthesis and is often used in the acute-care setting. PAB levels that range from 15 mg/dL to 5 mg/dL reflect mild to moderate protein depletion. Levels below 5 mg/dL are considered reflective of severe protein depletion. Total lymphocyte count (TLC) is sometimes used as a nutritional marker. In severe or prolonged malnutrition, immune proteins are depleted, and the TLC is decreased.

PATIENT PROBLEMS ASSOCIATED WITH NUTRITIONAL PROBLEMS

Patient problems are derived from assessing the patient during a comprehensive health history and physical examination, during a patient interview, or while carrying out nursing interventions. The patient's problems subsequently become the basis for the plan of care and goals for nursing care. Box 7.2 lists patient problems associated with a primary nutritional problem and diagnoses that commonly have a nutritional component.

EVIDENCE-BASED STRATEGIES TO IMPROVE NUTRITION

Alterations in nutrition require a plan of care that specifically addresses the nutritional problem. Nursing interventions related to nutrition include instruction and counseling regarding a diet adequate in a specific nutrient or nutrients, calories, and

> **BOX 7.2 Patient Problems Associated With Nutritional Problems**
>
> **Primary Nutritional Problem**
> - Intake, restricted calorie
> - Intake, excessive calorie
> - Weight loss
> - Weight gain
>
> **Nutritional Component**
> - Electrolyte abnormalities
> - Potential for aspiration
> - Diarrhea
> - Dehydration
> - Diminished swallowing
> - Impaired ability to feed self
> - Potential for diminished GI motility

fluids. Therapeutic diets have been modified to include more or less than the recommended amounts for a specific nutrient or nutrients. They are usually prescribed to manage or treat a chronic disease or illness. Therapeutic diets include those restricted in sodium, protein, cholesterol, total calories, fat, or gluten. Therapeutic diets also may include modifications in the texture of foods, such as a low-fiber or high-fiber diet, mechanical soft diet, pureed diet, or clear liquid diet. Finally, therapeutic diets may include specialized nutrition such as parenteral nutrition, enteral tube feeding, or oral supplements.

Oral supplements are often prescribed for patients unable to ingest adequate protein or calories because of early satiety or fatigue during eating. By adding a concentrated liquid oral supplement to the meal plan, the patient may improve protein or overall caloric intake. However, food consumption is always preferable to meal replacement or supplementation. If this is not possible, between-meal snacks of liquid caloric supplements can increase energy intake (Morley, 2011a). Commercial oral supplements are available at most pharmacies and grocery stores without a prescription. Additionally, supplements are available as soups, nutrient bars, and smoothies.

Components of a Healthy Diet

The United States Department of Agriculture's MyPlate method (USDA, https://www.myplate.gov/life-stages/older-adults) is an illustrative tool for demonstrating what constitutes a healthy diet and appropriate portion size. The USDA MyPlate (Fig. 7.1) divides a plate into quarters, with one-fourth for grains, one-fourth for protein, and the remaining half for vegetables and fruits. Older adults not eating close to these estimations should be advised that their nutrient intake might be inadequate, and action needs to be taken (Crogan, 2018).

In collaboration with the USDA, the Department of Health and Human Services (HHS) compiles and publishes nutritional guidelines every 5 years. The most recent guidelines were published in 2020 (USDA, 2020). The guidelines fit within five broad categories:

- Eat a variety of nutrient-dense foods and manage portion sizes
- Shift current food and drink choices to healthier alternatives
- Maintain a healthy diet throughout your life

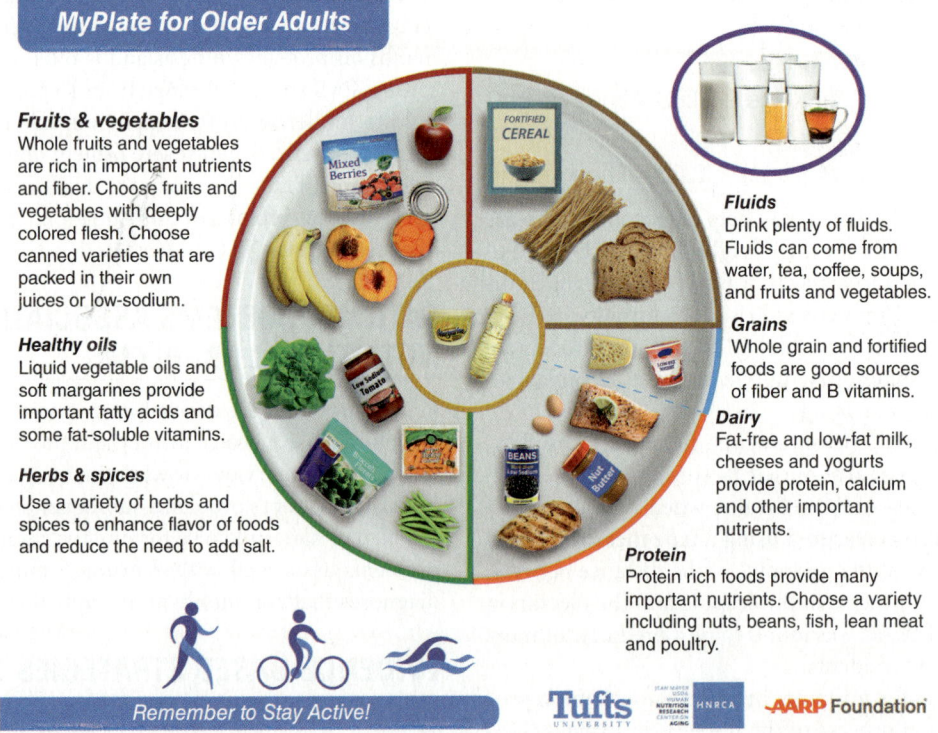

Fig. 7.1 MyPlate for Older Adults. ("My Plate for Older Adults" Copyright 2016 Tufts University, all rights reserved. "My Plate for Older Adults" graphic and accompanying website were developed with support from the AARP Foundation. "Tufts University" and "AARP Foundation" are registered trademarks and may not be reproduced apart from their inclusion in the "My Plate for Older Adults" graphic without express permission from their respective owners.)

- Limit caloric intake from added sugars and saturated fats, and reduce intake of sodium
- Support others in healthy eating

The guidelines pertain to all Americans. A healthy person should eat a variety of vegetables, fruits (preferably whole fruits), grains (half of which should be whole grains), fat-free or low-fat dairy, protein from various sources, and a limited amount of oils. Caffeinated drinks are limited to three to five 8-ounce cups of coffee daily.

Even though older adults' nutritional requirements are generally similar to those of the rest of the population, they can become more difficult to meet because of the physiologic, psychological, and social changes associated with older age. The nurse can be instrumental in encouraging older adults to eat a well-balanced diet, which can affect their overall health, independence, and QoL.

Dysphagia

Dysphagia is prevalent in older adults (Doan et al, 2022). About 30% of community-dwelling elderly, almost 50% of hospitalized older adults, and more than 50% of nursing-home residents are affected by some form of dysphagia. Dysphagia often affects nutritional status and may occur because of a cerebrovascular accident (CVA), oral or neck cancer treatment, or a neuromuscular or neurologic disorder. Dysphagia is usually identified as either oropharyngeal or esophageal, designating the phase in which the dysfunction occurs. In the oropharyngeal phase, food is chewed and mixed with saliva and then is moved posteriorly, triggering the pharyngeal swallow reflex. This triggering moves the bolus down the pharynx. During the pharyngeal swallow, the larynx closes, and the epiglottis redirects the bolus around the airway, protecting the respiratory tract. The esophageal phase begins when the bolus enters the esophagus at the cricopharyngeal juncture or upper esophageal sphincter. Peristaltic waves propel the bolus through the esophagus to the stomach (National Institute on Deafness and Other Communication Disorders [NIDCD], 2010). Because swallowing is a complex voluntary/involuntary event, the specific etiologies of dysphagia are multiple and diverse. The nurse plays a pivotal role in the early detection of swallowing problems to prevent complications from dysphagia, such as aspiration.

A videofluoroscopic swallowing study (VFSS) is the gold standard for detecting aspiration. Roughly 50% of older adults with dysphagia experience aspiration. Nearly 60% experience silent aspiration, where solids or liquids aspirate into the airways, but the person does not cough or experience shortness of breath due to an impaired cough reflex. Older adults who experience silent aspiration are at increased risk for respiratory infection, aspiration pneumonia, and death (Chen et al, 2021).

Depending on the type of dysphagia, the speech and language therapist (SLT) or occupational therapist (OT) will develop specific recommendations for care. Correct positioning while eating is paramount for safe eating and swallowing. To prevent aspiration, an upright position with the arms and feet supported, the head midline in a neutral position, and the chin slightly tucked is recommended. The upright position should be maintained for at least 30 minutes after eating (Gillen, 2016).

In 2019, the Academy of Nutrition and Dietetics (AND), the Association of Nutrition and Foodservice Professionals (ANFP), and the American Speech-Language-Hearing Association (ASHA) adopted the International Dysphagia Diet Standardization Initiative (IDDSI) framework to standardize terminology and definitions for texture-modified and thickened liquids to improve the safety and care of persons with dysphagia. Table 7.2 identifies the type of diet and provides a description and rationale for using the specific diet.

TABLE 7.2 Food Texture Modifications for Dysphagia

Food Level	Description/Characteristics	Physiologic Rationale for Level of Thickness
0 = Thin	Flows like water Fast flow Can drink through any type of cup or straw as appropriate for age and skills	Functional ability to safely manage liquids of all types
1 = Slightly thick	Thicker than water Requires a little more effort to drink than thin liquids Flows through a straw or syringe	Used in adult populations where thin drinks flow too fast to be controlled safely, these slightly thick liquids will flow at a slightly slower rate
2 = Mildly thick	Flows off a spoon Sippable, pours quickly from a spoon, but slower than thin drinks Mild effort is required to drink this thickness through standard bore straw (standard bore straw = 0.209 inch or 5.3 mm diameter)	If thin drinks flow too fast to be controlled safely, these mildly thick liquids will flow at a slightly slower rate May be suitable if tongue control is slightly reduced
3 = Liquidized, moderately thick	Can be drunk from a cup Moderate effort is required to suck through a standard bore or wide bore straw (wide bore straw = 0.275 inch or 6.9 mm) Cannot be piped, layered, or molded on a plate because it will not retain its shape Cannot be eaten with a fork because it drips slowly in dollops through the prongs Can be eaten with a spoon No oral processing or chewing required – can be swallowed directly Smooth texture with no "bits" (lumps, fibers, bits of shell or skin, husk, particles of gristle or bone)	If tongue control is insufficient to manage mildly thick drinks (Level 2), this liquidized/moderately thick level may be suitable Allows more time for oral control Needs some tongue propulsion effort Pain on swallowing

Continued

TABLE 7.2 Food Texture Modifications for Dysphagia—cont'd

Food Level	Description/Characteristics	Physiologic Rationale for Level of Thickness
4 = Pureed, extremely thick	Usually eaten with a spoon (a fork is possible) Cannot be drunk from a cup because it does not flow easily Cannot be sucked through a straw Does not require chewing Can be piped, layered, or molded because it retains its shape, but should not require chewing if presented in this form Shows some very slow movement under gravity but cannot be poured Falls off spoon in a single spoonful when tilted and continues to hold shape on a plate No lumps Not sticky Liquid must not separate from solid	If tongue control is significantly reduced, this category may be easiest to control Requires less propulsion effort than minced and moist (level 5), soft and bite-sized (Level 6), and regular easy to chew (Level 7) but more than liquidized/moderately thick (Level 3) No biting or chewing is required Increased oral and/or pharyngeal residue is a risk if too sticky Any food that requires chewing, controlled manipulation, or bolus formation are not suitable Pain on chewing or swallowing Missing teeth, poorly fitting dentures
5 = Minced and Moist	Can be eaten with a fork or spoon Can be eaten with chopsticks in some cases, if the individual has very good hand control Can be scooped and shaped (e.g., into a ball shape) on a plate Soft and moist with no separate thin liquid Small lumps visible within the food Adult, ≤4 mm width and no longer than 15 mm in length Lumps are easy to squash with tongue	Biting is not required Minimal chewing is required Tongue force alone can be used to separate the soft small particles in this texture Tongue force is required to move the bolus Pain or fatigue on chewing Missing teeth, poorly fitting dentures
6 = Soft and bite-sized	Can be eaten with a fork, spoon, or chopsticks Can be mashed/broken down with pressure from fork, spoon, or chopsticks A knife is not required to cut this food but may be used to help load a fork or spoon Soft, tender, and moist throughout but with no separate, thin liquid Chewing is required before swallowing "Bite-sized" pieces as appropriate for size and oral processing skills Adults, 15 mm = 1.5 cm pieces (no larger than)	Biting is not required Chewing is required Food piece sizes designed to minimize choking risk Tongue force and control is required to move the food and keep it within the mouth for chewing and oral processing Tongue force is required to move the bolus for swallowing Pain or fatigue on chewing Missing teeth, poorly fitting dentures
7 = Easy to chew	Normal, everyday foods of soft/tender textures that are developmentally and age appropriate Any method may be used to eat these foods Sample size is not restricted at Level 7; therefore, foods may be of a range of sizes Smaller or greater than 15 mm = 1.5 cm pieces (adults) Does not include: hard, tough, chewy, fibrous, stringy, crunchy, or crumbly bits, pips, seeds, fibrous parts of fruit, husks, or bones May include "dual consistency" or "mixed consistency" foods and liquids if also safe for Level 0, and at clinician discretion; if unsafe for Level 0 thin, liquid portion can be thickened to clinician's recommended thickness level	Requires the ability to bite soft foods and chew and orally process food for long enough that the person forms a soft, cohesive ball/bolus that is "swallow ready" Does not necessarily require teeth Requires the ability to chew and orally process soft/tender foods without tiring easily May be suitable for people who find hard and/or chewy foods difficult or painful to chew and swallow This level could present a choking risk for people with clinically identified increased risk of choking because food pieces can be of any size Restricting food piece sizes aims to minimize choking risk (e.g., Level 4 pureed, Level 5 minced and moist, Level 6 soft and bite-sized have food piece size restrictions to minimize choking risk) This level may be used by qualified clinicians for developmental teaching, or progression to foods that need more advanced chewing skills If the person needs supervision to eat safely, before using this texture level consult a qualified clinician to determine the person's food texture needs and meal time plan for safety People can be unsafe to eat without supervision due to chewing and swallowing problems and/or unsafe mealtime behaviors; examples of unsafe mealtime behaviors include not chewing very well, putting too much food into the mouth, eating too fast or swallowing large mouthfuls of food, and inability to self-monitor chewing ability; clinicians should be consulted for specific advice for patient needs, requests, and requirements for supervision Where mealtime supervision is needed, this level should only be used under the strict recommendation and written guidance of a qualified clinician

TABLE 7.2   Food Texture Modifications for Dysphagia—cont'd

Food Level	Description/Characteristics	Physiologic Rationale for Level of Thickness
7 = Regular	Normal, everyday foods of various textures that are developmentally and age appropriate Any method may be used to eat these foods Foods may be hard and crunchy or naturally soft Sample size is not restricted at Level 7; therefore, foods may be of a range of sizes ≥15 mm = 1.5 cm pieces (adults) Includes hard, tough, chewy, fibrous, stringy, dry, crispy, crunchy, or crumbly bits Includes food that contains pips, seeds, pith inside skin, husks, or bones Includes "dual consistency" or "mixed consistency" foods and liquids	Ability to bite hard or soft foods and chew them for long enough that they form a soft, cohesive ball/bolus that is "swallow ready" An ability to chew all food textures without tiring easily An ability to remove bone or gristle that cannot be swallowed safely from the mouth
Transitional foods (Levels 5, 6, and 7)	Food that starts as one texture (e.g., firm solid) and changes into another texture specifically when moisture (e.g., water or saliva) is applied, or when a change in temperature occurs (e.g., heating)	Biting not required Minimal chewing required Tongue can be used to break these foods once altered by temperature or with addition of moisture/saliva May be used for developmental teaching or rehabilitation of chewing skills (e.g., rehabilitation of chewing function post stroke)

Note: **Only information related to adults is provided.** The IDDSI Framework and Descriptors are licensed under the Creative Commons Attribution-Sharealike 4.0 International License https://creativecommons.org/licenses/by-sa/4.0/IDDSI 2.0 | July, 2019.
Disclaimer: Although descriptions are provided, use IDDSI Testing methods to decide if the food meets IDDSI Level. See *IDDSI Testing Methods* document or https://iddsi.org/framework/food-testing-methods/.
Data from the International Dysphagia Diet Standardisation Initiative (IDDSI). (2019). *IDDSI Framework and Descriptors 2.0*. Retrieved from https://iddsi.org/framework/food-testing-methods/.

BOX 7.3   The Utility of Tube Feedings in End-Stage Renal Disease

Nasogastric Tube (NG)
- For short-term use or short-term life expectancy
- Dysphagia secondary to:
  - CVA
  - Tumors obstructing swallowing
  - Inflammatory masses
  - Drug irritation
  - Gastric esophageal reflux disease (GERD)
- Significant change of condition secondary to infection, delirium

Percutaneous Endoscopic Gastrostomy (PEG)
- For long-term use or life expectancy >6 months
- Chronic neurologic causes: MS, ALS, Parkinson disease, traumatic brain injury (TBI)
- Weight loss of aging, anorexia
- Severe dysphagia, unable to swallow safely
- Cognitively impaired, dementia

Feeding Tubes and Advanced Dementia
When eating difficulties occur in older adults with advanced dementia, the American Geriatrics Society (2014) does not recommend the use of feeding tubes. Instead, careful hand-feeding should be offered with a patient-centered approach. Previous expressed wishes and an individual's surrogate decision-maker should be considered in any decisions regarding tube feeding. Often, families are concerned they will starve their loved one if they fail to place a feeding tube. Nursing homes, hospitals, and other care settings should promote shared and informed decision-making and honor preferences concerning tube feeding, as religious beliefs, cultural background, and ethnicity all play a role in the decision to place a tube for feeding (Ijaopo & Ijaopo, 2019).

The best available evidence concerning long-term placement of tube feedings indicates there is no beneficial effect on nutritional outcomes or healing of pressure injuries or other wounds. There is no improvement in overall well-being as the person with tube feeding is deprived of the joy of eating and the socialization associated with meals. The risk for aspiration pneumonia is not reduced with feeding tube placement; in fact, some studies indicate the risk for aspiration and death is twice as likely to occur in persons with tube feeding as opposed to those with careful hand-feeding (Ijaopo & Ijaopo, 2019). Finally, Ijaopo and Ijaopo (2019) reported that many nursing-home residents who had a feeding tube placed pulled it out within two weeks of insertion, resulting in hospitalization and replacement.

Specialized Nutritional Support

Specialized nutrition is used when a patient cannot ingest, digest, or absorb nutrients. The decision to initiate an enteral tube feeding is a complicated, collaborative decision made by the patient, health-care provider, and family or surrogate. Common indications for enteral tube feeding include conditions where a patient cannot swallow foods, for example, following a CVA or with myasthenia gravis, amyotrophic lateral sclerosis (ALS), and multiple sclerosis (MS) (Box 7.3).

Enteral nutrition is also used when the upper GI tract is obstructed, as in cancer or severe congenital esophageal stenosis. A feeding tube is placed below the area of obstruction; feeding tubes may be placed into the stomach or the intestine. The tubes are placed through the nose (nasogastric or nasointestinal), directly into the stomach (gastrostomy, PEG, or radiology-assisted gastrostomy), or directly into the jejunum (jejunostomy or percutaneous endoscopic jejunostomy).

Enteral formulas include standard (whole protein and complex carbohydrate), modified protein (peptide), and elemental (amino acid) formulas. Some enteral formulas have added soluble or insoluble fiber. Disease-specific formulas are also available for the dietary treatment of diseases, for example, reduced protein for patients receiving renal dialysis, increased lipid percentage of total calories for patients with diabetes and pulmonary disease, and increased percentage of branched-chain amino acids for patients with hepatic disease. Specialized enteral formulas are considerably more expensive than standard formulas and should be used only when indicated. Short-term enteral feeding is often used after surgery, traumatic injury, and burns.

Parenteral nutrition consists of an intravenous (IV) solution that includes dextrose, amino acids, vitamins, minerals, electrolytes, trace elements, and water. A lipid emulsion is commonly added to produce a total nutrient admixture but may be given by separate infusion. The dextrose and lipids provide calories to support metabolic needs, whereas amino acids are administered to meet daily protein requirements.

Parenteral nutrition is indicated when the GI tract cannot be used for enteral feeding or cannot absorb adequate nutrients to maintain health. Diseases and conditions typically associated with the need for parenteral nutrition include severe inflammatory bowel disease, fistula, acute pancreatitis, and massive bowel resection. Parenteral nutrition is administered through a vascular access device such as a central venous catheter, tunneled catheter, peripherally inserted central catheter, or implanted port. Most parenteral nutrition solutions are hypertonic and must be administered into a large central vein.

Patients receive enteral and parenteral nutrition in various health-care settings or at home. Nurses educate home-care patients about the use and care of their access devices, administration of the enteral formula or parenteral solution, use of an enteral or IV pump, management of common problems associated with specialized feeding, and signs and symptoms of complications. Although specialized nutrition is prescribed to patients of all ages, a large percentage of the patients who receive enteral tube feeding and parenteral nutrition are older adults (Box 7.4).

> **BOX 7.4 Evidence-Based Prevention: Can Nutritional Interventions Aid in the Prevention of Dementia?**
>
> It is estimated the world's population of persons living with dementia will increase to 152.8 million cases by 2050. Because no treatment or cure is known to affect the course of dementia, identifying risk factors, and implementing prevention strategies are current objectives. Modifiable risks affecting vascular health include physical inactivity, smoking, hypertension, diabetes, and obesity (GBD 2019 Dementia Forecasting Collaborators, 2022). Interestingly, adherence to a healthy diet appears to delay cognitive decline and positively affects brain function. The Mediterranean diet includes whole grains, fruit, vegetables, nuts, seeds, olives, legumes, and more fish and seafood than poultry, dairy, or eggs, and low consumption of red meat. Olive oil is the main source of fat, and moderate wine intake is allowed (Jennings et al, 2020). Researchers have linked the Mediterranean diet with lower risk for cognitive decline and beneficial effects on global cognition in middle-aged and elderly individuals who are cognitively healthy (Jennings et al, 2020; Limongi et al, 2020; Rodrigues et al, 2020).

SUMMARY

Malnutrition in older adults is often unrecognized, and its prevalence increases with age. Targeting modifiable factors will be crucial to effective treatment and prevention of malnutrition. Nurses must understand the role of vitamins and mineral supplements in their patients' overall diets to get a clear picture of their health and pharmaceutical history.

The older adult population is increasingly becoming a larger percentage of the total population, and the percentage of older adults will peak around 2030 with the aging of the Baby Boomer generation. Malnutrition is detected through nutritional screening and nutritional assessment. Anthropometrics, diet history, and laboratory studies are components of nutritional assessment. Specialized nutrition therapies such as parenteral nutrition and enteral tube feeding may nourish patients unable to ingest, digest, or absorb nutrients. The nurse and the interdisciplinary team play an important role in identifying alterations in nutrition and developing nursing interventions that restore nutritional adequacy. The nurse collaborates with the physician, nurse practitioner, dietitian, pharmacist, and other health-care team members to promote the patient's nutritional health.

KEY POINTS

- Malnutrition in older adults is often unrecognized, and the prevalence increases with age.
- Poverty is the most significant cause of weight loss and malnutrition in older adults.
- The interactions between drugs and nutrients may affect drug metabolism, absorption, digestion, or excretion.
- Older adults are at a greater risk of dehydration due to several factors, including an age-related decrease in sensitivity to thirst, a decrease in TBW resulting in an increased risk for dehydration with small changes in fluid intake, diminished kidney function, which causes the kidneys to be less effective at conserving BW, exposure to prescription drugs which

- affect BW, and mobility problems which affect the ability to obtain fluids.
- Micronutrients, such as vitamin D, calcium, and B_{12}, are commonly found to be deficient in older adults.
- Despite the availability of many validated nutritional screening tools, malnutrition often remains undiagnosed and can lead to prolonged hospital stays, frequent readmissions, and an increase in morbidity and mortality.
- Poor oral health in older adults is linked to protracted states of suffering and pain and functional, nutritional, aesthetic, and psychologic issues.
- Nutritional screening is an abbreviated assessment of nutritional risk factors that identifies patients needing a more comprehensive assessment and nutritional interventions.
- A nutritional assessment is a comprehensive evaluation of a patient's nutritional status. It typically includes data collection in the following areas: demographic and psychosocial data, medical history, dietary history, anthropometrics, drugs and laboratory values, and a physical assessment.
- Weight loss is considered clinically significant when there is involuntary loss of 10% or more of usual body weight within 6 months, or involuntary loss of ≥5% or more of usual body weight in 1 month; involuntary loss or gain of 10 pounds within 6 months; BMI less than 18.5 kg/m^2 or greater than 25 kg/m^2.
- In addition to a complete history and physical assessment, patients at nutritional risk require a more specific evaluation of their dietary intake patterns. Information that is typically part of a diet history includes the number of meals and snacks per day; chewing or swallowing difficulties; gastrointestinal problems or symptoms that affect eating; oral health and denture use; history of diseases or surgery; activity level; use of drugs; appetite; need for assistance with meals and meal preparation; and food preferences, allergies, and aversions.
- Height and weight are the mainstays of anthropometric measurements.
- No single laboratory test is diagnostic of malnutrition. Several tests that reflect protein synthesis may also reflect nutritional status.
- Even though older adults' nutritional requirements are generally similar to those of the rest of the population, they can become more difficult to meet because of the physiologic, psychologic, and social changes associated with older age. The nurse can be instrumental in encouraging older adults to eat a well-balanced diet, which can affect their overall health, independence, and QoL.
- Dysphagia is a problem that often affects nutritional status and may occur because of a CVA, oral or neck cancer treatment, or a neuromuscular or neurologic disorder.
- In 2019, the AND, the ANFP, and the ASHA adopted the IDDSI framework to standardize terminology and definitions for texture-modified and thickened liquids and improve the safety and care of persons with dysphagia.
- Specialized nutrition is used when a patient cannot ingest, digest, or absorb nutrients. The decision to initiate an enteral tube feeding is a complicated, collaborative decision made by the patient, health-care provider, and family or surrogate.
- Nurses have the opportunity and responsibility to assess nutritional status and should collaborate with other health-care team members to formulate a comprehensive and coordinated nutritional care plan.

CLINICAL JUDGMENT EXERCISES

1. A 68-year-old with COPD has been referred to home-health nursing services for medication instruction and respiratory assessment. During the nurse's first visit, the following information is obtained: overweight for height by about 30 pounds, weight loss of 10 pounds over the past 2 months, reports shortness of breath while eating, and unable to get to the grocery store (relies on a neighbor for assistance). How would this information relate to developing a nursing plan of care?
2. An 80-year-old who is 5 foot, 4 inches tall, weighs 152 pounds, and is in generally good health records the following 24-hour intake:

   Breakfast: 1 glass orange juice, 2 slices whole wheat toast, 1 tablespoon butter
   Lunch: ½ cup cottage cheese, 1 bag cheese curls, ½ peanut butter and jelly sandwich, 1 cup tea
   Dinner: 1 cup wheat flakes cereal, ½ cup skim milk
   Snack: 1 candy bar, 1 cup ice cream

   Analyze this patient's diet. What conclusions, if any, can be made about dietary status based on this 24-hour recall?
3. A 72-year-old is a practicing vegetarian who does not eat fish but does eat eggs. The person's health-care provider has recommended an increased intake of protein. What recommendations can the nurse offer?

REFERENCES

American Geriatrics Society Ethics Committee and Clinical Practice and Models of Care Committee. (2014). American Geriatrics Society feeding tubes in advanced dementia position statement. *Journal of the American Geriatrics Society, 62*(8), 1590–1593. doi:10.1111/jgs.12924.

Bakhtiari, A., Pourali, M., & Omidvar, S. (2020). Nutrition assessment and geriatric associated conditions among community dwelling Iranian elderly people. *BMC Geriatrics, 20*(1), 278. doi:10.1186/s12877-020-01668-8.

Barichella, M., Cereda, E., Cassani, E., Pinelli, G., Iorio, L., Ferri, V., et al. (2017). Dietary habits and neurological features of Parkinson's disease patients: Implications for practice. *Clinical Nutrition, 36*(4), 1054–1061. doi:10.1016/j.clnu.2016.06.020.

Becker, N., Hafner, T., Pishnamaz, M., Hildebrand, F., & Kobbe, P. (2022). Patient-specific risk factors for adverse outcomes following geriatric proximal femur fractures. *European Journal of Trauma and Emergency Surgery, 48*(2), 753–761.

Becker, N., Hafner, T., Pishnamaz, M., Hildebrand, F., & Kobbe, P. (2022). Patient-specific risk factors for adverse outcomes following geriatric proximal femur fractures. *European Journal of Trauma and Emergency Surgery, 48*(2), 753–761.

Besora-Moreno, M., Llauradó, E., Tarro, L., & Solà, R. (2020). Social and economic factors and malnutrition or the risk of malnutrition in the elderly: A systematic review and meta-analysis of observational studies. *Nutrients, 12*(3), 737. doi:10.3390/nu12030737.

Brownie, S. (2013). Nutritional wellbeing for older people. *Journal of the Australian Traditional Medicine Society, 19*(3), 140–145.

Burr, M. L., & Phillips, K. M. (1984). Anthropometric norms in the elderly. *British Journal of Nutrition, 51*(2), 165–169. doi:10.1079/bjn19840020.

Burris, M., Kihlstrom, L., Arce, K. S., Prendergast, K., Dobbins, J., McGrath, E., et al. (2021). Food insecurity, loneliness, and social support among older adults. *Journal of Hunger & Environmental Nutrition, 16*(1), 29–44. doi:10.1080/19320248.2019.1595253.

Chalcraft, J. R., Cardinal, L. M., Wechsler, P. J., Hollis, B. W., Gerow, K. G., Alexander, B. M., et al. (2020). Vitamin D synthesis following a single bout of sun exposure in older and younger men and women. *Nutrients, 12*(8), 2237. doi:10.3390/nu12082237.

Chen, S., Kent, B., & Cui, Y. (2021). Interventions to prevent aspiration in older adults with dysphagia living in nursing homes: A scoping review. *BMC Geriatrics, 21*(1), 429. doi:10.1186/s12877-021-02366-9.

Coll, P. P., Lindsay, A., Meng, J., Gopalakrishna, A., Raghavendra, S., Bysani, P., et al. (2020). The prevention of infections in older adults: Oral health. *Journal of the American Geriatrics Society, 68*(2), 411–416. doi:10.1111/jgs.16154.

Crogan, N. L. (2017). Nutritional problems affecting older adults. *Nursing Clinics of North America, 52*(3), 433–445. doi:10.1016/j.cnur.2017.04.005.

Crogan, N. L. (2018). Dysphagia and malnutrition. In K. Mauk (Ed.), *Gerontological nursing: Competencies for care* (4th ed., pp. 577–600). Burlington, MA: Jones & Bartlett.

Davies, N. (2011). Promoting health ageing: The importance of lifestyle. *Nursing Standard, 25*(19), 43–50. doi:10.7748/ns2011.01.25.19.43.c8270.

De Stefani, F., Pietraroia, P. S., Fernandes-Silva, M. M., Faria-Neto, J., & Baena, C. P. (2018). Observational evidence for unintentional weight loss in all-cause mortality and major cardiovascular events: A systematic review and meta-analysis. *Scientific Reports, 8*(1), 15447. doi:10.1038/s41598-018-33563-z.

Doan, T. N., Ho, W. C., Wang, L. H., Chang, F. C., Nhu, N. T., & Chou, L. W. (2022). Prevalence and methods for assessment of oropharyngeal dysphagia in older adults: A systematic review and meta-analysis. *Journal of Clinical Medicine, 11*(9), 2605. doi:10.3390/jcm11092605.

Docherty, N. G., Delles, C., D'Haese, P., Layton, A. T., Martínez-Salgado, C., Vervaet, B. A., et al. (2021). Haemodynamic frailty - A risk factor for acute kidney injury in the elderly. *Ageing Research Reviews, 70*, 101408. doi:10.1016/j.arr.2021.101408.

Edmonds, C. J., Foglia, E., Booth, P., Fu, C. H. Y., & Gardner, M. (2021). Dehydration in older people: A systematic review of the effects of dehydration on health outcomes, healthcare costs and cognitive performance. *Archives of Gerontology and Geriatrics, 95*, 104380. doi:10.1016/j.archger.2021.104380.

Gaddey, H. L., & Holder, K. K. (2021). Unintentional weight loss in older adults. *American Family Physician, 104*(1), 34–40.

GBD 2019 Dementia Forecasting Collaborators. (2022). Estimation of the global prevalence of dementia in 2019 and forecasted prevalence in 2050: An analysis for the Global Burden of Disease Study 2019. *The Lancet Public Health, 7*(2), e105–e125. doi:10.1016/S2468-2667(21)00249-8.

Gillen, G. (2016). *Stroke rehabilitation: A function-based approach* (4th ed.). St. Louis: Elsevier.

Greene, G. W., Lofgren, I., Paulin, C., Greaney, M. L., & Clark, P. G. (2018). Differences in psychosocial and behavioral variables by dietary screening tool risk category in older adults. *Journal of the Academy of Nutrition and Dietetics, 118*(1), 110–117. doi:10.1016/j.jand.2017.06.365.

Ijaopo, E. O., & Ijaopo, R. O. (2019). Tube feeding in individuals with advanced dementia: A review of its burdens and perceived benefits. *Journal of Aging Research, 2019*, 7272067. doi:10.1155/2019/7272067.

Isautier, J. M. J., Bosni, M., Yeung, S. S. Y., Trappenburg, M. C., Meskers, C. G. M., Whittaker, A. C., et al. (2019). Validity of nutritional screening tools for community-dwelling older adults: A systematic review and meta-analysis. *Journal of the American Medical Directors Association, 20*(10), 1351.e13–1351.e25. doi:10.1016/j.jamda.2019.06.024.

Jennings, A., Mulligan, A. A., Khaw, K., Luben, R. N., & Welch, A. A. (2020). A Mediterranean diet is positively associated with bone and muscle health in a non-Mediterranean region in 25,450 men and women from EPIC-Norfolk. *Nutrients, 19*(4), 1154. doi:10.3390/nu12041154.

Khoury, C., Samot, J., Helmer, C., Rosa, R. W., Georget, A., Dartigues, J. F., et al. (2022). The association between oral health and nutritional status in older adults: a cross-sectional study. *BMC Geriatrics, 22*(1), 499. doi:10.1186/s12877-022-03133-0.

Klatsky, A. L., Zhang, J., Udaltsova, N., Li, Y., & Tran, H. N. (2017). Body mass index and mortality in a very large cohort: Is it really healthier to be overweight? *The Permanente Journal, 21*, 16–142. doi:10.7812/TPP/16-142.

Lacey, J., Corbett, J., Forni, L., Hooper, L., Hughes, F., Minto, G., et al. (2019). A multidisciplinary consensus on dehydration: Definitions, diagnostic methods and clinical implications. *Annals of Medicine, 51*(3-4), 232–251. doi:10.1080/07853890.2019.1628352.

Limongi, F., Siviero, P., Bozanic, A., Noale, M., Veronese, N., & Maggi, S. (2020). The effect of adherence to the Mediterranean diet on late-life cognitive disorders: A systematic review. *Journal of the American Medical Directors Association, 21*(10), 1402–1409. doi:10.1016/j.jamda.2020.08.020.

Mac Giolla Phadraig, C., Farag, M., McCallion, P., Waldron, C., & McCarron, M. (2020). The complexity of tooth brushing among older adults with intellectual disabilities: Findings from a nationally representative survey. *Disability and Health Journal, 13*(4), 100935. doi:10.1016/j.dhjo.2020.100935.

Mentes, J. (2006). Oral hydration in older adults: greater awareness is needed in preventing, recognizing, and treating dehydration. *American Journal of Nursing, 106*(6), 40–50. doi:10.1097/00000446-200606000-00023.

Morley, J. E. (2011a). Undernutrition: A major problem in nursing homes. *Journal of the American Medical Directors Association, 12*(4), 243–246. doi:10.1016/j.jamda.2011.02.013.

Morley, J. E. (2011b). Assessment of malnutrition in older persons: A focus on the Mini Nutritional Assessment. *The Journal of Nutrition, Health & Aging, 15*(2), 87–90. doi:10.1007/s12603-011-0018-4.

Mueller, C., Compher, C., Druyan, M. A., & American Society for Parenteral and Enteral Nutrition (A.S.P.E.N.) Board of Directors. (2011). A.S.P.E.N. clinical guidelines: Nutrition screening, assessment, and intervention in adults. *JPEN Journal of Parenteral and Enteral Nutrition, 35*(1), 16–24. doi:10.1177/0148607110389335.

National Council on Aging. (2023). *Get the facts on healthy aging*. NCOA. Retrieved from https://www.ncoa.org/article/get-the-facts-on-healthy-aging. Accessed July 31, 2023.

National Institute on Deafness and other Communication Disorders (NIDCD). (2010). *Dysphagia*. NIH Pub. No., 13–4307. U.S. Department of Health and Human Services, National Institutes of Health.

Norman, K., Haß, U., & Pirlich, M. (2021). Malnutrition in older adults—Recent advances and remaining challenges. *Nutrients, 13*(8), 2764. doi:10.3390/nu13082764.

Rashid, I., Tiwari, P., & Lehl, S. S. (2020). Malnutrition among elderly a multifactorial condition to flourish: Evidence from a cross-sectional study. *Clinical Epidemiology and Global Health, 8*(1), 91–95. doi:10.1016/j.cegh.2019.05.001.

Rodrigues, B., Asamane, E. A., Magalhães, R., Sousa, N., Thompson, J. L., & Santos, N. C. (2020). The association of dietary patterns with cognition through the lens of neuroimaging—a systematic review. *Ageing Research Reviews, 63*, 101145. doi:10.1016/j.arr.2020.101145.

Rolf, K., Santoro, A., Martucci, M., & Pietruszka, B. (2022). The association of nutrition quality with frailty syndrome among the elderly. *International Journal of Environmental Research and Public Health, 19*(6), 3379. doi:10.3390/ijerph19063379.

Schlanger, L. E., Bailey, J. L., & Sands, J. M. (2010). Electrolytes in the aging. *Advances in Chronic Kidney Disease, 17*(4), 308–319. doi:10.1053/j.ackd.2010.03.008.

Seifter, J. L., & Chang, H. Y. (2017). Extracellular acid-base balance and ion transport between body fluid compartments. *Physiology, 32*(5), 367–379. doi:10.1152/physiol.00007.2017.

Shalit, N., Tierney, A., Holland, A., Miller, B., Norris, N., & King, S. (2016). Factors that influence dietary intake in adults with stable chronic obstructive pulmonary disease. *Nutrition & Dietetics, 73*(5), 455–462. doi:10.1111/1747-0080.12266.

Spanemberg, J. C., Cardoso, J. A., Slob, E. M. G. B., & López-López, J. (2019). Quality of life related to oral health and its impact in adults. *Journal of Stomatology, Oral and Maxillofacial Surgery, 120*(3), 234–239. doi:10.1016/j.jormas.2019.02.004.

Storbeck, T., Qian, F., Marek, C., Caplan, D., & Marchini, L. (2022). Dose-dependent association between xerostomia and number of medications among older adults. *Special Care in Dentistry, 42*(3), 225–231. doi:10.1111/scd.12662.

U.S. Department of Agriculture (USDA). (2020). *Dietary guidelines for Americans 2020-2025*. Retrieved from https://www.dietaryguidelines.gov/sites/default/files/2020-12/Dietary_Guidelines_for_Americans_2020-2025.pdf. Accessed July 31, 2023.

Volicer, L., Seltzer, B., Rheaume, Y., Fabiszewski, K., Herz, L., Shapiro, R., et al. (1987). Progression of Alzheimer-type dementia in institutionalized patients: A cross-sectional study. *Journal of Applied Gerontology, 6*(1), 83–94. doi:10.1177/073346488700600107.

World Health Organization. (2022). *Ageing and health*. Retrieved from https://www.who.int/news-room/fact-sheets/detail/ageing-and-health. Accessed July 31, 2023.

8

Sleep and Activity

Chiquesha Davis, DNP, MSN, CMSRN, RN-BC

http://evolve.elsevier.com/Yeager/gerontologic/

LEARNING OBJECTIVES

On completion of this chapter, the reader will be able to:
1. Identify three age-related changes in sleep.
2. Describe the features of insomnia.
3. Discuss four factors influencing sleep in older adults.
4. Discuss two sleep disorders.
5. List four components of a sleep history.
6. Describe the effects of lifestyle changes on sleep and activity in older adults.
7. Discuss the benefits of physical activity for older adults.
8. Identify three characteristics of meaningful activities for older adults with dementia.

WHAT WOULD YOU DO?

What would you do if you were faced with the following situations?
- A new patient is admitted to your hospital floor. At bedtime, they ask for "that little pill I buy at Target that helps me sleep." How would you respond?
- Following the death of their partner, your 68-year-old patient asks what they can do to remain active. How would you respond?

Sleep and activity are two universal, dichotomous functions of all human beings. Sleep is a natural, periodically recurring, physiologic state of rest for the body and mind; sleep is a state of inactivity or repose required to remain active. Activity includes things we do while awake, for example, personal care, daily tasks, exercise, and recreation. The type, amount, and intensity of the activities pursued vary widely among individuals according to personal choice, lifestyle, and health status.

SLEEP AND OLDER ADULTS

Biologic Brain Functions Responsible for Sleep

Regulation of sleep and wakefulness occurs primarily in the hypothalamus, which contains both a sleep center and a wakefulness center. The thalamus, limbic system, and reticular activating system (RAS) are controlled by the hypothalamus and influence sleep and wakefulness. The hypothalamus consists of several masses of nuclei, interconnected with other parts of the nervous system, and is located below the thalamus, where it forms the floor and part of the lateral walls of the third ventricle. Sleep is a state of consciousness characterized by the physiologic changes of reduced blood pressure, pulse rate, and respiratory rate, along with a decreased response to external stimuli.

Stages of Sleep

Normal sleep is divided into five stages: rapid eye movement (REM) sleep and four stages of non-REM sleep (NREM) (Table 8.1). NREM sleep accounts for about 75% to 80% of sleep. The remaining 20% to 25% of sleep is REM sleep. A night's sleep begins with NREM sleep and continues with a period of REM sleep. The body cycles through NREM and REM stages approximately four to six times a night, averaging 90 minutes for each cycle (Memar & Faradji, 2018).

The first stage is the wake stage or stage W. This stage depends on whether the eyes are open or closed. N1 (formerly stage 1) of NREM sleep is the lightest level of sleep. During N1 an individual can be easily awakened. Sleep progressively deepens during N2 (formerly stage 2). In N3, or slow wave sleep (formerly stages 3 and 4), the deepest level of sleep is reached. Muscles are relaxed and breathing becomes slower in N3 or Slow Wave Sleep (SWS). In REM sleep, the brain becomes active and dreams may occur.

Variations in the REM and NREM sleep stages occur with advancing age. REM sleep is interrupted by more frequent nocturnal awakenings, and the total amount of REM sleep is reduced. During REM, brain waves may appear fast and desynchronized on an electroencephalogram (EEG), similar to the state of being awake (MacDowell, 2023).

TABLE 8.1 Normal Stages of Sleep

Stages	Type of Sleep	Selected Characteristics
NREM Sleep		
Wake/alert	Wake/relaxed wakefulness	Easily awakened
N1 (Formerly stage 1)	Lightest stage of sleep	Easily awakened Between being awake and falling asleep
N2 (Formerly stage 2)	Medium deep sleep	Onset of sleep Becoming disengaged from surroundings Regular breathing and heart rate Body temperatures drop
N3/slow wave sleep (Formerly stages 3 and 4)	Deepest sleep	Relaxed muscles Slowed pulse Awakened with moderate stimuli Restorative sleep Body movement rare Awakened with vigorous stimuli
REM Sleep	Active sleep	Rapid eye movement Body becomes immobile and relaxed Provides energy to the brain Dreaming occurs

REM = Rapid eye movement; *NREM* = non–rapid eye movement.
Modified from Touhy, T., & Jett, K. (2020). *Ebersole & Hess' Toward healthy aging* (10th ed.). St. Louis: Elsevier.

Sleep and Circadian Rhythm

The sleep-wake cycle follows a circadian rhythm, which is roughly a 24-hour period. The hypothalamus controls many circadian rhythms, which include the release of certain hormones during sleep (e.g., growth hormone [GH], follicle-stimulating hormone [FSH], and luteinizing hormone [LH]). Numerous factors may gradually strengthen or weaken the sleep and wake aspects of circadian rhythm, including altered patterns of alertness, mood, and performance across the day, which can interfere with social and professional life (Quera Salva et al, 2017). Changes in the circadian and homeostatic processes may result in a decrease in nighttime sleep and an increase in daytime napping that accompanies the normal aging stages (Li et al, 2018; Ryden & Alessi, 2022).

Insomnia

Insomnia, or the inability to sleep, is a complex phenomenon. Reports of insomnia include difficulty falling asleep, difficulty staying asleep, frequent nocturnal awakenings, early morning awakening, and daytime somnolence. Insomnia may be transient, short-term, or chronic (WebMD Editorial Contributors, 2021b). Transient insomnia lasts only a few nights and is related to situational stresses. Short-term insomnia usually lasts less than a month and is related to acute medical conditions (e.g., postoperative pain) or psychological conditions (e.g., grief).

Chronic insomnia lasts more than a month and is related to age-related changes in sleep, medical or psychological conditions, or environmental factors. Insomnia may affect the older adult's quality of life (QoL) with increased incidence of falls, depression and anxiety, cognitive impairment, institutionalization, and mortality (Berkley et al, 2020).

Age-Related Changes in Sleep

Many older adults experience changes in sleep, which are considered "normal" age-related changes (Box 8.1). However, some healthy older adults sleep as well as younger adults and do not experience these common changes (Patel et al, 2018). The sleep changes experienced by many older adults include advanced sleep timing, shortened nocturnal sleep duration, increased frequency of daytime naps, increased number of nocturnal awakenings and time spent awake during the night, decreased SWS, and other changes (Li et al, 2018). Sleep latency, a delay in the onset of sleep, increases with age. More than 30% of females report taking more than 30 minutes to fall asleep; for men, this number is under 15%. Older adults report that it takes longer to fall asleep at the start of the night and after being awakened during the night. Because the time spent awake in bed trying to fall asleep increases, sleep efficiency decreases. Sleep efficiency is the relative percentage of time in bed spent asleep. For young adults, sleep efficiency is approximately 90%. However, older adults have decreased sleep efficiency over time, with 18.6% decline between 40 and 100 years of age (Didikoglu et al, 2020).

Nocturnal awakenings contribute to an overall decrease in the average number of hours of sleep. The frequency of nocturnal awakenings increases with age; older adults may wake up four or more times per night. The interruptions of sleep contribute to the perception that the amount of sleep is inadequate or of poor quality. If the person has little difficulty falling back to sleep, the decrease in the number of hours of sleep may be slight. However, some older adults report increased periods of wakefulness after nocturnal awakening. The reasons for nocturnal awakening include the need for bladder voiding, spontaneous waking, feeling thirsty, hearing a noise, disturbance by children, co-sleepers, pain, hunger pangs, or breathing problems (Thomas, 2019). Early morning awakening and the inability to fall back to sleep may be related to changes in circadian rhythm or to any of the reasons for nocturnal awakening.

Daytime sleepiness is often reported by older adults and may be caused by frequent nocturnal awakening or other sleep disturbances. However, in some older adults, daytime sleepiness

BOX 8.1 Age-Related Changes in Sleep

- Increased sleep latency
- Reduced sleep efficiency
- Increased nocturnal awakenings
- Increased early morning awakenings
- Increased daytime sleepiness

suggests underlying disease. It is associated with functional impairment and depression, and contributes to the increased risk of motor vehicle accidents. Daytime sleepiness occurs in up to 20% of older adults and usually coexists with multiple adverse health conditions, including cognitive impairment, cardiovascular events, and increased mortality risk (Li et al, 2018). Daytime sleepiness may also be caused by drug side effects (e.g., antiarrhythmics, clonidine, selective serotonin reuptake inhibitors [SSRIs], and antihistamines).

Daytime napping is common in older adults and does not necessarily indicate problems with nighttime sleep. Naps, that is, voluntary and involuntary episodes of daytime sleep, occur throughout the day. Fan, McPhillips, and Li (2018) found that having a habit of napping may be protective for cognitive function and concluded that napping could have favorable cognitive effects.

Although some of the sleep changes experienced by older adults are related to aging, other sleep changes are associated with chronic disease and other health problems. When patterns of sleep are examined, an increase in light sleep is seen as deep sleep declines. The loss of deep sleep is associated with stages 3 and 4 of sleep (see Table 8.1). This sleep disturbance may be a normal part of aging caused by changes in the reticular formation (RF) in the brain (Friedman, 2010). When older adults describe the changes in their sleep patterns as they have aged, they offer nurses valuable clues. Their descriptions indicate health problems (actual or potential), safety concerns, and possible interventions to improve sleep quality.

Factors Affecting Sleep

Proper sleep is essential for a person's sense of well-being and health. Sleep is often defined subjectively and linked to an individual's feelings on awakening. A good night's sleep is described as one that refreshes, restores, and leaves a person ready for the coming day's activities. Feeling tired and less alert after a poor night's sleep may lead to a less active and productive day. Factors that influence sleep quality in older adults include the following, alone or in combination: environment, pain, lifestyle, dietary influences, drug use, medical conditions, depression, and dementia. Nursing interventions can modify these factors and promote a good night's sleep.

Environment

The environment can positively or negatively influence a person's quality and amount of sleep. For older adults, environments conducive to sleep include low levels of stimuli, dimmed lights, silence, and comfortable furniture (Rosto, 2001).

Home environments. The home environment supports a good night's sleep by its very familiarity. The bed and bedding, the people, and the noises are all familiar. The routines leading up to bedtime are natural and individualized.

Hospitals and long-term care facilities. The environment of a healthcare institution may detract from the quality of sleep. Not only are these environments unfamiliar, they also typically have bright lights, noisy people and machines, limited privacy and space, and uncomfortable mattresses. Physical discomfort or pain may be caused by invasive procedures such as Foley catheterization, intravenous (IV) line placement, venipuncture, mechanical ventilation, and discomfort or pain from equipment such as oxygen masks, casts or traction devices, and monitors. The hospital patient or long-term care facility resident is often awakened to receive drugs and treatments or to be assessed for changes in vital signs and condition. Nocturnal awakenings for incontinence care or for other care procedures such as repositioning and skin care interrupt the normal sequence of sleep stages (Nagel et al, 2003). Fear of the unexpected or unknown may also keep older adults awake in healthcare institutions. The quality of sleep in institutional settings improves as nursing interventions address (1) the scheduling of procedures and care activities to avoid unnecessary awakenings, (2) modification of environmental factors to promote a quiet, warm, relaxed sleep setting, and (3) orientation of older adults to the institutional setting.

Noise. Environmental noise potentially interferes with sleep in all healthcare settings. The consequences of environmental noise may include (1) sleep deprivation, (2) alteration in comfort, (3) pain, and (4) stress or difficulty concentrating, which may interfere with the enjoyment of activities. Sources of noise include personnel, roommates, visitors, equipment, and routine activities in the nursing unit. Interventions to reduce environmental noise include closing the doors of patient and resident rooms when possible, adjusting the volume control on telephones, rescheduling nighttime cleaning routines, and reminding staff and visitors to speak quietly. Some older adults may appreciate headphones to provide relaxing music and block background noise. Headphones will also reduce noise from late-evening television watching. Noise reduction may include asking the facility's maintenance staff to clean and lubricate the wheels on all of the unit's utility carts. Reducing environmental noise in institutions involves cooperation among employees from other departments, visitors, and nurses.

Lighting. Most individuals are accustomed to sleeping in darkened rooms. The lights in hallways and nurses' stations in some healthcare institutions interfere with the sleep of patients and residents. The nurse should assess environmental lighting in the institutional setting for glare, brightness, and uneven levels of illumination. Selectively dimming the institution's lights at night may promote better sleep. However, safety concerns must be considered. Nightlights in rooms, bathrooms, and hallways may be a safe compromise—promoting sleep by reducing the glare of bright lights while allowing enough light to see.

Temperature. Falling asleep and staying asleep are difficult when a person is cold. Older adults may wake during the night because of a nighttime reduction in core body temperature related to reduced metabolic rate and muscle activity. Being too warm will also disrupt sleep, but some older adults sleep better if simple measures are used to keep them warm. The ambient temperature of the bedroom should be no lower than 65°F (Harding et al, 2019). Several lightweight thermal blankets and flannel sheets (both fitted and flat) make for a warmer bed. Flannel pajamas or nightgowns, bed socks, and nightcaps help sleepers stay warm. If bed socks are worn, slippers should be used when out of bed to prevent slipping on uncarpeted floors. Heating devices such as heating pads or hot water bottles should be avoided so that the fragile skin on the feet and lower legs is not exposed to thermal injuries.

Pain and Discomfort

Body pain, acute or chronic, interferes with falling asleep and staying asleep. Nursing interventions to relieve pain begin with assessment of the location, intensity, onset and duration, quality, and any aggravating or alleviating factors. The effect of pain on older adults' lifestyle, including sleep quality, should also be assessed. Both nonpharmacologic and pharmacologic measures may be used to relieve pain. When body pain interferes with sleep, analgesics are more effective for sleep promotion than sedative or hypnotic drugs. However, alterations in pharmacokinetics (PK) common to older adults taking drugs make careful selection of analgesics important. Drugs with long half-lives linger longer in many older adults. Small initial doses that may be titrated upward to achieve analgesia may be better tolerated than generous initial doses. Attention must be paid to common side effects such as constipation.

Even without any report of body pain, some older adults find just being in bed uncomfortable. For the older individual whose discomfort prevents sleeping in a standard bed, comfortable chairs may be a solution. Reclining chairs with soft cushions may be more comfortable for individuals with congestive heart failure (CHF) or severe chronic obstructive pulmonary disease (COPD). The rhythmic motion of a rocking chair may comfort some individuals and thus promote sleep. If being out of bed is not feasible, modifying the bed with extra pillows to support painful limbs and promote comfortable body positioning or using special mattresses (e.g., air or water mattresses) may be effective. Nighttime garments should be made of a soft material such as cotton and should not be restrictive to allow freedom of movement. The use of lightweight blankets avoids adding weight to sensitive body areas.

Lifestyle Changes

Loss of a partner. Widowhood is a common life event in the older adult population. Loss of a partner is much more common among older females than among older males. Twenty-four percent (24%) of older adults are widowed (United States Census Bureau, 2017). Loss of a bed partner may make sleep psychologically less comforting. Widowed older adults describe the strangeness of going to bed alone after many years of marriage (WebMD Editorial Contributors, 2022a). This change in bedtime routine may interfere with the onset of sleep. If the widowed older adult experiences depression, the depression should be treated.

Retirement. Retirement brings about changes in schedule and activities. For decades, the work schedule influenced older adults' times for going to bed and awakening; retirement removes that variable. The structure of a day in retirement is not imposed by the demands of a job. The work activities that caused fatigue may have ceased. Getting a good night's sleep is no longer necessary to be restored from the day's work and prepared for the next day's efforts. The activities that remain are personal care activities, activities around the house, recreational activities, and any new activities adopted with the coming of retirement. These changes create the potential for alterations in sleep (WebMD Editorial Contributors, 2022a). Some retired older adults may follow the same schedule they observed while working. It is familiar and feels comfortable. However, other retired older adults find their days and nights without structure. In the absence of old routines, sleep is disturbed. Unless other activities replace work activities, retired older adults may not feel fatigued at the end of the day or sleepy at bedtime. Sleep may also be disturbed by the uncertainties that come with retirement. Questions about family relationships, finances, and future activities may lead to sleep-disturbing stress.

Relocation. Some older adults experience relocation, or a change of residence, from their house or apartment to the home of their children or siblings, a retirement community, assisted-living facility, or nursing facility. Sleep is adversely affected by the transition to these unfamiliar surroundings. Deciding to move from the familiar place of residence to another residence, even if that other residence is desirable and the relocation voluntary, engenders stress during the time of decision-making, during the actual move, and during the time of adjustment to the new residence. The unfamiliar environment of the new residence also contributes to disturbed sleep. As older adults become accustomed to a new residence, sleep should improve.

Having a roommate. Having a roommate (or a bed partner) may interfere with sleep. Some sleep-related problems occur in long-term care facilities when roommates do not get along with one another because of different interests or lifestyles. For example, one older adult may watch television to fall asleep, and the other may find this disruptive to sleep. The nursing staff must make every effort to review significant psychosocial interests with residents and to match roommates accordingly. Ideally, residents should be allowed to select roommates with whom they share common interests. The roommate or bed partner who snores loudly, sleepwalks, talks in his or her sleep, or has restless leg syndrome (RLS) is also a cause of sleeplessness. Treatment must be directed toward the cause of the roommate's problem; if treatment is impossible or ineffective, separate bedrooms may be needed.

Dietary Influences

Sleep is influenced by what we eat and drink. Popular caffeine-containing beverages (e.g., coffee, tea, hot chocolate, energy drinks, and soda) make falling asleep more difficult for some older adults. The effects of caffeine include restlessness, nervousness, insomnia, tremors, reduced peripheral vascular resistance, increased heart rate, and relaxation of airway smooth muscle (ASM).

The standard advice is to avoid caffeine-containing beverages for several hours before going to bed. This diminishes the likelihood that the stimulant effect of caffeine will interfere with falling asleep and staying asleep. Other sources of caffeine include chocolate, some over-the-counter (OTC) pain analgesics, and cold remedies (Dopheide, 2020). Some herbal products also contain caffeine. Alternative choices for late-evening beverages are fruit juices, milk, and water.

Alcohol occupies an equivocal position among beverages that influence sleep. Many adults include alcohol as part of their normal lifestyle and continue to do so in their advancing years. They enjoy a glass of wine or other cocktail with an evening meal. Small amounts of alcoholic beverages may cause a slight drowsiness or relaxation that promotes falling asleep. However, with larger amounts of alcohol, older adults appear to be more vulnerable to alcohol-related brain aging and decrease in REM sleep (Zhang et al, 2021). The diuresis caused by alcohol-induced inhibition of antidiuretic hormone (ADH) secretion leads to nocturnal awakenings for urination. When discussing the use of alcohol with older adults, the nurse must determine how they define a "small" or "large" amount of alcohol and the circumstances of alcohol use. These details of alcohol use vary from group to group and from culture to culture.

Fluid intake in the evening and immediately before going to bed is associated with nocturia. Although nocturia may have other causes such as urinary retention related to benign prostatic hypertrophy (BPH) or diuretic therapy for heart failure, many older adults reduce the kind and volume of fluid intake in the evening. However, it is important that older adults, who as a group are at risk for inadequate fluid intake and dehydration, not reduce the total amount of liquids consumed in 24 hours.

Hunger and thirst may be causes of sleeplessness. Bedtime snacks and small amounts of liquids may provide the touch of comfort that promotes sleep. Warm snacks containing protein are better at bedtime than cold snacks (Pacheco & Guo, 2023). Milk, eggnog, creamed soup, or flavored gelatin may all be served hot to provide warmth and calories. Pudding, custard, or tapioca may be more palatable than crackers or graham crackers. For older adults with diabetes, bedtime snacks should be included in their special diets. Falling back to sleep after awakening during the night with a dry mouth is facilitated when a cup of water is available close to the bed.

Depression
Depression among older adults is a treatable condition that is frequently accompanied by insomnia. Patients awaken in the early morning and are unable to return to sleep. Patients may also report excessive daytime somnolence. Evaluation and treatment are essential if depression is suspected.

Dementia and Disturbed Sleep
Older adults with Alzheimer's disease or other dementias may experience disturbed sleep. Increased confusion at night, nocturnal wandering, disruptive vocalizations, and agitation have been reported. The causes of the sleep disruption may be no different from causes that disturb sleep in any older adult. However, cognitive impairment complicates assessment, intervention, and evaluation. The nurse may not receive a clear response when asking about sleep or any conditions that contribute to insomnia. Instead, nurses must anticipate the needs of older adults with dementia. Interventions include reducing confusion with an explanation of what is expected of the older adult ("Now it's time to sleep"), identification of the place for sleeping ("This is your bed"), and reassurance that going to bed is the right thing to do ("Your bed is ready for you"). Assisting older adults with dementia to perform bedtime routines redirects their behavior. Nocturnal wandering behaviors may signal a need that cannot be expressed verbally, for example, hunger, thirst, or the need to go to the bathroom. Wandering may also be an expression of pain or of a need for exercise. Once the meaning of the wandering is discerned, appropriate interventions follow naturally (Rowe, 2003). Drugs such as sedatives or antipsychotics should be avoided because of their side effects, which may worsen confusion, interfere with safe ambulation, and alter the sleep-wake cycle.

Sleep Disorders and Conditions
The two most common sleep disorders experienced by older adults are sleep apnea and periodic limb movements in sleep (PLMS). Both disorders are seen with excessive daytime sleepiness (EDS) and reports of insomnia. However, PLMS is essentially a benign condition, whereas the hypoxia related to sleep apnea might lead to serious consequences.

Sleep Apnea
During sleep, individuals with sleep apnea experience recurrent episodes of cessation of respiration. These apneic episodes may last from 10 seconds to 2 minutes. The number of apneic episodes may range from 10 to more than 100 per hour of sleep (Ryden & Alessi, 2022). The incidence of sleep apnea increases with age, and it is more common in males than in females. Complications related to sleep apnea include cardiac disease, hypertension (HTN), stroke, obesity, headaches, irritability, depression and anxiety, sexual dysfunction, daytime sleepiness, and difficulty with memory, thinking, and concentration. Persons with sleep apnea are also at increased risk for automobile or work-related accidents (Nabili & Marks, 2023).

The three major types of sleep apnea are central sleep apnea (CSA), obstructive sleep apnea (OSA), and complex sleep apnea syndrome (CompSAS). In CSA, a cessation of respiratory efforts, both diaphragmatic and intercostal, occurs. CSA is usually accompanied by daytime fatigue, nocturia and nighttime awakening, morning headaches, poor memory and concentration, and moodiness. Risk factors associated with CSA include CHF, hypothyroidism, chronic kidney disease (CKD), neurologic diseases, and damage to the brainstem. Treatment consists of managing underlying associated risk factors, weight loss, avoidance of alcohol and sleeping pills, sleeping on the side, and using sprays to maintain open nasal passages. Continuous positive airway pressure (CPAP) treatment may be beneficial for those with CSA, especially those with associated CHF (WebMD Editorial Contributors, 2022b).

OSA is more common in older adults than CSA (Osorio et al, 2021). In OSA, air flow ceases because of complete or partial airway obstruction; respiratory efforts increase in an attempt to open the airway. Factors associated with OSA include excessive weight, narrowed airway, HTN, chronic nasal congestion, and enlarged tonsils (Mayo Clinic Staff, 2023). Additionally, smoking, HTN, and cardiac risk factors increase the likelihood of developing OSA. Older adults with OSA report daytime fatigue; waking with a headache, sore throat or dry mouth, and confusion; trouble concentrating and irritability; and sexual dysfunction. The families of older adults with OSA describe loud snoring and choking or gasping sounds during the person's sleep. Treatment consists of weight loss, avoidance of alcohol and sleeping pills, propping oneself on the side using pillows, and using sprays to maintain open nasal passages. CPAP prevents collapse of the airway during sleep (see the Nursing Care Plan box). Other options include mandibular advancement devices (MADs) that prevent the tongue from blocking the throat and surgery (somnoplasty, uvulopalatopharyngoplasty (UPPP), mandibular or maxillary advancement surgery, or nasal surgery) (WebMD Editorial Contributors, 2021a).

NURSING CARE PLAN

Sleep Pattern Disturbance

Clinical Situation

Mr. V is a 79-year-old single white male who is admitted to the nursing facility for convalescence after a tracheotomy for OSA. Before hospitalization, he was living alone on the third floor of an apartment complex for older adults. He describes himself as limited in activities such as driving, traveling, and cooking because of respiratory distress. He reports daytime fatigue associated with grooming, dressing, feeding, and toileting. He admits to sleeping poorly, with several nighttime awakenings and general fatigue all day long, which prompts him to take a daytime nap.

Medical history includes HTN, obesity, COPD, severe PVD with a stage II venous stasis ulcer of the lower leg, and recent tracheotomy for OSA.

While at the nursing facility, Mr. V tells you that he plans on discharging himself home in 1 to 2 weeks. He is observed to need assistance in mobility and uses a wheelchair to wheel himself around his room. He refuses to go to the dining room and requests to have a refrigerator in his room. He eats all his meals in his room and rarely socializes with any resident or staff member. His pastimes include playing solitaire in his room and watching television. He is a retired sales representative, having worked in the business for more than 40 years.

Analyze Cues and Prioritize Hypotheses (Patient Problems)
- Altered sleep pattern resulting from obesity and reduced activity level

Generate Solutions [Planning]
- Patient will identify personal lifestyle habits contributing to sleep pattern disturbance.
- Patient will achieve weight loss of 1 pound (lb) per week.
- Patient will eat a well-balanced diet, as evidenced by food diary.
- Patient will participate in one group activity a day.
- Patient will walk 100 feet twice daily, increasing distance to tolerance.
- Patient will report increased length of uninterrupted periods of sleep.

Take Actions (Nursing Interventions)
- Teach relationship between weight and sleep pattern, and importance of losing weight to improve sleep pattern.
- Explore with patient motivators to lose weight; reinforce as needed.
- Teach about the United States Department of Agriculture's (USDA's) food guidance system, MyPlate (http://www.choosemyplate.gov/), and assist him in identifying nutritious foods.
- Teach use of food diary for self-monitoring.
- Offer nutritious foods as snacks.
- Encourage patient to increase level of activity on the unit by increasing mobility and engaging in nonsedentary activities; review a list of available activities with patient. Offer to accompany patient on a walk on the unit to his tolerance at least twice a day to help with wound healing and weight reduction.
- Introduce patient to fellow residents on the unit who share common interests.
- Encourage patient to join other residents in activities to tolerance.
- Explore with patient his likes or dislikes, previous hobbies, and level of activity during middle adulthood.
- Schedule an activity with the patient that will be part of his daily routine.
- Discourage daytime napping; instead, replace it with a stimulating activity.
- Teach patient to monitor pulse, to watch for symptoms of respiratory distress when engaging in activities on the unit, and to stop if respiratory distress occurs or an increase in heart rate causes adverse symptoms.
- Offer praise and positive reinforcement when he performs a nonsedentary activity and when weight loss is achieved.
- Observe patient during sleep for signs of OSA such as loud snoring or periods of apnea. Observe for daytime fatigue and somnolence.
- Encourage patient to assume a side-lying position for sleep.
- Discuss with patient plans for discharge and explore alternative living arrangements, including residence on a first-floor apartment, especially if mobility is impaired.

CompSAS occurs when persons treating OSA with CPAP are found to also have CSA during initial therapy. Persons present with excessive fatigue, sleepiness, and depression; these symptoms are secondary to unresponsiveness to CPAP. Risk factors include cardiovascular and cerebrovascular diseases, as well as use of opioid drugs. Prevalence may be as high as 20% and increases with age; it is predominant in men. Maintaining adherence to CPAP may improve CompSAS after 8 to 12 weeks. However, adherence is problematic because of poor initial response to therapy. Other contemporary treatment methods can be used, such as adaptive servo ventilation (ASV) which automatically adjusts to a person's respiration on a breath-by-breath basis or bi-level positive airway pressure (BPAP) treatment with controlled respiratory frequency (Pal'man, 2019).

Periodic Limb Movement in Sleep

Approximately 30% of older adults experience periodic limb movement in sleep (PLMS) (Cleveland Clinic, 2023). In PLMS, repetitive kicking leg movements occur throughout the night, most often during non-REM sleep, and may occur every 5 to 90 seconds; each kick causes a brief disruption of sleep. Some older adults are unaware of their leg movements; others wake up and have difficulty falling back to sleep. Older adults with PLMS report insomnia and EDS. Their bed partners report being kicked during the night. Drugs such as dopamine agonists (DAs), anticonvulsants, benzodiazepines, and narcotics are accepted pharmacologic therapies for PLMS. First-line pharmacologic therapy is DAs. Additionally, patients are encouraged to eliminate caffeine-containing products (e.g., tea, chocolate, and coffee) from their diet; they should also discuss the use of antidepressants with their healthcare provider, as these drugs may worsen symptoms (Cleveland Clinic, 2023). If the movements are frequent, the nurse may suggest that older adults sleep alone to allow their bed partners less disturbed nights' sleep (Ancoll-Israel, 2004).

> ### EVIDENCE-BASED PRACTICE
> #### Natural Light on Sleep Quality of Older Adults in Nursing Homes
>
> **Background**
> Fifty percent (50%) of older adults report sleep problems. Typically, sleep problems are treated with pharmacologic and nonpharmacologic interventions. Nonpharmacologic interventions have included stimulus control, sleep hygiene education, sleep restriction, relaxation techniques, cognitive behavior therapy, and light therapy.
>
> **Sample/Setting**
> The sample encompassed 61 older adults (30 in experimental group; 31 in control group) residing in the T. R. Ministry of Family and Social Services Narlidere Nursing Home YBRM in Turkey. Subject ages ranged from 75 to 84 years; 63.3% were female, 53.3% were widowed, and 56.7% were high-school graduates.
>
> All subjects were given the Pittsburgh Sleep Quality Index (PSQI) at baseline. The PSQI has 18 scorable questions, which are grouped into seven components. Each question can receive a score of 0 to 3. The sum of the component scores is the total PSQI score, ranging from 0 to 21; the higher the score, the poorer the sleep quality.
>
> **Methods**
> Experimental group subjects were taken to the garden of the nursing home for exposure to natural sunlight between 8 a.m. to 10 a.m. each morning for 5 days. They remained in the garden for at least 30 minutes but no longer than 120 minutes. Experimental subjects were provided brochures on health sleep habits. After 5 days, the experimental subjects repeated the PSQI.
>
> The control subjects remained in their rooms, the canteen, or the nursing-home living rooms while the experimental subjects were in direct sunlight. They, too, retook the PSQI after 5 days and received a copy of the healthy sleep habits brochure after retaking the PSQI.
>
> **Findings**
> Significant differences were found between the experimental group and control group across most of the components of the PSQI (subjective sleep quality, sleep latency, sleep duration, sleep activity, sleep disturbance, and daytime function) between baseline and day 5 ($P<.001$). A strong, positive relationship was found between sunlight exposure time and sleep duration, regular sleep activity, and daytime dysfunction ($P<.001$). There was no significant difference in global sleep quality score for those in the sunlight at least 30 minutes vs. those in the sunlight for at least 100 minutes.
>
> **Implications**
> Natural sunlight therapy can significantly improve sleep quality. This nonpharmacologic intervention is effective and has the potential to help prevent polypharmacy in nursing-home residents with insomnia.

Data from Duzgun, G., & Akyol, A. D. (2017). Effect of natural sunlight on sleep problems and sleep quality of the elderly staying in the nursing home. *Holistic Nursing Practice, 31*(5), 295–302.

Components of the Sleep History

A complete sleep history begins with the patient's report of their sleep pattern and sleep-related problems (Box 8.2). The quality of sleep is usually described along a continuum of poor, fair, good, or excellent. The quantity of sleep refers to the amount of sleep in a 24-hour period, including daytime naps. Quantity may be difficult to calculate, especially for the patient with frequent nocturnal awakenings who cannot recall whether sleep occurred after awakening. The nurse should determine when the patient retires for bed, falls asleep, and usually awakens. The number of nocturnal awakenings and length of time awake at night are important to review with the patient. If a patient retires at 9 p.m., does not fall asleep until 11 p.m., arises at 4 a.m., and takes a daytime nap from 4 p.m. to 5 p.m. daily, this individual has slept a total of 6 hours. Information about a person's typical bedtime rituals or practices should also be obtained.

The older adult is likely to seek additional help in achieving satisfaction with sleeping habits. If the older adult is too tired or fatigued to perform normal activities, the sleep problem may be viewed as disruptive to the daily routine and may require further evaluation. The nurse should ascertain whether the older adult experiences daytime sleepiness or has a strong desire to nap.

A patient's activities before bedtime and their exercise and activity patterns provide additional information about sleep habits. In general, strenuous activity should be avoided at least 2 hours before bedtime. The nurse should identify what the patient does to relax before bedtime, for example, reading or

> ### BOX 8.2 Sleep History Components
> - Sleep quality
>   - The self-report of the older adult, described as poor, fair, good, or excellent
> - Sleep quantity
>   - The number of hours asleep per 24 hours, including daytime naps
> - Bedtime routines
> - Place of sleep
> - Characteristics of the bed, bedding, and bedroom environment
> - Food and fluid intake in the evening and at bedtime
> - Use of alcohol and caffeine-containing beverages
> - Drugs (prescription and nonprescription)
> - Characteristics of the sleep disturbance
>   - Difficulty falling asleep
>   - Difficulty staying asleep
>   - Frequent nocturnal awakenings
>   - Early morning awakening
>   - Daytime sleepiness
> - The older adult's account of the reasons for the disturbed sleep

drinking a warm beverage. The nurse should question the patient having difficulty with sleep about the consumption of alcohol, caffeinated beverages, sedative-hypnotics, OTC drugs, and other practices before bedtime.

Questions about the type of bed in which the person sleeps are also important. Does the patient sleep in the same bed every night? Is it comfortable? Is the mattress soft, and does it provide adequate support? Some individuals who are unable to sleep in a recumbent position because of medical problems may be able to sleep in a semirecumbent position in a lounge chair or recliner. Patients who are unable to fall asleep in the supine position and who need several pillows or cushions in bed require further medical evaluation for CHF, pulmonary disease, or musculoskeletal problems (Spieker & Motzer, 2003). Common problems that cause pain and discomfort in bed include COPD; rheumatologic problems such as osteoporosis; degenerative joint disease of the spine, hips, or neck; and rheumatoid arthritis (RA). Nocturia occurring several times in the course of one night must be further evaluated. Older males with prostate enlargement need to urinate several times during the night. Older adults with CHF or urinary tract infections (UTIs) may also have nocturia.

Further Assessment of Sleep

A sleep diary kept by the older adult is helpful in recalling the amount of sleep, bedtime routines, and possible symptoms of disturbed sleep over a 24-hour period. The type and quantity of activities are also noted in the diary for the same 24-hour period. To complete the sleep diary, the older adult may need the assistance of a family member or the nurse. The nurse may suggest measures to help patients enter information in the diary, for example, video-recorded entries for patients with visual impairment or difficulty writing.

Sleep laboratories specialize in treating patients with primary sleep disorders. Patients are asked to spend the night so that a sleep study can be administered. This often includes polysomnography (PSG), which provides data about the stages of sleep and ventilation, and an EEG for graphic tracing of the variations in the brain's electric force. Physicians specially trained in sleep disorders evaluate the history and objective findings, including a review of basic sleep hygienic measures, to arrive at a diagnosis and treatment plan.

Additional information about sleep may be collected with the use of questionnaires. The Epworth Sleepiness Scale (ESS) (Fig. 8.1) measures feelings of sleepiness or tiredness at specific

The Epworth Sleepiness Scale (ESS)

How likely are you to doze off or fall asleep in the following situations, in contrast to feeling just tired? This refers to your usual way of life in recent times. Even if you have not done some of these things recently try to work out how they would have affected you. Use the following scale to choose the **most appropriate number** for each situation:

0 = would **never** doze
1 = **slight chance** of dozing
2 = **moderate chance** of dozing
3 = **high chance** of dozing

SITUATION	CHANCE OF DOZING (0–3)
Sitting and reading	
Watching television	
Sitting inactive in a public place (e.g. a theater or meeting)	
As a passenger in a car for an hour without a break	
Lying down to rest in the afternoon when circumstances permit	
Sitting and talking to someone	
Sitting quietly after a lunch without alcohol	
In a car, while stopped for a few minutes in the traffic	
TOTAL SCORE	

SCORE RESULTS:

1–6	Congratulations, you are getting enough sleep!
7–8	Your score is average
9 and up	Very sleepy and should seek medical advice

Fig. 8.1 Epworth Sleepiness Scale. (From Johns, M. W. [1991]. A new method for measuring daytime sleepiness: The Epworth Sleepiness Scale. *Sleep, 14,* 540–545.)

times. The ESS also measures sleepiness, but it measures it in terms of sleep propensity, the likelihood of falling asleep at a particular time. The person completing the ESS considers the effectiveness of examining patients' sleepiness in a range of different situations and indicates the likelihood (low-to-high) that they would fall asleep in those situations (Rozgonyi et al, 2021). Another instrument is the PSQI, which subjectively measures sleep quality and includes five additional questions for the bed partner. Additional sleep instruments to facilitate sleep assessment may be used (University of Pittsburgh Center for Sleep and Circadian Science [CSCS], n.d.).

Getting a Good Night's Sleep

Whether sleep is disturbed by the environment, diet, drugs, lifestyle changes, or sleep disorders, the first step in developing interventions to improve the amount and quality of sleep is taking a thorough sleep history. Supplementing the sleep history are measurement tools to assess sleep quality and quantity, direct observation of the older adult during sleep, a sleep diary, and diagnostic studies such as EEG monitoring, and sleep study evaluation. After assessment, interventions to improve sleep usually begin with basic sleep hygiene measures.

Sleep Hygiene

Basic sleep hygiene includes those activities that foster normal sleep and that can be practiced by individuals on a routine basis. The goal of sleep hygiene measures is to achieve normal sleep. Failure to reinforce habits, routines, and attitudes to obtain sufficient sleep can influence health, emotional well-being, and cognitive functioning (Tagler et al, 2017). Sleep hygiene measures emphasize stable schedules and bedtime routines, a sleep-friendly environment, avoidance of any substances that would interfere with sleep, regular exercise (but not immediately before trying to sleep), and stress reduction.

Retiring at the same time every night and awakening at the same time every morning help establish a routine. A patient may condition himself or herself to such a routine over time. Likewise, limiting the amount of time spent in bed to only the time spent sleeping establishes a routine for sleep. Retiring to the same location such as the bedroom, and not a couch or chair on some nights, also helps solidify the routine. If unable to fall asleep, the person should get up and move to another area to perform other activities until sleepy. Eliminating noise and creating a darkened environment promotes sleep. Limiting daytime napping and having warm beverages and light nutritious snacks at bedtime are additional measures that promote sleep.

Avoiding caffeinated beverages, sleeping pills, and alcohol may reduce the chances of sleep-related breathing disorders (SBDs). The basic measures to help reduce episodes of OSA include losing weight, sleeping on one's side or stomach, avoiding central nervous system (CNS) depressants such as sedative-hypnotics and alcohol, and treating any obvious nasal or upper airway diseases.

Fostering Normal Sleep in Homebound Older Adults

It is important for the nurse to assess risk factors (e.g., environment, pain, or equipment such as a Foley catheter) that predispose homebound older adults to sleep disturbances. Review all drugs to identify those that may interfere with sleep patterns. Instruct caregivers and homebound older adults on activities that foster normal sleep, such as avoiding caffeinated beverages and alcohol. Assist with environmental changes that foster normal sleep, such as using a rocking chair or taking a warm bath. It must be kept in mind that worry and anxiety concerning safety and welfare may be obstacles to sleep in older adults. A system of notification and monitoring to link older adults living alone with the outside world is important to promote their sense of security.

Nonpharmacological Therapies to Promote Sleep

In addition to sleep hygiene measures, the American Academy of Sleep Medicine (AASM) recommends other nonpharmacologic interventions to promote sleep. Among these measures are relaxation therapies, stimulus control therapy, sleep restriction therapy, and cognitive behavioral therapy. Relaxation therapies reduce either somatic arousal or cognitive arousal. Progressive muscle relaxation is one example of a therapy to reduce somatic arousal. Cognitive arousal is reduced by attention-focusing therapies such as guided imagery or meditation. Stimulus control therapy attempts to reestablish the bedroom environment as the stimulus for sleep by banning activities from the bedroom that are not related to a good night's sleep. Examples of such activities include eating and watching television. Stimulus control therapy is helpful for individuals with sleep-onset insomnia. Sleep restriction therapy limits the amount of time spent in bed. Individuals stay in bed only for the number of hours they estimate as their average time asleep, plus 15 minutes. Cognitive behavioral therapy helps the person with insomnia to address factors, such as stress, that interfere with sleep (Siebern et al, 2012).

Drugs Used to Promote Sleep

Although nonpharmacological measures are the treatment of choice of insomnia, drug therapy may be necessary for a short time. Most drugs traditionally used to promote sleep (tranquilizers and sedative hypnotics) are listed as drugs to avoid on the updated 2023 Beers Criteria for Potentially Inappropriate Medication Use in Older Adults. These drugs carry the risk of physical dependence, increased risk of cognitive impairment, delirium, and falls. Additionally, the nonbenzodiazepine receptor agonist hypnotics are also drugs to avoid in older adults due to the high risk for delirium falls and increased emergency department (ED) visits and hospitalizations. One antihistamine, diphenhydramine, which is a component of many OTC sleep aids, also makes the 2023 Beers Criteria for Potentially Inappropriate Medication Use in Older Adults. This drug should be avoided in older adults as tolerance develops when used as a hypnotic, and users face an increased risk of confusion and reduced clearance, which can lead to toxicity (American Geriatrics Society [AGS], 2019).

Doxepin, which is used to treat depression, anxiety, and sleep disorderes, should not be used in doses higher than 6 mg per day as it is highly anticholinergic, and patients have increased risk for orthostatic hypotension (OH). Mirtazapine and trazodone, both used to treat depression, should be used with caution, as patients may experience significant hyponatremia (American Geriatrics Soceity [AGS], 2019). Two drugs, ramelteon (a melatonin agonist) and suvorexant (an orexin receptor antagonist), currently have no restrictions for use in older adults; however, these drugs carry the same side effect profile as other sleep aids. Ramelteon is indicated for use in patients who have difficulty falling asleep; suvorexant helps patients both fall asleep and stay asleep (Mayo Clinic Staff, 2022) (see Patient/Family Teaching box). Pharmacologic treatment of insomnia should be short-term—no more than 1 or 2 weeks.

> **PATIENT/FAMILY TEACHING**
> *Treating Insomnia with Drugs*
>
> - Take the sleeping pill when all evening activities are completed, and you are ready to go to bed.
> - Only take a sleeping pill when you can get a full night's sleep (7–8 hours).
> - Be aware of side effects; if you feel sleepy or dizzy during the day, call your health-care provider.
> - Never mix alcohol and sleeping pills.

Data from Mayo Clinic. (2022). *Prescription sleeping pills: What's right for you?* MayoClinic.org [website]. Retrieved from https://www.mayoclinic.org/diseases-conditions/insomnia/in-depth/sleeping-pills/art-20043959.

Complementary and Alternative Medicines

Various complementary and alternative medicines (CAMs) have been recommended as aids for securing a good night's sleep. Unlike prescription drugs, the composition of these compounds is not readily available, and their side effects and interactions with prescription or OTC drugs have not been fully explored (Box 8.3). Some herbal remedies contain active ingredients that resemble prescription and OTC drugs, increasing the risk for drug-drug interaction (DDI) (Romero et al, 2017).

> **BOX 8.3 Tips for Older Adults Using Herbal and Homeopathic Remedies**
>
> 1. Before treating any symptom with a nonprescription product, make sure no conditions requiring medical attention exist.
> 2. Discuss the use of any nonprescription product with your physician and other health-care providers.
> 3. Be cautious about viewing herbal or homeopathic products as a substitute for prescribed drugs.
> 4. Use single-ingredient products rather than combinations.
> 5. Observe for beneficial and harmful effects.
> 6. Report any possible side effects to your physician for evaluation.
> 7. Seek information from objective sources rather than relying on promotional materials and package information.
> 8. Check any warnings on the label or package, and check for information from additional sources.
> 9. Consider the fact that herbal and homeopathic products are not required to meet standards for safety and efficacy.
> 10. Be skeptical about exaggerated claims—if it sounds too good to be true, it probably is!

From Miller, C. A. (1996). Alternative healing products. *Geriatric Nursing, 17*(3):145–146.

One CAM, melatonin, has undergone scientific study, demonstrating some effectiveness in healthy adults, decreasing sleep latency and increasing sleep duration when used for 3 months or less. However, as with other CAMs, it is unregulated, and caution is advised with its use (Bruce, 2022).

ACTIVITY AND OLDER ADULTS

Activity, as discussed in this chapter, includes routine daily activities, diversional activities, and physical exercise. Changes occur in the activities pursued by older adults as they age or experience acute or chronic illness. Other changes in activities occur in response to major lifestyle changes such as retirement, relocation, or loss of a spouse. Specialized activities to meet the needs of older adults with Alzheimer's disease or a related dementia are also available. Whether cared for at home or in a long-term-care facility, the older adult with dementia benefits from an activity program that includes both diversional activities and activities of daily living (ADLs) that promote independence. Physical exercise deserves special attention because of its health-promoting benefits for all older adults. Although the activities pursued by a particular older adult are influenced by his or her preferences, situation, and health, some general considerations for activity in older adults do exist. In some settings, nurses participate in planning activities, adapting activities to the older adult's current situation, and evaluating the effects of activities on health.

Activities of Daily Living

ADLs include the things that most adults do every day, often without special attention or effort. Until something happens to interfere with normal daily routines, little thought may be given to bathing, dressing, eating, or attending to elimination needs. However, with advancing age and changes in health and circumstances, activities that once were accomplished with ease may require modified approaches or the assistance of others. In addition to providing direct assistance with ADLs, nurses assist older adults in the modification of routines and the use of assistive devices that help maintain independence. Nurses also support and advise family members and friends who assist the older adult with ADLs.

Basic ADLs include the everyday personal care tasks related to hygiene, nutrition, and elimination. Remaining independent in these activities is highly prized by older adults. Dependency in basic ADLs increases the risk of relocation to a long-term-care facility or to the home of a family member. To remain independent in basic ADLs, older adults use assistive devices and modify their care routines. Handheld shower sprays, raised toilet seats, sturdy grab bars in bathrooms, plate guards, and built-up handles on toothbrushes and eating utensils are examples of assistive devices. Clothing with Velcro instead of buttons, ties that can be clipped on rather than tied, and shoes that can be slipped on rather than laced are examples of modifications to help with dressing. However, for some older adults, the amount of assistance needed with personal care exceeds their ability to modify routines and the capacity of family members and friends to help. Home-care nurses may supplement the care provided by family members and friends, or relocation to a long-term-care facility may be necessary.

Instrumental ADLs (IADLs) include activities such as driving, shopping, cooking, housekeeping, and using a telephone. Older adults modify their approaches to IADLs because of commonly experienced changes in aging such as reduced strength, impaired vision, or impaired hearing. Assistive devices make the tasks of cooking or housekeeping easier and safer. Driving may be restricted to familiar areas and daylight hours. Family members, friends, or paid caregivers may help with shopping and other tasks. During episodes of acute illness or recovery from hospitalization, additional help may be needed. If sufficient assistance with IADLs is available in the home, relocation to a long-term-care facility is not necessary.

Physical Exercise

Physical activity is important for older adults to maintain health, preserve the ability to perform ADLs, and improve general QoL. The benefits of physical activity include prevention of CHF and diabetes, reduction in elevated blood pressure, reduced risk of osteoporosis, promotion of appropriate weight, reduction in depressed mood, reduced cancer risk, and promotion of more restful sleep (Schoenborn et al, 2006). Exercise preserves mobility and reduces the risk of falls by promoting muscle strength and joint flexibility.

Older adults exercise for a variety of reasons (Schoenborn et al, 2006). They exercise to have fun, to socialize with friends and neighbors, and to simply feel better. Exercise is used to reduce stress, to promote relaxation, and, together with a good nutritional program, to control weight. The Centers for Disease Control and Prevention (CDC) (2023) recommends moderate-intensity aerobic exercise for 150 minutes a week. The activity may be divided into smaller segments of at least 10 minutes' duration. To measure the appropriate intensity while walking, the "talk test" may be used. The person exercising should be able to carry on a conversation while walking. Breathing may be slightly labored, but a conversation should still be possible. The walker should not be out of breath. Muscle strengthening should be done at least 2 days per week. Older adults with restricted abilities because of medical conditions should perform physical activity within their limitations.

If the older adult has not been exercising every day, starting with only 5 minutes of exercise each day and gradually working up to 20 minutes or 30 minutes a day is appropriate (Schoenborn et al, 2006). A gradual progression in an exercise program for older adults who have been sedentary is recommended. A sedentary lifestyle is not unusual for older adults. In one study, physical activity and sedentary behavior were measured in adults over the age of 60. Results indicate older adults average 10 minutes to 106 minutes per day in moderate physical activity. Activity declines with age; those over 80 averaged 5 minutes to 60 minutes of moderate physical activity per day. Females were more active than males. Older adults spent an average of 8.5 hours per day in sedentary behavior, with those over 80 spending the most time in sedentary behavior (Evenson et al, 2012).

In addition to recommending gradual increases in the amount of exercise time for older adults who have not been exercising regularly, the nurse may pass along other safety tips. Drinking water before and after exercise is important because of fluid loss during exercise. Clothing worn for exercise should allow for easy movement and perspiration. Athletic shoes should provide both support and protection. Outdoor exercise should be avoided in extremely hot or extremely cold weather. Enclosed shopping malls are sheltered places for walking during the extremes of weather or when there are concerns about neighborhood safety. Exercising with a partner provides both encouragement to continue exercising and safety. Older adults should be advised to modify or stop exercising if they experience arthritis, back pain, knee problems, or chest discomfort.

Activity as Affected by Lifestyle Changes

Retirement, relocation, and the loss of a partner influence older adults' activity levels and the types of activities they choose. Many older adults directly experience these lifestyle changes; others experience them indirectly when a partner retires or is admitted to a long-term-care facility.

Retirement

Retirement represents a major lifestyle change for older adults. During most of their lives, older adults have gone to work or watched a partner go to work each day. With retirement, the daily schedule changes. The hours spent on the job and in transit to and from the job are no longer committed. For couples where only one individual has worked, the partner's daily routine is affected by the other individual now being home. If the partner is still working outside the home when the individual retires, they now find themselves at home alone. For the unmarried retired person, retirement may be a transition from a companionable work setting to a lonely, empty house. Key issues for the retired older adult are replacing work with meaningful activities and replacing work-related friends with new acquaintances.

Activities in retirement may be chosen to be meaningful and to meet socialization needs. Past interests influence choices about activities. If past interests have focused only on work-related topics, retirement choices may be restricted unless the retired older adult develops new areas of interest. Finances may also impose practical restrictions on the types of activities chosen. Health status issues such as limited mobility, limited endurance, or sensory deficits may also restrict activity choices. However, for many older adults, retirement is a time to become involved in activities that could not be pursued while working because of time and energy constraints. Many older adults volunteer in community organizations, return to school for the joy of learning, or even start second careers. Nurses are empathetic listeners to accounts of the changes retirement brings and sources of information about different activities available.

Relocation

Relocation is movement from one place of residence to another. Relocation may be from the long-time home in a cold climate to a house or apartment in a warmer part of the country. Older adults may also move from their home to the home of their children or grandchildren. Still other older adults may move to a retirement community or an assisted-living or long-term-care facility. Regardless of the destination, relocation is always an uprooting and a disordering of usual routines. Even when the move is from an unpleasant or unsafe situation, a risk still exists that relocation may adversely affect well-being.

Relocation disrupts usual patterns of activity. Adaptations that maintained independence in ADLs may no longer function. The walk through a familiar neighborhood for exercise may no longer be possible. The new community or long-term-care facility will have different options for activities. New social networks can be established. The nurse's role during relocation is to support efforts to become accustomed to new situations and opportunities and to monitor the effect of relocation stress on health.

Activity programming in long-term-care facilities is the responsibility of activity directors. A sufficient variety of activities is provided to allow residents to have choices. Although residents are encouraged to participate in a variety of activities, they always have the right to determine the degree of their participation. The activity preferences of each resident are assessed on admission. The individualized care plan includes activities that are appropriate for the resident. Individual (one-on-one activities) and small- and large-group activities are typically provided (Fig. 8.2). Some facilities provide mechanisms for residents to participate in planning future activities and for families and friends of the residents to be part of the activity program (Box 8.4).

Loss of a Partner

The loss of a partner disrupts both joint activities and those activities where one individual supported the other. If death is preceded by an illness, activities are altered before death. During the period of grief, activities may be reduced. For example, the

> ### BOX 8.4 Examples of Activities in Long-Term Care Facilities
>
> **Exercise**
> - Walking programs (indoor, outdoor)
> - Dancing (balloon, square, line)
> - T'ai chi (or similar disciplines)
>
> **Spectator Activities**
> - Television (selected programming, including telecourses)
> - Video movies
> - Live performances at the facility
>
> **Participative Activities**
> - Cards, bingo, and board games
> - Adapted versions of bowling and volleyball
> - Adaptations of TV game shows (*Jeopardy, Wheel of Fortune*)
> - Yard games such as croquet, miniature golf, bocce ball, and horseshoes
> - Field trips to museums, sports events, restaurants, shopping malls, and parks
> - Picnics and barbecues
> - Fishing
>
> **Creative Activities**
> - Art projects (painting)
> - Crafts (woodworking, stitchery)
> - Gardening (indoor or outdoor)
> - Cooking or planning menus for special meals at the facility
> - Music (vocal or instrumental performances by residents)
> - Writing a newsletter for the facility
>
> **Intergenerational Activities**
> - Visits from children's groups
> - Adopting (and being adopted by) a schoolroom or scout troop
>
> **Pets and Other Animals**
> - Domestic animals kept at the facility (dogs, cats, rabbits, songbirds, parrots, fish, sheep, goats, llamas, chickens, ducks, and geese)
> - Other animals brought to the facility by zoos or conservation groups (owls, hawks, chimpanzees, and nonvenomous snakes)

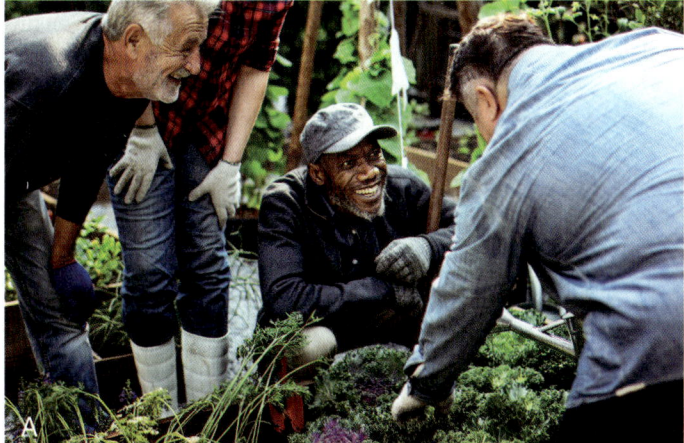 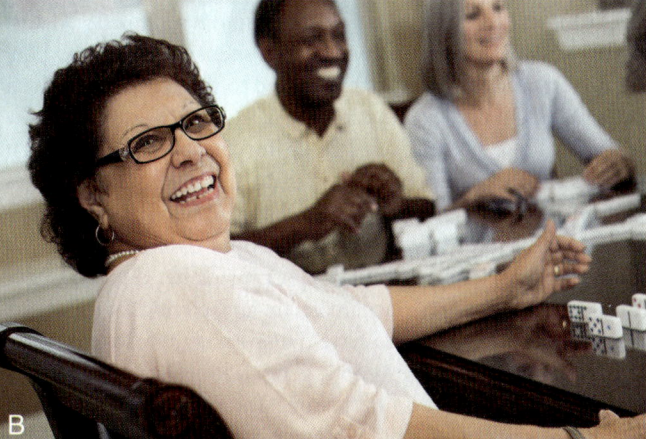

Fig. 8.2 Recreational activities are important for older adults. (A, From iStockphoto.com/Rawpixel; B, From iStockphoto.com/SDI Productions.)

older adult may not feel up to participating in an exercise class. However, part of the process of grief and recovery from grief is the adoption of a new pattern of life. That new pattern includes new activities but also includes the resumption of former activities, although these may be altered by the absence of the spouse.

Nurses assist older adults who have experienced the loss of a partner by listening attentively and supporting the development of new activities. Some of these new activities may require learning new skills such as handling finances, cooking, laundry, or car maintenance. Other activities may involve making new friends. Information from nurses about available programs and services may help with the acquisition of new skills and the re-establishment of social connections. During the period of adjustment after the loss of a partner, nurses also monitor the patient's physical and mental health, remembering that stress may lead to alterations in health.

Activity Affected by Alzheimer Disease and Other Dementias

Alzheimer disease and other dementias affect an estimated 6.7 million people in the United States (Alzheimer's Association, 2023). As Alzheimer disease progresses, cognitive impairment increases, adversely affecting the ability to participate in routine daily activities. The older adult with advancing dementia also loses the ability to initiate diversional activities and to participate in activities that were once enjoyed. Caregivers gradually assume more responsibility for monitoring behavior, performing basic personal care tasks, and providing opportunities for physical exercise, cognitive stimulation, and entertainment.

At the heart of planning activities for an older adult with dementia is the desire to preserve the remaining physical and cognitive abilities and to promote independence. Activities should draw on assets rather than deficits and should maximize the remaining abilities (Alzheimer's Association, 2017a). When planning activities, nurses or other caregivers must consider the extent of cognitive impairment, any concomitant physical constraints caused by aging or other diseases, and safety concerns.

Activities for older adults with dementia should be meaningful (Alzheimer's Association, 2017a). A meaningful activity has a purpose. The purpose may be to exercise arthritic joints or simply to have fun, but the activity should not be aimless. Meaningful activities are also voluntary. No one is compelled to participate. Instead, individuals are invited to participate and given encouragement and explanations of the activity. Meaningful activities foster a sense of well-being for the participants. If an older adult with dementia is stressed by the activity or indicates discomfort, that person should be allowed, or assisted, to stop or leave the activity. Activities should also be consistent with the older adult's social status and support his or her dignity. Older adults may choose to participate in an activity that appears childish, but they must also have the option to refuse to participate. Activities should promote good feelings, not feelings of embarrassment, distress, or failure. To successfully plan and implement activities for older adults with dementia, nurses and other caregivers must be flexible, patient, and sensitive to the environment (Alzheimer's Association, 2017b). Communication is enhanced when the nurse or other caregiver speaks to the older adult as one adult to another and assumes the older adult will understand. If the older adult does not understand, repetition or rephrasing may be necessary, but it is best to begin with the positive expectation that the older adult will understand. Scolding, addressing the older adult as a child, or issuing negative instructions ("Don't …") should be avoided (Alzheimer's Association, 2017b).

As cognitive impairment increases, the older adult with dementia requires more supervision and assistance with personal care activities such as bathing, dressing, grooming, toileting, oral hygiene, and eating. Personal care activities are best accomplished in regular routines that involve simple, single-step instructions and visual cues. The environment should be quiet, soothing, uncluttered, and unhurried. To promote independence and preserve functional ability, nurses should encourage older adults with dementia to do the personal care tasks, or parts of tasks, that are within their abilities.

Physical exercise for the older adult with dementia is important for general physical well-being, but exercise may also reduce agitation or wandering. The rhythmic movement of a rocking chair may reduce agitation. Going for a walk may redirect the impulse to wander. Whether the benefit is from the change of setting, the removal of the older adult from a provocative stimulus, or the physical effects of walking, the end result is often an older adult who appears more comfortable. Exercise is also important for preserving muscle strength, flexibility, and ambulation. Other activities providing physical exercise include dancing, marching in place or swinging the arms to music, and gardening.

Older adults with dementia gradually lose the ability to select diversional activities, yet when diversional activities are provided, they appear to enjoy themselves and participate to the extent of their abilities. Activities for older adults with dementia range from playing simple games to dancing to watching birds at a bird feeder. Activities may include simple housekeeping tasks such as dusting or folding towels. Activities may be one-on-one activities such as taking a walk with a caregiver or group activities such as attending a church service.

Activities that tap into the older adult's past-life experiences and interests may stimulate memory. Older adults with dementia may enjoy reminiscing, in groups or individually, because long-term memory may be preserved in the early stages of dementia. Activities that involve making or growing things evoke pride in the self and in accomplishments. Even in later stages of dementia, an object or a song may evoke a memory. Song lyrics or the familiar motions of cooking, painting, or playing the piano may be remembered when many other things have been forgotten.

The benefits of activity for older adults include the promotion of health and the preservation of independence. Nurses help older adults adapt their activities to the situations that arise in the later years. Nurses also work with older adults to identify new activities. Whether the activities involve daily activities, physical exercise, or diversion, older adults and nurses should work together to design and select activities that improve the QoL.

> **HOME CARE**
>
> 1. Assess risk factors (e.g., environment, pain, or depression) that would predispose homebound older adults to sleep disturbances.
> 2. Review all drugs to identify those that may interfere with homebound older adults' sleep patterns.
> 3. Instruct caregivers and homebound older adults on activities that foster normal sleep, for example, avoidance of caffeinated beverages and alcohol.
> 4. Assist caregivers and homebound older adults with environmental changes that foster normal sleep, for example, using a rocking chair or taking a warm bath.
> 5. Remember that anxiety concerning safety and welfare may be an obstacle to sleep. A system of notification and monitoring to link older adults living alone with the outside world is important to promote a sense of security.

SUMMARY

Sleep and activity are two halves that make a whole day. Without sleep, we are not restored from the previous day's efforts and today's activities are slowed by fatigue. Without activities, we face going to bed without feeling the necessity of rest. Without the appropriate balance of rest and activity, we are at risk of alterations in health. Nurses, by recognizing the changes that come with age and with alterations in health status, are able to assist older adults with their sleep and activity needs.

KEY POINTS

- The sleep changes experienced by many older adults include increased sleep latency, decreased sleep efficiency, increased awakening in the night, increased early morning awakening, and increased daytime sleepiness.
- Some of the sleep changes experienced by older adults are associated with chronic disease and other health problems.
- Factors influencing sleep quality include environmental factors, pain, lifestyle changes, diet, drug use, medical conditions, depression, and dementia.
- OSA and PLMS are two common sleep disorders that may result in EDS and reports of insomnia.
- The first step in developing interventions to improve the amount and quality of sleep is a thorough sleep history.
- The sleep history includes questions about sleep amount and quality, bedtime routines, the sleep environment, activities, diet, and drugs.
- Direct observation of the older adult during sleep, reports from a roommate or bed partner, a sleep diary, measurement instruments to assess sleep quality and quantity, and diagnostic studies in a sleep laboratory may be used to supplement the sleep history.
- Sleep hygiene measures include activities that promote sleep, emphasis on stable schedules, bedtime routines, a sleep-friendly environment, avoidance of substances that interfere with sleep, exercise, and stress reduction.
- Activities pursued by a particular older adult are influenced by that individual's preferences, lifestyle, and health.
- With advancing years and changes in health and lifestyle circumstances, performance of ADLs may require modified approaches or the assistance of others.
- Physical exercise is important for older adults to maintain health, preserve the ability to perform ADLs, and improve the general QoL.
- Safe exercise requires gradual increases in the amount of exercise for older adults who have not been exercising regularly, adequate hydration before and after exercise, and suitable clothing and footwear.
- Retirement, relocation, and the loss of a spouse influence the ways older adults are active and the types of activities that they pursue.
- The goals of activities for older adults with Alzheimer's disease and other dementias include preservation of physical and cognitive abilities and promotion of independence.

CLINICAL JUDGMENT EXERCISES

1. A nursing facility resident tells you they have not been sleeping well and asks to have the provider order a sleeping pill. What questions should be asked to assess the resident's sleep quality and quantity? Due to the drawbacks of the use of sedatives and hypnotics, what other interventions should be suggested to improve their sleep?
2. An older adult comes to the clinic accompanied by their partner. The partner reports the patient is snoring loudly every night and is always falling asleep during the day. However, the patient denies snoring, but admits that they are often very sleepy during the day. Which is the most likely sleep disorder the patient is experiencing? What additional data should be gathered to support diagnosis of this sleep disorder? What recommendations should be made to the patient?
3. After checking the blood pressure of an older adult at a senior citizens health fair, the individual asks about starting an exercise program. They have not been exercising, but some of their friends have told them that they should start to exercise regularly. What recommendations should be given to the individual? What precautions should be included with the recommendations?

REFERENCES

Alzheimer's Association. (2017a). *Activities at home: Planning the day for a person with middle or late stage dementia.* Retrieved from https://www.alz.org/media/Documents/alzheimers-dementia-activities-at-home-ts.pdf. Accessed July 27, 2023.

Alzheimer's Association. (2017b). *Behaviors: How to respond when dementia causes unpredictable behaviors.* Retrieved from https://www.alz.org/documents/national/brochure_behaviors.pdf. Accessed July 27, 2023.

Alzheimer's Association. (2023). *2023 Alzheimer's disease facts and figures: Special report.* Retrieved from https://www.alz.org/media/documents/alzheimers-facts-and-figures.pdf. Accessed July 27, 2023.

American Geriatrics Society (AGS). (2019). American Geriatrics Society 2019 Updated AGS Beers Criteria® for potentially inappropriate medication use in older adults. *Journal of the American Geriatrics Society, 67*(4), 674–694. doi: 10.1111/jgs.15767.

Ancoll-Israel, S. (2004). Sleep disorders in older adults. A primary care guide to assessing 4 common sleep problems in geriatric patients. *Geriatrics, 59*(1), 37–41.

Berkley, A. S., Carter, P. A., Yoder, L. H., Acton, G., & Holahan, C. K. (2020). The effects of insomnia on older adults' quality of life and daily functioning: A mixed-methods study. *Geriatric Nursing (New York, N.Y.), 41*(6), 832–838. doi:10.1016/j.gerinurse.2020.05.008.

Bruce, D. F. (2022). *Natural sleep aids and remedies.* WebMD [website]. Retrieved from https://www.webmd.com/women/natural-sleep-remedies#1. Accessed July 27, 2023.

Centers for Disease Control and Prevention (CDC). (2023). *How much physical activity do older adults need?* Retrieved from https://www.cdc.gov/physicalactivity/basics/older_adults/. Accessed July 27, 2023.

Cleveland Clinic. (2023). *Periodic limb movements of sleep (PLMS).* Retrieved from https://my.clevelandclinic.org/health/diseases/14177-periodic-limb-movements-of-sleep-plms. Accessed July 27, 2023.

Didikoglu, A., Maharani, A., Tampubolon, G., Canal, M. M., Payton, A., & Pendleton, N. (2020). Longitudinal sleep efficiency in the elderly and its association with health. *Journal of Sleep Research, 29*(3), e12898. doi:10.1111/jsr.12898.

Dopheide, J. A. (2020). Insomnia overview: Epidemiology, pathophysiology, diagnosis and monitoring, and nonpharmacologic therapy. *The American Journal of Managed Care, 26*(Suppl. 4), S76–S84. doi:10.37765/ajmc.2020.42769.

Evenson, K. R., Buchner, D. M., & Morland, K. B. (2012). Objective measurement of physical activity and sedentary behavior among US adults aged 60 years or older. *Preventing Chronic Disease, 9*, E26. doi:10.5888/pcd9.110109.

Fan, F., McPhillips, M. V., & Li, J. (2018). 0720 Daytime napping and cognition in older adults. [Abstract]. *SLEEP, 41*(Suppl. 1), A267–A268.

Friedman, S. (2010). Pain, temperature regulation, sleep, and sensory function. In K. L. McCance, S. E. Huether, V. Brashers, & N. Rote (Eds.), *Pathophysiology: The biological basis for disease in adults and children* (6th ed.). St. Louis: Elsevier.

Harding, E. C., Franks, N. P., & Wisden, W. (2019). The temperature dependence of sleep. *Frontiers in Neuroscience, 13*, 336. doi:10.3389/fnins.2019.00336.

Li, J., Vitiello, M. V., & Gooneratne, N. S. (2018). Sleep in normal aging. *Sleep Medicine Clinics, 13*(1), 1–11. doi:10.1016/j.jsmc.2017.09.001.

MacDowell, R. (2023). *The 4 stages of sleep – cycles, phases, and improvement.* Sleepopolis [website]. Retrieved from https://sleepopolis.com/education/stages-sleep-cycles/#what-are-process-s-and-process-c. Accessed July 27, 2023.

Mayo Clinic Staff. (2023). *Obstructive sleep apnea.* Mayo Clinic [website]. Retrieved from https://www.mayoclinic.org/diseases-conditions/obstructive-sleep-apnea/symptoms-causes/syc-20352090. Accessed July 27, 2023.

Mayo Clinic Staff. (2022). *Prescription sleeping pills: What's right for you?* Mayo Clinic [website]. Retrieved from https://www.mayoclinic.org/diseases-conditions/insomnia/in-depth/sleeping-pills/art-20043959. Accessed July 27, 2023.

Memar, P., & Faradji, F. (2018). A novel multi-class EEG-based sleep stage classification system. *IEEE Transactions on Neural Systems and Rehabilitation Engineering, 26*(1), 84–95. doi:10.1109/TNSRE.2017.2776149.

Nabili, S. N., & Marks, J. W. (2023). *Sleep apnea.* MedicineNet [website]. Retrieved from https://www.medicinenet.com/sleep_apnea/article.htm. Accessed July 27, 2023.

Nagel, C. L., Markie, M. B., Richards, K. C., & Taylor, J. L. (2003). Sleep promotion in hospitalized elders. *Medsurg Nursing, 12*(5), 279–290.

Osorio, R. S., Martínez-García, M. Á., & Rapoport, D. M. (2021). Sleep apnoea in the elderly: A great challenge for the future. *The European Respiratory Journal, 59*(4), 2101649. doi:10.1183/13993003.01649-2021.

Pacheco, D., & Guo, L. (2023). *Healthy bedtime snacks to eat before sleep.* Sleep Foundation [website]. Retrieved from https://www.sleepfoundation.org/nutrition/healthy-bedtime-snacks. Accessed July 27, 2023.

Pal'man, A. D. (2019). Complex sleep apnea. *Neuroscience and Behavioral Physiology, 49*(1), 48–53.

Patel, D., Steinberg, J., & Patel, P. (2018). Insomnia in the elderly: A review. *Journal of Clinical Sleep Medicine, 14*(6), 1017–1024. doi:10.5664/jcsm.7172.

Quera Salva, M. A., Hartley, S., Léger, D., & Dauvilliers, Y. (2017). Non-24-hour sleep-wake rhythm disorder in the totally blind: Diagnosis and management. *Frontiers in Neurology, 8*, 686. doi:10.3389/fneur.2017.00686.

Romero, K., Goparaju, B., Russo, K., Westover, M. B., & Bianchi, M. T. (2017). Alternative remedies for insomnia: A proposed method for personalized therapeutic trials. *Nature and Science of Sleep, 9*, 97–108. doi:10.2147/NSS.S128095.

Rosto, L. (2001). Sleep and the elderly. *Advance On-line Editions for Providers of Post-Acute Care, 4*(6), 27. https://brieflands.com/articles/semj-106830.

Rowe, M. A. (2003). People with dementia who become lost. *The American Journal of Nursing, 103*(7), 32–39. doi:10.1097/00000446-200307000-00016.

Rozgonyi, R., Dombi, I., Janszky, J., Kovács, N., & Faludi, B. (2021). Low test–retest reliability of the Epworth Sleepiness Scale within a substantial short time frame. *Journal of Sleep Research, 30*(4), e13277. doi:10.1111/jsr.13277.

Ryden, A., & Alessi, C. (2022). Sleep disorders. In J. B. Halter, J. G. Ouslander, S. Studenski, K. P. High, S. Asthana, M. A. Supiano, et al. (Eds.), *Hazzard's geriatric medicine and gerontology* (8th ed., pp. 643–664). New York: McGraw-Hill.

Schoenborn, C. A., Vickerie, J. L., Powell-Griner, E., & Centers for Disease Control and Prevention National Center for Health Statistics. (2006). Health characteristics of adults 55 years of age and over: United States, 2000–2003. *Advance Data, 370*, 1–31.

Siebern, A. T., Suh, S., & Nowakowski, S. (2012). Non-pharmacological treatment of insomnia. *Neurotherapeutics, 9*(4), 717–727. doi:10.1007/s13311-012-0142-9.

Spieker, E. D., & Motzer, S. A. (2003). Sleep-disorder in patients with heart failure: Pathophysiology, assessment, and management. *Journal of the American Academy of Nurse Practitioners, 15*(11), 487–493. doi:10.1111/j.1745-7599.2003.tb00337.x.

Tagler, M. J., Stanko, K. A., & Forbey, J. D. (2017). Predicting sleep hygiene: A reasoned action approach. *Journal of Applied Social Psychology, 47*(1), 3–12. doi:10.1111/jasp.12411.

Thomas, L. (2019). *Causes of nocturnal awakenings*. News-Medical.net [website]. Retrieved from https://www.news-medical.net/health/Causes-of-Nocturnal-Awakenings.aspx. Accessed July 27, 2023.

United States Census Bureau. (2017). *Facts for features: Older Americans Month: May 2017*. Retrieved from https://www.census.gov/newsroom/facts-for-features/2017/cb17-ff08.html. Accessed July 27, 2023.

University of Pittsburgh Center for Sleep and Circadian Science (CSCS). (n.d.). *Measures and study instruments*. Retrieved from https://www.sleep.pitt.edu/instruments/. Accessed July 27, 2023.

WebMD Editorial Contributors. (2022a). *How to sleep better as you get older*. WebMD [website]. Retrieved from https://www.webmd.com/sleep-disorders/aging-affects-sleep#2. Accessed July 27, 2023.

WebMD Editorial Contributors. (2022b). *Central sleep apnea*. WebMD [website]. Retrieved from http://www.webmd.com/sleep-disorders/guide/central-sleep-apnea. Accessed July 27, 2023.

WebMD Editorial Contributors. (2021a). *Obstructive sleep apnea (OSA)*. WebMD [website]. Retrieved from https://www.webmd.com/sleep-disorders/sleep-apnea/understanding-obstructive-sleep-apnea-syndrome. Accessed July 27, 2023.

WebMD Editorial Contributors. (2021b). *Insomnia*. WebMD [website]. Retrieved from https://www.webmd.com/sleep-disorders/insomnia-symptoms-and-causes. Accessed July 27, 2023.

Zhang, R., Tomasi, D., Manza, P., Shokri-Kojori, E., Demiral, S. B., Feldman, D. E., et al. (2021). Sleep disturbances are associated with cortical and subcortical atrophy in alcohol use disorder. *Translational Psychiatry, 11*(1), 428. doi:10.1038/s41398 021-01534-0.

9

Safety

Jerilyn W. Bumpas, DNP, MSN, RN and Jennifer J. Yeager, PhD, MSN, RN

http://evolve.elsevier.com/Yeager/gerontologic/

LEARNING OBJECTIVES

On completion of this chapter, the reader will be able to:
1. Identify the nurse's role in the promotion of safety for older adults.
2. Name various community, state, and federal safety-related resources for older individuals.
3. Identify safety hazards in the health-care setting that may lead to litigation.
4. Differentiate between intrinsic and extrinsic causes of falling in older adults.
5. Identify common treatable causes of falling in older adults.
6. Implement the nursing standard of practice for patients experiencing falls.
7. Use home safety tips to prevent burns, accidental poisoning, smoke inhalation, and foodborne illnesses among community-dwelling older adults.
8. Differentiate between hypothermia and hyperthermia and the nursing needs of each.
9. Identify disaster planning resources.
10. Differentiate among the various types of elder abuse.
11. List clinical syndromes and conditions that could impair older individuals and lead to safety hazards on the roadway.
12. Describe the pros and cons of having firearms in the homes of older adults.

WHAT WOULD YOU DO?

What would you do if you were faced with the following situations?
- Your 75-year-old nursing home resident was found on the floor in a sitting position, near the foot of the bed. After determining the resident had not sustained any head trauma or change in mental status nor sustained any apparent breaks, what would be your next steps?
- Your 80-year-old patient arrives at the clinic, using a rolling walker. They are not accompanied by their caregiver, as usual. Upon questioning, you determine the patient drove themselves to their appointment. How would you determine whether the individual was safe to drive? What would you do if it was determined they should not be driving?

Feeling safe and secure in one's living environment is essential for everyone. With aging comes a need to maintain peace of mind while engaging in daily activities. Perceived security and safety affect the confidence to carry out daily tasks. Safety is a broad concept that refers to security and preventing accidents or injuries. When working with older adults, the gerontological nurse must provide a standard of care that promotes safety and prevents foreseeable accidents or injuries while also respecting individuals' autonomy to make decisions. This standard of care should pervade all aspects of the nurse's health-care relationships with older adults.

Unintentional injury is one of the top 15 causes of death across all age groups (Murphy et al, 2021). Violent crimes, including homicide, are another concern for all Americans, including older adults. Violent crimes such as homicide remain a significant concern as rates are not declining. In fact, between 2019 and 2020, there was a 30% increase in homicide, the largest in US history (National Center for Health Statistics, 2021).

Part of the nurse's role in ensuring safety is educating older adults so they can make informed choices. Education affords the opportunity to weigh benefits versus risks and to choose the best option in a given situation. When patients cannot make informed choices, family members or significant others are sought as advocates for the patients. If patients cannot make informed choices and no family members are available, the nurse must use nursing judgment and follow acceptable standards of care to promote safety and security.

Previous authors: Debra L. Sanders, PhD, RN, GCNS-BC, FNGNA; Ramesh C. Upadhyaya, RN, CRRN, MSN, MBA, PhD-C, and Deb Bagnasco Stanford, MSN, RN, CCRN

This chapter presents common problems that jeopardize patient safety and lead to accidents, injuries, and even death. These include falls, restraint use, accidental injuries, crime and victimization, elder abuse, vulnerability to temperature changes, disasters, and dangers in the home environment. Attention will be given to safety tips and interventions for injury prevention.

FALLS

Overview and Magnitude of the Problem

Falls are common, threaten the independence of older adults (Rubenstein, 2022), and "are the leading cause of fatal and nonfatal injuries for older Americans" (National Council on Aging [NCOA], 2023, para. 1) in the United States. Over three million older adults are treated in the emergency department for falls annually. One in five falls results in a serious injury. In terms of serious injuries, falls are the leading cause of hip fractures, with more than 300,000 occurrences annually. Additionally, more than 800,000 older adults are hospitalized annually after a fall because of a head injury or hip fracture. Deaths from falls increased 30% between 2007 and 2016 in those over the age of 65 (CDC, 2021a).

Hip fractures occur in females about three times more often than in males. Females lose bone density faster than males, in part because the drop in estrogen levels that occurs with menopause accelerates bone loss. However, males also can develop dangerously low levels of bone density (Mayo Clinic Staff, 2022a).

Interventions designed to modify risk factors can reduce the frequency of falls. Programs targeting high-risk older adults have incorporated interventions aimed at medication modification, environmental improvements, and behavioral modification.

Not all falls are preventable; therefore, the goal for older adults with frequent falls is fall reduction, prevention of serious injury, and modification of significant risk factors.

Because falls are multifactorial, not all older adults fall due to the same factors. For instance, older adults may lose their balance and fall when hurrying to answer the telephone and then experience a second fall the next morning, getting up from bed too quickly. In this example, two distinct causes of falling are present, and both can be modified through education and behavioral modification. Thus, a comprehensive assessment must be performed because falls tend to be multifactorial in this age group. A comprehensive assessment includes a detailed history and physical examination.

Patient education is the cornerstone of fall prevention and management. The gerontological nurse must explore patient beliefs and misconceptions about falling. Older individuals may consider falling to be a normal part of the aging process. For some, it is an expectation of growing old. Individuals who hold these stereotypes must be educated about the normal aging process, which is distinct from diseases and the adverse effects of medications. It is important to tell older adults that the cause of falling can most often be determined by a health-care professional who has expertise in fall assessment and that falls can be reduced and even prevented through some simple interventions

---

BOX 9.1 General Fall Prevention Guidelines

General Care
- Wear low-heeled shoes with small wedge platforms.
- Wear leather- or rubber-soled shoes.
- Leave nightlights on at night.
- Keep items within reach to avoid overreaching.
- Check the tips of canes and walkers for evenness.
- Have the last step painted a different color, indoors, and outdoors.
- Dangle the legs between positional changes and rise slowly.
- Avoid the use of alcohol.
- Avoid rushing.
- Avoid risky behavior such as standing on ladders unaided.

Steps and Floor Surfaces
- Be careful to avoid slippery floors and frayed carpets.
- Watch for the last step when descending the stairs.
- Count the number of steps as a cue while ascending and descending the stairs.
- Install and use sturdy banisters on both sides of staircases.
- Tack down throw rugs or remove them entirely.
- Remove obstacles in the path of traffic.
- Use carpeting that has color contrast on landing surfaces.

Bathroom
- Have grab bars installed in the tub and shower and near the toilet.
- Avoid throw rugs; have carpeting installed.
- Avoid bar soaps; use liquid soap from a dispenser mounted in the shower.

(Box 9.1). Staff development programs and continuing education must also address the normal aging process, the adverse effects of medications, and the treatable causes of falling. Once the patient and staff's knowledge of falling improves, fall rates should improve.

Definition of Falling

It is important for the gerontological nurse to recognize that older individuals define falling in numerous ways and are influenced by perceptions of aging and disease, and the context of the situation. For instance, older individuals may not perceive a slip that results in a fall to the floor as an actual "fall"; rather, it may be termed a *slip, trip,* or *accident,* but not a *fall.* Box 9.2 illustrates some common reasons older adults give to explain a fall. The falling event needs to be reviewed in detail to determine whether the person fell to the ground. Moreover, how individuals define falling is likely to influence the reporting of falls. A *fall* "is defined as an event which results in a person coming to rest inadvertently on the ground or floor or other lower level" (World Health Organization [WHO], 2021, para. 1). An example of this is a sudden and unexpected drop from standing upright into a seat or onto the floor. Injuries such as

---

BOX 9.2 Common Explanations for Falling Given by Older Adults

- "I think I slipped."
- "I don't remember what happened."
- "I was in a hurry."
- "I tripped."
- "I lost my balance."

bruising, sprains, strains, or fractures may result from minimal height drops.

Key initial assessment points include level of consciousness (determining if loss of consciousness occurred), circulation, airway, and breathing. After treating acute injuries, a head-to-toe assessment of all body systems, including orthostatic vital signs (Lovence, n.d.), should occur. History-taking should be detailed enough for the examiner to envision the details leading to the fall and incorporate a detailed drug review.

Meaning of Falling

The health-care professional may equate a fall with a decline in patient health or function, a worsening of a patient's condition, or a marker of future decline. Falls may be a nonspecific presenting sign of an acute change in an older adult's condition. Conditions contributing to falls include constipation, urinary tract infection, pneumonia, and dehydration (Kelly, 2019; Scottish Government, 2023).

Normal Age-Related Changes Contributing to Falling

Numerous age-related changes predispose older adults to falling, especially when these changes affect functional ability and give rise to sensory impairment or gait and balance instability. This section highlights the salient age-related changes associated with falling, along with nursing interventions directed at modifying the effect of these changes to prevent falling. Normal age-related changes in organ function may contribute to an intrinsic risk for falling (Boltz et al, 2021).

Vision

Structural changes in eye shape and crystalline lens flexibility accompany the aging of the eye. Inflexibility of the lens causes presbyopia, a reduction in the eye's accommodation for changes in depth, as when ascending or descending the stairs. If older individuals are experiencing presbyopia, instruction must be given for them to carefully watch door edges, curbs, and landing steps, which signal a change in height. Additionally, because of the tendency for the crystalline lens to become cloudy and form a cataract with advancing years, eye glare may occur and cause temporary visual disturbances. This effect is particularly evident outdoors on sunny days or indoors as bright light reflects off shiny floors. Instruction must be given to older individuals with this problem to wear wide-brimmed hats or sunglasses to shield the eyes from the glare effect and to shade indoor windows with drapes or blinds to minimize the effects of sun glare.

Hearing

An age-related change affecting the inner ear is atrophy of the ossicle, which causes changes in sound conduction, including a loss of high-tone frequencies called *presbycusis*. Other age-related changes include an amplification of background noise and a decrease in directional hearing. The vestibular system is an integral part of maintaining balance and, to a large degree, is dependent on intact hearing. Therefore, older individuals with hearing impairments are more susceptible to falling when feedback to the brain is altered.

Assessment of hearing difficulties begins during the initial interview. In some individuals with significant hearing loss, it becomes necessary to use alternative forms of visual cues to signal where their feet and bodies are in space so that they can maintain stability. For instance, when hearing loss cannot be corrected, one aim of managing hearing problems is to introduce vibratory or visual cues to compensate for hearing loss. The use of bells on shoelaces causes a vibratory sense that can be felt by older adults when a foot is placed on the ground. Nursing interventions include instructing older patients to observe foot placement on the floor by literally "watching their step" and to be especially cognizant of environmental conditions such as floor surfaces.

Cardiovascular Factors

One of the most common problems facing older adults is the loss of tissue elasticity, which affects the arteries. This lack of elasticity leads to decreased tissue recoil, resulting in changes in blood pressure with position changes. Older adults who lie supine and then get up quickly are likely to experience the effects of a lack of tissue elasticity when blood pressure drops and a feeling of lightheadedness develops. It is important to educate older individuals to change position slowly and to dangle their legs for a few minutes when arising from a supine position. Older adults should be encouraged to wait between position changes and to hold onto the side of the bed or other furniture should lightheadedness occur, or use a single bed rail specifically manufactured to assist older adults in getting in and out of bed.

Musculoskeletal Factors

The bones of aging individuals, particularly the weight-bearing joints, undergo "wear and tear," which causes loss of supportive cartilage. As a result, joints may become unstable and "give way," leading to a fall. In many instances, osteoarthritis occurs in the weight-bearing joints, causing pain with weight-bearing and further eroding joint stability. Interventions are directed at identifying and correcting problems using antiinflammatory agents, prescribed activity and exercise, braces, joint replacement, or all of these measures. If joint pain develops and remains untreated, it may cause older adults to become sedentary or immobile. This phenomenon of disuse and muscle atrophy contributes to muscle weakness. This cycle of pain, reduced mobility, disuse, and atrophy may become a vicious one unless interrupted by regular mobility and pain control using topical or systemic medication. Nursing interventions are directed at encouraging, supervising, or assisting with regular ambulation; appropriate use of ambulation aids; joint range of motion; and modalities such as ice, hot packs, and physical therapy.

Another normal age-related musculoskeletal change is the reduction in steppage height, which may place older adults at risk for tripping, especially when door edges are not visible or carpeting is frayed. The gerontological nurse's role is to identify these changes and offer suggestions for improvement, depending on the cause. In some cases, an assistive device may have to be employed to aid mobility and avoid further joint damage.

Neurologic Factors

One of the most universal age-related changes affecting the neurologic system is a slowing in reaction time. It takes older individuals a longer time to respond both verbally and physically to changes in position. Older adults who lose their balance can right themselves to an upright position, provided the musculoskeletal strength of hips, ankles, and shoulders is adequate. However, those with functional impairments and diseases, muscle weakness, or adverse effects from medications might lose their postural stability and fall. For these individuals, uneven surfaces in the environment, such as steps, sidewalks, and curbs, may lead to loss of footing and subsequent falls. Nursing interventions for those with impaired righting reflexes include monitoring mobility for signs of unsteadiness and offering supervision and assistance when needed. In an effort to promote autonomy, it is important to allow older patients to continue to perform their usual activities independently and safely.

When independent activity is no longer possible, older adults require a physical therapy evaluation for the use of a walking aid such as a straight cane, stationary walker, or posterior walker. Nursing interventions also include the use of chair or bed alarms or call buttons worn around the neck to signal that assistance is needed. Shoes should be inspected for sturdy heels that are low and preferably wedge type. Observation of an older adult patient's ability to walk is crucial. For instance, is the walking path straight, or does the patient deviate from it? Does the patient trip when walking because of inappropriate shoes? For some older adults with gait disorders, rubber soles, such as those on sneakers worn on high-pile carpeting, may hinder and result in shuffling or stumbling while walking. Leather soles are preferable, as are those that are low-heeled and have laces, providing extra ankle and foot support.

Fall Risk

Overall, most published research on falls and falling pertains to determining fall risk. Antecedents (e.g., diseases such as stroke, delirium, dementia, or urinary incontinence) that lead to falls have been clearly defined (Box 9.3). However, many individuals with these disease-related risk factors do not fall. Thus, fall risk is not determined solely based on the number and kind of diseases but also on how these risk factors influence an older adult's functional ability, specifically in the areas of mobility, transferring, and negotiating within the environment.

Fall risk is best determined by observing mobility. It may be categorized according to intrinsic (illness or disease-related) or extrinsic (environmental) risk (CDC, 2017a).

A risk for falling according to these categories differs from the intrinsic or extrinsic causes of falling. *Risk* is determined by the clinician and is a term that reflects a judgment based on a thorough evaluation of a patient, known hazards for falling, and foreseeable events. Older patients at "risk" for falling may not experience a fall at all. Numerous extrinsic risks for falling exist, for example, lack of color contrast on curbs, poor lighting, frayed carpeting, and unsteady furniture. Intrinsic risks for falling include conditions such as orthostatic hypotension, blindness, or advanced dementia. The presence of these risk factors, however, does not mean that an older patient will actually fall—just that he or she is *likely* to fall given certain circumstances. In fact, some individuals at risk for falling, as evidenced by these risk factors, do not fall. Some of the circumstances that may lead to falling in older adults include unsteady gait or balance instability, delirium or side effects of medications causing unsteadiness, and an inability to right themselves when the footing is lost, or balance is unstable.

As mentioned, the risk for falling is different from actual intrinsic or extrinsic causes of falling. In the latter case, a fall has occurred and is the result of either intrinsic disease, extrinsic environmental causes, or a combination of the two. These falls will likely occur among those deemed at "risk for falling." The workup seeks to identify the underlying cause so that it can be treated, thus ultimately preventing or reducing recurrent falls. One aim of fall management is the reduction of risk factors to promote safety while respecting patient autonomy. Because falling is individually determined and not always preventable or predictable, it is important to avoid classifying patients according to the clinician's perception of their risk for falling (i.e., high versus low risk). As previously discussed, falling does not necessarily occur among individuals at greatest risk. The effect of functional ability is significant as it relates to older individuals who fall. Research has shown that an individual with frailty and physical functional limitations is at the greatest risk for falling.

Intrinsic Risk

Intrinsic risk for falling refers to the combined effect of normal age-related changes, concurrent disease, and adverse drug effects. Age-related changes can impair gait, balance, stability, and cognition (Rubenstein, 2022). This requires the gerontological nurse to assess an older individual's gait and balance and determine whether impairment exists. Measurement tools have

---

> **BOX 9.3 Treatable Causes of Falling in Older Adults**
>
> - Orthostatic hypotension
> - Dehydration
> - Profound anemia
> - Cardiac arrhythmia (e.g., bradyarrhythmia, tachyarrhythmia, sick sinus syndrome)
> - Overdosing with medication or alcohol
> - Urinary tract infection
> - Vitamin B_{12} deficiency
> - Osteoporosis
> - Hypoglycemia
> - Seizures
> - Carotid hypersensitivity
> - Carotid stenosis
> - Delirium[a]
>
> [a]Mental status is an important determinant of fall risk. Changes in mental status, such as those incurred with delirium, may cause older individuals to have difficulty negotiating within the environment. Delirium causes individuals to misperceive sensory input and stimuli and objects in the environment.

Instructions: Client is seated in a hard, armless, chair. The following maneuvers are tested:

1. Sitting balance
   - 0 = Leans or slides in chair
   - 1 = Steady and safe

2. Arise
   - 0 = Unable without help
   - 1 = Able, but uses arm to help
   - 2 = Able without use of arms

3. Attempts to arise
   - 0 = Unable without help
   - 1 = Able, but requires more than one attempt
   - 2 = Able to arise in one attempt

4. Immediate standing balance (first 5 seconds)
   - 0 = Unsteady (e.g., staggers, moves feet, marked trunk sway)
   - 1 = Steady, but uses walker or cane or grabs another object for support
   - 2 = Steady without walker, cane, or other support

5. Standing balance
   - 0 = Unsteady
   - 1 = Steady, but has a wide stance (i.e., medial heels >4 inches apart) or uses a cane, walker, or other support
   - 2 = Narrow stance without support

6. Nudge (with subject at maximum position with feet as close together as possible. Examiner pushes lightly on client's sternum three times with palm of the hand).
   - 0 = Begins to fall
   - 1 = Staggers, grabs, but catches self
   - 2 = Steady

7. Eyes closed (with subject at maximum position as in #6)
   - 0 = Unsteady
   - 1 = Steady

8. Turn 360°
   - 0 = Discontinuous steps
   - 1 = Continuous steps
   - 0 = Unsteady (e.g., grabs, staggers)
   - 1 = Steady

9. Sit down
   - 0 = Unsafe (e.g., misjudges distance, falls into chair)
   - 1 = Uses arms or does not use a smooth motion
   - 2 = Safe, smooth motion

_____ / 16 **Balance score**

Fig. 9.1 Tinetti Balance and Gait Evaluation. (From Fortinsky, R., Iannuzzi-Sucich, M., Baker, D., Gottschalk, M., King, M., Brown, C., et al. [2004]. Fall-risk assessment and management in clinical practice: Views from healthcare providers. *Journal of the American Geriatrics Society, 52*[9], 1522–1526.)

TABLE 9.1 Treatable Causes of Gait and Balance Abnormalities

Physical Examination Finding	Possible Associated Gait or Balance Impairment
Peripheral neuropathy	Inability to feel feet on the floor
Charcot joint	Foot instability, foot pain, or both
Loss of proprioception	Foot placement on floor altered
Hemiparesis	Leaning to one side; gait instability
Hammer toe	Foot pain during weight bearing
Decreased steppage height	Shuffling gait; tripping

been developed to rate both gait and balance. These tools identify key components of gait, such as step length and height, step symmetry, and path. Important areas of balance assessment include sitting and standing balance, turning, and the ability to sit without losing balance. The Tinetti Gait and Balance Test instruments are measurement tools that quantitatively score gait and balance. These tools have been tested through clinical research and hold acceptable validity and reliability ratings (Tinetti, 1986) (Fig. 9.1).

Additionally, other assessment tools employ a combination of measures, such as gait, balance, vestibular evaluation, and functional performance (CDC, 2017a).

Before managing gait or balance impairments with assistive aids or physical therapy, older individuals require medical workups for treatable causes of gait and balance abnormalities (Table 9.1).

Extrinsic Risk

Various indoor and outdoor environmental hazards may predispose individuals to falling (CDC, 2017a).

Research has found that older people continue to perform the same types of risk-taking behaviors in their later years of life as in their younger years. Modifying risky behaviors in the face of functional impairment may prevent accidental falls in and around the home. Because 6 of every 10 falls occur in the home, instruction in home safety tips should be incorporated into health encounters with older individuals who experience falls (National Institute on Aging, 2022a).

The modification of environmental risk factors is also critical for fall prevention. Environmental hazards are those that contribute to accidental falls. Research has found that about 31% of falls can be prevented by environmental changes (Campani et al, 2021). The key areas that require evaluation for safety are steps, floor surfaces, edges and curbs, lighting, and grab rails; nursing interventions are directed at environmental assessment of the indoor living space in these key areas. Whenever possible, uneven steps should be repaired or at least have a sturdy handrail to hold onto for support. Floor surfaces should have low-pile carpeting in good repair. Tears should be sewn to prevent shoe heels from becoming caught. Throw rugs should be eliminated because they are a tripping hazard. Curbs and cement landing surfaces should be painted with a contrasting color to outline edges. Lighting should be adequate in high-traffic and dimly lit areas. On a more global scale, a community effort to notify the local Housing Commission of areas needing improvement is an important step in the design of future homes that are safe for older adults.

Steps. The last step of a staircase is the most cited place where falls occur in the home. The last step is a problem area, primarily because of visual changes or functional impairment. Handrails should be present on both sides of a staircase or series of steps. The handrail typically ends at the second-to-last step; if a person descending the stairs is using the handrail as a guide for the landing surface, it will place the individual at the second-to-last step.

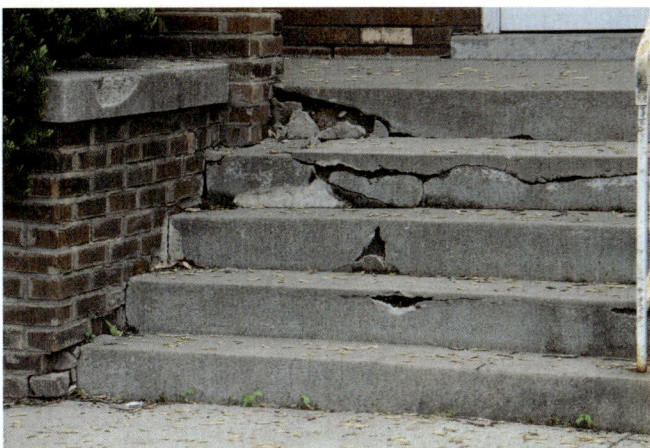

Fig. 9.2 Uneven stairs with missing handrail. (From SBSArtDept/iStockphoto.com.)

> **BOX 9.4 Conditions Associated With Greatest Risk for Serious Injury**
>
> - Mental status changes (e.g., those related to delirium and dementia)
> - Osteoporosis
> - Gait or balance instability
> - Concurrent fractures (e.g., of the hip, pelvis, humerus, or ulna)
> - Restraint use

Interventions to correct this include educating patients about this situation, teaching individuals to count the steps (i.e., keeping a mental tally of the number of steps ascending or descending), and reinstalling handrails that meet the individual's needs. Another problem regarding the staircase is the unevenness of steps (Fig. 9.2). Observation and correction of this phenomenon may be the first step toward fall prevention in the home.

Floor surfaces. Floors that have been waxed or polished are common slippery surfaces that are a safety risk for older adults, especially persons with visual impairments. Heels may be caught in frayed or torn carpeting. Throw rugs may cause tripping or sliding (if on a hardwood or tile surface). It is generally advisable to tack down throw rugs or remove them altogether. Floor surfaces should also be clutter-free, as clutter can lead to tripping and accidental falls.

Edges and curbs. Edging that lacks a contrasting color may lead to falls because surfaces tend to blend. In the home's interior, carpeting on the staircase and landing surface that are the same color may lead to falling. In the exterior of the home, concrete steps that are homogeneous in color may lead to misperceptions and subsequent falling. Uneven pavement outdoors may cause falling. Curbs that are not clearly marked with a bold contrast in color may also cause falling. Simple modifications include painting the outdoor steps a contrasting color at the landing surface and using carpet borders in a contrasting color (or adhesive tape) to distinguish changing indoor surfaces.

Lighting. Dimly lit rooms can be difficult for aging eyes and those with low vision or impaired vision. Bright lights may lead to glare and temporary visual impairment. Lighting should ideally be evenly distributed and consistent in brightness. Diffuse overhead lighting is often preferable to one bright light source.

Grab bars or rails. Grab bars and rails aid those with functional impairments and serve those who accidentally slip in the tub or shower. Grab bars to steady balance should be placed around the toilet, in the shower, or in the tub. Grab bars should be strategically placed to be most beneficial for the person with the impairment. Misplaced grab bars, which cause older people to reach, may actually lead to falls. Tubs and showers should have adhesive mats and be well-lit, and the use of bar soaps should be avoided, as they may lead to slipping and accidental falls during showering.

Risk for Serious Injury

As many as one-third of older individuals who fall are at risk for serious physical injury (Box 9.4). It is vital for the gerontological nurse to identify these individuals because they possess intrinsic risk factors that can be identified and often modified to prevent serious injury. Additionally, recognition and treatment of these individuals are part of the gerontological nurse's role in preventing foreseeable accidents. Serious injuries such as hip fractures, head trauma, and internal bleeding occur in as many as 30% of older adults who fall (WHO, 2021).

More than 95% of hip fractures are caused by falling, usually by falling sideways (CDC, 2021a).

A high mortality rate is associated with hip fractures, and the cost of their treatment places great economic strain on society for rehabilitation and other ancillary services (CDC, 2021a; NCOA, 2023).

Additionally, the use of physical restraints may increase the risk for serious injury. Individuals who are physically restrained may injure themselves when attempting to remove the restraints. Incidents of strangulation and asphyxiation have been reported secondary to restraint use. The elevation of both side rails may cause demented or delirious older adults to fall in their attempts to climb over the side rails. These individuals are at risk for serious injury because of the height of the fall; thus the effect is greater than if the side rails had not been elevated. Physical restraint use does not prevent falls and should never be employed as a "safety precaution" (American Academy of Nursing, 2018; Texas Health and Human Services, n.d.)

Reducing the Risk for Serious Injury

Behavioral modification is a broad term for interventions that alter behavior to achieve positive outcomes. The gerontological nurse is in a pivotal position to educate older individuals, especially those at risk for serious injury from falling, about fall prevention measures. Older individuals' knowledge base and receptivity to changing behavior are important aspects for the gerontological nurse to assess before initiating a teaching program. Specific teaching points will vary individually, but general guidelines for fall prevention and home safety may be illustrated through a pictorial display of high-risk environmental hazards or by issuing a handout with teaching points. Specific interventions can be reinforced as they relate to those conditions most likely to result in serious injury (Table 9.2).

Behavioral modification and instruction—for example, teaching an older patient with orthostatic hypotension to rise slowly or an individual with dizziness who moves too quickly to slow down—may not be as easy as it seems. Behavior modification first requires older patients to recognize behaviors that are contributing to problems. Often, the causes and effects of these

TABLE 9.2 Behavioral Interventions to Prevent Serious Injury

Condition	Patient Interventions
Osteoporosis	Take medications prescribed for increasing bone mineral density.
	Take vitamin D and calcium supplements.
	Eat well-balanced, nutritious meals high in calcium.
	Perform moderate weight-bearing exercises on a routine basis.
	Avoid smoking.
	Avoid excessive alcohol ingestion.
	Avoid strain on the spine (e.g., heavy lifting, bending).
Gait instability	Wear footwear with nonskid soles.
	Use mobility aids and assistive devices, as prescribed.
	Make deliberate attempts to scan the environment while walking to look for possible hazards.
	Participate in an exercise program that includes muscle strengthening and gait training.
	Make environmental modifications, as needed.
Balance instability	Change positions slowly and carefully.
	Stabilize position before moving.
	Use mobility aids and assistive devices, as prescribed.
	Assume a seated position during high-risk activities such as bathing and dressing.

behaviors need to be pointed out to patients in a clear and concise manner. However, this is not a foolproof method because falls might not occur while patients try to modify their behaviors. The patient's earlier behavior may thus be negatively reinforced, and he or she may feel justified in continuing to perform those same behaviors. Behavioral modification requires older patients to make conscious attempts, whenever a behavior is performed, to change or alter it. Much of what the nurse teaches must be remembered for later action; the use of notes and tape recorders as daily reminders may help.

Disease or condition modification to reduce the risk for serious injury from falls includes appropriate treatment of the actual disease. In the case of osteoporosis, agents to prevent bone demineralization and build bone mass are prescribed and used with calcium and vitamin D supplements. The nurse plays a key role in teaching patients with osteoporosis about the importance of calcium-rich foods and ways to incorporate these foods into the diet daily. Teaching about the risk factors associated with the development of osteoporosis is also important.

In cases of delirium, condition modification includes a determination of the underlying etiology; unless the cause is identified and treated, the condition will not resolve, and patients will remain at increased risk for serious injury from a fall. It is imperative for the nurse to recognize that the etiology is often multifactorial, thus requiring a variety of interventions based on the identified causes. While the delirium resolves, injury can be prevented through additional nursing interventions, including padding of side rails, increased surveillance, assistance with activities of daily living (ADLs), and measures to promote a calm and reassuring environment.

Fall Antecedents and Fall Classification

Falling occurs when persons are upright and walking, termed *ambulatory*, or when they are sitting or lying down, termed *nonambulatory*. Falls may also be considered serious or nonserious, depending on the consequences for patients. Individuals who fall but not to the ground and those who catch themselves are experiencing "near falls," and those who fall to the ground are experiencing true falls. Falling may be classified according to the cause of the fall (intrinsic, extrinsic, or situational), the frequency of falling, and the timing of falling in relation to other diseases. Most falls in older adults are *multifactorial* in etiology, a combination of intrinsic and extrinsic factors. Because so many different circumstances lead to falls in older adults (Tables 9.3 and 9.4), it is important to determine the type of fall according to a classification system (Rubenstein, 2022) (Box 9.5).

TABLE 9.3 Factors Contributing to Falls

Functional Impairment	Disorder
Blood pressure regulation	Anemia
	Arrhythmias
	Cardioinhibitory carotid sinus hypersensitivity
	Chronic obstructive pulmonary disease
	Dehydration
	Infections (i.e., pneumonia, sepsis)
	Metabolic disorders (i.e., diabetes, thyroid disorders, hypoglycemia, hyperosmolar states)
	Neurocardiogenic inhibition after micturition
	Postural hypotension
	Postprandial hypotension
	Valvular heart disorders
Central processing	Delirium
	Dementia
	Stroke
Gait	Arthritis
	Foot deformities
	Muscle weakness
Postural and neuromotor function	Cerebellar degeneration
	Myelopathy (i.e., due to cervical or lumbar spondylosis)
	Parkinson disease
	Peripheral neuropathy
	Stroke
	Vertebrobasilar insufficiency
Proprioception	Peripheral neuropathy (i.e., due to diabetes mellitus)
	Vitamin B_{12} deficiency
Otolaryngologic function	Acute labyrinthitis
	Benign paroxysmal positional vertigo
	Hearing loss
	Meniere disease
Vision	Cataract
	Glaucoma
	Macular degeneration (age-related)

From the MSD Manual Professional Version, edited by Sandy Falk. Copyright © 2024 Merck & Co., Inc., Rahway, NJ, USA and its affiliates. All rights reserved. Available at https://www.msdmanuals.com/professional. Accessed May 2024.

TABLE 9.4 Drugs That Contribute to Risk of Falls

Drug	Mechanism
Aminoglycosides	Direct vestibular damage
Analgesics (especially opioids)	Reduced alertness or slow central processing
Antiarrhythmics	Impaired cerebral perfusion
Anticholinergics	Confusion/Delirium
Antihypertensives (especially vasodilators)	Impaired cerebral perfusion
Antipsychotics	Extrapyramidal syndromes, other antiadrenergic effects, reduced alertness, or slow central processing
Diuretics (especially when patients are dehydrated)	Impaired cerebral perfusion
Loop diuretics (high dose)	Direct vestibular damage
Psychoactive drugs (especially antidepressants, antipsychotics, and benzodiazepines)	Reduced alertness or slow central processing

From the MSD Manual Professional Version, edited by Sandy Falk. Copyright © 2024 Merck & Co., Inc., Rahway, NJ, USA and its affiliates. All rights reserved. Available at https://www.msdmanuals.com/professional. Accessed May 2024.

BOX 9.5 Etiology of Falls

- Intrinsic factors (age-related decline in function, disorders, and adverse drug effects)
- Extrinsic factors (environmental hazards)
- Situational factors (related to the activity being done, e.g., rushing to the bathroom)

Thus, classifying falls will often aid in determining their underlying causes. It is important to note that individuals may experience any one of these types of falls singularly or in combination. Because falls are often unpredictable and, therefore not always preventable, the clinician needs to start the evaluation with the goal of identifying and managing those that are treatable (Rubenstein, 2022).

Fall Consequences
Physical Injury

The incidence of fall-related injuries spans from trivial trauma such as skin tears and sprains to serious injuries such as hip fractures, internal bleeding, or subdural hematomas. Each year, thousands of older Americans fall in their homes. Many of them are seriously injured, and some become disabled. It is estimated that every 20 minutes, an older adult dies from a fall (National Safety Council [NSC], 2022; NCOA, 2023).

Research investigations have found that cognitive impairment (CI), gait and balance impairment, low body mass index, and at least two chronic conditions were factors independently associated with serious injury during a fall (Dellinger, 2017).

Among older adults, most fall-related injuries are considered minor. Perhaps because of the low incidence of serious injuries, older individuals often do not perceive falling as a problem that warrants a report or a medical evaluation.

Serious injury from falling is more likely to occur among those with osteoporosis. Bones weakened by osteoporosis, particularly weight-bearing bones such as the femur, are more susceptible to breakage. Injury prevention measures to reduce the impact of falling, for example, lowering the distance an older patient might fall to the ground and even using padding over the bony prominences of the hips, are required. Undergarments such as girdles with extra padding over the high-risk bony prominences have been designed for females. Individuals with osteoporosis should also be prescribed medications to increase bone mineral density and strength over time. Exercise can aid in increasing bone mass.

Psychologic Trauma

Older individuals who fall may or may not experience psychologic trauma after the fall. Many factors influence the development of post-fall trauma, including personality, depression, anxiety, and stress-related syndromes. Overall, little research has been done to elucidate the incidence, prevalence, and occurrence of post-fall psychologic trauma. One significant consequence of falling may be fear of falling again or fear of being unable to get up independently after a fall. Both these conditions have been researched more extensively than other psychologic traumas associated with the post-fall period. This well-recognized "post-fall syndrome" sets the stage for subsequent falls and resultant injury (CDC, 2021a).

Fear of falling appears to occur variably in the older adult population. Some research has shown that if older persons express a fear of falling, they may avoid activities and become physically dependent (CDC, 2021a).

The gerontological nurse's role is to determine whether fear of falling or other psychological trauma has occurred after the fall. The best time to elicit this information is during history taking with older individuals who fall. The nurse focuses on how confident the older adults are in performing activities that might predispose them to falling. One exception to consider is an older adult who falls when nonambulatory, as in the case of a fall from bed. In this case, confidence may be unaffected during mobility. Box 9.6 presents issues related to a fear of falling.

Defining and measuring fear of falling. An older adult's fear of falling may be assessed in several ways. One method is to ask

BOX 9.6 Fear of Falling (FOF) Issues

1. FOF is higher among females than males.
2. FOF increases as aging progresses.
3. FOF is more prevalent in community-dwelling older adults.
4. FOF is more prevalent in older adults living alone.
5. FOF is decreased when social support is consistent.
6. FOF is a modifiable risk factor for falling.
7. FOF is lowered with the consistent use of ambulatory devices (cane, walker) when balance impairment is present.
8. FOF is reduced when home modifications (e.g., rails, grab bars) are made in appropriate (polypharmacy, balance deficit, history of falls, visual impairment, increased age, and certain chronic diseases) residences.

the older individual open-ended questions such as, "How do you define fear of falling, and what does it mean to you?" Responses will provide insight into the patient's perception of falling and give direction for intervention (Medline Plus, 2021).

While interviewing an individual who falls, the nurse may also assess his or her fear of falling by simply asking the respondent to quantify fear using a visual analog scale that measures (on a 100-millimeter [mm] line) perception of how fearful the patient is during ambulation.

Some researchers have operationally defined fear of falling as low-perceived self-efficacy in avoiding falls during nonhazardous ADLs. The Tinetti Falls Efficacy Scale (FES) lists a series of questions, on a Likert scale, related to how confident the person is during activities such as walking, reaching into cabinets, or hurrying to answer the telephone. This tool is based on Bandura's self-efficacy theory and is reported as a measure of fear of falling self-efficacy or confidence (Tinetti, 1986).

History

The underlying cause of falling will most often be identified during the health history. Because a tendency to underreport symptoms exists, the gerontological nurse must be sure to ask about key symptoms that could be related to a treatable cause or causes of falling. At the onset of the interview, an older individual should be informed that falling is not a result of normal aging. Therefore, information about the fall onset, location, activity associated with the fall, and other details is essential to the evaluation. It is important to elicit the patient's own words about the circumstances surrounding the fall. Inquiries should be made about fall frequency and what usually happens immediately before a fall. SPLATT helps in further evaluation (Ang et al, 2020; Oregon Department of Human Services, 2022):

- **S**ymptoms at the time of the fall
- **P**revious fall or near fall
- **L**ocation of the fall
- **A**ctivity at the time of the fall
- **T**ime of the fall
- **T**rauma, physical or psychologic

A fall history depends on fall recall and intact memory. If the patient who falls has dementia or delirium, it is advisable to seek additional information from witnesses or significant others. Often, a fall diary may be helpful in retrieving detailed information about the fall that the individual may have forgotten. Key symptoms to inquire about are related to diseases known to cause falls. Every older adult needs to be asked about key symptoms that will help further identify the fall's underlying cause. If these symptoms occurred at the time of the fall or precipitated the fall, it is likely that a treatable cause does exist (Table 9.5).

A postfall assessment tool can help evaluate the circumstances surrounding the fall and attempt to plan for future fall prevention (Fig. 9.3).

Physical Examination

The physical examination of an individual who falls includes a focused examination based on the patient's presenting complaints in addition to the sensory, cardiovascular, musculoskeletal, and neurologic systems. Many treatable causes of falling may be identified on physical examination. Sensory input originates from visual, auditory, tactile, cardiovascular, and motor response systems. Sensory inputs from vision and hearing, proprioception of the distal lower extremities, and the peripheral sensory system all provide stimuli for the brain to process regarding the maintenance of balance. The cardiovascular system is also critical because blood pressure regulation aids in homeostasis. Changes in apical heart rate, such as bradycardia, tachyarrhythmias, or irregular rhythms, may alter cerebral perfusion, affecting balance. A drop in blood pressure when a patient goes from supine to standing may lead to falling because of cerebral hypoperfusion, as blood pools in the lower extremities.

Assessment of the motor function includes muscle strength testing; particular attention should be paid to hip and knee extension, and ankle dorsiflexion. Research indicates that poor ankle function adversely affects the ability to maintain balance during a fall (Hernández-Guillén et al, 2021). Manual muscle-strength testing identifies weakness in particular muscle groups, which can then be targeted for exercise. Gait analysis includes the evaluation of footwear, the base of support, limb stability, and clearance. The neurologic examination focuses on position and vibratory sense, including the Romberg test and cranial nerve assessment. Refer to an assessment textbook for details regarding the examination of older adults.

Physical examination should identify any findings that might explain a patient's symptoms. For instance, if a patient complains of dizziness when getting up in the morning, the nurse should check orthostatic blood pressure. Other causes of dizziness for older adults include carotid artery hypersensitivity, cervical arthritis, carotid stenosis, and positional vertigo, all of which may cause dizziness with head movement and may often be reproduced during a physical examination.

Special Testing

A few tests will aid the nurse in further evaluating gait and balance. One helpful test for static balance is the sternal nudge. This is a test of the righting reflex and is done with two persons and the patient. One examiner stands in front of the patient and

TABLE 9.5 Key Symptoms to Elicit During History Taking From Patients Who Have Fallen

Symptom	Associated Medical Condition
Sudden onset of visual or hearing loss	Stroke
Sudden leg weakness (unilateral)	Stroke
Lower extremity weakness (bilateral)	Arthritis
Dizziness	Vertigo, labyrinthitis
Light-headedness with standing	Orthostatic hypotension
Tremors or confusion	Hypoglycemia, hypoxia
Loss of consciousness	Syncope
Involuntary loss of urinary or bowel function immediately after the fall	Seizure
Difficulty breathing or shortness of breath	Arrhythmia
Palpitations	Arrhythmia

FALLS MANAGEMENT – POST FALL ASSESSMENT TOOL

Resident		Age	Room #
Admit Date	Admit Dx		Current Dx
Date of Fall	Day of Week		Time AM PM
Assigned caregiver(s) (Name and title)			

1. Was this fall observed?   ❏ Yes ❏ No   *If yes*, by whom: _____
   (name and title)

2. Was the resident identified as "high risk" prior to the fall?   ❏ Yes ❏ No

3. Resident vital signs

Usual vital signs *before* the fall:	BP Lying:	Pulse:
	BP Sitting:	Pulse:
	BP Standing:	Pulse:
Vital signs *just after* the fall:	BP Lying:	Pulse:
	BP Sitting:	Pulse:
	BP Standing:	Pulse:

4. Does the resident have a history of falling?   ❏ Yes ❏ No   *If yes*, list dates of all previous falls for the past 12 months:

DATE/TIME OF FALL	DATE/TIME OF FALL

5. List any life safety measures in place prior to this current fall:

6. Ask the following question of the resident "immediately" after the fall: WHY DO YOU THINK YOU FELL?

7. Ask the following questions of the resident immediately after the fall:

	Yes	No		Yes	No
Were you hungry?			Did you need to use the bathroom?		
Were you in pain?			Other:		
Were you bored?					

8. What footwear did the resident have on?

❏ Barefoot   ❏ Shoes   ❏ Slippers   ❏ Other:

9. What was the resident doing at the time of the current fall?

	Yes	No	Other:
Getting out of bed?			
Going to the bathroom?			
Looking for something?			
Getting up from a chair?			
Going to the dining room?			

Fig. 9.3 Postfall assessment tool. (From the Best Practice Committee of the Health Care Association of New Jersey. [2012]. Falls management—post fall assessment tool. In *Falls Management Guideline*. Retrieved from https://www.hcanj.org/files/2013/09/hcanjbp_fallmgmt13_050113_2.pdf.)

10. Location of this current fall (check all that apply):

Activity room	Day room	Shower	Other:
Bathroom	Dining room	Toilet	
Bed room	Hall	Transferring	
Commode	Outside	Wheelchair	

11. Was a restraint used during this fall?

None	Waist restraint	Other:
Geri Chair	Vest restraint	
Side rails	Mittens	
Wrist restraint	Lap board	

12. If a restraint was present during the fall, was it properly applied prior to the fall? ☐ Yes ☐ No
If no, please describe:

13. Mechanical/Assistive Devices:

What *mechanical devices* were in use?	✓		Yes	No
Chair alarm		Was chair alarm working at time of fall?		
Bed alarm		Was bed alarm working at time of fall?		
Mobility monitor		Was monitor working at time of fall?		
What *assistive devices* were in use?	✓		Yes	No
Cane ☐ straight ☐ hemi ☐ quad		Was cane in good repair?		
Crutches		Were crutches in good repair?		
Walker		Was walker in good repair?		
Wheelchair		Was wheelchair in good repair?		
Geri-chair		Was Geri-chair in good repair?		
Lap board		Was lap board in good repair?		

14. Mental status of resident (check all that apply):

Mental status *prior to* the fall:	YES	NO	Mental status *after* the fall:	YES	NO
Alert			Alert		
Oriented			Oriented		
Disoriented/confused			Disoriented/confused		
Unable to follow directions			Unable to follow directions		
Other:			Other:		

15. Physical status of resident prior to the fall (check all that apply):

Physical status *prior to* fall	Yes	No	NA	Physical status *prior to* fall	Yes	No	NA
Unsteady gait				Impaired mobility/transfer			
Visual impairment				Glasses on			
Hearing impairment				Hearing aid in/working			
Weakness/fatigue				Recent acute illness			
Hearing impairment				Recent change in lab values (Hgb/Hct, blood sugar, O_2, etc.)			
Dizziness				Other:			
Pain							

Fig. 9.3.—cont'd

16. Environmental status at the time of the fall (check all that apply):

Environmental status *at time* of fall	Yes	No	NA	Environmental status *at time* of fall	Yes	No	NA
Call bell within reach				Call bell on at time of fall			
Bed locked				Room light on			
Wheelchair locked				Floor wet			
Night light on				Patterned carpet/throw rugs			
Uneven floor surfaces				Power/phone/TV cords out			
Glare on floor				Other:			

17. Medication Status

	Yes	No	NA		Yes	No	NA
Diuretic				Cardiac			
Antihypertensive				Antibiotic			
Psychotropic				Other:			
Laxative							

18. List all new medications prescribed/administered to resident in the past 7 days:

19. Describe the general health of the resident in the hours, days, and weeks before the fall:

20. Is there a need to re-educate the resident, family, staff: ❑ Yes   ❑ No

21. Has the resident's care/service plan been updated?   ❑ Yes   ❑ No

Additional notes:

_____   _____
Signature/title of person completing form   Date

Fig. 9.3.—cont'd

one behind; the examiner in front pushes on the patient's sternum to displace the patient. If the patient begins to fall, the test is considered positive. A test result is deemed "negative" when the patient can maintain a standing balance despite the nudge.

Tests of dynamic balance include observance of the patient walking and changing position. Additional balance tests include the administration of the Tinetti Assessment Tool for Balance (see Fig. 9.1). The Timed Up and Go (TUG) measures the patient's mobility. The patient is instructed to:

1. Stand up from the chair.
2. Walk to the line on the floor at your normal pace.
3. Turn.
4. Walk back to the chair at your normal pace.
5. Sit down again.

Results ≥12 seconds indicate the older adult is at risk for falling (CDC, 2017b).

Management

Managing falls is challenging for the nurse, especially when older individuals experience multiple or recurrent falls. In these cases, it is helpful to identify a pattern, if any, of the falling. Similarities in antecedents that lead to falling or specific symptoms might help identify the underlying cause. The goals of management are to identify the underlying cause, to reduce the incidence of recurrent falling, and to prevent serious injury (Agency for Healthcare Research and Quality [AHRQ], 2017; Boltz et al, 2021).

Several aids for monitoring and preventing falls are available. A fall diary helps to monitor fall occurrences, injuries, and patterns. Community-dwelling older patients may use a fall diary to jot down all the important information that led to the fall, occurred during the fall, or followed the fall. This information is extremely useful in determining the antecedents and consequences of falling. Fall diaries are inexpensive or may be created by the nurse simply by using a pen, paper, and ruler (Box 9.7).

For institutionalized older individuals at risk for serious injury from bed or chair falls, bed or chair alarms help alert the nurse when movement is initiated. A sensor is attached to a patient and to the chair or bed via a long, thin wire. When the patient attempts to get up, the wire falls off the sensor and signals an alarm. These alarms are noninvasive and do not restrict voluntary movement in any way. The alarm is loud and may startle an older adult, so it is important to alert the patient and family about the noise to be expected when the alarm is triggered. In the corridors of hospitals and nursing facilities, video surveillance cameras help staff view ambulatory patients around the corner or in distant areas. These cameras are prohibited, however, in areas such as patient rooms because of privacy laws. Other safety aids include safety belts in wheelchairs and the "lap buddy," which is a soft foam cushion that fits on the patient's lap and wraps underneath the armrests of a wheelchair. However, if patients cannot voluntarily remove these devices, they are considered restraining devices. If the use of these aids fits the criteria for "restraint" for a particular patient, then the clinical guidelines for restraint use must be instituted. Health-care providers must ensure that the use of these aids is the least restrictive alternative available for the patient and that the aids do not replace observation or inhibit purposeful activity.

The aging process and the effects of disease result in changes that affect the host. Injury prevention aims to alter factors that impinge on the host by maximizing patient health and functional status, reducing unnecessary medications, and altering risk-taking behaviors. These combined efforts will reduce the risk for unintentional injuries. Alterations in the environment through the elimination of environmental hazards will reduce accidental injuries in the older patient's home. Improved technology through research seeks to alter the transfer of energy and thus modify those agent-related factors contributing to injuries in older adults. One such example is the alteration in energy transfer by using super-soft mats and floor surfaces designed to absorb the effect of a falling body and redistribute its mass. Thus when an older patient falls on a special floor surface, the rate of injury is likely to be lower than on a conventional surface.

It is advisable to discuss the possibility that falling will result in serious injury and how to reduce the potential for such injury with all older patients at risk for falls and those at risk for serious injury from a fall. Patients should be given the choice of reducing mobility to prevent serious injury or continuing ambulation, knowing that the risk for serious injury is present. Patient autonomy should be promoted and respected; it is the patient's choice. In instances in which patients are demented or unable to make informed choices, discussion with the families or guardians is required. In any event, the goal of the gerontological nurse is to promote safety.

Fall and injury prevention modalities have received much attention in recent years. Evidence suggests that certain activities and programs may improve flexibility and balance, thus preventing injury. Evidence-based fall programs such as A Matter of Balance (MaineHealth, n.d.), Healthy Steps for Older Adults (Pennsylvania Department of Aging, n.d.), or Fit and Strong! (University of Illinois at Chicago Institute for Health Research and Policy, n.d.) are examples of program strategies that may improve fall prevention outcomes. Other programs can be found on the National Council on Aging website https://ncoa.org/article/evidence-based-falls-prevention-programs.

Moreover, following the recommendations presented in Box 9.8 and the Nursing Care Plan to reduce falling is advisable. The Emergency Treatment box gives recommendations for treating a patient who has fallen.

BOX 9.7 Designing a Fall Diary

1. Gather several sheets of 8½- × 11-inch paper.
2. Across the longest margin, write or type the headings "Date," "Time of Fall," "Activity at the Time of Fall," "Symptoms," and "Injury."
3. Instruct patients to write, in the space underneath each heading, the information pertaining to each fall soon after the fall occurs.
4. At the bottom of the fall diary, include an "Emergency Contact Number" for patients to call in case a fall results in serious injury.
5. Instruct patients who have experienced a fall to keep a record of the fall events and to bring it to the health-care provider's office at the next scheduled appointment.

BOX 9.8 Fall and Injury Prevention Strategies

Physical Modifications
- Cushion the landing surface.
- Use specialized tile that absorbs the impact of falls.
- Pad the floor.
- Cushion bony prominences.
- Use padding around high-risk bony prominences.
- Gain weight (if appropriate).
- Lower the distance to the floor surface.
- Use low-rise beds.
- Use futon beds or a mattress on the floor.
- Sit during dressing and shaving, whenever possible.
- Sit in a shower chair instead of standing in a tub.
- Avoid high heels; use wedge heels or flat shoes.

Behavioral Modifications
- Slow the pace of activities.
- Avoid risk-taking behaviors such as climbing on ladders, if feeling unsteady.
- Rise slowly and dangle the legs before changing position.
- Pay attention to the environment, terrain, and uneven or slippery surfaces.

Environmental Safety
- Have the curbs and edges painted in different colors.
- Have intravenous (IV) tubing removed in the hospital setting.
- Have urinary catheter and drainage bag removed.
- Have grab bars or rails installed.
- Use the "Lifeline" for fall detection.
- Set a predetermined schedule for "checking in" with neighbors or friends.

NURSING CARE PLAN

Risk for Injury: Fall

Clinical Situation

An older adult is admitted to the hospital from home with acute congestive heart failure secondary to aortic stenosis and new-onset pneumonia. Medical history includes osteoporosis and a hip fracture three years ago. The patient experiences shortness of breath with minimum exertion despite a recent diuresis and the loss of 10 pounds. The patient is receiving IV diuretics and antibiotics. Vital signs include a temperature of 98 F, a pulse of 100 beats per minute at rest, respirations of 26 breaths per minute at rest, and a blood pressure of 90/60 mm Hg; pulse oximetry while receiving 2 liters (L) of oxygen is 90%. The patient insists on walking by themselves to the bathroom to "stay independent." As a result of the diuretic, they must rush to the toilet to prevent urinary incontinence. The patient reports urgency due to diuretic use and dizziness upon standing.

Analyze Cues and Prioritize Hypotheses (Patient Problems)
- Injury risk: fall risk related to altered mobility, urinary urgency, and treatment modalities secondary to osteoporosis and respiratory compromise

Generate Solutions (Planning)
- Patient will maintain autonomy and independence while avoiding falls during the hospital stay.

Take Actions (Nursing Interventions)
- Observe patient during basic ADLs, instructing her regarding ways to conserve energy while still encouraging independence.
- Check blood pressure and pulse, supine and standing, to determine whether orthostatic hypotension exists.
- Keep immediate environment free of obstacles.
- Instruct patient to dangle legs before standing up from a supine position.
- Place call light within reach to encourage patient to call for assistance.
- Provide temporary use of bedside commode to limit exertional activities while still encouraging independence; instruct in the use of safe transfer procedures.
- Monitor electrolyte, blood urea nitrogen, and serum creatinine levels for evidence of drug-induced dehydration.
- Weigh patient daily to monitor fluid status.
- Monitor intake and output.
- Provide nonskid slippers.
- Eliminate IV tubing and use saline well so that tripping over clear tubing is avoided.
- Don't forget to include checking for outdoor hazards: decks, sand, and uneven surfaces.

EMERGENCY TREATMENT

Mr. J is an 84-year-old found lying on the floor in his bedroom in a residential care facility. He says, "I just fell down, but I feel okay." Closer examination reveals a large hematoma over the right temporal area and swelling of the right ankle and lower extremity. Mr. J's distal dorsalis pedis artery pulse on the right is obscured by the edema. A right lower-extremity fracture is suspected. To stabilize the patient, the nurse carries out the following interventions:

1. Immobilize suspected fractured extremity with a splint or board and flexible bandage
2. Apply ice to the right lower extremity and right temporal area
3. Check apical pulse immediately to ascertain whether an arrhythmia occurred, resulting in the fall; monitor vital signs, especially blood pressure and apical pulse
4. Conduct neurologic assessment and inquiry about a postfall headache
5. Check environment for any spills or hazards that could have led to the fall
6. Take health history for symptoms of medical conditions that could have led to the fall, for example, syncope, seizures, or vertigo
7. Contact emergency transportation to move the patient to the local emergency department for radiography and evaluation

SAFETY AND THE HOME ENVIRONMENT

Environmental hazards in the homes of older adults are common. These hazards are found in all living areas and entrances to homes of community-living older adults. Hazards have been observed less frequently in housing that is age-restricted to older adults (NSC, n.d.) or has been remodeled or designed with older adults in mind. Especially injurious hazards are those associated with temperature-regulating equipment and household chemicals. The equipment includes fire, heat, and ventilation sources, and the chemicals include household cleaners, herbicides, and pesticides (NSC, n.d.).

Burn Injuries in the Home
Burns

Residential fires are directly related to the increase in deaths of older adults as a result of burns to the body. Although hot food or beverages often cause scald burns, they do not account for the large percentage of deaths from burns. Home maintenance is associated with older adults living in older homes with limited resources for needed repairs and thus risk for fire (U.S. Fire Administration [USFA], 2018).

The major cause of scald burns is the temperature of the hot water coming from the faucets. Scalds resulting from bathing or showering were caused by hot-water tank temperatures exceeding 140°F (60° C). At temperatures of 150 F, only two seconds of exposure is needed to produce third-degree burns. Scalds can be prevented by turning down the thermostat on the household water heater to 120°F (Martin, 2018). However, it should be noted that if someone in the house has chronic respiratory disease or a suppressed immune system, the temperature should be set at 140°F to prevent the growth of *Legionellae* bacteria (Blok, 2023).

The nurse should instruct older adults to use a meat thermometer and a container with a padded or safety handle to check the hot-water temperature in the kitchen and bathroom. Water should be allowed to run until steam is noted, and the container is then filled. After the thermometer registers a stable temperature, the hot-water tank controls are adjusted accordingly. The temperature should not be above 120°F.

Cigarette Smoking

Home fires occur more frequently at night, and deaths are attributed to smoke injury more often than burns. Smoking materials are often the source of home fires (Hall & Evarts, 2022).

Smoking in the home has been associated with the dangers of secondhand smoke for many years. Smoking in bed or in a chair has also resulted in the deaths of numerous older adults from unintentional home fires. The environmental hazards of cigarette smoking include the careless disposal of cigarette butts and cigarettes dropped onto cloth surfaces (e.g., stuffed furniture, curtains, carpets, and clothing). Multiple injuries and deaths have been attributed to older persons falling asleep while smoking (Hall & Evarts, 2022).

The nurse should prepare an instructional plan to offer to older adults who smoke and review the materials with them on a quarterly basis to refresh the safety steps associated with smoking at home. These include the smoking safety instructions listed in Box 9.9.

Several types of fire extinguishers are available, but the best type for home use is a multipurpose dry chemical ABC-type extinguisher. ABC extinguishers generally use monoammonium phosphate as the active chemical and can put out most common fires (Will, 2022).

Fireplace Hazards

The risk for starting a residential fire exists when a wood or gas fireplace is used. Wood fireplaces need to be cleaned of ash and soot buildup regularly when used during winter and in geographic areas where cold weather persists for many months. When ash and other wood debris accumulate over time, the flue may become blocked, causing the smoke or flames to enter the living area instead of exiting through the chimney or vent. All chimneys, vents, and flues need to be checked annually for patency. The ash and wood debris must be removed to prevent blocking the exit of fire and smoke. If proper cleaning is not done regularly, the resulting inhalation of smoke may lead to substantial airway damage and pulmonary complications (Hall & Evarts, 2022).

Persons using natural gas fireplaces should avoid placing flammable objects and furniture close to the firebox. Gas fireplaces can be a source of carbon monoxide (CO) poisoning, so CO detectors should be on every floor of the house. It is recommended that natural gas fireplaces be inspected annually (Smyth, 2022).

The nurse should discuss fireplace safety and maintenance with older adults who acknowledge using fireplaces and suggest having the flues checked for blockages on a routine basis. Setting at least an annual date in early autumn will establish a routine.

BOX 9.9 Smoking Safety Instructions

- Never smoke in bed.
- Ensure mattress meets the 1973 Federal Mattress Flammability Standard.
- Do not put ashtrays on the arms of sofas or chairs.
- Use large, deep ashtrays with wide lips. Although smaller ashtrays may be more attractive, they are not safe. Cigarettes can roll off the edge, and the ashes can easily be blown away.
- Water down your ashes. Empty ashtrays into either the toilet or an airtight metal container. Warm ashes dumped in waste cans can smolder for hours, and then ignite into fire.
- Do not leave cigarettes, cigars, or pipes unattended. Extinguish all smoking materials before you walk away.
- If you begin to feel drowsy while watching television or reading, extinguish your smoking materials in a safe container.
- Close a matchbook before striking and hold it away from your body. Set your cigarette lighter on a "low" flame to prevent burns.
- If friends or relatives who smoke have paid you a visit, be sure to check on the floor and around chair cushions for ashes that may have been dropped accidentally.
- Do not discard cigarettes in vegetation such as mulch, potted plants or landscaping, peat moss, dried grasses, leaves or other things that could ignite easily.

Based on Smoke and Home Fire Safety. NPFA Public Education Division. ©NFPA 2016.

Kitchen Hazards

Between 2015 and 2019, fires caused by cooking were the leading cause of home structure fires and related injuries and the second leading cause of fire deaths. Cooking caused an average of 169,400 home fires per year. These fires caused an annual average of 540 deaths, 4670 injuries, and $1.2 billion in property damage (Hall & Evarts, 2022).

The nurse should instruct older adults living alone about the possibility of fires. Patients with mild dementia need to be evaluated for their ability to cook safely because of their forgetfulness. Instruct older adults to remember three basic rules:

1. Be on the lookout for potential hazards.
2. Doing things correctly can prevent accidents (no shortcuts).
3. Use protective equipment when needed (e.g., potholders, oven mitts, etc).

Space Heaters

A space heater may be overturned by accident, causing a fire that may not be noticed until it fully engulfs the home. All space heaters should have a safety mechanism that turns the unit off as soon as it changes position (e.g., falls forward or backward). This safety device can shut off the heater and prevent the ignition of a fire in carpeting, curtains, or upholstery (Hall & Evarts, 2022).

The nurse should recommend that older adults have home inspections; programs are often available through local fire departments. When space heaters are used, an emergency shutoff must be operable. The equipment housing and the electrical cords must be intact. The cords must be appropriate for the electrical outlets being used (i.e., a three-prong plug cannot be placed in a two-prong adapter, which negates a grounded outlet).

Fire Safety Tips

Local fire districts nationwide encourage families to keep fire extinguishers, smoke detectors, and CO detectors in their homes. Home fire drills are recommended for all families, but especially for households with older adults. Box 9.10 lists safety tips to protect the home from fire hazards. Identification of exits and a plan for meeting outside the building are necessities for independent older persons or couples living alone in a private residence (Hall & Evarts, 2022).

The nurse should instruct older adults and families with older adult members regarding prevention measures (USFA, 2018).

Common home fire hazards include flammable liquids (e.g., gasoline, acetone, and paint thinner), combustible liquids (e.g., lighter fluid, turpentine, and kerosene), overloaded or worn electrical circuits, rubbish and trash stored near a heat source, Christmas trees and lighting that are frayed or have poor insulation, and natural gas leaks (USFA, 2018; Hall & Evarts, 2022).

Other Injuries in the Home

Knife Injuries

The use of knives, particularly in the kitchen, provides the potential for injury. The nurse should instruct older adults in six basic rules (American Knife & Tool Institute, 2023):

1. When using knives, always cut *away* from the body and on a proper cutting surface.
2. Keep the blades sharp and clean.

BOX 9.10 Safety Tips to Protect the Home From Fire

- Maintain smoke alarms.
- Develop and practice a fire escape plan.
- Have home fire sprinklers installed.
- Never smoke in bed.
- Put your cigarette or cigar out at the first sign of feeling drowsy while watching television or reading.
- Use deep ashtrays and put out your cigarettes completely.
- Do not walk away from lit cigarettes and other smoking materials.
- Never leave cooking unattended.
- Always wear short or tight-fitting sleeves when you cook. Keep towels, potholders, and curtains away from flames.
- Never use the range or oven to heat your home.
- Double-check the kitchen before you go to bed or leave the house.
- Keep fire in the fireplace by making sure you have a screen large enough to catch flying sparks and rolling logs.
- Space heaters need space. Keep flammable materials at least three feet away from heaters.
- When buying a space heater, look for a control feature that automatically shuts off the power if the heater falls over.

Data from U.S. Fire Administration. (2018). *Fire safety for older adults.* Retrieved July 28, 2023, from https://www.usfa.fema.gov/downloads/pdf/publications/fa_221.pdf.

---

3. Keep the knife grips clean.
4. Never leave knives lying in water because this may injure an unsuspecting person washing dishes.
5. Always point the cutting edge away from the hand when wiping blades.
6. If a knife should fall, do not try to catch it; pick it up after it has fallen.

Carbon Monoxide Poisoning

CO poisoning presents as a viral illness with headaches, sleepiness, fatigue, confusion, and irritability. Higher CO levels can cause nausea, vomiting, irregular heartbeat, impaired vision and coordination, and death (Verbanas, 2021).

CO toxicity from heating oil or natural gas may occur during the winter months. Furnaces that do not have flues checked for patency may be one cause of this silent killer. The condition of furnace venting should be checked annually just before the furnace is turned on for the home heating season (CDC, n.d.).

Power interruptions during cold weather increase the risk for unintentional CO poisoning. Often, power outages occur during severe winter storms. This may create a need for alternative heating methods. Methods associated with CO exposure are gasoline generators, propane or kerosene heaters, and charcoal grills. Warnings regarding the use of alternative heating methods during power outages should become part of all home safety instructions. Older adults should be educated to ensure generators are at least 20 feet away from the house and to never use the stove to heat their house or to use charcoal-burning devices for heat inside the home (Verbanas, 2021).

> **BOX 9.11 Carbon Monoxide Poisoning: Prevention Guidelines**
>
> - **Do** have your heating system, water heater, and any other gas, oil, or coal burning appliances serviced by a qualified technician every year.
> - **Do** install a battery-operated CO detector in your home, and check or replace the battery when you change the time on your clocks each spring and fall. If the detector sounds, leave your home immediately and call 9-1-1.
> - **Do** seek prompt medical attention if you suspect CO poisoning and are feeling dizzy, light-headed, or nauseous.
> - **Do not** use a generator, charcoal grill, camp stove, or other gasoline or charcoal-burning device inside your home, basement, garage, or near a window when outside.
> - **Do not** run a car or truck inside a garage attached to your house, even if you leave the door open.
> - **Do not** burn anything in a stove or fireplace that is not vented.
> - **Do not** heat your house with a gas oven.
>
> Modified from Centers for Disease Control and Prevention, & National Center for Environmental Health. (2017). *Prevention guidelines: You can prevent carbon monoxide exposure.* Retrieved January 4, 2023, from https://www.cdc.gov/co/pdfs/guidelines.pdf.

The nurse should include a recommendation for the installation of a CO detector in all home safety programs. Box 9.11 lists ways to prevent CO in the home.

Household Chemical Emergencies

Most homes have products that contain hazardous chemicals, including hair spray and spray deodorant, nail polish and polish remover, cleaning products and furniture polishes, antifreeze or motor oil, batteries, fluorescent light bulbs, paint thinners, herbicides, and insecticides. Older adults should be instructed to store hazardous household chemicals safely (U.S. Department of Homeland Security, 2022):

- Only store household chemicals in places where children can't get to them. Lock or childproof cabinets and storage areas if you have children in your home.
- Keep products containing hazardous materials in their original containers and never remove the labels unless the container is corroding. Corroding containers should be repackaged and clearly labeled.
- Never store hazardous products in food containers.
- Never mix household hazardous chemicals or waste with other products. Some chemicals, such as chlorine bleach and ammonia, may react, ignite, or explode.
- Never use hair spray, cleaning solutions, paint products, or pesticides near an open flame.
- Clean up any chemical spills immediately. Allow the fumes in the rags to evaporate outdoors, then dispose of them by wrapping them in a newspaper and placing them in a sealed plastic bag in your trash can.
- Dispose of hazardous materials correctly.

Symptoms of toxic poisoning include difficulty breathing, irritation of the eyes, skin, throat, or respiratory tract, changes in skin color, headache or blurred vision, dizziness, clumsiness or lack of coordination, and cramps or diarrhea. If someone is experiencing toxic poisoning symptoms or has been exposed to a household chemical, call the national poison control center at 800-222-1222 (U.S. Department of Homeland Security, 2022).

Portable Electric Cooling Fans

Older fans that have metal blades and limited shrouds can be dangerous, particularly if they tip over. Additionally, if a box fan (designed to fit in a window) falls over, the restricted airflow can lead to the electric motor overheating and catching fire. It is important that all fan power cords are free of damage, do not create a tripping hazard, and are not run through doorways, draped over furniture, or in/near water. Older adults should be educated about additional safety precautions, including turning the fan off immediately if a burning smell is noted and not leaving the fan running if they leave the home (Minnesota Commerce Department, n.d.).

It is important to educate older adults that although fans may make them feel cooler if they are outside and the temperature is above 95°F, it increases their risk for heat stroke. Fans work to cool us by evaporating sweat. By doing so, they cause the body to lose water faster. If that water is not replaced (by drinking or directly spraying the skin with a spray bottle), dehydration and heat stroke can occur. This is more of a problem in very hot and arid heat wave conditions (Hospers et al, 2020; Schultz, 2019).

> **EVIDENCE-BASED PRACTICE**
>
> *Promoting Older Adult Fall Prevention Education and Awareness in a Community Setting: A Nurse-Led Intervention*
>
> **Background**
>
> Falls are one of the most expensive conditions to treat. The Centers for Disease Control and Prevention estimate the financial burden to surpass $65 billion in 2020. As people age, it takes longer to recover from falls. Fall risk is increased by sensory disorders, polypharmacy, and weakness. "The implementation of fall prevention toolkits (FPTs), such as fall risk screenings and fall prevention education (FPE), have become progressively important in reducing fall incidences. Nurses have a greater role and responsibility to care for the aging population. The purpose of this project was to implement an FPT to adults age 65 and older that attended mobile interprofessional education (IPE) community clinics" (para 1).
>
> **Sample/Setting**
>
> A convenience sample was obtained from a mobile IPE clinical site. Thirty (30) participants completed both baseline and follow-up assessments. The participants were predominantly female (73.3%). Fifty percent (50%) were independent, community-dwelling older adults.
>
> **Methods**
>
> This mixed-methods project used pretest/posttests and an open-ended participant feedback survey. "The Missouri Alliance for Home Care 10-question survey and components of the CDC's Stopping Elderly Accidents, Deaths, and Injuries (STEADI) FPE were used to assess and educate participants on fall risks and fall prevention" (para 2). Survey data was collected at baseline and one month; at the one-month follow-up, additional data was gathered with open-ended questions.

> **EVIDENCE-BASED PRACTICE—cont'd**
>
> **Findings**
> In both fall-risk assessment tools, lower scores indicated a lower fall risk; both fall-risk assessment tool mean scores decreased over the one-month period. Additionally, six participants reported falling in the three months before the FPE; during the one-month follow-up period, two participants reported falling.
>
> **Implications**
> Future FPE implementation projects should consider providing items such as double-sided tape and nonskid mats and portable lights to the participants; many of the participants were low income and had difficulty obtaining the resources necessary to improve home safety. Future projects should be longer than one month to incorporate balance and strengthening exercises.

Data from Chidume, T. (2021). Promoting older adult fall prevention education and awareness in a community setting: A nurse-led intervention. *Applied Nursing Research, 57,* 151392.

Foodborne Illnesses

Food handling, preparation, and consumption behaviors associated with foodborne diseases are common in the homes of older adults. Fruits and vegetables are available all year in most parts of the United States because of the long-distance trucking industry. These foods are shipped from unknown locations, where pesticides and other sprays may have been used. Therefore, washing fruits, vegetables, and hands before beginning food preparation is a must to prevent foodborne illnesses. Ground meat and ground poultry are more perishable than most foods. In the danger zone between 40° F and 140° F, bacteria multiply rapidly. Because bacteria cannot be seen, smelled, or tasted, ground meats should be kept cold to keep them safe. Safe handling and storage are necessary when preparing ground meat and poultry (CDC, 2022a).

Cleaning all surfaces before and after food preparation is essential for preventing the spread of bacteria and fungi common on raw foods. Common household bleach diluted with tap water may be sprayed and wiped off preparation surfaces after cleaning with soap and water. Cleaning procedures should be done after each different type of food is prepared (CDC, 2022a).

SEASONAL SAFETY ISSUES

Older adults are at particular risk for environmental temperature-induced illnesses. Predisposing medical conditions and side effects from a variety of medications may render older persons vulnerable to heat- or cold-related symptoms ranging from weakness, dizziness, and fatigue to exhaustion, coma, and death.

The nurse should prepare seasonal information materials on the dangers of hyperthermia or hypothermia for all older adults living independently. Additionally, the nurse should identify patients at risk for illnesses associated with temperature extremes and promote ways of initiating a neighborhood watch program for dangerous climatic changes.

Health-care facilities, including acute, subacute, and long-term care, need to have oversight of environmental conditions for safe patient care and living. In some areas of the United States, climatic changes may develop rapidly and unexpectedly, especially as seasons change from cold to hot or the reverse. Nurses acting as patient advocates should work with physicians and management of the health-care facility to maintain environmental temperature and humidity levels conducive to patient well-being.

Hypothermia and Hyperthermia in Older Adults

With aging, thermoregulatory mechanisms undergo physiologic changes, placing the older individual at risk for the inability to manage extreme temperatures. The hypothalamus is responsible for regulating the body temperature. Although no significant age-related changes occur in this organ, the hypothalamus depends on the sensory functions to transmit sensory information. These sensory functions undergo changes with aging, and older persons may be unable to effectively manage changes in temperature.

Hypothermia

Hypothermia is defined as a core body temperature of less than 95°F (35°C). The two categories of hypothermia are primary and secondary hypothermia. Primary, or exposure, hypothermia follows exposure to low temperature or immersion accidents with intact thermoregulation. Secondary hypothermia is most often seen in patients with chronic illnesses, alcohol or substance abuse, and extreme age (Mayo Clinic Staff, 2022b; Li et al, 2021).

Hypothermia in the United States has approximately a 21% mortality rate. This rate increases with severe hypothermia to about 40%. It is estimated that about 700 people die of hypothermia each year in the United States (CDC, 2019).

At rest, an individual produces 40 to 60 kilocalories (kcal) of heat per square meter of body surface area. Heat production increases with movement, and shivering increases the rate of heat production by two to five times.

The body loses heat through various mechanisms. Under dry conditions, heat is lost via radiation (55% to 65%). However, evaporation is the dominant mechanism of heat loss with medical alterations in the body, especially when the person receives drugs that hinder perspiration. Conduction and convection account for about 15% of heat loss, and respiration accounts for the remainder (Mayo Clinic Staff 2022b; Li et al, 2021).

Changes in the environment drastically affect the way heat is lost. The hypothalamus controls the thermoregulation mechanism, and alterations in the central nervous system (CNS) may impair this mechanism.

Risk factors. Primary hypothermia is caused by environmental exposure; no underlying medical conditions contribute to this process. Secondary hypothermia is associated with an underlying medical condition that prevents the body from conducting normal thermoregulation. The causes and risk factors include the following:
- Accidental immersion in cold water
- Exposure to cold temperature
- Drastic changes in the environmental temperature
- Alcohol and substance abuse
- Excessive heat loss or impaired production

- Burns, psoriasis, or other desquamating skin conditions that contribute to heat loss
- Surgery and trauma, especially cardiac surgery
- Nutritional deficiency
- Sepsis
- Spinal cord injury with poikilothermy
- Stroke
- Anoxia
- Uremia
- Hypoglycemia
- Adrenal insufficiency and hypothyroidism
- Drugs (benzodiazepines, opiates, alcohol, barbiturates, clonidine, and lithium)

Clinical manifestations. In its early stages, hypothermia, like other conditions in older adults, presents in a nonspecific manner. Findings include fatigue, apathy, confusion, lethargy, shivering, numbness, slurred speech, impaired coordination, and possible coma. As the core temperature drops below 95°F (35°C), the individual's clinical picture appears more like a disorder. For this reason, nurses need to become familiar with the clinical manifestations of hypothermia in older adults. Early signs of hypothermia include confusion, impaired gait, fatigue, lethargy, and combativeness. As the core temperature drops, the signs and symptoms worsen. When an older adult's temperature drops below 93°F (34°C), cardiac arrhythmias occur, particularly bradyarrhythmia, as well as flattening of the T or P waves and atrial fibrillation. Death is usually the result of lethal arrhythmias or respiratory arrest (Li et al, 2021). Peripheral vasoconstriction occurring with hypothermia may also lead to increases in kidney perfusion and a subsequent increase in urine output referred to as *cold diuresis.*

Diagnostic findings. The most objective finding for the diagnosis of hypothermia is a measured core temperature below 95°F (35°C). In addition to physical findings, individuals may manifest changes in their acid–base balance. Initially, the individual hyperventilates, which leads to respiratory alkalosis. As the hypothermia progresses, the metabolic rate drops and metabolic and respiratory acidosis ensues. As a result of these stresses on the body, glucose and white blood cell levels become elevated. Coagulopathy may be seen as a result of prolonged hypothermia. Thyroid-stimulating hormone and corticotropin should also be assessed. Toxicology screening is performed to rule out the presence of opiates or illicit substances as the causative factor. Chest radiography is necessary to rule out patchy infiltrates or signs of pneumonia. Computed tomography of the head is done to rule out concomitant conditions.

Management. The therapeutic management of hypothermia depends on the core temperature. If hypothermia is mild, passive external rewarming with insulated coverings and moving the older adult to a warm environment are indicated. Active external rewarming is useful in mild to moderate hypothermia without cardiac symptoms. This rewarming includes warming blankets, head coverings, heating lamps, and warm water immersion. Moderate to severe hypothermia requires active core-rewarming techniques such as warm IV fluids, warm humidified oxygen, and warm gastric and bladder irrigation. Peritoneal dialysis and pleural lavage are reserved for cases with cardiac instability (Li et al, 2021). In older patients with comorbid conditions, the mortality rate after moderate to severe hypothermia may be greater than in the general population (by ≥50%), depending on the severity at presentation and the underlying disease (Li et al, 2021).

Hyperthermia

Hyperthermia is a disorder affecting the thermoregulatory mechanism in which patients have a core body temperature greater than 105°F (40.6°C). Hyperthermia causes severe CNS dysfunction and hot, dry skin. The most severe and life-threatening heat illness in older persons is heat stroke. This condition is most often seen in debilitated individuals and usually presents differently from the exertional heat stroke seen in the young.

The body should be able to produce and dissipate heat to balance the core temperature. Core heat develops as a result of cellular metabolism. When the environmental temperature exceeds the core temperature, the body's thermoregulatory mechanism activates heat loss via dissipation. Dissipation occurs via the skin, one of the most important elements in body heat regulation (Schraga & Kates, 2022).

In response to elevated core temperature, the hypothalamus activates efferent fibers of the autonomic nervous system to stimulate vasodilation of the skin vessels, which leads to perspiration. This form of heat dissipation is achieved via the convection and evaporation mechanisms. Heat in the body can only be generated by activity occurring in the muscular system. For body temperature to increase, the rate of heat production has to exceed the rate of heat loss. Consequently, hyperthermia occurs when excessive metabolic production of heat, excessive ambient heat, or the inability to dissipate heat overwhelms the thermoregulatory mechanism.

Risk factors. Risk factors leading to hyperthermia are either physiologic or environmental but usually work in combination. Older individuals are unable to increase their cardiac output for heat dissipation. This condition and poorly ventilated homes lacking air conditioning during heat waves increase the probability of heat stroke. Combining environmental conditions with a sedentary lifestyle, disabilities, poor hydration, and prescription medications that impair the ability to tolerate heat (e.g., diuretics, antihypertensives, neuroleptics, and anticholinergics) may also hasten the development of heat stroke (National Institute on Aging, 2022b).

Additional factors that cause or predispose older adults to hyperthermia are as follows:

- Disorders leading to excessive heat production
- Malignant hyperthermia associated with anesthesia
- Thyrotoxicosis (hormonal hyperthermia)
- Salicylic acid intoxication
- Delirium tremens
- Extensive use of occlusive clothing
- Dehydration
- Cerebrovascular accident
- Alcohol abuse (ethanol)
- Heat syncope and heat exhaustion

Clinical manifestations. Anhidrosis (lack of perspiration) is the most common manifestation of hyperthermia other than a core temperature >105°F (40.6°C). Most clinical manifestations occur because of altered CNS function and range from confusion to coma. Additional neurologic signs of hyperthermia include hallucinations, combativeness, bizarre behaviors, and syncope. Extensive evaluation is required to rule out possible psychiatric alterations contributing to this phenomenon.

Management. Monitoring core temperature and performing complete neurologic and physical assessments in older persons with hyperthermia is important. The main objective is to bring the temperature down immediately. Interventions used to decrease body temperature include the following:

- Spraying or sponge bathing the individual with cool water (approximately 90°F [32°C])
- Placing a fan near the patient to circulate cool air
- Decreasing the room temperature
- Placing ice packs on the groin and axillae together with cooling blankets

The nurse should use protective cream on the older adult to prevent skin burns from the cooling blanket and provide a lightweight gown and bed coverings for the individual. Bed rest should be maintained to decrease muscle activity and subsequent heat production. Antipyretic medications may be administered, as ordered, to facilitate patient comfort. Administering oral and IV fluids is essential to maintain adequate hydration.

More invasive medical techniques used to treat hyperthermia include peritoneal and gastric lavage with ice water. Precautions need to be taken before conducting these interventions. The airway needs to be protected, and no surgery should be scheduled. Benzodiazepines may be used to manage shivering (Schraga & Kates, 2022).

By understanding the risk factors for developing thermoregulatory disorders, the nurse is better equipped to develop strategies to prevent these alterations in older persons.

DISASTERS

Floods, tornadoes, earthquakes, hurricanes, wildfires, earthquakes, and drought are common natural disasters that may require evacuations and protection of personal property. Man-made disasters include industrial accidents, shootings, mass violence, and acts of terrorism. These traumatic situations may overwhelm communities and drain resources (Substance Abuse and Mental Health Services Administration [SAMHSA], 2023). In 2017 alone, three Atlantic hurricanes (Irma, Maria, and Harvey) were declared major disasters. 2017 also brought devastating fires – a major disaster was declared in Northern California in October due to fast-moving wildfires (Federal Emergency Management Agency [FEMA], 2022).

Natural and man-made disasters affect thousands of people each year. In 2021, 1 in 10 homes were affected by natural disasters, with costs nearing $57 billion in property damage (Jacobson, 2022). These traumatic events cause major loss of life and destruction of property. Although many people who experience these disasters recover with family and community help, others experience emotional distress. These persons experience anxiety, worry, difficulty sleeping, and depression (SAMHSA, 2023).

Additionally, disasters result in those with chronic health conditions experiencing disruptions and challenges in obtaining medications and equipment. Power outages can disrupt treatment for chronic conditions (i.e., dialysis). Disability increases the risk of injury and death as the person is less likely to evacuate when a disaster occurs (Merdjanof, 2021).

Chronic health conditions, cognitive decline, and limited social networks adversely affect older adults during disaster. However, older adults with lower educational levels and fixed/limited income, in addition to these factors, are most vulnerable during disasters due to limited preparedness. Emergency preparedness is an effective and low-cost intervention to reduce vulnerability (Merdjanof, 2021). Nurses are uniquely positioned to intervene in this area, assisting older adults in developing an emergency plan that addresses their individual needs, including medical care and a designated contact person to check on them during emergencies. Part of making a disaster preparedness plan involves making a plan for pets. Have an emergency evacuation plan for pets, and have them microchipped. Pets left behind may end up lost, injured, or dead. For those with large animals, plan and evacuate them early, if possible. Ensure all animals have identification (U.S. Department of Homeland Security, 2023). Further information about pets and farm animals during a disaster is available at https://www.ready.gov/pets.

Finally, older adults should create a 72-hour emergency supply kit that contains a list of important contacts and copies of important documents kept in a waterproof/Ziplock bag (i.e., power-of-attorney, copies of ID and insurance cards). Basic supplies to last three days should also be in the kit (i.e., nonperishable food, water, a flashlight, extra batteries, cash, and clothing). The kit should be checked every six months to ensure everything is present and up to date. Finally, the older adult should be able to lift/move the kit. This means it must be in a bag with wheels (Merdjanof, 2021). Further information on making a disaster supply kit can be found at https://www.ready.gov/kit.

STORAGE OF MEDICATIONS AND HEALTH CARE SUPPLIES IN THE HOME

Most older adults take medications regularly. The storage of medications at home may become a safety and drug-effectiveness issue. Some storage areas in the home are not safe for keeping medications. The windowsill in the bathroom or kitchen is frequently used to shelve medication bottles. Most drugs degrade when left in direct sunlight, with or without excessive heat. Heat changes the chemical makeup of specific compounds in the medication, and moisture is considered an undesirable element for solid-based drugs such as tablet-form medications.

The nurse should review the home conditions and instruct patients to identify those places that are undesirable areas for medication storage (e.g., kitchens, bathrooms, laundry rooms, basements, and windowsills) (Skidmore-Roth, 2023). Patients should be instructed to appropriately dispose of all outdated prescriptions when new ones are written. The most common disposal method for outdated or unused medications is to flush them down the toilet. Instructions for older adults on throwing away old medications must explicitly direct them to dispose of them in the toilet, not trash or garbage containers.

If healthcare has been delivered in the home setting, dressings and other medical supplies may remain after treatment ends. Patients should be instructed on how to dispose of used wound dressings and needles or syringes according to local health department regulations. Dressings and bandages touched by infectious disease drainage require special disposal instructions by home-care nurses. When home care is provided, the nurse should provide and collect biohazard containers for contaminated dressings and sharp objects (e.g., needles and syringes). The nurse should also prepare instructional material related to safety and using sharp objects that may be left with patients after home care is discontinued. These sharp objects must not be disposed of among regular paper trash in home trash collection. Arrangements for disposal should be made through the local health department or hospital.

CRIME PREVENTION

Older adults who live alone often become targets of crime. Over the past few years, assaults and homicides against adults over the age of 60 have increased. Often, the crimes committed against older adults are perpetrated by someone they know and trust; roughly 50% of homicides of older adults were committed by a family member or friend. African American, American Indian, Alaskan Native, or Hispanic older adults experience higher rates of violent injury and homicide (Galvin, 2019). Older adults should be taught basic crime prevention tips (Shuman, 2023):

- Have deadbolts installed on your doors, and keep all doors and windows locked.
- Draw the curtains at night, and keep the outside and inside of your house well-lit.
- Install motion sensor lights outside and use automatic timers on lamps.
- Install a peephole in your door.
- Do not leave extra keys in obvious places outside.
- If possible, install a home security system.
- If you live in a building with an elevator, do not remain in an elevator with a stranger if you feel unsafe. Do not buzz anyone in unless you know who they are.

In addition to these tips, older adults should be taught never to allow unsolicited contractors to enter their homes, regularly review their will, power-of-attorney, and property titles, and monitor all accounts for abnormal withdrawals. When traveling, older adults should carry as few cards as possible (identity and credit) and avoid carrying large amounts of cash. And, although older adults should be encouraged to carry cell phones with them for help in emergencies, they should be instructed not to talk or text while walking and shopping (Shuman, 2023).

Older adults should be educated about the risk for phone scams. Common scams include (Shuman, 2023):

- The caller announces that you won the lottery.
- A law enforcement officer says you must pay bail for a family member.
- A hospital calls you to pay for a family member's emergency operation.
- The Internal Revenue Service (IRS) claims that you owe back taxes, and if you don't pay over the phone, they will seize your property.
- A utility company claims you have unpaid bills, and your services are due to be cut off.
- A person calls, posing as a grandchild, and asks for help with a financial problem.

Scamming is not limited to phone calls. Older adults should also be educated about cybercrimes, email phishing scams, social media risks, and the risks associated with online dating (Shuman, 2023).

AUTOMOBILE SAFETY

Maintaining independence after retirement includes traveling to shopping centers and health-care providers' offices, visiting family and friends, and participating in recreational activities. A decline in an older adult's ability to drive safely may result in losing driving privileges. This decline may result from presbyopia, decreased dark adaptation, decreased depth perception, susceptibility to glare, and the general slowing of reflexes and cognitive processing (Muché & McCarty, 2023).

Because driving is a complex skill that involves rapid cognitive and psychomotor coordination and because many older adults have age-related changes or illnesses or take medications that slow their responses to road conditions, automobile safety eventually becomes an issue. In drivers who have experienced a stroke, vision and attention essential for safe driving are often impaired. The severity of these deficits could influence driving behaviors (Muché & McCarty, 2023).

Operating a motor vehicle often requires quick reflexes and reaction time, especially in hazardous road conditions. As response time diminishes with advancing age, health-care professionals and their patients must address driving safety issues.

When a functional assessment strongly indicates a driving safety issue, discussion regarding driving cessation may become necessary. Because an older adult's lack of driving may burden other family members, this discussion is best done in the presence of significant others viewed as trustworthy by the patient. States laws and policies differ as to mandatory reporting of high-risk individuals and licensing provisions. The nurse must be aware of the significance that driving has for older adults. If driving is an important quality-of-life issue for an older person and he or she wants to continue to drive, the nurse should provide the following guidelines for safe travel:

- Preplan the route of travel.
- Bring someone else to assist in navigation.
- Maintain space between oneself and the vehicle in front.
- Avoid night driving.
- Continue to wear appropriate hearing aids and glasses while driving.
- Avoid driving in poor weather conditions (e.g., ice, snow, rain, or fog).
- Keep the automobile's maintenance records up to date.
- Avoid driving if medications warn against using mechanical devices while under the influence of the drug.

If the older adult must stop driving, the nurse needs to teach the patient and family to plan ahead to stay active and continue doing what they enjoy. The shift from driver to passenger can mean (National Highway Traffic Safety Administration [NHTSA], n.d.):

- Rides with friends and family
- Taxis
- Shuttle busses or vans
- Public buses, trains, and subways
- Walking
- Para-transit services (special services for people with disabilities)

It is important for older adults to discover any community volunteer programs that offer free or low-cost travel (NHTSA, n.d.).

The issues of quality of life, personal autonomy, and safety dictate that older adults need to be supported in their desire to continue to drive automobiles. As the number of drivers older than the age of 70 continues to grow, new ways of evaluating driving safety while supporting personal autonomy are needed (CDC, 2022b; NHTSA, n.d.).

ABUSE AND NEGLECT

One in six community-dwelling adults over the age of 60 experienced abuse in the past year. In the setting of long-term care, the incidence is higher. Abuse increased during the COVID-19 pandemic (WHO, 2022). *Abuse* is defined by the WHO as "a single or repeated act, or lack of appropriate action, occurring within any relationship where there is an expectation of trust, which cause harm or distress to an older person. This type of violence constitutes a violation of human rights and includes physical, sexual, psychologic, and emotional abuse; financial and material abuse; abandonment; neglect; and serious loss of dignity and respect" (WHO, 2022, Overview section). Factors that increase the risk for abuse include functional dependence/disability, poor physical health, CI, poor mental health, and low income (WHO, 2022). Strategies to mitigate the risk for abuse include caregiver interventions to relieve the burden of caregiving, money management programs for older adults at risk for financial abuse or exploitation, helplines and emergency shelters, and multidisciplinary teams to address individual risk factors (WHO, 2022).

Domestic violence is considered a "hidden problem"; survivors experience physical and emotional abuse out of fear of retaliation. In response to this problem, the Family Violence Prevention and Services Act (FVPSA) was enacted in 1984 and reauthorized seven times (Billings, 2022). Common types of abuse include (CDC, 2021b):

- *Physical abuse* is when an elder experiences illness, pain, injury, functional impairment, distress, or death because of the intentional use of physical force and includes acts such as hitting, kicking, pushing, slapping, and burning.
- *Sexual abuse* involves forced or unwanted sexual interaction of any kind with an older adult. This may include unwanted sexual contact or penetration or noncontact acts such as sexual harassment.
- *Emotional or psychologic abuse* refers to verbal or nonverbal behaviors that inflict anguish, mental pain, fear, or distress on an older adult. Examples include humiliation or disrespect, verbal and nonverbal threats, harassment, and geographic or interpersonal isolation.
- *Neglect* is the failure to meet an older adult's basic needs. These needs include food, water, shelter, clothing, hygiene, and essential medical care.
- *Financial abuse* is the illegal, unauthorized, or improper use of an elder's money, benefits, belongings, property, or assets for the benefit of someone other than the older adult.

In nearly 60% of abuse and neglect cases, a family member was identified as the perpetrator. The spouse or adult child of the abused or neglected older adult was identified as responsible in two-thirds of the cases. Older adults who are abused, exploited, or neglected are at an increased risk for death (Kaplan, 2023).

Abuse results in physical and emotional trauma. Victims of abuse are fearful and anxious. They often have trust issues. They may have physical injuries ranging from cuts, scratches, bruises, and welts to head injuries and broken bones, leading to lasting disability and persistent pain (CDC, 2021b).

Forensic nursing is a specialty whose nurses care for victims of trauma, violence, and abuse while collecting and preserving evidence of the crimes for the legal system. Forensic nursing represents the response of nurses to the rapidly changing health-care environment and to the global challenges of caring for victims and perpetrators of intentional and unintentional injuries (American Nurses Association [ANA], 2017). Through continued support, these nurses aid the healing process and provide information to prevent further victimization. For further information on this nursing specialty, see https://www.forensicnurses.org/page/WhatisFN.

FIREARMS

Nearly one-half of older adults own a firearm (Betz et al, 2020; Price & Khubchandani, 2021). In a study examining the use of advance planning by older adult gun owners to transfer their firearms to someone else, the researchers discovered the participants owned an average of three firearms, and 18% reported carrying a loaded handgun during the previous month. More than half of the participants in the study had a plan in place to transfer firearms if they were no longer able to handle them or died (Betz et al, 2020). A firearm in the home offers both benefits and risks (Gani et al, 2017; Price & Khubchandani, 2021). Community training programs for the care and safe use of legal firearms have addressed gun safety issues for several decades. Firearms are associated with high rates of suicide among older males and females; between 2010 and 2018, the use of firearms to commit suicide increased by nearly 50%. Suicides using firearms among older adults were the third leading cause of injury-related death. Risk factors for using a firearm to commit include physical illnesses, mental illness, and social factors (Price & Khubchandani, 2021).

HOME CARE

1. Assess the home environment for the presence of hazards and risk factors that predispose homebound older adults to falls.
2. Carefully assess the physical status of homebound older adults for risk factors that predispose them to falls (i.e., examine feet, gait, vision, posture, muscle control, and memory).
3. Instruct caregivers and homebound older adults on tools and techniques to maximize independent functioning.
4. Assist caregivers and homebound older adults in planning a safe environment for the older adults based on the identified risks and hazards.
5. Emphasize the value of physical therapy in assessing the home setting; determine what environmental adaptations should be made to make it safer and easier for homebound older adults.
6. Teach older adults the effects of prescribed medications, focusing on the potential risks associated with falling. Instructions to decrease the effects of orthostatic hypotension, for example, rising slowly and waiting one to two minutes before standing are important in preventing falls.
7. For frail older adults, ensure that emergency phone numbers are located in accessible locations throughout the home; identify emergency call buttons or boxes and alarms.
8. Assess community-dwelling older adults' homes for hazards associated with fire and heat, chemicals, food handling, storage of medications and health-care supplies, and firearms, and instruct or make recommendations to promote a safe, hazard-free environment.
9. Assess the temperature of the home environment during seasons of extremely high or low temperatures. Refer homebound older adults to area energy-assistance programs, if indicated, or to other community agencies that provide heating and cooling assistance.
10. Be alert to signs of abuse and neglect of homebound older adults by caregivers. If abuse or neglect is suspected, follow the reporting laws of the given state.

SUMMARY

Safety encompasses many aspects of an older person's internal and external environments. The challenge for the nurse caring for older patients is to conduct individualized safety assessments, identify age-related risk factors that affect safety, and develop interventions aimed at preventing harm and injury.

Fall-related injuries are common among older adults. Before planning nursing interventions or preventive measures, it is essential to identify some of the more common risk factors, which include environmental issues and existing health conditions.

Nurses must also consider non–fall-related injuries such as burns, poisoning with CO or pesticides, seasonal safety issues with hyperthermia and hypothermia, disasters, motor vehicle accidents, crimes and abuse, and suicide. Gerontological nurses are on the cutting edge for developing nursing interventions and seeking research opportunities highlighting safety issues among independent older adults. Patient assessment and education concerning safety matters must be incorporated into every discharge plan and, in the case of primary care, into each clinic or office visit. The most challenging step to promoting safety in the homes of older adults is the prevention of injuries and illnesses from environmental hazards.

KEY POINTS

- Safety and freedom from harm are essential to an older adult's well-being.
- A direct correlation exists between an older person's sense of autonomy and his or her sense of personal safety.
- Risk factors contributing to falls in older adults include sensory impairment, CI, unsafe living environments (e.g., poor lighting, staircases and walkways in poor repair or without handrails, lack of grab bars in bathrooms, unsecured or worn rugs, and unstable furniture), and a history of falls.
- Thorough and accurate assessment of fall risk factors is essential.
- Methods for preventing falls in older adults may include exercise programs, alarms, and safer environmental conditions.
- As a leading cause of injury in older adults, burns may occur from scalds associated with bathing, cooking, fireplace hazards, use of space heaters, and careless smoking in the home. Chemical burns or injuries may occur when household chemicals, including pesticides and herbicides, are mixed or stored.
- CO poisoning is preventable through maintenance and repair of heating sources in the home and detection with properly placed CO detectors.
- Foodborne illnesses may be prevented by carefully cleaning all foods before cooking and cleaning the food preparation area before, during, and after meal preparation.
- With aging, thermoregulatory mechanisms undergo physiologic changes, placing the older individual at risk for inability to manage extreme temperatures.
- Hypothermia is a core body temperature of less than 95°F (35°C).
- Primary hypothermia is caused by environmental exposure; no underlying medical conditions contribute to this process.
- Secondary hypothermia is associated with an underlying medical condition that prevents the body from conducting normal thermoregulation.
- Hyperthermia is a disorder affecting the thermoregulatory mechanism in which the core body temperature is greater than 105°F (40.6°C).
- Anhidrosis (lack of perspiration) is the most common manifestation in hyperthermia other than a core temperature greater than 105°F (40.6°C).
- Operating a motor vehicle is often a basic factor in an older adult's independence. However, with this independence comes an increased risk for accidents, mainly due to decreased visual acuity and peripheral vision.

- Many older adults are victims of abuse, usually from a relative. Risk factors include poor health, physical or mental dependency, and advanced age.
- The maintenance of firearms in the homes of older adults may present special problems. The safety of the equipment, the need for its use, the ability to manage firearms, and the safety of others in the home must be considered.
- Nurses must be aware of the risk factors associated with safety hazards and injury in older adults and implement the necessary methods to prevent injuries.

CLINICAL JUDGMENT EXERCISES

1. An older adult is hospitalized for management of diabetes. History includes functional urinary incontinence and poor vision from diabetes. The nursing staff often observes the patient climbing over the side rails at night en route to the bathroom. They are quite agitated during this time. The nursing assistant requests that you obtain an order for a body restraint at night to prevent the patient from falling out of bed. Should this patient be restrained to prevent injury? Should restraints be ordered? Why, or why not? What other information is relevant to this case? What nursing interventions could be tried before considering a restraint?
2. An older adult is hospitalized in a medical–surgical unit and shares a room with another older adult. You see them sitting on the edge of the bed with their feet dangling about two feet from the floor. The patient has two IV lines and a Foley catheter. The Foley catheter is hanging on the floor beneath their feet as they sit on the edge of the bed. The bed is next to a window, which is usually left open. In the middle of the night, the patient climbs over the side rails to get out of bed and walks barefoot to the bathroom about 30 feet away. They tell you they hang onto their IV pole to steady themself and drag their Foley catheter bag alongside. What environmental hazards can you identify, and what environmental modifications could you make to improve her safety?
3. You are a home-care nurse visiting an older adult in their small second-story apartment following discharge from the hospital after having had two toes amputated because of frostbite injuries. During your initial visit, you note that they live in a two-room, dimly lit, musty-smelling apartment. Stacks of newspapers and old mail are scattered in both rooms. The temperature is noted to be 68°F on the wall thermostat. Cold drafts can be felt around the large window in the bedroom. List the safety hazards in this apartment and identify nursing interventions that will improve the patient's living conditions.

REFERENCES

Agency for Healthcare Research and Quality (AHRQ). (2017). *The falls management program: A quality improvement initiative for nursing facilities*. Rockville, MD: AHRQ. Retrieved from https://www.ahrq.gov/patient-safety/settings/long-term-care/resource/injuries/fallspx.html. Accessed July 28, 2023.

American Academy of Nursing. (2018). *Twenty-five things nurses and patients should question*. Retrieved from https://aann.org/uploads/about/AANursing-Choosing-Wisely-List__4_19_18___1_.pdf. Accessed July 28, 2023.

American Nurses Association (ANA). (2017). *Forensic nursing: Scope and standards of practice* (2nd ed.). Silver Spring, MD: ANA.

American Knife & Tool Institute. (2023). *Knife safety key points (SASS)*. Retrieved from https://www.akti.org/education/teach-children-knife-safety/. Accessed January 4, 2023.

Ang, G. C., Low, S. L., & How, C. H. (2020). Approach to falls among the elderly in the community. *Singapore Medical Journal, 61*(3), 116–121. doi:10.11622/smedj.2020029.

Betz, M. E., Azrael, D., Johnson, R. L., Knoepke, C. E., Ranney, M. L., Wintemute, G. J., et al. (2020). Views on firearm safety among caregivers of people with Alzheimer disease and related dementias. *JAMA Network Open, 3*(7), e207756. doi:10.1001/jamanetworkopen.2020.7756/.

Billings, K. C. (2022). *Family violence prevention and services act (FVPSA): Background and funding*. Congressional Research Service. Retrieved from https://crsreports.congress.gov/product/pdf/R/R42838. Accessed July 28, 2023.

Blok, A. (2023). *Set your water heater to this exact temperature to save money this winter*. CNET [website]. Retrieved from https://www.cnet.com/home/energy-and-utilities/set-your-water-heater-to-this-exact-temperature-to-save-money-this-winter/. Accessed July 28, 2023.

Boltz, M., Capezuti, E. A., Zwicker, D., & Fulmer, T. (2021). *Evidence-based geriatric nursing protocols for best practice* (6th ed.). New York: Springer.

Campani, D., Caristia, S., Amariglio, A., Piscone, S., Ferrara, L. I., Barisone, M., et al. (2021). Home and environmental hazards modification for fall prevention among the elderly. *Public Health Nursing, 38*(3), 493–501. doi:10.1111/phn.12852.

Centers for Disease Control and Prevention (CDC). (2022a). *Four steps to food safety: Clean, separate, cook, chill*. Retrieved from https://www.cdc.gov/foodsafety/keep-food-safe.html. Accessed July 28, 2023.

Centers for Disease Control and Prevention (CDC). (2022b). *Older adult drivers*. Retrieved from https://www.cdc.gov/injury/features/older-driver-safety/index.html. Accessed July 28, 2023.

Centers for Disease Control and Prevention (CDC). (2021a). *Facts about falls*. Retrieved from https://www.cdc.gov/falls/facts.html. Accessed July 28, 2023.

Centers for Disease Control and Prevention (CDC). (2021b). *Fast facts: Preventing elder abuse*. Retrieved from https://www.cdc.gov/violenceprevention/elderabuse/fastfact.html. Accessed July 28, 2023.

Centers for Disease Control and Prevention (CDC). (2019). *Prevent hypothermia & frostbite*. Retrieved from https://www.cdc.gov/disasters/winter/staysafe/hypothermia.html. Accessed July 28, 2023.

Centers for Disease Control and Prevention (CDC). (2017a). *Fact Sheet: Risk factors for falls.* Retrieved from https://www.cdc.gov/steadi/pdf/Risk_Factors_for_Falls-print.pdf. Accessed July 28, 2023.

Centers for Disease Control and Prevention (CDC). (2017b). *Assessment: Timed Up & Go (TUG).* Retrieved from https://www.cdc.gov/steadi/pdf/TUG_test-print.pdf. Accessed July 28, 2023.

Centers for Disease Control and Prevention. (n.d.). *Carbon monoxide (CO) poisoning.* Retrieved from https://www.cdc.gov/co/pdfs/Flyer_Danger.pdf. Accessed July 28, 2023.

Chidume, T. (2021). Promoting older adult fall prevention education and awareness in a community setting: A nurse-led intervention. *Applied Nursing Research, 57,* 151392.

Dellinger, A. (2017). Older adult falls: Effective approaches to prevention. *Current Trauma Reports, 3*(2), 118–123. doi:10.1007/s40719-017-0087-x.

Federal Emergency Management Agency (FEMA). (2022). *Historic disasters.* Retrieved from https://www.fema.gov/disaster/historic. Accessed July 28, 2023.

Galvin, G. (2019). *Violence against older Americans on the rise.* U.S. News & World Report [website]. Retrieved from https://www.usnews.com/news/health-news/articles/2019-04-04/violence-against-older-americans-on-the-rise-cdc-says. Accessed July 28, 2023.

Gani, F., Sakran, J. V., & Canner, J. K. (2017). Emergency department visits for firearm-related injuries in the United States, 2006-2014. *Health Affairs, 36*(10), 1729–1738. doi:10.1377/hlthaff.2017.0625.

Hall, S., & Evarts, B. (2022). *Fire loss in the United States during 2021.* Quincy, MA: National Fire Protection Association. Retrieved from https://www.nfpa.org/News-and-Research/Data-research-and-tools/US-Fire-Problem/Fire-loss-in-the-United-States. Accessed July 28, 2023.

Hernández-Guillén, D., Tolsada-Velasco, C., Roig-Casasús, S., Costa-Moreno, E., Borja-de-Fuentes, I., & Blasco, J. M. (2021). Association ankle function and balance in community-dwelling older adults. *PLoS One, 16*(3), e0247885. doi:10.1371/journal.pone.0247885.

Hospers, L., Smallcombe, J. W., Morris, N. B., Capon, A., & Jay, O. (2020). Electric fans: A potential stay-at-home cooling strategy during the COVID-19 pandemic this summer? *The Science of the Total Environment, 747,* 141180. doi:10.1016/j.scitotenv.2020.141180.

Jacobson, L. (2022). *Natural disasters hit roughly 1 in 10 American homes in 2021.* CNBC [website]. Retrieved from https://www.cnbc.com/2022/02/17/natural-disasters-such-as-fires-hurricanes-hit-1-in-10-us-homes-in-2021.html. Accessed July 28, 2023.

Kaplan, D. B. (2023). Elder abuse. In *Merck manual professional edition.* Merck & Co., Inc. Retrieved from https://www.merckmanuals.com/professional/geriatrics/elder-abuse/elder-abuse?query=abuse%20older%20adult. Accessed July 28, 2023.

Kelly, K. (2019). Infection masquerading as a fall in the elderly. *The journal of urgent care medicine.* Retrieved from https://www.jucm.com/infection-masquerading-as-a-fall-in-the-elderly/. Accessed July 28, 2023.

Li, J., Silverberg, M. A., Decker, W., & Edelstein, J. A. (2021). *Hypothermia.* Medscape [website]. Retrieved from https://emedicine.medscape.com/article/770542. Accessed July 28, 2023.

Lovence, K. (n.d.). *Post-fall care nursing algorithm.* RNJournal [website]. Retrieved from http://rn-journal.com/journal-of-nursing/post-fall-care-nursing-algorithm. Accessed July 28, 2023.

MaineHealth. (n.d.). *Fall prevention. A matter of balance.* MaineHealth.org [website]. Retrieved from https://www.mainehealth.org/healthy-communities/healthy-aging/matter-of-balance. Accessed July 28, 2023.

Martin, T. (2018). *How to adjust the temperature of your water heater.* CNET [website]. Retrieved from https://www.cnet.com/home/smart-home/how-to-adjust-the-temperature-of-your-water-heater/. Accessed July 28, 2023.

Mayo Clinic Staff. (2022a). *Hip fracture.* Mayo Clinic [website]. Retrieved from https://www.mayoclinic.org/diseases-conditions/hip-fracture/symptoms-causes/syc-20373468. Accessed July 28, 2023.

Mayo Clinic Staff. (2022b). *Hypothermia.* Mayo Clinic [website]. Retrieved from https://www.mayoclinic.org/diseases-conditions/hypothermia/symptoms-causes/syc-20352682. Accessed July 28, 2023.

MedlinePlus. (2021). *Fall risk assessment.* Bethesda, MD: MedlinePlus [website]. Retrieved from https://medlineplus.gov/lab-tests/fall-risk-assessment/. Accessed July 28, 2023.

Merdjanof, A. A. (2021). Climate, disasters, and extreme weather events: Vulnerability, resources, and interventions for lower-income older adults. *Generations Journal, 45*(2), 1–10.

Minnesota Commerce Department. (n.d.). *Fans: The first line of cooling.* MN.gov [website]. Retrieved from https://mn.gov/commerce-stat/pdfs/fans-the-first-line-of-cooling.pdf. Accessed July 28, 2023.

Muché, J. A., & McCarty, S. (2023). *Geriatric rehabilitation.* Medscape [website]. Retrieved from https://emedicine.medscape.com/article/318521. Accessed July 28, 2023.

Murphy, S. L., Kochanek, K. D., Xu, J., & Arias, E. (2021). Mortality in the United States, 2020. *NCHS Data Brief,* (427), 1–8.

National Center for Health Statistics. (2021). *The record increase in homicide during 2020.* Centers for Disease Control and Prevention [website]. Retrieved from https://www.cdc.gov/nchs/pressroom/podcasts/2021/20211008/20211008.htm. Accessed July 28, 2023.

National Council on Aging (NCOA). (2023). *Get the facts on falls prevention.* NCOA.org [website]. Retrieved from https://www.ncoa.org/article/get-the-facts-on-falls-prevention. Accessed July 28, 2023.

National Highway Traffic Safety Administration (NHTSA). (n.d.). *Older drivers.* Retrieved from https://www.nhtsa.gov/road-safety/older-drivers. Accessed July 28, 2023.

National Institute on Aging. (2022a). *Preventing falls at home: Room by room.* Retrieved from https://www.nia.nih.gov/health/fall-proofing-your-home. Accessed July 28, 2023.

National Institute on Aging. (2022b). *Hot weather safety for older adults.* Retrieved from https://www.nia.nih.gov/health/hot-weather-safety-older-adults. Accessed July 28, 2023.

National Safety Council (NSC). (2022). *Home and community overview.* Injury Facts. Retrieved from https://injuryfacts.nsc.org/home-and-community/home-and-community-overview/introduction/. Accessed July 28, 2023.

National Safety Council (NSC). (n.d.). *Fall safety: Take steps to remain independent longer.* Retrieved from https://www.nsc.org/home-safety/safety-topics/older-adult-falls. Accessed July 28, 2023.

Oregon Department of Human Services. (2022). *Self-study program. 723J: Fall prevention.* Oregon.gov [website]. Retrieved from https://www.oregon.gov/dhs/SENIORS-DISABILITIES/PROVIDERS-PARTNERS/Documents/0723J-Fall-Prevention-Modified.pdf. Accessed January 4, 2023.

Pennsylvania Department of Aging. (n.d.). *Healthy steps for older adults - fall prevention.* Retrieved from https://acl.gov/sites/default/files/programs/2017-03/HSOA-Intervention-Summary-Report.pdf. Accessed July 28, 2023.

Price, J. H., & Khubchandani, J. (2021). Firearm suicides in the elderly: A narrative review and call for action. *Journal of Community Health, 46*(5), 1050–1058. doi:10.1007/s10900-021-00964-7.

Rubenstein, L. Z. (2022). Falls in older people. In *Merck manual professional version*. Merck & Co., Inc. Retrieved from https://www.merckmanuals.com/professional/geriatrics/falls-in-older-people/falls-in-older-people. Accessed July 28, 2023.

Schraga, E. D., & Kates, L. W. (2022). *Cooling techniques for hyperthermia*. Medscape [website]. Retrieved from https://emedicine.medscape.com/article/149546. Accessed July 28, 2023.

Scottish Government. (2023). *Causes of falls*. NHS Inform [website]. Retrieved from https://www.nhsinform.scot/healthy-living/preventing-falls/causes-of-falls. Accessed July 28, 2023.

Shuman, T. (2023). *Crime prevention tips for senior citizens*. Seniorliving.org [website]. Retrieved from https://www.seniorliving.org/safety/crime-prevention-tips/. Accessed July 28, 2023.

Skidmore-Roth, L. (2023). *Mosby's 2022 nursing drug reference* (35th ed.). St. Louis, MO: Elsevier.

Smyth, D. (2022). *Toxic fumes & the gas fireplace*. eHow [website]. Retrieved from https://www.ehow.com/facts_7501086_toxic-fumes-gas-fireplace.html. Accessed July 28, 2023.

Substance Abuse and Mental Health Services Administration (SAMHSA). (2023). *Types of disasters*. Retrieved from https://www.samhsa.gov/find-help/disaster-distress-helpline/disaster-types. Accessed July 28, 2023.

Texas Health and Human Services. (n.d.). *Physical restraint reduction*. Retrieved from https://www.hhs.texas.gov/providers/long-term-care-providers/nursing-facilities-nf/quality-monitoring-program/evidence-based-best-practices/physical-restraint-reduction. Accessed July 28, 2023.

Schultz, J. (2019). Doctors say avoid box fans in this heatwave — they may do more harm than good. News San Diego. Retrieved from https://www.10news.com/lifestyle/doctors-say-avoid-box-fans-in-this-heatwave-they-may-do-more-harm-than-good. Accessed October 23, 2024.

Tinetti, M. E. (1986). Performance-oriented assessment of mobility problems in elderly patients. *Journal of the American Geriatrics Society, 34*(2), 119–126. doi:10.1111/j.1532-5415.1986.tb05480.x.

University of Illinois at Chicago Institute for Health Research and Policy. (n.d.). *Fit & Strong!* Retrieved from www.fitandstrong.org. Accessed July 28, 2023.

U.S. Department of Homeland Security. (2023). *Prepare your pets for disasters*. Ready.gov [website]. Retrieved from https://www.ready.gov/pets. Accessed July 28, 2023.

U.S. Department of Homeland Security. (2022). *Household chemical emergencies*. Ready.gov [website]. Retrieved from https://www.ready.gov/household-chemical-emergencies. Accessed July 28, 2023.

U.S. Fire Administration (USFA). (2018). *Fire safety for older adults*. Emmitsburg, MD: USFA. Retrieved from https://www.usfa.fema.gov/downloads/pdf/publications/fa_221.pdf. Accessed July 28, 2023.

Verbanas, P. (2021). *Carbon monoxide poisoning risk rises during winter storms*. Rutgers The State University of New Jersey [website]. Retrieved from https://www.rutgers.edu/news/carbon-monoxide-poisoning-risk-rises-during-winter-storms. Accessed July 28, 2023.

Will, J. (2022). *Why you should replace your fire extinguishers*. Consumer Reports [website]. Retrieved from https://www.consumerreports.org/home-garden/fire-extinguishers/why-you-should-replace-your-fire-extinguishers-a1635637699/. Accessed July 28, 2023.

World Health Organization (WHO). (2022). *Abuse of older people*. Retrieved from https://www.who.int/news-room/fact-sheets/detail/abuse-of-older-people. Accessed July 28, 2023.

World Health Organization (WHO). (2021). *Falls*. Retrieved from https://www.who.int/news-room/fact-sheets/detail/falls. Accessed July 28, 2023.

10

Sexuality and Aging

Linda A. Bub, MSN, RN, GCNS-BC, NPD-BC

http://evolve.elsevier.com/Yeager/gerontologic/

LEARNING OBJECTIVES

On completion of this chapter, the reader will be able to:
1. Identify the myths surrounding sexuality and aging.
2. Identify reasons for nurses' hesitancy in talking about sexuality and intimacy with older adults.
3. Describe the normal changes of aging in the male and female urogenital systems.
4. Describe the pathologic problems of the aging male and female urogenital systems.
5. Identify issues surrounding persons with dementia and their expression of sexuality.
6. Discuss barriers to older adults' sexual expression and the ways to overcome these barriers.
7. Conduct a sexuality and intimacy assessment of an older adult.
8. Identify two nursing diagnoses applicable to older adults' sexual or intimate expression.
9. Plan nursing interventions to assist older adults in fulfilling their need for sexuality and intimacy.

WHAT WOULD YOU DO?

What would you do if you were faced with the following situations?
- An older adult neighbor confides in you that they have started a new relationship with an individual they met through a dating app. They live in another state, and your neighbor has invited them to come to their house. What do you do?
- The nursing home you work at recently developed a protocol for sexuality and intimacy for residents. You have been asked to create an in-service on this protocol for the employees. What do you do?
- Your older adult patient in the clinic is a recent widower and shyly tells you about their new relationship with a younger individual in their apartment complex. The patient states that they feel things are easier at their age because there is no need to worry about pregnancy. How do you respond?

OLDER ADULT NEEDS FOR SEXUALITY AND INTIMACY

Sexuality is an important aspect of health, general well-being, and quality of life. Human sexuality includes intimate activity as well as sexual knowledge, beliefs, attitudes, and values. Sexual activity not only provides pleasure for older adults but may also help maintain healthy self-esteem. Sexual activity can help each partner express love, affection, and loyalty. It can also enhance personal growth, creativity, and communication. The current older generation, predominately Baby Boomers, is more open about sex and expects that their care providers are willing and able to discuss this topic with them.

Sexuality is an important aspect of overall wellness and happiness in older adults (Smith et al, 2019). Older adults can adapt to the aging process through other acts of intimacy that they are able to enjoy and are less concerned with the frequency of intimacy (Skałacka and Gerymski, 2019). Most older adults are willing to discuss their sexual health and wellbeing, but unfortunately, it is often initiated by the older adult (Agochukwu-Mmonu et al, 2021). Nursing needs to get more comfortable having these conversations if we are to support the overall wellness of our patients, especially with the large number of older adults currently in the health care system.

THE IMPORTANCE OF INTIMACY AMONG OLDER ADULTS

Many older adults are starting to share with their providers their needs for sexual intimacy, but unfortunately, health care professionals are not trained in how to discuss or incorporate this into the care of this population (Agochukwu-Mmonu et al, 2021). One reason for this is that society continually equates sexuality with sexual intercourse. However, according to the World Health Organization (n.d.),

> Sexual health is fundamental to the overall health and well-being of individuals, couples and families, and to the social and economic development of communities and countries. Sexual health, when viewed affirmatively, requires a positive and respectful approach to sexuality and sexual relationships, as well as the possibility of having pleasurable and safe sexual experiences, free of coercion, discrimination, and violence. The ability of men and women to achieve sexual health and well-being depends on their:
> - access to comprehensive, good-quality information about sex and sexuality;
> - knowledge about the risks they may face and their vulnerability to adverse consequences of unprotected sexual activity;
> - ability to access sexual health care;
> - living in an environment that affirms and promotes sexual health.

If sexuality among older adults is viewed as a need for intimacy, society and health care professionals may be more comfortable helping older adults meet those needs.

Females outlive males. The Administration for Community Living (2022) reports females reaching age 65 have an additional 20.8 years of life expectancy and males an additional 18.2 years. The ratio of older females is 125 females for every 100 males. This often leaves older females without sexual partners. The loss of a partner does not necessarily mean that older females do not have continuing sexual needs. The Michigan State University National Poll on Aging found that 40% of those aged 65–80 were sexually active (Agochukwu-Mmonu et al, 2021). The benefits of sexual health for overall health include enjoyment of life, improved mental health, lower risks of certain cancers, and decreased fatal coronary events (Smith et al, 2019). Despite the discomfort most health professionals feel with this topic, it is imperative that health care professionals value the sexual needs of older adults. The next study is going on currently, and it will be interesting to see if the pandemic had any influence on how participants answered or patterns of behavior.

Almost half of the older adult population experiences some sexual dysfunction, ranging from erectile dysfunction (ED) and premature climax among males to lack of desire, decreased vaginal lubrication, pain, and the inability to reach orgasm among females. A recent study looking at older adults and the impact of society demonstrated three themes: changing bodies, media, and society, and "feeling the same inside" (Towler et al, 2021). The need to look and feel younger, along with the idea that sexual intercourse is the main form of intimacy, has created a booming business focused on treating sexual problems. Older adults that focus on sexual problems as part of their natural aging experience less distress (Sinković and Towler, 2019).

Just like younger Americans, older adults are the most likely to be single (not married and living with a partner or in a committed relationship), 41% for younger adults and 36% for older adults. In younger groups, males are far more likely to be single than females (51% male vs. 32% female); in older adults, it is the exact opposite (21% single males and 49% single females). For older adult singles, "just like being single" and "having more important priorities right now" are the most common reasons for not dating, and "feeling like I am too old" is shared by 25% (Brown, 2020). Understanding the changes over time is important for open and nonjudgmental discussions with patients.

The pandemic has positively impacted the use of technology among older adults. AARP conducted a recent study of technology and older adults and found that older adults are using all forms of technology, have almost tripled how much they spend on technology, and see it as an important aspect of their daily lives (Kakulla, 2021). Familiarity with technology has afforded many older adults the option of online dating to find a partner. In the survey *How Seniors and Millennials Date: A New Comparative Study on Dating Habits* (MedicareAdvantage.com, 2023), older adults answered questions on dating apps and other ways to meet other singles, as well as thoughts on age. The key findings are as follows:
- Almost 30% of seniors (55+) have gone on a date with someone they met through online dating.
- Older adults are less likely to say that looks are extremely important than millennials.
- Older males are much more likely to say that age is not important than females over 55.
- Millennials are more likely to be intimate on a first date than seniors.

Older adults participate in a variety of sexual practices depending on functional ability, including kissing, embracing, petting or fondling, masturbation, and intercourse (vaginal, oral, or anal) (Smith et al, 2019). Masturbation is a method through which both males and females may feel sexually fulfilled in the absence of partners. The literature has established that in addition to older adults' ongoing need to express their sexuality through traditional sexual methods, the human need to touch and to be touched must also be fulfilled. A person's need for intimacy and closeness to another does not end at any age.

Touch is an important component of nursing care and should be incorporated into nursing interventions to achieve quality outcomes. Touch is part of nonverbal communication. It can express empathy, comfort, and reassurance and can promote trust. Touch is important to a person's well-being and sense of self. However, the perception of touch and the need for touch vary between individuals and cultures. Touch may also have different meanings based on a person's past experiences. Touch can be interpreted as disrespectful, sexual, patronizing, or threatening. When touching, ask permission to provide nursing care or comfort and reassurance. If the older adult cannot express their wishes concerning touch, ask family members about their preferences. Always avoid touching in a manner that can be misinterpreted (Catlin, n.d.).

For older adults who reached young adulthood before 1959, sexuality was hidden behind closed doors for much of their lives. Coupled with the idea that older adults do not need or desire intimacy, this makes conversations uncomfortable. Therefore, an assessment of an older adult's sexuality may be the first opportunity they have to discuss sexuality openly. Embarrassment, shyness, and apprehension in this area are common. In addition, the patient may view the normal changes of aging as embarrassing or indicative of illness and may be reluctant to discuss these matters with a nurse. Understanding attitudes and myths about aging will help the nurse assess and intervene to sensitively promote the older adult's need for sexuality and intimacy.

NURSING'S RELUCTANCE TO MANAGE THE SEXUALITY OF OLDER ADULTS

Nursing's attitude toward older adult sexuality and intimacy is complicated and can be influenced by multiple factors, including the nurses' own beliefs about sexuality, religious beliefs, the support of management, the type of behaviors the older adult is expressing (more loving), and where the behavior or activity occurs (Aguilar, 2017; Thys et al, 2019). The staff with more positive attitudes towards sexuality included those who were older, had a higher level of education, and had more experience. Negative attitudes or feeling uncomfortable were associated with younger staff, less support from management, and more erotic types of intimacy (Aguilar, 2017; Thys et al, 2019).

Older adults that had self-reports of fair/poor health had lower rates of satisfaction with their sexual health (Smith et al, 2019). Older adults have a decline in their sexual expression, drive, or desire that includes an overall decline in the frequency of sexual activities, ability to have an erection (males), or become sexually aroused (females) (Jackson et al, 2019). Most older adults are interested in discussing this with their provider but are the instigators of this conversation, not the provider (Smith et al, 2019). Nurses are in a key position to address newly developed or potential sexual dysfunction during patient interactions. However, because of discomfort, myths, ageism, and a lack of training in sexual health, these problems are often ignored. The result is that the needs of older adults with newly developed or chronic sexual dysfunction are ignored, leading to loneliness and a lack of intimacy (Aguilar, 2017).

NORMAL CHANGES OF THE AGING SEXUAL RESPONSE

Nurses must understand the normal urogenital changes associated with aging. Knowledge about these normal changes helps nurses work more confidently with older adults, enabling them to compensate for these changes, assisting them to understand these changes, and recognizing when possible pathologic changes occur.

To assess sexual function in older adults, healthcare providers need to understand the sexual response cycle, which includes the physical and emotional changes leading to orgasm and how the cycle can change with aging. The four stages of the sexual response cycle for both females and males are: 1) desire or libido, 2) arousal or excitement, 3) orgasm, and 4) resolution. Sexual dysfunction can occur at any one of these stages and can include sexual desire disorders, sexual arousal disorders, ED, premature ejaculation, orgasm disorders, and sexual pain disorders. Sexual dysfunction is a common disorder but is often not diagnosed. Sexual dysfunction can occur in any phase of the sexual response, with a partner or alone, throughout life, once or repeatedly, and with one partner or with certain partners (Cleveland Clinic, 2023). This knowledge will give the healthcare provider the background to talk openly and honestly with the patient and partner(s).

Physiologic Changes

The orgasm response changes with aging. Dysfunctions include anorgasmia, premature ejaculation, and retarded ejaculation. In addition, a longer period of stimulation is typically required for both males and females to reach orgasm. The refractory period after orgasm is also longer for both males and females.

In older adults, the reduced availability of sex hormones in both genders results in less rapid and less extreme vascular responses to sexual arousal (Wise and Crone, 2006). Although some older adults view this gradual slowing as a decline in function, others do not consider it an impairment because it merely results in them taking more time and creativity in their sexual health (Smith et al, 2019).

There are two main changes in sexual function in males with aging: ED and ejaculatory dysfunction (Slack and Aziz, 2020). The refractory period between ejaculations is long. Andropause has several physical, sexual, and emotional symptoms. Serum sex hormone-binding globulin (SHBG) concentrations gradually increase due to age, making less free testosterone. Testosterone levels diminish with age from a reduction in testosterone production and metabolic clearance. These hormonal changes lead to a loss of libido, decreased muscle mass and strength, alterations in memory, diminished energy and well-being, increased sleep disturbance, and possibly osteoporosis secondary to a decrease in bone mass. Currently, new studies are being conducted with a focus on the role of endogenous sex hormones on the health outcomes of older males, including heart attacks, strokes, cardiovascular deaths, cancer, dementia, and psychosocial and behavioral impacts in the Androgens in Men Study (AIMS) (Yeap et al, 2020).

ED is a persistent difficulty in achieving and maintaining a sufficient erection to have satisfactory sexual intercourse. Prevalence ranges from 2% in males less than 40 years of age to half of males aged 40–70 and 85% of those over the age of 80 (Salas-Huetos et al, 2019). Causes of ED include increasing age; structural abnormalities of the penis; the adverse effects of drugs; psychological disorders; substance use disorders; surgery, trauma, and radiation of the pelvis; and vascular, neurologic, and endocrine disorders. It is most common to have more than one cause of ED, and it is treatable (Ellsworth, 2022).

The use of medications such as phosphodiesterase 5 (PDE 5) inhibitors (e.g., sildenafil citrate, tadalafil, and vardenafil hydrochloride) has increased public awareness of the prevalence of ED among males in the United States. When appropriately prescribed, these medications may be effective in treating ED in older males and, therefore, may enhance the quality of life in older adults.

Up to 85% of postmenopausal females experience sexual dysfunction. Sexual dysfunction in older females encompasses loss of sexual desire, problems with arousal, an inability to achieve orgasm, and painful intercourse. Three areas have been found to influence female sexual health. They include biologic (i.e., age, genitourinary syndrome of menopause (GSM) status, physical health, and hormones), psychological (i.e., mental health, personality, satisfaction with life, and self-esteem), and interpersonal (i.e., partner availability, quality of relationships, and social support) factors (Mernone et al, 2019).

Genitourinary Syndrome of Menopause

GSM comprises three areas of clinical symptoms that include genital, sexual, and urinary symptoms (Nappi et al, 2019). Genital symptoms include dryness, burning, and irritation; sexual symptoms include dyspareunia or painful intercourse; and other dysfunctions such as decreased lubrication, thinning of the vaginal wall, decreased elasticity, and decreased vaginal rugae. Urinary symptoms occur in approximately 50%–75% of females and include urgency, overactive bladder, incontinence, dysuria, and recurrent urinary tract infections (Nappi et al, 2019; Vesco et al, 2021).

Many older females experience *dyspareunia*, painful intercourse, or pain with attempted intercourse, which may result in a decreased desire to participate in sexual activity. Forty percent of sexually active females between the ages of 55 and 75 experience painful sexual intercourse. Dyspareunia can be classified as primary (pain experienced with the first attempt at intercourse) and secondary (pain after intercourse). Causes include sexually transmitted infections, bladder diseases, anatomic changes, decreased hormones or diabetes, external creams, soaps, or douches (Kellogg Spadt and Kusturiss, 2016).

Recent studies have focused on the impact of GSM on the lives of females over 55. Females in these studies have shared that it has a negative impact on their daily lives, their sexuality, intimate relationships, self-esteem, emotional wellbeing, social life, and quality of life. (Moral et al, 2018). Most females in the study saw the physical symptoms of GSM as normal aging and did not pursue treatment. When seeking a gynecologist's opinion, 70% received treatment (Moral et al, 2018). This has a profound message: treating GSM is an important factor in the wellbeing of females over 55.

PATHOLOGIC CONDITIONS AFFECTING OLDER ADULTS' SEXUAL RESPONSES

Illness, Surgery, and Medication

Sexual function is a process that depends on the neurologic, endocrine, and vascular systems. Lifestyle factors that can influence sexual function include smoking, alcohol consumption, activity, psychological health, weight, and diet (Salas-Huetos et al, 2019). Many chronic illnesses common to older adults can affect sexual function (Box 10.1).

Surgeries may also affect an older adult's sexual responses. Some of these surgeries include coronary artery bypass surgery, hysterectomy, mastectomy, prostatectomy, orchiectomy, and the removal of the anus and the rectum. In addition, many drugs adversely affect sexuality (Table 10.1).

Human Immunodeficiency Virus

Adults over the age of 50 account for 48% of those living with the human immunodeficiency virus (HIV). In 2019, 15% of persons newly diagnosed with HIV were over the age of 65.

BOX 10.1 Conditions That Affect Sexual Function

Cardiac Conditions
Congestive heart failure
Myocardial infarction
Angina
Arrhythmias
Hypertension

Endocrine Conditions
Diabetes mellitus
Hypothyroidism

Genitourinary Conditions
Prostatitis
Cystitis and urethritis
Chronic renal failure
Incontinence

Immune Conditions
Human immunodeficiency virus (HIV) infection and acquired immunodeficiency syndrome (AIDS)
Cancer

Musculoskeletal Conditions
Arthritis
Chronic pain

Neurologic Conditions
Parkinson disease
Dementia
Stroke
Depression

Respiratory Conditions
Chronic emphysema
Bronchitis
Sleep apnea

Surgery
Hysterectomy
Mastectomy
Prostatectomy

Data from Merghati-Khoei, E., Pirak, A., Yazdkhasti, M., & Rezasoltani, P. (2016). Sexuality and elderly with chronic diseases: A review of the existing literature. *Journal of Research in Medical Sciences, 21,* 136.

When older adults are found to be HIV-positive, they tend to be diagnosed later in the course of the illness (Centers for Disease Control and Prevention [CDC], 2021a). Additionally, older adults living with HIV have four times higher rates of comorbidity compared to younger adults, including illnesses such as cardiovascular disease, malignancies, osteoporosis, frailty, and disability, as well as noncommunicable diseases (Roomaney et al, 2022). Polypharmacy and uncertainties in treating comorbidities in those with HIV are still impacting the overall health of this population (Roomaney et al, 2022).

The availability of drugs to treat ED has extended the sexual lives of many males. Increasingly larger numbers of older adults have substance use disorders (e.g., alcohol, illicit drugs, and

TABLE 10.1 Drugs Affecting Sexuality

Drug Class	Example	Effect on Sexuality
Diuretics	Thiazide diuretics Potassium sparing diuretics	Decreased libido Erectile dysfunction Decreased vaginal lubrication
Antihistamines	Diphenhydramine Chlorpheniramine	Erectile dysfunction
Histamine blockers	Histamine-2 antagonists	Decreased libido Erectile dysfunction
Antipsychotics	Phenothiazines First-generation antipsychotics Atypical antipsychotics	Decreased libido Erectile dysfunction
Antidepressants	Tricyclic antidepressants Tetracyclic antidepressants (mirtazapine) Selective serotonin reuptake inhibitors Monoamine oxidase inhibitors Bupropion hydrochloride	Decreased libido Decreased ejaculate Delayed ejaculation
Antihypertensives	Alpha-blockers Beta-blockers Centrally acting agents	Decreased libido Erectile dysfunction Lack of orgasm Decreased ejaculate
Alcohol		Erectile dysfunction Decreased sexual response in females
Antianxiety medications	Benzodiazepines	Decreased libido Erectile dysfunction
Antiepileptics	Carbamazepine Valproic acid Phenytoin	Decreased libido Erectile dysfunction
Hormones	GnRH agonists GnRH antagonists Androgen receptor inhibitors Estrogen	Decreased libido
Tobacco		Erectile dysfunction Decreased vaginal lubrication
Recreational drugs	Alcohol Amphetamines Barbiturates Cocaine Marijuana Heroin Nicotine	Erectile dysfunction
Statins		Research is conflicting, but they may lower testosterone
Drugs for BPH	Finasteride	Decreased libido Erectile dysfunction Abnormal ejaculation
Opioids		Decreased libido

BPH, Benign prostatic hyperplasia; *GnRH,* gonadotropin-releasing hormone.
Data From Stratton, K. L. (2023). *Drugs that may cause erection problems.* Medline Plus [website]. Retrieved from https://medlineplus.gov/ency/article/004024.htm; Ulrich, A., & Gragnolati, A. B. (2022). *11 medications that may be affecting your sex life.* GoodRx [website]. Retrieved from https://www.goodrx.com/drugs/side-effects/these-drugs-may-be-affecting-your-sex-life.

recreational use of prescription drugs). These factors, combined with an underestimation of personal risk, mean many older adults engage in behaviors that put them at risk for HIV infection. Older adults are often not using a condom with sexual activity; in studies, more than 90% of males over the age of 50 did not use a condom with a date or casual partner, and 70% did not use a condom with someone who was a stranger (Karpiak and Lunievicz, 2017). It is important to understand the risk for HIV and STIs, and it should not be assumed that older adults are not having sex and, if they do, that they are using protection. Health care providers should communicate clearly and openly with patients and their partners to minimize complications.

Age-related changes also increase the risk of HIV infection. For example, age-related thinning of the vaginal mucosa and subsequent vaginal tissue disruption and age-related reductions in immune function place older adults at increased risk for HIV infection. Older adults who contract HIV are more likely to be diagnosed late in the disease, experience progression more quickly, and often have much more complicated care (McMillan et al, 2018).

Malignancies

Breast cancer, one of the leading cancers affecting older females, has clear implications for self-esteem and sexual functioning. Dysphoria from the disease, fears of death, and disfigurement may diminish sexual desire before treatment begins. With the growing older adult population, invasive breast cancer rates will double by 2030. Identifying those biases against older females for treatment of breast cancer can impact their lives as well as their sexual intimacy. 2021 was the first year that guidelines were published for mammography for survivors over 75 (Freedman et al, 2021). Breast cancer is the second most deadly cancer for females behind lung/bronchus cancer, and the rates of death have declined in the last few decades (CDC, 2021b).

Prostate cancer is the most common new cancer in males and the second leading cause of death from cancer behind lung cancer in males in the United States (CDC, 2021b). The risk of developing prostate cancer increases with age. When cancer has not spread outside of the prostate, a radical prostatectomy may be performed; it involves the removal of the prostate gland and some surrounding tissue, leading to a disruption of surrounding nerves, veins, and arteries. In 25% to 90% of males, radical prostatectomy results in impotence in up to 90% of males (Bratu et al, 2017); additionally, roughly 50% experience incontinence. The introduction of robot-assisted laparoscopic techniques has reduced sexual dysfunction; however, males may need to wait 2 to 3 years for maximum function to return. Phosphodiesterase inhibitors, prosthetic devices, and vacuum constriction devices (penile rehabilitation, or PR) are available to treat ED after treatment for prostate cancer, with varying rates of success depending on adherence to the PR (Albaugh et al, 2019).

Colorectal cancer is the fourth most common cancer in the United States and the fourth leading cause of cancer death (CDC, 2021b). Sexual function is impaired by colon cancer, resulting in a significant decrease in sexual satisfaction and an increase in sexual problems. This is not limited to the patient but can impact the partner as well (Stulz et al, 2020).

Dementia

The need for companionship and intimacy does not fade just because a person is diagnosed with dementia. As dementia progresses and changes in cognition and judgment occur, some individuals experience a decrease in sexuality, whereas others may experience sexual disinhibition. Many older adults with dementia long for physical closeness and seek out physical touch; however, their intentions may be misinterpreted as sexual in nature. Masturbation continues to be a source of pleasure for both males and females with dementia. Still, a lack of privacy in institutional settings can lead caregivers to believe the behavior is inappropriate. Inappropriate sexual behavior (ISB) can be distressing for caregivers, both family and members of the health care team. Some actions labeled as inappropriate may be caused by confusion or misidentification, such as undressing in public or kissing and touching a caregiver (D'cruz et al, 2020). Approximately 7%–25% of females and males with dementia may exhibit some form of sexually inappropriate behavior (D'cruz et al, 2020). Alzheimer dementia has a lower rate, with vascular dementias having a typically higher prevalence. ISB can be overt or implied and can be classified into four areas: inappropriate sex talk, sexual acting out, implied sex acts, and false sexual allegations (D'cruz et al, 2020).

The management of ISB includes nonpharmacologic and pharmacologic management. Nonpharmacologic management includes an evaluation of the environment (under or over stimulation), clothing (uncomfortable), temperature, and avoiding contact with the family member, caregiver, or patient that the older adult is directing the behavior towards (D'cruz et al, 2020). Behavioral management includes offering alternatives if the older adult is seeking intimacy, such as soft toys to cuddle, a change in clothing that has zippers or buttons in the back, and distraction or guiding the individual away from the source of stimulation (D'cruz et al, 2020). Residential facilities should have policies in place that address the need for intimacy and sexual expression. Offering time to debrief and share management techniques is important to help staff and family deal with the needs of the dementia patient.

Pharmacologic interventions may become necessary when the behaviors become harmful or detrimental to safe care. Selective serotonin reuptake inhibitors, gabapentin, carbamazepine, beta-blockers, and cholinesterase inhibitors have been used for their known side effects of decreased libido and ED, with varying degrees of success. Hormonal agents (e.g., antiandrogens and estrogens) have been successful in treating some persons with dementia with sexually disinhibited behavior, but controversy surrounds their use as it is considered *chemical castration* (De Giorgi and Series, 2016).

ENVIRONMENTAL AND PSYCHOSOCIAL BARRIERS TO SEXUAL PRACTICE

Sexual dysfunction may signal other psychosocial disorders, such as depression, delirium, and dementia. Sexuality may also be affected by anxiety concerning partner availability and lifestyle issues. Substance use disorders (SUD), including smoking, alcohol, and illicit or recreational drug use, are often associated with sexual dysfunction. The growing Baby Boomer generation has created concern that, over time, the number of older adults using substances to cope with mental and physical impairments, loneliness, and other medical conditions will continue to rise. This will further complicate the adverse effects of SUD, chronic medical conditions, and prescription drug use (Mattson et al, 2017).

Patients with dementia should be given special attention to ensure their safety when they decide to engage in sexual relationships. Health care professionals working with cognitively impaired older adults need to determine whether the individual is consenting to sexual activity. Determine if the older adult with dementia is a willing and active participant. If they are unable to give consent or are inactive, the surrogate decision-maker should be involved, and the activity will need to be stopped (D'cruz et al, 2020).

LESBIAN, GAY, BISEXUAL, AND TRANSGENDER OLDER ADULTS

Lesbian, gay, bisexual, transgender, queer, intersex, and asexual (LGBTQIA) older adults have spent much of their lives hiding their sexual preference and gender identity, not only from family and the rest of society but also from their healthcare providers. Older adults who are LGBTQIA face many health disparities, including victimization, psychological distress, disability, discrimination, and a lack of access to appropriate health services. They are also more likely to experience chronic illness and disability (e.g., cancer, obesity, hypertension, hypercholesterolemia, arthritis, cardiovascular disease, and diabetes) and delay treatment for health issues compared with older adults who are heterosexual. Older adults who are LGBTQIA are more likely to be more vulnerable to social isolation and loneliness due to a lifetime of discrimination and victimization (Goldsen, 2018).

Despite stereotypes, nurses need to recognize that LGBTQIA is an acceptable expression of sexuality for both males and females. Nurses should examine their own personal beliefs about LGBTQIA intimacy and ensure they do not prevent older adults from fulfilling their sexual needs. Self-examination will allow nurses to develop a therapeutic relationship with older adults who are LGBTQIA without the interference of personal feelings. The patients' partners should be encouraged to participate in the sexual assessment and planning when appropriate. Nurses should also remember that no information about the sexual orientation of patients should be shared with a patient's family unless permission has been given. See Box 10.2 for questions that can be added to an assessment.

NURSING CARE GUIDELINES FOR SEXUALITY AND AGING

Recognize Cues (Assessment)

As demonstrated throughout this chapter, sexual health is integral to the overall health of the older adult; therefore, it is essential to obtain a sexual history (Table 10.2). However, one of the greatest obstacles in assessing the sexuality of older adults occurs at the beginning of the assessment. Gathering sexual history becomes easier with experience. One challenge nurses

BOX 10.2 Questions on Sexuality

- Are you currently sexually active? If so, with one or more than one partner?
- Male or female partner? Or both?
- Are your sexual desires being met?
- Do you have any questions or concerns about your sexual function? About your partner's sexual function?
- What kind of information would you like?

TABLE 10.2 Evaluating Sexual Risk in Older Adults

Normalizing the discussion	• I am going to ask you a few questions about your sexual health. Sexual health is important to overall health, and I ask all my patients these questions.
Broaching the topic	• Before we begin, do you have any questions or concerns you want to discuss? • Tell me about your sex life. • When you say you have had sex, can you expand on that? • Who are your sexual partners? Males, females, or both?
Asking about partners	• Tell me about the number of sex partners within the past 3 months. • Where do you meet your partners? • Have you been pressured or coerced to have sex? • Have you ever gone online to meet partners for sex? • How well do you know your sexual partners? • What do you know about the human immunodeficiency virus (HIV) status of your partners? • How does your partner's HIV status affect your sexual behavior? • Have you noticed symptoms in your partner that are causing you concern?
Asking about sexual activity	• What sexual activities do your sexual partners engage in? • Do you have oral sex? Vaginal sex? Anal sex? • Do you select partners based on HIV status? • Do you ever get drunk or high before you have sex?
Asking about prevention methods	• What do you do to protect yourself during sex? • Do you use condoms when having sex? How often? With what types of sex? • What has been your experience with using condoms? • What factors or situations get in the way of using condoms?

Data from Centers for Disease Control and Prevention (CDC). (2022). *Discussing sexual health with your patients.* Retrieved from https://www.cdc.gov/stophivtogether/library/topics/prevention/brochures/cdc-lsht-prevention-brochure-clinicians-quick-guide-discussing-sexual-health-your-patients.pdf.

face is helping older adults develop and sustain the intimate relationships they desire. This involves active assessment, including actively reviewing health concerns and conditions that affect sexual functioning. Although discomfort in this area is understandable, increased proficiency comes with experience. Healthy sexuality depends on good communication between the health professional and the patient. Nurses are in a pivotal position to begin this communication. The PLISSIT model has been used to assess and manage the sexuality of adults since 1976. PLISSIT is an acronym for **P**ermission, **L**imited **I**nformation, **S**pecific **S**uggestions, and **I**ntensive **T**herapy. The model offers suggestions for initiating and maintaining a discussion of sexuality with older adults. The PLISSIT model can be used in a variety of clinical settings with additional assessment questions (Smyth, 2018). A simple sexual history performed by nurses may include questions such as those found in Box 10.2.

The goal of the model is to gather information, allow the client to express their sexuality in a safe environment, and not feel uninhibited (Smyth, 2018). The healthcare provider should complete a detailed sexual history. The goal of the assessment, regardless of the model used, is to gather information that allows patients to express sexuality safely and feel uninhibited by normal or pathologic problems.

It is common for nurses and nursing students to feel uncomfortable and embarrassed when assessing the sexual desires and functions of any patient, but even more so for older patients. Nonetheless, a sexual assessment should be performed as a routine part of the nursing assessment. Knowledge, skill, and a sense of comfort are necessary for the nurse to assess the sexuality of older adults. Nurses may take several steps to create a nonthreatening environment conducive to communication:

- Provide a quiet, private meeting place, and avoid interruptions during the discussion.
- Sit at eye level with the patient and ask questions in a manner that is not threatening.
- Avoid using terms that may suggest they are making assumptions about sexual behavior or orientation.
- Avoid medical terminology and the use of slang words.

Other components of the sexual history–taking process include reviewing medications and medical conditions that may contribute to sexual dysfunction. In addition, the nurse should review the older adult's early experiences, if they are willing to share. A physical assessment, including an examination of the breasts and genital tissue, is an essential part of the sexual assessment. Laboratory tests may be useful in determining reductions in hormone levels that may contribute to decreased libido, or ED. Box 10.3 lists laboratory tests relevant to a sexual assessment of older adults.

The nurse should also obtain information on sexual preferences. This should be followed by an assessment of the patient's living environment. The nurse should determine where the patient plans to engage in sexual activity. In acute and long-term care settings, the environment should be assessed for privacy and safety. This enables older adults to proceed with sexual activity safely and comfortably. In the community setting, the environment should be assessed for safety and the availability of adaptive equipment such as side rails, medical trapezes, and specialized beds, which may be needed to enable older adults to participate in sexual activity safely within the home.

The nursing staff should be cognizant of indications of sexual interest in older adults. Overt gestures of sexuality in public areas or hints of sexual interest during conversations with patients should not be ignored or punished; they should be viewed as an indication of sexual interest between two older adults.

BOX 10.3 Laboratory Tests to Guide Sexual Assessment

- Total serum testosterone
- Serum luteinizing hormone
- Serum prolactin
- Prostate-specific antigen (after risk and benefits have been reviewed)
- Chemistry panel
- Thyroid-stimulating hormone
- Hemoglobin A1c
- Lipid profile
- Urinalysis
- Complete blood count
- Estradiol
- Follicle-stimulating hormone
- Vitamin B_{12} and folate

EVIDENCE-BASED PRACTICE

Exploration of Knowledge, Attitudes, and Experiences with Sexual Expression in Nursing Homes

Background
The Baby Boomers were part of the 1960s sexual revolution and considered sexuality and sexual expression of vital importance. By 2030, 58 million Baby Boomers will be between the ages of 66 and 84, with increasing numbers of them in need of nursing home services. This systematic review of the literature was conducted to "explore the knowledge, attitudes, and experiences of administrators, care staff, relatives, community-dwellers, and residents toward older people's sexuality and sexual expression in nursing homes" (p. 471).

Sample/Setting
The cumulative Index to Nursing and Allied Health Literature (CINAHL) and PubMed databases were searched for quantitative studies using the keywords sexuality *or* intimacy, older people *or* older age *or* residents, long-term care *or* nursing home, and attitudes *or* knowledge *or* experience. Articles were limited to those published between January 2000 and November 2016 and excluded if they were not written in English. Twelve research articles met the selection criteria.

Methods
The Preferred Reporting Items for Systematic Reviews and Meta-Analysis (PRISMA) was used to help summarize the selection process and compare data.

Findings
Sexual expression in older adults is a need that should be supported in nursing homes. Positive attitudes toward sexuality in the nursing home environment were correlated with increased knowledge of sexuality and aging. Positive predictors among care providers included age, level of education, and years of experience. Barriers to addressing the sexual needs of residents included a lack of privacy and staff discomfort.

Implications
Failure to thoroughly assess the sexual needs of older adults and include them in the treatment plan can lead to a lack of intimacy and loneliness. Health care personnel must meet the needs of nursing home residents and accommodate their values and expectations.

Data From Aguilar, R. A. (2017). Sexual expression of nursing home residents: Systematic review of the literature. *Journal of Nursing Scholarship, 49*(5), 470–477.

Among older adults, an added risk factor is cognitive impairment, which may hinder a patient's decision-making abilities. Before a sexual relationship commences, it may be appropriate for the nurse to meet with both patients individually and together to discuss their intentions and expectations regarding the sexual relationship. In so doing, the patients' fears and apprehensions may be expressed, and their questions answered. In addition, such a discussion may reveal whether one patient is being coerced into the relationship or is not mentally competent to decide to enter such a relationship.

A cognitive assessment such as the Montreal Cognitive Assessment, or whatever your practice setting uses, should be performed as part of the assessment of older adults. The information gained from this assessment is useful if the nurse suspects that patients are cognitively impaired and unable to make decisions to participate in sexual relationships. If the cognitive assessment does not provide sufficiently clear information regarding patients' decision-making abilities, a more thorough assessment by a psychologist may be necessary to prevent anyone from taking advantage of these patients.

Analyze Cues and Prioritize Hypotheses (Patient Problems)

Several patient problems pertain to older adults experiencing sexual problems. Sexual dysfunction applies to older adults who express concern about meeting their need for sexuality and intimacy. Factors related to this patient problem include fear, lack of opportunity, misconceptions, pain, and embarrassment (see Nursing Care Plan on Sexual Dysfunction: Drugs).

NURSING CARE PLAN
Sexual Dysfunction: Drugs

Clinical Situation
Mr. J, a 76-year-old retired electrical engineer, comes to the clinic complaining of headaches that have been increasing in severity over the past several months. His initial assessment shows severe hypertension. During the nursing assessment, it is revealed that Mr. J is a widower and lives alone. However, he has a female friend who visits him often, and they have sexual intercourse every 1 to 2 weeks. To date, he has not experienced any problems with his sexual performance. He was prescribed a beta-blocker to control his hypertension.

Analyze Cues and Prioritize Hypotheses (Patient Problems)
- Reduced sexual expression resulting from potential side effects from antihypertensive medication

Generate Solutions (Planning)
- The patient will not experience a disruption in meeting his need for sexuality and intimacy.

Take Actions (Nursing Interventions)
- Instruct the patient on the normal aging changes in sexual functioning.
- Instruct the patient that ED is not a normal aging change and may be a side effect of his antihypertensive medication.
- Instruct the patient to notify his health care provider if ED or any other sexual problem is noticed.
- Instruct the patient concerning the proper and consistent use of condoms to prevent sexually transmitted infections.

Sexual dysfunction would also be an applicable diagnosis for an aging female experiencing dyspareunia or decreased or absent sexual desire (see Nursing Care Plan on Sexual Dysfunction: Privacy).

NURSING CARE PLAN
Sexual Dysfunction: Privacy

Clinical Situation
Mr. K is a 78-year-old retired boxer who has resided at a nursing facility for 3 years. He has Parkinson disease and uses a walker. He is generally happy and pleasant. Mrs. P is an alert 75-year-old widow who was admitted to the facility 1 month ago after a stroke left her wheelchair-bound and unable to perform her activities of daily living (ADLs) independently. She was upset when she arrived at the nursing facility and had some difficulty adjusting to her new home.

Over the past 2 weeks, a close relationship has developed between these two residents. Mrs. P has been happier than she was on admission, and both residents appear to have a new sense of energy and enthusiasm for life. Recently, the nursing staff has noticed sexual expression and signs of intimacy between the two in public areas.

Analyze Cues and Prioritize Hypotheses (Patient Problems)
- Reduced sexual expression results from a lack of privacy.

Generate Solutions (Planning)
- Patients will be free to pursue their sexual relationship in private

Take Actions (Nursing Interventions)
- Perform a sexual assessment of both patients.
- Provide a climate in which both can openly discuss the situation and respond with trust and confidence.
- Pay close attention to verbal and nonverbal cues while listening. Provide reassurance, as needed.
- Meet with both patients individually to assess each one's desire regarding sexual activity and each one's degree of competence.
- Assess the level of comfort in discussing the topic and issues, alone or with each other present, and provide opportunity for both.
- Provide teaching on the normal changes of the aging sexual system (see Box 10.1 and the Patient/Family Teaching boxes).
- Compensate for any physical disabilities assessed.
- Implement precautions against the spread of sexually transmitted infections.
- Find a safe, private location for the couple to pursue their sexual interests.

Other potential appropriate patient problems include:
- Anxiety
- Reduced sexual expression
- Need for health education
- Discomfort
- Reduced self-concept

Generate Solutions (Planning)

The nurse should develop an individualized care plan that includes the information elicited during history taking, physical assessment, and discussion about specific sexual relationships. This plan should (1) compensate for the physical disabilities of older adults, (2) prevent the spread of infection, (3) provide for the emotional well-being of older adults, (4) satisfy the needs of family members when possible, and (5) ensure patient safety.

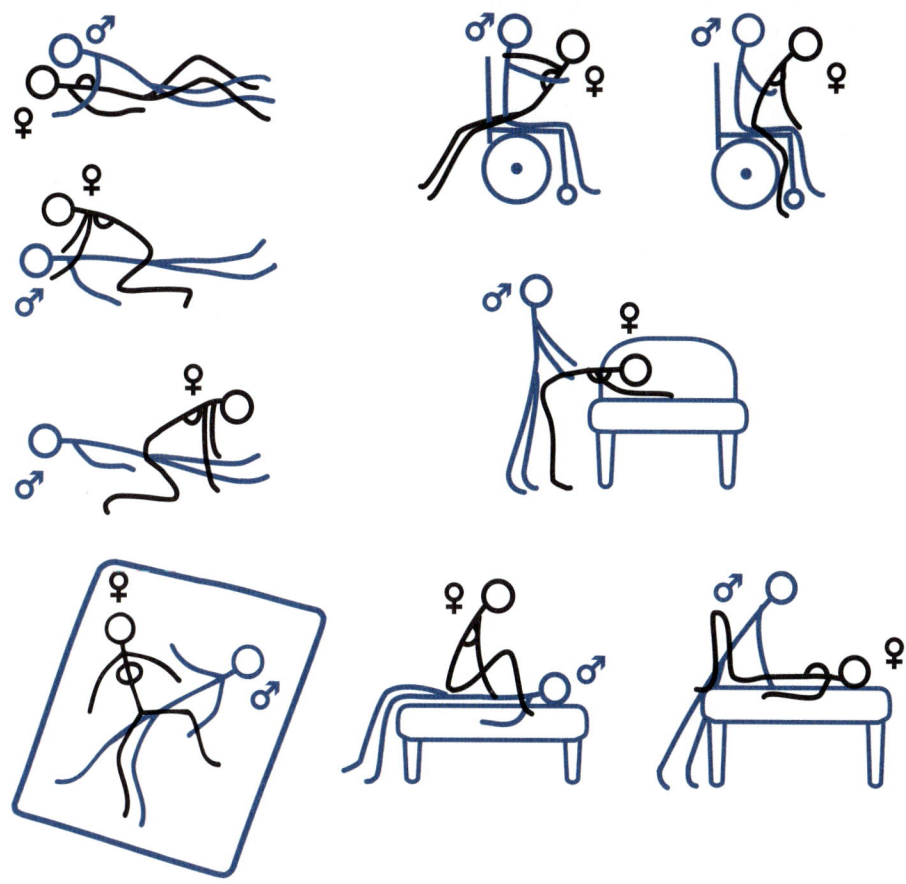

Fig. 10.1 Coital positioning for older couples.

The expected outcomes of the care plan should result from specific, time-limited goals aimed at restoring or promoting the patient's sexual satisfaction.

Expected outcomes include, but are not limited to, the following:
1. The patient attains a satisfactory level of sexual activity, as evidenced by the resumption of sexual activity at a level acceptable to the patient.
2. The patient verbalizes their sexual concerns and discusses them with their significant other.
3. The patient explores various sexual activities and practices to attain sexual satisfaction.
4. The patient verbalizes their feelings about sexual performance.

Take Actions (Nursing Interventions)

Older adults should be provided with information, education, and direction to assist them in creating and sustaining intimate relationships. Education starts with discussing changes associated with aging. Teaching and reassurance by the nurse that some changes are a normal part of aging helps patients understand their bodies and feel comfortable learning how to compensate for these changes (see Patient/Family Teaching boxes). Teaching regarding coital positioning for couples with physically disabling conditions is often a necessary intervention (Fig. 10.1).

> **PATIENT/FAMILY TEACHING**
> ### Normal Changes of the Aging Female Sexual System
> Instruct female patients that, with aging, the following occur:
> - Vaginal secretions diminish; the use of an artificial water-based lubricant helps decrease discomfort.
> - The vagina becomes shorter and does not expand to accommodate the penis. Some discomfort may be experienced, so the use of alternative positions for intercourse (see Fig. 10.1) may help decrease discomfort.
> - Orgasmic contractions are fewer and may be accompanied by painful uterine contractions. However, these generally do not indicate pathologic problems.
> - Vaginal irritation and clitoral pain are common and do not signify illness.
> - The breasts lose tone, and the areolar area does not enlarge as much.
> - Infrequent rectal sphincter contractions, which do not interfere with orgasm, and postcoital need to void may be experienced.

> **PATIENT/FAMILY TEACHING**
> ### Normal Changes of the Aging Male Sexual System
> Instruct male patients that, with aging, the following occur:
> - The penis may take longer to become firm and may not be as firm as at a younger age; therefore, a longer period of foreplay should be planned.
> - Ejaculation may take longer to achieve, may be less intense, and may be shorter in duration. The patient should conserve strength and not work hard at the beginning of intercourse, which could result in tiring before climax.

Continued

> **PATIENT/FAMILY TEACHING—cont'd**
> - The erection diminishes more quickly after climax, so if condoms are being used, the patient should plan to withdraw immediately after climax.
> - It takes longer to achieve a second orgasm, so the patient should plan to resume foreplay or use this time to touch or talk.
> - Rectal sphincter contractions may be experienced, but these do not interfere with orgasm.

When sexual intercourse is not the preferred method of intimacy or is not possible for an older couple, the couple may be taught alternative methods of intimacy in the form of touch. Touch is a means of expressing intimacy and closeness that may fulfill older patients' sexual needs and desires. Touch is best fulfilled by finding a comfortable environment in which an older adult couple can expose parts of their bodies to each other as they feel comfortable. A shower or bath may be enjoyable. The couple should be taught to move their fingertips slowly or lightly over each other's skin while enjoying the closeness of the other person. Massage therapy, books, and videos may provide older adults with a way of touching that results in the fulfillment of sexual desires. The use of sex toys may be suggested to help the older adult(s) achieve orgasm and feel a sense of intimacy. Soft music may make the environment more conducive for older couples.

Proper precautions need to be implemented to prevent sexually transmitted infections. Low-risk behaviors such as practicing monogamous relationships, reducing the number of partners, and consistent use of condoms (male and female types) should be encouraged (see Box 10.4).

If an older adult is concerned about their family's feelings regarding a sexual relationship, further counseling should be provided and should include the family, when possible. At this time, family members may bring forth their concerns regarding the relationship, and the older adult may answer them with a nurse present. It is important for the older adult's family to understand and accept their decisions about any relationships. However, if no amenable agreement between the older adult and family can be reached, the older adult's needs must be the nurse's primary consideration.

As discussed previously, older adults with cognitive impairment may display ISB, such as exposure or advances toward other patients and staff. It is important for the nurse to manage these behaviors while maintaining the dignity of these older adults. Ignoring the behavior or punishing the older adult does not curtail the behavior. A thorough assessment of mental status and sexuality is necessary to isolate the cause of the behavior. Inappropriate behavior is best managed by determining the root cause of the behavior (e.g., pain, discomfort, or hyperthermia) and redirecting the older adults' sexual interest toward socially acceptable behaviors, which may be accomplished by providing a quiet place for masturbation and viewing sexually explicit materials (magazines or videos).

Acute and long-term care facilities should make proper arrangements for privacy during older adults' sexual experiences. The physical facilities within each setting vary. The ideal situation is to set up a room with a pleasant environment, which can be used for a variety of activities but may also be reserved by older adults for private visits with a spouse or partner. In most settings, this may not be possible; thus, patient rooms may be used if the nursing staff gains permission from the patient's roommate and plans alternate activities for them.

In any setting, patient safety should be maintained. The call lights should be easily accessible. Side rails on the bed should be used, if necessary, and the room should be situated such that the nursing staff is aware when it is in use. Although the patients' privacy is important, they should not be left alone in any situation in which they may injure themselves.

In a community setting, adaptive equipment such as hospital beds, side rails, or a medical trapeze may be needed to allow patients to function safely. Based on the information gathered from the assessment, the nurse may assist patients in acquiring the equipment. The nurse may also need to demonstrate safe transfer processes to ensure that patients are able to transfer and function, independently or with the help of their partner. See Box 10.5 for strategies that may enhance sexual function in older patients.

Staff education about the sexuality and intimacy of older adults should include recognition of cues, desires, and interest in sexual

> **BOX 10.4 Sexually Transmitted Infections (STIs) in Older Adults**
>
> STIs are not just happening in younger populations. As of 2018:
> - 20% of new cases of chlamydia infections happened in those over age 50.
> - Syphilis cases in older adults increased by 50%.
> - 17% of new HIV cases are in older adults.
> - Currently, 1.2 million people are living with HIV; 50% are over age 50.
>
> Data from ACRIA, New York State Department of Health (NYSDOH) AIDS Institute, New York State Office for the Aging (NYSOFA). (2020). *Older adults and sexual health: a guide for aging services providers*. Retrieved July 28, 2023 from https://www.health.ny.gov/diseases/aids/general/publications/docs/sexual_health_older_adults.pdf.

> **BOX 10.5 Strategies to Maintain Sexual Health**
>
> **Open Communication with Your Doctor**
> Have sexual health be a part of annual checkups
> Ask about drug side effects that impact sexual health
> Ask for testing for STIs
>
> **Talk to Your Partner**
> Be open in intimate relationships
> Look for a licensed therapist if needed
>
> **Live Healthy**
> Eat well
> Exercise regularly
> Moderate alcohol intake
> Eliminate tobacco use
> Healthy weight
> Practice stress-reducing activities
>
> Data from the National Council on Aging. (2021). *Sexual health for older adults. How do you maintain sexual health after 50?* NCOA.org [website]. Retrieved July 28, 2023 from https://www.ncoa.org/article/how-do-you-maintain-sexual-health-after-50.

activity and intimacy. Staff should recognize that older adults may use and have access to pornographic material, especially through the Internet. The use of sex toys to help achieve orgasm should be normalized. The education of nursing staff also needs to address eliminating stereotypes. Open discussion of attitudes and sexual issues among staff may help increase comfort in dealing with older patients' sexual issues. Case studies and other learning tools, such as trivia games, may be effective means of education. Education should also be available to the family. The training should begin by discussing and dispelling the myths surrounding older adults' sexual desires and activities. The training should include normal changes associated with older males and females and how to compensate for specific physical disabilities. Healthcare providers should have a focus on wellness and overall health to make both the patient and the provider more comfortable with this topic (Agochukwu-Mmonu et al, 2021).

Training should conclude with discussion groups to allow staff and family to discuss their own feelings about sexuality and its role in the lives of older adults. Role-playing may be an effective technique to gain an understanding of the effect of the staff and family's personal values on older adults.

Evaluate Outcomes (Evaluation)

Evaluation of concerns related to sexuality and intimacy is based on the patient's achievement of established expected outcomes. Older adults may attain a satisfying level of sexual activity that is compatible with functional capacity with the help of sound, sensitive nursing interventions. When sexual functioning cannot be restored, alternatives should be explored. The use of touch and massage may be an alternative to sexual intercourse and may help older adults achieve sexual satisfaction. Although many stereotypes hinder the ability of professionals to promote sexuality among older adults, older adults can and should be allowed to achieve satisfactory sexual outcomes with the full support of health care professionals. Proper documentation is important to communicate the interventions and progress toward meeting the expected outcomes.

> **HOME CARE**
> 1. Assess sexual patterns in homebound older adults who have chronic conditions.
> 2. Provide information regarding sexual positions or sexual function to accommodate environmental barriers (e.g., a Foley catheter) to both homebound older adults and their partners.
> 3. Foster a supportive environment for homebound older adults and their partners to discuss sex-related fears, concerns, and feelings.
> 4. Explain pathologic conditions that may adversely affect sexuality (e.g., diabetes).
> 5. Teach safe sexual practices to homebound older adults and their partners.
> 6. Teach alternative methods of intimacy to both homebound older adults and their partners based on identified sexual dysfunctions or alterations.

SUMMARY

The need for sexuality and intimacy continues throughout a person's life span. It is the nurse's role to dispel societal myths surrounding sexuality and aging and to enable older adults to reach their sexual potential. After thorough assessment and management of the normal and pathologic changes in the aging urogenital system, older adults can pursue sexuality as desired, resulting in the highest quality of life attainable.

KEY POINTS

- Sexual desire and interest persist throughout the life span of people into older adulthood.
- Nurses are often influenced by myths surrounding the sexual practices of older adults, and many lack the knowledge and training to work with older adults who experience sexual dysfunction.
- Normal, age-related changes in the urogenital system may interfere with an older adult's expression of sexuality.
- Pathologic problems with the aging sexual response are often related to illnesses and medication.
- Older adults with dementia may display ISB and may not be competent to participate in sexual relationships.
- Environmental barriers in the home and in acute and long-term care settings may prevent older adults from meeting their needs for sexual intimacy.
- All older adults should receive a sexual assessment so that normal and pathologic changes can be identified.
- Older adults should be taught about the normal changes of aging in the urogenital systems, and the means to compensate for these changes (i.e., topical estrogen to relieve the symptoms of vaginal atrophy).
- Interventions used to assist older adults in adapting to age-related changes include manipulation of the environment and the procurement of assistive equipment and devices needed to continue to function sexually.
- Touch is an alternative to sexual intercourse and provides the intimacy needed by some older adults.

CLINICAL JUDGMENT EXERCISES

1. A 74-year-old female patient is asking about painful sexual intercourse with her 72-year-old long-term partner. She has asked her friends about it but has not been to find out how to minimize the pain. What suggestions do you have for her on this important matter?

2. A gay married couple resides in a long-term care facility where you work. They have told you that they do not feel comfortable trying to have sexual intimacy because of the reactions of some of the staff. How should you respond? Discuss your feelings about this situation.

REFERENCES

Administration for Community Living. (2022). *2021 profile of older Americans*. Washington, DC: U.S. Department of Health and Human Services. Retrieved from https://acl.gov/aging-and-disability-in-america/data-and-research/profile-older-americans. Accessed August 12, 2024.

Agochukwu-Mmonu, N., Malani, P. N., Wittmann, D., Kirch, M., Kullgren, J., Singer, D., et al. (2021). Interest in sex and conversations about sexual health with health care providers among older U.S. adults. *Clinical Gerontologist*, 44(3), 299–306. doi:10.1080/07317115.2021.1882637.

Aguilar, R. A. (2017). Sexual expression of nursing home residents: systematic review of the literature. *Journal of Nursing Scholarship*, 49(5), 470–477. doi:10.1111/jnu.12315.

Albaugh, J., Adamic, B., Chang, C., Kirwen, N., & Aizen, J. (2019). Adherence and barriers to penile rehabilitation over 2 years following radical prostatectomy. *BMC Urology*, 19(1), 89. doi:10.1186/s12894-019-0516-y.

Bratu, O., Oprea, I., Marcu, D., Spinu, D., Niculae, A., Geavlete, B., et al. (2017). Erectile dysfunction post-radical prostatectomy – a challenge for both patient and physician. *Journal of Medicine and Life*, 10(1), 13–18.

Brown, A. (2020). A profile of single Americans. In *Nearly half of U.S. adults say dating has gotten harder for most people in the last 10 years*. Washington, DC: Pew Research Center. Retrieved from https://www.pewresearch.org/social-trends/2020/08/20/a-profile-of-single-americans/. Accessed August 12, 2024.

Catlin, A. (n.d.). *How skilled human touch can transform person-centered dementia care*. Compassionate Touch® white paper. Hurst, TX: AGE-u-cate™ Training Institute.

Centers for Disease Control and Prevention (CDC). (2021a). Diagnoses of HIV infection in the United States and dependent areas 2019: National profile. Retrieved from https://www.cdc.gov/hiv/library/reports/hiv-surveillance/vol-32/content/national-profile.html#Diagnoses. Accessed August 12, 2024.

Centers for Disease Control and Prevention (CDC). (2021b). *Leading causes of death – females – all races and origins – United States, 2017*. Retrieved from https://www.cdc.gov/women/lcod/2017/all-races-origins/index.htm. Accessed July 28, 2023.

Cleveland Clinic. (2023). *Sexual response cycle*. ClevelandClinic.org [website]. Retrieved from https://my.clevelandclinic.org/health/articles/9119-sexual-response-cycle. Accessed August 12, 2024.

D'cruz, M., Andrade, C., & Rao, T. S. S. (2020). The expression of intimacy and sexuality in persons with dementia. *Journal of Psychosexual Health*, 2(3-4), 215–223. doi:10.1177/2631831820972859.

De Giorgi, R., & Series, H. (2016). Treatment of inappropriate sexual behavior in dementia. *Current Treatment Options in Neurology*, 18(9), 41. doi:10.1007/s11940-016-0425-2.

Ellsworth, P. I. (2022). *Erectile dysfunction (ED, impotence)*. MedicineNet [website]. Retrieved from https://www.medicinenet.com/erectile_dysfunction_ed_impotence/article.htm. Accessed August 12, 2024.

Freedman, R. A., Minami, C. A., Winer, E. P., Morrow, M., Smith, A. K., Walter, L. C., et al. (2021). Individualizing surveillance mammography for older patients after treatment for early-stage breast cancer: Multidisciplinary expert panel and International Society of Geriatric Oncology Consensus Statement. *JAMA Oncology*, 7(4), 609–615. doi:10.1001/jamaoncol.2020.7582.

Goldsen, K. F. (2018). Shifting social context in the lives of LGBTQ older adults. *The Public Policy & Aging Report*, 28(1), 24–28. doi:10.1093/ppar/pry003.

Jackson, S. E., Firth, J., Veronese, N., Stubbs, B., Koyanagi, A., Yang, L., et al. (2019). Decline in sexuality and wellbeing in older adults: A population-based study. *Journal of Affective Disorders*, 245, 912–917. doi:10.1016/j.jad.2018.11.091.

Kakulla, B. (2021). *Personal tech and the pandemic: Older adults are upgrading for a better online experience*. AARP.org [website]. Retrieved from https://www.aarp.org/research/topics/technology/info-2021/2021-technology-trends-older-americans.html. Accessed August 12, 2024.

Karpiak, S. E., & Lunievicz, J. L. (2017). Age is not a condom: HIV and sexual health for older adults. *Current Sexual Health Reports*, 9, 109–115. doi:10.1007/s11930-017-0119-0.

Kellogg Spadt, S., & Kusturiss, E. (2016). Female sexual function and aging. *Topics in Geriatric Rehabilitation*, 32(3), 193–198. doi:10.1097/TGR.0000000000000115.

Mattson, M., Lipari, R. N., Hays, C., & Van Horn, S. L. (2017). *A day in the life of older adults: substance use facts*. The CBHSQ Report. Rockville, MD: Center for Behavioral Health Statistics and Quality, Substance Abuse and Mental Health Services Administration. Retrieved from https://www.samhsa.gov/data/sites/default/files/report_2792/ShortReport-2792.html. Accessed August 12, 2024.

McMillan, J. M., Krentz, H., Gill, M. J., & Hogan, D. B. (2018). Managing HIV infection in patients older than 50 years. *CMAJ*, 190(42), E1253–E1258. doi:10.1503/cmaj.171409.

MedicareAdvantage.com. (2023). *How seniors and millennials date: a new comparative study on dating habits*. Retrieved from https://www.medicareadvantage.com/senior-dating-survey#:~:text=Millennials%20were%20found%20to%20make,to%20just%2039%25%20of%20millennials. Accessed August 12, 2024.

Mernone, L., Fiacco, S., & Ehlert, U. (2019). Psychobiological factors of sexual functioning in aging women – findings from the Women 40+ Healthy Aging Study. *Frontiers in Psychology*, 10, 546. doi:10.3389/fpsyg.2019.00546.

Moral, E., Delgado, J. L., Carmona, F., Caballero, B., Guillán, C., González, P. M., et al. (2018). The impact of genitourinary syndrome of menopause on well-being, functioning, and quality of life in postmenopausal women. *Menopause*, 25(12), 1418–1423. doi:10.1097/GME.0000000000001148.

Nappi, R. E., Martini, E., Cucinella, L., Martella, S., Tiranini, L., Inzoli, A., et al. (2019). Addressing vulvovaginal atrophy (VVA)/genitourinary syndrome of menopause (GSM) for healthy aging in women. *Frontiers in Endocrinology, 10*, 561. doi:10.3389/fendo.2019.00561.

Roomaney, R. A., van Wyk, B., & Pillay-van Wyk, V. (2022). Aging with HIV: Increased risk of HIV comorbidities in older adults. *International Journal of Environmental Research and Public Health, 19*(4), 2359. doi:10.3390/ijerph19042359.

Salas-Huetos, A., Muralidharan, J., Galiè, S., Salas-Salvadó, J., & Bulló, M. (2019). Effect of nut consumption on erectile and sexual function in healthy males: A secondary outcome analysis of the FERTINUTS randomized controlled trial. *Nutrients, 11*(6), 1372. doi:10.3390/nu11061372.

Sinković, M., & Towler, L. (2019). Sexual aging: A systematic review of qualitative research on the sexuality and sexual health of older adults. *Qualitative Health Research, 29*(9), 1239–1254. doi:10.1177/1049732318819834.

Skałacka, K., & Gerymski, R. (2019). Sexual activity and life satisfactioin in older adults. *Psychogeriatrics, 19*(3), 195–201. doi:10.1111/psyg.12381.

Slack, P., & Aziz, V. M. (2020). Sexuality and sexual dysfunctions in older people: A forgotten problem. *BJPsych Advances, 26*(3), 173–182. doi:10.1192/bja.2019.80.

Smith, L., Yang, L., Veronese, N., Soysal, P., Stubbs, B., & Jackson, S. E. (2019). Sexual activity is associated with greater enjoyment of life in older adults. *Sexual Medicine, 7*(1), 11–18. doi:10.1016/j.esxm.2018.11.001.

Smyth, C. (2018). *Sexuality assessment for older adults. Try This: General Assessment Series. Issue #10*. The Hartford Institute for Geriatric Nursing, New York University Rory Meyers College of Nursing. Retrieved from https://hign.org/sites/default/files/2020-06/Try_This_General_Assessment_10.pdf. Accessed August 12, 2024.

Stulz, A., Lamore, K., Montalescot, L., Favez, N., & Flahault, C. (2020). Sexual health in colon cancer patients: a systematic review. *Psychooncology, 29*(7), 1095–1104. doi:10.1002/pon.5391.

Thys, K., Mahieu, L., Cavolo, A., Hensen, C., Dierckx de Casterlé, B., & Gastmans, C. (2019). Nurses' experiences and reactions towards intimacy and sexuality expressions by nursing home residents: A qualitative study. *Journal of Clinical Nursing, 28*(5-6), 836–849. doi:10.1111/jocn.14680.

Towler, L. B., Graham, C. A., Bishop, F. L., & Hinchliff, S. (2021). Older adults' embodied experiences of aging and their perceptions of societal stigmas toward sexuality in later life. *Social Science & Medicine, 287*, 114355. doi:10.1016/j.socscimed.2021.114355.

Vesco, K. K., Leo, M. C., Bulkley, J. E., Beadle, K. R., Stoneburner, A. B., Francisco, M., et al. (2021). Improving management of the genitourinary syndrome of menopause: Evaluation of a health system–based, cluster-randomized intervention. *American Journal of Obstetrics and Gynecology, 224*(1), 62.e1–62.e13. doi:10.1016/j.ajog.2020.07.029.

Wise, T., & Crone, C. (2006). Sexual function in the geriatric patient. *Clinical Geriatrics, 14*(12), 17–26.

World Health Organization. (n.d.). *Sexual health: Overview*. WHO.int [website]. Retrieved from https://www.who.int/health-topics/sexual-health#tab=tab_1. Accessed August 12, 2024.

Yeap, B. B., Marriott, R. J., Adams, R. J., Antonio, L., Ballantyne, C. M., Bhasin, S., et al. (2020). Androgens In Men Study (AIMS): Protocol for meta-analyses of individual participant data investigating associations of androgens with health outcomes in men. *BMJ Open, 10*(5), e034777. doi:10.1136/bmjopen-2019-034777.

11

Pain

Jennifer Mundine, EdD, MSN, RN, CNE

http://evolve.elsevier.com/Yeager/gerontologic/

LEARNING OBJECTIVES

On completion of this chapter, the reader will be able to:
1. Define the concept of pain, including types and sources.
2. Describe the consequences of unrelieved pain in older adults.
3. Discuss the goals of pain management in older adults.
4. Identify barriers that affect the assessment of pain or its management in older adult patients.
5. Describe the effect of pain on the quality of life (QoL) of older adult patients.
6. Identify factors that may affect the older adult's pain experiences.
7. Use a pain assessment tool to rate patients' pain intensity.
8. Describe the use of pharmacologic and nonpharmacologic therapies for older adults with pain.

WHAT WOULD YOU DO?

What would you do if you were faced with the following situations?
- You are on a memory unit with 13 residents. You were told in the report that all residents have been calm, purposefully wandering, eating, and drinking fluids today. At dinner, one resident begins crying when brought from their room and continues to become more upset as they walk. What would you do?
- On a skilled long-term care (LTC) unit of 16 residents, a resident who recently had a knee replacement presents with confusion, different from his normal presentation of alertness. As the day progresses, he becomes increasingly confused and meets criteria for being delirious. The resident will not allow anyone to examine him and retreats to his room. What would you do?
- You check on your mother every day, and each day she begins to present differently. Today, she does not want to go with you to the park, and you notice dishes are in the sink, her bed is not made, and she cancelled a bridge game with her friends yesterday. You notice she is walking hesitantly, and you ask if she is in pain. She says, "A little." What do you do?

Pain is a common experience for many older adults. Of adults aged 65 and older, 52.3% reported bothersome pain, with 75% having pain in more than one location (Hulla et al, 2017). Adults aged 65 and older are the fastest-growing segment of the U.S. population. Adults aged 85 and older are projected to increase by 118% by 2040 (Administration for Community Living [ACL], 2022). Aging has demonstrated increases in the risk for pain secondary to high rates of chronic and acute conditions; 45% of older adults on Medicare have at least 4 chronic conditions (Horgas, 2017). Before the mid-1990s, literature on pain in older adults was scarce (Horgas, 2017). However, significant efforts have been made to address and improve pain in older adults (Horgas, 2017). "Assessment and management of pain is a responsibility of all health professionals and is within the scope and standards of an registered nurse's (RN's) practice" (Arnstein et al, 2017, p. 21).

Pain has long been recognized as a symptom of something else in the body. Although pain has often been referred to as the *fifth vital sign*, in 2019 (original statement in 2016), The Joint Commission (TJC) continued to communicate it DOES NOT endorse this concept, preferring to encourage nonpharmacologic individualized interventions and appropriate prescribing of pharmacologic measures, in accordance with the patient's care, treatment, and services (The Joint Commission, 2018).

Pain should not be felt when all body systems are working together well. These are facts, whereas pain, as an expectation of aging, is a myth. Persistent, chronic pain is associated with isolation, greater costs, suffering, and disability (Domenichiello and Ramsden, 2019). When approaching pain management in older adults, consideration of physical, psychologic, social, and coping must be used to facilitate a pain management approach (Ho, 2019).

Pain is underrecognized, highly prevalent, and undertreated in older adults, especially in those with impaired cognition. After age 60, the incidence rate of pain more than doubles. Older adults are more vulnerable when having pain, which also contributes to increased risk for overall vulnerability. An older adult is more at risk for double jeopardy when experiencing pain (Schofield and Gibson, 2021). Many health-care practitioners have encountered older adults only in an emergency room (ER) or in hospitals,

---

Previous authors: Joanne Alderman, MSN, APRN-CNS, RN-BC, FNGNA; Jacqueline Kayler DeBrew, PhD, MSN, RN; and Ramesh C. Upadhyaya, RN, CRRN, MSN, MBA, PhD-C.

where they need unusually intense medical or nursing treatment; this is not an optimal way to understand that the conditions of these patients / residents are not representative of normal aging. However, older adults are at high risk for pain-inducing situations during their lifespan because of the alteration of the pain experience. The pain experience in older adults is altered due to changes in processing mechanisms and degeneration of circuits, decreasing pain tolerance (Dagnino and Campos, 2022).

UNDERSTANDING PAIN

Definition

McCaffery (1979) further stated that *pain* is "whatever the experiencing person says it is, existing whenever he or she says it does." Booker and Haedtke (2016) identify *uncontrolled pain* as a rational reason for an older adult's hospital admission. The definition by Aronoff (2002) is more specific: "a subjective, personal, unpleasant experience involving sensations and perceptions that may or may not relate to bodily or tissue damage." *Pain* is also defined as an unpleasant sensory and emotional experience (Merskey and Bogduk, 1994). "Pain is a complex biopsychosocial disease" which affects all aspects of an older adult's function (Schwan et al, 2019, p. 548). In 2020, the International Association for the Study of Pain (IASP) revised the definition of pain as "an unpleasant sensory and emotional experience associated with, or resembling that associated with, actual or potential tissue damage (Raja et al, 2020, p. 1976).

Pain may be classified as *acute* or *chronic*. Acute pain is defined by rapid onset and relatively short duration and is a sign of a new health problem requiring diagnosis and analgesia. Treatment usually involves treating the underlying disease or injury and using short-term analgesics. In contrast, chronic or persistent pain continues after healing or is not amenable to a cure. This pain usually has no autonomic signs and is associated with longstanding functional and psychologic impairment. The older adult is most likely to suffer from chronic pain due to neuropathies, post-surgery, post-cancer, cardiovascular diseases, arthritis, and other chronic disease processes (Schwan et al, 2019). In June 2018, the World Health Organization (WHO) updated the classifications of chronic pain to reflect the significance of chronic pain better (Scholz, 2019) (Box 11.1).

Scope of the Problem of Pain

Although pain is not part of normal, healthy aging, pain is a common problem among older adults, and persistent physical pain is widespread in the older population (AGS, 2009). It is estimated that 25% to 50% of community-dwelling older adults experience significant pain problems (Park and Hughes, 2012; Reid et al, 2011). Adults 65 to 85 years old are at a higher risk for developing persistent pain, especially when enduring severe, acute pain. This risk supports the importance of focused assessments, prevention, and prompt pain treatment in older adults (Arnstein et al, 2017). Pain is even greater in older adults in nursing homes, where it has been shown that 70% to 80% of residents have substantial undertreated pain (AGS, 2009; Robinson, 2010; Schofield, 2010).

Stereotyping older adults as having less pain because of their age contributes to less-frequent pain assessment and, consequently, less appropriate and effective treatment for the pain. Older adults commonly report less pain because they do not want to be complainers, fear having to undergo more tests and medical treatments, and fear losing their independence (AGS, 2009). Additionally, older adults have been told that they will have pain sometime in their later years. Thus, they become resigned to the experience of pain. The fear that pain will be seen as a reason for having to give up independent living is associated with a reluctance to express pain freely to nonfamily members. Older adults may be ambivalent about the benefit of any action for their pain. Some of these responses by older persons may be attributed to health-care practitioners saying, "What do you expect at *your* age?" which supports the belief that nothing can be done to control or stop the pain.

Compounding this problem is the fact that older patients have been systematically excluded from clinical trials of analgesic drugs even though they are more likely to experience the side effects of analgesic medications. Research groups do not want comorbid conditions confounding the findings of a single medication or treatment.

Consequences of Unrelieved Pain

"Persistent intense pain can harm an individual's mind, body, spirit, and social interactions, resulting in disability, financial hardships, despair, and medical frailty" (Arnstein et al, 2017). Schwan et al (2019) found that chronic pain in older adults "reduces mobility, is associated with depression and anxiety, and can disrupt familial and social relationships" (p. 547). Consequences of persistent pain also include decreased socialization, sleep disturbance, decreased or impaired ambulation, prolonged recovery periods, increased use of health-care resources, premature death, and increased health-care costs which have all been documented with the presence of pain in older patients (AGS, 2009). The prevalence of pain in older adults who also have hypertension (HTN) is increased when not treated properly and will also affect HTN control (Li et al, 2022). Unrelieved pain has been shown to result in increased frailty in comparison with older adults who do not have pain (Otones Reyes et al, 2019). Pain may make getting to the bathroom so difficult that it leads to incontinence. Constipation may also be related to unrelieved pain when the person changes their diet, decreases activity, and has difficulty getting to a toilet before the urge passes (Jansen, 2008). Untreated pain may result in the older adult being unable to participate in self-care or health promotion (HP) activities (Bishop and Morrison, 2007). Pain combined with cognitive impairment (CI), feeling as if they are a burden to others, and pain-related disability may drive the older adult to consider or attempt suicide (Arnstein et al, 2017). Pain may go untreated if the older adult has dementia or other CIs (Herr et al, 2010).

Assessing and managing pain in older adults poses unique challenges to health-care professionals. The nurse caring for older adults in pain must understand the special needs of this diverse population. Although older adults are at risk for chronic disease (45% of Medicare beneficiaries have at least 4 chronic conditions [Horgas, 2017]) and the often painful conditions that accompany those ailments, their pain is often underrecognized

BOX 11.1 Primary and Secondary Chronic Pain Classifications

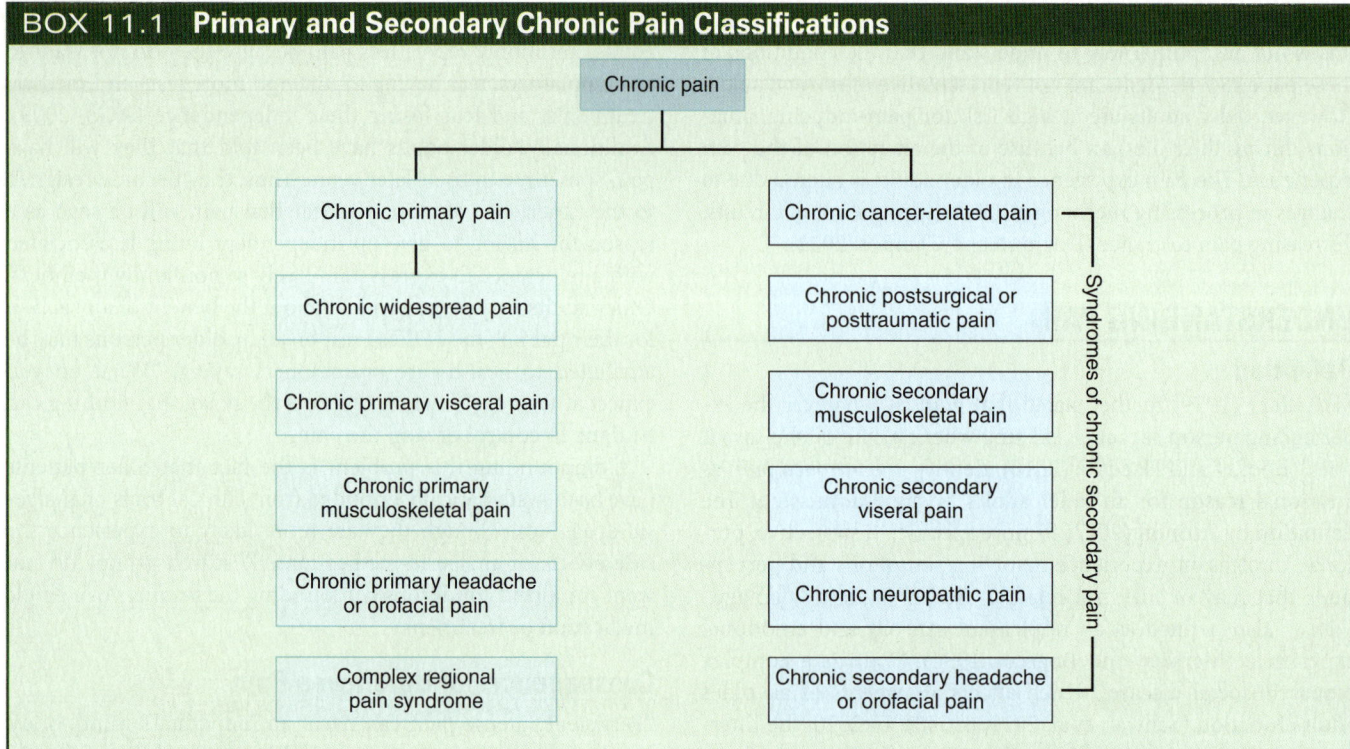

Chronic Primary Pain (CPP)
Chronic Widespread Pain (CWP)
Diffuse pain in at least 4 of 5 regions of the body: Fibromyalgia.

Complex Regional Pain Syndrome (CRPS)
Pain usually in the limbs, occurring after an injury, that is significantly greater than it should be. Involves sensory changes, abnormal skin temperature, impaired movement, changes in hair, skin and sweating. CRPS type 1: due to illness or injury (i.e., fracture or soft tissue injury); CRPS type 2 due to nerve injury in the limb.

Chronic Primary Headache and Orofacial Pain (OFP)
Pain in the head, face, and mouth that lasts for at least 2 hours per day: chronic migraine, chronic tension-type headache (CTTP), burning mouth syndrome (BMS), and chronic primary temporomandibular disorder (TMD).

Chronic Primary Visceral Pain (CPVP)
Pain stemming from specific internal organs: CPVP, chronic pelvic pain syndrome (CPPS), chronic primary epigastric pain syndrome, interstitial cystitis and chronic primary painful bladder syndrome (IC-PBS), chronic primary abdominal pain syndrome (CAP).

Chronic Primary Musculoskeletal Pain (CPMP)
Pain in the muscles, bones, joints, and tendons: low back pain (LBP), cervical pain, thoracic pain, limb pain.

Chronic Secondary Pain
Chronic Cancer-Related Pain (CRP)
Pain caused by cancerous tumors, metastases, and cancer treatment.

Chronic Postsurgical or Posttraumatic Pain (CPSP)
Pain that develops or intensifies following surgery (i.e., spinal surgery, herniotomy, hysterectomy, amputation, thoracotomy, breast surgery, or arthroplasty) or tissue injury (i.e., burn, whiplash, or musculoskeletal injury).

Chronic Secondary Musculoskeletal Pain (CMP)
Pain that comes from the bones, joints, muscles, spine, and related soft tissues, including persistent inflammation from autoimmune disease, structural changes of osteoarthritis (OA) and spondylosis; and diseases of the nervous system including multiple sclerosis (MS), Parkinson's disease (PD) and peripheral neuropathy (PN).

Chronic Secondary Visceral Pain (CSVP)
Pain from internal organs caused by mechanical factors (i.e., kidney stones, intestinal blockage or restricted blood flow and compression); vascular mechanisms, and persistent inflammation of the internal organs.

Chronic Neuropathic Pain (CNP)
Pain due to a lesion or disease in the part of the nervous system involved in sensory information. Chronic central neuropathic pain (CCNP) can be caused by spinal cord injury (SCI), injury to the brain, stroke, or MS. Chronic peripheral neuropathic pain (CPNP) can be caused by injury to the peripheral nerves, polyneuropathy, and radiculopathy.

Chronic Secondary Headache or Orofacial Pain (OFP)
Pain caused by all secondary head, face, and mouth pain (i.e., chronic dental pain, chronic trigeminal neuralgia (CTN), headache, or OFP caused by a secondary disorder (i.e., inflammation, injury, or central nervous system (CNS) disease.

Data from Dellwo, A. (2021). *Primary and secondary chronic pain classifications*. Verywell Health [website]. Retrieved from https://www.verywellhealth.com/primary-and-secondary-chronic-pain-classifications-5118466#toc-chronic-primary-pain.
Image modified from Treede, R.D., Rief, W., Barke, A., et al. (2019) Chronic pain as a symptom or a disease: The IASP classification of chronic pain for the International Classification of Diseases (ICD-11). *Pain*, 160(1), 19–27.

and untreated, leading to poor outcomes (Arnstein et al, 2017). Therefore, accurate and ongoing assessment is essential for managing pain in older adults. Goals for pain management in older adults include the following:
- Listening to the older adult and paying close attention
- Relief from pain
- Control of chronic disease conditions causing pain
- Maintenance of mobility and functional status
- Promotion of self-care and maximum independence
- Improved QoL

These goals can be achieved by educating patients, families, and health-care professionals, as well as through good nursing care.

PATHOPHYSIOLOGY OF PAIN IN OLDER ADULTS

Pain has multiple components that affect one's physical and psychosocial functioning. Although older adults develop more chronic diseases as they age, pain does not need to be an expectation of normal aging. Understanding pain physiology and theories is essential to effective pain management in older adults.

The three major components of the nervous system that cause the sensation and perception of pain are (1) the afferent pathways (reception), (2) the central nervous system (CNS; perception), and (3) the efferent pathways (reaction). The afferent pathways have nociceptors and are found on the skin. The nerve endings distributed in the skin are Pacinian corpuscles that mediate sensation, including pain, pressure, and itching. Stimulation of these nerve endings by vibrations from massage or sound waves may reduce the perception of pain in conditions such as chronic rheumatoid arthritis (RA). The free nerve endings of nociceptors are sensitive to mechanical, thermal, electrical, or chemical stimuli, and are responsible for transmitting sensory pain information. This stimulation flows through peripheral sensory nerves (afferent pathways) to the spinal cord. A painful stimulus (e.g., a pinprick) sends an impulse to a nociceptor (a receptor for painful stimuli) along a peripheral nerve fiber, which enters the gray matter of the spinal cord. Nociceptors terminate in the spinal cord (McCaffery and Pasero, 1999). Here, the nociceptor stimulation flows to the brain through a series of relay neurons.

When the pain stimulus or signal reaches the CNS, it is evaluated and interpreted in the limbic system, reticular formation, thalamus, hypothalamus, medulla, and cerebral cortex. The brain's interpretation is based on both physical and psychologic factors. Modulation of the pain stimulus may occur in the gray matter, the dorsal horn of the cord. Here, transmission occurs from the nociceptor to the spinothalamic tract (STT) neuron. Substance P, a neurotransmitter, facilitates transmission of the stimulus from the afferent (peripheral) neuron across the synapse to the STT neuron. Uninhibited by drugs or other modalities, the pain impulse travels to the brain's cerebral cortex, where the brain interprets the quality of pain, processing past experiences with pain, knowledge of pain, and cultural associations related to pain perception. The interpretation is relayed back through the peripheral nervous system (efferent) pathways, which are fibers connecting the reticular formation, midbrain, and substantia gelatinosa of Rolando (SGR). Pain modulation occurs in the efferent neural pathways and may involve chemical factors of neuropeptides, which may increase the sensitivity of the afferent pain receptors to noxious stimuli. These pathways result in the sensation and perception of pain (Huether and McCance, 2017).

Perception of Pain in Older Adults

Although not completely understood, it is accepted that pain perception differs in older adults compared to younger people (McCleane, 2008). Aging can have opposite influences on the sensory dimension versus the affective dimension. Reduction of and increased excitability can occur in the pain pathways from peripheral changes in aging (Yezierski, 2012). Lautenbacher et al (2017) noted in their meta-analysis that pain thresholds increase with pain, but the only alteration in pain perception supported in the literature was to heat stimulation (nociception in superficial tissues). This change predisposes older adults to bruising, injury, and burns.

BARRIERS TO EFFECTIVE PAIN MANAGEMENT IN OLDER ADULTS

Seeking pain treatment is a barrier for older adults. Supporting the findings of Niederstrasser and Atridge (2022), Makris et al (2015) found negative attitudes toward pain treatment, especially in terms of perceived lack of efficacy and concerns over adverse side effects, as well as addiction, the belief in the inevitability of pain in old age, and reports of pain perceived as of lower importance compared to other comorbidities may explain why older adults are reluctant to seek pain treatment. Up to 75% of older adults experience persistent pain due to chronic conditions (Molten and Terrill, 2014). Many barriers impede the assessment and management of pain in older adults. Some of these barriers are related to nursing care, some are related to efforts on the part of the prescriber, and some are related to the older adult and their beliefs about pain and aging. Although not considered a normal part of aging, many health-care professionals, as well as older patients and their family members, continue to believe that pain is a natural occurrence of aging and chronic disease. This belief may lead to underreporting of pain and may prevent accurate pain assessment and appropriate use of pain-relief measures. Effective treatment of pain (acute or chronic) is essential for this population, as unrelieved pain may lead to altered immune function, functional decline, postoperative complications, CI, depression, and sleep disturbance (Horgas, 2017) (Fig. 11.1).

Accurate assessment and pain management are also inhibited when older patients underreport their pain. Older patients may underreport pain because they believe that stoicism and refusal to "give in" to the pain are appropriate behaviors or attitudes. Pain assessment may also be hindered by older patients who do not report pain because they "don't want to bother anyone," or they believe their report of pain will not be believed.

Older adults with cancer may fear the meaning of pain and its implications of worsening disease and possible death. Patients experiencing cancer-related pain may believe that this is a natural outcome of cancer and cannot be relieved. These

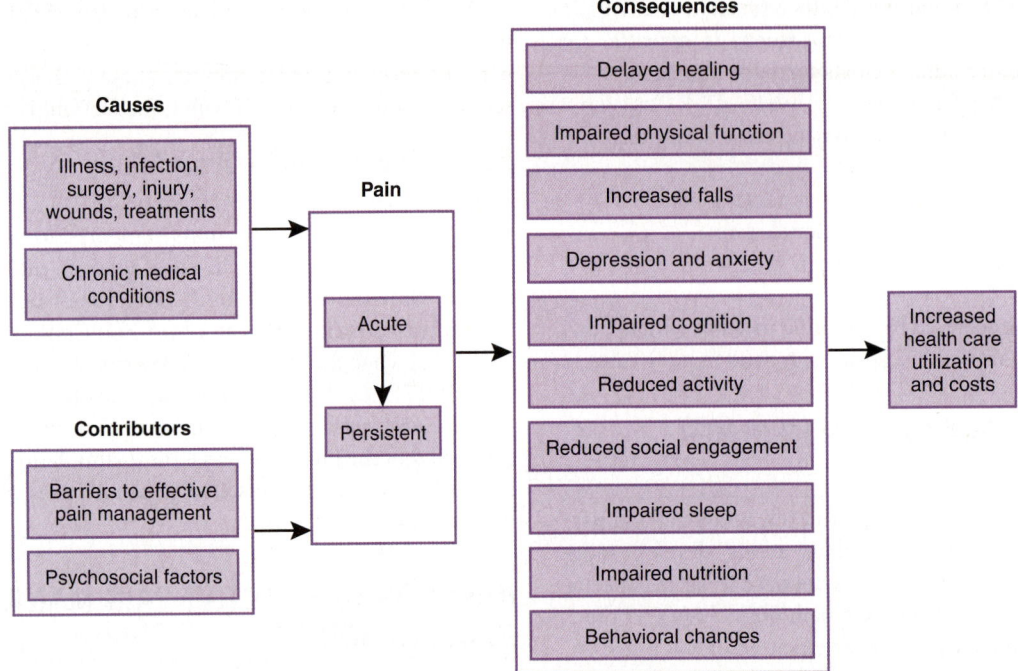

Fig. 11.1 Conceptual model of the causes and consequences of pain in older adults. (From Horgas, A. L. [2017]. Pain assessment in older adults. *Nursing Clinics of North America, 52*[3], 377).

patients and their family members needlessly suffer from the patients' experiences of pain. Inadequate access to diagnostic services is another barrier to appropriate pain assessment for older residents of nursing facilities and frail older adults in the community. Often, it is difficult to schedule appointments and arrange transportation so that a family member or health-care professional can accompany the patient to a diagnostic testing facility. Furthermore, many older adults do not have children who live near them and have lost their social networks (Robinson, 2010; Molten and Terrell, 2014).

The nurse's lack of knowledge regarding adequate pain assessment is also viewed as a barrier. Nurses should be knowledgeable of assessment techniques and how to adapt these techniques, as well as standardized tools to use when assessing an older adult's pain. When using any pain assessment tool, the nurse must evaluate each patient's ability to give accurate responses with that tool. A second tool may help confirm the value obtained with the first tool. The Hartford Institute for Geriatric Nursing (HIGN) (Flaherty, 2019) has found that commonly used pain assessment tools, such as the Faces Pain Scale-Revised (FPS-R), are valid and reliable for use with older adults, even those with mild-to-moderate CIs. The AGS (2009) found that the patient's self-report is the most accurate and reliable indicator of pain intensity and experience.

However, the compromised ability of people with moderate-to-severe dementia to report their pain clearly or consistently is challenging. Persons with dementia are consistently undermedicated. The Pain Assessment in Advanced Dementia (PAINAD) scale developed by Warden et al (2003) is a simple, valid, and reliable tool for assessing pain in people with dementia in both community and hospital settings (Gabrick, 2016) (Table 11.1).

PAINAD assesses the person with dementia in the following categories on a 0 to 10 scale:
1. Breathing
2. Negative vocalization
3. Facial expression
4. Body language
5. Consolability

Additionally, the person with dementia should be asked if they have pain, and the nurse should ask the family if their family member's behavior is customary or changed. A behavior change could indicate pain (Horgas, 2017).

PATIENT / FAMILY TEACHING
Controlling Pain through a Team Approach

The best way to control pain is through a team approach involving the patient, the family, and the nurse and physician. In the long-term care (LTC) and LTC skilled areas, inclusion of the social worker and the Department of Therapy would be beneficial to the resident. In addition to a patient telling the others the extent of his or her pain, he or she should be asked the following:
- Where is your pain located?
- When did the pain start?
- Describe the pain. Is it sharp? Dull? Throbbing? Burning?
- Does the pain come and go, or is it constant?
- What makes the pain worse?
- What makes the pain better?
- What medications are you taking for pain?
- Are you using any other methods such as relaxation, a heating pad, or a cold pack to relieve your pain? Do they seem to help?

Always ask about the presence of pain when examining an older adult. Collaborate with patient / resident, family, and staff regarding probable atypical presentations of pain inclusive of changes in function or gait, increased confusion, new behavior of withdrawal, and new or increased agitation.

TABLE 11.1 Pain Assessment in Advanced Dementia (PAINAD)

Items	0	1	2	Score
Breathing (independent of vocalization)	Normal	Occasional labored breathing Short period of hyperventilation	Noisy labored breathing Long period of hyperventilation Cheyne-Stokes respirations	
Negative vocalization	None	Occasional moan or groan Low level of speech with a negative or disapproving quality	Repeated troubled calling out Loud moaning or groaning Crying	
Facial expression	Smiling or inexpressive	Sad, frightened, frown	Facial grimacing	
Body language	Relaxed	Tense Distressed pacing Fidgeting	Rigid Fists clenched Knees pulled up Pulling or pushing away Striking out	
Consolability	No need to console	Distracted or reassured by voice or touch	Unable to console, distract, or reassure	
TOTAL				

From Warden, V., Hurley, A. C., Volicer, L. (2003). Development and psychometric evaluation of the Pain Assessment in Advanced Dementia (PAINAD) scale. *Journal of the American Medical Directors Association, 4*(1), 9–15.

PAIN ASSESSMENT

Pain assessment begins when the nurse accepts the person's report of pain and takes that report seriously. Assessment is essential in differentiating acute life-threatening pain from long-standing chronic pain (Herr et al, 2010). Otherwise, disease progression and acute injury may go unrecognized and be attributed to preexisting disease or illness. Table 11.2 identifies components of the clinical assessment of pain in older adults.

Pain assessment should include a thorough history and a physical examination. These assessments are especially important for older adults because effective pain management often treats underlying disease or illness appropriately. Multidisciplinary consultation is indicated when the underlying disease is unknown (AGS, 2009; Linton and Lach, 2007).

The following are general principles on pain assessment from the AGS Panel on Persistent Pain in Older Persons (AGS, 2009):

- No biologic markers for the presence of pain exist.
- The patient's report is the most accurate and reliable evidence of pain and its intensity.
- Patients with mild-to-moderate CI may be assessed using simple questions and screening tools.
- Older adults may be reluctant to report pain despite substantial impairments.
- Older adults may expect pain with aging.
- Older adults may use words like *discomfort, aching,* and *hurting* rather than *pain.*
- Older adults may see pain as a metaphor for serious disease or death.
- Older adults may feel pain represents "God's will" or atonement for "bad" deeds.
- Assess patients for evidence of chronic pain.
- Recognize pain significantly affecting functional ability or QoL as a significant problem.
- For patients with cognitive or language impairments, observe nonverbal pain behaviors, recent functional changes, and vocalizations (e.g., groans and cries).
- For patients with cognitive or language impairments, seek caregiver reports and input. Seek specialist consultation for patients with debilitating psychiatric problems, substance abuse problems, or intractable pain.
- Monitor patients with chronic pain by recording pain intensity, medication use, response, and associated activities in a pain log or diary.
- Reassess all patients with chronic pain regularly for improvement, deterioration, positive or negative effects of medications, and complications of treatment. Use the same pain instruments at each patient visit.

Pain Assessment and Culture

Pain is an individual experience. A patient's pain intensity and distress are related to cultural factors, past pain experiences, individual attributes, and pain threshold. Nurses must take an individual approach with each patient, incorporating his or her cultural beliefs and practices when assessing and managing pain. It is vitally important our pain assessments are culturally sensitive and that pain management is provided in a culturally competent manner. The U.S. Census Bureau reports that the racial and ethnic composition of the U.S. is rapidly changing. Between 2010 and 2019, the White population decreased by 8.6%, populations identifying as either Latino or Hispanic grew by 18.5%, Black or African American population increased by more than 88%, and Asian American populations grew by 6%; American Indian and Alaskan native populations grew by 27% and 160%,

TABLE 11.2 Assessment of Pain in Older Adults

History	Physical Examination	Assessment of Other Variables
Medical History Acute illnesses Chronic illnesses Previous surgeries Timed events leading to present pain complaint	**Routine Examination**	**Pertinent Laboratory Data and Tests** Depression Scales Beck Depression Inventory (BDI) Zung Self-Rating Depression Scale (SDS) Geriatric Depression Scale (GDS)

	Musculoskeletal Examination
	Neuromuscular:
	  weakness
	  hyperalgesia
	  numbness
		Cognitive Assessment
		Mini-Mental State Examination (MMSE)
		Short Portable Mental Status Questionnaire (SPMSQ)
		Philadelphia Geriatric Center Morale Scale (PGCMS)

Pain History Intensity Character Frequency Pattern Location Precipitating factors Relieving factors Alleviating factors	**Signs of Trauma** Bruises Inflammation Tenderness Guarding Swelling	**Functional Assessment** Katz Activities of Daily Living (ADL) Lawton Instrumental Activities of Daily Living (IADL) Stanford Health Assessment Questionnaire (HAQ) Barthel Index of ADL Fulmer SPICES Assessment
History of Trauma Recent falls Other injuries	**Functional Performance** Range of motion (ROM) Timed Up-and-Go (TUG) Test Tinetti Gait and Balance Test	**Psychosocial Assessment** Finances Social networks Dysfunctional relationships
Medication History Prescription Over-the-counter Herbal or natural Side effects		**Pain Assessment Scales** Visual analog scale Word descriptor scale Numeric scale Faces scale
Pain Medications Drugs that worked Drugs that did not work Prescription or over-the-counter Natural remedies Side effects		**QoL Measures** Dartmouth Primary Care Cooperative Information Project (COOP Project) Profile of Mood States (POMS) Pain / Quality of Life Scale (QOLS)
Previous Pain Experiences		

From American Geriatrics Society. (2002). The management of persistent pain in older persons. *Journal of the American Geriatrics Society, 50*(6), S205–S224.

respectively (Jones et al, 2021). Cultural aspects of pain management affect the provider, the nurse, and the patient as they all are met with the challenges of assessment and management of pain while trying to understand language and communication nuances. The Agency for Healthcare Research and Quality (AHRQ) (2020) has developed a toolkit to help health-care providers understand their patients' health beliefs and customs (Box 11.2).

The experience of pain is influenced by "personal values, cultural traditions, physiologic injury, disease, and life stage" (Booker et al, 2022, p. 48). Cultural beliefs and pain-coping strategies include praying, catastrophizing and dramatization, distraction, reinterpreting pain and its intensity, ignoring, seeking support, and using physical activity or work to cope (Orhan et al, 2018). It is important for us to be aware of cultural differences related to the management of pain and, at the same time, avoid stereotyping and if a patient will respond to pain in a certain way based on their cultural background (Narayan, 2010).

Health-care professionals should include educational materials on pain developed in collaboration with a specified cultural group. Health-care professionals must understand the difference between what is culturally sensitive versus what is linguistically appropriate. Culturally sensitive materials consider the subtle nuances of culture; they go beyond simple translation (Lasch, 2000). Additionally, the knowledge that collaboration is needed to understand differences in the ways pain is experienced and expressed by various cultures is needed from health-care professionals (Lovering, 2006).

"Respecting cultural norms promotes a feeling of being valued" (Narayan, 2010). One model that provides a collaborative way to

BOX 11.2 Learn From Patients

- **Respectfully ask patients** about their health beliefs and customs and note their responses in their medical records. Address patients' cultural values specifically in the context of their health care. For example:
  - "I would like to be respectful—what do you like to be called and what pronouns do you use?"
  - "Tell me about the things that are important to you. What should I know that would help us work together on your health?"
  - "Lots of people visit providers outside of the clinic. Who else do you visit about your health?"
  - "Tell me about the foods you eat at home so we can develop a plan together to help you reach your goal of losing weight."
  - "Your condition is very serious. Some people like to know everything that is going on with their illness, whereas others may want to know what is most important but not necessarily all the details. How much do you want to know? Is there anyone else you would like me to talk to about your condition? What do you call your problem? What do you think caused it? How do you think it should be treated?"
- Do not stereotype. Understand that each person is an individual and may or may not adhere to certain cultural beliefs or practices common in his or her culture. Do not make assumptions based on group affiliations or how people look or sound. Asking patients themselves is the best way to ensure you know how their culture may impact their care.

From Agency for Healthcare Research and Quality. (2020). *Health literacy universal precautions toolkit, 2nd edition*. Rockville, MD: AHRQ. Retrieved from https://www.ahrq.gov/health-literacy/improve/precautions/tool10.html.

educate the patient is the LEARN model (Ladha et al, 2018). Separated into its individual letters, this mnemonic represents:

Listen: Ask questions to help you understand why a certain practice is meaningful or important.
Explain: If a certain practice is harmful, explain why.
Acknowledge: Discuss differences and similarities between practices; be careful not to disparage cultural practices.
Recommend: Recommend a course of action that meets both your patient's needs and health-care standards.
Negotiate: Assess learning needs and provide effective education to reach a mutually agreeable plan of care.

Pain Assessment Tools

Pain assessment tools assist health-care professionals in objectively and accurately measuring a patient's report of pain and any relief or change in that pain. Pain assessment tools include the Functional Pain Scale (FPS), such as a 0 to 10 scale, where 0 means *no pain* and 5 means *intolerable* (Table 11.3); visual analog scales (VAS); descriptive pain intensity scales, using descriptions such as "no pain," "a little pain," "a lot of pain," and "too much pain"; pain diaries; and pain logs. An example of a pain diary is illustrated in Fig. 11.2.

A patient's report of pain should also be evaluated for its intensity and the amount of distress it causes. Pain intensity is a measure of the amount of pain that the patient is experiencing and is measured by a numeric rating scale (NRS), such as the 0 to 10 scale. The numeric pain rating scale translates the patient's report of pain into a number that provides the health-care professional with an objective description of the patient's pain. An NRS score ≥4 should trigger a comprehensive pain assessment

TABLE 11.3 Functional Pain Scale (FPS)

Score	Description of Pain by Patient Function
0	No pain
1	Tolerable (and does not prevent any activities)
2	Tolerable (but does prevent some activities)
3	Intolerable (but can use telephone, watch TV, or read)
4	Intolerable (cannot use telephone, watch TV, or read)
5	Intolerable (and unable to verbally communicate because of pain)

From Gloth, F. M., Scheve, A. A., Stober, C. V., Chow, S., & Prosser, J. (2001). The Functional Pain Scale (FPS): Reliability, validity, and responsiveness in a senior population. *Journal of the American Medical Directors Association, 2*(3), 110–114.

(Flaskerud, 2015). This measure of pain can then be used to gauge relief, given the assumption that the number is lower after treatment of the pain. These measures should be documented in the patient's chart.

A note of caution concerning the use of the NRS. Studies show using the NRS is ineffective, in isolation, to determine the need for analgesics, as anxiety, depression, and anger affect scores. Using multidimensional tools is more effective. The Overall Benefit of Analgesic Score (OBAS) is a reliable indicator of pain intensity, adverse effects of analgesia, and patient satisfaction with analgesia than the NRS (Box 11.3). Another reliable tool is the Clinically Aligned Pain Assessment Tool (CAPA). In studies, patients and nurses preferred the CAPA to the NRS (Table 11.4) (Scher et al, 2018).

History

The nurse should carefully question and thoroughly assess a patient's report of pain. This is especially important in older adults because of their tendency to have multiple sources of pain from different chronic problems simultaneously. Acute pain is often attributed to chronic illness; however, it should be evaluated with the knowledge that older adults often demonstrate an altered presentation of common acute illnesses, including "silent" myocardial infarctions and "painless" intraabdominal emergencies. Additionally, chronic pain is characterized by variable intensity and character and thus is often overlooked.

Linton and Lach (2007) suggested that questions should address the onset (acute or chronic), location (localized, referred, subcutaneous, or visceral), duration (constant or intermittent), intensity (have the older adult rate the pain on a standardized scale), characteristics (stabbing, shooting, sore, grinding, gnawing, achy, lightening, burning, etc), aggravating and alleviating factors, and self-treatment (use of heat, cold, immobilization, elevation, or medication) or other prescribed treatments that either helped or did not help. Various physical assessment books recommend using the mnemonic "P, Q, R, S, T, U" to assist in remembering how to ask questions regarding pain. The root word for the mnemonic may differ from text to text, but the meaning is similar: P = pattern of pain; Q = quality of pain; R = what relieves the pain; S = what stimulates the pain; T = timing, duration, and frequency of the pain; and U = what do you do that has worked and what have you not tried that was suggested or tried that did not work.

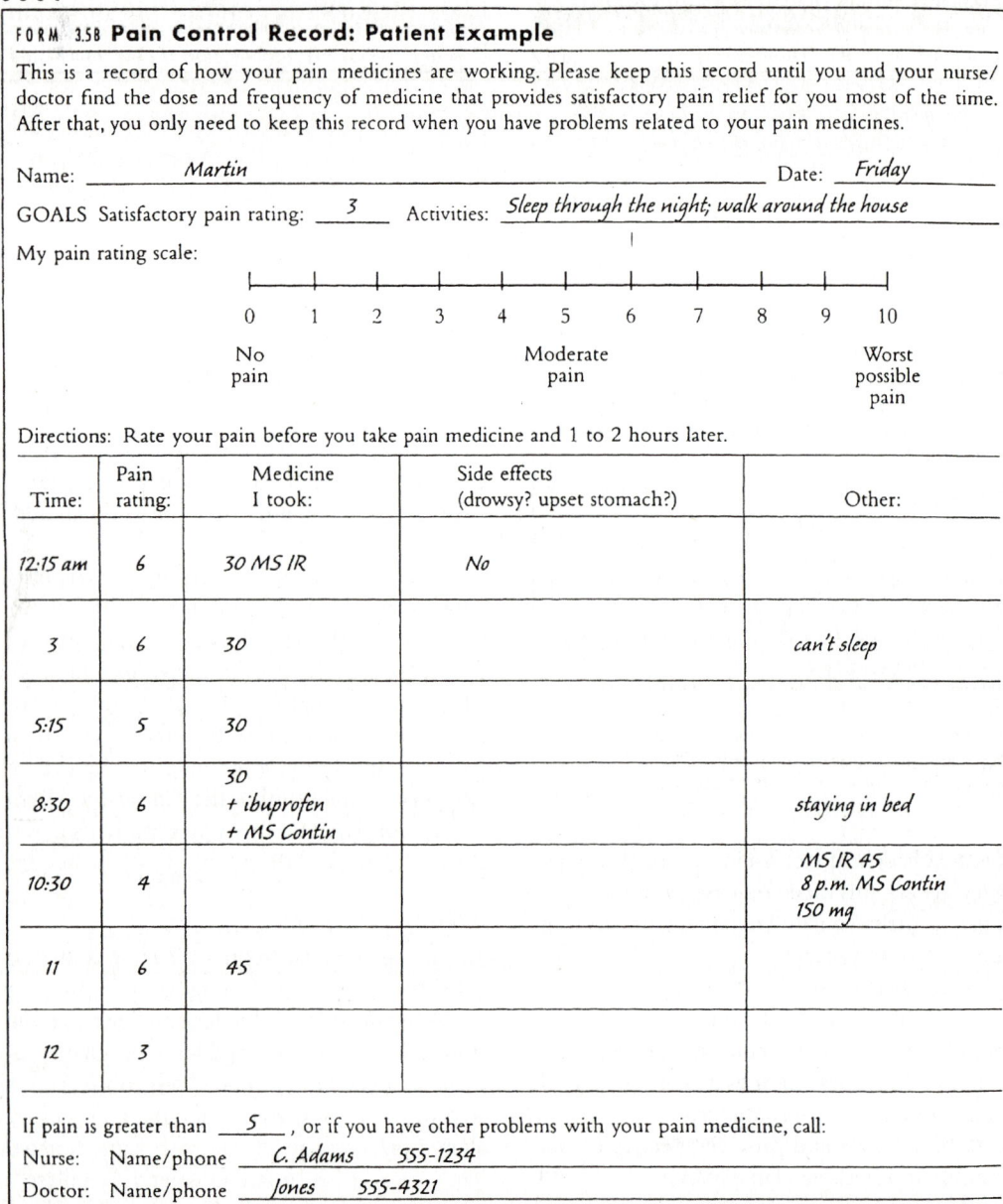

Fig. 11.2 Daily pain diary. (From McCaffery, M., & Pasero, C. [1999]. *Pain: Clinical manual* [2nd ed.]. St. Louis, MO: Mosby.)

Physical Examination

Pain assessment for older adults includes a comprehensive physical examination of body systems, as many older adults experience painful traumatic and degenerative problems. Additionally, a thorough neurologic assessment includes an evaluation for autonomic, sensory, or motor deficits; these may indicate neuropathic conditions or nerve injuries. Depression and cognitive screening should be included as well.

Evaluation for Functional Impairment

Impaired functional status is a major problem for older adults. An evaluation of an older adult's level of function is important so that mobility and independence can be maximized. Functional status evaluation includes assessing ADLs, ambulation, psychosocial well-being, and overall QoL. Standardized tools are available to assess functional status and have been proven effective with older adults. These include tools such as the Katz index

BOX 11.3 The Overall Benefit of Analgesic Score (OBAS)

1. Please rate your current pain at rest on a scale between 0=minimal pain and 4=maximum imaginable pain
2. Please grade any distress and bother from vomiting in the past 24 h (0=not at all to 4=very much)
3. Please grade any distress and bother from itching in the past 24 h (0=not at all to 4=very much)
4. Please grade any distress and bother from sweating in the past 24 h (0=not at all to 4=very much)
5. Please grade any distress and bother from freezing in the past 24 h (0=not at all to 4=very much)
6. Please grade any distress and bother from dizziness in the past 24 h (0=not at all to 4=very much)
7. How satisfied are you with your pain treatment during the past 24 h (0=not at all to 4=very much)

To calculate the OBAS score, compute the sum of scores in items 1–6 and add '4-score in item 7'. For example, a patient with minimal pain (NRS=0), severe vomiting (NRS=4), and no itching, sweating, and freezing who is slightly dizzy (NRS=1) and is not very satisfied with his postoperative pain treatment (NRS=1) has an OBAS of 8. Note that a low score indicates high benefit.

From Lehmann, N., Joshi, G.P., Dirkmann, D., Weiss, M., Gulur, P., Peters, J., et al. (2010). Development and longitudinal validation of the overall benefit of analgesia score: A simple multi-dimensional quality assessment instrument. *British Journal of Anaesthesia, 105*(4), 511–518.

TABLE 11.4 The Clinically Aligned Pain Assessment Tool (CAPA)

Question	Response
Comfort	Intolerable
	Tolerable with discomfort
	Comfortably manageable
	Negligible pain
Change in pain	Getting worse
	About the same
	Getting better
Pain control	Inadequate pain control
	Partially effective (effective, just about right)
	Fully effective (would like to reduce medication [why?])
Functioning	Can't do anything because of pain
	Pain keeps me from doing most of what I need to do
	Can do most things, but pain gets in the way of some
	Can do everything I need to do
Sleep	Awake with pain most of night
	Awake with occasional pain
	Normal sleep

Adapted with permission from Donaldson, G., & Chapman, C.R. (2013). Pain management is more than just a number. University of Utah Health/Department of Anesthesiology, Department of Anesthesiology, Salt Lake City, Utah.

of ADLs, the Lawton scale of IADLs (Ward and Reuben, 2022), and the Fulmer SPICES assessment (Wallace and Fulmer, 1998). The presence and intensity of pain may restrict functional activities. A functional evaluation includes assessing factors that contribute to or help alleviate pain. Functional status can be significantly improved through aggressive pain management. It is important to assess for new or different causes of pain; it should not be assumed that increased pain represents an exacerbation of a previous diagnosis. It is also imperative that the nurse assesses the older person for the cause of a complaint of pain and does not simply attribute it to age. Aging does not cause pain; disease and injury do.

Evaluation of QoL

Pain is not an isolated phenomenon; it is an experience that influences all dimensions of an individual's QoL. Pain assessment should include an evaluation of the effect of pain on a patient's QoL. Practitioners can quickly assess their patients' or residents' QoL by asking, "How is life for you?" "Are you doing and enjoying what you want to do and enjoy?" and "Has there been a recent change in your life activities?" Such questions may be as effective and accurate as more scientific tools that are impractical for daily practice.

Evaluation for Depression

Pain assessment of older adults also includes an evaluation for depression. A high incidence of depression is associated with chronic pain. Persistent depression affects a person's ability to cope with the pain, so it must be treated. Anxiety may also affect the management of chronic pain, especially if the outcome of the chronic problem is uncertain. The Geriatric Depression Scale (GDS) is a valid and reliable tool that can be used to screen for depression in an older adult.

NURSING CARE GUIDELINES FOR OLDER ADULTS WITH PAIN

Pharmacologic Treatment

As the administrators of drugs, nurses play a major role in ensuring that older adults have their pain treated safely, effectively, and efficiently. Nurses must be knowledgeable about the physiologic changes of aging that may alter drug absorption, metabolism, and excretion in older adults. Changes that require ongoing assessment of a patient's response to a drug, with subsequent adjustments in dose and dosing intervals or prescribed drug, are as follows:

- Changes in physiologic factors, such as decreased gastric acid production and gastrointestinal (GI) motility
- Changes in body composition, such as decreased total body water, lean body mass, and serum protein and increased body fat
- Changes in organ function, such as decreased hepatic blood flow and reduced glomerular filtration rate (GFR)

These changes, especially those in liver and renal function, may increase the risk for accumulation of lipid-soluble drugs such as fentanyl and may slightly delay the onset of action and increase the risk for accumulating agents used to control pain (AGS, 2009). Age-related changes in absorption, distribution, metabolism, and elimination demand that prescribers be conservative, especially as recommendations for age-adjusted doses are rarely available for most analgesics (AGS, 2009).

Analgesic drugs may be classified into 2 categories: nonopioid and opioid. Additionally, many adjuvant drugs are useful in the management of pain in older adults.

The World Health Organization (WHO) developed its original 3-step analgesic ladder in 1986. The original ladder was unidirectional, moving from nonsteroidal antiinflammatory drugs (NSAIDs) and ending with strong opioids. The new, 4-step approach (Fig. 11.3) includes recommendations for treating persistent pain, with or without the combination of opioids, and includes interventional and minimally invasive procedures. The new approach is intended to be bidirectional, allowing for de-escalation when pain is resolved (Anekar and Cascella, 2022). The WHO analgesic ladder helps guide nurses' decisions when determining how to medicate an older adult in pain after completing a pain assessment. Guidelines state that pain medications should be given around the clock to anticipate the patient's pain rather than waiting for the patient to ask for it.

Nonopioid Analgesics

Analgesics are used as a first-line approach to pain management. Acetaminophen, ibuprofen, and naproxen are examples of nonopioid analgesics. These drugs block pain by inhibiting pain reception at the local level. As with all medications, their use by older adults must be continuously monitored. Acetaminophen seems well tolerated by older adults and does not affect platelet function. It is the drug of choice for relieving mild-to-moderate musculoskeletal pain (AGS, 2009). The maximum dosage of all consumed acetaminophen is 3000 milligrams (mg) in 24 hours unless under the care of a health-care provider. Acetaminophen has few side effects and is probably the safest nonopioid for most people. Acetaminophen is as effective as aspirin in its analgesic and antipyretic properties but less effective than aspirin in its anti-inflammatory properties. Although acetaminophen has not been associated with renal or gastric problems, it may result in hepatic toxicity in patients with a history of alcohol abuse or after the ingestion of persistently high doses. Older adults should be cautioned to be aware of "hidden" acetaminophen in over-the-counter products such as cold remedies or sleep aids.

NSAIDs are especially effective for treating mild-to-moderate arthritic pain and other inflammatory disorders. NSAIDs have been associated with a variety of adverse side effects in older adults, including stomach ulcers, renal insufficiency, and a tendency to bleed. The most common complaint associated with NSAIDs is indigestion. Indigestion may be reduced with antacid use or food consumption timed to coincide with analgesic intake. However, health-care professionals must remember that GI irritation may occur without symptoms. Severe ulceration may result in perforation and extensive bleeding. The older adult's response to the medication must be evaluated closely. NSAIDs should be avoided in high doses, for long periods, in patients with abnormal renal function, and in patients with a history of ulcer disease or bleeding (AGS, 2009).

Opioid Analgesics

Opioids are usually prescribed for patients with mild-to-moderate pain that is poorly tolerated or cannot be adequately managed with a nonopioid analgesic. Clinical experience suggests that older adults are particularly sensitive to the effects of opioid analgesics because they experience a higher peak and longer duration of pain relief (AGS, 2009).

Because older adults may be more sensitive to opioids, clinicians should follow the advice to "Start low and go slow" and monitor patients until the drug is titrated for adequate pain relief. Problems with opioids usually involve those with long half-lives, such as methadone or levorphanol. The half-life of an opioid is defined as the time it takes for the drug to decrease to half its initial plasma concentration. Plasma levels of drugs that have long half-lives rise slowly over several days after the initiation of a dosing schedule. Thus, the risk for delayed toxicity is much greater with

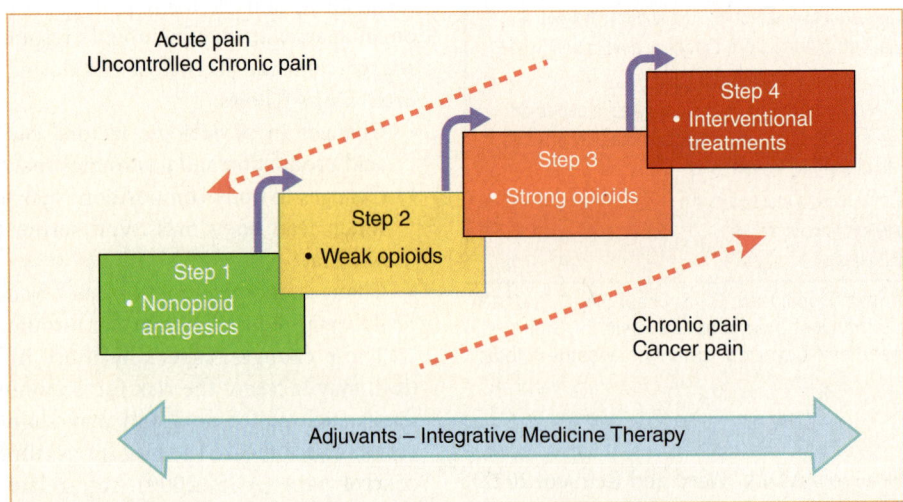

Fig. 11.3 A depiction of the revised WHO's pain-relief ladder. In addition to providing a bidirectional approach, the additional "interventional" step 4 includes invasive and minimally invasive treatments. (Redrawn from Mestdagh, F., Steyaert, A., & Lavand'homme, P. [2023]. Cancer pain management: A narrative review of current concepts, strategies, and techniques. *Current Oncology, 30*[7], 6838-6858.)

these drugs than with drugs having shorter half-lives. Codeine, hydromorphone, and morphine, in appropriate doses, can be used safely in older adults with pain (see Nursing Care Plan box).

Moderate-to-severe pain may be relieved with opioids such as hydrocodone, oxycodone, hydromorphone, oxymorphone, or immediate-release morphine.

NURSING CARE PLAN
Prostate Cancer with Bone Metastases

Clinical Situation

Mr. K is a 77-year-old retired telephone company executive who has been admitted to the local hospital-based home-care program. Mr. K had always been in good health until diagnosed with prostate cancer 2 years ago. He and his wife have enjoyed an active social life. His 4 adult children live in cities throughout the United States. The couple does not have any church affiliation. Mr. and Mrs. K have been married for 10 years and live in a mobile-home park in the desert. They also own a condominium in the city but do not have any resources for support in that neighborhood. Three (3) years ago, they acquired a puppy named Max. Up until the last 2½ months, Mr. K had taken morning and evening walks with Max throughout the neighborhood and local park.

In the last 2 months, Mr. K has noted a great deal of pain in his legs and back. He has lost 35 pounds in the past month. He tires easily and is unable to walk outside his home or for distances longer than 25 feet without resting. Mr. K's first wife died 20 years ago from breast cancer. Mr. K relates how she suffered intensely from the effects of chemotherapy and severe pain. He had refused all treatment for his cancer until 6 months ago, when he started receiving hormone therapy. He has refused to take the long-acting opioid prescribed by his physician because he does not want "to get hooked." Mr. K rates his pain as a 9 on a scale of 0 to 10, with 0 meaning *no pain* and 10 meaning *the worst pain*. Mrs. K is having difficulty caring for him and dealing with his impending death.

Analyze Cues and Prioritize Hypotheses (Patient Problems)
- Need for health teaching from inadequate knowledge of pain management
- Self-care deficit from inadequate control of pain and decrease in ADLs
- Potential for injury resulting from reduced mobility resulting from pain

Generate Solutions (Planning)
- The patient will report 2 ways to control pain with a level of 3 or below at rest and with activity, as evidenced by self-report.
- The patient will control pain to participate in ADLs.
- The patient will maintain ADLs and other physical activities, as able.

Take Actions (Nursing Interventions)
- Discuss general pain content information with the patient and caregivers.
- Elicit the patient's description of his pain, including the quality of the pain, its location, and its precipitating and relieving factors.
- Identify the intensity of the patient's pain by using a pain assessment tool.
- Identify the distress the patient experiences in relation to his pain.
- Evaluate the patient's current use of pharmacologic and nonpharmacologic pain relief methods.
- Discuss the patient's fear of addiction and the need to maintain control of his life and remain alert and functional.
- Implement the use of a self-care pain management log, including the use of a pain rating scale.
- Instruct the patient and his wife about around-the-clock scheduling for analgesics.
- Discuss the current pain management regimen and plans for further treatment with the patient's physician
- Identify the patient's current fecal elimination pattern.
- Explain the physician's prescription for a stool softener.
- Discuss the use of a mild laxative if bowel movement has not occurred after 2 days.
- Encourage a fluid intake of at least 8 glasses of water each day.
- Modify the patient's diet to increase his intake of high-fiber foods.
- Discuss the effect of analgesics on fecal elimination with the patient.
- Reinforce the fact that although constipation is an expected side effect of opioids, it can be prevented
- Instruct the patient to take analgesic medications on a regular basis
- Identify activities important to the patient that he would like to maintain.
- Encourage him to take short walks with his dog and sit in the dining room for his meals.
- Encourage use of a self-care log.
- Instruct the patient about energy conservation and about the need to space activities with periods of rest.
- Evaluate the environment to determine the need for equipment for ambulation or other activities.

Side effects. Common side effects of opioids include nausea, vomiting, constipation, and urinary retention, especially in individuals with prostatic hypertrophy. Older adults are more sensitive to sedation and respiratory depression, probably because of altered distribution and excretion of medications. This is especially true in opioid-naïve patients, that is, those who have not had earlier exposure to opioids. Fentanyl patches should never be given to patients who are opioid-naïve because of the high risk for severe adverse reactions. If oral opioids are not successful and higher doses have been tried without success, a smaller dose of fentanyl may be tried with upward titrations until the correct level is found. Most nurses will never be involved in this titration determination but may be involved in assessing the pain response after the provider makes an increase.

Constipation as a side effect of opioid use is of particular concern in older patients because many of them have preexisting bowel conditions. It is good practice to start a patient on a bowel program when initiating opioid treatment (see Patient / Family Teaching box). Careful assessment of bowel habits, including the use of stool softeners and laxatives and the dietary intake of high-fiber foods, is essential when a patient is using opioids. The health-care professional must emphasize to the patient and his or her family the importance of being proactive, preventing constipation rather than waiting for it to occur. To deal with the side effects of constipation, the Oncology Nursing Society (ONS) recommends the following (Becze, 2020).

- Hydration
- Modify diet; add high-fiber foods (see Nutritional Considerations box)
- Maintain or increase activity levels
- Use of prophylaxis medications

PATIENT / FAMILY TEACHING
What Can You Do for Constipation?

Opioid analgesics cause constipation in most people. The following suggestions help prevent constipation from becoming a problem and causing discomfort:
- Eat foods high in fiber, for example, uncooked fruits and vegetables, and whole grain breads and cereals.
- Add 1 or 2 tablespoons of unprocessed bran to foods.
- Drink plenty of liquids—8 to 10 glasses per day.
- Eat foods that have helped relieve constipation in the past.
- Plan your bowel movement for the same time each day, if possible.
- Try to use the toilet or bedside commode for fecal elimination.
- Have a hot drink about 30 minutes before the planned time for a bowel movement.
- Consult with a physician about using a bulk laxative such as psyllium (Metamucil) or any other laxative or stool softener.

Modified from American Cancer Society and National Cancer Institute. (2019). *Cancer pain control: Support for people with cancer.* Retrieved from https://www.cancer.gov/publications/patient-education/pain-control. Accessed September 21, 2022.

NUTRITIONAL CONSIDERATIONS
High-Fiber Foods to Relieve Constipation

- Oatmeal, bran, whole wheat, rye
- Apples, pears, strawberries, peaches, plums, citrus
- Beans, dry beans
- Peas, cabbage, root vegetables, fresh tomatoes, green beans, carrots

Although nausea and vomiting caused by opioid use usually disappear after a few days of taking the medication, clinicians must take a preventive approach to treat these side effects. As with all medications, antiemetics must be evaluated for their effectiveness in controlling nausea and vomiting in older adults, as well as for side effects such as sedation. The nurse should advise patients and family members that sedation may occur because of the antiemetic. If nausea persists beyond a few days of starting the opioid, a new opioid should be tried (AGS, 2009).

Sedation and impaired cognitive performance should be anticipated when starting opioids (AGS, 2009). The sedation usually decreases in 1 to 3 days. If it does not, the patient must be informed orally and in writing that the health-care provider should be notified. Sedation may also be related to sleep deprivation resulting from unrelieved pain. A fact that must be stressed is that sedation may occur without adequate pain relief. This type of rest does not result in the expected rejuvenation offered by sleep. Nurses should monitor for respiratory depression (<8 breaths per minute or oxygen saturation of <90% [AGS, 2009]), especially during rapid, high-dose escalations. Table 11.5 identifies analgesics that should be avoided in older adults.

Adjuvant Medications

Adjuvant medications, defined as drugs without intrinsic analgesic properties, help treat certain types of chronic pain. Adjuvant drugs include anticonvulsants, antidepressants, and some sedatives. The treatment of underlying depression or mood disorders may enhance other pain management strategies.

Anticonvulsants, drugs usually used to treat seizures, are often helpful in controlling painful conditions such as postherpetic neuralgia, diabetic neuropathy, and phantom limb pain. An anticonvulsant useful in the treatment of older adult patients that has few side effects is gabapentin. Medications in this category include zonisamide, tiagabine, pregabalin, and milnacipran. Anticonvulsants may cause blood dyscrasias; therefore, laboratory data must be obtained on a regular basis. For older adults, some sedatives or tranquilizers may cause side effects such as increased confusion and constipation. The use of these drugs in older adults must be continuously monitored. Tricyclic antidepressants (TCAs) are useful in treating neuropathic pain but do not seem to be effective in the case of musculoskeletal pain; higher doses are needed for therapy superimposed on cancer pain. Desipramine hydrochloride seems to be better tolerated by older adults, with fewer anticholinergic side effects compared with certain other drugs, such as amitriptyline. However, TCAs may cause constipation, blurred vision, dry mouth, urinary retention, and sedation; those with glaucoma and benign prostatic hypertrophy should avoid them. TCAs have been known to cause arrhythmias, cognitive changes, orthostatic hypotension, and falls. Selective serotonin reuptake inhibitors (SSRIs) seem to have relatively low side-effect profiles. Newer combination drugs of selective norepinephrine reuptake inhibitors (SNRIs) and SSRIs are helping to achieve better results in additional pain relief and antidepressant effects. These drugs appear to block pain transmission pathways (AGS, 2009).

Adjuvant drugs alter or modulate the perception of pain. They may be used alone or with other pain drugs (Portenoy et al, 2022). The nurse must notify patients and their family members when these adjuvant drugs are used to treat the patient's pain. Clinical experience has shown that a patient may

TABLE 11.5 Opioids to Avoid in Pain Management of Older Adults

Drug	Precautions	Potential Solutions
Meperidine	Metabolite (normeperidine) may accumulate and cause confusion, agitation, and seizure activity, especially among patients with renal impairment.	No advantages to either oral or parenteral meperidine exist over other opioid drugs.
Pentazocine	Mixed opioid agonist or antagonist activity often leads to central nervous system excitement, confusion, and hallucinations.	Avoid all use in frail older adults.
Levorphanol	The optimal analgesic dose varies widely among patients. Doses should be titrated to treat pain or for prevention. Use with caution in patients with hypersensitivity reactions to morphine, hydrocodone, hydromorphone, oxycodone, or oxymorphone.	For use in relief of moderate-to-severe pain.

Modified from American Geriatrics Society. (2015). American Geriatrics Society 2015 Updated Beers Criteria for Potentially Inappropriate Medication Use in Older Adults. *Journal of the American Geriatrics Society, 63,* 2227–2246.

discontinue the analgesic when an adjuvant drug is added. The patient / resident may also take an adjuvant drug, such as an antidepressant, without realizing that it is being used in conjunction with the analgesic to treat pain. As with all analgesics, the nurse must continue to assess the patient / resident's reports of pain and the effectiveness and side effects of the adjuvant drug.

The combined use of pharmacologic and nonpharmacologic pain management therapies works well in older adults. Individually, most of the nondrug therapies work well only with mild pain. With moderate pain, drug therapy must complement the other therapies. Clinical experience suggests that many of these techniques are effective in individual cases. As with all treatment modalities, the individual response must be evaluated.

Complementary and Alternative Medicine

Complementary and alternative medicine (CAM) and *integrative medicine* are gaining new ground in health care. These terms, however, may be confusing and are often used interchangeably despite having different meanings. The National Center for Complementary and Alternative Medicine (NCCAM) suggests using the term to describe products and practices in addition to mainstream medical practices (http://nccam.nih.gov/health/whatiscam). These practices fall into 2 subgroups: (1) natural products and (2) mind and body practices. Natural products include herbals and botanicals, as well as vitamins and minerals. Capsicum is commonly used for pain control, particularly because it can be used as a cream and applied directly to painful areas. Mind and body practices include acupuncture, massage therapy, meditation, movement therapies, relaxation techniques, spinal manipulation, tai chi, healing touch, and yoga. Nurses should be aware of these alternative therapies and assess their use and effectiveness in their patients.

Heat and Cold

Heat is useful in decreasing pain and discomfort (see the Evidence-Based Practice box). It increases blood flow to the skin and superficial tissues, increases oxygen and nutrient delivery, and decreases joint stiffness by increasing the elasticity of muscles (Nazario, 2021). Hot-water bottles, heating pads, compresses, tub baths, soaks, and heat lamps can be used to deliver heat. Patients and caregivers must be cautious of thermal burns when using these items. Temperature and length of use are important to determine before use.

Cold reduces inflammation, edema, and pain, especially after an acute injury such as a fall. It may reduce muscle spasms not relieved by heat therapy (Nazario, 2021).

Visualization or Imagery

This is a state of pleasure and peace achieved by creating a vivid picture in one's mind. This picture might be the setting sun, a serene forest, or rolling waves of water. It might be recalled from the past or a new experience imagined. It transports the patient to another place and uses all five senses (Giacobbi et al, 2015).

Progressive Muscle Relaxation

Progressive muscle relaxation (PMR) involves tensing one muscle group at a time, in a specific order, followed by relaxation.

EVIDENCE-BASED PRACTICE

Warm Blankets to Reduce Pain Among Nursing Home Residents

Background
More than 80% of nursing-home residents are reported to experience pain and agitation. Additionally, alterations in thermal regulation experienced by the older adult contribute to discomfort. Best practices strategies in pain management include nonpharmacologic interventions as they have few adverse effects. The purpose of this quality improvement project was to determine (a) frequency of warmed blankets used for pain, agitation, or thermal discomfort; (b) changes in pain, agitation, mood, or as-needed (PRN) use of analgesics when a warmed blanket is used; and (c) changes in pain, agitation, PRN analgesic use over a 1-month period between those provided a warm blanket and those who did not.

Sample / Setting
Of the 141 eligible nursing-home residents in a skilled LTC facility, residents in the intervention group ($n = 34$) received a warm blanket for pain, agitation, or thermal discomfort.

Method
Warm blankets (from warmers set to 150°F) were placed over residents with pain, agitation, or thermal discomfort. The Revised FPS-R, PAINAD, and the Brief Agitation Rating Scale (BARS) and documentation in the electronic health record (EHR) were used to gather data.

Findings
Short-term significant decreases in pain and agitation were found after 20 minutes in 83% of residents treated when warm blankets were used. Long-term changes included fewer reports of pain ($P = .040$), severity of pain ($P = .009$) and use of analgesics ($P = .011$).

Implications
Limitations to this project include a small treatment group, and there was variability in the warmth of blankets by the time they were placed on residents, and in the amount of clothing worn by participants. However, data indicates using warm blankets show promise in a short-term reduction in pain and agitation, and thermal discomfort, and long-term reductions in pain, analgesic use. "Warmed blankets are a low-cost intervention with a high potential for bringing comfort to nursing home residents" (p. 530).

Data from Kovach, C.R., Putz, M., Guslek, B., & McInnes, R. (2019). Do warmed blankets change pain, agitation, mood or analgesic use among nursing home residents? *Pain Management Nursing, 20,* 526-531.

It is usually done lying down in a quiet, often darkened room. It can be accomplished with soft music in the background. Relaxation tapes can be found in many bookstores (Nazario, 2020). Patients should be instructed to do the following (Martin, 2021):

- While inhaling, contract 1 muscle group (for example, your upper thighs) for 5 to 10 seconds, then exhale and suddenly release the tension in that muscle group.
- Give yourself 10 to 20 seconds to relax, then move on to the next muscle group (for example, your buttocks).
- While releasing the tension, focus on the changes you feel when the muscle group is relaxed. Imagery may be helpful in conjunction with the release of tension, such as imagining that stressful feelings flow out of your body as you relax each muscle group.

- Gradually work your way up the body, contracting and relaxing muscle groups.

PMR has been used to treat headaches, cancer pain, high blood pressure, and gastric distress (Stöppler, 2022).

Distraction

Distraction can be almost anything that takes one's mind off of pain. It can include radio, television, videos, music, memories, humor, pet therapy, or projects such as games or puzzles. This is usually used with mild pain, but it can be used with pain medication.

Exercise

Exercise and physical therapy prevent stiffness, maintain function, relieve muscle spasms, and increase the sense of well-being. Patients and residents should obtain medical consultation before instituting physical therapy. Many patients and residents need pretreatment analgesic medication shortly before starting the regimen.

Peripheral Nerve Stimulation

Peripheral nerve stimulation (PNS) is a technique for managing chronic pain in which electrical leads are placed subcutaneously into the area of a person's pain. It may be used to treat a variety of painful conditions, such as neuropathic pain and migraines. Helm et al (2021) conducted a systematic review of the effectiveness and safety of PNS. They determined there is evidence of its effectiveness in treating refractory peripheral nerve injury, noting that roughly 50% of persons using PNS experienced sustained pain relief. The authors also determined some evidence to support the use of PNS for cluster headaches, but no studies have been conducted to determine its efficacy in OA. Adverse events (AEs) associated with the use of PNS are minor.

Music Therapy

Music therapy may be incorporated into many of the other therapies presented here. Furthermore, it has been used extensively in clinical practice with older adults, and research has demonstrated its therapeutic benefits on health and QoL (González-Ojea et al, 2022). The music should be appreciated by the patient and at a volume that the patient can control.

Hypnosis

Hypnosis incorporates cognitive modalities such as deep concentration, imagery, and breathing exercises. Hypnosis "involves relaxation, focused attention and targeted verbal suggestion to alter perceptual experience and behavior" (Thompson et al, 2019, p. 298). The effectiveness of hypnosis in the reduction of pain is supported by the literature (Thompson et al, 2019).

Education

Education is a cognitive therapy that involves teaching a patient about pain and the role of cognition in pain perception. The patient learns to track the pain and record episodes of pain and distress. The nurse helps the patient/resident interpret the thoughts that accompany pain. Relaxation is incorporated to divert attention from the pain of the body. The goal is to help a patient/resident develop some mastery over his or her pain.

Planning Pain Relief

The primary consideration when selecting pain relief methods is individualized planning. Patients vary greatly in their medication requirements, choices of nonpharmacologic interventions, and prior pain experiences. Patients should be involved in choosing pain management methods and should share responsibility for implementing pain relief measures. Active involvement of patients / residents and family caregivers is essential to successfully implementing pain management regimens. This applies to both pharmacologic and nonpharmacologic pain relief measures.

> **HOME CARE**
>
> 1. The nurse caring for homebound older adults should know the effects pain has on functional status and QoL.
> 2. The home-care nurse should evaluate a patient's / resident's pain at each home visit.
> 3. The nurse should assess factors that may influence effective pain control in homebound older adults (e.g., motor, cognitive, and functional impairments).
> 4. When using a pain assessment tool, a home-care nurse must evaluate a homebound older adult's ability to use the tool.
> 5. Caregivers are an important source of information to the nurse when he or she assesses homebound older adults with pain.
> 6. The nurse should instruct homebound older adults and their caregivers on adjunctive therapies that can be used with analgesics to enhance pain management.
> 7. The nurse should assess and identify barriers for homebound older adults and caregivers related to pain and its management.
> 8. The nurse should encourage around-the-clock pain management to provide optimal pain control.

SUMMARY

Pain continues to be underrecognized and undertreated in older adults despite dramatic increases in the knowledge of pain and pain management. Pain in patients in nursing facilities is a large problem. Older adults suffer many painful chronic illnesses such as arthritis and cancer. When conducting assessments, the practicing nurse must look for pain in older adult patients / residents and be alert for chronic diseases that may cause pain. Many excellent pharmacologic treatments for pain and many routes of administration are available today; thus, it is possible to individualize care for each patient. Although pharmacology is the main therapy for most chronic illnesses, many alternative and complementary therapies are available that will benefit the nurse's older adult patients / residents. For further information, see the list of websites at the end of this chapter.

KEY POINTS

- Pain often remains underrecognized and undertreated in older adults, mainly because of limited gerontological pain research. Therefore, nurses must have a special understanding and conduct an accurate and ongoing assessment of the needs of this population regarding pain.
- Goals for pain management in older adults include controlling chronic disease conditions that cause pain, maintaining mobility and functional status, promoting maximum independence, and improving QoL.
- Barriers to effective pain management in older adults include the misconception that intolerance to pain is age-related, underreporting of pain, lack of access to diagnostic services, cognitive and functional impairment, the inability to communicate pain effectively through pain behavior scales, fear of addiction, and inadequacies in pain education.
- Accurate and ongoing assessment and a thorough understanding of pain physiology are essential for effective pain management in older adults.
- The nurse's clinical assessment of older adults' pain includes many important components: medical history; pain history; history of trauma, medications, and previous pain experiences; physical examination; examination for signs of trauma; musculoskeletal system examination; assessment of range of motion; and assessment of functional impairments. A variety of tools and scales are available for these assessments.
- QoL assessment is a vital part of pain assessment in older adults. This assessment may include sleeping, ADL function, pain, social relationships, and other pertinent areas. Different areas will have different values based on an individual's preferences.
- Pharmacologic pain management includes the use of analgesics, opioid analgesics, and adjuvant drugs. Nonpharmacologic therapies include methods using cold or heat, relaxation or distraction, imagery, peripheral nerve stimulation, and hypnosis. For pain management to be effective, the nurse must continually assess a patient's / resident's response to pain when employing any of these methods.
- A standard assessment scale that differentiates between pain intensity and pain distress in older adult patients / residents is useful for nurses when planning successful pain interventions. Consistent use of this tool, coupled with accurate record keeping, helps promote effective pain management.
- Family members often play an integral role in the pain management of older adults. Family members may provide insight into older adult's pain experiences by offering the nurse information that the patients may not be willing or able to share accurately.

CLINICAL JUDGMENT EXERCISES

1. A 91-year-old female with a small bowel obstruction is admitted to the hospital from an LTC facility. She also has a history of dementia and is incoherent. Discuss how you would revise your assessment and evaluation techniques in managing her pain.

2. What criteria should you use to determine whether an older adult patient requires an adjustment in dose or dosing interval or a change in the drug prescribed for pain management?

REFERENCES

Administration for Community Living (ACL). (2022). *2021 profile of older Americans.* Washington, DC: US Department of Health and Human Services. Retrieved from https://acl.gov/aging-and-disability-in-america/data-and-research/profile-older-americans. Accessed January 9, 2023.

Agency for Healthcare Research and Quality (AHRQ). (2020). *Health literacy universal precautions toolkit, 3rd edition.* Rockville, MD: AHRQ. Retrieved from https://www.ahrq.gov/health-literacy/improve/precautions/tool10.html. Accessed February 6, 2023.

American Geriatrics Society (AGS). (2009). The management of persistent pain in older persons. *Journal of the American Geriatrics Society, 57*(8), 1331–1346. doi:10.1111/j.1532-5415.2009.02376.x.

Anekar, A. A., & Cascella, M. (2022). WHO analgesic ladder. In *StatPearls* [Internet]. Treasure Island, FL: StatPearls Publishing. Retrieved from https://www.ncbi.nlm.nih.gov/books/NBK554435/. Accessed January 9, 2023.

Arnstein, P., Herr, K. A., & Butcher, H. K. (2017). Evidence-based practice guideline: Persistent pain management in older adults. *Journal of Gerontological Nursing, 43*(7), 20–31. doi:10.3928/00989134-20170419-01.

Aronoff, G. M. (2002). Drawing the line between pain management and addiction. *Psychopharmacology Update, 12*(9), 1.

Becze, E. (2020). *Manage cancer treatment-related constipation with ONS Guidelines.* ONS.org [website]. Retrieved from https://voice.ons.org/news-and-views/manage-cancer-treatment-related-constipation-with-ons-guidelinestm. Accessed September 21, 2022.

Bishop, T. F., & Morrison, R. S. (2007). Geriatric palliative care—part 1: Pain and symptom management. *Clinical Geriatrics, 15*(1), 25–32.

Booker, S. Q., & Haedtke, C. (2016). Controlling pain and discomfort, part 1: Assessment in verbal older adults. *Nursing, 46*(2), 65–68. doi:10.1097/01.NURSE.0000473408.89671.52.

Booker, S. Q., Baker, T. A., Epps, F., Herr, K. A., Young, H. M., & Fishman, S. (2022). Interrupting biases in the experience and management of pain. *The American Journal of Nursing, 122*(9), 48–54. doi:10.1097/01.NAJ.0000874120.95373.40.

Dagnino, A. P. A., & Campos, M. M. (2022). Chronic pain in the elderly: Mechanisms and perspectives. *Frontiers in Human Neuroscience, 16*, 736688. doi:10.3389/fnhum.2022.736688.

Domenichiello, A. F., & Ramsden, C. E. (2019). The silent epidemic of chronic pain in older adults. *Progress in Neuropsychopharmacology & Biological Psychiatry, 93*, 284–290. doi:10.1016/j.pnpbp.2019.04.006.

Flaherty, E. (2019). *Pain assessment for older adults.* Hartford Institute for Geriatric Nursing General Assessment Series, issue 7. Retrieved from https://hign.org/consultgeri/try-this-series/pain-assessment-older-adults. Accessed September 21, 2022.

Flaskerud, J. H. (2015). Pain, culture, assessment, and management. *Issues in Mental Health Nursing, 36*(1), 74–77. doi:10.3109/01612840.2014.932873.

Gabrick, J. (2016). *PAINAD scale offers alternative to assessing pain in the dementia patient.* JEMS.com [website]. Retrieved from https://www.jems.com/patient-care/painad-scale-offers-alternative-to-assessing-pain-in-the-dementia-patient/. Accessed September 21, 2022.

Giacobbi, Jr., P. R., Stabler, M. E., Stewart, J., Jaeschke, A. M., Siebert, J. L., & Kelley, G. A. (2015). Guided imagery for arthritis and other rheumatic diseases: A systematic review of randomized controlled trials. *Pain Management Nursing, 16*(5), 792–803. doi:10.1016/j.pmn.2015.01.003.

González-Ojea, M. J., Domínguez-Lloria, S., & Pino-Juste, M. (2022). Can music therapy improve the quality of life of institutionalized elderly people? *Healthcare, 10*(2), 310. doi:10.3390/healthcare10020310.

Helm, S., Shirsat, N., Calodney, A., Abd-Elsayed, A., Kloth, D., Soin, A., et al. (2021). Peripheral nerve stimulation for chronic pain: A systematic review of effectiveness and safety. *Pain and Therapy, 10*(2), 985–1002. doi:10.1007/s40122-021-00306-4.

Herr, K., Bursch, H., Ersek, M., Miller, L. L., & Swafford, K. (2010). Use of pain-behavioral assessment tools in the nursing home: Expert consensus recommendations for practice. *Journal of Gerontological Nursing, 36*(3), 18–29. doi:10.3928/00989134-20100108-04.

Ho, L. Y. W. (2019). A concept analysis of coping with chronic pain in older adults. *Pain Management Nursing, 20*(6), 563–571. doi:10.1016/j.pmn.2019.03.002.

Horgas, A. L. (2017). Pain assessment in older adults. *The Nursing Clinics of North America, 52*(3), 375–385. doi:10.1016/j.cnur.2017.04.006.

Huether, S., & McCance, K. (2017). *Understanding pathophysiology* (6th ed.). St. Louis: Elsevier.

Hulla, R., Vanzzini, N., Salas, E., Bevers, K., Garner, T., & Gatchel, R. J. (2017). Pain management in the elderly. *Practical Pain Management, 17*(1), 24–32.

Jansen, M. P. (2008). Pain in older adults. In M. P. Jansen (Ed.), *Managing pain in the older adult* (pp. 3–16). New York: Springer.

Jones, N., Marks, R., Ramirez, R., & Ríos-Vargas, M. (2021). *2020 census illuminates racial and ethnic composition of the country.* United States Census Bureau. Retrieved from https://www.census.gov/library/stories/2021/08/improved-race-ethnicity-measures-reveal-united-states-population-much-more-multiracial.html. Accessed January 9, 2023.

Ladha, T., Zubairi, M., Hunter, A., Audcent, T., & Johnstone, J. (2018). Cross-cultural communication: Tools for working with families and children. *Paediatrics & Child Health, 23*(1), 66–69. doi:10.1093/pch/pxx126.

Lasch, K. E. (2000). Culture, pain, and culturally sensitive pain care. *Pain Management Nursing, 1*(3 Suppl. 1), 1–22. doi:10.1053/jpmn.2000.9761.

Lautenbacher, S., Peters, J. H., Heesen, M., Scheel, J., & Kunz, M. (2017). Age changes in pain perception: A systematic-review and meta-analysis of age effects on pain and tolerance thresholds. *Neuroscience and Biobehavioral Reviews, 75*, 104–113. doi:10.1016/j.neubiorev.2017.01.039.

Li, C. Y., Lin, W. C., Lu, C. Y., Chung, Y. S., & Cheng, Y. C. (2022). Prevalence of pain in community-dwelling older adults with hypertension in the United States. *Scientific Reports, 12*(1), 8387. doi:10.1038/s41598-022-12331-0.

Linton, A. D., & Lach, H. W. (2007). *Matteson & McConnell's gerontological nursing: Concepts and practice.* St. Louis: Elsevier.

Lovering, S. (2006). Cultural attitudes and beliefs about pain. *Journal of Transcultural Nursing, 17*(4), 389–395. doi:10.1177/1043659606291546.

Makris, U. E., Higashi, R. T., Marks, E. G., Fraenkel, L., Sale, J. E. M., Gill, T. M., et al. (2015). Ageism, negative attitudes, and competing co-morbidities—why older adults may not seek care for restricting back pain: A qualitative study. *BMC Geriatrics, 15*, 39. doi:10.1186/s12877-015-0042-z.

McCaffery, M. (1979). *Nursing management of the patient with pain* (2nd ed.). Philadelphia: Lippincott Williams & Wilkins.

McCaffery, M., & Pasero, C. (1999). *Pain: Clinical manual* (2nd ed.). St. Louis: Mosby.

McCleane, G. (2008). Pain perception in the elderly patient. *Clinics in Geriatric Medicine, 24*(2), 203–211. doi:10.1016/j.cger.2007.12.008.

Merskey, H., & Bogduk, N. (Eds.). (1994). *Classification of chronic pain* (2nd ed.). Seattle: IASP Press.

Molten, I. R., & Terrill, A. L. (2014). Overview of persistent pain in older adults. *The American Psychologist, 69*(2), 197–207. doi:10.1037/a0035794.

Martin, L. (2021). *What is progressive muscle relaxation (PMR)?* Medical News Today [website]. Retrieved from https://www.medicalnewstoday.com/articles/progressive-muscle-relaxation-pmr. Accessed October 7, 2024.

Narayan, M. C. (2010). Culture's effects on pain assessment and management. *The American Journal of Nursing, 110*(4), 38–47. doi:10.1097/01.NAJ.0000370157.33223.6d.

Nazario, B. (2021). *When should I use heat or ice for pain?* WebMD [website]. Retrieved from https://www.webmd.com/pain-management/when-use-heat-ice. Accessed September 21, 2022.

Niederstrasser, N. G., & Attridge, N. (2022). Associations between pain and physical activity among older adults. *PloS One, 17*(1), e0263356. doi:10.1371/journal.pone.0263356.

Orhan, C., Van Looveren, E., Cagnie, B., Mukhtar, N. B., Lenoir, D., & Meeus, M. (2018). Are pain beliefs, cognitions, and behaviors influenced by race, ethnicity, and culture in patients with chronic musculoskeletal pain: A systematic review. *Pain Physician, 21*(6), 541–558.

Otones Reyes, P., García Perea, E., & Pedraz Marcos, A. (2019). Chronic pain and frailty in community-dwelling older adults: A systematic review. *Pain Management Nursing, 20*(4), 309–315. doi:10.1016/j.pmn.2019.01.003.

Park, J., & Hughes, A. K. (2012). Nonpharmacological approaches to the management of chronic pain in community dwelling older adults: A review of empirical evidence. *Journal of the American Geriatrics Society, 60*(3), 555–568. doi:10.1111/j.1532-5415.2011.03846.x.

Portenoy, R. K., Ahmed, E., & Keilson, Y. Y. (2022). Cancer pain management: Role of adjuvant analgesics (coanalgesics). In J. Abrahm & S. Shah (Eds.), *UpToDate.* Waltham, MA: UpToDate, Inc. Retrieved from https://www.uptodate.com/contents/cancer-pain-management-role-of-adjuvant-analgesics-coanalgesics. Accessed January 9, 2023.

Raja, S. N., Carr, D. B., Cohen, M., Finnerup, N. B., Flor, H., Gibson, S., et al. (2020). The revised International Association for the Study of Pain definition of pain: Concepts, challenges, and compromises. *Pain, 161*(9), 1976–1982. doi:10.1097/j.pain.0000000000001939.

Reid, M. C., Bennett, D. A., Chen, W. G., Eldadah, B. A., Farrar, J. T., Ferrell, B., et al. (2011). Improving the pharmacologic management of pain in older adults: Identifying the research gaps and methods to address them. *Pain Medicine, 12*(9), 1336–1357. doi:10.1111/j.1526-4637.2011.01211.x.

Robinson, P. (2010). Pharmacological management of pain in older persons. *The Consultant Pharmacist, 25*(Suppl. A), 11–19.

Scher, C., Meador, L., Van Cleave, J. H., & Carrington Reid, M. (2018). Moving beyond pain as the fifth vital sign and patient satisfaction scores to improve pain care in the 21st century. *Pain Management Nursing, 19*(2), 125–129. doi:10.1016/j.pmn.2017.10.010.

Schofield, P. (2010). "It's your age": The assessment and management of pain in older adults. *Continuing Education in Anaesthesia, Critical Care & Pain, 10*(3), 93–95.

Schofield, P., & Gibson, S. (2021). *Pain in older adults.* International Association for the Study of Pain (IASP) [website]. Retrieved from https://www.iasp-pain.org/resources/fact-sheets/pain-in-older-adults/. Accessed September 21, 2022.

Scholz, J. (2019). Finally, a systematic classification of pain (the ICD-11). *Practical Pain Management, 19*(3). Retrieved from https://www.practicalpainmanagement.com/resources/clinical-practice-guidelines/finally-systematic-classification-pain-icd-11. Accessed February 6, 2023.

Schwan, J., Sclafani, J., & Tawfik, V. L. (2019). Chronic pain management in the elderly. *Anesthesiology Clinics, 37*(3), 547–560. doi:10.1016/j.anclin.2019.04.012.

Stöppler, M. C. (2022). *Progressive muscle relaxation for stress and insomnia.* WebMD [website]. Retrieved from https://www.webmd.com/sleep-disorders/muscle-relaxation-for-stress-insomnia. Accessed January 9, 2023.

The Joint Commission. (2018). *Pain assessment and management standards for nursing care centers.* R3 Report, Issue 21. Retrieved from https://www.jointcommission.org/-/media/tjc/documents/standards/r3-reports/r3_21_pain_standards_ncc_12_21_18_final.pdf. Accessed September 29, 2022.

Thompson, T., Terhune, D. B., Oram, C., Sharangparni, J., Rouf, R., Solmi, M., et al. (2019). The effectiveness of hypnosis for pain relief: A systematic review and meta-analysis of 85 controlled experimental trials. *Neuroscience and Biobehavioral Reviews, 99,* 298–310. doi:10.1016/j.neubiorev.2019.02.013.

Wallace, M., & Fulmer, T. (1998). Fulmer SPICES. An overall assessment tool of older adults. *Journal of Gerontological Nursing, 24*(12), 3. doi:10.3928/0098-9134-19981201-03.

Ward, K. T., & Reuben, D. B. (2022). Comprehensive geriatric assessment. In K. E. Schmader & J. Givens (Eds.), *UpToDate.* Waltham, MA: UpToDate, Inc. Retrieved from https://www.uptodate.com/contents/comprehensive-geriatric-assessment. Accessed January 9, 2023.

Warden, V., Hurley, A. C., & Volicer, L. (2003). Development and psychometric evaluation of the Pain Assessment in Advanced Dementia (PAINAD) scale. *Journal of the American Medical Directors Association, 4*(1), 9–15. doi:10.1097/01.JAM.0000043422.31640.F7.

Yezierski, R. P. (2012). The effects of age on pain sensitivity: Preclinical studies. *Pain Medicine, 13*(Suppl. 2), S27–S36. doi:10.1111/j.1526-4637.2011.01311.x.

WEBSITES

American Academy of Hospice and Palliative Medicine (AAHPM). http://aahpm.org.

American Academy of Pain Medicine (AAPM). http://www.painmed.org.

American Geriatrics Society (AGS). https://www.americangeriatrics.org.

American Pain Society (APS). https://painmed.org/american-pain-society/.

International Association for Hospice and Palliative Care (IAHPC). https://hospicecare.com/home/.

National Hospice and Palliative Care Organization (NHPCO). https://www.nhpco.org.

International Association for the Study of Pain (IASP). https://www.iasp-pain.org.

World Health Organization (WHO). http://www.who.int/en/.

12

Infection and Inflammation

Mary B. Winton, PhD, MSN, RN

http://evolve.elsevier.com/Yeager/gerontologic/

LEARNING OBJECTIVES

On completion of this chapter, the reader will be able to:
1. Describe aging-related alterations in the immune system.
2. Describe nutritional factors that influence immune status.
3. Describe psychosocial factors that influence immune status.
4. Describe the effect of lifestyle factors on immune status.
5. Describe the effect of drugs on immune status.
6. Identify strategies to prevent health-care-associated infections, community-acquired infections, or both.
7. Incorporate nutritional, psychosocial, and lifestyle factors into a nursing care plan.

WHAT WOULD YOU DO?

What would you do if you were faced with the following situations?
- After a review of facility weights, you determine your 72-year-old resident has lost more than 5% of their weight in the past 6 months. What effect does weight loss have on the older adult's immune system? Knowing this, what would you do?
- You are discharging your patient home and ask if they have had their influenza vaccine. They respond, "No, I don't get that anymore; it doesn't help anyway." How would you respond?

The immune system has two primary functions: (1) to discriminate between that which is self and that which is nonself and (2) to remove from the body that is recognized as nonself. This system comprises antibodies, cells, chemicals, proteins, lymphoid tissue, bone marrow, and the spleen (Huether et al, 2020). Furthermore, this system interacts with the neurologic and endocrine systems in a highly complex manner to modulate the human immune response. Psychological and behavioral factors may mediate immunologic function. Awareness of the effect of mood, activity-level, stress, and nutrition on the capacity of the immune system to provide optimal protection is increasing.

This chapter examines age-related changes in the immune system and the influence of other factors, such as psychosocial and nutritional status, on the immune status of older adults. Cancer, autoimmune diseases (ADs), human immunodeficiency virus (HIV), and significant health-care-associated pathogens are also discussed.

IMMUNOLOGIC THEORY

The immune system is a network of specialized cells, tissues, and organs that protect the body against invading organisms. Its primary role is to differentiate self from nonself, protecting the organism from attack by pathogens. As a person ages, the immune system becomes less effective. The term immunosenescence has been given to this age-related decrease in function (Berben et al, 2021).

Essential components of the immune system include the innate and adaptive immune systems. The innate system releases inflammatory chemicals in response to pathogens (Berben et al, 2021). With aging, the functions of neutrophils and monocytes are altered, decreasing immune function among the elderly. Decreases in the innate immune system may alter the adaptive immune system.

The adaptive immune system consists of T-lymphocytes, responsible for cell-mediated immunity, and B-lymphocytes, the antibodies responsible for humoral immunity (Berben et al, 2021). Both T- and B-lymphocytes may respond to an invasion of an organism, although one may provide more protection than the other, depending on the situation. The changes that occur with aging are most apparent in T-lymphocytes, although changes also occur in the functioning capabilities of B-lymphocytes. Accompanying these changes is a decrease in the body's defense against foreign pathogens; this manifests as an increased vulnerability to infectious diseases, a decreased effectiveness of vaccinations, the development of autoimmune disorders, and an increase in age-related inflammatory diseases (Aiello et al, 2019; Bulut et al, 2020; Oh et al, 2019).

The changes in the immune system cannot be explained by an exact cause-and-effect relationship, but they do seem to increase with advancing age. These changes include a decrease in the humoral immune response, often predisposing older adults to (1) decreased resistance to a tumor cell challenge and the development of cancer, (2) decreased ability to initiate the immune process and mobilize the body's defenses against aggressively attacking pathogens, and (3) heightened production of autoantigens, often leading to an increase in autoimmune-related diseases.

Immunodeficient conditions such as HIV infection and immune suppression in organ transplant recipients have demonstrated a relationship between immunocompetence and cancer development. HIV infection has been associated with the development of cancer (i.e., Kaposi sarcoma and Merkel cell carcinoma; D'Arcy et al, 2021; Engels, 2017). Recipients of organ transplants are five times more likely to develop cancer than the rest of the population (Furst, 2022).

AGE-RELATED CHANGES IN THE IMMUNE SYSTEM

Older adults are at an increased risk for infectious diseases and chronic inflammation because of age-related changes to the immune system (Haynes, 2020). The effectiveness of vaccinations is also decreased among older adults. Some researchers believe that much of the illness seen in older adults may directly result from changes in "both cell-mediated and antibody-mediated immune response" (Townsend, 2008). Scientists have tried to determine whether the diminished immunocompetence noted with advancing age results from decreased numbers of immune cells or merely decreased functioning of the cells. However, because immunocompetence is affected by numerous other factors, it has been difficult to isolate changes related to age alone. Atrophy of the thymus, which occurs naturally with aging, affects T-lymphocyte function. Diminished cellular (T-cell–mediated) and humoral (B-lymphocyte) immunity have been associated with aging. Box 12.1 summarizes age-related changes in the immune system (Haynes, 2020). Cell-mediated immunity is the ability of the host to differentiate between self and nonself. Diminished cell-mediated immunity in older adults is generally associated with diminished T-cell response. With aging, B-cells demonstrate reduced antibody response.

As age increases, so does the production of autoantibodies. This predisposes older adults to an increase in ADs. The mechanism underlying this issue is felt to be alteration in both T- and B-cell function (Agrawal et al, 2012). The skin is the largest immunologically active system of the body and the body's first line of defense. Normal microbial flora on the skin (e.g., *Propionibacterium acnes* and *Staphylococcus aureus*) prevent pathogenic bacteria from flourishing (Grice and Lambris, 2013). With aging, the skin becomes more fragile and prone to breakdown or abrasion, thus disrupting the defensive mechanisms and providing a portal of entry for bacteria.

FACTORS AFFECTING IMMUNOCOMPETENCE

Nutritional Factors

Nutritional and dietary status is of critical importance to immune function. This is especially true in the older adult population. Older adults are at high risk for nutritional deficits;

> **BOX 12.1 Age-Related Changes In the Immune System**
>
> **Innate Immune System**
> Increased cytokine production
> Decreased cellular production
> Decreased cellular phagocytic activity
> Decreased antigen-presenting cells
> Decreased bactericidal activity
>
> **Adaptive Immune System**
> Decreased total number of B-cells
> Decreased antibody production after vaccinations
> Increased number of T-helper cells
> Decreased number of suppressor T-cells
> Increased number of T-memory cells
> Increased number of T-regulatory cells
> Decreased T-cell responsiveness
> Decreased CD_4 and CD_8 cells
>
> **Lymphoid Tissue**
> Atrophy of the thymus gland
> Decreased thymus activity
> Atrophy or hypertrophy of some lymph nodes
>
> **Mechanical Barriers**
> Decreased effectiveness of physical barriers due to changes in skin and mucous membranes

at least one-third of individuals over 65 have nutritional deficiencies. Risks associated with developing a health-care-associated infection include poor nutrition, unintentional weight loss, low serum albumin (ALB) levels, decreased fluid intake, poor oral hygiene, and altered mental status. Factors contributing to this tendency toward inadequate nutrition include altered taste, social isolation, physical inability to prepare food, altered absorption, and poverty. Older adults should consult with their health-care providers and have a thorough assessment of their dietary intake done before beginning nutritional supplementation. When adequate amounts of vitamins and minerals are consumed in the diet, supplementation is unnecessary and may lead to toxicity.

Malnutrition

Significant deprivation of protein, calories, or other vitamins and minerals has resulted in altered immune function. Along with other age-related changes in the immune system, this deprivation increases susceptibility to infectious disease. Restoring nutritional balance can improve the immune status of older adults (Alam et al, 2019).

Iron and Trace Element Deficiency

The most common nutritional deficiency in older adults is iron. Iron is necessary for proper immune function (Alam et al, 2019). Iron deficiency increases morbidity and risks for infectious disease. Low iron levels also contribute to decreased functioning of neutrophils, macrophages, and B- and T-cells. Additionally, iron deficiency contributes to a delayed responsiveness to antigens.

Zinc affects many aspects of the immune system (Alam et al, 2019). A prolonged zinc deficiency leads to impaired cell-mediated immunity, wound healing, and protein synthesis (Lin et al, 2017). Patients with decreased zinc levels experience an increase in the number of infections and the needed healing time.

Psychosocial Factors

Awareness is growing of the potential effect of psychosocial factors on immune status. These factors include chronic and acute stress, depression, bereavement, and social relationships. Recognition that such factors influence immune status is relatively recent, and our understanding of the nature of these relationships is constantly changing. Therefore, the clinical relevance of these changes remains a source of investigation and controversy.

Older adults experience many psychosocial changes that potentially affect immune status and must be considered. Older adults work through bereavement as they lose family and friends. Additionally, they experience a shrinking sphere of social relationships and exhibit a high incidence of depression.

Depression

Depression has also been associated with decreased immune function. This is significant because approximately 13.5% of older adults requiring home healthcare and 11.5% who are hospitalized are diagnosed with major depression (CDC, 2022a). Furthermore, adults over 65 represent more than 16% of the population (Administration for Community Living, 2021). Some evidence suggests that the negative effect of depression on the immune system increases with age. Thus older adults who are depressed may be at risk for more immune deficiencies than younger individuals with depression.

Drugs

Various drugs may affect the immune system; these include immunosuppressants and immunoenhancers. Many drugs given for therapeutic purposes have an immunosuppressant effect. Some of these drugs include corticosteroids, cyclosporine, and chemotherapeutics for cancer. Corticosteroids such as prednisone are given for a variety of reasons, including treatment of autoimmune processes (e.g., rheumatoid arthritis [RA]). Individuals receiving corticosteroids, those taking cyclosporine after transplantation to reduce the risk for organ rejection, or individuals taking anticancer drugs have an altered immune response and are at higher risk for infection.

Complementary and Alternative Medications

Some individuals take complementary and alternative medications (CAMs) to bolster their immune system (e.g., *Echinacea*, garlic, ginger, St. John's wort). However, CAM products are not thoroughly tested and vary significantly based on growing conditions and harvesting methods. Additionally, some CAMs are harmful and may negatively affect the immune system (e.g., *Bupleurum*, glucosamine, red yeast rice, and cascara sagrada) or interact with prescription drugs. Patients should be advised to discuss all herbal supplementation with their health-care provider.

Infections

The importance of investigating infections in older adults cannot be overstated. Infections, including COVID-19, pneumonia, influenza, and septicemia, are one of the 15 leading causes of death in persons over 65 (CDC, 2021a). Infections in older adults often present with atypical signs and symptoms, which can lead to delayed treatment (Esme et al, 2019). The immune system enables the body to defend itself against disease-causing micro-organisms and other foreign bodies; it is vital to human survival. However, this system exhibits a diminished ability to provide such protection with aging. Considering the immune system's fundamental importance in maintaining health, a clear understanding of age-related changes is crucial.

THE CHAIN OF INFECTION

For an infection to occur, a reservoir of infectious disease, a portal of entry, and a susceptible host must be present (Huether et al, 2020). The source of an infectious disease is the reservoir or substance from which the infectious agent was acquired. The source may be a person's own microbial flora (endogenous) or something in the environment (exogenous), such as water, air, food, soil, or another person. Infectious diseases passed from other animal species to humans are called *zoonoses,* for example, cat-scratch fever and rabies. Infections acquired in the health-care setting are called *health-care-associated infections*, and those acquired outside the health-care facility are called *community-acquired infections.* The source of transmission may be feces, blood, and other body fluids. Infections may be transmitted from person to person through shared inanimate objects (fomites) contaminated by infected body fluids. Examples of infections transmitted through this mechanism include *Clostridium difficile* infection from a commode or other contaminated surface and HIV infection from the use of shared needles by intravenous (IV) drug users.

The portal of entry is how a pathogen enters the body and gains access to tissues, where it may multiply and cause disease. The portal of entry may be skin penetration, direct contact, ingestion, or inhalation. Any disruption or penetration in the integrity of the skin and mucous membranes is a potential portal of entry. The break may be accidental (e.g., an abrasion or burn), the result of a medical procedure (e.g., surgery or catheterization), or the result of direct inoculation from animal or arthropod bite (e.g., Lyme disease or malaria). In direct contact, pathogens are transmitted from infected tissues or secretions to exposed intact mucous membranes. Sexually transmitted infections (STIs) such as gonorrhea and chlamydia are examples of direct contact transmission. The oral cavity and gastrointestinal tract are the most efficient portals of entry. Pathogens are ingested and successfully compete with normal bacterial flora to cause infection. Cholera, food poisoning, and hepatitis A are examples of diseases that occur through ingestion. Pathogens must survive the low pH and enzymes of the gastric acid secretions to establish infection. People with reduced gastric acidity (because of disease or drugs) are more susceptible to this mode of infection.

Many pathogens invade the body through the respiratory tract and cause diseases such as influenza, the common cold, and bacterial pneumonia. The portal of entry does not limit the site of infection. Ingested pathogens may penetrate the mucosa, disseminate through the circulatory system, and cause disease in other organs. Hepatitis A and vancomycin-resistant enterococci (VRE) are examples of ingested pathogens causing infection in the liver and bloodstream. Genetic, constitutional, and other nonspecific factors in the host determine whether a pathogen will succeed in causing infection and clinical disease.

COMMON PROBLEMS AND CONDITIONS

The immune deficiencies among older adults make this population more vulnerable to both infection and cancer. As people age, the likelihood of autoimmune antibodies being found in serum increases, which suggests an increased likelihood of autoimmune processes. However, whether such autoimmune processes are age-related is still being investigated (Watad et al, 2017).

Individuals with diminished immune function are susceptible to numerous infections. Some of the more common infections in older adults include influenza, pneumonia, tuberculosis, urinary tract infections (especially in females), and shingles (herpes zoster). Medical management of infections consists primarily of determining the source of the infection and appropriate prescribing of antimicrobials.

COVID-19, Influenza, and Pneumonia

COVID-19 is the third leading cause of death among older adults; and pneumonia and influenza are ranked as the tenth leading causes of death (CDC, 2021a). The predominant portal of entry for COVID-19 and influenza is the inhalation of small droplets transmitted through sneezing, coughing, or talking. Closed populations, such as those in long-term care facilities, provide an ideal setting for transmission. The social environment in these institutions also facilitates transmission through group activities, communal dining rooms, and rehabilitation activities.

The most effective measure to control COVID-19 and influenza is vaccinating individuals at high risk. COVID-19 and influenza vaccinations are a Medicare-covered benefit for older adults, yet of the population 65 years or older, only 95% was vaccinated against COVID-19 (CDC, 2022b) and 75.2% against influenza (CDC, 2021b) during the 2020–2021 season. Other strategies to control the health-care-associated spread of COVID-19 and influenza include the early identification and grouping of infected patients, careful hand washing, and use of barrier precautions when handling bodily substances, especially respiratory secretions.

Multiple pathogens cause community-acquired pneumonia, the most common being *Streptococcus pneumoniae, Haemophilus influenzae,* atypical bacteria (i.e., *Chlamydia pneumoniae, Mycoplasma pneumoniae, Legionella sp*), and viruses (Sethi, 2024). Early recognition and treatment of bacterial pneumonia leads to recovery, although antibiotic resistance is becoming problematic. The pneumococcal vaccine is recommended for everyone over 65; in 2020 67%.5 of older adults were vaccinated (CDC, 2022c).

Older adults are more susceptible to community-acquired pneumonia than younger populations (Almirall, Serra-Prat, Bolibar, & Balasso, 2017). In addition to advanced age, other major risk factors include smoking, excessive alcohol intake, chronic lung disease, dysphagia, chronic heart disease, cancer, and persons with poor nutritional status. Changes in lung function that come with aging enable inhaled microorganisms to survive and multiply. Social environments such as congregate housing, communal dining rooms, religious organizations, crowded shopping centers, adult day care centers, or nursing facilities place older adults at risk for exposure and infection. However, social isolation is not recommended because of its negative psychological consequences. Older adults should be encouraged to select activities that reduce the risk for infection during the colder months.

Infection-control measures should be in place to reduce the risk for illness. Hand-washing, monitoring fluids and nutritional intake, and proper disposal of bodily secretions help to manage the spread of infection when it does occur (Eliopoulos, 2005). Older adults and their families should be instructed to seek early medical attention for subtle changes that may signal the onset of infection. For example, pneumonia may be signaled by confusion or tachypnea, with no other findings. Many older adults present with atypical or diminished signs and symptoms (Esme et al, 2019). Nursing care of older patients must be attentive to ensure early detection of subtle changes.

Cancer

Neoplasms occur with greater frequency in older adults. Common types include lung, breast, and prostate cancers. However, the potential for numerous other forms of cancer should not be overlooked.

The presence of cancer reveals a decreased immune response. Cancer cells are normally detected by the immune system and eliminated after being recognized as abnormal cells. It is only when the immune system fails to carry out this function that cancer occurs. However, cancer and treatment for cancer may induce additional immune deficits.

For example, cancer is often accompanied by a decrease in appetite, which increases the possibility of malnutrition. Furthermore, anticancer drugs often deplete immune cells, causing further immune system decline. Because many of these drugs have the greatest effect on rapidly dividing cells, the cells of the immune system are attacked concurrently with the cancer cells. Each patient's response to treatment is individual; decisions about treatment need to be personalized. The prognosis for cancer is highly variable depending on the time of diagnosis, the patient's general health, and the type of cancer.

Autoimmunity

Older adults may have ADs such as RA; however, these cannot be considered solely age-associated. Older adults with ADs are more likely to take immunosuppressants as treatment, increasing the immune deficits accompanying aging. Therefore these older adults carry higher infection risks than older adults without AD. Criteria for identifying AD include (1) evidence of autoimmune reaction, (2) determination that immunologic findings are not secondary to another condition, and (3) lack of other identified causes for the disorder.

Systemic Lupus Erythematosus

Systemic lupus erythematosus (SLE) may affect many parts of the body, including the joints, skin, kidneys, heart, lungs, blood vessels, and brain. The most common symptoms are extreme fatigue, painful or swollen joints, unexplained fever, skin rashes, and kidney problems. The antinuclear antibody (ANA) test is one of the more specific tests for SLE. There is no cure for SLE. The management objective is to control the severity of symptoms and prevent a flare. The warning signs of a flare are increased fatigue, pain, rash, fever, stomach discomfort, headache, and dizziness. Patients must monitor their health and learn to recognize symptoms of disease activity. Avoiding the sun, exercising, complying with drugs, limiting stress, and having regular health-care visits are important.

Rheumatoid Arthritis

RA is characterized by inflammatory polyarthritis of unknown cause. Symptoms include morning stiffness lasting for hours, tenderness, pain on motion, limited range of motion, and joint deformity in the small joints of the hands and feet. Extraarticular signs are pulmonary (e.g., pleuritis and pneumonitis), cardiac (e.g., pericarditis and myocarditis), renal (e.g., amyloidosis), and ocular (e.g., scleritis); rheumatoid (subcutaneous) nodules also develop. The course of RA is highly variable; most people develop progressive functional limitations and physical disability. Patients with RA have a higher mortality rate than the general population. In addition to physical therapy, first-line drugs for RA are nonsteroidal antiinflammatory drugs (NSAIDs). These drugs reduce inflammation, pain, and swelling. During arthritis flare-ups or when NSAIDs are ineffective, patients may be treated with short bursts of corticosteroids. Because of their side effects, corticosteroids should not be used for long periods in high doses. Patients with RA may need drugs to slow joint destruction. These drugs are known as *disease-modifying antirheumatic drugs* (DMARDs) and may take months to demonstrate a therapeutic effect. Newer DMARDs include biologic agents (e.g., adalimumab) and targeted synthetic DMARDs (e.g., baricitinib).

HIV INFECTION IN OLDER ADULTS

HIV infection is an underrecognized problem among the older adult population. As of 2022, 54% of those diagnosed with HIV were adults over age 50; persons newly diagnosed accounted for 16% (HIV.gov, 2024). To complicate matters, upon a diagnosis of HIV, 35% of people aged 50 and over had late-stage HIV. This means that treatment is started much later for an already weakened immune system.

Risk factors for HIV are the same as people of other ages and include unprotected sexual intercourse and sharing needles (NIH, 2024). Age-related factors in older adult females include atrophy to the vaginal membrane, causing tears. Older adults are less concerned about pregnancy; therefore condoms are less likely to be used during sexual intercourse.

As mentioned earlier, HIV is not diagnosed among older adults until the late stage. Health-care providers usually do not consider older adults at risk for acquiring HIV; testing is not offered to older adults. Many older adults are embarrassed or afraid to be tested. When older adults complain of some of the signs and symptoms of HIV, many people attribute them to age-related conditions (NIH, 2024). Complications from HIV and its pharmacologic therapy arise because of the aging immune system. The immune system cannot eliminate the HIV residing in macrophages, lymphoid tissue, or the brain. The disease progresses more rapidly because the immune system's regenerative capacity is diminished and not all replacement cells are fully functional (Mpondo, 2016).

Major implications for nursing practice exist. In assessing older adults, nurses must complete a thorough sexual history. Nurses need to discuss HIV and risk behaviors for acquiring HIV. Older adults should be taught the proper use of condoms and how and when to get tested for HIV.

SIGNIFICANT HEALTHCARE-ASSOCIATED PATHOGENS

Clostridium difficile

C. difficile is a common pathogen causing health-care-associated infection (HAI). The presence of *C. difficile* alone does not indicate infection. The disease occurs when this organism is allowed to flourish when the normal bowel flora is disturbed. *C. difficile* produces toxins, which can damage the lining of the intestines, resulting in hemorrhaging and frequent profuse, watery diarrhea (Mayo Clinic Staff, 2023). The hallmark diarrhea is caused by a motility-altering factor that stimulates peristalsis. Older adults are at an increased risk for *C. difficile* infection because of a decreased immune system and the altered normal intestinal flora (Donskey, 2017). Other risk factors include unnecessary use of proton pump inhibitors and antibiotics.

C. difficile is transmitted from person to person, primarily from the hands of health-care workers (Donskey, 2017). Consistent hand-washing between contacts with patients and the use of gloves when handling body substances such as feces are imperative. Patients with *C. difficile* should be placed in private rooms with their own bathrooms or commodes.

Treatment includes replacing fluid and electrolytes and discontinuing current antibiotic therapy, followed by treatment with oral vancomycin or fidaxomicin. For serious infections, a combination treatment with oral vancomycin and metronidazole may be used (Mayo Clinic Staff, 2023). For patients who experience recurrent *C. difficile* infections that do not respond to antibiotics, fecal microbiota transplant can be considered (Mayo Clinic Staff, 2023). Other treatments include antibody-based therapy and probiotics.

Vancomycin-Resistant Enterococcus

Vancomycin-resistant enterococcus (VRE) was first identified in the United States in 1989. Multiple factors predispose a person to infection with VRE, but colonization precedes most infections

(Beale and Durward-Diioia, 2022). Since the advent of vancomycin, its use has increased dramatically because of many factors, including increases in the incidence of methicillin-resistant *Staphylococcus aureus* (MRSA). Risk factors for VRE acquisition include advanced age, antibiotic use, alcoholism, and dementia (Mathis et al, 2019).

VRE is transmitted from person to person and by contact with contaminated surfaces and equipment (CDC, 2019a). To control the transmission of VRE, health-care workers must perform hand hygiene with soap and water for a minimum of 20 seconds. Nurses can use alcohol-based hand sanitizer that contains a minimum of 60% alcohol and rub on hands and fingers until they are dry. Dedicated equipment (e.g., stethoscopes) is required for infected patients. Colonized and infected patients should be isolated in private rooms or grouped with other infected patients in the acute care setting. Barrier precautions, gloves, and gowns should be implemented for patient care. Antibiotics are not used in asymptomatic persons with colonization; symptomatic patients should be treated with antibiotics indicated through culture and sensitivity.

Methicillin-Resistant *Staphylococcus aureus*

In the early 1940s, when penicillin became available, *S. aureus* was highly susceptible to antibiotic treatment; however, resistant strains developed quickly (Turner et al, 2019). *S. aureus* resistant to methicillin was first discovered in the 1960s. Since the 1990s, MRSA rapidly spread into the community.

Like VRE, MRSA is transmitted from person to person and by contact with contaminated surfaces and equipment (Popovich et al, 2021). Risk factors for acquiring MRSA include older adults, persons who are frequently in crowded situations (e.g., military personnel in barracks), skin-to-skin contact, and those who share equipment or supplies (e.g., needles) (CDC, 2019b). Control of MRSA focuses on health-care worker hand-washing to reduce transmission. Health-care workers should wear gloves for all contact with patients who are either colonized or infected. MRSA-positive patients should be placed in private rooms. Antibiotics are not used in persons with colonization without symptoms; symptomatic patients should be treated with antibiotics indicated through culture and sensitivity.

Extended Spectrum β-Lactamase-Positive *Escherichia coli*

E. coli usually does not cause harm in otherwise healthy individuals. However, in persons with decreased immune systems (i.e., older adults), infections with *E. coli* are common. They are one of the most common pathogens for urinary tract infections (UTIs) (Amarsy et al, 2019). Asymptomatic bacteriuria is also common among older adults; cultures are positive for *E. coli* but the patients are without symptoms of infection. Overdiagnosing UTI among older adults is also common because of multiple comorbidities and impaired cognition, resulting in inappropriate use of antibiotics. The misuse of antibiotics leads to antibiotic resistance. Microbes, such as *E. coli*, can produce extended-spectrum β-lactamases (ESBLs), which are enzymes that can negatively affect the effectiveness of antimicrobials containing β-lactam rings (i.e., penicillins and cephalosporins) (CDC, 2019c).

Persons at risk for ESBL-positive *E. coli* include those who are exposed to healthcare, including hospitals, long-term care facilities, and home healthcare (CDC, 2019c). Microbes with ESBLs have also been found among those who have traveled abroad. ESBL microbes are spread from person to person through contaminated hands and surfaces and through consuming contaminated food and water. Nurses can help mitigate the spread of ESBLs by proper hand hygiene with soap and water. Alcohol-based hand sanitizer should be used when soap and water are not readily available. Older adults who are infected with ESBL-producing microbes may need to be hospitalized and treated with IV antibiotics, such as carbapenems.

NURSING CARE GUIDELINES FOR INFECTION

Recognize Cues (Assessment)

With such a spectrum of possible infections, clinical assessment varies widely. However, health-care workers must remember some crucial aspects of assessing older adults for infection (Box 12.2). Older adults with decreased immune function may not exhibit classic symptoms of infection. The diminished inflammatory response may lead to false-negative results for skin tests used in the diagnosis of disease, for example, the purified protein-derivative skin test for tuberculosis (Byng-Maddick and Noursadeghi, 2016). Similarly, redness, swelling, or inflammation may be reduced with infections. These reduced responses are even more likely to occur in people with diseases or drug treatments that further suppress the immune system, such as cancer patients or those taking immunosuppressants.

Another classic example of a reduced response to infection is the absence of fever. With an infection, the immune response provokes local or systemic fever. In younger adults, an elevated temperature is an indicator of infection. However, older adults with decreased immune function may not have a fever, or their fever may be blunted (Esme et al, 2019). Symptoms of pain may

---

BOX 12.2 Assessment of Individuals at High Risk for Infection

Subjective
Obtain history:
- Previous infections
- Predisposing illnesses
- Drugs
- Vaccinations
- Living environment
- Lifestyle factors (e.g., smoking, activity level, and chemical exposures)
- Social support system

Objective
Assess for signs and symptoms of infection:
- Fever: high grade or low grade
- Inflammation: pronounced or slight
- Pain: slight or severe
- Malaise, fatigue
- Turbidity, odor, and amount of body fluids
- Complete blood cell count with differential

also be reduced or absent. Thus, infection in these older adults may progress to the life-threatening stage before it is detected.

Because of this reduced immune response, mild symptoms such as a low-grade fever must be taken seriously. Close observation is needed to detect subtle symptoms. Changes in the behavior of patients (e.g., increased malaise, fatigue, or poor oral intake) may indicate the onset of infection (Esme et al, 2019). Furthermore, older adults may have normal or decreased white blood cell (WBC) count with infection (Compté et al, 2018).

In addition to observed data, subjective and historical data are valuable when evaluating older adults with infection. A history of previous episodes of infection, including the timing, nature, and severity of the infection, is important. Infections in older adults often recur. Information regarding exposure to others with infections may also be helpful. Older adults are more susceptible to infection, especially if they live in environments conducive to spreading pathogens. Such environments include nursing facilities, hospitals, and crowded environments, where strict hygiene standards are difficult to maintain. Immunization records also provide important information that needs to be obtained.

It is also important to determine other disease processes for which patients may currently be receiving treatment. Persons with cancer may be experiencing assaults on their immune systems from the disease and treatment. Older adults with ADs may be receiving antiinflammatory and immunosuppressant drugs. Individuals with HIV infection experience an extreme assault on their immune system. All of these make older adults more prone to a variety of infections.

A thorough drug history is necessary to detect the potential for drug-related immunosuppression. This record should include prescription and over-the-counter (OTC) drugs, herbs, and other dietary supplements. Patients receiving drugs with immunosuppressant qualities are more prone to infections. Additionally, information on the use of alcohol, tobacco, and other drugs, as well as exposure to toxic substances, should be obtained.

Knowledge about a patient's lifestyle may provide invaluable information in developing a care plan. Information should include a thorough nutritional history and activity and exercise habits. An understanding of an individual's social support system should be acquired, and indicators of life stressors should be elicited. A classic life stressor is bereavement, especially the loss of a spouse. However, the loss of friends and other family members should not be overlooked. Even the loss of a home or relocation to another place may result in a sense of bereavement.

Analyze Cues and Prioritize Hypotheses (Patient Problems)

Several patient problems may be applicable to older patients who either have infections or are at high risk for developing infections. The risk factors determined during the assessment indicate potential patient problems. For example, many older adults are either inadequately or inappropriately nourished. Thus, a hypothesis of "impaired nutritional status" is likely. People with cancer may be malnourished because of lack of appetite or side effects resulting from drugs. Poor nutrition may also be attributed to a self-care deficit in preparing and eating food; older adults sometimes have difficulty preparing their own meals. These difficulties may be related to various problems, such as visual deficits, arthritis, or depression. Regardless of the cause, older adults are at higher risk for infection if these self-care deficits result in poor nutrition.

The hypothesis "potential for infection" applies to both those at risk for developing an infection and those with existing infections. The presence of an infection indicates that the immune system is already challenged, which increases the likelihood of a secondary infection. For instance, it is not unusual for an individual with viral influenza to develop a secondary bacterial infection of pneumococcal pneumonia.

A hypothesis of "teaching about infection" is also a possibility. Knowledge deficits may be in immunizations, nutrition, or protection against infection from oneself or others. Patients may be unaware of their nutritional needs or the relationship between nutritional and immune status. Older adults may be more likely to consume appropriate foods if they have this knowledge. Similarly, older adults may be unaware of available vaccinations or the benefits such vaccinations may hold for them. Older individuals need information on ways to reduce their risk for developing infections.

Finally, "impaired socialization" may be a relevant hypothesis associated with the individual at risk for infection because social support has also been associated with immune status.

Generate Solutions (Planning)

In planning care for older patients, the health-care team and patients must set goals together. Goals must be congruent with realistic expectations and with patients' desired outcomes. For individuals at increased risk for infection, goals include avoiding primary or secondary infection and maintaining or improving immune status. A careful assessment of patient knowledge in infection prevention, maintenance of immune status, and health practices determines the goals for patient teaching.

In setting nutritional goals, nurses might find a consultation with a registered dietitian appropriate. They must consider patients' dietary preferences and financial ability to buy food (if not in an institutional setting). An outcome might be that a patient consumes a well-balanced, high-calorie diet daily. Patients with cancer may have even more extreme nutritional needs. An outcome for these individuals might be that they stabilize body weight and then gradually increase it to 1 pound every 3 weeks. Another outcome may be that a patient performs self-care activities with minimum energy expenditure and risk of injury. For patients with activity deficits, an appropriate goal might be to participate in 15 minutes of moderate exercise three times a week. The exact target goal for exercise should be established in consultation with the primary care provider and possibly achieved through physical therapy.

Take Actions (Nursing Interventions)

Nursing management of older adults with alterations in immunity focuses on preventing and recognizing infections. Interventions addressing these are targeted at (1) preventing exposure to infections, (2) enhancing the immune system to enable patients to better resist infections, and (3) recognizing early signs and symptoms of infections. Totally preventing exposure to pathogens is impossible, especially because one source of pathogens is the body's own natural flora. However, infection can be minimized for individuals with diminished immune capacity. During times of epidemics such as during the influenza season, the patient should try to avoid places with crowds of people. Visitors should be screened for infections in an institutional or home setting. If contact is unavoidable, infected visitors may be given a mask to wear to minimize potential contamination of the patients. Any catheters, IV fluids, or similar therapeutic devices should be carefully assessed for signs of irritation or inflammation. Teaching patients to drink at least 2000 milliliters (mL) of fluids a day, unless contraindicated, will aid in preventing UTI and constipation. Additionally, teaching stress management techniques to promote immune system function may be indicated. Finally, hygiene standards should be rigorously maintained, especially for patients experiencing treatment-induced immune suppression, as is seen with some anticancer drugs. In addition to normal bathing, careful attention should be paid to oral and perineal care. Both patients and caregivers should be alert for changes in the color, consistency, and odor of body fluids to detect the onset of infections.

Nutritional Interventions

Other measures may be taken to strengthen the immune system to better enable patients to resist infection. As previously mentioned, optimal nutritional status is important. Although all nutritional needs of healthy older adults may be met through normal dietary intake, many older adults have dietary deficiencies. In patients with cancer, nutritional deficits may be extreme. After assessment, efforts should be made to resolve detected deficiencies. In institutional settings, dietary supplements and frequent meals may be supplied (see the Evidence-Based Practice box). Food may be prepared specifically to suit the patients' tastes and needs. For older adults in the community, it is helpful to have services such as Meals on Wheels (MOW), assistance with food preparation, or the ability to visit a senior center nutrition site. Liquid food supplements or OTC vitamins are other alternatives. However, these may be beyond the financial resources of some patients.

The inability to feed oneself is another barrier to proper nutrition. Individuals feeding patients in the home or institutional setting must ensure that the patients receive a balanced, nutritional diet. Family members or care providers may need special instruction on how to accomplish this with patients.

Psychosocial Interventions

A variety of modalities based on the relationships between psychosocial factors and immunity are available, and their use may enhance immunocompetence. These include relaxation and visualization, social support, and exercise.

Exercise programs should be tailored to suit individual abilities. For patients with physical debility, exercise programs should be tailored to meet their needs and interests. Possible exercises include walking, dancing or dancelike movements, water exercises, or swimming. Developing exercise programs that are moderately difficult rather than strenuous for older individuals is important.

New treatment modalities are developed as the relationships between immune status and psychosocial variables are explored. Modalities currently being explored include biofeedback, therapeutic touch, and hypnosis.

> **EVIDENCE-BASED PRACTICE**
>
> ### Effect of Probiotics on C. difficile Infection
>
> **Background**
> C. diff is a leading cause of infectious diarrhea. The incidence has tripled in the last decade. C. diff-associated diarrhea leads to increased morbidity, mortality, longer hospitalizations, and increased cost.
>
> **Sample/Setting**
> Following specified inclusion and exclusion criteria, five studies were selected for inclusion in the systematic review. Inclusion criteria included participants 60 years or older, patients in acute and postacute care facilities on, or intending to start, antibiotics therapy. Additionally, participants took probiotic capsules or probiotic-containing food products compared with placebo. The five studies included 3461 participants, whose mean age was over 70 years.
>
> **Method**
> Two independent reviewers assessed the selected experimental designed studies for methodological quality using critical appraisal instruments from the Joanna Briggs Institute (JBI). Data were extracted from the papers using the standardized data extraction tool from the JBI Meta-Analysis of Statistics Assessment and Review Instrument.
>
> **Findings**
> Of the five studies, only one found statistically significant results between participants receiving probiotics and those receiving placebo. The other studies demonstrated no effect on the incidence of C. diff infection. However, across the studies, the type of probiotic treatment was inconsistent, as well as the strain of bacteria, method of administration and dose.
>
> **Implications**
> Probiotics were not found to be more effective than placebo for reducing C. diff infection in hospitalized older adults. More studies need to be completed examining dose, frequency, method of administration, length of administration, and number of strains of bacteria administered. Nurses should strive to be knowledgeable about the treatments with the best supporting evidence for their patients.

Data from Vernaya, M., McAdam, J., & Hampton, M. D. (2017). Effectiveness of probiotics in reducing the incidence of Clostridium difficile-associated diarrhea in elderly patients: A systematic review. *JBI Database of Systematic Reviews and Implementation Reports, 15*(1), 140–164.

Evaluate Outcomes (Evaluation)

Monitoring the success of interventions is based on the patient's responses in meeting their goals and outcomes. One standard for evaluation is whether a patient contracts an infection through contact with others or by their own flora. Improving or at least maintaining immune status may be more difficult for some patients because the understanding of both the immune system and the concomitant changes that occur with aging is incomplete. Furthermore, many individuals are enduring severe assaults on their immune systems. Persons with cancer receive anticancer drugs that may destroy the immune response. In persons with HIV, the immune system is directly targeted by viral attack. Interventions such as diet, exercise, and psychosocial enhancement are rarely sufficient in overcoming such odds, although unexplained recoveries have been known to occur. For most situations, it may be unreasonable to expect a return to normal status for immunocompromised individuals. However, any improvement in immune status, or even maintenance, may allow older patients to live better lives (see the Nursing Care Plan boxes).

NURSING CARE PLAN

Pneumococcal Pneumonia

Clinical Situation

An 80-year-old patient is admitted to the hospital for treatment of pneumococcal pneumonia, which was developed while the patient had influenza. The patient lives alone in a low-rent housing development in a large city, having moved there two years ago after the death of the patient's partner. Without the partner's income, the patient was unable to afford the rent on their previous home. The nearest family member lives 75 miles away and rarely visits. The patient's former neighbors, who live across town, are unable to visit because of the distance and because of their own debilities. The patient is 20% underweight for height and is anemic. WBC count is high. Other lab values are as follows: red blood cell count, 3.7/milliliter (mL); hematocrit, 34%; hemoglobin, 10.8; WBC count, 18,200/mL; and ALB, 2.6 grams per deciliter (g/dL).

Analyze Cues and Prioritize Hypotheses (Patient Problems)
- Potential for infection resulting from compromised immune status
- Impaired nutrition resulting from low income, transportation difficulties
- Impaired socialization resulting from loss of friends and limited contact with family
- Teaching about infection resulting from influenza and pneumococcal vaccination because of new experience

Generate Solutions (Planning)
- The patient will not experience additional infections as evidenced by (1) WBC count returning to normal limits, (2) afebrile state, and (3) other vital signs being within normal limits.
- The patient will verbalize knowledge of infection prevention strategies.
- The patient will have adequate nutrition as demonstrated by (1) weight gain of half-pound per week, (2) an increased hemoglobin level, and (3) an increased serum protein level.
- The patient will consume a well-balanced, sufficient-calorie diet, as evidenced by (1) calorie counts showing an intake of at least 1800 calories per day and (2) consumption of food from all food groups, including protein sources, breads, fruits and vegetables, and dairy products.
- The patient will acquire social contacts desirable to her, as evidenced by (1) spending time each week with others and (2) voicing satisfaction with social contacts.
- The patient will identify the advantages of the influenza and pneumococcal vaccines.

Take Actions (Nursing Interventions)
- Screen all visitors with infection who may come into direct contact with the patient.
- Provide family and visitors with information on transmission of infection.
- Explain to the patient that they may be at risk for additional infections because of their depressed immune status and should limit their exposure to additional pathogens. Observe for slight increases in temperature every 4 hours or more often, as needed.
- Be aware that the patient may develop subtle or undetected signs and symptoms of infection and that slight changes in temperature may be highly significant.
- Observe for increased respiratory difficulty.
- Auscultate the patient's lungs at every shift and as needed.
- Have the patient report any sore throat.
- Monitor dietary intake using calorie counts.
- Teach what constitutes a well-balanced diet that is high in protein.
- Ensure adequate intake of vitamins and trace minerals through diet or supplements.
- Encourage the patient to eat foods that include vitamins and minerals, as well as trace minerals such as zinc and magnesium.
- Provide vitamin and mineral supplements in addition to the high-protein diet, if needed.
- Arrange for MOW on discharge or facilitate attendance at a nutrition site to provide better nutrition after discharge.
- Contact religious affiliations or other organizations to include the patient in their social gatherings to help re-establish a social support system.
- Assess the patient's level of stress to determine whether an easily accessible, low-exertion relaxation program is indicated. (A relaxation program may provide an easily accessible, low-exertion intervention with an immune benefit.)
- Plan a program of graduated exercise designed to fit the patient's tolerance.
- Contact social services or a local senior citizen center to identify center activities and transportation.
- Contact area organizations or religious affiliations for information about activities.
- Collaborate with the patient to develop a plan of action.
- Provide information for the patient regarding the COVID-19 and influenza vaccine: (1) COVID-19 and influenza could be serious, life-threatening conditions in older people; (2) routine immunizations are important; (3) the signs and symptoms of COVID-19 and influenza can be similar, which include weakness, coughing, headaches, a sudden increase in temperature, aches, chills, and occasional vomiting; and (4) pneumonia is a common complication of respiratory infections, such as COVID-19 and influenza.
- Refer the patient to their primary care provider for specific advice regarding recuperation time before taking the vaccine.
- Provide information for the patient on the pneumococcal vaccine.
- Inform the patient that the vaccine should not be administered soon after having pneumonia.
- Refer the patient to their primary care provider for the specific timing of administration after any illness.

NURSING CARE PLAN

Effects of Chemotherapy

Clinical Situation

A 68-year-old patient is receiving chemotherapy after a modified radical mastectomy for breast cancer. Although the patient was previously well nourished, stomatitis developed which made eating painful and their appetite has decreased. In addition, the chemotherapy has decreased total WBC count to 2000. The patient lives at home with their partner. The patient receives chemotherapy on an outpatient basis but is visited daily by a home-health nurse to maintain the indwelling peripherally inserted central catheter (PICC).

NURSING CARE PLAN—cont'd

Analyze Cues and Prioritize Hypotheses (Patient Problems)
- Potential for infection resulting from suppressed immune system
- Impaired nutrition resulting from inability to eat secondary to side effects of chemotherapy

Generate Solutions (Planning)
- The patient will not develop an infection, as evidenced by (1) no change in behavior (2) no sudden elevation in WBC count, (3) no white patches to mouth, tongue, or throat, and (4) no redness or irritation around wounds or catheters.
- The patient will demonstrate what constitutes adequate dietary intake of proteins, vitamins, and minerals, as evidenced by (1) developing a weekly meal plan and (2) maintenance of body weight.

Take Actions (Nursing Interventions)
- Teach the patient to minimize exposure to pathogens and to screen visitors with contagious infections.
- Explain the need to maintain careful hygiene (e.g., daily shower and proper oral, foot, and perineal care).
- Use sterile technique when working with PICC.
- Monitor the patient's mouth and throat for signs of infection such as white patches or redness; teach the patient to report the same to the nurse.
- Auscultate the lungs at each visit.
- Teach the patient to monitor body fluids for alterations in color, odor, or consistency.
- Encourage fluid intake of at least 2000 milliliters per day unless otherwise indicated.
- Teach the patient to eat small, frequent meals, rich in protein, vitamins, and minerals.
- Teach the patient about food sources high in calories, protein, vitamins, and minerals.
- Have the patient take food supplements to increase intake, if needed.
- Teach the importance of eating nutrient-dense foods (e.g., those with high nutritional content in small volumes).
- Acquire an oral anesthetic to treat stomatitis.
- Teach the patient how to prepare bland foods of moderate temperature.
- Provide an example meal plan.

HOME CARE

1. Assess nutritional and dietary status to ensure proper immune functioning in homebound older adults.
2. Instruct older adults and caregivers about the need to receive a balanced nutritional diet and the role of vitamin supplements in promoting proper immune functioning.
3. An altered emotional state may lead to decreased immune functioning in homebound older adults.
4. Vaccinations are imperative for homebound older adults (e.g., annual influenza vaccine, COVID-19 vaccine, and pneumococcal vaccine).
5. Assess and report any signs of impaired immunity (e.g., fever and changes in WBC count).
6. Bedridden or immunocompromised older adults are at high risk for infections. Instruct older adults and caregivers about ways to protect the older adults from infection from themselves and others.
7. Tailor an exercise program for homebound or bedridden older adults to enhance their immune system and to prevent infection.
8. Assess how homebound older adults manage personal hygiene and teach them the importance of hand-washing.
9. Practice appropriate cleaning and maintenance of humidifiers, catheters, respiratory equipment, and other devices used in home care–related treatment.
10. Develop a plan for alternative care in case a caregiver develops an infection.

SUMMARY

This chapter explored age-related changes in the immune system. The influences of other factors, such as psychosocial influences and nutrition, on the immune status of older adults were also discussed. Discussions on cancer, ADs, HIV, and significant health-care-associated pathogens in older adults were also presented.

A key role of the nurse in caring for older adults in all settings is to recognize the potential for infection in this population and develop care plans to prevent infection and promote its early detection. Because of the increased risk of morbidity and mortality associated with infection in this age group, immunizations and interventions specific to various body systems should be implemented for those identified as susceptible to infection.

KEY POINTS

- With aging, the immune response diminishes.
- The diminished immune response reduces the normal responses to infection, such as fever, which makes infection in older adults more difficult to detect.
- Nutrition, especially regarding protein, vitamins, and trace minerals, substantially affects immune status.
- Activity has a substantial effect on immune status. Even moderate amounts of daily exercise may enhance immune status.
- Interventions dealing with infection and decreased immune response must address nutrition, exercise, mood, stress, and physical protection.

CLINICAL JUDGMENT EXERCISE

1. Your neighbor is a 72-year-old patient whose partner died last year. Since the partner's death, the patient has become sedentary and withdrawn. Feeling concerned about the patient, you decide to visit the patient. The patient explains that they have been ill off and on for the past few weeks and does not understand why they keep getting sick. The patient reports losing faith in doctors. Recognizing that depression and a sedentary lifestyle may have altered the immune response, how might you intervene to help?

REFERENCES

Administration for Community Living. (2021). *2020 profile of older Americans*. Washington, DC: U.S. Department of Health and Human Services. Retrieved from https://acl.gov/sites/default/files/aging%20and%20Disability%20In%20America/2020Profileolderamericans.final_.pdf. Accessed August 12, 2024.

Agrawal, A., Sridharan, A., Prakash, S., & Agrawal, H. (2012). Dendritic cells and aging: consequences for autoimmunity. *Expert Review of Clinical Immunology, 8*(1), 73–80. doi:10.1586/eci.11.77.

Aiello, A., Farzaneh, F., Candore, G., Caruso, C., Davinelli, S., Gambino, C. M., et al. (2019). Immunosenescence and its hallmarks: How to oppose aging strategically? A review of potential options for therapeutic intervention. *Frontiers in Immunology, 10*, 2247. doi:10.3389/fimmu.2019.02247.

Alam, I., Almajwal, A. M., Alam, W., Alam, I., Ullah, N., Abulmeaaty, M., et al. (2019). The immune-nutrition interplay in aging - facts and controversies. *Nutrition and Healthy Aging, 5*(2), 73–95. doi:10.3233/NHA-170034.

Almirall, J., Serra-Prat, M., Bolibar, I., & Balasso, V. (2017). Risk factors for community-acquired pneumonia in adults: A systematic review of observational studies. *Respiration, 94*, 299–311. doi:10.1159/000479089.

Amarsy, R., Guéret, D., Benmansour, H., Flicoteaux, R., Berçot, B., Meunier, F., et al. (2019). Determination of *Escherichia coli* phylogroups in elderly patients with urinary tract infection or asymptomatic bacteriuria. *Clinical Microbiology and Infection, 25*(7), 839–844. doi:10.1016/j.cmi.2018.12.032.

Beale, J. W., & Durward-Diioia, M. (2022). Clinical considerations in the approach to vancomycin-resistant Enterococci: A narrative review. *International Journal of Medical Students, 10*(2), 202–209. doi:10.5195/ijms.2022.1010.

Berben, L., Floris, G., Wildiers, H., & Hatse, S. (2021). Cancer and aging: Two tightly interconnected biological processes. *Cancers, 13*(6), 1400. doi:10.3390/cancers13061400.

Bulut, O., Kilic, G., Domínguez-Andrés, J., & Netea, M. G. (2020). Overcoming immune dysfunction in the elderly: Trained immunity as a novel approach. *International Immunology, 32*(12), 741–753. doi:10.1093/intimm/dxaa052.

Byng-Maddick, R., & Noursadeghi, M. (2016). Does tuberculosis threaten our ageing populations? *BMC Infectious Diseases, 16*, 119. doi:10.1186/s12879-016-1451-0.

Centers for Disease Control and Prevention (CDC). (2019a). *Vancomycin-resistant Enterococci (VRE) in healthcare settings*. Retrieved from https://www.cdc.gov/hai/organisms/vre/vre.html. Accessed July 28, 2023.

Centers for Disease Control and Prevention (CDC). (2019b). *Methicillin-resistant staphylococcus aureus* (MRSA). Retrieved from https://www.cdc.gov/mrsa/community/index.html#. Accessed July 28, 2023.

Centers for Disease Control and Prevention (CDC). (2019c). *ESBL-producing Enterobacterales in healthcare settings*. Retrieved from https://www.cdc.gov/hai/organisms/ESBL.html. Accessed July 28, 2023.

Centers for Disease Control and Prevention (CDC). (2021a). *About underlying cause of death, 1999-2020*. CDC Wonder [database]. Retrieved from https://wonder.cdc.gov/ucd-icd10.html. Accessed August 12, 2024.

Centers for Disease Control and Prevention (CDC). (2021b). *Flu vaccination coverage, United States, 2020-2021, influenza season*. Retrieved from https://www.cdc.gov/flu/fluvaxview/coverage-2021estimates.htm. Accessed August 12, 2024.

Centers for Disease Control and Prevention (CDC). (2022a). *Depression is not a normal part of growing older*. Retrieved from https://www.cdc.gov/aging/depression/index.html. Accessed July 28, 2023.

Centers for Disease Control and Prevention (CDC). (2022b). *COVID-19 vaccinations in the United States*. COVID Data Tracker [database]. Atlanta, GA: US Department of Health and Human Services, CDC. Retrieved from https://covid.cdc.gov/covid-data-tracker/#vaccinations_vacc-total-admin-rate-total. Accessed August 12, 2024.

Centers for Disease Control and Prevention (CDC). (2022c). *Vaccination coverage among adults in the United States, national health interview survey, 2019-2020*. Retrieved from https://www.cdc.gov/vaccines/imz-managers/coverage/adultvaxview/pubs-resources/vaccination-coverage-adults-2019-2020.html. Accessed August 12, 2024.

Compté, N., Dumont, L., Bron, D., De Breucker, S., Praet, J. P., Bautmans, I., et al. (2018). White blood cell counts in a geriatric hospitalized population: A poor diagnostic marker of infection. *Experimental Gerontology, 114*, 87–92. doi:10.1016/j.exger.2018.11.002.

D'Arcy, M. E., Castenson, D., Lynch, C. F., Kahn, A. R., Morton, L. M., Shiels, M. S., et al. (2021). Risk of rare cancers among solid organ transplant recipients. *Journal of the National Cancer Institute, 113*(2), 199–207. doi:10.1093/jnci/djaa078.

Eliopoulos, C. (2005). Immunity. In C. Eliopoulos (Ed.), *Gerontological nursing*. Philadelphia, PA: Lippincott.

Engels, E. A. (2017). Cancer in solid organ transplant recipients: There is still much to learn and do. *American Journal of Transplantation, 17*(8), 1967–1969. doi:10.1111/ajt.14140.

Esme, M., Topeli, A., Yavuz, B. B., & Akova, M. (2019). Infections in the elderly critically-ill patients. *Frontiers in Medicine, 6*, 118. doi:10.3389/fmed.2019.00118.

Furst, J. (2022). *Solid organ transplant patients are at higher risk of skin cancer and require coordinated care, Mayo Clinic researchers find*. Mayo Clinic News Network [website]. Retrieved from https://newsnetwork.mayoclinic.org/discussion/solid-organ-transplant-patients-are-at-higher-risk-of-skin-cancer-and-require-coordinated-care-mayo-clinic-researchers-find/. Accessed August 12, 2024.

Grice, E., & Lambris, J. (2013). *Immune system, skin microbiome "complement" one another, finds Penn Medicine study*. PennMedicine

News [website]. Retrieved from https://www.pennmedicine.org/news/news-releases/2013/august/immune-system-skin-microbiome. Accessed August 12, 2024.

Haynes, L. (2020). Aging of the immune system: Research challenges to enhance the health span of older adults. *Frontiers in Aging, 1*, 602108. doi:10.3389/fragi.2020.602108.

HIV.gov. (2024). *Aging with HIV*. HIV.gov [website]. Retrieved from https://www.hiv.gov/hiv-basics/living-well-with-hiv/taking-care-of-yourself/aging-with-hiv. Accessed August 12, 2024.

Huether, S. E., McCance, K. L., & Brashers, V. L. (Eds.). (2020). *Understanding pathophysiology* (7th ed.). St. Louis, MO: Elsevier.

Lin, P. H., Sermersheim, M., Li, H., Lee, P. H. U., Steinberg, S. M., & Ma, J. (2017). Zinc in wound healing modulation. *Nutrients, 10*(1), 16. doi:10.3390/nu10010016.

Mathis, B., Haïne, M., Girard, R., & Bonnefoy, M. (2019). Risk factors for vancomycin-resistant enterococcus acquisition during a large outbreak in patients aged 65 years and older. *BMC Geriatrics, 19*(1), 377. doi:10.1186/s12877-019-1398-2.

Mayo Clinic Staff. (2023). *C. difficile infection*. MayoClinic.org [website]. Retrieved from https://www.mayoclinic.org/diseases-conditions/c-difficile/symptoms-causes/syc-20351691. Accessed August 12, 2024.

Mpondo, B. C. T. (2016). HIV infection in the elderly: arising challenges. *Journal of Aging Research, 2016*, 2404857. doi:10.1155/2016/2404857.

National Institutes of Health (NIH). (2024). *HIV and specific populations*. HIVinfo.NIH.gov [website]. Retrieved from https://hivinfo.nih.gov/understanding-hiv/fact-sheets/hiv-and-older-people. Accessed August 12, 2024.

Oh, S. J., Lee, J. K., & Shin, O. S. (2019). Aging and the immune system: the impact of immunosenescence on viral infection, immunity and vaccine immunogenicity. *Immune Network, 19*(6), e37. doi:10.4110/in.2019.19.e37.

Popovich, K. J., Green, S. J., Okamoto, K., Rhee, Y., Hayden, M. K., Schoeny, M., et al. (2021). MRSA transmission in intensive care units: Genomic analysis of patients, their environments, and healthcare workers. *Clinical Infectious Diseases, 72*(11), 1879–1887. doi:10.1093/cid/ciaa731.

Sethi, S. (2024). *Community-acquired pneumonia*. Merck Manual [website]. Retrieved from http://www.merckmanuals.com/professional/pulmonary-disorders/pneumonia/community-acquired-pneumonia. Accessed August 12, 2024.

Townsend, M. C. (2008). *Essentials of psychiatric mental health nursing* (4th ed., pp. 581–609). Philadelphia, PA: FA Davis.

Turner, N. A., Sharma-Kuinkel, B. K., Maskarinec, S. A., Eichenberger, E. M., Shah, P. P., Carugati, M., et al. (2019). Methicillin-resistant *Staphylococcus aureus:* An overview of basic and clinical research. *Nature Reviews Microbiology, 17*(4), 203–218. doi:10.1038/s41579-018-0147-4.

Watad, A., Bragazzi, N. L., Adawi, M., Amital, H., Toubi, E., Porat, B. S., et al. (2017). Autoimmunity in the elderly: Insights from basic science and clinics - a mini-review. *Gerontology, 63*(6), 515–523. doi:10.1159/000478012.

PART IV

Diagnostic Studies and Pharmacologic Management

13

Laboratory and Diagnostic Tests

Donna Leake Hamby, DNP, RN, APRN, ACNP-BC

http://evolve.elsevier.com/Yeager/gerontologic/

LEARNING OBJECTIVES

On completion of this chapter, the reader will be able to:

1. Identify key laboratory values that increase or decrease with aging.
2. Describe the effect of aging on the erythrocyte sedimentation rate (ESR).
3. Name 2 drugs that can interfere with potassium excretion and affect serum potassium levels.
4. Explain the difference between serum creatinine concentrations in younger adults and older adults.
5. Explain the relationship between bacteria in urine and urinary tract infections (UTIs) in older adults.
6. Relate the significance of troponin levels to diagnosing cardiac emergencies.
7. Explain the relationship of the brain natriuretic peptide (BNP) to chronic heart failure (CHF).
8. Discuss the role of laboratory tests in determining thyroid function in older adults.
9. Describe the nurse's role in interpreting laboratory values in older adults.

WHAT WOULD YOU DO?

What would you do if you were faced with the following situations?

- An older adult patient had labs drawn during an office visit. The basic metabolic panel (BMP) returned with a potassium level of 3.2 and a sodium level of 138. What information would you tell the patient when you call her with the lab results?

- Your new admission to the nursing home, comes in with routine, baseline laboratory work, which includes a urinalysis (UA) that is nitrite negative, leukocyte esterase negative, and 80,000 colony-forming units (CFUs) per milliliter of bacteria. What would you do?

Aging is a progressive process that is along a continuum from 65 years of age to 100+ years. The aging process that leads to a decline or weakening in the body's physical structure varies among individuals. The greater the change in general health, the greater the association with a decline in function and vulnerability to illness and disease, as well as the potential for increased mortality (Harper et al, 2022). The gerontological nurse needs to consider the effect of laboratory and diagnostic testing on an older adult's overall health and well-being. For example, with aging, subcutaneous tissue is decreased, and the fragility of veins is increased. As a result, one may see that a frail older adult is more likely to have increased bruising and discomfort after a venous blood drawing.

It is also important for the nurse to have a basic understanding of commonly ordered tests, especially if a patient is anxious. Anxiety may range from concerns about the costs of tests, the blood draw procedure, the concern for privacy, to concerns about the test results. Commonly ordered laboratory and diagnostic tests evaluate selected hematologic blood and urine chemistry components of the body's overall function, with reference ranges for younger and older adults. These reference ranges may vary from institution to institution and in the literature (Table 13.1). Research on older adults has linked changes related to aging and disease when frailty occurs. Frailty is biologic cell dysfunction that leads to weakness, weight loss, neurodegeneration, poor endurance, and inflammation that sequentially triggers physical dysfunction, cognitive impairment (CI), and multiple chronic diseases, along with additional geriatric syndromes (Ferrucci and Walston, 2022). When interpreting laboratory values and deciding the best course of treatment, the older adult should be viewed holistically; signs, symptoms, and test results should all be considered, and decisions should not be made based only on laboratory results.

TABLE 13.1 Hematology Tests

Name	Adult Normal	Older Adult Normal	Significance of Deviations
Red blood cells (RBCs)	4.2–6.1 million/unit	Unchanged with aging	*Low:* hemorrhage, anemia, chronic illness, kidney failure, pernicious anemia (PA) *High:* high altitude, polycythemia (PV), dehydration
Hemoglobin	12–18 grams per deciliter (g/dL)	Values may be slightly decreased	*Low:* anemia, cancer, nutritional deficiency, kidney disease *High:* PV, heart failure (HF), chronic obstructive pulmonary disease (COPD), high altitudes, dehydration
Hematocrit	37%–52%	Values may be slightly decreased	*Low:* anemia, cirrhosis, hemorrhage, malnutrition, rheumatoid arthritis (RA) *High:* PV, severe dehydration, severe diarrhea, COPD
White blood cells (WBCs) (total)	5.0–10.0 thousands/cubic millimeter (mm^3)	Unchanged with aging	*Low:* drug toxicity, infections, autoimmune disease (AD), dietary deficiency *High:* infection, trauma, stress, inflammation
Neutrophils	55%–70%	Unchanged with aging	*Low:* dietary deficiency, overwhelming bacterial infections, viral infections, drug therapy *High:* physical and emotional stress, trauma, inflammatory disorders
Eosinophils	1%–4%	Unchanged with aging	*Low:* increased adrenosteroid production *High:* parasitic infections, allergic reactions, AIDs
Basophils	0.5%–1%	Unchanged with aging	*Low:* acute allergic reactions, stress reactions *High:* myeloproliferative disease (MPD)
Monocytes	2%–8%	Unchanged with aging	*Low:* drug therapy (predisposition) *High:* chronic inflammatory diseases, tuberculosis (TB), chronic ulcerative colitis (UC)
Lymphocytes	20%–40%	Unchanged with aging	*Low:* leukemia, sepsis, systemic lupus erythematosus (SLE), chemotherapy, radiation *High:* chronic bacterial infections, viral infections, radiation, infectious hepatitis
Folic acid	5–25 nanograms per milliliter (ng/mL)	Unchanged with aging	*Low:* malnutrition, folic acid anemia, hemolytic anemia, alcoholism, liver disease, chronic kidney disease (CKD) *High:* PA
Vitamin B$_{12}$	160–950 picograms per milliliter (pg/mL)	Unchanged with aging	*Low:* PA, inflammatory bowel disease (IBD), atrophic gastritis (AG), folic acid deficiency *High:* leukemia, PV, severe liver dysfunction
Total iron-binding capacity (TIBC)	250–460 micrograms per deciliter (mcg/dL)	Unchanged with aging	*Low:* hypoproteinemia, cirrhosis, autoimmune hemolytic anemia (AIHA), PA *High:* PV, iron-deficiency anemia (IDA)
Iron (Fe)	60–180 mcg/dL	Unchanged with aging	*Low:* insufficient dietary iron, chronic blood loss, inadequate absorption of iron *High:* hereditary hemochromocytosis (HH), AIHA, hepatitis, iron poisoning
Uric acid	4–8.5 mg/dL	May be slightly increased	*Low:* lead poisoning *High:* gout, increased ingestion of purines, CKD, hypothyroidism
Prothrombin time (PT)	11–12.5 seconds (sec)	Unchanged with aging	*High:* liver disease, vitamin K deficiency, warfarin ingestion, bile duct obstruction (BDO), salicylate intoxication
Partial thromboplastin time (PTT)	60–70 sec	Unchanged with aging	*Low:* early stages of disseminated intravascular coagulation (DIC), metastatic cancer *High:* coagulation factor deficiency (CFD), cirrhosis, vitamin K deficiency, heparin administration
D-dimer	<0.4 mcg/mL (<0.4 mg/L SI units)	Unchanged with aging	*High:* deep vein thrombosis (DVT), DIC, pulmonary embolism (PE), recent surgery, sepsis
Platelets	150,000–400,000/mm^3	Unchanged with aging	*Low:* hemorrhage, thrombocytopenia, SLE, PA, chemotherapy, infection *High:* malignancy, PV, RA, IDA

Data from Pagana, K. D., Pagana, T. J., & Pagana, T. N. (2019). *Mosby's diagnostic and laboratory test reference* (14th ed.). St. Louis: Elsevier.

HEMATOLOGIC TESTING

Hematopoiesis is the development of the blood cellular components to maintain a steady state in the peripheral circulation (Bertschi, 2021). Blood is composed of erythrocytes (red blood cells [RBCs]), leukocytes (white blood cells [WBCs]), and specialized cell fragments (platelets), within a fluid matrix called plasma. The test used to assess the blood components is the complete blood count (CBC). A CBC with differential may be ordered, which means the specifics of the WBCs, as well as the RBCs and platelets are also measured.

Red Blood Cells

RBCs, or erythrocytes, are non-nucleated biconcave disks that carry molecules of hemoglobin (Hb). Hb allows the transport and exchange of oxygen (O) and carbon dioxide (CO_2). The average lifespan of an erythrocyte is 120 days. Although aging does not affect the lifespan of an erythrocyte, replenishment after bleeding may be delayed because of a decrease in hematopoietic tissue occupying the marrow of the long bones (Bertschi, 2021).

RBCs are necessary for maintaining O and CO_2 transport. A reduction in the number of circulating RBCs, a decrease in the quality or quantity of Hb, a decrease in the volume of packed cells (hematocrit), or a combination of these factors is classified as anemia. Anemia may be attributed to (1) impaired erythrocyte production, (2) blood loss, (3) increased erythrocyte destruction, (4) dietary deficiency, (5) genetic disorders, or (6) a combination of these causes. Anemia is a clinical sign, not a disease process itself. Signs of anemia may go unnoticed if the anemia is mild, or the patient may experience overt symptoms such as fatigue, shortness of breath, and paresthesia. In older adults, common symptoms are falls, slower walking speed, decreased mobility, and even depression (Ershler et al, 2021). It is important to not ignore vague symptomatology and vague clinical presentation as an older adult's complaints of "old age" and fail to assess properly.

Other conditions involving erythrocytes are related to increased cell numbers and abnormalities in the cells themselves. Overproduction of RBCs is known as polycythemia (PV). This may occur secondarily because of hypoxia caused by COPD or HF. In sickle cell anemia (HbSS), the RBCs become abnormal in shape and surface composition because of a genetic defect in the Hb. Additional diagnostic testing is usually performed by a specialist.

White Blood Cells

WBCs, or leukocytes, are another type of cell present in blood. Their major function is defense against foreign substances. WBCs function mainly in the interstitial fluid. Leukocytes consist of neutrophils, lymphocytes, monocytes, eosinophils, and basophils. A decrease in leukocytes in older adults may be related to drugs or a severe infection. Drugs that may cause a decrease in leukocytes include antibiotics, anticonvulsants, antihistamines, antimetabolites, cytotoxic agents, analgesics, phenothiazines, and diuretics (Pagana et al, 2019).

An increase in leukocytes is generally seen in the presence of infections. However, a WBC count may be only moderately elevated in older adults when an infection, such as pneumonia, is present. Other typical symptoms of infection, such as fever, pain, and lymphadenopathy, may be minimal or absent in older adults with infections (Ershler et al, 2021). Consequently, the nurse must be alert for other signs and symptoms of infection, such as the sudden onset of confusion or lethargy. Pharmacologic agents have also been associated with an increase in leukocytes. These drugs include allopurinol, aspirin, heparin, steroids, and triamterene (Pagana et al, 2019).

Neutrophils, eosinophils, and basophils are produced in the bone marrow and possess similar structures of segmented nuclei and many membrane-bound granules. Their primary function is phagocytosis (i.e., ingesting and destroying invading microorganisms and cellular debris). In addition, the basophil's cytoplasmic granules contain powerful chemicals such as histamine, bradykinin, leukotrienes, and prostaglandins, which contribute to the activation of the inflammatory response (Bertschi, 2021). The monocyte, the largest of the leukocytes, is produced in bone marrow and differs in appearance from neutrophils, eosinophils, and basophils. The monocyte has a single nucleus and can destroy large bacterial organisms and virally infected cells by phagocytosis (Pagana et al, 2019).

Lymphocytes, the smallest of the leukocytes, are classified into 2 types: B- and T-Lymphocytes have large nuclei and relatively little cytoplasm. Originating in bone marrow and the thymus, lymphocytes are housed in the lymph nodes, spleen, and tonsils. Lymphocytes do not act as phagocytes but rather produce antibodies and other specific defenses against antigens (Pagana et al, 2019).

Aging does not appear to affect the function of neutrophils, although the ability of bone marrow to release and store these cells is reduced. Lymphocytes of older adults have shown impaired function in vitro and are suspected to be the cause of a reduction in antibody response in later life (Bertschi, 2021). It is suspected that there is a decline in monocyte function, given the increased susceptibility to infections and the increased incidence of malignancies in older adults. The remaining leukocytes, eosinophils, and basophils have shown no evidence of being affected by aging.

Leukocytes are necessary for the body's resistance and response to infections, cancers, and other foreign substances. The nursing implications regarding infections and malignancies include recognizing subtle and sometimes altered responses to infections and diseases in older adults. Educating older adults about the importance of participating in cancer screening programs and maintaining immunization status throughout life is essential.

Folic Acid

Folic acid is one of the 8 B vitamins that make up the B-complex group. Folic acid is a water-soluble vitamin that functions as a *coenzyme*, which means it is inactive unless linked to an enzyme. Folic acid is necessary for the normal functioning of RBCs and WBCs. A decrease in folic acid may indicate macrocytic anemia, thiamine-responsive megaloblastic anemia (TRMA), and liver and renal disease. Alcohol and various other drugs are known to interfere with the absorption of folate. Some drugs have also been shown to decrease folic acid levels. These include anticonvulsants, antimalarials, and methotrexate (Pagana et al, 2019). However, the effect of aging on folate is still debatable because of differences in defining the lower limits of "normal" and the different methods used to determine folate levels (Puga et al, 2021).

Because of the relationship between nutrition and alcohol consumption and folic acid levels, it is important for the gerontological nurse to assess nutritional intake, including alcohol consumption habits. Elevated levels of folic acid may be seen in people with PA who do not have an adequate amount of vitamin B_{12} to metabolize folic acid. Therefore, folic acid levels should be tested in conjunction with the assessment of vitamin B_{12} levels (Pagana et al, 2019).

Vitamin B_{12}

Vitamin B_{12}, or cobalamin, is a water-soluble vitamin that is part of the B-complex group of vitamins. Vitamin B_{12} deficiency is present in nearly a quarter of older adults. Common causes of deficiency include malabsorption secondary to gastric bypass (GB), pancreatic disease, ileocecal resection (ICR) or inflammation, and prolonged use of certain medications such as proton pump inhibitors (PPIs), colchicine, cholestyramine, histamine 2 (H_2) blockers, or metformin (MTF). Strict vegetarian or vegan diets may also lead to vitamin B_{12} deficiency (Puga et al, 2021). Malabsorption of vitamin B_{12} may be caused by the effect of antibodies on gastric parietal cell antibodies (GPCAbs) and a decrease in intrinsic factor, the underlying cause of PA. The prevalence of PA increases significantly with aging (Puga et al, 2021).

Vitamin B_{12} is important for normal erythrocyte maturation (Kehoe et al, 2019) and acts as a coenzyme with folic acid. The synthesis of nucleic acids, and therefore the structure of deoxyribonucleic acid (DNA), depends on adequate vitamin B_{12} intake (Mandaviya et al, 2019). Vitamin B_{12} deficiency may lead to demyelination of the dorsal and lateral spinal columns, which, in turn, may lead to paresthesia of the feet, disequilibrium, and loss of vibratory sensation in the fingers. Low vitamin B_{12} levels may also lead to fatigue, weakness, and memory loss.

Total Iron-Binding Capacity

Total iron-binding capacity (TIBC) measures the amount of iron and the amount of available transferrin in the serum (Ershler, 2019). Transferrin is a protein in the plasma that collects iron and transports it to the bone marrow for incorporation into Hb. Increased TIBC and transferrin levels may indicate iron-deficiency anemia (IDA), whereas their decreased levels may indicate anemia caused by chronic disease.

Iron

Iron is found in the Hb of the RBCs. When iron-containing foods are ingested, iron is absorbed by the small intestine and transported to the plasma (Pagana et al, 2019). Iron is necessary for controlling protein synthesis in the mitochondria and for generating energy in the cells (Bertschi, 2021). Serum iron levels show progressive decreases in both genders with advancing age, although the ability to absorb iron appears to remain intact (Ershler, 2019). IDA is the most common form of anemia seen in older adults. However, despite the decreases in serum iron levels seen with aging, anemia in older adults is not a normal consequence of aging. The gerontological nurse should assess older adults for poor dietary intake of iron-containing foods and occult or chronic blood loss (Kehoe et al, 2019).

Uric Acid

Uric acid is a product of purine catabolism and is excreted by the kidneys. Age-related changes in uric acid levels are significantly different between the genders. Because estrogen is thought to promote the excretion of uric acid, elevated levels are rarely seen in females before the onset of menopause (Yang and Cao, 2022). There is an age-related risk associated with elevated levels of uric acid greater than 4.8 mg/dL for mortality (Ungar et al, 2022).

Problems with uric acid may be a result of faulty excretion (e.g., kidney disease), overproduction of uric acid, or the presence of other substances that compete for excretion sites (e.g., ketoacids) (Pagana et al, 2019). Elevated uric acid levels are seen in patients with gout. Gout, a common condition in older adults, involves a disturbance in the body's control of uric acid production or excretion. Excess uric acid accumulates in the body's fluids, especially blood and synovial fluids, forming crystals in high concentrations. These crystals deposit in the connective tissue of the body, causing painful, inflamed joints. Thiazide diuretics, caffeine, low-dose aspirin, and antiparkinsonian drugs are also common causes of increased uric acid levels in older adults (Pagana et al, 2019).

Prothrombin Time

Prothrombin is a plasma protein that is converted to thrombin in the first step of the clotting cascade. Clotting is necessary to prevent the loss of vital body fluids that occurs when blood vessels rupture (Capecchi et al, 2021). In addition to measuring prothrombin time (PT), health-care professionals also measure the activity of fibrinogen and coagulation factors V, VII, and X. The results of the PT laboratory test reveal how effectively the vitamin K-dependent coagulation factors of the extrinsic and common pathways of the coagulation cascade are performing. An increased PT is seen in liver disease, vitamin K deficiency, bile duct obstruction (BDO), and salicylate intoxication. Some drugs, including allopurinol, cephalothins, cholestyramine, clofibrate, and certain antibiotics, may also cause an increase in a patient's PT. Digitalis and diphenhydramine may cause decreased PT levels (Pagana et al, 2019).

Older adults are often prescribed the drug warfarin after open-heart surgery and in cases of chronic atrial fibrillation (AFib). Warfarin interferes with the production of vitamin K-dependent coagulation factors, thereby decreasing the chance of thrombus formation. Warfarin may interact with many medications, especially those often taken by older adults (Pagana et al, 2019). Gerontological nurses should help patients understand the importance of keeping their appointments for PT checks and consulting their health-care providers before taking any over-the-counter (OTC) medications or supplements. Monitoring a patient's PT level can assess the adequacy of warfarin therapy. The PT value is traditionally reported in seconds and includes a value called the international normalized ratio (INR). INR is a mathematical "correction" of the results of the 1-stage PT and was created to standardize results caused by a variation in laboratory reagents. The INR should be between 2.0 and 3.0 for most thrombosis and embolus conditions, and between 3.0 and 4.0 for patients with a history of recurrent venous thromboembolism (VTE) or mechanical heart valves (Dorgalaleh et al, 2021) (see Nutritional Considerations box).

> **NUTRITIONAL CONSIDERATIONS**
>
> Vitamin K is used in emergency situations to counteract the increased coagulation times that sometimes occur when patients receive warfarin. The nurse should be aware that foods high in vitamin K may affect clotting times and counteract the prescribed therapy. Foods such as turnip greens, broccoli, cabbage, spinach, and liver, which are high in vitamin K, should be eaten in moderate amounts while receiving anticoagulant therapy.

Data from Leavitt, A. D., & Price, E. (2022). Disorders of hemostasis, thrombosis, & antithrombotic therapy. In M. A. Papadakis, S. J. McPhee, M. W. Rabow, & K. R. McQuaid (Eds.), *Current medical diagnosis & treatment 2022* (61st ed., pp. 548–581). New York: McGraw Hill.

Partial Thromboplastin Time

Partial thromboplastin time (PTT) refers to the measurement of the common pathway of clot formation. Heparin may inactivate prothrombin, so the PTT is a good indicator of the adequacy of anticoagulation therapy. The effect of heparin on the body is faster than that of warfarin, but the effects are shorter. Nursing considerations include monitoring for bleeding and correct administration of the heparin dosage (Capecchi et al, 2021).

D-dimer Test

A D-dimer is a fragment produced during the degradation of a clot. The D-dimer test may be ordered when a person has symptoms of thrombus, embolus, or disseminated intravascular coagulation (DIC). Results are interpreted when combined with clinical information and other laboratory data. Age, vascular disease, and kidney or hepatic disease may affect test results (Capecchi et al, 2021).

Erythrocyte Sedimentation Rate

The erythrocyte sedimentation rate (ESR) test measures the time that RBCs take to settle in normal saline over 1 hour. The measured values are reported in millimeters (mm). The test does not relate to one specific condition or disorder but does indicate the presence of inflammation, so it is useful in monitoring the course of inflammatory activity in autoimmune diseases (ADs), infections, and cancers. Elevated rates may indicate infections, inflammatory diseases, malignancies, renal disease, or tissue trauma. Further testing and physical assessment are needed for a diagnosis (Surana and Kasper, 2022).

C-Reactive Protein

C-reactive protein (CRP) is a marker present in the acute phase of an inflammatory response. CRP is useful in assessing patients with tissue injuries (e.g., myocardial infarction [MI]), ADs, or bacterial infections. CRP does not usually rise with viral infections (Pagana et al, 2019). CRP is used with other diagnostics to determine cause; this test is not used alone for treatment considerations (Cush, 2022).

Platelets

Platelets are small, irregular bodies, also known as *thrombocytes*, that are essential for clotting. They are formed in bone marrow and stored in the spleen. Vascular injury triggers platelet activation and aggregation, along with the activation of the coagulation system to stop the bleeding (Weitz, 2022).

Decreases in platelet counts (to less than 100,000 per cubic millimeter [mm^3]) require investigation. In a condition known as myelodysplastic syndrome (MDS), pancytopenia is noted in more than half the patients diagnosed. Pancytopenia is present when the levels of RBCs, WBCs, and platelets are all below normal. Most often, individuals diagnosed with MDS are older than 60. Treatment consists of managing symptoms, preventing infection and bleeding, and slowing disease progression. This condition has been known to progress to acute leukemia (Young, 2022). At platelet levels below 20,000/mm^3, the nurse should observe for spontaneous bleeding. If the patient's levels are 40,000/mm^3 or below, prolonged bleeding may occur after certain procedures (Pagana et al, 2019).

In assessing patients for potential or hidden blood losses, nurses have traditionally questioned patients about the color and consistency of their stools. The gerontological nurse, however, must recognize that older adults who take iron supplements have changes in bowel habits and stool color, which may not necessarily indicate the presence of occult blood. When preparing older adults for fecal occult blood testing, it is important to instruct them to stop iron supplements 3 days before testing.

COMPONENTS OF BLOOD CHEMISTRY TESTING

A basic metabolic panel (BMP) measures electrolytes, glucose, and kidney function. This test is most often used to make treatment decisions, such as the need for fluids (Katzman et al, 2020). A comprehensive metabolic panel (CMP) involves additional elements and is used to determine liver function or nutritional status. Current terminology labels for these chemical analyses may vary in name from institution to institution. Nurses should learn the terminology specific to their workplace and be able to identify the individual tests contained in each package.

Electrolytes

Electrolytes are inorganic substances that include acids, bases, and salts. In solutions, electrolytes break up to form positively or negatively charged particles known as ions. Positively charged ions are known as cations; negatively charged ions are called anions. Compounds formed from acids and bases are known as salts. Blood testing may include measurement of the amount of an electrolyte in the circulating blood (Mount, 2022). Although many types of electrolytes may be tested, only the most common are discussed here.

Older adults may have serious problems with electrolyte imbalance. Dehydration is the most common form of electrolyte disorder that occurs in older adults, and it is usually attributed to excess loss of water or altered fluid intake. Excess water loss may be caused by infections such as pneumonia and cystitis or by environmental conditions. Altered fluid intake may result from an age-related decrease in thirst sensation in older adults or a result of decreased functional ability that limits the intake of fluids (Mount, 2022).

Sodium

The test for sodium (Na^+) measures the amount of sodium in circulating blood and is an index of body water deficit or excess. Sodium regulation is important for the maintenance of blood pressure, the transmission of nerve impulses, and the regulation of body fluid levels in and out of the cells. This movement of sodium affects blood volume, which is tied to the thirst mechanism and total body fluids (Mount, 2022). Although sodium is also present in intracellular fluid, the majority resides in extracellular fluid, which makes it the major cation of extracellular fluid. Serum sodium levels describe the balance between ingested sodium and that excreted by the kidneys (Pagana et al, 2019). Aging changes in the kidney, such as a decreased glomerular filtration rate (GFR) and a decrease in the number of functioning nephrons, can mean that an older adult has difficulty maintaining homeostasis in the presence of sodium depletion or overload (Table 13.2). Because of the intrinsic loss in function, kidneys have a decreased renin–angiotensin–aldosterone response (RAAS) and may not respond appropriately; thus, further sodium losses may occur (Mount, 2022). A normal sodium level is necessary for maintaining the extracellular fluid balance (osmolarity).

The occurrence of hyponatremia (a low sodium level) increases with age. Most cases are related to the kidneys' inability to excrete free water because of decreased basal levels of renin and aldosterone. Vague symptoms such as malaise, confusion, headache, and nausea may also progress to coma and seizures. It is important, however, to determine whether an older adult has a low sodium level but normal osmolarity; this is known as hypertonic hyponatremia. In these cases, the osmolarity remains normal or high because of excess amounts of other osmolytes in the blood, such as glucose, triglycerides, or plasma proteins. By determining the underlying cause and providing appropriate treatment, the health-care provider can take steps to ensure the return of the sodium level to normal (Mount, 2022).

Gerontological nurses must understand the goal of treatment for patients with fluid and sodium disorders. In patients with fluid deficiencies, the nurse can help identify reasons for a given condition, for example, restrictions in mobility, visual disturbances, urinary incontinence, and swallowing disorders. Hypernatremia (a high sodium level) may be caused by the infusion of high-sodium solute fluids, excessive water loss, prolonged diarrhea and vomiting, and decreased oral intake. Hypernatremia is often seen in hospitalized older adults; some cases are present on admission, whereas others are the consequence of hospitalization. Symptoms are similar to those of hyponatremia, and the most common neurologic signs are those of lethargy and weakness, progressing to altered consciousness and coma. The pathophysiology behind the neurologic signs is thought to be neuronal cell dehydration (Robertson and Bichet, 2022).

Potassium

Potassium (K^+) is present in both the intracellular and extracellular fluids. Most potassium is found within the cell, and minute amounts are found in the extracellular fluid. This extracellular amount is measured by serum testing. Potassium imbalances in older adults are caused by the same changes in the renal system as those affecting sodium. Salt substitutes, used by many older adults with hypertension (HTN) or CHF, are high in potassium and should be used with caution. Many drugs, such as potassium-sparing diuretics, angiotensin-converting enzyme inhibitors (ACEIs), and angiotensin receptor blockers (ARBs), used in conjunction with potassium supplements may cause hyperkalemia in older adults (Mount, 2022). In addition, nonsteroidal anti-inflammatory drugs (NSAIDs) interfere with potassium excretion (Lim et al, 2021). Hypokalemia may be caused by gastrointestinal (GI) loss and the use of diuretics. Potassium imbalance may predispose older adults to tachyarrhythmias and potentiate digitalis toxicity (Mount, 2022). Because OTC drug use has increased, it is important for the gerontological nurse to carefully assess an older adult's prescriptions, OTC, and complementary and alternative drug history (see Emergency Treatment box).

> ### ✚ EMERGENCY TREATMENT
> ### *Abnormal Laboratory Values: Potassium*
>
> **Hypokalemia**
> - If asymptomatic, the test may be repeated before treatment:
>   - K^+ between 3 mEq/L and 3.5 mEq/L is seldom symptomatic
> - Monitor for neuromuscular and cardiac effects of hypokalemia:
>   - Skeletal muscle weakness
>   - Smooth muscle atony
>   - Dysrhythmias
> - Observe for signs of digitalis toxicity.
> - A maximum oral replacement is 40–80 mEq/day if renal function is normal.
> - The maximum safe rate for intravenous (IV) replacement is 20 mEq/hr.
>   - Maximal concentration of 40 mEq/100 mL should be used with an infusion pump
> - Repeat the K^+ level after replacement therapy and until values are normal.

Data from Mount, D. B. (2022). Fluid and electrolyte disturbances. In J. Loscalzo, A. Fauci, D. Kasper, S. Hauser, D. Longo, & J. Jameson (Eds.). *Harrison's principles of internal medicine* (21st edition). New York: McGraw Hill, pp 338-355.

Potassium, like sodium, maintains cell osmolarity, muscle function, and the transmission of nerve impulses, as well as regulating acid–base balance. Cardiac muscle is particularly sensitive to serum concentrations of potassium. Hyperkalemia may cause muscle twitching, arrhythmias, and GI symptoms (Mount, 2022). Hypokalemia may occur because of excessive loss of potassium through the GI tract, usually by vomiting. Symptoms include muscle weakness, confusion, and the absence of bowel sounds. When replacing potassium in older adults, the nurse must take care to prevent hyperkalemia.

TABLE 13.2 Blood Chemistry

Test Name	Adult Normal	Older Adult Normal	Significance of Deviation
Sodium	136–145 milliequivalents per liter (mEq/L)	Unchanged with aging	Low: decreased intake, diarrhea, vomiting, diuretic administration, CKD, CHF, peripheral edema, ascites High: increased intake, Cushing's syndrome, extensive thermal burns
Potassium	3.5–5 mEq/L	Unchanged with aging	Low: deficient intake, burns, diuretics, Cushing's syndrome, insulin administration, ascites High: excessive dietary intake, kidney failure, infection, acidosis, dehydration
Chloride	98–106 mEq/L	Unchanged with aging	Low: overhydration, CHF, vomiting, chronic gastric suction, chronic respiratory acidosis (CRA), hypokalemia, diuretic therapy High: dehydration, Cushing's syndrome, kidney dysfunction, metabolic acidosis, hyperventilation
Calcium	9–10.5 milligrams per deciliter (mg/dL)	Tends to stay the same or decrease	Low: kidney failure, vitamin D deficiency, osteomalacia, malabsorption High: Paget's disease of the bone (PDB), prolonged immobilization, lymphoma
Phosphorus	3–4.5 mg/dL	Slightly lower	Low: inadequate dietary ingestion, chronic antacid ingestion, hypercalcemia, alcoholism, osteomalacia, malnutrition High: kidney failure, increased dietary intake, hypocalcemia, liver disease
Magnesium	1.3–2.1 mEq/L	Decreases by 15% between the third and eighth decades	Low: malnutrition, malabsorption, alcoholism, CKD High: CKD, ingestion of magnesium-containing antacids or salts, hypothyroidism
Fasting glucose	70–105 mg/dL	Increase in the normal range after age 50	Low: hypothyroidism, liver disease, insulin overdose, starvation High: diabetes mellitus (DM), acute stress response, diuretic therapy, corticosteroid therapy
Amylase	60–120 Somogyi units/dL	Slightly increased in elderly	High: acute pancreatitis, perforated bowel, acute cholecystitis, diabetic ketoacidosis
Glycosylated hemoglobin (HbA$_{1c}$)	2.2%–4.8%	Unchanged with aging	Low: hemolytic anemia, CKD High: newly diagnosed diabetes, poorly controlled diabetes, nondiabetic hyperglycemia
Total protein	6.4–8.3 grams per deciliter (g/dL)	Unchanged with aging	Low: liver disease, malnutrition, ascites High: hemoconcentration
Albumin	3.5–5 g/dL	Decreases slightly with aging	Low: malnutrition, liver disease, overhydration High: dehydration
Blood urea nitrogen (BUN)	7–22 mg/dL	May be slightly higher	Low: liver failure, overhydration, malnutrition High: hypovolemia, dehydration, alimentary tube feeding, renal disease
Creatinine	0.7–1.5 mg/dL	A decrease in muscle mass may cause decreased values	Low: debilitation, decreased muscle mass High: reduced renal blood flow, diabetic neuropathy (DPN), urinary tract obstruction (UTO)
Creatinine clearance	87–107 milliliters per minute (mL/min)	Values decrease by 6.5 mL/min/decade of life due to a decline in glomerular filtration rate (GFR)	Low: CKD, CHF, cirrhosis High: high cardiac output syndromes
Cholesterol (total)	> 200 mg/dL	Increases until about middle age but decreases thereafter (or can increase abruptly in females)	Low: malabsorption, malnutrition, cholesterol-lowering medication, PA, liver disease, MI High: hypercholesteremia, hyperlipidemia, hypothyroidism, uncontrolled DM
High-density lipoprotein (HDL)	> 45 mg/dL	Unchanged with aging	Low: familial low HDL, liver disease, hypoproteinemia High: familial HDL lipoproteinemia, excessive exercise
Low-density lipoprotein (LDL)	60–180 mg/dL	Increases with aging after menopause	Low: hypolipoproteinemia High: hypothyroidism, alcohol consumption, chronic liver disease (CLD), Cushing's syndrome
Alkaline phosphatase	30–120 units/L	Slightly higher	Low: hypothyroidism, malnutrition, PA High: cirrhosis, healing fracture, Paget's disease
Aspartate transaminase (AST)	0–35 units/L	Values are slightly higher	Low: acute kidney injury (AKI), diabetic ketoacidosis (DKA), chronic kidney dialysis High: MI, hepatitis, cirrhosis, multiple traumas, AIHA
Creatine kinase (CK)	30–170 units/L	Unchanged with aging	High: diseases or injuries affecting heart muscle, skeletal muscle, and brain

Data from Pagana, K. D., Pagana, T. J., & Pagana, T. N. (2019). *Mosby's diagnostic and laboratory test reference* (14th ed.). St. Louis: Elsevier.

Chloride

Chloride (Cl⁻) is mostly present in the fluid outside the cell; it is the major anion in the extracellular fluid. Chloride is closely tied to sodium; losses and excesses in sodium affect chloride levels (Pagana et al, 2019). Chloride levels have not been shown to change with aging (see Table 13.2).

Calcium

The serum calcium (Ca^{++}) level measures only the amount of calcium in the blood, which is about 1% of the body's total calcium. Approximately 99% of the body's calcium is found in bones and teeth (Mount, 2022). Changes in calcium regulation occur with aging; however, due to homeostatic mechanisms within the body, there is no resultant alteration in serum calcium levels. The loss of calcium from bones maintains the normal calcium level in the blood, but the resulting bone loss secondary to calcium leaching may lead to osteoporosis (Lindsay and Samuels, 2022). Calcium is important in blood clotting, conduction of nerve impulses, enzyme activity, and especially muscle contraction and relaxation (Mount, 2022). Calcium levels measure free calcium as well as calcium that is protein-bound with albumin. Therefore, any change in albumin level also affects calcium (Pagana et al, 2019).

Calcium metabolism is one of the factors that determines phosphorus levels; an inverse relationship is present. A decrease in calcium may cause an increase in phosphorus, and vice versa. Parathyroid hormone (PTH) also affects phosphorus levels by affecting the resorption of phosphorus in the kidneys (Pagana et al, 2019). PTH acts on plasma membrane receptors of the nephrons of the kidneys to increase the resorption of calcium and decrease the resorption of phosphorus (Potts, Jr. and Jüppner, 2022).

Phosphorus

Phosphorus (phosphate) is a mineral found mostly in bones in combination with calcium. Phosphorus is generally well absorbed from the small intestine in the presence of vitamin D. Long-term use of antacids, which bind to phosphorus, may interfere with absorption. Additionally, the kidneys excrete excess phosphorus from the blood; in the setting of kidney disease, hyperphosphatemia may develop. Phosphorus plays an important role in the maintenance of homeostasis (as a component in DNA and ribonucleic acid [RNA]); the metabolism of fats, carbohydrates, and proteins; and the transfer of energy stored as adenosine triphosphate (ATP) (Bringhurst et al, 2022). In older adults, phosphorus levels are slightly lower in comparison with younger adults (see Table 13.2).

Magnesium

Magnesium plays a significant role in the enzymatic processes needed for energy production. The most important sites of function are muscles and nerves. Approximately one-half of the body's magnesium is contained in bones. With aging, GI absorption of magnesium decreases and excretion of magnesium by the kidneys increases; these changes, coupled with a lower dietary intake of magnesium, put the older adult at risk of hypomagnesemia (Bringhurst et al, 2022) (see Table 13.2).

TABLE 13.3 Diagnosis and Classification of Diabetes

	HbA$_{1c}$	Fasting Plasma Glucose	Oral Glucose Tolerance Test
Diabetes	≥ 6.5%	≥ 126 mg/dL	≥ 200 mg/dL
Prediabetes	5.7–6.4%	100–125 mg/dL	140–199 mg/dL
Normal	< 5.7%	< 100 mg/dL	< 140 mg/dL

HbA$_{1c}$, glycohemoglobin; *mg/dL*, milligrams per deciliter
Data from American Diabetes Association; Professional Practice Committee. (2022). Standards of Medical Care in Diabetes—2022. *Diabetes Care, 45*(Supplement 1), S3.

Glucose

Glucose is used for energy by the cells. Blood glucose tests are evaluated on the basis of the time the blood was drawn and the duration of fasting. The American Diabetes Association (ADA) updated diabetes management guidelines in 2022 (Table 13.3).

In addition to patient symptoms, the 4 methods of diagnosing diabetes are as follows:

1. *Fasting plasma glucose (FPG).* Blood is drawn after fasting for 8 hours. A fasting plasma ≥126 mg/dL is indicative of diabetes.
2. *Oral glucose tolerance test (OGTT).* A person fasts for at least 8 hours; then, 2 hours after the person drinks a liquid containing 75 grams of glucose dissolved in water, blood sugar is tested. This test is typically used to diagnose gestational diabetes; a 2-hour plasma glucose ≥ 200 mg/dL is indicative of diabetes.
3. *Glycohemoglobin (hemoglobin A$_{1c}$; HbA$_{1c}$).* This is a blood test that checks the amount of glucose bound to Hb. A test is used to diagnose diabetes and monitor therapy. It provides an average of blood glucose levels over the previous 2–3 months. An A$_{1c}$ ≥ 6.5% is indicative of diabetes.
4. *Random blood sugar.* This test measures blood glucose without fasting. A random glucose measurement ≥200 mg/dL, combined with symptoms of hyperglycemia, is indicative of diabetes.

The American Diabetes Association (2022) recommends screening for prediabetes and type 2 diabetes mellitus (T2DM) starting at age 35 years. This should not preclude screening older adults. Glucose metabolism alters with aging; older adults develop reduced insulin effectiveness and islet cell dysfunction. This results in a higher incidence of diabetes in older adults. In older adults with diabetes, hypoglycemia is harder to recognize. Neurologic symptoms of hypoglycemia (e.g., dizziness and visual disturbances) are more common than autonomic symptoms (e.g., palpitations and sweating) (Hernandez et al, 2019).

Amylase

Amylase is an important enzyme in the catabolism of carbohydrates in the intestine. The acinar units of the pancreas produce it. Amylase levels are tested to aid in the diagnosis and management of pancreatitis and other pancreatic diseases. Elevated levels may occur secondary to damage to or disease of the pancreas or obstruction of the pancreatic duct. Elevated amylase levels may also be seen in nonpancreatic disorders such as perforated ulcers, perforated or necrotic bowel, or those secondary to medications. Decreased amylase levels may be found with chronic pancreatitis, pancreatic insufficiency, or cystic fibrosis (CF) (Pagana et al, 2019) (see Table 13.2).

Total Protein

Protein makes up a significant portion of colloidal osmotic pressure (COP). Protein is also a major component in muscle, enzymes, hormones, transport vehicles, and Hb. Total protein testing measures the amount of albumin and globulin in the plasma. This test is performed to identify nutritional problems (Pagana et al, 2019).

Albumin and Prealbumin

Serum albumin levels are used to monitor nutritional status and liver and kidney disease. Albumin levels decrease with age. Low albumin levels (<3.5 grams per deciliter [g/dL]) have been associated with increased mortality in hospitalized patients (Akirov et al, 2017). Additionally, when albumin is insufficient to sustain sufficient COP to counterbalance hydrostatic pressure, edema develops. Low albumin levels are also associated with chronic diseases, including diabetes, hyperthyroidism, and CHF. Finally, low levels of albumin are found in patients with burns, CHF, acute infections, and thyrotoxicosis. High albumin levels are associated with blood loss and dehydration (Hoffer et al, 2022).

Prealbumin and hypoalbuminemia indicate systemic inflammation, which leads to muscle catabolism and anorexia (Hoffer et al, 2022). It is a measurement of protein status over the short term and is a more accurate measurement of malnutrition because of its short half-life of 1.9 days. Plasma prealbumin levels are useful in monitoring therapy with total parenteral nutrition (Pagana et al, 2019).

Blood Urea Nitrogen

The measurement of urea in blood is known as the blood urea nitrogen (BUN) test. Urea is a major waste product of protein catabolism and a result of ammonia conversion in the liver. Urea is excreted from the body by the kidneys. BUN levels are indicative of both liver and kidney function. Values for older males are slightly higher than the adult normal levels of 7–22 milligrams per deciliter (mg/dL). In older females, BUN levels are also increased, but less than in older males (Pagana et al, 2019) (see Table 13.2).

Creatinine

Creatinine is another end-product of protein metabolism. A rise in a patient's BUN and creatinine levels is indicative of kidney disease. The physiologic decline in the GFR in older adults is not generally accompanied by a rise in the creatinine level secondary to a decrease in muscle mass with aging. Therefore, the creatinine level in an older adult should not be considered an independent indicator of renal function as it would be in a younger individual. It should, instead, be used to calculate the creatinine clearance for a more realistic indication of renal function in older adults (Pagana et al, 2019).

Creatinine Clearance

Creatinine clearance is the measure of the GFR, estimated from serum creatinine (SCr) and urine creatinine levels. A 24-hour urine test is required along with a serum level within the same 24-hour period. To allow for changes with aging that are not reflected in the creatinine level, many primary care providers use the Cockcroft and Gault formula to estimate creatinine clearance:

Creatinine clearance (milliliters per minute [mL/min])

$$= \frac{140 - \text{Age (in years)} \times \text{Weight (in kilograms [kg])}}{72 \times \text{Serum creatinine (\%mg/dL)}}$$

(For females, multiply the result by 0.85.)

An alternative method of calculating creatinine clearance is the Modification of Diet in Renal Disease (MDRD) formula:

$$\text{MDRD} - \text{GFR} = 186(\text{SCr})^{1.154} \times (\text{age})^{0.203}(0.742 \text{ if female})(1.210 \text{ if Black})$$

Neither method of calculating GFR is without variation; however, the MDRD is currently the method of choice. The gerontological nurse should recognize the importance of creatinine clearance as a reflection of an older adult's overall health status. Creatinine clearance decreases an average of 6.5 mL/min each decade of life after age 20. The older adult's response to medications, especially newly prescribed drugs, should be monitored because impaired renal function may precipitate side effects that could otherwise be overlooked (Pagana et al, 2019).

Triglycerides

Triglycerides are the principal lipids found in circulating blood bound to a protein; they are transported by low-density lipoproteins (LDLs) and very-low-density lipoproteins (VLDLs). Triglycerides are produced in the liver from glycerol and fatty acids found in the blood. When the triglyceride level in the blood reaches its peak, the excess is deposited in the fatty tissue for later release as energy between meals (Pagana et al, 2019).

Total Cholesterol

Cholesterol is a steroid compound that helps stabilize the membranes of the body's cells. It is also the major lipid associated with cardiovascular disease (CVD). The liver metabolizes cholesterol and binds it to LDLs and high-density lipoproteins (HDLs) for transport in the bloodstream (Pagana et al, 2019). Total cholesterol levels are a combination of LDL and HDL levels in the bloodstream. The National Cholesterol Education Program (NCEP) recommends that total cholesterol levels be kept at less than 200 mg/dL. However, it is important to evaluate cholesterol in relation to HDL, LDL, and triglyceride levels, not in isolation.

High-Density Lipoprotein

HDL, referred to as "good cholesterol," carries greater amounts of protein and lesser amounts of lipids, hence the term *high density*. HDL's role is to take cholesterol to the liver for degradation. A high HDL level (>60 mg/dL) is considered healthy; it is protective against heart disease (Pagana et al, 2019).

Low-Density Lipoprotein

LDL, referred to as "bad cholesterol," carries cholesterol from the liver to the body. The LDL level is calculated from the total cholesterol level, HDL level, and fasting triglycerides with the use of the following equation:

$$\text{LDL cholesterol} = \text{Total cholesterol} - \text{HDL cholesterol} - (\text{Triglyceride level} \div 5)$$

Patients with established heart disease and another risk factor such as smoking are recommended to have the LDL cholesterol level at less than 70 mg/dL. Those at high risk but without established disease are recommended to have their LDL level at less than 100 mg/dL. Patients considered at moderate risk for heart disease should maintain the LDL level at less than 130 mg/dL, and those at low risk for heart disease should have the LDL level at less than 160 mg/dL (Pagana et al, 2019).

Brain Natriuretic Peptide

The brain natriuretic peptide (BNP) is a neurohormone secreted from the cardiac ventricles in response to ventricular stretching and pressure overloading. This test helps diagnose and treat patients with CHF. Studies have shown that an elevated BNP level is highly sensitive and specific for the diagnosis of CHF. Plasma levels of BNP are significantly elevated in patients with CHF and left ventricular dysfunction (LVD); however, the values cannot be used to differentiate between systolic and diastolic CHF. Additionally, the BNP cannot be used to monitor CHF (Pagana et al, 2019).

Alkaline Phosphatase

Alkaline phosphatase (ALP) is an enzyme found in many tissues, although it has its highest concentrations in the liver and bone. Testing for ALP is used to identify liver and bone disorders. Testing of the ALP level in older adults is often used in the biochemical assessment of Paget's disease and other bone diseases (Pagana et al, 2019) (see Table 13.2).

Aspartate Aminotransferase

Aspartate transaminase (AST) measures the enzyme of the same name, which is found in muscles and in the liver and kidneys. It is primarily used to diagnose liver disease. A threefold to fivefold increase in AST may be indicative of hepatotoxicity from drugs such as isoniazid, rifampin, ethambutol, and pyrazinamide (Pagana et al, 2019).

Creatine Kinase

Creatine kinase found in brain tissue (CK-BB) is present in cardiac and skeletal muscles, the brain, and the lungs. CK-BB is primarily found in the lungs and brain, whereas CK found in the heart muscle (CK-MB) is associated with cardiac muscle cells. CK found in the muscle (CK-MM) is normally found in circulating blood, and the level rises with damage to skeletal muscle. CK levels rise and peak at specific intervals during MI, and these levels may be used to determine the amount of myocardial damage; however, this test has largely been replaced by troponin. CK may also be ordered when a person has experienced physical trauma, such as crushing injuries or extensive burns, or to diagnose rhabdomyolysis (Pagana et al, 2019).

Lactate Dehydrogenase

Lactate dehydrogenase (LDH) is an enzyme found in the muscles, brain, liver, kidneys, and RBCs. LDH may be isolated into 5 isoenzymes. These isoenzymes help clarify the site of release of the LDH and assist the nurse in assessing and monitoring specific complications related to the site of injury. Patterns of LDH elevation can be used to monitor injuries to the heart, lungs, and liver (Pagana et al, 2019).

Troponin

The troponin test measures the levels of certain proteins in the blood that are released when cardiac muscle has been damaged. Troponins (troponin I or troponin T) are the preferred tests for a suspected heart attack because they are more specific for detecting heart injury compared with other tests. These indices appear 2–8 hours after a decrease in the oxygenation of cardiac muscle caused by occlusion of the cardiac vessels. Levels may remain elevated up to 2 weeks after an MI. This test may also be ordered when a patient has worsening angina or acute coronary syndrome (ACS) without ST elevation (Pagana et al, 2019).

Thyroid Function Tests

Testing of thyroid function includes the assessment of two hormones secreted by the thyroid gland: thyroxine (T_4) and triiodothyronine (T_3). Thyroid function tests (TFTs) are a means of screening for hypothyroidism or hyperthyroidism and for monitoring the effectiveness of thyroid suppression or hormone replacement therapy (HRT). T_4 and T_3 are generally elevated in hyperthyroidism and decreased in hypothyroidism. Thyroid-stimulating hormone (TSH), a hormone secreted by the pituitary gland, is also usually tested when thyroid function is investigated; TSH is elevated in hypothyroidism and decreased in hyperthyroidism (Table 13.4). Higher-than-normal TSH levels are most often caused by an underactive thyroid gland (hypothyroidism), which may result from AD, treatment for hyperthyroidism,

TABLE 13.4 Thyroid Testing

Test Name	Adult Normal	Older Adult Normal	Significance of Deviations
Thyroxine (T_4)	4–12 micrograms per deciliter (mcg/dL)	Slightly decreased	Low: hypothyroidism, malnutrition, kidney failure, cirrhosis High: hyperthyroidism, hepatitis
Triiodothyronine (T_3)	75–220 nanograms per deciliter (ng/dL)	Slightly decreased	Low: hypothyroidism, pituitary insufficiency, protein malnutrition, kidney failure, liver diseases High: hyperthyroidism, hepatitis, hypoproteinemia
Thyroid-stimulating hormone (TSH)	2–10 microunits/mL	Unchanged with aging	Low: pituitary dysfunction, hyperthyroidism High: primary hypothyroidism

Data from Pagana, K. D., Pagana, T. J., & Pagana, T. N. (2019). *Mosby's diagnostic and laboratory test reference* (14th ed.). St. Louis: Elsevier.

radiation therapy or thyroid surgery, or certain medications (e.g., lithium). Lower-than-normal levels may be caused by an overactive thyroid gland (hyperthyroidism), which may result from Graves' disease, toxic nodular goiter, thyroiditis, or certain drugs (e.g., glucocorticoids and opioids) (Pagana et al, 2019).

Prostate-Specific Antigen

The prostate-specific antigen (PSA) test measures the amount of PSA, a protein produced in the prostate and found in the blood. High levels of PSA may indicate the presence of prostate cancer. However, other conditions, such as an enlarged or inflamed prostate, may also cause an increase in PSA levels. Before any prostate screening is initiated, the gerontological nurse needs to ensure that the patient understands the risks and benefits associated with the results: Would the diagnosis and treatment of prostate cancer improve or worsen the person's QoL? Would he want treatment in the event that cancer was found? The risk of prostate screening may outweigh the benefit for males age 75 and older, including those with less than 10 years' life expectancy (Pagana et al, 2019).

URINALYSIS

Urinalysis (UA) includes testing for the presence of protein, glucose, bacteria, blood, ketones, and leukocytes in the urine (Pagana et al, 2019). It also involves studying the sample for properties of specific gravity and the potential of hydrogen (pH). Urine is a waste product formed by the kidneys and consists of 95% water. The composition of urine may inform a health-care professional of the status of many body systems. When blood passes through the kidneys, water, nitrogen compounds, toxins, and electrolytes are filtered, reabsorbed, and secreted. The amounts retained or excreted affect the body's homeostasis.

Protein

Protein in urine (proteinuria) is considered an abnormal finding and indicates damage to the kidneys' glomeruli (Table 13.5). Its presence warrants further investigation to determine the presence of kidney disease, amyloidosis, or multiple myeloma (MM) (Pagana et al, 2019).

Glucose

Normally, glucose is not present in urine. When the blood sugar levels exceed 180 mg/dL, the kidneys release some of the excess glucose from the blood into the urine. Glucose may also be found in urine when the kidneys are damaged or diseased (Pagana et al, 2019).

Bacteria

Although occasional trace amounts of bacteria (bacteriuria) may normally appear in urine, significant amounts, defined as greater than 100,000 colony forming units (CFUs) per milliliter of urine, indicate infection. The gerontological nurse should assess older adults for symptoms of urinary incontinence, flank pain, fever, voiding frequency, burning, and suprapubic or low back pain (LBP). However, common symptoms may be absent in most older adults, and symptoms such as confusion, the new onset of incontinence, lethargy, nocturia, and anorexia may be the first indication of an underlying UTI. Females are more prone to lower UTIs compared with males because of the shorter urethra and its proximity to the vagina and anus. Significant numbers of older adults are asymptomatic, even when bacteria are found in urine (Perry and Landi, 2022).

TABLE 13.5 Urine Chemistry

Test Name	Adult Normal	Older Adult Normal	Significance of Deviations
Color	Yellow or amber	Same	Straw-colored urine indicates dilution
Appearance	Clear	Same	Cloudy urine may indicate the presence of pus, casts, blood, and bacteria
Specific gravity	1.005–1.030	Values decrease with aging	*Low:* overhydration, kidney failure, diuresis, hypothermia *High:* dehydration, water restriction, vomiting, diarrhea
Potential of hydrogen (pH)	4.6–8.0	Same	*Acidic urine:* diarrhea, metabolic acidosis, DM, respiratory acidosis, emphysema *Alkaline urine:* respiratory alkalosis, metabolic alkalosis, vomiting, gastric suctioning, diuretic therapy, urinary tract infection (UTI)
Protein	1–8 milligrams per milliliter (mg/mL)	Same	*Positive:* DM, CHF, SLE, malignant HTN
Glucose	Negative	Same	*Positive:* DM, Cushing's syndrome, severe stress, infection, drug therapy
Ketones	Negative	Same	*Positive:* uncontrolled DM, starvation, excessive aspirin ingestion, high-protein diet, dehydration
Blood	Negative	Same	*Positive:* kidney trauma, kidney stones, cystitis, prostatitis
Leukocyte esterase	Negative	Same	*Positive:* possible UTI
Bacteria	Negative	May be seen in older adults without symptoms; evaluate for pyuria and symptoms	*Positive:* UTI

Data from Pagana, K. D., Pagana, T. J., & Pagana, T. N. (2019). *Mosby's diagnostic and laboratory test reference* (14th ed.). St Louis: Elsevier.

Leukocyte Esterase

The presence of leukocytes in urine (pyuria) is more indicative of UTI, and a positive leukocyte esterase indicates the need for microscopic examination, urine culture, and sensitivity testing (Pagana et al, 2019).

Nitrites

The nitrite test is used, in conjunction with leukocyte esterase, in the diagnosis of UTI. Nitrites occur when certain bacteria (e.g., *Escherichia coli*, Proteus spp., and *Klebsiella pneumoniae*) produce the enzyme reductase, which converts urinary nitrates to nitrites. If the test is positive, a urine culture should be obtained (Pagana et al, 2019).

Ketones

The presence of ketones, the result of fatty acid breakdown, in urine is another abnormal finding. When overaccumulation of ketones occurs in the blood, the excess is excreted in urine. Causes of ketones in urine include diabetic ketoacidosis, a low-carbohydrate diet, starvation or fasting, and severe vomiting (Pagana et al, 2019).

pH

The pH of the urine sample indicates the acid or base value of the urine, which reflects the body's homeostatic state. The normal range for urine pH is 4.6–8.0. Drugs that increase urine pH include acetazolamide, potassium citrate, and sodium bicarbonate; drugs that may decrease urine pH include ammonium chloride, thiazide diuretics, and methenamine. Urine pH can be helpful in the identification of renal calculi, which are acid or base in origin, depending on the underlying substances that form the stones: acidic urine is associated with xanthine, cystine, uric acid, and calcium oxalate stones; and alkaline urine is associated with calcium carbonate, calcium phosphate, and magnesium phosphate stones. Prevention and treatment of calculi are aimed at changing the urine to the reverse pH of the stone's composition (Pagana et al, 2019).

Blood

The presence of blood in the urine (hematuria) is always an abnormal finding. The cause may be renal obstruction from calculi, trauma to the kidneys, inflammation, infection, or malignancy. Blood may be grossly apparent or occult, giving urine a cloudy or pink hue on visual inspection (Pagana et al, 2019).

COMPONENTS OF ARTERIAL BLOOD GAS TESTING

Arterial blood gas (ABG) testing involves drawing a sample of blood from an artery, usually from the radial or brachial artery. Components of ABG testing are pH, oxygen, and (CO_2) content; oxygen saturation; and bicarbonate level (Table 13.6). It is important that the health-care provider and laboratory personnel be aware of supplemental oxygenation at the time of blood draw (i.e., the type of air being breathed [room air or other], the amount of oxygen support, and the type of oxygen delivery device). Pulse oximetry is a reliable alternative to ABG testing when the percentage of oxygen saturation in the blood needs to be determined. The use of pulse oximetry is less painful and less expensive, and results are immediately available (Pagana et al, 2019).

Partial Pressure of Oxygen

Age-related changes such as a decrease in chest wall recoil, a decrease in alveolar surface area, and less effective oxygen (O_2)-to-CO_2 exchange all contribute to potential changes in oxygenation with aging. In the absence of disease, however, respiratory function remains adequate in older adults. Partial pressure of oxygen (PaO_2) indirectly measures arterial oxygen content. It can be used to monitor the effectiveness of oxygen therapy (Pagana et al, 2019).

pH of the Blood

pH measures the hydrogen ion (H^-) concentration in the bloodstream. A pH of less than 7.0 is called *acid pH*, and a pH greater than 7.0 is called *basic pH* (alkaline) (Naureckas and Solway, 2022). pH is influenced by vomiting, diarrhea, lung function, endocrine function, and kidney function (see Table 13.6).

Bicarbonate

Carbon dioxide (CO_2) in blood exists in the form of bicarbonate (HCO_3^-); therefore, the CO_2 blood test really is a measure of blood bicarbonate level. The HCO_3^- test is used to monitor conditions that affect blood bicarbonate levels, including kidney diseases, lung diseases, and metabolic conditions. The normal adult range is 21–28 mEq/L (Naureckas and Solway, 2022).

TABLE 13.6 Arterial Blood Gases

Test Name	Adult Normal	Older Adult Normal	Significance of Deviations
pH	7.35–7.45	Same	*Low:* respiratory or metabolic acidosis *High:* respiratory or metabolic alkalosis
PaO_2	80–100 mm Hg	Decreases 25% between 30 and 80 years old	*Low:* cardiac or respiratory disease
$PaCO_2$	35–45 mm Hg	Same	*Low:* respiratory alkalosis *High:* respiratory acidosis
O_2 saturation	95%–100%	95%	*Low:* impaired gas exchange
HCO_3^-	21–28 mEq/L	Same	*Low:* metabolic acidosis *High:* metabolic acidosis

HCO_3-, bicarbonate; *mEq/L*, milliequivalents per liter; *mm Hg*, millimeters of mercury; $PaCO_2$, partial pressure of arterial carbon dioxide; PaO_2, partial pressure of arterial oxygen.
Data from Pagana, K. D., Pagana, T. J., & Pagana, T. N. (2019). *Mosby's diagnostic and laboratory test reference* (14th ed.). St Louis: Elsevier.

> **EVIDENCE-BASED PRACTICE**
> *Reducing the Treatment of Asymptomatic Bacteriuria*
>
> **Background**
> As many as 25% to 50% of older females and 15% to 40% of older males who are asymptomatic and residing in long-term care (LTC) facilities have bacteria in their urine when tested. Bacteria in urine are rare in the younger population but increase in adults after the age of 60. Causes range from urinary and fecal incontinence to declining cell-mediated immunity. In patients with diabetes, there is also glucosuria. Asymptomatic bacteria is the presence of a significant quantity of bacteria without the physiologic symptoms. There are challenges about whether or not treat.
>
> **Sample / Setting**
> Zalmanovici et al. (2015) conducted a systematic review of all randomized control and quasi-random control trials evaluating the effectiveness of antibiotics for the treatment of UTIs.
>
> **Methods**
> The study participants were 18 years of age or older and were outpatient or institutionalized. Studies that included antibiotic treatment, placebo, or no treatment were included. Excluded were pregnant females, patients with catheters, or those who had received any urologic surgery. There were older adults in geriatric facilities. The process for the systematic review involved searching multiple databases, reviewing abstracts, selecting studies to review, and then analyzing the studies for bias. Measurements of the combined results were analyzed to evaluate the validity of the results.
>
> **Findings**
> Out of 340 studies, 9 studies with 1614 participants were selected that met the criteria. The results indicated no evidence of clinical benefit from treating asymptomatic bacteriuria. For the symptomatic UTIs, there was no development of complications from the antibiotics used for treatment, and the bacteria were cleared. These findings did not include any patients diagnosed with sepsis.
>
> **Implications**
> Treating asymptomatic bacteria is not recommended; however, patients should be assessed (recognize cues) often for any potential symptoms with planning care (generating solutions) for urinary and fecal incontinence as well as any other possible contributing factors.

Data from Zalmanovici Trestioreanu, A., Lador, A., Sauerbrun-Cutler, M. T., & Leibovici, L. (2015). Antibiotics for asymptomatic bacteriuria. *Cochrane Database of Systematic Reviews, 4*(4), CD009534.

Oxygen Saturation

Oxygen saturation (O_2 sat %) measures how much of the Hb in the RBCs carries oxygen. The normal adult value for oxygen saturation is greater than 95%. Levels below 90% are low. Conditions affecting lung function (e.g., pneumonia, COPD) alter oxygen saturation (Naureckas and Solway, 2022).

THERAPEUTIC DRUG MONITORING

Therapeutic drug monitoring measures the blood level of certain drugs at specified intervals to monitor the therapeutic drug concentration. Individuals absorb, metabolize, and excrete drugs at different rates based upon their age, gender, diet, general state of health, genetic makeup, and other drugs they are taking. Therapeutic drug monitoring is typically used with drugs that have a narrow therapeutic index, which is a small difference in the drug plasma level between therapeutic and toxic levels (Nicoll and Lu, 2017). Examples include theophylline, valproic acid, and phenytoin. Drug monitoring is performed in older adults receiving antibiotics (e.g., aminoglycosides and glycopeptides).

SUMMARY

In providing age-specific and age-appropriate health care, gerontological nurses must recognize that individuals do not respond in the same way to similar experiences. Although many laboratory values compensate for age-related changes in older adults, an older adult must be considered within the total context of a person with unique responses to diseases. Laboratory tests and their results should be considered an adjunct to the detection and treatment of illness, not in isolation from the presenting clinical picture.

KEY POINTS

- The ESR rises approximately 10 mm–20 mm in older adults; this is considered a normal age-related change.
- Potassium-sparing diuretics and NSAIDs may interfere with potassium excretion.
- Older adults may have hyponatremia in the presence of normal osmolarity, indicating the presence of other osmolarities in excess in the blood.
- Renal and hepatic system functioning may be reflected in the BUN level.
- Hypokalemia may potentiate digitalis toxicity in older adults.
- Comparable serum creatinine levels in younger adults and older adults are not indicators of comparable kidney function.
- Urine testing for glucose in older adults is considered unreliable in view of age-related changes in renal function.
- Thyroid disease may be present in older adults without the overt symptoms typically seen in younger adults with thyroid disorders.

- Older adults may be asymptomatic in the presence of bacteriuria.
- Pyuria is more indicative of a symptomatic UTI than the presence of bacteria in the urine of older adults.
- The "normal" oxygen saturation in older adults may be 95% or greater in arterial blood.

CLINICAL JUDGMENT EXERCISES

1. When evaluating the laboratory data for a 73-year-old male, you note that his HDL is 60 and his LDL is 140. He has a history of coronary artery disease (CAD). What conclusion, if any, can be drawn from these findings? Should the data be reported to the physician?
2. You are making home visits to an 82-year-old female recently discharged from the hospital, and she reports feeling tired, cold, and light-headed when standing. The daughter reports that she is only eating soup and tomato sandwiches. A CBC laboratory result came in this morning. What labs and drug prescriptions would you assess (recognize cues) and analyze (analyze cues) to correlate to the symptoms for reporting to the physician?

REFERENCES

Akirov, A., Masri-Iraqi, H., Atamna, A., & Shimon, I. (2017). Low albumin levels are associated with mortality risk in hospitalized patients. *American Journal of Medicine*, 130(12), 1465.e11–1465.e19. doi:10.1016/j.amjmed.2017.07.020.

American Diabetes Association, & Professional Practice Committee. (2022). Standards of Medical Care in Diabetes—2022. *Diabetes Care*, 45(Suppl. 1), S3. doi:10.2337/dc22-Sppc.

Bertschi, L. A. (2021). CE: Back to basics: The complete blood count. *The American Journal of Nursing*, 121(1), 38–45. doi:10.1097/01.NAJ.0000731656.00453.12.

Bringhurst, F., Kronenberg, H. M., & Liu, E. S. (2022). Bone and mineral metabolism in health and disease. In J. Loscalzo, A. Fauci, D. Kasper, S. Hauser, D. Longo, & J. Jameson (Eds.), *Harrison's principles of internal medicine* (21st ed., pp. 3157–3168). New York: McGraw Hill.

Capecchi, M., Scalambrino, E., Griffini, S., Grovetti, E., Clerici, M., Merati, G., et al. (2021). Relationship between thrombin generation parameters and prothrombin fragment 1 + 2 plasma levels. *International Journal of Laboratory Hematology*, 43(5), e248–e251. doi:10.1111/ijlh.13462.

Cush, J. J. (2022). Approach to articular and musculoskeletal disorders. In J. Loscalzo, A. Fauci, D. Kasper, S. Hauser, D. Longo, & J. Jameson (Eds.), *Harrison's principles of internal medicine* (21st ed., pp. 2844–2853). New York: McGraw Hill.

Dorgalaleh, A., Favaloro, E. J., Bahraini, M., & Rad, F. (2021). Standardization of prothrombin time/international normalized ratio (PT/INR). *International Journal of Laboratory Hematology*, 43(1), 21–28. doi:10.1111/ijlh.13349.

Ershler, W. B. (2019). Unexplained anemia in the elderly. *Clinics in Geriatric Medicine*, 35(3), 295–305. doi:10.1016/j.cger.2019.03.002.

Ershler, W. B., Groarke, E. M., & Young, N. S. (2021). Hematology in older persons. In K. Kaushansky, M. A. Lichtman, J. T. Prchal, M. Levi, L. J. Burns, & D. C. Linch (Eds.), *Williams hematology* (10th ed., pp. 121–136). New York: McGraw Hill.

Ferrucci, L., & Walston, J. D. (2022). Frailty. In J. B. Halter, J. G. Ouslander, S. Studenski, K. P. High, S. Asthana, M. A. Supiano, et al. (Eds.), *Hazzard's geriatric medicine and gerontology* (8th ed., pp. 615–632). New York: McGraw Hill.

Harper, G. M., Witt, L. J., & Landefeld, C. S. (2022). Geriatric disorders. In M. A. Papadakis, S. J. McPhee, M. W. Rabow, & K. R. McQuaid (Eds.), *Current medical diagnosis & treatment 2022* (61st ed., pp. 51–67). New York: McGraw Hill.

Hernandez, L., Leutwyler, H., Cataldo, J., Kanaya, A., Swislocki, A., & Chesla, C. (2019). Symptom experience of older adults with type 2 diabetes and diabetes-related distress. *Nursing Research*, 68(5), 374–382. doi:10.1097/NNR.0000000000000370.

Hoffer, L., Bistrian, B. R., & Driscoll, D. F. (2022). Enteral and parenteral nutrition. In J. Loscalzo, A. Fauci, D. Kasper, S. Hauser, D. Longo, & J. Jameson (Eds.), *Harrison's principles of internal medicine* (21st ed., pp. 2539–2545). New York: McGraw Hill.

Katzman, B. M., Bryant, S. C., & Karon, B. S. (2020). Is it time to remove total calcium from the basic and comprehensive metabolic panels? Assessing the effects of American Medical Association—approved chemical test panels on laboratory utilization. *Clinical Chemistry*, 66(11), 1444–1449. doi:10.1093/clinchem/hvaa203.

Kehoe, L., Walton, J., & Flynn, A. (2019). Nutritional challenges for older adults in Europe: Current status and future directions. *The Proceedings of the Nutrition Society*, 78(2), 221–233. doi:10.1017/S0029665118002744.

Lim, C. C., Ang, A. T. W., Kadir, H. B. A., Lee, P. H., Goh, B. Q., Harikrishnan, S., et al. (2021). Short-course systemic and topical non-steroidal anti-inflammatory drugs: Impact on adverse renal events in older adults with co-morbid disease. *Drugs & Aging*, 38(2), 147–156. doi:10.1007/s40266-020-00824-4.

Lindsay, R., & Samuels, B. (2022). Osteoporosis. In J. Loscalzo, A. Fauci, D. Kasper, S. Hauser, D. Longo, & J. Jameson (Eds.), *Harrison's principles of internal medicine* (21st ed., pp. 3191–3208). New York: McGraw Hill.

Mandaviya, P. R., Joehanes, R., Brody, J., Castillo-Fernandez, J. E., Dekkers, Koen, F., et al. (2019). Association of dietary folate and vitamin B-12 intake with genome-wide DNA methylation in blood: A large-sclae epigenome-wide association analysis in 5841 individuals. *The American Journal of Clinical Nutrition*, 110(2), 437–450. doi:10.1093/ajcn/nqz031.

Mount, D. B. (2022). Fluid and electrolyte disturbances. In J. Loscalzo, A. Fauci, D. Kasper, S. Hauser, D. Longo, & J. Jameson (Eds.), *Harrison's principles of internal medicine* (21st ed., pp. 338–355). New York: McGraw Hill.

Naureckas, E. T., & Solway, J. (2022). Disturbances of respiratory function. In J. Loscalzo, A. Fauci, D. Kasper, S. Hauser, D. Longo, & J. Jameson (Eds.), *Harrison's principles of internal medicine* (21st ed., pp. 2133–2139). New York: McGraw Hill.

Nicoll, D., & Lu, C. (2017). Therapeutic drug monitoring & pharmacogenetic testing: principles and test interpretation. In D. Nicoll, C. M. Lu, & S. J. McPhee (Eds.), *Guide to diagnostic tests* (7th ed., pp. 221–234). New York: McGraw Hill.

Pagana, K. D., Pagana, T. J., & Pagana, T. N. (2019). *Mosby's diagnostic and laboratory test reference* (14th ed.). St. Louis: Elsevier.

Perry, L. A., & Landi, A. J. (2022). Should you treat asymptomatic bacteriuria in an older adult with altered mental status? *Journal of Family Practice, 71*(5), E8–E10. doi:10.12788/jfp.0420.

Potts, Jr., J. T., & Jüppner, H. (2022). Disorders of the parathyroid gland and calcium homeostasis. In J. Loscalzo, A. Fauci, D. Kasper, S. Hauser, D. Longo, & J. Jameson (Eds.), *Harrison's principles of internal medicine* (21st ed., pp. 3169–3190). New York: McGraw Hill.

Puga, A. M., Ruperto, M., Samaniego-Vaesken, M., Montero-Bravo, A., Partearroyo, T., & Varela-Moreiras, G. (2021). Effects of supplementation with folic acid and its combinations with other nutrients on cognitive impairment and Alzheimer's disease: A narrative review. *Nutrients, 13*(9), 2966–2021. doi:10.3390/nu13092966.

Robertson, G. L., & Bichet, D. G. (2022). Disorders of the neurohypophysis. In J. Loscalzo, A. Fauci, D. Kasper, S. Hauser, D. Longo, & J. Jameson (Eds.), *Harrison's principles of internal medicine* (21st ed., pp. 2918–2925). New York: McGraw Hill.

Surana, N. K., & Kasper, D. L. (2022). Approach to the patient with an infectious disease. In J. Loscalzo, A. Fauci, D. Kasper, S. Hauser, D. Longo, & J. Jameson (Eds.), *Harrison's principles of internal medicine* (21st ed., pp. 941–947). New York: McGraw Hill.

Ungar, A., Rivasi, G., Di Bari, M., Virdis, A., Casiglia, E., Masi, S., et al. (2022). The association of uric acid with mortality modifies at old age: Data from the uric acid right for heart health (URRAH) study. *Journal of Hypertension, 40*(4), 704–711. doi:10.1097/HJH.0000000000003068.

Weitz, J. I. (2022). Antiplatelet, anticoagulant, and fibrinolytic drugs. In J. Loscalzo, A. Fauci, D. Kasper, S. Hauser, D. Longo, & J. Jameson (Eds.), *Harrison's principles of internal medicine* (21st ed., pp. 924–940). New York: McGraw Hill.

Yang, M., & Cao, S. (2022). Gender and age specific differences in the association of thyroid function and hyperuricemia in Chinese: A cross sectional study. *International journal of endocrinology, 2022*, 2168039. doi:10.1155/2022/2168039.

Young, N. S. (2022). Bone marrow failure syndromes including aplastic anemia and myelodysplasia. In J. Loscalzo, A. Fauci, D. Kasper, S. Hauser, D. Longo, & J. Jameson (Eds.), *Harrison's principles of internal medicine* (21st ed., pp. 792–801). New York: McGraw Hill.

14

Drugs and Aging

Patti A. Parker, PhD, RN, ACNS, ANP, GNP, BC, GS-C

http://evolve.elsevier.com/Yeager/gerontologic/

LEARNING OBJECTIVES

On completion of this chapter, the reader will be able to:
1. Describe the characteristics of drug use in older adults.
2. List at least four classes of drugs best avoided by older adults.
3. Identify potential risk factors for adverse drug reactions.
4. Describe the pharmacokinetic and pharmacodynamic changes associated with aging and the implications for drug therapy and misuse.
5. Recognize significant drug–drug, drug–food, and drug–disease interactions, giving specific examples for each.
6. State the effect drugs may have on an older adult's quality of life.
7. Describe issues related to the optimum use of antipsychotics, sedatives, hypnotics, cardiovascular agents, antimicrobials, and analgesics.
8. Anticipate the effects of the increased availability of nonprescription and herbal remedies on patient self-management.
9. Identify risk factors for nonadherence and suggest strategies to improve adherence.
10. List the key components of assessing older adults for substance use disorder (SUD).
11. Identify the key multidisciplinary and nursing interventions for older adults with SUD.

WHAT WOULD YOU DO?

What would you do if you were faced with the following situations?
- Your resident is in the Alzheimer unit at your facility. Your resident has been having issues with insomnia and agitation. The following drugs are prescribed:
  - Docusate 240 mg PO (by mouth) every HS (hour of sleep) (constipation)
  - Melatonin 3 mg PO every day (insomnia)
  - Trazodone 75 mg PO every HS (agitation)
  - Mirtazapine 15 mg PO every HS (depression)
  - Sertraline 100 mg PO once daily (depression, obsessive-compulsive disorder, and anxiety)
  - Singular 10 mg PO every day (asthma)
  - Gabapentin 600 mg PO three times per day (neuropathy)
  - Acetaminophen 650 PO every 6 hours PRN (as needed [headache])

  Are any of the drugs prescribed for your resident on the Beers list? What are the drug–drug interactions your resident may be experiencing, if any?
- You are precepting a 20-year-old nursing student. When reviewing the admission history they completed on a new 78-year-old patient, you notice questions about SUD were omitted. When questioned, the student states, "I didn't feel comfortable asking the questions; they are an older adult, so I doubt it's an issue with them anyway." How would you respond?

OVERVIEW OF DRUG USE AND PROBLEMS

Demographics of Drug Use

Drugs have an important role in the management of conditions and the maintenance of well-being in older adults. At least 96% of community-dwelling adults aged 65–74 take prescription or over-the-counter (OTC) drugs. Of these, 87% regularly take prescription drugs, 38% take OTC drugs, and 64% take dietary supplements. The prevalence of drug use increases in those 75 years of age or older (Qato et al, 2016).

Drugs may be vital for health and well-being, but all drugs carry risks. For older adults, these risks may be dangerous and even life-threatening. To ensure optimal health outcomes, it is important to understand how aging and its associated conditions affect drug processes and actions.

Changes in Drug Response With Aging

Aging alters the dynamic processes drugs undergo to produce therapeutic effects. These alterations involve pharmacokinetics (what the body does to the drug) and pharmacodynamics (what the drug does to the body).

Pharmacokinetic Changes: What the Body Does to the Drug

When a drug is taken, it begins a journey of four phases: (1) absorption, (2) distribution, (3) metabolism, and (4) excretion. What the body does to the drug during the four phases of this journey is known as *pharmacokinetics*. The normal physiologic changes that occur with aging alter pharmacokinetics. This section explores the pharmacokinetic changes that occur with aging. A summary of important age-related

TABLE 14.1 Age-Related Changes in Pharmacokinetics

Variable	Result	Consequence
Absorption Gastric pH increased Decreased small bowel surface area Slowed gastric emptying	Alters the absorption of drugs requiring acidic environment	Decreased absorption of calcium carbonate Early release of enteric coated drugs
Distribution Decreased serum albumin Increased alpha-1-acid glycoprotein Increased body fat Decreased total body water	Increased volume of distribution for highly lipophilic drugs (e.g., diazepam) Rapid decreases in serum albumin may enhance drug effects (e.g., phenytoin and warfarin)	Increase in drug elimination half-life Increased serum levels of unbound drug
Hepatic Metabolism Decreased hepatic metabolism via the cytochrome P-450 enzyme system Decrease in first pass metabolism (decreases 1%/year after age 40)	Drug clearance may decrease by 30%–40%	May lead to higher circulating drug levels (e.g., nitrates, propranolol, phenobarbital, nifedipine)
Renal Excretion Decreased creatinine clearance (average roughly 8 mL/minute/1.73 m^2/decade)	Serum creatinine typically stays the same due to decreased muscle mass and decreased physical activity	Dosage may need to be decreased or the frequency of dosing decreased (e.g., levofloxacin, nitrofurantoin, hydrochlorothiazide)

Data from Burchum, J. R., & Rosenthal, L. D. (2022). *Lehne's pharmacology for nursing care* (11th ed.). St. Louis, MO: Elsevier.

physiologic alterations that affect pharmacokinetics is presented in Table 14.1.

Absorption refers to the movement of a drug from the site of administration to the systemic circulation. Primary alterations in absorption occur with drugs taken orally or via feeding tubes. Drugs administered orally first need to enter the stomach and intestines. With aging, the risk of decreased secretion of gastric acid, slowed gastric emptying, and decreased gastrointestinal motility exists. Although these effects may *slow* the absorption of oral drugs, they do not substantially affect the *amount* of drug absorption that occurs; therefore, age-related changes in the absorption of most drugs are usually insignificant (Ruscin and Linnebur, 2021); however, the first dose of a new drug may take longer to take effect (Drenth-van Maanen et al, 2020). Topical drugs also face barriers to absorption. Reduction in subcutaneous fat associated with integumentary changes of aging alters topical drug absorption. These changes may impair absorption of some drugs administered as lotions, creams, ointments, and patches (Flammiger and Maibach, 2006).

Distribution refers to the movement of the drug from systemic circulation to the site of action. Distribution is affected by relative amounts of total body water, fat content, and protein binding. Total body water decreases with aging; decreased total body water results in higher concentrations of water-soluble drugs. Water-soluble drugs tend to stay in circulation longer, leading to higher drug concentration levels. To decrease the risk of toxicity, smaller doses of water-soluble drugs such as digoxin, lithium, metoprolol, and aminoglycosides may be needed for older adults (Aymanns et al, 2010). Older adults have decreased lean body mass and an increased percentage of fat compared with young adults. The increase in fat composition offers increased storage capability for fat-soluble drugs. As a result, fat-soluble drugs such as benzodiazepines and certain anesthetics (e.g., halothane and thiopental) may have extended half-lives (Ruscin and Linnebur, 2021). A final area of concern regarding distribution involves drugs that are highly protein-bound. Drugs of this type, for example, warfarin, phenytoin, furosemide, and naproxen, tend to bind primarily to albumin, a protein in the plasma, and only become active when unbound. With age, particularly for malnourished or frail adults, albumin levels may drop as much as 15%–25% (Kaufman, 2013), resulting in increased free drug availability for action. Decreased protein available for binding may result in toxicity and difficulty maintaining stable drug levels (Ruscin and Linnebur, 2021).

Metabolism refers to the biotransformation of drugs into metabolites that are more easily excreted. Less commonly, metabolism will convert inactive drugs, known as *prodrugs,* to an active form. Metabolism is accomplished through either phase I reactions (oxidation, reduction, demethylation, or hydrolysis via the cytochrome P [CYP] 450 enzyme system) or phase II reactions (glucuronidation, acetylation, conjugation, or sulfation). Recent research has demonstrated that aging does not appear to affect phase II processes. Furthermore, although some isoenzymes (e.g., CYP2C19, which has a role in metabolizing diazepam, naproxen, omeprazole, and propranolol) are reduced with aging, others remain unchanged, are variable, or affect only those older adults who are malnourished or frail (Drenth-van Maanen et al, 2020). In addition, with aging, a decrease in hepatic blood flow occurs (Drenth-van Maanen et al, 2020). This is particularly relevant in relation to first-pass metabolism. *First-pass metabolism* is a process in which drugs absorbed from the stomach or intestines first enter the portal circulation of the liver, and a portion is metabolized (inactivated) before reaching the systemic circulation. A decrease in hepatic blood flow may result in a decrease in the amount of a drug inactivated before entering the systemic circulation, resulting in a greater amount of active drug and thus increasing the risk that standard doses of drugs may result in toxic effects (Drenth-van Maanen et al, 2020; Ruscin and Linnebur, 2021). The implications of these alterations are that the metabolism of some drugs may be slowed, leading to a prolonged drug half-life and an increased risk of drug accumulation and toxic effects; however, this cannot be generalized to all older adults. Individualization of drug regimens and close monitoring for signs and symptoms of toxic effects and complications are necessary while dosing is adjusted.

Excretion, the elimination of drugs from the body, occurs primarily via the kidneys. When renal function is decreased, half-life increases, and drugs may accumulate to toxic levels. This has important implications for older adults, as renal function typically decreases with aging, especially for those who have conditions such as hypertension or heart disease (Shi et al, 2008). Renal function varies from patient to patient, so it is important to evaluate renal function on an individual basis. A serum creatinine level is commonly used as a screening test for renal function; however, serum creatinine is affected by nutritional status, protein intake, and muscle mass (Ruscin and Linnebur, 2021). Therefore, in older adults, the best indicator of renal function is the glomerular filtration rate (GFR). Two methods of calculating GFR are deemed acceptable for use in older adults: (1) the Modification of Diet in Renal Disease 6 (MDRD6) formula, and (2) the Cockcroft and Gault formula (CG). The MDRD6 slightly overestimates GFR and includes albumin in its calculation; the CG slightly underestimates GFR and is easier to calculate (Raman et al, 2017; Drenth-van Maanen et al, 2013).

Current nephrology guidelines now include the use of the CKD-EPI equation (Chronic Kidney Disease Epidemiology Collaboration) and Cystatin C as viable methods to estimate renal function in older adults. All of these methods can be used to provide a more accurate measure of renal function that can be used to adjust drug dosing and ensure safe prescribing (Raman et al, 2017; Drenth-van Maanen et al, 2013).

Nursing management associated with altered pharmacokinetics rests primarily on careful patient monitoring to assess the adequacy of the drug level to achieve the desired effect and identify adverse drug reactions and events that create problems for the patient. Each drug manifests toxicity in different ways, so it is essential that the nurse become familiar with the signs and symptoms of toxicity for each drug a patient takes so toxicity can be detected in the early stages. It is also important for the nurse to understand therapeutic drug monitoring. For some drugs (e.g., digoxin), a serum drug level is measured; other drugs (e.g., warfarin) are monitored through diagnostic tests evaluating drug effects (e.g., international normalized ratio [INR]). If evidence of toxicity exists, the nurse will need to assess the patient and promptly notify the provider. The nurse should anticipate an adjustment in the drug dosage.

Pharmacodynamic Changes: What the Drug Does to the Body

Physiologic changes associated with aging may also alter how the older adult's body responds to drugs. *Pharmacodynamics*, that is, what the drug does to the body, is the term used to explain the body's response to a drug. Age-related changes affect all substances involved in pharmacodynamics: enzymes, receptors on cell surfaces, carrier molecules, and protein transporters in cell membranes (Kim and Parish, 2017; Kim and Parish, 2021; Kim et al, 2018; Shi et al, 2008). As a result, drug sensitivity may be either increased (e.g., increased anticholinergic effects of tricyclic antidepressants [TCAs]) or decreased (e.g., decreased response to beta-blockers [BBs]). In both respects, the altered sensitivity is unrelated to the drug level. Furthermore, the bodily processes that maintain homeostasis (autonomic control and reflex activity) become less responsive; consequently, the older adult may be less able to tolerate certain drugs. As with nursing actions related to pharmacokinetics, the nurse must assess individual responses to drugs so they can be adjusted to optimize patient outcomes.

Inappropriate Drugs for Older Patients

Because of age-related changes in pharmacokinetics and pharmacodynamics, some drugs and drug classes are less likely to be tolerated by older adults. To identify problematic drugs, expert panels developed screening tools and lists detailing inappropriate drugs for older adults. The most well-known of these is the *Beers Criteria for Potentially Inappropriate Medication Use in Older Adults,* originally formulated in 1991 (Beers et al, 1991). American Geriatrics Society (AGS) Beers Criteria Update Expert Panel made the most recent update in 2023 (AGS, 2019). The National Committee for Quality Assurance recently made changes to the *Healthcare Effectiveness Data and Information Set (HEDIS): Use of High-Risk Medications in the Elderly and Potentially Harmful Drug-Disease Interactions in the Elderly* to maintain alignment with the 2023 revised Beers Criteria (http://www.ncqa.org).

The Beers list is quite extensive. Readers are asked to review this list directly at https://agsjournals.onlinelibrary.wiley.com/doi/epdf/10.1111/jgs.18372. It is not included in this text.

The Beers list has been widely disseminated in the literature since its initial development; however, the use of potentially inappropriate drugs in older adults remains a significant problem. A study conducted by Clark and colleagues (2020) found that potentially inappropriate medication (PIM) use was associated with a 17% increase in hospitalizations, a 26% increase in ER visits, and an 18% increase in outpatient health care visits. In addition, this study revealed that 34% of older adults in a community setting continue to be prescribed potentially inappropriate drugs, despite recent attention to the problem. The most widely prescribed categories of PIMs were antispasmodics, antidepressants, barbiturates, hypnotics, androgens, estrogens, digoxin, and metoclopramide. Although the Beers Criteria provide important information regarding potentially inappropriate drugs, it is important to recognize that drugs considered appropriate and frequently prescribed for older adults may also carry serious drug-related risks. Of these, only digoxin is included in the Beers Criteria, where it is categorized as moderate risk. Thus, it is important to remember that all drugs are potentially harmful and must be weighed in terms of benefit versus risk.

Drugs and Quality of Life

In addition to evaluating drugs in terms of benefit versus risk, it is also important to weigh them in terms of desired versus undesired outcomes. It is natural to assume that a drug is appropriate if it achieves the desired outcome. For example, if an antihypertensive drug such as metoprolol adequately maintains blood pressure within normal parameters or if a prokinetic drug such as metoclopramide promotes adequate gastric emptying to decrease gastroesophageal reflux, they would generally be perceived as appropriate drugs. However, if metoprolol causes erectile dysfunction or if metoclopramide causes tardive dyskinesia, the patient's quality of life may decrease compared with the extent of the benefit provided by the drug.

Drugs may have various detrimental effects on cognition, emotion, ambulation, continence, and other essential functions. These negative effects on an older adult's quality of life must be carefully considered as part of pharmacologic therapy. Some patients may prefer to endure a condition rather than suffer an adverse effect from its treatment. Generally, alternative drugs or interventions may be used. If one uses the earlier example, an angiotensin-converting enzyme inhibitor (ACEI) will be less likely to cause erectile dysfunction compared with the Beta-blockers (BB), and the patient's gastroesophageal reflux may be managed with drugs that decrease acidity. For this reason, if a patient refuses a drug, rather than simply charting a drug as refused, the nurse should elicit the patient's perspective so that a more appropriate intervention may be implemented. When other options are not advisable, it is generally important to honor the patient's wishes. Patient-centered therapeutic management considers the patient's beliefs and goals regarding quality of life to be tantamount to those of the provider and is necessary to ensure optimal outcomes.

Pharmacologic Contributors to Risk

Many factors may increase the risk of poor outcomes for older adults who require pharmacologic therapy. Among the most important risk factors are drug interactions, polypharmacy, and substance misuse.

Drug Interactions

Drugs may interact with other drugs and with food. Some drugs may even interact with disease processes. It is important for the nurse to be aware of potential interactions so that harmful patient outcomes can be avoided.

Drug–drug interactions occur in a variety of ways. Perhaps the most common interaction is the result of altered metabolism via the CYP450 hepatic enzyme system. Some drugs can induce or inhibit the activity of various CYP isozymes, which results in increased or decreased biotransformation of drugs. If the biotransformation is accelerated, the affected drug will be inactivated prematurely; however, if the biotransformation is decelerated, the drug may accumulate to toxic levels. Drugs may also interact indirectly through opposing or antagonistic actions. For example, in a patient who has both asthma and hypertension, a BB given to control hypertension may oppose the actions of a beta-agonist given to dilate the bronchi. Some drug–drug interactions occur in other ways. For example, some laxatives may cause rapid transit of an orally administered drug through the gastrointestinal system so that it is not adequately absorbed. Drugs may also interact chemically. This is more readily seen in intravenous solutions in which incompatible drugs may crystallize when mixed; however, it may also occur when certain oral drugs are taken together. Table 14.2 lists examples of significant drug–drug interactions.

Drug–food interactions are less common than drug–drug interactions but still increase risk. Drug metabolism or effects may be altered when combined with certain foods. For example, potentially dangerous interactions may occur when certain drugs are taken with grapefruit juice because a chemical found in grapefruit juice inhibits metabolism by 3A4 isoenzymes of the CYP450 enzyme system. The 3A4 isoenzymes are responsible for the first-pass metabolism of many drugs; therefore, as a result of inhibited metabolism, drugs normally metabolized by 3A4 isoenzymes, for example, lovastatin, rivaroxaban, and calcium channel blockers (CCBs), may accumulate to high or even toxic levels. See Table 14.3 for examples (Bailey et al, 2013).

Drug–disease interactions may exacerbate patients' conditions or hinder healing. These drugs are generally contraindicated in patients with coexisting underlying diseases. For example, 13% of African American males and 20% of African American females are carriers of a gene that may cause a deficiency in the enzyme glucose-6-phosphate dehydrogenase (G6PD). If a patient with this deficiency takes certain drugs, such as sulfonamides or aspirin, erythrocyte hemolysis may occur (Nagalla and Besa, 2023). Table 14.4 lists examples of drug–disease interactions.

Education is an essential component of any risk prevention program. Nurses should provide patients with information regarding the risk of potentially dangerous interactions among all of the drugs they are taking: prescription, OTC, and complementary and alternative drugs. It may be helpful to provide the patient with a list of acceptable OTC drugs for common problems such as mild pain or constipation. A "safe OTC drug list" may be a useful tool for health care providers to review with patients before completing the office visit (Table 14.5).

TABLE 14.2 Common Drug–Drug Interactions in Older Adults

Drug–Drug Combination	Potential Effect
Warfarin and aspirin	Increased risk of bleeding
Digoxin and quinidine sulfate	Increased risk of digoxin toxicity
Hydrochlorothiazide and SSRIs	Increased risk of hyponatremia
Hydrochlorothiazide and glyburide	Increased risk of hypoglycemia
Levodopa and clonidine	Decreased antiparkinsonian effect
Hydrochlorothiazide and NSAIDs	Decreased diuretic and antihypertensive effects of thiazides
Lithium and furosemide	Increased risk of lithium toxicity
Simvastatin and gemfibrozil	Increased risk of myopathy, rhabdomyolysis, and other adverse effects
Prednisone and phenobarbital	Decreased steroid effect
Ginkgo with aspirin	Increased bleeding risk

NSAIDs, nonsteroidal anti-inflammatory drugs; *SSRIs*, selective serotonin reuptake inhibitors

TABLE 14.3 Common Drug–Food Interactions in Older Adults

Food	Drug	Potential Effect
Caffeine	Theophylline	Increased potential for theophylline toxicity
Vitamin K foods: broccoli, Brussels sprouts, kale, parsley, spinach	Warfarin	Decreased effect of drug and inhibiting anticoagulation
Food	Many antibiotics	Reduced absorption rate of drug
Dairy products	Tetracycline	Prevent the body from absorbing calcium
Tyramine foods: aged cheese, wines, pickled herring, chocolate	Monoamine oxidase inhibitors (MAOIs) (phenelzine, tranylcypromine), selegiline, St. John's wort	May precipitate a hypertensive crisis
Grapefruit juice	Benzodiazepines, calcium channel blockers, cyclosporine, estrogen, statin drugs, DOACs	Altered metabolism and elimination can increase the concentration of drugs

DOACs, direct acting oral anticoagulants

Polypharmacy

Polypharmacy is the term currently used to indicate taking five or more medications each day (Masnoon et al, 2017) (see Evidence-Based Practice box). Older adults are vulnerable to polypharmacy because many have one or more chronic conditions requiring multiple drugs (Fig. 14.1). To complicate matters, patients may see more than one provider and may have prescriptions filled at more than one pharmacy (Walckiers et al, 2015). Additional contributors to polypharmacy include the use of OTC and alternative medicines or supplements in the treatment of conditions (Qato et al, 2016). As a result, the patient may end up taking duplicate drugs, similar drugs from the same drug class, and drugs that are contraindicated when taken together.

TABLE 14.4 Common Drug–Disease Interactions in Older Adults

Disease	Drug	Potential Effect
Chronic kidney disease	NSAIDs	Worsening kidney function
Heart failure	First-generation CCBs (e.g., verapamil) NSAIDs	Cardiac decompensation; fluid retention
Dementia	Anticholinergics Benzodiazepines TCAs Barbiturates	Worsening memory due to decreased acetylcholine transmission
Diabetes	Corticosteroids	Hyperglycemia
Falls	Benzodiazepines TCAs Typical antipsychotics Sedative hypnotics SSRIs	Increased risk of fall and fracture
Parkinson disease	Metoclopramide Prochlorperazine	Worsening Parkinson symptoms
Peptic ulcer disease	Aspirin NSAIDs	Increased risk of bleeding
Seizures	Bupropion Opioids	Decreased seizure threshold
Constipation	Anticholinergics	Worsening constipation
Benign prostatic hyperplasia	Anticholinergics Decongestants	Urinary retention

CCBs, calcium channel blockers; *NSAIDs,* nonsteroidal anti-inflammatory drugs; *SSRIs,* selective serotonin reuptake inhibitors; *TCAs,* tricyclic antidepressants.

EVIDENCE-BASED PRACTICE

Management of Potentially Inappropriate Drugs in Vulnerable Populations

Background
Nearly 40% of Medicare beneficiaries have four or more chronic illnesses, leading to duplicate testing, conflicting treatments, and poor coordination of drug therapy. African Americans face a higher incidence of chronic disease than Caucasians.

Sample/Setting
The sample encompassed 400 community-dwelling, underserved, older adults who self-identified as African Americans in Los Angeles County. The mean age was 73.5 years; 20% were over the age of 80. The majority (65%) were females. A few were married or lived with a companion (20%). Participants averaged five comorbid diseases; 19% reported at least eight comorbidities.

Methods
Polypharmacy is defined by a number of drugs prescribed for participants for a "single, or several, coexisting diseases" (p. 2). Participants were recruited from 16 predominantly African American churches. They were asked to bring all OTC and prescription drugs used over the previous 2 weeks. The 2012 Beers for PIMs was used to identify PIMs for each participant. Pain was evaluated using the Short-Form McGill Pain Questionnaire-2, scoring pain on a 0 (none) to 10 (worst) imaginable scale. Comorbidity was identified by self-report. The number of health care providers and drug costs were identified by self-report. Participants were also asked to self-identify alcohol and tobacco use.

Findings
Most participants (92%) had a primary care provider and averaged seven scheduled visits over the previous 12 months. Many had more than one prescriber (38%) and used more than one pharmacy (28%). Of the participants, 23% took at least eight drugs per day; 37% took five to seven drugs per day; and 40% took zero to four drugs per day. Twenty-seven percent took drugs classified as "avoid" on the Beers list; 43% took drugs classified as "use conditionally." Females were prescribed more drugs (81% taking five or more drugs) than males (65% taking five or more drugs).

Implications
Polypharmacy and the use of PIMs are issues among underserved African Americans, particularly among females. Innovative strategies to improve coordination among multiple providers and pharmacies are necessary to improve the quality of care provided to underserved populations.

Data from Bazargan, J., Smith, J., Movassaghi, M., Martins, D., Yazdanshenas, H. Mortazavi, S. S., et al. (2017). Polypharmacy among underserved older African American adults. *Journal of Aging Research, 2017,* 6026358.

TABLE 14.5 A List of Safe Over-the-Counter Drugs

If You Have	Generally, Avoid Over-the-Counter Medicines Containing	Examples	Because	Safer Alternatives
Asthma or lung disease	Ephedrine Epinephrine Extra theophylline Pseudoephedrine Caffeine	Bronkaid Primatene Sudafed NoDoz, DeWitt's pills	May cause insomnia, nervousness, and irregular heartbeats, especially when taking prescription asthma medicines	Ask your doctor
	Aspirin/salicylates (if you have an aspirin allergy)	Ecotrin	May cause an allergic reaction (e.g., wheezing, itching, and hives)	Acetaminophen
	NSAIDs (if you have an aspirin allergy)	Nuprin Motrin Advil Aleve	May increase risk of asthma exacerbation	Ask your doctor
Blood clots (and are taking blood thinners)	Aspirin/salicylates	Ecotrin, Vanquish, Alka-Seltzer, Pepto-Bismol	May cause bleeding	Acetaminophen
	NSAIDs	Nuprin Motrin Advil Aleve	May cause bleeding	Ask your doctor
Heart problems (high blood pressure, heart failure, abnormal heartbeat)	Sodium, salt Ephedrine Epinephrine/pseudoephedrine Caffeine	Alka-Seltzer, antacids Bronkaid Primatene, Sudafed NoDoz	May worsen your condition	Acetaminophen, nasal sprays, nonmedicated throat lozenges
Diabetes	Liquids or syrups containing alcohol or sugar	Emetrol and many cough or cold syrups	May alter blood sugar	Sugar-free, sugarless, or alcohol-free liquids
	Ephedrine	Bronkaid	May alter blood sugar	Ask your doctor
	Epinephrine	Primatene	May alter blood sugar	Ask your doctor
	Aspirin/salicylates	Ecotrin and Pepto-Bismol	May decrease blood sugar if taking oral diabetes pills to lower sugar	Acetaminophen
Seizures	Aspirin/salicylates	Ecotrin	May change levels of prescription seizure medicines	Acetaminophen
	Antihistamines (depressant medicine)	Benadryl, Unisom	May add to the drowsiness caused by prescription seizure medicines	Ask your doctor
	Decongestants	Ephedrine Pseudoephedrine	May lower the seizure threshold	Ask your doctor
Stomach ulcers	Aspirin/salicylates	Ecotrin	May worsen your ulcers	Acetaminophen
	NSAIDs	Nuprin Motrin Advil Aleve	May worsen your ulcers	Ask your doctor

Note: These are general suggestions and should be discussed with your doctor. They may want to change this list or may add suggestions to fit your individual needs. *Always* read the label on nonprescription (over-the-counter) medicines before purchasing, and have a pharmacist assist you if you are not sure what choice to make.
NSAIDs, nonsteroidal anti-inflammatory drugs.

Although only advanced practice nurses can prescribe drugs, other nurses play a vital role in decreasing the number of drugs taken by older adults. Whenever an older patient is seen with a new symptom, the nurse should consider whether the new problem could be caused by a drug the patient is taking (Walckiers et al, 2015). If the problem is significant, the prescriber may prefer to discontinue the drug causing the problem rather than prescribe another drug to treat the problem. The nurse may also employ nonpharmacologic interventions, whenever possible. For example, methods such as relaxation therapy and chronotherapy (an intervention combining wake therapy, bright-light therapy, and sleep scheduling) have been shown to be effective nonpharmacologic interventions for the management of insomnia in older adults (Joshi, 2008). Lifestyle changes such as weight loss, dietary modifications, and an exercise plan may reduce the need for additional drugs to control hypertension (Verma et al, 2021).

Drug Errors: Human and Economic Burdens

The Centers for Disease Control and Prevention (2010) report that 1.3 million emergency department visits and more than 350,000 hospitalizations occur each year in the United States

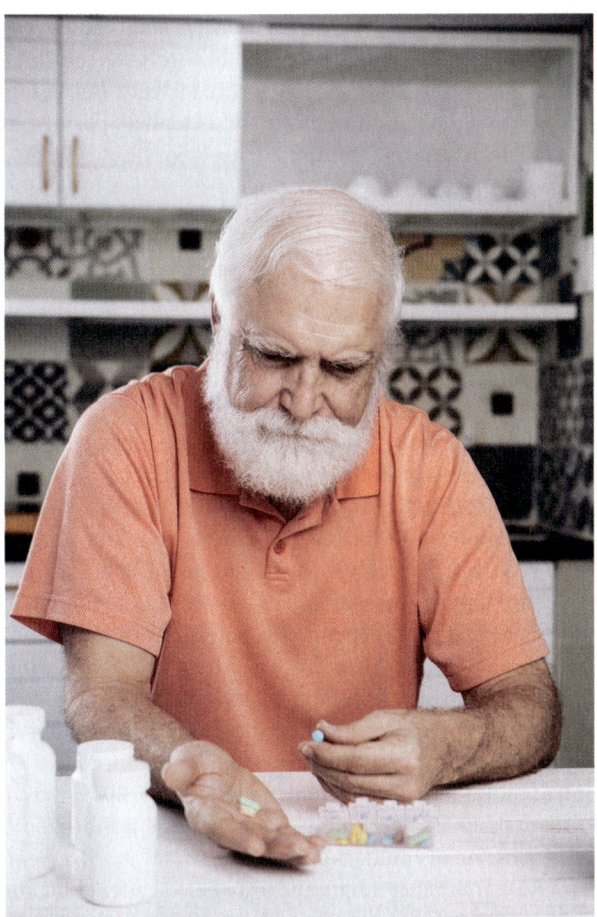

Fig. 14.1 Older adults' concurrent use of many prescription drugs may lead to polypharmacy. (©DragonImages/iStock/Thinkstock.)

secondary to drug errors, resulting in $3.5 billion in added medical costs. Older adults are disproportionately affected. They identified the following as potential causes:
- New drug development.
- New uses for older drugs.
- Aging American population.
- Increased use of drug therapy for disease management and prevention.
- Expansion of insurance coverage for prescription drugs.

The U.S. Food and Drug Administration (2019) uses the National Coordinating Council for Medication Error Reporting and Prevention (NCCMERP) definition of a medication error:

"a medication error is any preventable event that may cause or lead to inappropriate medication use or patient harm while the medication is in the control of the health care professional, patient, or consumer. Such events may be related to professional practice, health care products, procedures, and systems, including prescribing; order communication; product labeling, packaging, and nomenclature; compounding; dispensing; distribution; administration; education; monitoring; and use." (para. 2)

Because this definition is both comprehensive and complex, an examination of its component parts may help best understand it.

The first part of the definition—"A medication error is any preventable event that may cause or lead to inappropriate medication use or patient harm ..."—speaks to the outcome of a drug error. The injuries resulting from patient harm are commonly referred to as adverse drug events.

The second part of the definition—"... while the medication is in the control of the healthcare professional, patient, or consumer"—addresses the person who manages the drug storage, dosage, schedule, and disposal. Of concern to older adults are the findings of a 20-year study in which researchers identified a marked increase in fatal drug errors among those who take their drugs at home (Spiesel, 2008). This has increased, in part, because of a trend toward shorter hospital stays. As a result, patients are taking drugs at home that were previously closely monitored in a hospital setting. Additionally, the development of new drugs has resulted in an increase in drugs prescribed, which has resulted in an increase in the number of prescriptions for drugs (Spiesel, 2008) as well as an increase in OTC drugs. When patients take OTC drugs, they may not be aware of allergies, contraindications, or interactions with prescribed drugs. Further, many patients may keep drugs long after they have expired rather than dispose of them (Wendling, 2006).

The final part of the definition—"Such events may be related to professional practice, healthcare products, procedures, and systems, including prescribing; order communication; product labeling, packaging, and nomenclature; compounding; dispensing; distribution; administration; education; monitoring; and use"—details the various means by which a drug error may occur. Nurses are involved in processes related to order communication and drug administration, education, monitoring, and use. Errors in order communication commonly occur when verbal orders are poorly communicated or misunderstood (Wakefield et al, 2008). Errors in administration involve what have often been referred to as the six *rights of drug administration:* (1) the right drug, (2) in the right dose, (3) at the right time, (4) via the right route, (5) to the right patient, and (6) with the right documentation (Burchum and Rosenthal, 2022). Drug errors related to education may occur when education is insufficient or unclear. The nurse's role in drug monitoring involves assessing the patient's response for both therapeutic and adverse effects (Burchum and Rosenthal, 2022); therefore, errors attributable to monitoring may include a failure to assess for inadequate therapeutic effect or, more likely, a failure to identify when a new problem is attributable to an adverse effect of a drug. Finally, errors related to drug use occur when drugs are not used as indicated; for example, drug misuse occurs when a prescribed opioid analgesic is given for sedation to aid sleep rather than for pain.

Interventions to decrease drug errors are receiving increased importance after the Institute of Medicine's (IOM) report on preventing drug errors (IOM, 2007). Strategies to reduce errors include the use of barcoded drug labels, error tracking, and public education. Additionally, the Food and Drug Administration (FDA) reviews drugs for look-alike or sound-alike names before marketing and has mandated standardized labeling for both prescription and OTC drugs (U.S. FDA, 2022).

COMMONLY USED DRUGS

Antipsychotics

Antipsychotic drugs are often prescribed for older adults despite evidence demonstrating their "limited efficacy and significant adverse effects" (Carnahan et al, 2017, p. 554). These drugs have been prescribed for hitting, yelling, and screaming; refusing care and wandering; and inconsolable crying, agitation, and aggression. However, research has demonstrated that these drugs do not help persons with dementia become more involved in their care, interact better with others, or stop inappropriate behavior. In fact, prescribing these drugs led to an increased risk for falls, fractures and breaks, incontinence, strokes, and death (Jeste and Maglione, 2013). In 2008, the FDA instituted boxed warnings for antipsychotics due to the increased risk of stroke and death in older adults with dementia (Yan, 2008). In 2012, the Centers for Medicare and Medicaid Services (CMS) collaborated with the nursing home industry to reduce inappropriate prescribing of antipsychotic drugs for residents. Since the inception of this initiative, antipsychotic prescribing has decreased from 23.9% in 2012 to 14.4% in 2021 (a 39.6% decrease in prescribing) (CMS, 2022). The Improving Antipsychotic Appropriateness in Dementia Patients educational program (IA-ADAPT) and CMS Partnership to Improve Dementia Care programs instituted in nursing homes provided evidence-based training and treatment algorithms for the implementation and documentation of nonpharmacologic interventions to manage older adults with behavioral and psychological symptoms of dementia (BPSD). Decreasing antipsychotic use in nursing homes has not been associated with an adverse effect on BPSD (Carnahan et al, 2017).

Anxiolytics and Hypnotics

Insomnia and anxiety are problems that plague older adults. Many drugs used to treat these problems have the potential for bothersome and potentially dangerous adverse effects when used in older adults. Because insomnia and anxiety often occur secondary to drug side effects or secondary to medical conditions such as dementia, thyroid abnormalities, or depression, proper diagnosis and treatment of the underlying causes of insomnia or anxiety may decrease the inappropriate use of these drugs. Nonpharmacologic interventions are often effective but tend to be underused (Snow et al, 2021; Moon, 2009); therefore, a trial of nonpharmacologic treatment is preferred before initiation of pharmacologic therapy in older adults.

Barbiturates have been prescribed for both insomnia and anxiety in the past, but their use has declined. These drugs are not recommended for older adults because of their narrow margin of safety and the risks of significant drug interactions and dependence.

Benzodiazepines, which are often prescribed for insomnia and anxiety, also carry concerns for older adults. Benzodiazepines with long half-lives; for example, diazepam, should be avoided because of the increased risk of toxicity. In addition, all benzodiazepines, including shorter-acting ones such as alprazolam, may cause excessive sedation, impaired memory, decreased psychomotor performance, and balance disturbances, and may lead to drug dependence (Calleo and Stanley, 2008). If a benzodiazepine is required, it is best to give the smallest dose possible and monitor closely for side effects. Because benzodiazepines should not be used for extended periods, it is important to assess the continued need for these drugs and discontinue them in a timely manner.

First-generation antihistamines, such as diphenhydramine, have been used for indications other than allergy, for example, the treatment of insomnia and anxiety. Antihistamines are potentially inappropriate drugs for use in older adults because these patients are more sensitive than younger patients to the anticholinergic adverse effects such as dry mouth, urinary retention, sedation, and even delirium (Patel et al, 2018).

Optimal treatment rests with alternative pharmaceuticals. For anxiety, non–central nervous system (CNS) depressants such as buspirone are effective agents. They take approximately 4 weeks to demonstrate a clinical response, so a benzodiazepine may be required for short-term management if the anxiety is severe (Burchum & Rosenthal, 2022). These drugs avoid many of the adverse effects and dependence potential of the benzodiazepines. Similarly, when sleep hygiene and other nonpharmacologic interventions for insomnia fail, short-term treatment with benzodiazepine receptor agonists (BZRAs), pyrazolopyrimidines, and melatonin receptor agonists are appropriate a short period of time alternatives for older adults (AGS, 2019; Burchum & Rosenthal, 2022). Melatonin, along with the nonbenzodiazepine options for insomnia, appears to have fewer adverse drug effects (ADEs) in older adults and may be considered for short-term use in some patients (Burchum & Rosenthal, 2022). The melatonin receptor agonist ramelteon, which is nonsedating, carries the least risk of falls; however, it may not be effective in some patients (Burchum & Rosenthal, 2022).

Antidepressants

Most antidepressants are effective for managing depression in older adults; however, some are better tolerated than others. Older TCAs have been used to treat depression as well as insomnia and neuropathic pain; however, significant side effects occur even in low doses and well before therapeutic levels are reached. As a treatment for insomnia, the TCAs are generally too sedating and may cause daytime somnolence. Additionally, TCAs possess anticholinergic side effects that may create problems for many older adults.

Selective serotonin reuptake inhibitors (SSRIs) are the antidepressants of first choice for older adults because these agents are better tolerated; however, they are not without risks. They may cause dose-related gastrointestinal disturbances, including gastrointestinal bleeding, and CNS arousal effects. Fortunately, most of the side effects of the SSRIs last only a few days.

Selection of an antidepressant is often based on side effect profiles, which differ among available agents (Table 14.6). For instance, mirtazapine has more potential for sedation compared with some of the SSRI antidepressants. It may also reduce anxiety and increase appetite; therefore, if the patient suffers from depressive symptoms of anxiety, insomnia, and lack of appetite, then mirtazapine may be an appropriate choice to help the patient sleep while also increasing appetite and reducing

TABLE 14.6 Antidepressants: Comparative Profiles				
Drug	Avoid in Older Adults	Anticholinergic Side Effects in Older Adults	Sedation	Orthostatic Hypotension
Tricyclics: Tertiary Amines				
Amitriptyline	√	++++	++++	++
Clomipramine	√	+++	+++	++
Doxepin	√	++	+++	++
Imipramine	√	++	++	+++
Trimipramine	√	++	+++	++
Tricyclics: Secondary Amines				
Desipramine	√	+	+	+
Nortriptyline	√	++	++	+
Protriptyline	√	+++	+	+
Selective Serotonin Norepinephrine Reuptake Inhibitors				
Venlafaxine		0	0	0
Desvenlafaxine		0	0	0
Duloxetine		0	0	0
Tetracyclics				
Maprotiline	√	++	++	+
Triazolopyridines				
Trazodone		+	++	++
Aminoketones				
Bupropion		++	++	++
Selective Serotonin Reuptake Inhibitors				
Fluoxetine	√	0/+	0	0/+
Paroxetine		+	0/+	0
Sertraline		0	0	0
Citalopram		0/+	0/+	0/+
Escitalopram		0/+	0/+	0/+
Fluvoxamine	√	0/+	0/+	0
Vortioxetine		0/+	0	0
Miscellaneous				
Nefazodone	√	0/+	++	+
Mirtazapine		++	+++	+

+++, Strong; ++, moderate; +, weak; 0, none.
Data from Dopheide, J. (2021). More than stressed out: Addressing anxiety and panic. *The Rx Consultant for Prescribers, 30*(9); and Burchum, J. R., & Rosenthal, L. D. (2022). *Lehne's Pharmacology for nursing care* (11th ed.). St. Louis, MO: Elsevier.

anxiety. A patient exhibiting depressive symptoms such as increased sleepiness, decreased affect, and decreased socialization may benefit from a more stimulating antidepressant such as sertraline or venlafaxine. Thus, the side effect profile of an antidepressant may be used to identify the most appropriate drug for a patient's depressive symptom pattern.

Cardiovascular Drugs

Heart disease remains the number one cause of death among older adults; stroke is the third leading killer. Nearly a third of persons over the age of 65 have hypertension. In the United States, the Joint National Committee on Prevention, Detection, Evaluation, and Treatment of High Blood Pressure (JNC), the American Heart Association (AHA), and the American College of Cardiology (ACC) are the foremost providers of evidence-based clinical guidelines to guide the management of hypertension. The drugs recommended for the management of hypertension are also used in the management of many other cardiovascular conditions.

The Eighth Report of the Joint National Committee on Prevention, Detection, Evaluation, and Treatment of High Blood Pressure (JNC 8) has been published to offer guidance for the management of hypertension. Lifestyle modification is advised as a primary method for preventing and treating hypertension (Whelton et al, 2018):

- Weight loss is recommended in adults who are overweight or obese.

- A heart-healthy diet that supports weight loss, reduces sodium, and supplements potassium is recommended (unless contradicted by co-morbid illness).
- Adult males should consume no more than 2 standard alcohol drinks per day and women 1.

If a pharmacologic agent is needed to treat hypertension, the JNC 8, AHA, and ACC current recommendations suggest chlorthalidone as first-line therapy for most patients based on outcome data from clinical trials (Whelton et al, 2018). The addition of a second drug is often determined by the drug's inherent benefits and risks. Those most commonly used for older adults are BBs, ACEIs, angiotensin receptor blockers (ARBs), and CCBs.

BBs have demonstrated improved mortality rates for patients with a history of cardiovascular disease. They decrease angina symptoms, cardiac workload, and oxygen demand through a reduction of heart rate, cardiac output, and atrioventricular conduction. This provides a cardioprotective effect for patients with a history of ischemia or myocardial infarction.

CCBs have a beneficial effect on decreasing cardiac workload through decreasing peripheral resistance. For this reason, they are an alternative for patients with severe reactive airway disease or with a high degree of heart blockage where a BB might be contraindicated.

ACEIs and ARBs also have demonstrated value in decreasing the chance of cardiac mortality in patients with heart failure. They also confer renal protection, which is particularly beneficial for patients with diabetes.

Because older adults are likely to have more comorbidities (e.g., diabetes, reduced kidney function, and heart disease), the most current recommendations suggest selecting hypertensive treatment based on comorbid conditions or compelling indications (Whelton et al, 2018). For example, a 70-year-old patient with hypertension and diabetes would benefit from thiazide-type diuretics and an ACEI or ARB, but if the patient had hypertension with ischemic heart disease, the optimal management may be with a thiazide diuretic with a BB.

The main concerns with the use of antihypertensive drugs in older adults are an increased risk of orthostatic hypotension and dehydration, especially with volume-depleting agents and vasodilators. The older adult might have reduced kidney function and a decreased ability to maintain fluid and electrolyte balance. In addition, some older adults may have a decreased appetite and sense of thirst, resulting in decreased oral intake of food and fluids and an increased risk of dehydration. Subsequently, it is not surprising that dehydration is common among older people and is a frequent reason for admission to the hospital. Assessing the adverse effects of antihypertensive therapy is essential to maintaining the health of older adults and reducing complications and hospitalizations.

In addition to drugs used in the management of hypertension and related disorders, many older adults are prescribed digoxin. Digoxin is sometimes used to treat heart failure because it increases the force of cardiac contraction, thereby increasing cardiac output; however, research has shown that it does not necessarily reduce morbidity and mortality (Ahmed et al, 2006). For this reason, its use in the management of heart failure has become controversial, and it is no longer considered first-line therapy. However, digoxin remains a beneficial agent for the management of atrial tachyarrhythmias because it slows the heart rate, allowing for adequate ventricular filling.

Antimicrobials

Infections in older adults may result in devastating health events because of decreased physiologic reserves. Urinary tract infections (UTIs) and respiratory infections (especially pneumonia and exacerbations of chronic lung diseases) are common and often lead to hospital admissions. A frail older person with UTI may experience significant mental status changes, weakness, and sepsis and may require extended hospitalization and weeks of rehabilitation to return to baseline functional status.

Pharmacologic treatment of infections has the potential to achieve cures, but problems related to their use persist. Because many older adults have reduced renal function, dosage adjustments may be needed for certain antibiotics, such as fluoroquinolones. Antibiotic resistance, an increasing problem, may hinder finding the right treatment mix for complicated infections. Common antibiotic side effects, such as diarrhea, may create significant and even dangerous shifts in fluids and electrolytes in older adults. Nausea may result in decreased intake, further contributing to this problem.

Opioid Analgesics

Certain patient groups, such as older adults and those with cognitive impairment, may experience unrecognized and/or chronic pain that goes untreated or undertreated. When an older adult is prescribed an opioid for an acute or chronic medical condition, they must be monitored closely. As part of normal aging, older adults have reduced renal function, even in the absence of renal disease. These age-related renal changes can lead to drug accumulation.

Older adults with liver dysfunction are at risk of drug accumulation; thus, the dose and frequency of the opioid must be adjusted for safety (Wu, 2018).

Because older adults often have multiple medical comorbidities, they may be on multiple medications, which puts them at risk for drug–drug interactions. Nurses and all members of the interprofessional care team should counsel older adults taking opioids not to save unused medications and to avoid using multiple health care providers (Wu, 2018).

When opioids are prescribed for older adults, the suggested starting dose should be 25%–50% less than the recommended adult starting dose. Immediate-release medications should be initiated and slowly titrated to minimize adverse drug effects (Holle, 2017). Nurses should closely monitor older adults taking opioids for dry mouth, drowsiness, nausea, and vomiting. These common side effects usually resolve over time. In addition, nurses should alert the patient about the constipating effects of the drugs and suggest a bowel regimen when opioids are initiated.

Nonprescription Agents

Older adults are the largest consumers of nonprescription drugs (Safari et al, 2022). They often use these drugs believing that if they are available over the counter, they are safe; however, many of the prescription drugs that have been reclassified to nonprescription status (e.g., nonsteroidal anti-inflammatory drugs [NSAIDs] and sedating antihistamines) have a potential for significant harm in older populations.

Older adults might not volunteer information about the use of OTC drugs (Safari et al, 2022). As a result, opportunities for drug-related education and checks for interactions with prescribed drugs or effects that may worsen the patient's current health status are missed. This need for education is complicated by the realization that many older adults have decreased visual acuity, cataracts, macular degeneration, and other visual problems that limit the ability to read finely printed labels and instructions (Pawaskar and Sansgiry, 2006). Further, one nationwide study found that 46% of patients taking prescription drugs also take nonprescription drugs, thus increasing the potential for drug–drug interactions (Qato et al, 2016).

The first challenge for nurses regarding nonprescription drugs is to remain informed about *all* the drugs patients are currently taking. It is necessary to verify that no contraindications or significant interactions with prescribed drugs exist. It is also important to caution patients against certain products that may interact negatively with other drugs or with their medical condition(s).

Dietary Supplements

Dietary supplements are an overarching category of drugs that include vitamins, minerals, herbal remedies, and alternative medicines. The use of dietary supplements is an established practice among many older adults. According to a recent study, more than half (63.7%) of older adults living in the United States take some sort of dietary supplement on a regular basis (Qato et al, 2016). The same study identified that more than half (71.7%) of older adults who take prescription drugs also take supplements, and this increases the potential for drug–drug interactions. The most common dietary supplements identified in this study were vitamins or minerals and system-specific remedies such as omega-3 fatty acids, garlic, and coenzyme Q-10 for cardiovascular problems; glucosamine–chondroitin for joint problems; and saw palmetto for prostate problems. Additional frequently used supplements identified in separate retrospective reviews of supplement use in older adults include vitamin D, ginkgo biloba, black cohosh, borage, evening primrose, flaxseed oil, dehydroepiandrosterone (DHEA), grapeseed extract, hawthorn, and St. John's wort (Wold et al, 2005; Gahche et al, 2017). A particularly troubling finding was the identification of supplement–drug interactions with 10 of the supplements and the potential of 142 interactions over the 6-year period.

Many additional concerns exist with regard to the use of dietary supplements. They are not regulated for safety and efficacy by the FDA in the same manner as prescription drugs, which undergo a rigorous drug approval process. As a result, the predictability of product quality and potency is lacking. Many herbs are available in their natural, unprocessed state, further complicating predictability. Beyond these concerns, the use and safety of these products in older adults, especially in older adults with comorbidities, have not been adequately studied.

Unfortunately, information regarding dietary supplements is often nebulous and misleading. To address the need for scientific research and authoritative information, the National Center for Complementary and Integrated Health (NCCIH) was established under the umbrella of the National Institutes of Health (NIH). NCCIH provides information to health care professionals as well as to the lay public on its website at https://www.nccih.nih.gov.

DRUG ADHERENCE

Drug regimens should be planned so that optimal dosing and scheduling will prevent drug interactions and other complications while promoting optimal well-being. Many patients, however, may omit drugs at times or alter drug dosages or schedules. This failure to stick to the agreed-upon drug regimen is called *nonadherence*. Although nonadherence occurs in all age groups, it is likely to create more problems in older adults, who tend to have chronic and often multiple illnesses requiring drug therapy.

The most common reasons for nonadherence in older adults include polypharmacy, decreased visibility, motor dexterity, and autonomy (Khairullah et al, 2018). Other contributors to nonadherence include fear, cost of medications, misunderstanding, lack of symptoms, mistrust, worry, and depression (AMA, 2023). In addition, cultural factors and health literacy can contribute to nonadherence (Li et al, 2008; Davis et al, 2006; Maniaci et al, 2008). By understanding the reasons for nonadherence, nurses are better equipped to identify adherence risks and take specific risk-targeted action to decrease this common problem.

Recent analysis finds that for 28% of older adults, prescription-related costs contribute to nonadherence (Bunis, 2019). Drugs may be expensive, and many older adults are on fixed incomes, requiring tight budgets. Even those with insurance to deflect the cost may not be able to afford the required deductible. To cope with high drug costs, some patients decrease or skip doses to make a prescription quantity last longer. Others resort to decreasing the amount of money spent on food or other needs so that they can afford drugs. For many, however, the costs are so high that prescriptions for necessary medicines are left unfilled (Madden et al, 2008).

Side effects and the fear that side effects may occur are other common reasons for nonadherence. If the side effects are perceived as significant or if they interfere with daily activities, patients may be tempted to avoid these effects by omitting the drug that causes them. Side effects are especially relevant if drug benefits are not obvious. Indeed, the patient's perception of the effectiveness and necessity of the drug plays an important role in adherence. Many of the drugs prescribed for chronic illnesses serve to keep the conditions from progressing but do not cure the illness. Patients who do not feel better may perceive that the drug is ineffective. If a drug is given to cure an illness, such as an infection, the patient may stop the drug prematurely once the symptoms resolve because of the erroneous belief that it is no longer needed.

Age-related changes that contribute to nonadherence may be functional or cognitive. Vision changes that occur with aging may affect the ability of the patient to read labels on drug containers or to distinguish one drug from another. Stiffness of joints coupled with decreased hand strength or tremors may make it difficult to open drug bottles. Swallowing difficulties are exacerbated by large tablets. For some older adults, mental status changes that affect the ability to think clearly and make reasoned judgments contribute to unintentional nonadherence. Similarly, memory impairment and forgetfulness increase the likelihood that drugs will not be taken as prescribed.

For older adults with complex or multiple chronic illnesses requiring several drugs, drug schedules may be complex. For example, some drugs should be taken on an empty stomach, whereas others should be taken with food. Some drugs should not be taken together because drug–drug interactions may occur. Still others require scheduling to coordinate with certain times of the day (e.g., at bedtime). Keeping up with complicated schedules, particularly when they conflict with everyday activities, may increase the probability of nonadherence.

Assessing for Risk Factors

Because the effects of nonadherence can be devastating, it is important for the nurse to be proactive in preventing nonadherence. Prevention begins with an assessment of risk factors. A simple checklist may be used to help identify areas of primary concern.

- Are the prescribed drugs costly, or does the cost of drugs present a substantial burden to the patient?
- Do the prescribed drugs have the potential for significant side effects, or does the patient experience troublesome side effects?
- Are drug schedules cumbersome, or do they interfere with the patient's daily activities or sleep?
- Does the patient have any conditions that would make opening bottles, manipulating individual tablets, or swallowing drugs difficult?
- Does the patient have difficulty reading and comprehending instructions?
- Does the patient believe that any of the prescribed drugs are ineffective or unnecessary?
- Does the patient have any cultural beliefs that would cause them to avoid reliance on drugs or regard certain drugs as inappropriate?

Each item checked indicates a potential contributor to nonadherence. For those items, the nurse needs to work further with the patient to correct any misunderstandings, establish necessary support services or networks, and advocate for patient-centered adjustments in the drug regimens.

Strategies for Improving Adherence

Many patients do not share information regarding nonadherence, so it is a mistake to assume that the patient takes drugs as prescribed or recommended. In clinic settings, the nurse should have the patient bring in all prescription and OTC drugs and any dietary supplements at the initial visit and at least every 6 months thereafter (Pham and Dickman, 2007). Nurses working in hospitals should adopt this policy for every admission or emergency department visit. When reviewing drugs, the nurse should ask the patient how each drug is taken and compare this information with the prescription label or to the drugs listed in the patient's record to see whether nonadherence is a concern.

Patient teaching is an essential intervention for addressing the problem of drug nonadherence; however, studies show that teaching alone is rarely sufficient to evoke change (Ruppar et al, 2008). To adequately address issues of drug nonadherence, nurses need to understand the factors that contribute to a patient's failure to take drugs as directed and to develop risk-specific assessments and interventions individualized to the patient. Interventions should also consider the resources available in the region where services are provided. For example, if the patient has difficulty paying for drugs, the nurse may provide the patient with a resource list of pharmacies offering low-cost generic discounts. If generic drugs are not available for a proprietary drug that is ordered, the nurse may need to check for patient assistance programs for the drug in question.

The nurse should encourage all patients to have prescriptions filled at the same pharmacy each time because this provides an extra way to discover problems. The nurse should also tailor the drug regimen to the patient's home schedule to cause the least disruption in daily life and give the patient a sense of control over the drugs. The regimen should be simplified as much as possible; multiple daily doses should be avoided where appropriate and feasible.

Reviewing the Drug List for Problems

Nurses confronted with a complex drug regimen for an older patient should determine the answers to the following questions:

- Is there a documented and appropriate indication for each drug present?
- Is a drug dosage appropriate for the patient's age, weight, and renal or liver function?
- Does the patient have a documented drug allergy to a drug?
- Are doses of a drug being scheduled appropriately?
- Is the duration of treatment appropriate?
- Is the chosen drug the best one for the patient?
- Are two or more similar drugs prescribed (i.e., therapeutic duplication)?
- Is the patient experiencing an adverse drug reaction?
- Is a potential drug–drug interaction present?
- Does a medical indication exist for the use of a drug when none is currently prescribed?
- Is the patient using OTC drugs appropriately?
- What herbal or alternative therapies are being used by the patient? Is the patient's health care provider aware of these?
- Is the patient taking the prescribed medications as the prescription is written?

> **HOME CARE**
>
> 1. During each home visit, assess both prescription and nonprescription drugs being taken by the homebound older adult.
> 2. Document and notify the primary health care provider of the homebound older adult's drug regimen and of multiple physician sources for drugs if present.
> 3. Teach the side effects and interactions of all OTC drugs to homebound older adults and their caregivers.
> 4. Collaborate with social workers to identify community resources for financial assistance with pharmaceutical needs.
> 5. Monitor drug levels and other appropriate laboratory values as appropriate (e.g., potassium or sodium).
> 6. Teach the homebound older adult to set up a daily or weekly schedule for drugs using a method or tool that fosters safe, independent administration.
> 7. Reduce the chance of drug errors by labeling or color-coding drug bottles.
> 8. Keep an accurate record of the homebound older adult's weight.
> 9. Teach drug safety in the home environment by instructing patients to do the following:
>   - Keep drugs in original, labeled containers.
>   - Follow appropriate guidelines for drug disposal; never dispose of drugs in the trash within reach of children.
>   - Never "share" drugs with friends or family members.
>   - Always finish a prescribed drug; do not save it for a future illness.
>   - Read labels carefully and follow all instructions.
> 10. Instruct older adults who have difficulty opening childproof containers to ask their health care providers for non–childproof containers when writing prescriptions.

SUBSTANCE USE DISORDERS

Many older adults enjoy leisure activities as a result of decreased work schedules and retirement. However, some are unable to enjoy leisure activities because of the emotional, physical, social, and economic effects of growing older. Use of illicit drugs such as cocaine, opiates, and marijuana, previously thought to be a problem among young adults, has become more prevalent in older adults as Baby Boomers, with a history of being more tolerant of such practices, reach retirement age. Among older persons, misused substances include alcohol, prescription and nonprescription drugs, and tobacco. Marijuana and cocaine are included in the category of nonprescription drugs.

More than a million older adults had a SUD in 2018 (978,000 with alcohol use disorder [AUD] and 161,000 with illicit drug use disorder). SUD has become a public health concern among older adults. The current number of older adults in the United States with SUD that are in need of treatment is 5.7 million (Dufort and Samaan, 2021). The emergence of SUD as a public health concern among older adults reflects, in part, the relatively higher drug use rates of the Baby Boomers compared with previous generations (SAMHSA, 2019; NIH, 2020). Older adults with SUD experience increased "physical and mental health issues, social and family problems, involvement with the criminal justice system, and death from drug overdose" (Mattson et al, 2017, para. 1) and adverse drug interactions with prescription and OTC drugs (Mattson et al, 2017).

Frequently, the symptoms of SUD are subtle or atypical, or they mimic symptoms of other age-related illnesses and remain undiagnosed. A patient's presenting symptoms may be erratic changes in affect, mood, or behavior; malnutrition; bladder and bowel incontinence; gait disturbances; and recurring falls, burns, and head trauma (Mattson et al, 2017; Kuerbis et al, 2014). Many older adults began to misuse alcohol late in life because of bereavement, retirement, loneliness, or physical and emotional illnesses. Denial is more intense in older adults because of cognitive and memory problems and shame. The most frequently misused prescription drugs are opioids, benzodiazepines, sedatives, tranquilizers, and stimulants, which may result in ataxia, falls, accidents, and cognitive impairments such as attention and memory problems (Kuerbis et al, 2014).

Definitions and Common Usage

Nurses must understand the definitions associated with SUD to correctly assess it and plan appropriate interventions for older adults. The *Diagnostic and Statistical Manual of Mental Disorders, Fifth Edition, Text Revision* (DSM-5-TR), published by the American Psychiatric Association is used in the diagnosis of patients with suspected SUD. Substance use disorders "occur when the recurrent use of alcohol and/or drugs causes clinically and functionally significant impairment, such as health problems, disability, and failure to meet major responsibilities at work, school, or home. According to the DSM-5, a diagnosis of substance use disorder is based on evidence of impaired control, social impairment, risky use, and pharmacological criteria ("Substance Use Disorders," n.d., para. 2).

Difficulty in Identification of SUD

The physiologic, psychological, and sociologic changes associated with aging make the identification and treatment of SUD in older adult patients difficult. Age-related psychological and sociologic changes and symptoms may be subtle or atypical and may mimic symptoms of SUD (Mohundro and Ramsey, 2003; Kuerbis et al, 2014). Often, clinicians and family members are hesitant to ask whether the older adult is having problems with the use or misuse of prescription drugs. Traditionally accepted ways of detecting problems with substances (e.g., time lost from work, legal problems, or decreased participation in important social activities) are not helpful for older adults because they generally have fewer activities and obligations (Savage, 2014; Yarnell et al, 2020).

Physiologic Changes

Patients with early-onset AUD appear to have a more severe course of illness. They make up about two-thirds of older adults with AUD, are predominantly male, and have more alcohol-related medical problems and psychiatric comorbidities. Patients with later-onset AUD tend to have a milder clinical picture and fewer medical problems because of the shorter exposure to alcohol. They are more affluent, include more females, and are likely to begin their alcohol use after a stressful event such as the loss of a spouse, job, or home (Yarnell et al, 2020).

Nurses should be aware of age-related physiologic changes in absorption, distribution, plasma protein binding, hepatic metabolism, and the elimination or clearance of a drug. The assessment of these changes in relation to substance use is essential in planning interventions to prevent or halt substance use and misuse in the older adult population.

Psychological Changes

Psychological changes in older adults result primarily from the numerous losses this age group experiences in a relatively short period of time. Roughly 6% of persons over the age of 65 drink heavily. Heavy drinking is often in response to bereavement, retirement, loneliness, relationship stress, and physical illness (Fig. 14.2).

Nurses should be aware of the misconception that select prescribed or OTC substances may help the patient deal with unmet psychological needs. For example, an older adult may become anxious if sleep has decreased to less than 8 hours and may seek sedatives. In addition, some older adults tend to use certain substances to mask negative feelings about themselves; they may eventually attribute some of their positive personality characteristics to substances. Examples of such substances include alcohol, benzodiazepines (e.g., diazepam), and cannabis. Patients who are prescribed benzodiazepines by a physician for a limited period of time may become dependent on the drug. An older adult who has become dependent may find another physician to prescribe the drug when the original physician discontinues it.

The nurse must also assess older adults for suicidal ideation. Patients should be asked whether they have had thoughts of harming themselves and whether they have a plan to carry out these thoughts. Advancing age and substance misuse are among the greatest risk factors for suicide. Suicide rates tend to increase with age in White males, and it should be noted that suicide is the 13th leading cause of death in older adults.

Sociologic Changes

Sociologic changes such as reduced income, transportation, and social support tend to place older adults at risk for SUD. Because of decreased finances and transportation, many older adults fill prescriptions through mail-order pharmacies. Mail-order pharmacies tend to increase the potential for drug misuse because of prescription errors, late arrivals, and large quantities of drugs. Social conditions such as low income, difficulty shopping, and a lack of socialization tend to affect the nutrition of older adults. The nurse should educate older adults about the dual effects of poor nutritional status and drug metabolism.

Sociologic changes are based on the cultural values and attitudes about substance misuse behaviors passed from one generation to another. A lower incidence of SUD is seen in cultures whose religious and moral values prohibit or limit their use. Older adults are targeted by advertisements for prescription and nonprescription drugs because they experience minor aches, pains, and major health problems. SUDs are symptomatic of the larger social problems among minority groups (e.g., poverty, substandard housing, inadequate health care, and lack of power). The lack of culturally competent care is an additional barrier to care for older adults with SUD.

NURSING CARE GUIDELINES FOR SUDs

Recognize Cues (Assessment)

The following section is a general overview of the key concepts in assessing and planning nursing interventions for SUD in the older adult population. Nurses should be aware of the specific assessment and nursing intervention strategies for AUD, misuse of prescription and nonprescription drugs, illicit drugs, and nicotine. SUDs in older adults are challenging in that they require expertise in gerontology, geriatrics, psychiatric mental health, and the specific presentation and management of disorders in this population.

Substance Use History

The DSM-5-TR criteria for SUD are developed for the general population, not specifically for the older adult population. Therefore, it is essential for the nurse to assess patients' medical and psychological histories. After the history-taking is completed, the nurse should identify the key medical and psychological manifestations of SUD.

Screening Tools

Many screening tools are available to assess alcohol use. The two most commonly used tools are the CAGE (**C**utdown, **A**nnoyed by criticism, **G**uilt about drinking, and **E**ye-opener drinks) (Mayfield et al, 1974) and the Michigan Alcoholism Screening Test (MAST) (Selzer, 1971). The Brief Michigan Alcoholism Screening Test (BMAST) is a modified form of the MAST (Pokorny et al, 1972). Frederick Blow developed the MAST–Geriatric Version (MAST-G) (Morton et al, 1996). Results indicate that the MAST-G is an instrument that is more reliable and valid in the older adult population compared with the MAST (Knight and Mjelde-Mossey, 1995). Even though further research is required to validate the use of these tools for the assessment of SUD besides AUD, positive clinical results have been demonstrated with the use of these tools, substituting the words *substance* or *prescription medication* for *drink*.

Patients undergoing detoxification from AUD should be assessed with the use of the Clinical Institute Withdrawal Assessment tool on an ongoing basis. The tool measures the severity

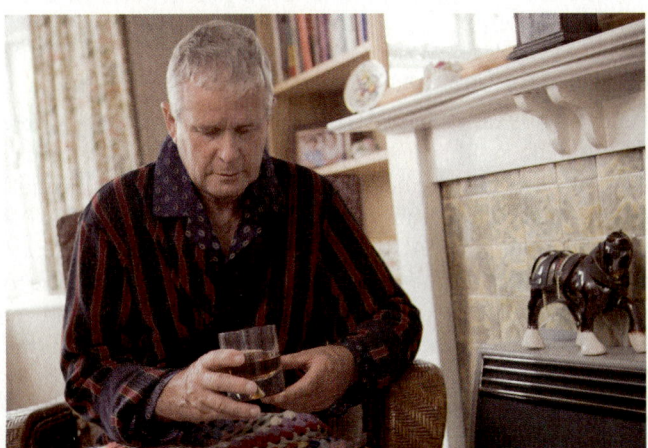

Fig. 14.2 Loneliness and hopelessness may be manifestations of AUD. (©BananaStock/Thinkstock.)

of alcohol withdrawal based on 10 common signs and symptoms: (1) nausea and vomiting; (2) tremor; (3) paroxysmal sweats; (4) anxiety; (5) agitation; (6–8) tactile, auditory, and visual disturbances; (9) headache; and (10) orientation. The maximum score is 67, and patients who score higher than 20 should be admitted to a hospital (Fontaine, 2008).

Nursing Caveats

In assessing older adults for SUD, the nurse must be aware of their own perceptions and attitudes regarding SUD in the older adult population. Many health care providers overlook the possibility that the presenting symptoms in an older adult may be related to SUD. It is important to have a healthy collaborative relationship with patients, showing respect for their values and choices.

Inherent changes in tissue and organ function are highly variable and individual. Hence, the response to drug therapy is just as variable and unpredictable in this population. The guiding principles are to "start low and go slow" when prescribing drugs; change or add only one drug at a time; review each drug to see whether the patient is still taking it; and determine the dose, frequency, and time.

Analyze Cues and Prioritize Hypotheses (Patient Problems)

The following list identifies patient problems that may be used for older adults with SUD:
- Inadequate family therapeutic management
- Anxiety
- Inadequate thermoregulation
- Confusion
- Inadequate coping
- Disrupted family routines
- Inadequate nutrition
- Reduced self-care ability (bathing, dressing, feeding, or toileting)
- Reduced body image
- Reduced sleep pattern
- Reduced social interaction
- Potential for self-directed violence
- Potential for outward-directed violence

Take Actions (Nursing Interventions)

Multidisciplinary interventions are appropriate for all individuals overcoming SUD because no single intervention is appropriate. Effective interventions attend to the multiple needs of individuals, not just their drug or substance use. Interventions must address medical, nursing, psychological, social, vocational, and legal problems.

Interventions and treatment options include brief therapy, intensive outpatient or inpatient treatment, and residential treatment. Brief therapy is usually provided by a trained professional in a community drug treatment center. Goal-setting, self-monitoring, and identifying high-risk situations are specific learned behaviors that help stop or reduce patients' substance misuse. Intensive outpatient programs allow patients to remain at home and continue working while they participate in treatment in an unrestricted setting for 4–5 hours every day. Intensive inpatient treatment is provided in the emergency department or acute care inpatient units to patients at risk of severe withdrawal symptoms, those who are psychiatrically disabled, and those who have not responded to less intensive treatment efforts. Residential treatment programs are downsizing and closing because third-party reimbursement is rapidly decreasing. Traditionally, treatment lasted 7–21 days and offered a safe and structured environment to those who lacked social and vocational skills and drug-free social supports to be abstinent in a less restricted setting (Fontaine, 2008).

Older adults resist referrals to SUD programs and are more comfortable with senior-oriented programs. Some are unable or unwilling to leave their homes; thus, programs should be specific for older adults and use special approaches such as slow-paced and emotionally supportive therapy instead of the confrontational style used with younger adults.

Acupuncture has been used to treat SUDs. It eases the symptoms of withdrawal, decreases the intensity of cravings, and decreases the number of relapses. Acupuncture is a safe and relatively low-cost form of treatment. However, more research is necessary before acupuncture or other complementary and alternative therapies can be recommended as treatment modalities for SUD (Junyue et al, 2021).

Evaluate Outcomes (Evaluation)

The evaluation of the treatment of older adults with SUD consists of the assessment of safe detoxification, adherence to the sobriety treatment plan, and outpatient support. Detoxification is safe if a patient has been weaned from the misused substance without seizures, delirium tremens (DTs), changes in vital signs, or other complications of withdrawal. Adherence is measured by noting if the patient is abstaining from substance use and attending meetings (e.g., Alcoholics Anonymous [AA] or Narcotics Anonymous [NA]) and individual or family group sessions. Finally, outpatient support is assessed to determine whether the patient maintains the relationship with a sponsor. A *sponsor* is someone who can be a mentor and support the patient during abstinence.

COMMONLY MISUSED SUBSTANCES IN OLDER ADULTS

Alcohol

Prevalence

AUD is difficult to assess because of the drug's legal status and socialization as a recreational activity in the United States. The difficulty in identifying AUD notwithstanding, the incidence of AUD identified in the older adult population in healthcare settings is 22%. The prevalence rate of alcohol misuse is projected to increase as more Baby Boomers reach retirement age (Kuerbis et al, 2014).

Some heavy drinkers with early-onset AUD survive into old age; others are late-onset drinkers who may have started drinking in late middle age and began to exhibit health problems related to AUD as they moved into older adulthood. Older adults who have used alcohol in the past without misuse may experience problems with alcohol consumption as changes occur in their bodies as a result of normal aging (e.g., decreased liver function or changes in body composition) (NIH, 2020).

Recognize Cues (Assessment)

Older adults with AUD may display symptoms of anxiety, nervousness, memory impairment, depression, blackouts, confusion, weight loss, and falls. In addition, the physical examination of an older adult may indicate the effects of alcohol on the various body systems. Table 14.7 shows age-related and alcohol-related changes in select body systems of older adults. The nurse should assess carefully for the following signs and symptoms: impaired sensations in the extremities, poor coordination, confusion, facial edema, alcohol on the breath, liver enlargement, jaundice, ascites, trembling or fidgeting, lack of attention to personal hygiene, and poor eating habits. Secondary problems may include malnutrition, cirrhosis, compromised hepatic function, osteomalacia because of a compromised metabolism of vitamin D, cardiomyopathy, atrophic gastritis, and a decline in cognitive status, especially with regard to memory and information processing. Laboratory evaluation should include assessment of liver function and levels of electrolytes, glucose, and magnesium, as well as electrocardiography (ECG) (Kuerbis et al, 2014).

AUD may not be accurately identified in older adults because many AUD symptoms, such as falls, bruises, cardiovascular problems, hypertension, and memory problems, may resemble other disease processes. Therefore, if an older adult displays these symptoms, it is imperative that the nurse assess for the possibility of alcohol misuse in addition to medical illness and disease.

After obtaining a health history and conducting a physical examination, the nurse should begin to assess specifically for AUD. The CAGE, MAST, MAST-G, or BMAST screening tools may help the nurse determine the amount and frequency of alcohol consumption. Input from family and friends should also be obtained. Family and friends may deny the problem; therefore, it is imperative that the nurse obtain the history of alcohol use in a detail-oriented, nonjudgmental manner (Pokorny et al, 1972; Knight and Mjelde-Mossey, 1995).

The nurse should be able to distinguish alcohol intoxication from alcohol withdrawal to apply the appropriate nursing interventions. Signs associated with alcohol intoxication include the scent of alcohol on the breath, slurred speech, lack of coordination, unsteady gait, nystagmus, impairment in attention or memory, and stupor or coma (APA, 2022). Assessment of the signs and symptoms of alcohol withdrawal is essential to providing the appropriate treatment and preventing DTs and seizures. Indications of alcohol withdrawal are elevated blood pressure, an elevated pulse, and autonomic hyperactivity. In addition, fever; increased hand tremors; insomnia; nausea and vomiting; transient visual, tactile, or auditory hallucinations or illusions; psychomotor agitation; anxiety; and grand mal seizures may occur (APA, 2022). Withdrawal symptoms begin 4–12 hours after alcohol use has been stopped or reduced. Symptoms tend to peak 48–72 hours after a patient's last drink (APA, 2022). It is important to assess older patients for the possibility of alcohol withdrawal if agitation, hallucinations, anxiety, or seizures develop 2 or 3 days after hospitalization (see Emergency Treatment box).

TABLE 14.7 Age- and Alcohol-Related Changes in Body Systems of Older Adults

Age-Related Changes	Corresponding Alcohol-Related Changes
Decline in liver function	Hepatotoxicity
Delayed neurologic conduction	An increase in Parkinson disease symptoms and altered balance
Idiopathic tremors	Tremors related to withdrawal
Predisposition to fall	Predisposition to fall
Loss of short-term memory	Impairment of short-term memory
Decreased glucose tolerance	Inhibition of glycogenesis
Decreased secretion of hydrochloric acid	Impaired absorption of nutrients
Slowed peristalsis	Impaired absorption of nutrients
Decreased saliva production	Impaired absorption of nutrients
Increase in cholesterol levels and cardiovascular disease	Increased plasma triglyceride levels Reduced total cholesterol and LDL levels
Less efficient cardiovascular function	Risk of congestive heart failure
Increased incidence of arthritis and gout	Increased uric acid levels
Decline in immunologic competence	Increased susceptibility to infection

Data from Coffey, C. E., & Cummings, J. L. (1994). *Textbook of geriatric neuropsychiatry*. Washington, D.C.: American Psychiatric Press; Solomon, K., Manepalli, J., Ireland, G. A., & Mahon, G. M. (1993). Alcoholism and prescription drug abuse in the elderly: St. Louis University Grand Rounds. *Journal of the American Geriatric Society, 41*, 57–69.

✚ EMERGENCY TREATMENT

Delirium Tremens

The following nursing interventions should be implemented for patients who experience DTs:
1. Assessment of vital signs.
2. Provision of a safe environment (padded side rails and decreased stimulation).
3. Close observation.
4. Administration of prescribed drugs such as benzodiazepines, BBs, clonidine, and anticonvulsant drugs.

Take Actions (Nursing Interventions)

Nursing interventions for older adults with AUD vary, depending on whether the patient is in detoxification or rehabilitation. Nurses should observe and document signs of withdrawal, provide an environment of low stimulation (e.g., dim lights and a quiet atmosphere), and initiate seizure precautions (e.g., padded side rails and the bed in the lowest position) during the detoxification process. In addition, the nurse should administer drugs such as benzodiazepines, BBs, and anticonvulsants, which are used to reduce symptoms of withdrawal and prevent complications. During the rehabilitation stage, recommended nursing interventions include patient education; continued administration of drugs; group, individual, and family therapy; and introducing the patient to the 12-Step Program. The nurse supports the patient with (1) education on the harmful effects of alcohol on the body and the effects of alcohol taken with prescription and nonprescription drugs, (2) various methods to overcome potential triggers for future substance misuse, and (3) plans to maintain sobriety in the community setting. The nurse should also educate family members on the potential changes in family dynamics resulting from the patient's sobriety. In addition, the nurse should encourage the recognition that SUD is a "family disease" and abstinence is affected by the family process. All family members need education to help identify triggers to avoid relapse and strategies for dealing with triggers (Fontaine, 2008; Mahgoub, 2009).

Many pharmacologic interventions have been used to inhibit drinking behaviors, with varying results. Drugs for recovery may include disulfiram, naltrexone, acamprosate, or topiramate. Disulfiram, when taken with alcohol, causes vomiting; naltrexone interferes with the pleasure derived from drinking; acamprosate reduces the craving for alcohol; and topiramate may alter the stimulating effects of alcohol. Thiamine may have to be added to improve nutritional status.

Evaluate Outcomes (Evaluation)

The evaluation of the treatment of an older adult patient with AUD includes safe detoxification, adherence to a treatment plan for sobriety, and outpatient support. Safe detoxification consists of weaning from alcohol without seizures, DTs, or other withdrawal complications. The nurse also assesses whether the patient is adhering to the sobriety protocol of abstinence and attendance at AA meetings and individual or family therapy. In addition, a continued relationship with the patient's sponsor and the patient's progress as reported by home health nurses provide the opportunity for evaluation of the patient's transition back into the community (Fontaine, 2008).

Prescription Drugs
Prevalence

The prevalence of misuse of prescription drugs among older adults is high. The number of drugs prescribed is directly correlated with the risk of their inadvertent misuse. As a result, the possibility of polypharmacy is high. Prescription drugs commonly used by independent older people are cardiovascular drugs, benzodiazepines, diuretics, cathartics, antacids, thyroidal drugs, and anticoagulants. Opioid and benzodiazepine dependence is a common occurrence, and the drugs may have been prescribed for long periods of time (Yarnell et al, 2020). The nurse may be the person who recognizes the possible existence of prescription drug misuse. The rapport between the nurse and the patient allows the patient to feel comfortable discussing drug use. Therefore, it is imperative that the nurse assess for prescription drug misuse in older adults.

Recognize Cues (Assessment)

The nursing assessment for prescription drug misuse in older adult patients is like the assessment used for AUD. The nurse should begin the assessment by taking a careful history using the CAGE, MAST, BMAST, or MAST-G screening tools (Morton et al, 1996). The nurse should remember to substitute the term *prescription drugs* for *alcohol*. In addition, the nurse should assess for a tendency to repeatedly lose prescriptions or pills (e.g., "I threw it away by accident," "I didn't think I would use them so I flushed them down the toilet"), prescriptions from multiple physicians, frequent emergency department visits, strong preferences for particular drugs (e.g., "Only X drug works for pain for me," "I'm allergic to Y, so I can only take X"), and above-average knowledge about drugs, as well as the severity of the complaint matching the clinical presentation. Finally, the nurse should assess the patient for signs associated with withdrawal, for example, anxiety, irritability, insomnia, fatigue, headache, tremors, sweating, dizziness, decreased concentration, nausea, depression, and visual or tactile hallucinations (Fontaine, 2008; Neushotz and Fitzpatrick, 2008; McNeely et al, 2021).

Take Actions (Nursing Interventions)

The interventions for prescription drug misuse are like the interventions associated with alcohol misuse. First, if prescription drug misuse is suspected, the nurse should ask the patient or a family member to bring in all drugs the patient is currently using and inform the physician so that a plan for safe detoxification can be established. The patient should be informed that, by bringing in all drugs currently being used, they are ensuring that the health care team can develop a comprehensive care plan to address the patient's needs. This also enables the health care provider to prevent any untoward drug interactions resulting from prescribing a new drug contraindicated because of an existing prescription. The nurse should document any signs of withdrawal, provide an environment of low stimulation, and implement seizure precautions. In addition, the nurse should administer, on a planned reduction schedule, any drugs prescribed to minimize withdrawal symptoms. Nutritional support interventions should also be implemented for patients with compromised nutritional status. Agents used to treat opioid dependence are methadone, buprenorphine, naloxone, and clonidine. Although these harm-reduction pharmacologic treatments are widely used for persons with opioid use disorders, no studies of the use of these drugs in the older adult population have been performed (Yarnell et al 2020). Finally, after discussion within the multidisciplinary team, concerns about prescription drug misuse and treatment options such as AA, NA, or individual or group therapy should be presented to the patient and family members in a patient-care conference (Fontaine, 2008).

Evaluate Outcomes (Evaluation)

The evaluation of nursing interventions for prescription drug misuse includes assessments of safe detoxification, participation in a rehabilitation treatment plan, and decreased drug-seeking behaviors. The nurse should also observe and document the patient's response to any teaching regarding appropriate drug use and the effects of drug misuse on the body.

Nicotine

Prevalence

Tobacco use disorder (TUD) is the single greatest cause of preventable disease and disability in the United States. TUD is a risk factor in 6 of the 13 leading causes of death in older adults. In the United States alone, approximately $50 billion is spent annually on medical costs attributed directly to tobacco use. Many tobacco users 50 years of age or older express the desire to quit; however, only those older adults with chronic illnesses tend to have the motivation to do so. Older adults who stop tobacco usage may improve quality of life and possibly increase life expectancy.

Recognize Cues (Assessment)

The nurse should thoroughly assess a patient's tobacco use pattern and look for signs of nicotine withdrawal. The CAGE questionnaire can be modified by substituting the word *smoking* for *alcohol* (Rustin, 2000). The patient's responses allow the nurse to plan appropriate interventions. Older adult patients should be monitored for signs of nicotine withdrawal such as depressed mood, insomnia, irritability, frustration, anger, anxiety, difficulty concentrating, restlessness, decreased heart rate, and increased appetite (APA, 2022).

Take Actions and Evaluate Outcomes (Nursing Interventions and Evaluation)

Nursing interventions for older adults with TUD include monitoring for signs of withdrawal, administration of nicotine replacement, behavior modification, and education. The type of nicotine replacement used is determined by the health care provider; options include gum, an inhaler, a lozenge, nasal spray, or a patch. The replacement period lasts from 6 weeks to several months and reduces the craving for cigarettes by weaning the patient from nicotine and preventing withdrawal symptoms. Patients who do not tolerate nicotine replacement may respond to bupropion or varenicline.

Cannabis

Prevalence

Recent analysis of data from the National Survey on Drug Use and Health (Han and Palamar, 2020) revealed that cannabis use among older adults increased from 0.4% in 2006 to 4.2% in 2018. This increase is thought to be related to recent changes in laws making cannabis more available and different attitudes and beliefs in current cohorts of older adults (Solomon et al, 2021).

Surveys suggest that older adults may use cannabis to treat common physical ailments and improve their general sense of well-being; the nurse should consider this perspective when doing a social history on all older adults (Agronin, 2021).

Recognize Cues (Assessment)

Older adults report using cannabis for pain, insomnia, epilepsy, glaucoma, inflammatory bowel disease, multiple sclerosis, post-traumatic stress disorder, and a variety of other medical comorbidities, but there are very few studies that have evaluated the safety and efficacy of medical or recreational cannabis in the older population (Solomon et al, 2021).

All older adults should be asked about their use of cannabis; the type and route of marijuana or CBD that is being used should be documented. In addition, the patient should be asked about the benefits and adverse reactions that they have experienced (Agronin, 2021).

Cannabis may present unique risks to older adults because of age-related changes, other comorbid medical problems, and other medications that they may be taking. There are no current studies that examine interactions between cannabis and other drugs in the older adult population.

Cannabis can cause a sedative effect and may potentiate the effects of sedatives or hypnotics. Cannabis, especially CBD, interacts with warfarin to prolong the INR. It is imperative that medication reconciliation be performed at each health care encounter and include all prescription, over the counter and herbal agents—whether they are legal or illegal. This process will assist in identifying potential drug interactions and untoward effects (Solomon et al, 2021).

Take Actions and Evaluate Outcomes (Nursing Interventions and Evaluation)

The psychoactive component of cannabis, Δ-9 tetrahydrocannabinol (THC), has been shown to reduce memory, attention, reaction time, and motor function in a dose-dependent fashion in older adults (Vo et al, 2018). The nurse should query the older adult in regard to driving issues, changes in mentation, changes in energy level, or alertness in an attempt to determine if the patient is experiencing any adverse effects from their cannabis usage. Oftentimes, the older adult is using cannabis to treat a medical malady that is not well controlled or is untreated by other prescription regimens. Because the science is evolving, we do not have data to ensure safety with the use of cannabis products. Surveillance and monitoring are paramount to reducing the risk of untoward side effects.

> ### PATIENT/FAMILY TEACHING
> #### Safe Use of Drugs
>
> - Know the name, amount, type, frequency, purpose, and side effects of both the prescription and nonprescription drugs that you are taking.
> - If you see more than one care provider, always bring all your drugs to every visit you make.
> - Never borrow drugs from anyone else or share your drugs with anyone else.
> - Make sure your family members can safely self-administer drugs; adequate vision, memory, judgment, and coordination are all essential.
> - Supervise drug administration for those people who cannot safely self-administer. Talk to the health care provider about simplifying the drug regimen by using a daily dosing schedule set for once or twice a day.
> - Never mix alcohol with *any* drug.
> - Use a single pharmacy for filling all prescriptions to reduce the potential for interactions as well as misuse.

Sustained-release bupropion is an effective aid in smoking cessation. The nurse should obtain a detailed patient history regarding the existence of any seizure disorder because bupropion is contraindicated in such cases, and another drug or technique should be recommended. Furthermore, the nurse must carefully assess the bupropion candidate for any history of alcohol misuse or head trauma; these patients are at increased risk for seizures. Varenicline, along with education and counseling, is also effective in helping people stop smoking. Varenicline is in a class of drugs called *smoking cessation aids*. It works by blocking the pleasant effects of nicotine on the brain. Some people have experienced changes in behavior, hostility, agitation, depression, suicidal ideation, and worsening of preexisting psychiatric illness while taking varenicline (American Cancer Society, 2020).

Evaluation of nursing interventions includes assessing for decreased use of tobacco, adherence to a plan to reduce tobacco use, and understanding of the effects that tobacco and nicotine have on the body.

FUTURE TRENDS

Current figures indicate as many as 7.2% of older adults use illicit drugs; prevalence is expected to increase as more Baby Boomers reach retirement age (Kuerbis et al, 2014). Older adults should be screened for drug misuse. A simple, one-question screen, "How many times in the past year have you used an illegal drug or used a prescription drug for nonmedical reasons?" has been shown to accurately identify individuals using drugs in the outpatient setting; however, a trial has not been conducted in older adults (Smith et al, 2010).

HOME CARE

1. Obtain a prescription drug inventory, including the physician's sources for all prescriptions.
2. Mail-order prescription suppliers send large quantities of drugs to homebound older adults, which predisposes them to drug wasting, overdosing, and other misuse.
3. Assess the number of caregivers involved with drug administration to prevent overdosing and other administration errors.
4. Drug use patterns of homebound older adults, including the administration of prescription drugs, OTC drugs, and home remedies, are influenced by cultural and ethnic health practices.
5. During the assessment of homebound older adults, include an inventory of the use of caffeine, nicotine, and alcohol.
6. Assess high-risk factors (e.g., social isolation and depression) that may predispose homebound older adults to SUD.
7. Assess for signs of SUD in homebound older adults.
8. Encourage caregivers to attend support groups such as AA to ease the burden of caring for a homebound older adult with SUD.

SUMMARY

Achieving positive therapeutic outcomes and reducing ADEs requires knowledge of age-related alterations that determine how older adults react to drugs, an understanding of the unique problems attributable to aging, and an awareness of resources to address problems and concerns related to drug use. Nurses must accept this responsibility if improved patient outcomes are to be realized.

The prognosis for untreated SUD in older adults is poor because of physiologic and psychological consequences. It is essential that nurses identify SUD in older adults and examine their own attitudes about SUD in this population. Early identification and intervention are essential for preventing misdiagnosis and ineffective, costly treatments. Nurses should recognize that older adults who misuse substances can be treated effectively. The first step in effective treatment is identification. After a problem is identified, a cost-effective treatment may be initiated to help an older adult return to a healthy lifestyle.

KEY POINTS

- Older adults consume a large proportion of pharmaceutical products. The use of inappropriate drugs results in significant morbidity and mortality and adds an economic burden to patients and the health care system.
- Older adults may be at risk for adverse drug reactions because of age-related changes, multiple chronic illnesses, polypharmacy, nonadherence, and a lack of knowledge.
- A reduction in drug dosage is often required for older adults whose ability to excrete drugs is decreased or whose renal or hepatic function is reduced.
- Knowledge of clinically important drug interactions is essential in planning alternative drug regimens and preventing potentially serious ADEs.
- Drug problems should always be suspected in patients experiencing overt or subtle changes in cognitive or physical function.
- Antipsychotic drugs should not be used by older adults with dementia.
- The nurse can play a key role not only in assessing patients for risk factors that may reduce adherence but also in developing strategies to reduce or eliminate these risks.
- For most drugs prescribed for older adults, it is necessary to start low, go slow, and periodically review drug regimens.
- The age-related physiologic changes of altered absorption, distribution, metabolism, and excretion affect drug usage and place older adults at an increased risk for SUD.
- Psychological changes, primarily a result of the numerous losses older adults may experience in a relatively short time, place them at an increased risk for SUD.
- Sociologic changes such as decreased finances, transportation, and social support, as well as sociocultural factors such as gender and race, may place older adult patients at risk for SUD.
- The substances most often misused by the older adult population are alcohol, prescription drugs, nonprescription drugs, nicotine, and caffeine.

- The nurse should assess older adult patients for key medical and psychological manifestations of SUD through their health history. Some of these key manifestations are falls, hypertension, memory loss, depressed mood, and social withdrawal.
- Screening tools such as the CAGE, MAST, MAST-G, and BMAST should be used to screen for SUD in older adult patients.
- Key nursing interventions for SUD in older adult patients include assessing for signs of withdrawal, administering appropriate drugs to provide safe detoxification, providing a safe environment, educating patients regarding harmful effects, and encouraging patients to participate in AA, NA, or individual, family, or group therapy.

CLINICAL JUDGMENT EXERCISES

1. An older adult with a history of congestive heart failure is taking many prescription drugs, including psyllium, digoxin, phenytoin, and cimetidine. They are 5 feet, 9 inches tall and weigh 139 pounds. Based on potential drug interactions, identify the relevant assessment priorities. What factors place this patient at risk for drug toxicity?
2. A home care nurse is seeing an older adult who is taking a complex drug regimen. They cannot remember when they last took several of their drugs, and their partner states they are confused by the recent switch of several drugs to other generic brands. What questions should the nurse ask to establish the patient's risk for nonadherence?
3. An older adult's child wonders if they should have their parent use ginkgo and other herbals to help with Alzheimer disease. How would you advise the adult child?
4. Compare nursing assessments and interventions for prescription drug, nonprescription drug, and alcohol misuse. How are they similar, and how are they different? How might assessment techniques be revised for the older adult population?
5. Analyze your own perceptions and attitudes regarding SUD in general. How do these perceptions and attitudes differ from those presented here regarding SUD in the older adult population? What factors and assumptions contribute to these perceptions?
6. How might the DSM-5 criteria for SUD be revised to specifically address the older adult population?

REFERENCES

Agronin, M. (2021). The age of cannabis has arrived: Issues for older adults. *Psychiatric Times*, 38(3), 18–19. Retrieved from https://cdn.sanity.io/files/0vv8moc6/psychtimes/1fa187081479c0a745b41127ad4288f11ec573cd.pdf/PSY0321_ezine.pdf. Accessed July 28, 2023.

Ahmed, A., Rich, M. W., Fleg, J. L., Zile, M. R., Young, J. B., Kitzman, D. W., et al. (2006). Effects of digoxin on morbidity and mortality in diastolic heart failure: The ancillary digitalis investigation group trial. *Circulation*, 114(5), 397–403. doi:10.1161/CIRCULATIONAHA.106.628347.

American Cancer Society. (2020). *Prescription medicines to help you quit tobacco*. Retrieved from https://www.cancer.org/healthy/stay-away-from-tobacco/guide-quitting-smoking/prescription-drugs-to-help-you-quit-smoking.html#. Accessed July 28, 2023.

American Geriatrics Society (AGS). (2023). American Geriatrics Society 2023 Updated AGS Beers Criteria® for potentially inappropriate medication use in older adults. *Journal of the American Geriatrics Society*, 71, 2052–2081. doi:10.1111/jgs.18372.

American Medical Association (AMA) Staff. (2023). *8 reasons patients don't take their medications*. Retrieved from https://www.ama-assn.org/delivering-care/patient-support-advocacy/8-reasons-patients-dont-take-their-medications. Accessed July 28, 2023.

American Psychiatric Association (APA). (2022). *Diagnostic and statistical manual of mental health disorders: Text revision (DMS-5-TR)*. Washington, DC: The Association.

Aymanns, C., Keller, F., Maus, S., Hartmann, B., & Czock, D. (2010). Review on pharmacokinetics and pharmacodynamics and the aging kidney. *Clinical Journal of the American Society of Nephrology*, 5(2), 314–327. doi:10.2215/CJN.03960609.

Bailey, D. G., Dresser, G., & Arnold, J. M. O. (2013). Grapefruit-medication interactions: Forbidden fruit or avoidable consequences? *CMAJ: Canadian Medical Association Journal*, 185(4), 309–316. doi:10.1503/cmaj.120951.

Beers, M. H., Ouslander, J. G., Rollingher, I., Reuben, D. B., Brooks, J., & Beck, J. C. (1991). Explicit criteria for determining inappropriate medication use in nursing home residents. *Archives of Internal Medicine*, 151(9), 1825–1832.

Bunis, D. (2019). *High prescription drug prices lead many consumers to ignore doctors' orders*. AARP [website]. Retrieved from https://www.aarp.org/politics-society/advocacy/info-2019/drug-prices-consumer-impact.html. Accessed July 28, 2023.

Burchum, J. R., & Rosenthal, L. D. (2022). *Lehne's pharmacology for nursing care* (11th ed.). St. Louis MO: Elsevier.

Carnahan, R. M., Brown, G. D., Letuchy, E. M., Rubenstein, L. M., Gryzlak, B. M., Smith, M., et al. (2017). Impact of programs to reduce antipsychotic and anticholinergic use in nursing homes. *Alzheimer's & Dementia*, 3(4), 553–561. doi:10.1016/j.trci.2017.02.003.

Calleo, J., & Stanley, M. A. (2008). Anxiety disorders in later life: Differentiated diagnosis and treatment strategies. *Psychiatric Times*, 25(8), 24–27. Retrieved from https://www.psychiatrictimes.com/view/anxiety-disorders-later-life. Accessed July 28, 2023.

Centers for Disease Control and Prevention (CDC). (2010). *Medication safety basics.* Retrieved from https://www.cdc.gov/medicationsafety/basics.html. Accessed July 28, 2023.

Centers for Medicare & Medicaid Services (CMS). (2022). *National partnership to improve dementia care in nursing homes: Antipsychotic medication use data report (April 2022).* Retrieved from https://www.cms.gov/files/document/antipsychotic-medication-use-data-report-2021q2-updated-01142022.pdf. Accessed July 28, 2023.

Clark, C. M., Shaver, A. L., Aurelio, L. A., Feuerstein, S., Wahler, Jr., R. G., Daly, C. J., et al. (2020). Potentially inappropriate medications are associated with increased healthcare utilization and costs. *Journal of the American Geriatrics Society, 68*(11), 2542–2550. doi:10.1111/jgs.16743.

Davis, T. C., Wolf, M. S., Bass, P. F., Thompson, J. A., Tilson, H. H., Neuberger, M., et al. (2006). Literacy and misunderstanding prescription drug labels. *Annals of Internal Medicine, 145*(12), 887–894. doi:10.7326/0003-4819-145-12-200612190-00144.

Drenth-van Maanen, A. C., Wilting, I., & Jansen, P. A. F. (2020). Prescribing medicines to older people—how to consider the impact of ageing on human organ and body functions. *British Journal of Clinical Pharmacology, 86*(10), 1921–1930. doi:10.1111/bcp.14094.

Drenth-van Maanen, A. C., Jansen, P. A. F., Proost, J. H., Egberts, T. C. G., van Zuilen, A. D., van der Stap, D., et al. (2013). Renal function assessment in older adults. *British Journal of Clinical Pharmacology, 76*(4), 616–623. doi:10.1111/bcp.12199.

Dufort, A., & Samaan, Z. (2021). Problematic opioid use among older adults: Epidemiology, adverse outcomes and treatment considerations. *Drugs & Aging, 38*(12), 1043–1053. doi:10.1007/s40266-021-00893-z.

Flammiger, A., & Maibach, H. (2006). Dermatological drug dosage in the elderly. *Skin Therapy Letter, 11*(8), 1–7.

Fontaine, K. L. (2008). *Mental health nursing* (6th ed.). Upper Saddle River, NJ: Pearson.

Gahche, J. J., Bailey, R. L., Potischman, N., & Dwyer, J. T. (2017). Dietary supplement use was very high among older adults in the United States in 2011–2014. *The Journal of Nutrition, 147*(10), 1968–1976. doi:10.3945/jn.117.255984.

Han, B. H., & Palamar, J. J. (2020). Trends in cannabis use: Use among older adults in the United States, 2015-2018. *JAMA Internal Medicine, 180*(4), 609–611. doi:10.1001/jamainternmed.2019.7517.

Holle, L. (2017). Pharmacist perspective on the CDC guideline for prescribing opioids for chronic pain. *Drug Topics, 161*(3), 54–65.

Institute of Medicine (IOM). (2007). *Preventing medication errors: Quality chasm series.* Washington, DC: The National Academies Press.

Jeste, D. V., & Maglione, J. E. (2013). Atypical antipsychotics for older adults: Are they safe and effective as we once thought? *Journal of Comparative Effectiveness Research, 2*(4), 355–358. doi:10.2217/cer.13.33.

Joshi, S. (2008). Nonpharmacologic therapy for insomnia in the elderly. *Clinics in Geriatric Medicine, 24*(1), 107–119. doi:10.1016/j.cger.2007.08.005.

Junyue, J., Siyu, C., Xindong, W., Qinge, X., Jingchun, Z., Liming, L., et al. (2021). Complementary and alternative medicine for substance use disorders: A scientometric analysis and visualization of its use between 2001 and 2020. *Frontiers in Psychiatry, 12*, 722240. doi:10.3389/fpsyt.2021.722240.

Kaufman, G. (2013). Prescribing and medicines management in older people. *Nursing Older People, 25*(7), 33–41. doi:10.7748/nop2013.09.25.7.33.e441.

Khairullah, A., Platt, B., & Chater, R. W. (2018). Medication nonadherence in older adults: Patient engagement solutions and pharmacist impact. *Pharmacy Times, 84*(11). Retrieved from https://www.pharmacytimes.com/view/medication-nonadherence-in-older-adults-patient-engagement-solutions-and-pharmacist-impact. Accessed July 28, 2023.

Kim, J., & Parish, A. L. (2017). Polypharmacy and medication management in older adults. *Nursing Clinics of North America, 52*(3), 457–468. doi:10.1016/j.cnur.2017.04.007.

Kim, J., & Parish, A. L. (2021). Nursing: Polypharmacy and medication management in older adults. *Clinics in Integrated Care, 8*, 100070. doi:10.1016/j.intcar.2021.100070.

Kim, L. D., Koncilja, K., & Nielsen, C. (2018). Medication management in older adults. *Cleveland Clinic Journal of Medicine, 85*(2), 129–135. doi:10.3949/ccjm.85a.16109.

Knight, B. G., & Mjelde-Mossey, L. A. (1995). A comparison of the Michigan Alcoholism Screening Test and the Michigan Alcoholism Screening Test–Geriatric Version in screening for higher alcohol use among dementia caregivers. *Journal of Mental Health and Aging, 1*(2), 147.

Kuerbis, A., Sacco, P., Blazer, D. G., & Moore, A. A. (2014). Substance abuse among older adults. *Clinics in Geriatric Medicine, 30*(3), 629–654. doi:10.1016/j.cger.2014.04.008.

Li, W. W., Wallhagen, M. I., & Froelicher, E. S. (2008). Hypertension control, predictors for medication adherence and gender differences in older Chinese immigrants. *Journal of Advanced Nursing, 61*(3), 326–335. doi:10.1111/j.1365-2648.2007.04537.x.

Madden, J. M., Graves, A. J., Zhang, F., Adams, A. S., Briesacher, B. A., Ross-Degnan, D., et al. (2008). Cost-related medication nonadherence and spending on basic needs following implementation of Medicare Part D. *JAMA, 299*(16), 1922–1928. doi:10.1001/jama.299.16.1922.

Mahgoub, N. (2009). An 80-year-old woman with alcohol problems. *Psychiatric Annals, 39*(1), 17. doi:10.3928/00485713-20090101-04.

Maniaci, M. J., Heckman, M. G., & Dawson, N. L. (2008). Functional health literacy and understanding of medications at discharge. *Mayo Clinic Proceedings, 83*(5), 554–558. doi:10.4065/83.5.554.

Masnoon, N., Shakib, S., Kalisch-Ellett, L., & Caughey, G. E. (2017). What is polypharmacy? A systematic review of definitions. *BMC Geriatrics, 17*(1), 230. doi:10.1186/s12877-017-0621-2.

Mattson, M., Lipari, R. N., Hays, C., & Van Horn, S. L. (2017). *A day in the life of older adults: Substance use facts.* The CBHSQ Report [website]. Rockville, MD: Center for Behavioral Health Statistics and Quality, Substance Abuse, and Mental Health Services Administration. Retrieved from https://www.samhsa.gov/data/sites/default/files/report_2792/ShortReport-2792.html. Accessed July 28, 2023.

Mayfield, D., McLeod, G., & Hall, P. (1974). The CAGE questionnaire: validation of a new alcoholism screening instrument. *The American Journal of Psychiatry, 131*(10), 1121–1123. doi:10.1176/ajp.131.10.1121.

McNeely, J., Adam, A., Rotrosen, J., Wakeman, S. E., Wilens, T. E., Kannry, J., et al. (2021). Comparison of methods for alcohol and drug screening in primary care clinics. *JAMA Network Open, 4*(5), e2110721. doi:10.1001/jamanetworkopen.2021.10721.

Mohundro, M., & Ramsey, L. A. (2003). Pharmacologic considerations in geriatric patients. *Advance for Nurse Practitioners, 11*(9), 21–22, 25–28.

Moon, M. A. (2009). Elderly with anxiety respond well to CBT. *Family Practice News, 39*(9), 18.

Morton, J. L., Jones, T. V., & Manganaro, M. A. (1996). Performance of alcoholism screening questionnaires in elderly veterans. *The*

American Journal of Medicine, 101(2), 153–159. doi:10.1016/s0002-9343(96)80069-6.

Nagalla, S., & Besa, E. C. (2023). *Glucose-6-phosphate dehydrogenase [D6PD] deficiency*. Medscape.com [website]. Retrieved from https://emedicine.medscape.com/article/200390-print. Accessed July 28, 2023.

National Institutes of Health (NIH), & National Institute on Drug Abuse. (2020). *Substance use in older adults*. DrugFacts. Retrieved from https://nida.nih.gov/publications/drugfacts/substance-use-in-older-adults-drugfacts. Accessed July 28, 2023.

Neushotz, L. A., & Fitzpatrick, J. J. (2008). Improving substance abuse screening and intervention in a primary care clinic. *Archives of Psychiatric Nursing, 22*(2), 78–86. doi:10.1016/j.apnu.2007.04.004.

Patel, D., Steinberg, J., & Patel, P. (2018). Insomnia in the elderly: A review. *Journal of Clinical Sleep Medicine, 14*(6), 1017–1024. doi:10.5664/jcsm.7172.

Pawaskar, M. D., & Sansgiry, S. S. (2006). Over-the-counter medication labels: Problems and needs of the elderly. *Journal of the American Geriatrics Society, 54*(12), 1955–1956. doi:10.1111/j.1532-5415.2006.00958.x.

Pham, C. B., & Dickman, R. L. (2007). Minimizing adverse drug events in older patients. *American Family Physician, 76*(12), 1837–1844.

Pokorny, A. D., Miller, B. A., & Kaplan, H. B. (1972). The brief MAST: A shortened version of the Michigan Alcoholism Screening Test. *The American Journal of Psychiatry, 129*(3), 342–345. doi:10.1176/ajp.129.3.342.

Qato, D. M., Wilder, J., Schumm, P. L., Gillet, V., & Alexander, G. C. (2016). Changes in prescription and over-the-counter medication and dietary supplement use among older adults in the United States, 2005 vs 2011. *JAMA Internal Medicine, 174*(4), 473–482. doi:10.1001/jamainternmed.2015.8581.

Raman, M., Middleton, R. J., Kalra, P. A., & Green, D. (2017). Estimating renal function in old people: an in-depth review. *International Urology and Nephrology, 49*(11), 1979–1988. doi:10.1007/s11255-017-1682-z.

Ruppar, T. M., Conn, V. S., & Russell, C. L. (2008). Medication adherence interventions for older adults: literature review. *Research and Theory for Nursing Practice, 22*(2), 114–147.

Ruscin, J. M., & Linnebur, S. A. (2021). Pharmacokinetics in older adults. In *merck manual professional version*. Merck & Co., Inc. Retrieved from https://www.merckmanuals.com/professional/geriatrics/drug-therapy-in-older-adults/pharmacokinetics-in-older-adults. Accessed October 23, 2024.

Rustin, T. A. (2000). Assessing nicotine dependence. *American Family Physician, 62*(3), 579–584, 591–592.

Safari, D., DeMarco, E. C., Scanlon, L., & Grossberg, G. T. (2022). Over-the-counter remedies in older adults: Patterns of use, potential pitfalls, and proposed solutions. *Clinics in Geriatric Medicine, 38*(1), 99–118. doi:10.1016/j.cger.2021.07.005.

Savage, C. (2014). The baby boomers and substance use—are we prepared? *Journal of Addictions Nursing, 25*(1), 1–3. doi:10.1097/JAN.0000000000000015.

Selzer, M. L. (1971). The Michigan alcoholism screening test: The quest for a new diagnostic instrument. *The American Journal of Psychiatry, 127*(12), 1653–1658. doi:10.1176/ajp.127.12.1653.

Shi, S., Mörike, K., & Klotz, U. (2008). The clinical implications of ageing for rational drug therapy. *European Journal of Clinical Pharmacology, 64*(2), 183–199. doi:10.1007/s00228-007-0422-1.

Smith, P. C., Schmidt, S. M., Allensworth-Davies, D., & Saitz, R. (2010). A single-question screening test for drug use in primary care. *Archives of Internal Medicine, 170*(13), 1155–1160. doi:10.1001/archinternmed.2010.140.

Snow, A. L., Loup, J., Morgan, R. O., Richards, K., Parmelee, P. A., Baier, R. R., et al. (2021). Enhancing sleep quality for nursing home residents with dementia: A pragmatic randomized controlled trial of an evidence-based frontline huddling program. *BMC Geriatrics, 21*(1), 281. doi:10.1186/s12877-021-02189-8.

Solomon, H. V., Greenstein, A. P., & DeLisi, L. E. (2021). Cannabis use in older adults: A perspective. *Harvard Review of Psychiatry, 29*(3), 225–233. doi:10.1097/HRP.0000000000000289.

Spiesel, S. (August 27, 2008). Medication error death rate up 500 percent [Radio broadcast episode]. In A. Chadwick (Editor and Host), *Health & science*. Washington, DC: National Public Radio.

Substance Abuse and Mental Health Services Administration (SAMHSA). (2019). *Results from the 2018 National survey on drug use and health: Detailed tables*. Rockville, MD: Center for Behavioral Health Statistics and Quality, Substance Abuse and Mental Health Services Administration. Retrieved from https://www.samhsa.gov/data/report/2018-nsduh-detailed-tables. Accessed July 28, 2023.

Substance Use Disorders. (n.d.). Retrieved from https://adultmentalhealth.org/substance-use-disorders/. Accessed October 7, 2024.

U.S. Food and Drug Administration (FDA). (2019). *Working to reduce medication errors*. Retrieved from https://www.fda.gov/drugs/information-consumers-and-patients-drugs/workingreduce-medication-errors. Accessed July 28, 2023.

U.S. Food and Drug Administration (FDA). (2022). *Information for consumers and patients—drugs*. Retrieved from https://www.fda.gov/drugs/resources-drugs/information-consumers-and-patients-drugs. Accessed October 23, 2024.

Verma, N., Rastogi, S., Chia, Y. C., Siddique, S., Turana, Y., Cheng, H. M., et al. (2021). Non-pharmacological management of hypertension. *Journal of Clinical Hypertension, 23*(7), 1275–1283. doi:10.1111/jch.14236.

Vo, K. T., Horng, H., Li, K., Ho, R. Y., Wu, A. H. B., Lynch, K. L., et al. (2018). Cannabis intoxication case series: The dangers of edibles containing tetrahydrocannabinol. *Annals of Emergency Medicine, 71*(3), 306–313. doi:10.1016/j.annemergmed.2017.09.008.

Wakefield, D. S., Ward, M. M., Groath, D., Schwichtenberg, T., Magdits, L, Brokel, J., et al. (2008). Complexity of medication-related verbal orders. *American Journal of Medical Quality, 23*(1), 7–17. doi:10.1177/1062860607310922.

Walckiers, D., Van der Heyden, J., & Tafforeau, J. (2015). Factors associated with excessive polypharmacy in older people. *Archives of Public Health, 73*, 50. doi:10.1186/s13690-015-0095-7.

Wendling, P. (2006). Doctors need to educate patients on proper disposal of old drugs. *Internal Medicine News, 34*(4), 50.

Whelton, P. K., Carey, R. M., Aronow, W. S., Casey, Jr., D. E., Collins, K. J., Himmelfarb, C. D., et al. (2018). 2017 ACC/AHA/AAPA/ABC/ACPM/AGS/APhA/ASH/ASPC/NMA/PCNA Guideline for the prevention, detection, evaluation, and management of high blood pressure in adults: A report of the American College of Cardiology/American Heart Association Task Force on Clinical Practice Guidelines. *Journal of the American College of Cardiology, 71*(19), e127–e248. doi:10.1016/j.jacc.2017.11.006.

Wold, R. S., Lopez, S. T., Yau, C. L., Butler, L. M., Pareo-Tubbeh, S. L., Waters, D. L., et al. (2005). Increasing trends in elderly persons' use of nonvitamin, nonmineral dietary supplements and concurrent use of medications. *Journal of the American Dietetic Association, 105*(1), 54–64. doi:10.1016/j.jada.2004.11.002.

Wu, A. (2018). Special considerations for opioid use in elderly patients with chronic pain. *US Pharmacist, 43*(3), 26–30.

Retrieved from https://www.uspharmacist.com/article/special-considerations-for-opioid-use-in-elderly-patients-with-chronic-pain. Accessed July 28, 2023.

Yan, J. (2008). FDA extends black-box warning to all antipsychotics. *Psychiatric News, 43*(14). Retrieved from https://psychnews.psychiatryonline.org/doi/full/10.1176/pn.43.14.0001.

Yarnell, S., Li, L., MacGrory, B., Trevisan, L., & Kirwin, P. (2020). Substance use disorder in later life—a review and synthesis of the literature of an emerging public health concern. *American Journal of Geriatric Psychiatry, 28*(2), 226–236. doi:10.1016/j.jagp.2019.06.005.

PART V

Nursing Care of Physiologic and Psychological Disorders

15

Integumentary Function

Patti A. Parker, PhD, RN, ACNS, ANP, GNP, BC, GS-C

http://evolve.elsevier.com/Yeager/gerontologic/

LEARNING OBJECTIVES

On completion of this chapter, the reader will be able to:
1. Discuss the primary functions of the integumentary system.
2. Identify normal, age-related skin changes.
3. Discuss common skin problems and conditions experienced by older adults and their associated nursing implications.
4. Describe common skin cancers that affect older adults.
5. Describe the risk factors for pressure-injury development.
6. Identify five pressure-injury preventive strategies endorsed by the National Pressure Injury Advisory Panel (NPIAP) and the current evidence-based guidelines.
7. State the three principles necessary for successful wound healing.
8. Conduct an assessment for a patient with impaired skin integrity.
9. Determine when to appropriately use antiseptics.
10. Describe the indications, contraindications, advantages, and drawbacks of various wound dressings.
11. Distinguish between arterial and venous lower extremity ulcers.

WHAT WOULD YOU DO?

What would you do if you were faced with the following situations?
- You are caring for an older adult patient in the critical care unit. The admitting diagnosis is heart failure (HF); the patient also has a history of diabetes type 2 mellitus (T2DM) and hypertension (HTN). The patient is ambulatory with standby assistance. How would you determine your patient's risk for a pressure injury? What is your patient's risk?
- Your 68-year-old patient with obesity and a history of chronic obstructive pulmonary disease (COPD) is admitted with pneumonia and is prescribed levofloxacin and prednisone. Your patient is at risk of developing acute skin conditions? How would the acute skin conditions be treated?

The integumentary system is the largest organ in the body. The primary function of the skin is to serve as a barrier against harmful bacteria and other threatening agents, which makes the skin the first line of defense for the immune system. Other major functions of the integumentary system include (1) preventing fluid loss or dehydration, (2) protecting the body from ultraviolet (UV) rays and other external environmental hazards, and (3) protecting underlying organs from injury. In addition, the skin provides thermal regulation of body temperature. Radiation, conduction, convection, and evaporation are facilitated by sensory perceptions that occur in the skin's nerve endings. The skin also assists in the regulation of blood pressure via its effects on cutaneous vessels, blood flow, and sodium retention (Lawton, 2019). The integumentary system reveals emotions such as anger, fear, or embarrassment through vasodilatation, which reddens the skin tissue. In the presence of the sun's UV rays, the skin synthesizes vitamin D, which is then used by other parts of the body. Subcutaneous (SQ) fat, the deepest layer of the integumentary system, provides insulation and acts as a caloric reservoir. Hair serves as body insulation and provides unique physical characteristics through its varying textures, shades, patterns, and colors.

A careful and thorough assessment of the integumentary system is essential when a physical assessment is performed on a patient. Skin assessment helps determine hydration status, potential for or actual infection, and other information about the individual (e.g., sun exposure, attention to personal appearance, and scars). Palpation of the skin identifies tender areas, nodules, and masses.

The value of the integumentary system is demonstrated by the high morbidity and mortality rates associated with extensive burns when all functions of the skin are greatly compromised. The overall state of health is affected by physical or emotional insults to this system, for example, loss of thermal regulation or fluid, impaired barrier protection, and other catastrophic changes in physical appearance and functioning.

AGE-RELATED CHANGES IN SKIN STRUCTURE AND FUNCTION

The integumentary system reflects changes associated with aging, which include graying hair, increased number and depth of wrinkles, loss of elasticity, and discoloration and thickening of the nails. Box 15.1 describes basic age-related skin changes.

Epidermis

The epidermis is the outermost layer of the skin. The replacement rate of the stratum corneum, the first layer of epidermis, declines by 50% as a person ages. This decline results in slower healing, reduced barrier protection, and delayed absorption of medications and chemicals placed on the skin. The area of contact between the epidermis and dermis decreases with age, which results in easy separation of these layers. Therefore, skin tears occur from harmless activities such as removing a bandage or pulling an older patient up in the bed. The older adult is more at risk for blistering skin diseases, such as bullous pemphigoid, because of this separation. Bruising occurs more easily because of these age-related skin changes. A thinner epidermis allows more moisture to escape and may compound previously existing skin problems. The number of melanocytes, which provide pigment and hair color, decreases with age, giving older adults less protection from UV rays, paler skin, and graying hair. Melanocytes also produce uneven pigmentation, causing the development of solar lentigos (or lentigines), also known as *age spots* or *liver spots*.

Dermis

The dermis decreases in thickness by approximately 20% with aging. It consists of strong connective tissue that contains the sweat glands, blood vessels, and nerve endings. With aging, sweat glands, blood vessels, and nerve endings decrease in number. These changes lead to diminished thermoregulatory function and inflammatory responses, decreased tactile sensation, reduced pain perception, and the development of wrinkles and sagging skin because of the loss of underlying tissue. Collagen, a fibrous protein that provides tensile strength within the dermis, stiffens and becomes less soluble.

Subcutaneous Fat

Aging results in a decreased amount of SQ tissue and a redistribution of fat to the abdomen and thighs. Breast tissue also changes and becomes more granular and atrophic. Because of a loss of padding supplied by SQ tissues, the risk for hypothermia, skin shear (see Pressure Injuries section later in this chapter for the definition and adverse effects of shear), and blunt trauma injury is greater. The loss of this protective padding increases the vulnerability of pressure points. Topical medication and dermal medication patch absorption may be increased because of the changes in the SQ tissue.

Dermal Appendages

With aging, fewer eccrine glands (sweat glands of the palms, feet, and forehead) and apocrine sweat glands (sweat glands of the axilla, scalp, face, and genital areas) exist, resulting in decreased body odor and reduced evaporative heat loss because of decreased sweating. The need for antiperspirants and deodorants is reduced. However, older adults are at greater risk of heat stroke because of a compromised cooling mechanism. Older adults should avoid heat exposure over long periods and in areas of high humidity. Hats with wide brims and cool, light, breezy sun-protective clothing should be worn when outdoors. It is important that older adults drink adequate fluid to maintain adequate hydration. Although more data are needed in this area (Scherer et al, 2016), the National Council on Aging (2021) recently released guidelines for hydration in older adults. These guidelines take into consideration the age-related attenuation of the body's ability to maintain extracellular electrolyte levels during exercise and heat (Meade et al, 2020).

Sebum oils the skin and provides an antimicrobial property. The sebaceous glands and pores become larger with aging. Nevertheless, many older adults experience dry skin (xerosis), which places them at a greater risk of infection because of an impaired immune response.

Hair thins, and its growth declines. A progressive loss of melanin occurs, resulting in graying of the hair. Heredity influences the onset of the graying process. Older females may have increased lip and chin hair while experiencing thinning of the hair on the head, axilla, and perineal area. Males lose scalp and beard hair and experience increased growth over the eyebrows and in the ears and nostrils. The increased hair in the ears predisposes males to cerumen impaction, which leads to impaired hearing. Changes in the patterns of hair growth and distribution as a person ages are thought to be hormone-related. Nails grow more slowly with age and become thick, brittle, and dull, developing longitudinal striation with ridges (Blume-Peytavi et al, 2016). These changes may affect a person's body image and self-concept (see Cultural Awareness box).

Dermatoporosis

Nearly 35% of older adults experience chronic skin fragility. This fragile skin is called *dermatoporosis*. The identifying features of dermatoporosis include atopic changes, actinic purpura, and white pseudoscars (Fig. 15.1). The skin appears nearly translucent. It occurs on sun-exposed areas of the extremities. Individuals with dermatoporosis frequently experience skin lacerations associated with increased bleeding and delayed healing (Dyer and Miller, 2018).

BOX 15.1 Age-Related Skin Changes

- Loss of thickness, elasticity, vascularity, and strength that may delay the healing process and increase the risk of skin tears and bruising
- Increased lentigines (brown-pigmented spots, or age spots)
- Loss of SQ tissue causes wrinkling and sagging of the skin, which may affect self-esteem, temperature control, and drug efficacy
- Loss of hair follicles along with thinning and graying
- Increased hair density in the nose and the ears, particularly in males, which may clog external ear canals and impair hearing
- Thicker nails with longitudinal lines
- Decreased sebaceous and sweat gland activity, which affects thermoregulation and decreases sweating
- Higher incidence of benign and malignant skin growths

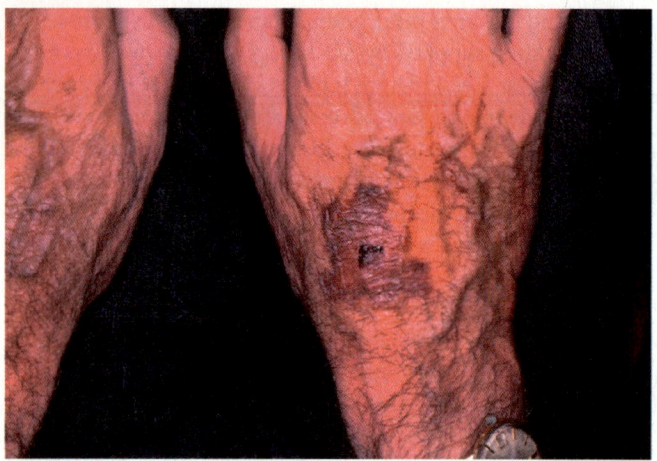

Fig. 15.1 Dermatoporosis. (From Wallach, D. [2013]. Dermatologie pour les gériatres. *NPG Neurologie – Psychiatrie – Gériatrie, 13*[78], 303–315.)

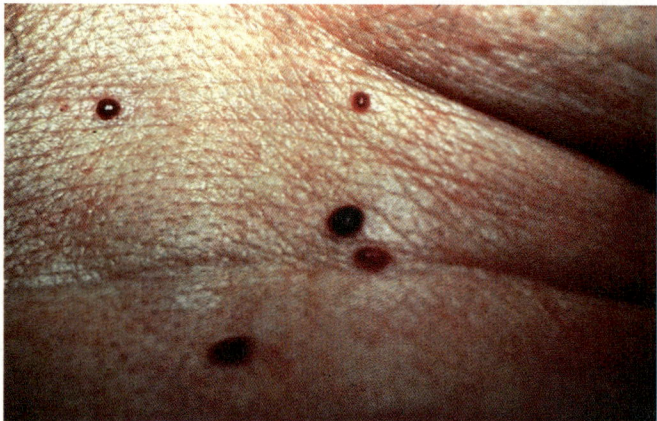

Fig. 15.2 Cherry angiomas. (From Ignatavicius, D. D., Workman, M. L., & Rebar, C. R. [2018]. *Medical-surgical nursing: Concepts for interprofessional collaborative care* [9th ed.]. St. Louis, MO: Elsevier.)

> ### 🌐 CULTURAL AWARENESS
> #### Skin Assessment in Darkly Pigmented Skin
>
> Prioritize the assessment of:
> - Skin temperature
> - Edema
> - Change in tissue consistency in relation to surrounding tissue
>
> Assess localized pain as part of every skin assessment:
> - Use natural light or halogen versus fluorescent, which gives the illusion of bluish tint
> - May not distinguish blanching; look for areas darker than surrounding skin, or taut, shiny, indurated areas
> - Light from a camera flash may enhance visualization
> - Check for localized changes in skin texture and temperature
> - Erythema may cause hyperpigmentation with no visible redness
> - May appear dark bluish-purple
> - Should be able to detect heat over an area of localized inflammation
> - Injured skin may have nonpitting edema with or without color changes

Data From Black, J., & Simende, A. (2020). Ten top tips: assessing darkly pigmented skin. *Wounds International, 11*(3), 8–11. Retrieved from https://www.woundsinternational.com/resources/details/ten-top-tips-assessing-darkly-pigmented-skin; and Zulkowski, K. (2011). *Conducting a comprehensive skin assessment*. Agency for Healthcare Research and Quality. [PowerPoint presentation]. Retrieved from https://www.ahrq.gov/sites/default/files/wysiwyg/professionals/systems/hospital/pressure_ulcer_prevention/webinars/webinar4_pu_skinassesst_final.pdf.

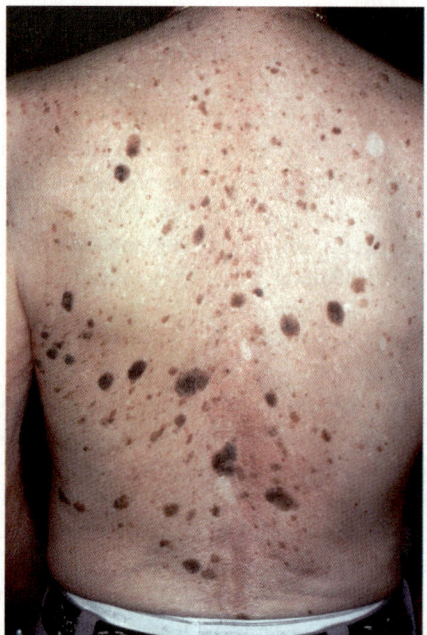

Fig. 15.3 Seborrheic keratosis. (From Micheletti, R. G., James, W. D., Elston, D. M., & McMahon, P. J. [2023]. Epidermal nevi, neoplasms, and cysts. In *Andrews' Diseases of the Skin Clinical Atlas* [2nd edition]. Philadelphia: Elsevier, pp 437-462.)

COMMON PROBLEMS AND CONDITIONS

Benign Skin Growths

Cherry Angiomas

Cherry angiomas are common, bright red, 1–5-millimeter (mm) superficial vascular lesions that begin around age 30 and increase in number with age. The cause of these lesions is unknown. They are red or deep purple dome-shaped papules (Fig. 15.2). Although they are most often found on the trunk, they may be located anywhere on the body and vary in number. Because cherry angiomas are new growths, patients are often concerned that they are malignant or indicate a serious health problem. Patients need to be reassured that cherry angiomas are benign growths resulting from increased vascularity in the dermis and occur in most people. These lesions need no treatment.

Seborrheic Keratoses

Seborrheic keratoses are benign lesions more commonly seen in older adults. These are scaly growths that have a "stuck-on," crumbly appearance that varies in color from tan to brown to black (Fig. 15.3). The lesions may be elevated and range in diameter from 2–3 mm. Characterized by slow growth; these lesions begin to appear later in life. The borders may be round and smooth or irregular and notched. To the untrained eye, these lesions may resemble a malignant melanoma, particularly when dark brown or black. They have a greasy feeling and often

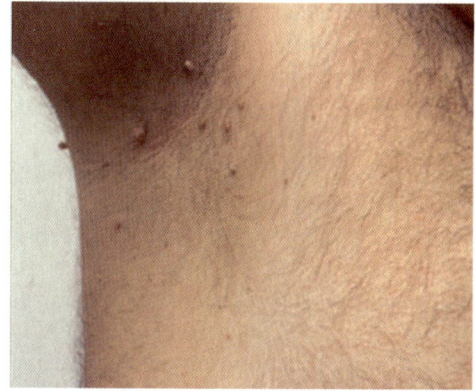

Fig. 15.4 Skin tags. (From Yuen, K. C. J., & Beckers, A. [2021]. Acromegaly: clinical description and diagnosis. In C. A. Stratakis, [Ed.]. *Gigantism and Acromegaly.* London: Elsevier, [pp 53-78.])

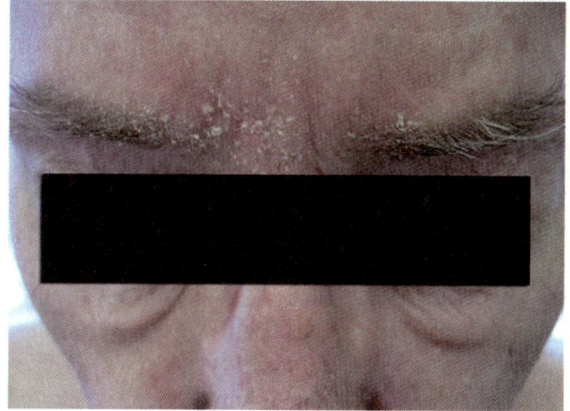

Fig. 15.5 Seborrheic dermatitis. (From Endo, J. Skin problems. In E. Flaherty, R. J. Ham, M. K. McNabney, J. F. Potter, G. A. Warshaw, & M. T. Heflin. [2022]. *Ham's primary care geriatrics: A case-based approach* [7th ed., pp. 532–551]. Philadelphia: Elsevier. Courtesy Dr. Robert Norman.)

occur in sun-exposed areas (face, neck, or trunk) but may appear anywhere on the body. The growths may be removed for cosmetic reasons (often related to self-esteem) or if they are irritated. If the lesion is "picked off," it will recur. Therefore, it is best to have a health care provider remove the growth if it is bothersome to the patient. Cryotherapy is effective, and the lesion usually sloughs off in a few weeks. Patients should be reassured that the growths are benign and are a commonly occurring skin manifestation.

Skin Tags (Acrochordons)

Skin tags are common stalk-like, benign tumors often found on the neck, axilla, eyelids, and groin, although they may occur anywhere on the body (Fig. 15.4). Beginning as early as age 20, these are tiny, flesh-colored, or brown excrescences that develop into a long, narrow stalk (up to 1 centimeter [cm]). As they mature, they can be easily removed with scissors, electrocautery, or liquid nitrogen. Skin tags are usually excised only at the request of the patient, usually for cosmetic reasons.

Inflammatory Dermatoses
Seborrheic Dermatitis

Seborrheic dermatitis is a common, chronic inflammation of the skin. The scalp, ear canals, eyebrows, eyelashes, nasolabial folds, axilla, breasts, chest, and groin are common sites (Fig. 15.5). The usual pattern of distribution begins at the hairline; it can involve the scalp and move down toward the eyebrows, progressing to the chest with a bilateral, symmetric presentation. It is more common in patients who have Parkinson disease or who have suffered a stroke.

In differentiating between dandruff and seborrheic dermatitis, it should be noted that *dandruff* is scaling without inflammation, and *seborrheic dermatitis* is an inflammatory response sometimes associated with scaling. With inadequate management, dandruff may evolve into seborrheic dermatitis. Seborrheic dermatitis appears as a white or yellow scale with a plaque-like appearance. An erythematous red base, indicating an inflammatory process, is *always* present. Mild itching is not uncommon. Medicated shampoos containing ketoconazole, ciclopirox, selenium sulfide, zinc pyrithione, coal tar, and salicylic acid are

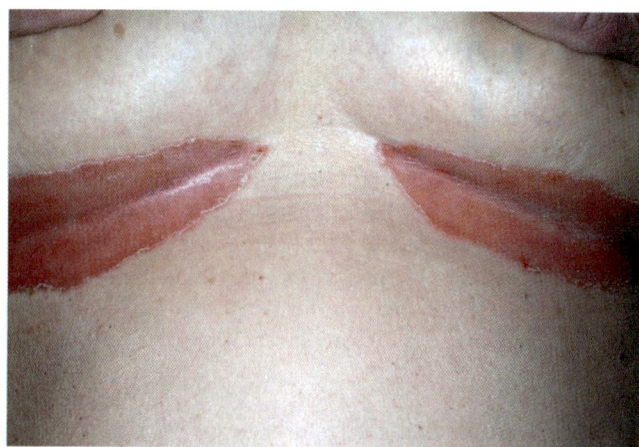

Fig. 15.6 Intertrigo. (From Miller, J. J., & Marks, Jr., J. G. [2019]. *Lookingbill and Marks' principles of dermatology* [6th ed., pp. 166–183]. Philadelphia: Elsevier.)

effective for seborrheic dermatitis of the scalp. Low-potency topical corticosteroids, such as hydrocortisone, desonide, and mometasone furoate, are effective for facial seborrheic dermatitis. Topical calcineurin inhibitors such as pimecrolimus and tacrolimus can be used in refractory cases as steroid-sparing agents (Clark et al, 2015; Elgash et al, 2019; Bholah et al, 2022).

Intertrigo

Intertrigo is a rash in the skin flexures (Fig. 15.6). This condition suggests inflammation or infection. Skin surfaces that are touching one another because of moisture, lack of ventilation, or friction are common etiologies. Bodily fluids such as fecal materials, urine, or sweat can worsen the inflammatory process (Oakley et al, 2018). It is usually found in the armpits, inner aspects of the thighs, skin folds of the breasts, and abdominal folds. The area is erythematous and may itch. Intertrigo often occurs in older adults who are obese or have diabetes. Medical management includes appropriate use of an antimicrobial agent (antifungal or antibacterial), a low-potency topical steroid, and keeping the skin clean and dry.

Psoriasis

Psoriasis is an autoimmune condition that affects 2%–3% (125 million people) of the world's population and approximately 2.2% (78 million) of the US population (Armstrong et al, 2021). The condition may affect persons of any age, although it often begins during early adulthood. Psoriasis is often associated with other diseases, such as cardiovascular disease, metabolic syndrome, hypertension, dyslipidemia, and Crohn's disease. Obesity and tobacco use are independent risk factors for developing psoriasis. Approximately one-third of patients with psoriasis have a first-degree relative affected by the disease; those developing the disease before age 40 have a stronger genetic component (Mercy et al, 2013; Burden-Teh et al, 2016). Once psoriasis begins, there are periods of remission and relapse with varying degrees of intensity. Currently, no known cure exists.

Clinically, psoriatic lesions are typically seen as well-circumscribed, pink plaques covered with silver-white, loosely adherent scales. These scaly plaques result from the accelerated replication of the dermis and epidermis in certain parts of the body. Psoriasis frequently affects the skin of the elbows, knees, scalp, lumbosacral areas, intergluteal cleft, and genitals. Changes in the nails occur in approximately 30% of patients and consist of yellow-brown discoloration with pitting, dimpling, separation of the nail plate from the underlying bed (oncolysis), thickening, and crumbling. Psoriasis is a reactive disorder. Triggers such as infection, smoking, climate, and hormonal factors may exacerbate an attack; other factors, such as sunlight, may decrease the severity of an attack. There are multiple forms of psoriasis, including plaque, nail, guttate, pustular, inverse, erythrodermic, and psoriatic arthritis.

Nursing Care Guidelines for Psoriasis

Recognize cues (assessment). Nursing assessment consists of recognizing the inflammatory dermatitis and noting its location, degree of erythema, itching, and scaling. The dermatitis should be examined for an erythematous base with yellow, white, or silvery scales or plaques. The nurse should inquire about itching, usual hygienic habits, and steps the patient has taken to control the scaly, erythematous dermatitis. Bedbound individuals are more likely to develop seborrheic dermatitis; therefore, targeting these patients for assessment, in addition to thorough cleansing of the scalp, hair, and skin, is a preventive strategy.

Analyze cues and prioritize hypotheses (patient problems). Patient problems for a patient with inflammatory dermatitis include the following:
- Reduced skin integrity resulting from an immunologic deficit (psoriasis)
- Reduced skin integrity resulting from bedbound states (seborrheic dermatitis)
- Reduced skin integrity resulting from the physiologic disease process (intertrigo)
- Distorted body image resulting from the psoriatic lesions

Generate solutions (planning). The goal of nursing management is to control the inflammatory process with maintenance therapy using topical agents and shampoo, as prescribed. Patient comfort is evidenced when medical treatment is performed according to advice. Expected outcomes include the following:
1. Skin lesions will remain free from infection.
2. The patient will experience resolution of the inflammatory process.
3. The patient will demonstrate increased knowledge of the condition, as evidenced by:
    - Verbalizing the rationale for regular and consistent skin care
    - Verbalizing knowledge of maintenance therapy
    - Verbalizing triggers inflammatory dermatitis
    - Demonstrating accurate application of topical medications

Take actions (nursing interventions). One crucial aspect of nursing management is to ensure proper use of an antiseborrheic shampoo containing zinc pyrithione, selenium sulfide, or ketoconazole. One successful strategy is to wet the hair, chest, axilla, and affected areas; apply the shampoo; and then proceed with the rest of the bath or shower. After cleansing the affected areas, the patient should apply the prescribed steroid cream, which decreases the inflammation and irritated red appearance of the skin. After inflammation and scaling have resolved, the patient should continue using selenium shampoo on the scalp twice a week as preventive maintenance therapy.

Nursing interventions for a patient with psoriasis consist of reinforcing the directions of the health care provider to optimize treatment and identify patient-specific triggers that may be avoided to decrease the severity of flare episodes. Because psoriasis varies in type and severity, treatment plans may use both prescription and over-the-counter (OTC) topical ointments. As with seborrheic dermatitis, a common therapy used to treat psoriasis is a topical steroid. Topical steroids, which may be OTC or prescription-strength ointments or creams, are not recommended for use on the facial, axillary, or perineal skin. Tazarotene is a *retinoid*, a group of drugs related to vitamin A. It should be applied only to the affected areas, and contact with the eyes, eyelids, and mouth should be avoided. Because the medication may result in photosensitivity, exposure to sunlight should be avoided. Psoriasis that affects >5% of the body's surface area; affects the palms, soles, and perineum; or is refractory to topical therapies is best treated with immune and/or biologic therapies under the care of a health care provider specializing in dermatology. These agents may be oral, SQ, or intravenous (IV) medications.

For those who are not candidates for immune modulators and have failed topical therapies, light therapy using ultraviolet B (UVB) rays has been shown to be beneficial when used in prescription light boxes. It is currently thought that ultraviolet A (UVA) light therapy used in combination with psoralen (an oral or topical medication) is the preferred method (called *PUVA*). The UV dosage is carefully monitored for exposure because the total exposure time has a set limit. With UVA light therapy, it is important to be aware of the potential risk of developing skin cancer. Many reports suggest that foods may trigger psoriasis attacks; therefore, approaches to diet modification and other homeopathic remedies abound in the patient resource literature. Patients should be encouraged to discuss with their health care team all remedies used. The nurse should teach the older adult patient, family members, and staff the causes of inflammatory dermatitis to alleviate anxiety and misconceptions. An explanation of treatment measures and the importance of follow-through will increase adherence and involvement in care. Symptom management is an area where nurses can have a positive effect on an older adult's quality of life.

Evaluate outcomes (evaluation). Nursing accountability and evaluation are supported through accurate, comprehensive charting that describes physical assessment and maintenance interventions. A weekly assessment of the lesions with a description of the response to treatment, including maintenance therapy, is performed. In addition, the nurse should address the response to teaching (e.g., verbalized understanding) as measured by patient, family, or staff adherence to treatment.

Pruritus

Pruritus is another term for itching that is so intense that it causes the patient to scratch the offending area. The most common cause of itching is dry skin, or xerosis. Atopic eczema, contact or other forms of dermatitis, urticaria, psoriasis, or bullous pemphigoid are other sources of pruritus. Infections and drug reactions can also be causative agents.

The mechanism of itching is not fully understood, but histamine is a known mediator of pruritus. Heat, sudden temperature changes, sweating, clothing, cleaning products such as soap, fatigue, and emotional stress may precipitate itching, and it may be more severe in the winter (De Oakley and de Menezes, 2016). Pruritus may be related either to a skin disorder or systemic disease; therefore, the complaint should not be dismissed and warrants a complete assessment. Pruritus may occur with other dermatologic conditions and with systemic disorders such as liver, kidney, hematologic, diabetes, and thyroid conditions (Oakley and de Menezes, 2016).

Nursing Care Guidelines for Pruritus

Recognize cues (assessment). A full skin assessment is warranted when a patient complains of pruritus. The patient is interviewed to determine the location, intensity, and onset of the itching. The nurse should inquire about any patterns of behavior that precipitate itching (e.g., anxiety, environmental exposures, or friction [rubbing the skin with a towel]) and obtain information about bathing practices and the kinds of soaps, detergents, and skin products used (Ständer et al, 2015). The nurse should also look for rashes, vesicles, scaling, and erythema; any of these suggests a skin disorder.

Analyze cues and prioritize hypotheses (patient problems). Patient problems for a patient with pruritus include the following:
- Potential for reduced skin integrity resulting from scratching
- Pain resulting from persistent burning and itching
- Anxiety resulting from role strain, family crisis, or other sources of the patient's anxiety
- Potential for infection resulting from impaired skin integrity

Generate solutions (planning). The goal of nursing management is to resolve pruritus without injury from scratching. Time should be planned to teach the patient and family about etiologic factors and the importance of not scratching. Expected outcomes include the following:
1. The skin will remain intact.
2. The patient will experience adequate periods of rest without symptoms of scratching.
3. The patient will obtain adequate pain relief, as evidenced by the verbalization of comfort and pain relief.

Take actions (nursing interventions). Nursing interventions are influenced by the cause of the pruritus. If dry, scaly skin (xerosis) is present with no lesions or erythema, the nurse should suggest that the patient apply emollients (e.g., Lubriderm, Moisturel, or Eucerin cream), which have more lanolin or oily substances than many commercial lotions. Emollients should be applied at least twice daily and immediately after bathing to trap moisture. The patient should gently pat the skin dry and avoid brisk drying with a towel. If the patient is unable to apply cream, the nurse should instruct the caregiver on its use. The patient should decrease the frequency of baths or showers to a maximum of every other day (see Patient/Family Teaching box). Antihistamines may be needed to relieve itching and prevent tissue breakdown from scratching, but they are to be used with caution because of their adverse effects in older adults.

The American Academy of Dermatology (AAD) has online educational materials for the public devoted to dry skin relieving interventions (AAD, 2023a).

PATIENT/FAMILY TEACHING
Prevention and Treatment of Dry Skin (Xerosis)

- Take short baths or showers (no more than 5–10 minutes) daily with warm (not hot) water.
- Use gentle fragrance-free cleansers.
- Gently pat (rather than rub) the skin dry.
- Apply skin moisturizer immediately after drying; use ointment or cream rather than a lotion.
- Skin care products should be unscented and alcohol-free.
- If needed, use a humidifier to add moisture to the air in the home.
- Apply sunscreen daily, especially when going outdoors.
- Wear fabrics such as cotton that allow the skin to breathe and use hypoallergenic laundry detergent.
- Stay hydrated by drinking at least 8 glasses of water daily, if not contraindicated by a medical condition (e.g., HF or renal disease).

Modified from Scott, S. (2012). Atopic dermatitis and dry skin. In D. Krinsky, R. Berardi, S. Ferreri, A. L. Hume, G. D. Newton, C. J. Rollins, et al. (Eds.), *Handbook of nonprescription drugs* (17th ed.). Washington, DC: American Pharmacists Association; and *Dermatologists' top 10 tips for relieving dry skin.* American Academy of Dermatology Aging SkinNet [website]. Retrieved from www.skincarephysicians.com/agingskinnet/winter_skin.html.

A diagnostic workup may be conducted to identify any systemic cause of persistent pruritus (e.g., cancer or diabetes). Anxiety or stress may be the source of itching. If so, the nurse should assess the patient's self-esteem and coping strategies and identify any family or role strain or other factors that may lead to anxiety. The nurse should also discuss stress management strategies and assist the patient in determining effective ones.

A referral to a community agency or counseling may be needed for continued support and guidance.

The older patient, family members, and staff need to be taught the management of pruritus and the need to prevent skin trauma from scratching. Treatment measures should also be explained to increase adherence and involvement in care. The causes of pruritus may be difficult to determine, and the expected effects of topical agents may be diminished because of the delayed absorption of medications placed on aging skin.

Evaluate outcomes (evaluation). Evaluation of interventions focuses on symptom relief, prevention of secondary complications, and, when possible, identification of the source of the pruritus. Nursing accountability is demonstrated through documentation of physical presentation such as erythema and intact skin with no lesions, hives, or rash; response to treatment measures; patient comprehension of teaching; and other nursing interventions.

Candidiasis

Candidiasis is an inflammatory process of the epidermis caused by a yeast-like fungus. There are more than one hundred subspecies of this fungus; however, the most common species that affect the skin are *Candida albicans, Candida tropicalis,* and *Candida glabrata.* Most recently, *Candida aureus* has become a pathogen of concern as it is often resistant to current available therapies (Flowers and Elston, 2020). *C. albicans* is a normally occurring flora in the mouth, vagina, and gut (moist habitats). Pregnancy, oral contraception, antibiotics, diabetes, topical and inhalant steroids, skin maceration, and immunocompromised conditions create an environment that fosters the development of yeast infections such as candidiasis. Candidiasis is most often seen in diaper-clad infants, patients with incontinence, and bedbound individuals, as well as in the moisture-prone areas of the body (e.g., skin folds and axillae).

Candidiasis is characterized by erythematous, denuded, or raw skin, usually surrounded by satellite papules or pustules (Fig. 15.7). Satellite lesions are a helpful diagnostic clue. Red, erythematous areas on the buttocks, perineum, or intertriginous areas of incontinent patients also have diagnostic significance. Scaling may also be present, usually at the borders (Flowers and Elston, 2020).

Nursing Care Guidelines for Candidiasis

Recognize cues (assessment). Nursing assessment includes inspection of the skin, particularly under any fat folds, where moisture will accumulate. A hallmark of candidiasis is a bright red erythema with satellite papules or pustules. Any breaks in the skin, which place the patient at greater risk for infection or further breakdown, should be noted. The patient may be the one to alert the nurse to the infection. The nurse should conduct a medication assessment to identify any medications that may have precipitated this fungal infection, for example, antibiotics or steroids. If the patient has diabetes, hyperglycemia may be present; therefore, the nurse should conduct a diet assessment to evaluate adherence and should check the blood sugar level. In some individuals with diabetes mellitus type 2, candidiasis infection may be the first clinical manifestation of hyperglycemia.

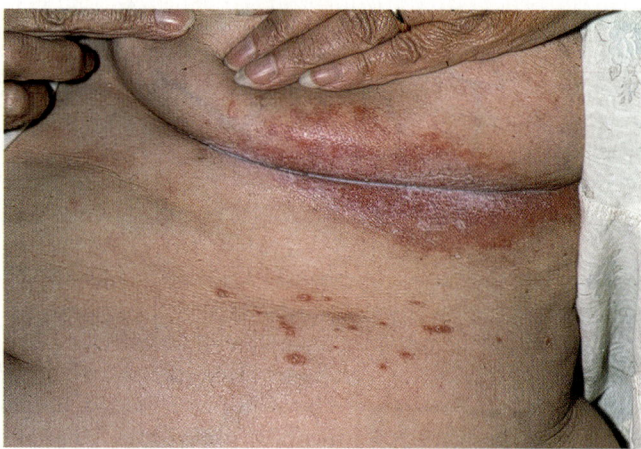

Fig. 15.7 Candidiasis. (From White, G. M., & Cox, N. H. [Eds.]. [2006]. *Diseases of the skin: A color atlas and text* [2nd ed.]. St. Louis: Mosby.)

Therefore, a thorough health history is warranted when a candidiasis infection is present.

Analyze cues and prioritize hypotheses (patient problems). Patient problems for a patient with candidiasis include the following:
- Reduced skin integrity results from poor control of moisture
- Inadequate toileting self-care
- Inadequate urinary elimination

Generate solutions (planning). The goals of nursing management are the prevention and resolution of candidiasis and, consequently, increased patient comfort. Expected outcomes include the following:
1. Skin lesions will be without evidence of infection and will heal.
2. The patient will perform self-care practices (within limitations) to keep the skin dry and clean.
3. The skin will regain its usual appearance without evidence of candidiasis.

Take actions (nursing interventions). The main nursing intervention is keeping the skin dry, especially the intertriginous areas. A patient's discomfort, costs, and nursing time are minimized through the use of preventive strategies such as drying the skin well (particularly the skin folds) after bathing or sweating episodes and changing the sheets as soon as possible after an episode of incontinence. After changing linens, the nurse should cleanse and dry the skin well and apply a zinc-based cream (such as Desitin or Calmoseptine) to the buttocks and perineal area. Cornstarch or powder, whether medicated or scented, is not recommended because of clumping. Creams are much more effective and efficient.

The nurse should teach the older adult patient, family members, and support staff to pat the skin dry; the nurse should also educate the staff and provide the scientific rationale for changing linen, cleansing the affected area, and using a moisture barrier such as zinc oxide or Desitin. The importance of prompt delivery of care after an incontinent episode must be stressed. It is important to keep topical antifungal agents on the infected area until healing is complete, which may take 2–3 weeks. If the yeast infection does not improve or appears worse, the health care provider should be informed so that an alternative agent can be considered.

Management protocols may be developed and approved by the employee's institution and medical and nursing staff with the intent of empowering the professional nurse to act immediately when candidiasis is present. This promotes high-quality care, patient comfort, a sense of professional pride, and a team approach. Nursing management is key to resolving a candidiasis infection.

Evaluate outcomes (evaluation). Evaluation of nursing management focuses on treatment efficacy and the rate of recurrence. The nurse must document how the infection responds to medical treatment and the maintenance therapy of keeping the skin dry and applying a moisture barrier. The effectiveness of patient care is supported by positive outcomes, adherence to preventive actions, and verbalized comprehension. If little improvement is seen in 2 weeks, the nurse should ensure that moisture control and the application of antifungal cream are being maintained. Consultation with the health care provider is needed when the response to therapy is poor; another agent may need to be prescribed.

Herpes Zoster (Shingles)

Herpes zoster, also known as *shingles,* is caused by the reactivation of the latent varicella zoster (chickenpox) virus (Fig. 15.8). The virus remains in the dorsal nerve endings after an episode of chickenpox, which is usually experienced in childhood. The main reason for recurrence is decreased immunity. Conditions that may impair the immune system are advanced age, stress or emotional upset, fatigue, or radiotherapy. An immunocompromised state caused by disease (e.g., human immunodeficiency virus [HIV], COVID-19, lymphoma, leukemia, and other malignancies) or drugs (e.g., chemotherapy and steroids) may also activate the latent virus. Chickenpox is highly contagious because it is an airborne virus. Herpes zoster is not as infectious; however, it may spread through direct contact with open sores. Therefore, it is not necessary to isolate a patient with herpes zoster. Cases of contracting chickenpox after personal exposure have been reported, but these have been in individuals who have not had chickenpox. Consequently, only health care personnel who have had chickenpox or have positive serum varicella titers should care for patients with herpes zoster (Centers for Disease Control and Prevention [CDC], 2023). As always, universal precautions should be followed.

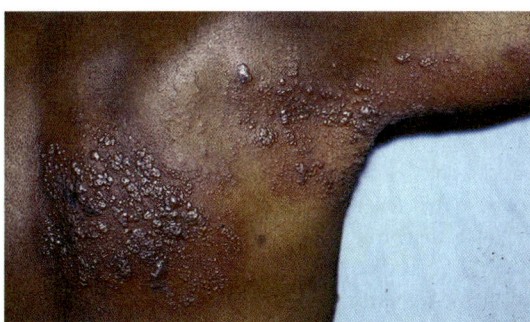

Fig. 15.8 Herpes zoster. (From Chen, H. M., Prundeanu Croitoru, A. G., Hu, S., Kamino, H., Ramos-e-Silva, M., & Busam, K. J. [2016]. Infectious diseases of the skin. In K. J. Busam [Ed]. *Dermatopathology* [2nd ed.]. Philadelphia: Elsevier, pp 102-180.)

Approximately 50% of herpes zoster cases involve the thoracic region, 15% involve the cranial dermatomes, and 10% affect the cervical and lumbar regions. Ophthalmic herpes zoster is referred to an ophthalmologist for evaluation and treatment because blindness could result from corneal scarring.

Herpes zoster often has prodromal symptoms of tingling, hyperesthesia, tenderness, and burning or itching pain along the affected dermatome. Vesicles follow the prodromal symptoms, with an erythematous base occurring within 3–5 days. A unilateral, bandlike, erythematous, maculopapular rash first occurs along the involved dermatome and rarely crosses the midline of the body. The rash develops into clustered vesicles (usually on an erythematous base) that become purulent, rupture, and crust. Debilitated older adults may have a prolonged and difficult course. For them, the eruption is typically more extensive and inflammatory, occasionally resulting in hemorrhagic blisters, skin necrosis, secondary bacterial infection, or extensive scarring, which is sometimes hypertrophic or keloidal (CDC, 2023). These vesicles are prone to secondary bacterial infections. This occurs more often in older adults. It may take up to 1 month for the crusting lesions to heal; mild cases resolve in 7–10 days. The average duration for herpes zoster is 3 weeks. Scarring and permanent or temporary pigment discoloration may occur, especially in severe cases. Lymphadenopathy and occasional temperature elevations are not uncommon. Postinfection paresthesia and meningoencephalitis may occur for 2–4 weeks when motor neurons and the central nervous system (CNS) are involved (Brizzi and Lyons, 2014).

The incidence of herpes zoster increases with age, most likely because of diminishing immune function. The older adult is also at a greater risk of developing postherpetic segmental pain. Dissemination is often seen in older adults or immunosuppressed patients. Disseminated herpes zoster, which is rare and occurs in only 2%–5% of patients, is more serious because of its systemic nature. In disseminated herpes zoster, satellite lesions appear outside the affected dermatome within 4–6 days after the initial eruption. Dissemination may be associated with fever, lymphadenopathy, headache, neck rigidity, and an increased risk of serious complications such as encephalitis, hepatitis, and pneumonitis (Dinulos, 2021).

One of the major complications from this acute viral infection is postherpetic neuralgia, which is pain that persists along the affected dermatome after resolution of vesicular lesions. Postherpetic neuralgia may last less than 1 year, but it may last a lifetime with little pain relief. It affects approximately 33% of patients aged 40 or older, and by age 70, the risk increases to 74%. Postherpetic neuralgia is more common in persons with trigeminal nerve involvement (CDC, 2023).

Postherpetic neuralgia is markedly reduced through vaccination for herpes zoster. The recombinant herpes zoster vaccine (Shingrix) is currently approved for adults aged 50 and older (Dinulos, 2021).

Nursing Care Guidelines for Herpes Zoster (Shingles)

Recognize cues (assessment). Nursing assessment begins with interviewing the patient to identify prodromal symptoms such as burning, itching, or tingling along a dermatome before rash development. The nurse should obtain a pertinent health history that addresses chickenpox history, medications, diabetes, malignancy with recent chemotherapy or radiotherapy, and HIV and other immunocompromised states, such as recent COVID-19 infection. The nurse should also identify persons with whom the patient has had close physical contact who have not had chickenpox or the chickenpox vaccine because they may be at risk of infection. The nurse should inspect the area of discomfort for the characteristic unilateral, bandlike, erythematous, maculopapular rash that may have clustered vesicles. Initially, the area may have a raised, erythematous rash before the vesicles appear. Intense pain is often associated with the rash, particularly in older adults. Based on the lesions and prescribed treatments, the nurse must determine the effect on the patient's mobility and capacity for activities of daily living (ADLs). Recommended treatment measures may require the assistance of another person.

Analyze cues and prioritize hypotheses (patient problems). Patient problems for a patient with herpes zoster include the following:
- Reduced skin integrity resulting from an immunologic deficit
- Potential for infection resulting from impaired skin integrity
- Disrupted sleep pattern resulting from impaired skin integrity or pain
- Pain resulting from inadequate pain relief from analgesia
- Need for health education resulting from a lack of previous exposure to disease processes and treatments

Generate solutions (planning). The goals of nursing management are pain relief and the prevention of secondary infections and scarring. Local skin care treatments may need to be taught to the patient or caregiver. The nurse must be alert to the possibility of long-term pain (postherpetic neuralgia) and the resulting depression. Expected outcomes include the following:
1. Skin lesions will remain free from necrotic tissue and infection.
2. The patient will experience adequate periods of restful sleep, as evidenced by:
   - No requests for pain medication during the night
   - Reports of uninterrupted sleep during the night and feeling well rested arose
3. The patient will obtain adequate pain relief, as evidenced by:
   - Verbalizing comfort and pain relief after taking an analgesic
   - Augmenting analgesic pain relief with the use of relaxation exercises, music diversion tapes, or guided imagery
4. The patient will demonstrate increased knowledge of their condition, as evidenced by:
   - Verbalizing significant and reportable signs and symptoms of infection
   - Verbalizing the rationale for regular, consistent use of analgesics
   - Correctly performing a return demonstration of lesion care and dressing change procedure

Take actions (nursing interventions). Nursing interventions consist of notifying the health care provider as soon as the characteristic rash and vesicles are identified, especially if they follow a dermatomal pattern. After a diagnosis is made, follow-through with medical and nursing management is paramount to patient comfort. Lesions should be monitored closely for the development of secondary bacterial infections, as evidenced by erythema, tenderness, or a purulent discharge. If satellite lesions develop outside the dermatome, especially if the patient is also experiencing headaches, neck rigidity, or pulmonary congestion, the health care provider must be notified immediately because this is indicative of disseminated herpes zoster (CDC, 2023).

The nurse should teach the older adult patient, family members, and staff the cause of shingles so that anxiety and misconceptions may be alleviated, and the nurse should explain the treatment measures to increase adherence and involvement in care. Herpes zoster may be very painful, so prompt administration of pain medications is crucial for patient comfort. For optimal pain control, patients should be instructed to inform the nurse when they experience the initial onset of pain before the pain becomes well entrenched. Effective pain management is one area in which nurses may have a positive effect on a patient's quality of life. If postherpetic neuralgia occurs, antidepressants are used as adjuncts to analgesics for control of pain.

Evaluate outcomes (evaluation). Evaluation of interventions focuses on pain control, with documented results of analgesics and adjunct therapies, and on prevention of secondary infection by frequent monitoring of the site. Many barriers to effective pain management in older adults exist, leading to frequent underrecognition and undertreatment of pain. If pain is not relieved, the health care provider should be consulted to obtain an alternative analgesic agent or adjunct drug therapy. The inflammatory response in an older adult may be diminished, even in the presence of a severe infection, so the nurse should be alert to even slight symptoms of a secondary bacterial infection. If evidence of cellulitis is noted, the health care provider should be informed to implement topical or oral antibiotic therapy. Documentation of assessment, the response to treatment measures, patient comprehension of teaching, and other nursing interventions demonstrate nursing accountability (see Nursing Care Plan: Herpes Zoster).

Premalignant Skin Growths: Actinic Keratosis

Actinic keratosis is a premalignant lesion of the epidermis caused by long-term exposure to UV rays. This precancerous lesion is more common in individuals with light complexions and occurs most commonly on the dorsum of the hands, scalp, outer ears, face, and lower arms. Treatment should be aggressive, and patients should be monitored closely to prevent progression to squamous cell carcinoma (SCC) (Oakley, 2015a).

Actinic keratosis begins in vascular areas as a reddish macule or papule that has a rough, yellowish-brown scale that may itch or cause discomfort (Fig. 15.9). During assessment, the nurse should be attuned to the rough surface of the lesion and its location and be particularly alert if a suspicious lesion occurs in a sun-exposed area. Patients should be cautioned to avoid sun exposure from 10 AM to 3 PM, wear protective clothing, and use sunscreen. The medical treatment of actinic keratosis is topical fluorouracil 5% cream and imiquimod 5% cream, topical 3%

NURSING CARE PLAN

Herpes Zoster

Clinical Situation

Mr. F. is a 72-year-old male who lives with his daughter and her husband. He has severe rheumatoid arthritis and hypertension. He takes ibuprofen, amlodipine, and atorvastatin. He has had both knees replaced in the past 5 years.

Mr. F. began to experience burning and pain 2 days ago, and this morning, he awoke with clustered vesicles on the left side of his torso, extending from the mid-back around to the midline of the anterior aspect of his chest. He went in to see his primary care physician. The provider ordered acyclovir, analgesics as needed for pain, and a topical antibiotic to prevent secondary infection.

Analyze Cues and Prioritize Hypotheses (Patient Problems)
- Potential for infection resulting from herpes zoster and open lesions

Generate Solutions (Planning)
- The patient will experience no secondary infection, as evidenced by no fever and other vital signs within normal limits, and will practice habits that decrease the risk of infection.

Take Actions (Nursing Interventions)
- Instruct the patient not to scratch or rub the affected area so as not to break vesicles, which would increase the risk of secondary infection.
- Assess vital signs, mental status, and skin lesions every shift to identify signs of infection (e.g., fever, tachycardia, erythema, tenderness, purulent discharge, and confusion).
- If the patient is febrile, ensure adequate hydration because a fever increases hydration needs.
- Tachycardia could precipitate HF from decreased cardiac output; monitor for shortness of breath, rales, edema, and other signs of cardiovascular compromise.
- If vesicle lesions rupture, implement topical treatment, noting the response.
- Ensure adequate nutrition to foster healing.
- Monitor food and fluid intake and ensure food preferences are being met.
- Be alert for vesicles outside of the involved dermatome, which could indicate disseminated herpes zoster; if vesicles appear, contact the physician or nurse practitioner immediately.
- Teach the patient, staff, and visitors the value of hand washing and proper disposal of dressing and treatment material as an infection control standard.
- Identify staff and visitors who have no known history of chickenpox or vaccine and inform them that they are not able to provide care for the patient because they may not have immunity to the varicella virus; isolation is not required. The infection control strategy is to take universal precautions.

---

diclofenac gel, ingenol mebutate 0.015% or 0.05% topical gel, and aminolevulinic acid 10% topical gel (Oakley, 2015a).

Nursing Care Guidelines for Actinic Keratosis

Recognize cues (assessment). Nursing assessment begins with the patient interview to determine risk factors such as the frequency of activities with sun exposure and the use of preventive practices (e.g., wearing a hat and long sleeves while outside). The skin should be inspected, and any rough lesions should be palpated and noted for location and texture. If hand lotion is used frequently, roughness will not be present; therefore, the nurse should look for an erythematous macule or papule. The nurse should refer patients to their primary care provider whenever a suspicious lesion is found. The nurse should also explain the value of treating skin cancer early, which may minimize scarring and disfigurement.

Analyze cues and prioritize hypotheses (patient problems). Patient problems for a patient with actinic keratosis include the following:
- Reduced skin integrity results from the removal of a lesion

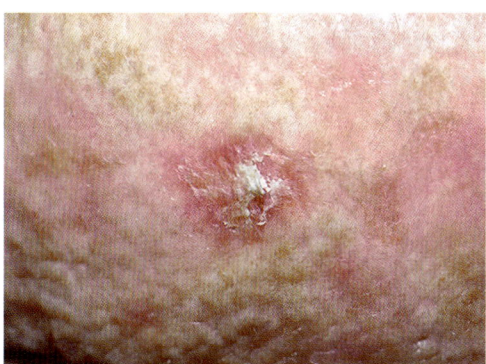

Fig. 15.9 Actinic keratosis. (From High, W. A., & Prok, L. D. [2021]. *Dermatology secrets* [6th ed.]. Philadelphia: Elsevier.)

- Potential for infection resulting from a break in skin integrity
- Distorted body image resulting from disfigurement and scarring resulting from the removal of a lesion

Generate solutions (planning). The goals of nursing management after the removal of premalignant lesions are the prevention of secondary infection and assistance in coping with any body image disturbance. Expected outcomes include the following:
1. The site of lesion removal will heal without evidence of secondary infection.
2. The patient will demonstrate no changes in body image perception.
3. The patient will demonstrate behavior change through the adoption of preventive skin care practices.

Take actions (nursing interventions). Nursing intervention consists of reinforcing the treatment regimen with the patient and family, monitoring the treated site to prevent secondary infection, providing support, and teaching preventive strategies. To lower a patient's anxiety and assist with body image changes, the nurse should explain the treatment, stressing that erythema and crusting are temporary. The resulting body image trauma from the treatment of many facial lesions may isolate an individual. The nurse should identify the patient's fears and discuss them in an open, reassuring manner.

Wounds should be assessed for the development of a bacterial infection, as evidenced by increased tenderness, increasing erythema around the treated site, purulent discharge, and possibly fever. In high-risk patients, topical treatment with an antibiotic ointment may be implemented prophylactically.

The nurse should teach older adult patients and family members the strategies necessary to prevent recurrence and stress the need to wear hats with wide brims and long-sleeved shirts to protect the skin from sun exposure. If an individual is going to be exposed to the sun, a sunscreen with a sun protection factor (SPF) of at least 40 should be applied (Dinulos, 2021).

Evaluate outcomes (evaluation). Evaluation of nursing management is supported by documentation addressing treatment progress, which includes a physical description, patient comprehension of educational information, and identification of and coping with any body image disturbances.

MALIGNANT SKIN GROWTHS

Basal Cell Carcinoma

Basal cell carcinoma (BCC) is the most common skin cancer and is more prevalent in fair-skinned, blond, or red-headed individuals with extensive previous sun exposure. It occurs more often in males than in females; however, this gender difference has decreased in recent years. BCC is most often found on the face and scalp, less often on the trunk, and rarely on the hands. It may also arise from scars or burns, particularly in older adults who have experienced chronic sun damage. BCC usually does not metastasize, but if left untreated, it may metastasize to the bone, lungs, and lymph nodes (Bader and Granick, 2022; Oakley, 2015b).

Typically, BCC appears as a pearly papule with a depression in the center, giving the lesion a doughnut-shaped appearance with telangiectasia on or around the lesion (Fig. 15.10). BCC may also appear as a blue-black pearly nodule (pigmented basal cell) or a red, scaly, or eczematous-appearing macule, usually on the thoracic area (superficially spreading BCC).

Squamous Cell Carcinoma

SCC is skin cancer arising from the epidermis, found most often on the scalp, outer ears, lower lip, and dorsum of the hands. SCC may also develop in chronic leg ulcers or open fractures and has a 20% incidence of metastasis, generally to regional lymph nodes. SCC accounts for 90% of lip lesions and occurs along the vermillion border of the lower lip. The etiologic factors of SCC may be UV rays, chemical carcinogens, and X-rays. SCC is more common in males and older adults, and the incidence increases with geographic proximity to the equator. Although SCC is less common in Black persons, "it carries a higher mortality rate, perhaps due to delayed diagnosis, because tumors are more likely to occur in sun-protected areas in these individuals" (Wells and Meyers, 2021; Oakley, 2015c; Ramji and Oakley, 2017).

SCC usually presents as a firm, elevated lump; it may have a thick, adherent scale with a center that is often ulcerated or crusted (Fig. 15.11). At first glance, SCC may even look like a wart. The base may be inflamed and red, and it usually bleeds easily. SCC may arise from actinic keratosis, which supports early detection and removal of such lesions. If tumors are ignored or left unattended, they may enlarge, creating significant disfigurement after surgical excision.

Melanoma

Melanoma is a malignant neoplasm of pigment-forming cells capable of metastasizing to any organ of the body, even before the lesion is noted; therefore, early detection is crucial. Invasive melanoma is the fifth most common cancer in males and females. If detected and treated before spreading to the lymph nodes, there is a 99% 5-year survival rate (American Cancer Society, 2022; Siegel et al, 2022).

The incidence of melanoma has doubled in recent years. Ninety-five percent of melanomas can be attributed to UV exposure. A genetic predisposition to melanoma also exists: 10% of patients have a parent or sibling with a history of melanoma. Individuals with a family history of melanoma should perform monthly skin self-examinations and have a professional skin evaluation at regular intervals (Beroukhim et al, 2020).

Individuals at high risk are fair-skinned, and their skin tends to burn rather than tan; have red or blond hair; have multiple

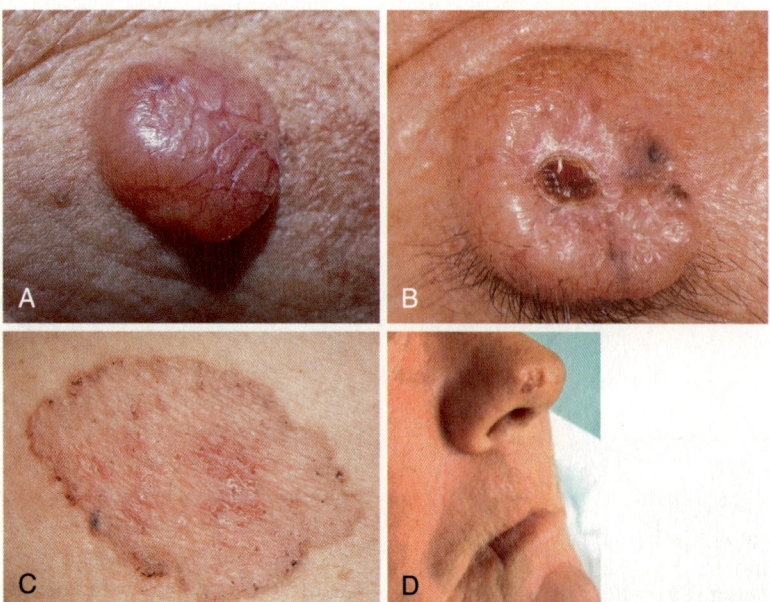

Fig. 15.10 Basal cell carcinoma. (From Lambert Smith, F., Hajar, T., & Brown, M. [2023]. Skin cancer. In M. A. Scholes, & V. R. Ramakrishnan [Eds.]. *ENT secrets* [5th ed., pp. 58–70]. Philadelphia: Elsevier. Courtesy Fitzsimons Army Medical Center.)

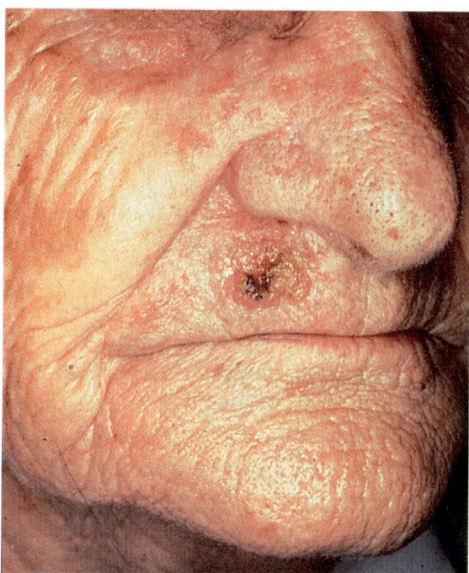

Fig. 15.11 Squamous cell carcinoma. (From Damjanov, I., Perry, K. D., & Perry, A. M. [2022]. *Pathology for the health professions* [6th ed.]. St. Louis: Elsevier.)

nevi; and tend to freckle. African Americans, Asians, and dark-skinned Whites are at less risk of developing melanoma; however, most melanomas found in these populations occur in skin areas not exposed to the sun, especially the periungual, palmar, and plantar surfaces. An individual with one melanoma is at risk of having another (Beroukhim et al, 2020).

Melanoma's clinical hallmark is an irregularly shaped nevus (mole), papule, or plaque that has undergone a change, particularly in color. The characteristic signs of most malignant melanomas are referred to as the *ABCDEs*: Asymmetry, Border irregularity, Color variation (red, white, and blue), and Diameter greater than 6 mm (Evolution) (Fig. 15.12). The lesion may itch or bleed; however, this is usually a later sign. A dermatologist or primary care provider should examine any mole or lesion that has irregularly shaped borders and has had a color change, usually to a darker color (AAD, 2023b).

Of the four types of melanomas, the most common is the *superficial spreading melanoma*, which is slower growing. Superficial spreading melanoma accounts for 70% of all melanomas, occurring most commonly on the trunk in males, the extremities in females, and the upper back in both. The mean age of diagnosis is in the mid-forties. A superficial melanoma is a slow-growing, flat, slightly elevated, pigmented papule or patch that has irregular borders and varied colors within the lesion (Seebacher, 2022).

Nodular melanoma occurs in 10%–15% of patients with melanoma and has the worst prognosis because it is usually invasive by the time it is diagnosed. Nodular melanoma is most often found on the trunk, legs, and arms; it may also occur on the scalp in males. The mean age at diagnosis is the fifth or sixth decade of life. Nodular melanoma is a hard, usually dark nodule arising from a preexisting mole (Dinulos, 2021).

Lentigo maligna occurs most often in the elderly. *Lentigo maligna* melanoma is a brown-tan macular lesion with varied pigmentation and highly irregular borders. It is found most often on chronically sun-exposed skin of the face, ears, arms, and upper trunk and remains superficial for some time, before becoming invasive (Dinulos, 2021).

Acral-lentiginous melanoma usually occurs on the palms of hands and soles of feet, as well as under fingernails/toenails. It is more common in older adults, and the mean age is 60 at the time of diagnosis. It is the most common melanoma found in Blacks and Asians; therefore, careful inspection of the foot soles, palms, and hands is warranted when caring for Black and Asian American patients. Acral-lentiginous melanoma resembles lentigo melanoma with its flat, irregular, discolored borders. It spreads superficially before becoming invasive (Dinulos, 2021; Brazen et al, 2020).

Nursing Care Guidelines for Malignant Skin Growths
Recognize Cues (Assessment)

Nursing assessment begins with interviewing the patient to determine how long the lesion(s) have been present and to identify risk factors such as chronic sun exposure and family history. The nurse should inspect and palpate the suspicious lesion, surrounding tissue, and lymph nodes (to identify possible metastasis). A dermatoscope (a magnifying glass–type device) may be useful for closely examining any lesion. When a suspicious lesion is identified, the nurse should promptly refer the patient to the primary care provider. The nurse should also explain that early treatment lessens the extent of scarring and possibly intervenes before metastasis. Additionally, the nurse should discuss the patient's feelings and fears about cancer.

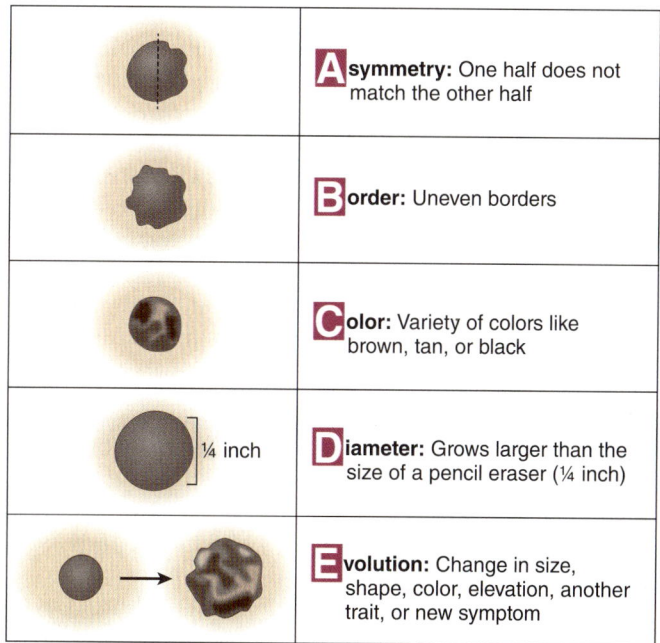

Fig. 15.12 The ABCDEs of melanoma: **A**symmetry, **B**order irregularity, **C**olor variation, **D**iameter over 6 mm, and **E**volution.

Analyze Cues and Generate Hypotheses (Patient Problems)

Patient problems for a patient with skin cancer include the following:

- Reduced skin integrity resulting from the removal of a cancerous lesion
- Fear of cancer, pain, or death resulting from having a cancerous skin lesion
- Potential for infection resulting from a break in skin integrity and a surgical wound
- Distorted body image resulting from disfigurement and scarring resulting from the removal of a cancerous lesion

Generate Solutions (Planning)

The goals of nursing management are to facilitate the referral of patients for treatment and removal of suspicious lesions, prevent secondary infections and metastasis, and address fears and feelings related to cancer; referrals to community resources should be made as indicated. The nurse must discuss the patient's and family's feelings about having a cancerous lesion so that any need for a community referral or educational material can be identified. Expected outcomes include the following:

1. The site of the excision will heal without evidence of infection.
2. The patient will verbalize fears related to the diagnosis and actively seek information and clarification.
3. The patient will identify community resources for support and additional information.
4. The patient will verbalize understanding of the treatment plan.
5. The patient will demonstrate increased knowledge of the condition, as evidenced by the adoption of preventive strategies.

Take Actions (Nursing Interventions)

Nursing management includes reinforcement of the treatment regimen by monitoring the wound for secondary infection (e.g., erythema, tenderness, and purulent discharge) and reinforcement of the caring component of nursing by discussing the patient's and family's feelings related to cancer. The nurse should identify and discuss the patient's and family's feelings about having a cancerous lesion and refer the patient to appropriate community resources if they are having difficulty coping or have a high level of anxiety. The nurse should also explain that a risk of metastasis exists and refer the patient to the American Cancer Society (https://www.cancer.org/), appropriate Internet resources, or the local library for additional information.

The nurse should teach the patient or family dressing care and signs of infection. Removal may result in scarring, especially if the lesion is large. Consequently, reassurance must be provided, and feelings related to body image changes should be addressed; the focus is on comfort, education, and emotional support. Preventive strategies such as avoiding suntanning beds, wearing hats with wide brims, wearing long sleeves, and using sunscreen should also be taught to both the patient and family. In addition, the patient and family members should have annual skin assessments because a hereditary tendency for occurrence exists.

Evaluate Outcomes (Evaluation)

Evaluation of nursing interventions focuses on monitoring for infection, the effectiveness of pain control measures, comprehension of patient education, and discussions related to body image changes and fears about cancer. If there is poor pain control or the development of an infection, the health care provider should be contacted for an alternative strategy. Documentation of assessment, the response to treatment measures, patient comprehension of teaching, and other nursing interventions demonstrate nursing accountability.

LOWER EXTREMITY ULCERS

Chronic leg ulcers are a common problem in older adults, occurring primarily from three causes: arterial insufficiency, venous hypertension, and diabetic neuropathy (Table 15.1). A brief overview of each etiologic factor and treatment follows. Greater emphasis is placed on venous ulcers because they are more prevalent in older adults and more challenging because of their chronicity.

Arterial Ulcers

Arterial or ischemic ulcers result from arterial insufficiency. Arterial insufficiency is also referred to as peripheral arterial occlusive disease (PAOD). Arteriosclerosis—thickening and hardening of the arterial wall—is the primary cause of the decreased blood flow that results in ischemia and eventually tissue death. Several risk factors, including obesity, diabetes, hyperlipidemia, and hypertension, may lead to arterial ulcers.

Pain with exercise, at night, or while resting is the most common sign of arterial insufficiency. Pain at rest indicates severely restricted arterial blood flow. The area proximal to (above) the painful area is usually the site of restricted blood flow. Pulses distal to the restriction may be present because of collateral circulation. The patient may also complain of cramping, burning, or aching. As the disease advances, the extremity develops

TABLE 15.1 Leg Ulcer Differentiation

Type	Primary Cause	Characteristics
Arterial ulcers	Arterial insufficiency; peripheral vascular disease	Located on the toes, feet, or lower third of the leg; irregularly shaped wound; thin, shiny, cool skin with a cyanotic hue, loss of hair, thickened toenails; pain with activity, rest, or at night
Venous ulcers	Venous hypertension	Located on the medial aspect of the lower third of the leg; irregularly shaped wound; either a flat or shallow crater; discoloration, varicosities, edema, and exudate; pain relieved with activity
Diabetic foot lesion	Neuropathy	Located on the plantar surface of the foot; circular, often deep wounds; decreased or absent vibratory sensation; painful; paresthesia

a cyanotic hue and becomes cool. The skin becomes thin, shiny, and dry, and has an associated loss of hair and thickened nails, all of which result from the diminished blood supply. Tissue anoxia leads to necrosis and poor healing. Arterial ulcers are usually located on the outer ankle, feet, and toes. The ulcerated area appears "punched out," with well-defined wound margins. The causes must be corrected so that oxygen and other nutrients are available to promote the healing of necrotic wounds. Treatment is usually surgical intervention with revascularization; if the disease is too advanced, amputation may be necessary.

Venous Ulcers

Venous ulcers, also known as stasis ulcers, are thought to arise secondary to chronic venous insufficiency. Venous ulcers affect roughly 1% of the general population, with the highest incidence in older adults. The incidence ranges from 0.73–3.12 per 1000 persons per year. The annual direct cost to manage each patient with this disease is estimated to be $5,527 per year (Kolluri et al, 2022). Chronic venous leg ulcers usually have an onset in early adulthood; however, peak prevalence is seen in people ages 70 or older. Venous ulcers occur more often in females than in males. Epidemiologic studies have revealed that 57%–80% of all lower leg ulcers are related to venous insufficiency, and 10%–25% have a combination of venous and arterial insufficiency.

Venous hypertension is the primary cause of venous ulcers. Valvular incompetence of the deep or perforating veins of the lower leg is present in most venous ulcer cases. Venous hypertension leads to a tortuous capillary system, which causes an accumulation of fibrinogen, leukocytes, and erythrocytes. The accumulation of erythrocytes in the tissue produces a brownish skin discoloration caused by the release of hemoglobin. Often, the discoloration (hemosiderin) and thickening of the skin (lipodermatosclerosis) are the first indications of venous hypertension. Capillary occlusion caused by the trapping of white blood cells (WBCs) results in the release of proteolytic enzymes, which foster fibrinogen leakage. The fibrin cuff creates a barrier that prevents or delays the exchange of oxygen and other nutrients, resulting in cell death. Anoxia and the trapping of growth factors are the primary causes of ulceration and poor healing. The fibrin cuff is irreversible, which sets the stage for frequent recurrence and makes venous ulcers a chronic disorder (Caesar and Coulson, 2020; Labropoulos, 2019).

The diagnosis of a venous ulcer is commonly based on clinical presentation. Venous ulcers are usually on the medial aspect of the lower leg, with flat or shallow craters and irregular borders, accompanied by varicosities, lipodermatosclerosis, hemosiderin deposit (reddish brown pigmentation), and itching. Venous ulcers generate a large amount of exudate and are usually surrounded by erythema and edema. Although it may be difficult, it is important to differentiate between venous ulcers and cellulitis.

It is well recognized that venous ulcers heal with prolonged elevation of the affected extremity; however, adherence is difficult. Research has demonstrated that compression therapy of at least 30–40 mm Hg at the ankle and distal lower leg decreases edema by compressing fluid through the fibrin cuff (Dissemond et al, 2016). The most common cause of recurrence is nonadherence to compression therapy. It is important to remember that compression therapy is intended for ambulatory patients. The older adult with dependent edema, not primary venous disease, does not tolerate compression well. Compression therapy is not a management option for arterial insufficiency; pain and cyanosis will occur from further impaired circulation.

Diabetic Foot Lesions

Risk factors for developing diabetic foot lesions are peripheral neuropathy, foot deformity, peripheral arterial disease, and a history of previous foot lesions. Adequately offloading footwear is a protective factor (Khan and Khardori, 2020). Older adults who live alone or who have mental confusion are at increased risk for foot lesions because they may not have the means to recognize a diabetic foot lesion or to follow up with appropriate treatment. A risk factor for lower extremity amputation is neuropathy, which is implicated in approximately 90% of diabetic foot lesions. This sensory loss is associated with a 15.5% relative risk of amputation. Therefore, individuals with diabetes and neuropathy are at risk of developing lower leg lesions, which may lead to an amputation.

Pain and temperature are usually the first sensations affected by neuropathy. The loss of the peripheral sensory feedback system impairs the patients' ability to feel tissue damage, inflammation, or injury. Lesions resulting from diabetic peripheral neuropathy tend to be bilateral, symmetric, and located on the plantar surface of the foot. Patients usually complain of pain and paresthesias; however, they also have diminished or absent vibratory and temperature sensations in the affected extremities. Pain relieved by walking is one diagnostic sign of neuropathy. Neuropathic lesions are usually not well perfused; in addition, a patient with diabetes may have arterial insufficiency, which compromises healing abilities (Volmer-Thole and Lobmann, 2016).

Treatment varies depending on the etiologic factors and wound condition. Patient education regarding how to minimize the risk of chemical, thermal, and mechanical trauma is the first line of defense against diabetic foot lesions. A physical examination of the foot should include testing for neuropathy and the identification of high foot pressures. An easy and inexpensive device for establishing neuropathy is the Semmes-Weinstein monofilament. Inability to feel the 5.07 monofilament indicates the patient is at risk for lesion development and needs orthotics (specially fitted shoes designed to prevent ulcers and decrease callous formation by redistributing weight) to offload pressure (Baraz et al, 2014). The nurse should stress to patients with diabetes, particularly if they have PAOD, that any trauma to the lower leg, ankles, or feet may lead to a lesion and possible amputation. They must protect their feet and lower legs with proper shoes and foot care. Orthotics may be helpful in preventing mechanical trauma. When an ulcer is present, a total contact cast may be applied to redistribute weight and minimize trauma, but it is contraindicated with cellulitis or excessive drainage. Some physicians use hyperbaric oxygenation in hopes of increasing oxygenation to the affected area; however, this treatment is controversial because of its questionable effectiveness in wounds with compromised circulation, such as diabetic foot lesions. The success of this strategy depends on the amount of circulation present in the affected area.

Nursing Care Guidelines for Lower Extremity Ulcers

Recognize Cues (Assessment)

Nursing assessment begins with the determination of the location and characteristics of lower leg ulcers and lesions. The nurse should determine wound dimensions, depth, and amount of exudate; palpate popliteal pulses at least every day if the patient is in an acute care setting and at every visit if they are in an ambulatory or home setting. Any discoloration or edema should be documented. The nurse should also ascertain if the patient experiences any pain or itching and how it has been managed. A nutritional assessment should be conducted, which includes the patient's weight, 24-hour diet recall, chewing abilities, and food preparation abilities. The nurse should determine whether shopping assistance is needed.

Analyze Cues and Prioritize Hypotheses (Patient Problems)

Patient problems for a patient with lower extremity ulcers and lesions include the following:
- Reduced skin integrity resulting from altered circulation
- Potential for infection resulting from open, chronic wounds

Generate Solutions (Planning)

The goal of nursing management is to facilitate healing without infection by promoting treatment adherence and by providing patient education regarding the disease process and treatment. The nurse should inform patients with venous ulcers that these ulcers are a chronic process. Time for patient education will be needed. Expected outcomes include the following:
1. Skin lesions will remain free from necrotic tissue and infection.
2. Edema in the lower extremities will be controlled.
3. Skin lesions will heal with minimal scarring.
4. The patient will be able to maintain a healed state for at least 6 months.

Take Actions (Nursing Interventions)

Nursing interventions for venous ulcers consist of keeping the legs elevated, implementing compression therapy, administering wound care, and educating the patient about the causes of lower extremity ulcers and lesions, the strategy of compression therapy, and specific wound care. The nurse must stress the need to maintain compression therapy to facilitate the healing of venous ulcers and avoid further breakdown.

Nursing interventions for arterial and diabetic ulcers often focus on complex wound care over long periods of time, after the patient has undergone surgical management to restore adequate oxygenation. These wounds are not treated with compression therapy.

Infection is difficult to determine because lower extremity ulcers and lesions often have erythematous bases with induration; however, if the patient develops a fever and tenderness surrounding the wound, the health care provider should be contacted. The nurse should determine whether any community services, such as home-delivered meals, grocery shopping assistance, and other support services, are needed. They should also identify and discuss the patient's feelings regarding chronic illness and body image changes, teach the patient with venous ulcers that they generate a large amount of exudate, and instruct on dressing changes.

Evaluate Outcomes (Evaluation)

Evaluation of nursing interventions focuses on prevention of further wound deterioration and infection, as well as the effectiveness of patient education. A return demonstration of wound care and compression therapy, if the wound is venous, is a concrete evaluation and ensures patient comprehension. Nursing accountability is demonstrated by documentation of assessment, the response to treatment measures, patient comprehension of teaching, and other nursing interventions.

PRESSURE INJURIES

Pressure injuries (previously referred to as *pressure ulcers*) have plagued humans for centuries. Hippocrates devised a debridement treatment with healing by secondary closure. Ambroise Paré, a sixteenth-century surgeon, published strategies for healing skin wounds that challenged the existing practice of pouring hot oil on the wound. These included increased nutrition and mobility, debridement, and the application of dressings (Levine, 1992).

It was not until the twentieth century that scientific research began to determine the cause and appropriate management of pressure injuries. In 1930, Landis determined that the average capillary pressure before which ischemia occurs is below 32 mm Hg. In the 1950s, Kosiak (1958) found that pressure applied to rabbits' ears over 2 hours would result in ulceration. Thus, the universal recommendation of turning every 2 hours was established. The first pressure injury risk assessment tool was designed and tested by Doreen Norton (1989) in the late 1950s but not disseminated until 1962, when she presented study findings at a conference.

In 1962, researchers first demonstrated that moisture, applied with occlusive dressings, increases epithelialization (the healing process) (Krasner, 1991). In 1972, a plastic occlusive dressing was shown to cut epithelialization time in half, which led to film dressings, followed by hydrocolloidal dressings.

This information explosion has resulted in varied terminology and beliefs. As a result, leading experts in pressure injury management and research formed the NPIAP in 1987, with the intent of improving prevention and management through education, legislation, standardization of staging criteria, and identification of research needs. The NPIAP held consensus conferences beginning in May 1988, the outcome of which included standardized staging criteria endorsed by the International Association for Enterostomal Therapists and the Agency for Healthcare Research and Quality (AHRQ). To standardize terms and ensure more accuracy related to the causation of the pressure injury, NPIAP decreed that *pressure injury* is a more appropriate term than *pressure ulcer* or *decubitus*. Therefore, the term *pressure injury* is used throughout this discussion.

Pressure injury prevention and management is one of four costly adverse events addressed in AHRQ's *Safety Program for Nursing Homes: On-Time Prevention*. The AHRQ has developed tools for nursing homes with electronic health records designed to improve clinical decision-making and prevent adverse events. For further information, see https://www.ahrq.gov/professionals/systems/long-term-care/resources/index.html.

Epidemiology of Pressure Injuries

The epidemiology of pressure injuries has been difficult to quantify and varies depending on sample size, definition of terms, and type of facility. Despite methodologic limitations, the incidence (new cases) and prevalence (over a specific period) rates of pressure injuries are sufficiently high to generate concern.

There are 2.5 million pressure injury cases that occur each year, amounting to $26.8 billion in actual costs per year. The average cost to heal a stage 3, stage 4, or unstable pressure injury is between $75,000 and $150,000 per patient (Padula and Delarmente, 2019). Since 2014, the rate of pressure injuries has increased by 6%, making it the only hospital-acquired condition that has increased rather than improved (AHRQ, 2019; NPIAP, 2021). Several groups have been identified as high-risk for the development of pressure injuries while hospitalized: quadriplegic patients, older patients with hip fractures, orthopedic patients who are immobile, and critical care patients.

The prevalence rate of pressure injuries in long-term care facilities is near 20%, resulting in an annual cost of $3.3 billion (Stone, 2020). Incidence rates vary among nursing care facilities because of the heterogeneous case mix and staffing patterns. Better data are needed to determine the degree of the problem in long-term care.

Etiology of Pressure Injuries

Pressure on soft tissue over bony prominences or other hard surfaces is the primary causative factor in pressure injury formation. However, other contributing factors exist and explain why the tissue of some individuals breaks down within 30 minutes of lying in the same position, whereas that of others does not break down for hours.

Pressure injuries begin at the point of contact between soft tissue and a hard surface (e.g., bone). Consequently, an inverted cone-shaped wound develops, with the largest area of breakdown being near the bone. Common bony prominences susceptible to pressure injury development are the sacrum, ischial tuberosity (especially in an upright sitting position in a chair or bed), lateral malleolus, trochanter, and heels (Fig. 15.13).

The intensity of pressure that leads to capillary closure, compounded by the duration of pressure and tissue tolerance, results in tissue anoxia, ischemia, edema, and eventually tissue necrosis. Immobility, decreased activity, and decreased sensory perception place individuals at risk for unrelieved pressure that generates tissue ischemia and death. Tissue tolerance is influenced by extrinsic factors—moisture, friction, and shearing—and intrinsic factors—poor nutrition, advanced age, hypotension, emotional stress, smoking, and skin temperature (Kirman and Geibel, 2022). The development of pressure injuries is a complex, synergistic phenomenon that makes prevention a challenge (Fig. 15.14).

Capillary pressure ensures the movement of blood through the capillary membrane, maintaining oxygenation and tissue nutrition. Capillary collapse may result from prolonged pressure, which leads to tissue anoxia, ischemia, reactive hyperemia (erythema), leakage of plasma into interstitial tissue, and microvascular hemorrhaging observable by nonblanchable erythema. If the pressure persists, tissue death will result. External pressure of 33 mm Hg, depending on the location and individual, may be enough to impair circulation (Kirman and Geibel, 2022).

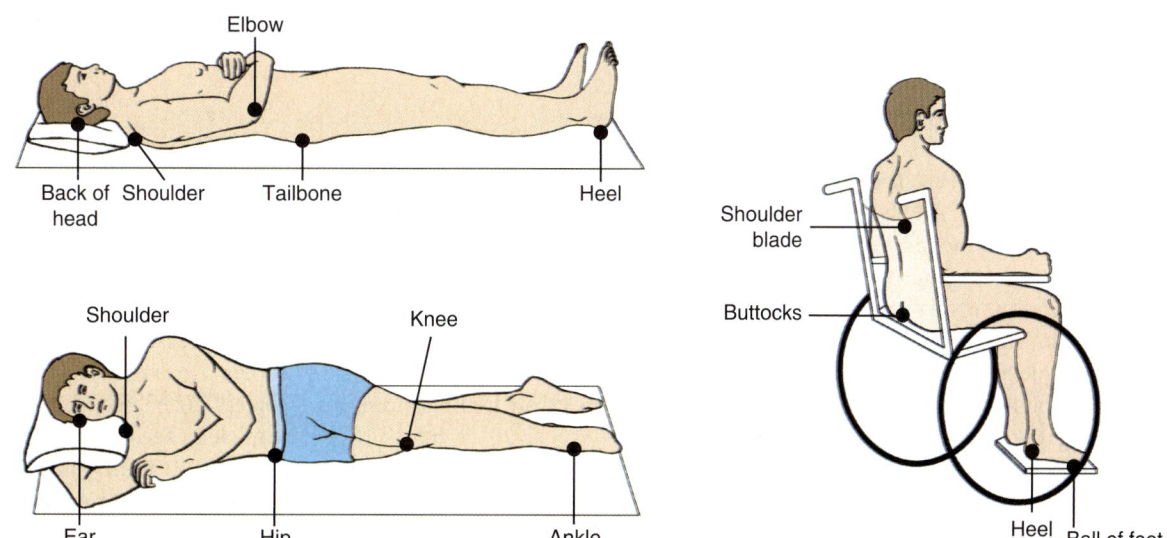

Fig. 15.13 Pressure points where pressure injuries often occur. (Adapted from deWit, S. C., & O'Neill, P. [2014]. *Fundamental concepts and skills for nursing* [4th ed.]. St. Louis, MO: Elsevier.)

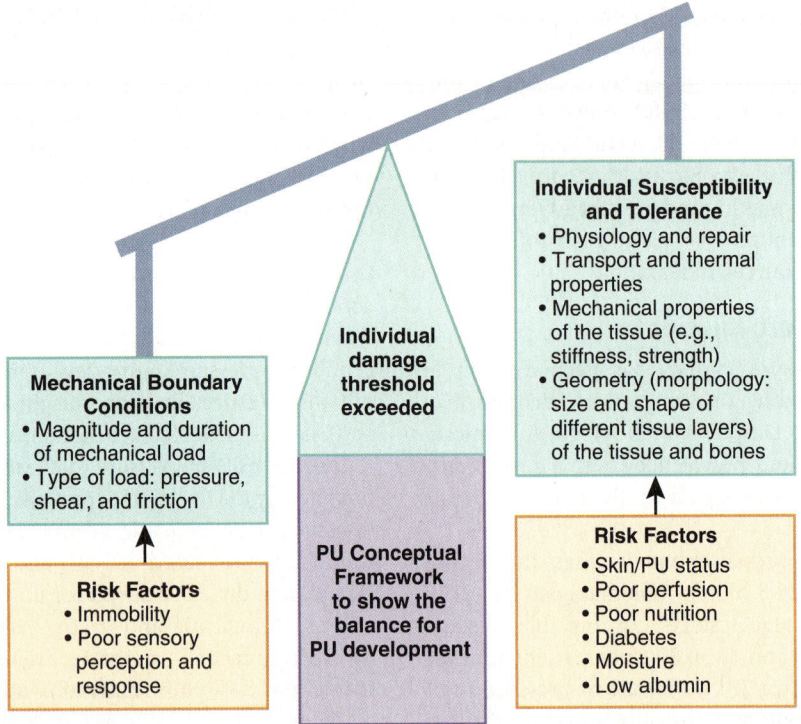

Fig. 15.14 Pressure ulcer conceptual framework. *PU*, pressure ulcer. (From Coleman, S., Nixon, J., Keen, J., et al. [2014]. A new pressure ulcer conceptual framework. *Journal of Advanced Nursing, 70*[10], 2222–2234.)

People with sensory impairment (paralysis or sedation) do not have a normal protective reflex, which is shifting weight in response to discomfort from capillary closure and tissue anoxia. This inability may explain the higher incidence of pressure injuries among individuals with paralysis or those undergoing long surgical procedures. Patients with altered mental status because of disease (e.g., dementia) or medication may have decreased pain or tissue anoxia perception. These individuals are at risk for pressure injury development.

Tissue tolerance, another major contributing factor in the development of a pressure injury, is defined as the ability of the skin and supporting structures to endure the effects of pressure. It is apparent, then, that poor tissue tolerance makes one more vulnerable to pressure intensity and duration, thus increasing the response to pressure. Shearing, friction, age-related changes in the integumentary system, low blood pressure, and nutritional status all influence tissue tolerance.

Shearing, which is the sliding of parallel surfaces, causes stretching and occlusion of the arterial supply, usually of the fascia and muscle. Shearing forces may decrease the blood supply, leading to tissue ischemia and necrosis (Fig. 15.15). The most common position for shearing is when the head of the bed is elevated, causing the body to slide downward. Resistance keeps the skin in place while gravity pulls the body toward the foot of the bed (Coleman et al, 2014; Oomens et al, 2010).

Friction, the rubbing of skin against another surface, primarily affects the epidermal and dermal layers, causing a superficial abrasion (e.g., a sheet burn) (Oomens et al, 2010). Restless

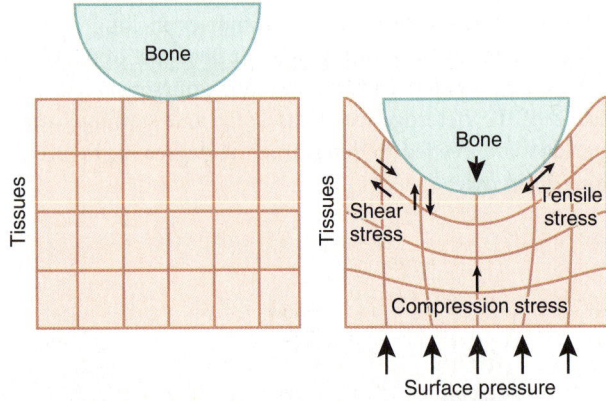

Fig. 15.15 Shear stress. (From International Review. [2010]. *Pressure ulcer prevention: Pressure, shear, friction, and microclimate in context. A consensus document.* London, UK: Wounds International.)

patients or those with persistent movements are at risk for friction injuries. However, when friction occurs concurrently with gravitational forces, shearing is the outcome.

Moisture from incontinence or profuse sweating may decrease tensile strength, alter skin resiliency to external forces, and exacerbate friction and shearing forces (Coleman et al, 2014; Oomens et al, 2010). Efforts should be made to keep the skin dry.

As many studies have revealed, nutritional status greatly influences the development of pressure injuries. Protein deficiency weakens tissue tolerance (i.e., the spring between the skin surface and bony prominences), making soft tissue more susceptible to breakdown when pressure intensity is prolonged.

Hypoproteinemia changes osmotic equilibrium, which leads to edema. Consequently, sluggish oxygenation and transportation create an environment for tissue breakdown and poor healing. Serum albumin levels below 3.5 g/dL (grams per deciliter) have a correlation with pressure injury development and poor wound healing (Dharmarajan and Ahmed, 2003). Proteins are also needed for collagen formation, granulation tissue formation, and immunologic response.

The incidence of pressure injuries is increased in older adults, particularly those older than age 70. With aging, the epidermis thins, elasticity decreases, and vessels degenerate, resulting in reduced blood flow. These age-related changes impair the early warning sign of erythema, delay crucial early immunologic responses, and impede the healing process, thereby making older adults at risk for pressure injury development.

Low blood pressure and dehydration may reduce circulation, especially in the microvasculature, which eventually leads to tissue ischemia. Systolic blood pressure below 90 mm Hg has been found to be a risk factor for pressure injury formation, presumably because of decreased peripheral circulation and subsequent ischemia (Cox, 2017). Another factor associated with pressure injury formation is elevated temperature, especially in older adults, possibly caused by increased oxygen demands in anoxic tissue (Coleman et al, 2013; Coleman et al, 2014; Jaul et al, 2018).

The formation of a pressure injury is a complex process involving many variables within the nurse's control (e.g., pressure, shearing, and moisture) as well as variables out of the nurse's control (e.g., malnutrition, low blood pressure, and paralysis). The principal mechanism of injury is loss of microcirculation through pressure compressing the microvessels or intrinsic factors causing soft tissue to become more vulnerable to lost blood supply.

Risk Assessment Tools

The success of pressure injury prevention depends on the early identification of at-risk patients. As recommended by the AHRQ clinical guidelines, a valid, research-based assessment tool should be used. For consistency and accuracy to be established, there should be written protocols specifying how to use the risk assessment tool, when to use it, and which health care team members should use it. A risk assessment should be conducted on all individuals who are bedbound, chairbound, incontinent, frail, disabled, or nutritionally compromised, or who have demonstrated altered mental status (Berlowitz et al, 2014). An assessment should be conducted on patients admitted to an acute care facility, rehabilitation hospital, nursing facility, home care agency, or other health care facility. Identified high-risk individuals should be reassessed at regular intervals if mobility or activity is impaired. The risk assessment should be repeated, and the care plan should be modified accordingly whenever a patient's condition changes. Examples of these changes include decreased mobility, eating less, a change in the serum albumin level or other abnormal laboratory findings, and mentation changes.

Numerous instruments have been designed to identify patients at risk for pressure injury formation. However, many tools have not been subjected to vigorous evaluation for reliability and validity testing. The Braden and Norton risk assessment tools, according to AHRQ clinical guidelines, have undergone the most extensive evaluations.

The Norton Risk Assessment Scale was the first such tool designed for use in a study investigating geriatric nursing problems in hospitals. Consequently, it has set the stage for more comprehensive assessment tools. The study began in the late 1950s, but results were not disseminated until a conference in 1962. At that time, it was believed that pressure injuries were the result of poor nursing care; however, additional research has revealed the problem to be much more complex. The Norton scale is simple to use and has only five assessment categories. Although the original research assessed nutritional status, it was not included in the scale because it was believed that the patient's general health reflected nutritional status. Norton (1989) indicates that nutritional status, including eating behaviors, would have been an important parameter to include. Patients with a score of 16 or lower on the Norton scale are at risk for pressure injury development (Fig. 15.16).

The Braden Scale for Predicting Pressure Sore Risk has been shown to be highly reliable when used by registered nurses (RNs) and is the most rigorously tested risk assessment tool (Berlowitz et al, 2014). The Braden scale assesses sensory perception rather than mental status. Assessing sensory perception

NORTON SCALE

		PHYSICAL CONDITION	MENTAL CONDITION	ACTIVITY	MOBILITY	INCONTINENT	
		Good 4	Alert 4	Ambulant 4	Full 4	Not 4	
		Fair 3	Apathetic 3	Walk/help 3	Slightly limited 3	Occasional 3	TOTAL
		Poor 2	Confused 2	Chairbound 2	Very limited 2	Usually/urine 2	SCORE
		Very bad 1	Stupor 1	Bedrest 1	Immobile 1	Doubly 1	
Name	Date						

Fig. 15.16 Norton risk assessment scale. Total score over 18: low risk; between 14 and 18: medium risk; between 10 and 14: high risk; less than 10: very high risk. (From Norton, D., McLaren, R., & Exton-Smith, A. N. [1962]. *An investigation of geriatric nursing problems in the hospital.* Center for Policy on Ageing. Reproduced with permission from the Centre for Policy on Ageing [formerly NCCOP], London, UK.)

is thought to be a more precise risk indicator because impaired sensation prevents an individual from sensing the need to change positions, which, in turn, would decrease pressure intensity (Braden and Bergstrom, 1989). As a rule, a patient scoring below 18 on the Braden scale is at high risk for skin breakdown.

A third tool available to assess pressure injury risk is the Waterlow Pressure Ulcer Scale, developed by Judy Waterlow in 1985. The scale has increased sensitivity and specificity when compared to the Norton Scale; however, the scale has not demonstrated reliability when used with patients who have a spinal cord injury. Administration time ranges from 5–10 minutes and covers eight categories: age, sex, body build, appetite, continence of urine and feces, mobility, skin appearance in risk areas, and special risks. Special risks include malnutrition, neurologic deficits, medication, recent surgery, or trauma. Each category is assigned weights for specific clinical indicators (Fig. 15.17A). Scores are summed; a score of 10–15 is at risk, 15–20 is high risk, and 20 and over is very high risk. Scores from the scale must be combined with clinical judgment to determine a person's true risk. In addition to the rating scale, the Waterlow comes with guidance on nursing care for the person at risk and wound assessment and dressing for those with pressure injuries (Serpa et al, 2009) (see Fig. 15.17B).

> ### EVIDENCE-BASED PRACTICE
> #### Critical Care Nurse Knowledge Related to Prevention and Staging of Pressure Injuries
> **Background**
> Pressure injuries in critical care are a continued challenge, often resulting from pressure, shearing forces, and bony prominences in susceptible individuals.
>
> **Sample/Setting**
> The sample encompassed 32 RNs employed in medical intensive care/coronary care, or surgical intensive care units at Veterans Affairs hospitals in the Midwestern United States.
>
> **Methods**
> Following a 2-year educational initiative, nurses on two critical care units were asked to complete the 72-item Pieper-Zulkowski Pressure Ulcer Knowledge Test (PZ-PUKT). The PZ-PUKT measures knowledge concerning wound descriptions, prevention/risk assessment, and staging. The test is true/false.
>
> **Findings**
> The mean age of participants was 44.8 years, and they were predominantly females. The overall mean subscale score for items focusing on pressure injury staging was 81%. The overall mean score for the prevention subscale was 70%. The cumulative mean score for all scales was 72%. Participants with 5–10 years' experience scored higher than those with 20 years or more experience, although this was not statistically significant.
>
> **Implications**
> Pressure injury knowledge was assessed in a small cohort of critical care nurses practicing in the Midwestern United States. Nurses participating in the study scored higher in pressure ulcer staging compared with pressure ulcer risk assessment and prevention. This study highlights the need for continued education to reduce gaps in nursing knowledge throughout a nurse's career.

Data From Miller, D. M., Neelon, L., Kish-Smith, K., Whitney, L., & Burant, C. J. (2017). Pressure injury knowledge in critical care nurses. *Journal of Wound, Ostomy, and Continence Nurses, 44*(5), 455–457.

Preventive Strategies

Prevention is the first line of defense against pressure injuries, which are costly health care problems that adversely affect a patient's quality of life. The professional nurse has a responsibility to identify patients at risk for pressure injuries and to implement research-based preventive strategies. Nurses, as front-line providers and managers of care, are key team members of the health care system who can influence the prevalence of pressure injuries and enhance the patient's quality of life. Nurses should mobilize the health care team when needs are identified by seeking a dietary consultation and alerting the health care provider when a patient is not eating sufficiently or when a patient develops nonblanchable erythema. Written preventive protocols endorsed (and embraced) by the health care team and institution empower the professional nurse to act independently and immediately when vulnerable patients are identified.

All at-risk individuals identified through the use of a risk assessment tool should have a daily skin inspection with close attention to bony prominences as recommended by AHRQ clinical guidelines. The NPIAP guidelines also recommend assessment for localized heat, edema, or induration. These signs are recommended as warning signs of pressure injury development on darkly pigmented skin because redness is not always possible to see. This routine assessment should be documented to demonstrate professional accountability so that preventive strategy outcomes can be evaluated. Another skin-related activity recommended by AHRQ clinical guidelines is to cleanse the skin of a patient with incontinence with a mild, nonirritating cleanser using warm—not hot—water at the time of soiling to minimize skin irritation and dryness. Moisturizers such as emollient lotions should be used to keep the skin from drying and cracking. It is best to apply the lotion immediately after bathing to increase the amount of moisture absorbed by the skin. Skin should not be rubbed or massaged over bony prominences because it may cause further deep tissue damage, especially if erythema is present (which already indicates injury) (Berlowitz et al, 2014; European Pressure Ulcer Advisory Panel, National Pressure Injury Advisory Panel and Pan Pacific Pressure Injury Alliance, 2019).

Proper turning and placement reduce the effects of pressure but not the intensity. It has been standard practice to turn patients a minimum of every 2 hours, which was endorsed in the AHRQ clinical guidelines. However, capillary closing pressure varies with each individual; therefore, the ideal strategy is to determine the turning schedule based on the development of erythema, which may precede ischemia. Currently, there is no strong evidence to support a 30-degree oblique angle versus a side-lying 90-degree angle to prevent pressure injury (Gillespie et al, 2014) (Fig. 15.18). To decrease pressure intensity on the heels, a patient should have a pillow or pillows under the calves to lift the feet and heels off the bed. Commercial devices also exist to suspend the heel, maintain or correct foot-ankle position, and protect the patient from neurosensory damage.

At-risk individuals should be placed on a pressure-reducing device in hopes of preventing the development of a pressure injury by decreasing pressure intensity. Pressure-reducing support surfaces such as mattress overlays, chair cushions or over-

WATERLOW PRESSURE ULCER PREVENTION/TREATMENT POLICY
RING SCORES IN TABLE, ADD TOTAL. MORE THAN 1 SCORE/CATEGORY CAN BE USED

BUILD/WEIGHT FOR HEIGHT	♦	SKIN TYPE VISUAL RISK AREAS	♦	SEX AGE	♦	MALNUTRITION SCREENING TOOL (MST) (Nutrition Vol.15, No.6 1999 - Australia)		
AVERAGE BMI =20–24.9	0	HEALTHY	0	MALE	1	A– HAS PATIENT LOST WEIGHT RECENTLY		B– WEIGHT LOSS SCORE
ABOVE AVERAGE BMI =25–29.9	1	TISSUE PAPER DRY	1 1	FEMALE 14–49	2 1	YES – GO TO B		0.5–5 Kg = 1
OBESE BMI >30	2	OEDEMATOUS CLAMMY, PYREXIA	1 1	50–64	2	NO – GO TO C UNSURE – GO TO C		5–10 Kg = 2 10–15 Kg = 3
BELOW AVERAGE BMI <20	3	DISCOLOURED GRADE1	2	65–74 75–80	3 4	AND SCORE 2		>15 Kg = 4 Unsure = 2
BMI = Wt(Kg)/Ht(m)²		BROKEN/SPOTS GRADE 2–4	3	81+	5	C-PATIENT EATING POORLY OR LACK OF APPETITE 'NO' = 0; 'YES' SCORE =1		NUTRITION SCORE If >2 refer for nutrition assessment/intervention

CONTINENCE	♦	MOBILITY	♦	SPECIAL RISKS				
COMPLETE/ CATHETERISED	0	FULLY	0	TISSUE MALNUTRITION	♦	NEUROLOGICAL DEFICIT		♦
URINE INCONT.	1	RESTLESS/FIDGETY	1	TERMINAL CACHEXIA	8	DIABETES, MS, CVA		4–6
FAECAL INCONT.	2	APATHETIC	2	MULTIPLE ORGAN FAILURE	8	MOTOR/SENSORY		4–6
URINARY + FAECAL INCONTINENCE	3	RESTRICTED BEDBOUND e.g., TRACTION	3 4	SINGLE ORGAN FAILURE (RESP, RENAL, CARDIAC)	5	PARAPLEGIA (MAX OF 6)		4–6
		CHAIRBOUND e.g. WHEELCHAIR	5	PERIPHERAL VASCULAR DISEASE	5	MAJOR SURGERY OR TRAUMA		
SCORE				ANAEMIA (Hb<8)	2	ORTHOPAEDIC/SPINAL		5
10+ AT RISK				SMOKING	1	ON TABLE >2 HR#		5
15+ HIGH RISK						ON TABLE >6 HR#		8
20+ VERY HIGH RISK				MEDICATION – CYTOTOXICS, LONG TERM/HIGH DOSE STEROIDS, ANTI-INFLAMMATORY MAX OF 4				

\# Scores can be discounted after 48 hours provided patient is recovering normally

© J Waterlow 1985 Revised 2005*
Obtainable from the Nook, Stoke Road, Henlade TAUNTON TA3 5LX
*The 2005 revision incorporates the research undertaken by Queensland Health.
www.judy-waterlow.co.uk

A

REMEMBER TISSUE DAMAGE MAY START PRIOR TO ADMISSION, IN CASUALTY. A SEATED PATIENT IS AT RISK ASSESSMENT (See Over) IF THE PATIENT FALLS INTO ANY OF THE RISK CATEGORIES, THEN PREVENTATIVE NURSING IS REQUIRED. A COMBINATION OF GOOD NURSING TECHNIQUES AND PREVENTATIVE AIDS WILL BE NECESSARY.
ALL ACTIONS MUST BE DOCUMENTED

PREVENTION
PRESSURE REDUCING AIDS

Special Mattress/beds:
- 10+ Overlays or specialist foam mattresses.
- 15+ Alternating pressure overlays, mattresses and bed systems
- 20+ Bed systems: Fluidised bead, low air loss and alternating pressure mattresses

Note: Preventative aids cover a wide spectrum of specialist features. Efficacy should be judged, if possible, on the basis of independent evidence.

Cushions: No person should sit in a wheelchair without some form of cushioning. If nothing else is available - use the person's own pillow. (Consider infection risk)
- 10+ 100 mm foam cushion
- 15+ Specialist gel and/or foam cushion
- 20+ Specialised cushion, adjustable to individual person.

Bed Clothing: Avoid plastic draw sheets, inco pads and tightly tucked in sheet/sheet covers, especially when using specialist bed and mattress overlay systems
Use duvet - plus vapour permeable membrane.

NURSING CARE
General HAND WASHING, frequent changes of position, lying, sitting. Use of pillows
Pain Appropriate pain control
Nutrition High protein, vitamins and minerals
Patient Handling Correct lifting technique - hoists - monkey poles Transfer devices
Patient Comfort Aids Real sheepskin - bed cradle
Operating Table Theatre/A&E Trolley 100 mm (4 ins) cover plus adequate protection

Skin Care General hygiene, NO rubbing, cover with an appropriate dressing

WOUND GUIDELINES
Assessment Odour, exudate, measure/photograph position

WOUND CLASSIFICATION - EPUAP
GRADE 1 Discolouration of intact skin not affected by light finger pressure (non-blanching erythema)
This may be difficult to identify in darkly pigmented skin

GRADE 2 Partial thickness skin loss or damage involving epidermis and/or dermis
The pressure ulcer is superficial and presents clinically as an abrasion, blister or shallow crater

GRADE 3 Full thickness skin loss involving damage of subcutaneous tissue but not extending to the underlying fascia
The pressure ulcer presents clinically as a deep crater with or without undermining of adjacent tissue

GRADE 4 Full thickness skin loss with extensive destruction and necrosis extending to underlying tissue.

Dressing Guide Use local dressings formulary and/or www.worldwidewounds

IF TREATMENT IS REQUIRED, FIRST REMOVE PRESSURE

B

Fig. 15.17 The Waterlow Pressure Ulcer Prevention/Treatment Policy card. **(A)** Front; **(B)** Back. (From White GM, Cox NH [eds]. [2006]. *Diseases of the Skin: A Color Atlas and Text* [2nd ed.] St. Louis, Mosby.)

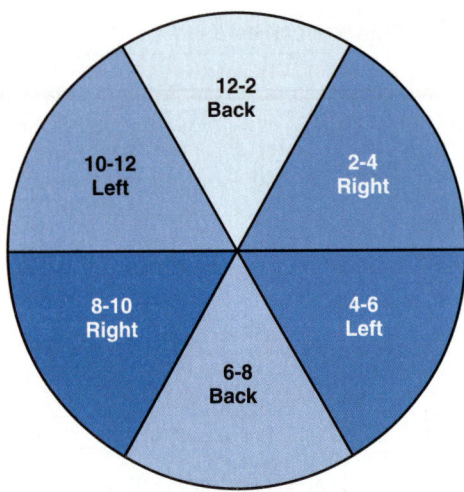

Fig. 15.18 Turning schedule for pressure injury prevention and treatment. (From Bryant, R., & Nix, D. [2016]. *Acute and chronic wounds: Current management concepts* [5th ed.]. St. Louis, MO: Elsevier.)

lays, and specialized beds redistribute weight over a larger area and reduce tissue–interface pressure. Tissue–interface pressure is the amount of pressure between the skin and resting surface (e.g., a mattress). It has been thought that if the tissue–interface pressure is 32 mm Hg or lower, capillary closure will not occur. However, this logic may be questioned because capillary closing pressures vary from one individual to another.

Mattress overlays reduce pressure, are usually economical with only a one-time charge, and are accessible in most environments. Overlays may be static (e.g., foam, gel, water, air, and low air loss) or dynamic (e.g., alternating air). Because the overlays are placed on top of a mattress, the height of the bed is increased, making it more difficult for patients to get in and out of the bed, which is a common patient and nurse complaint. The overlay may also decrease the protective height of bedside rails because the effective mattress height has increased. Some mattress overlays trap moisture and heat, which may be uncomfortable. Foam overlays should have a base height of at least 4 inches from the bottom to the *beginning* of the convolutions, not to the peak, and a stiffness of 25% of indentation load deflection (AHRQ, 2019). Foam overlays must also be examined regularly to assess their continued effectiveness (i.e., no obvious sagging) because their use is limited. Static air and water overlays must be checked regularly for proper inflation and must be cleaned periodically.

Specialty beds such as air-fluidized beds or low-air-loss beds are generally used for individuals who have multiple stage III and IV pressure injuries or who are at high risk after posterior grafts or flap procedures. These beds may, in fact, overheat a patient and may elevate the body temperature if not adequately controlled. Multiple hybrids of air-fluidized and low-air-loss beds exist, which enables the nurse to better match beds with patient needs. Specialty beds do not eliminate the need for meticulous nursing care. Patients must still be repositioned, assessed, and kept clean and dry.

The presence of skin moisture (whether the result of incontinence of urine or feces, perspiration, or wound exudate) should be minimized. If necessary, absorbent undergarments may be used to maintain a dryer skin surface. However, it is important to check these absorbent pads or undergarments frequently to determine whether new products are needed after significant wetting or any soiling. Topical barriers such as zinc oxide may be applied after cleansing and gently drying the skin (AHRQ, 2019). Indwelling Foley catheters should be used only on a short-term basis or avoided, if possible, because of the risk of urinary tract infections. Thought must be given to the reason for a catheter and whether the benefit of placement outweighs the risk of infection. Although most orders are for turning and repositioning every 2 hours, the primary care provider may need to be contacted to implement consistent scheduled checks before the 2-hour intervals. With the implementation of regular checks to keep skin clean and dry and the use of absorbent pads and topical barriers, catheter placement can be avoided, thus reducing patient risk.

Skin injury from friction or shearing forces can be avoided by using proper turning techniques and proper placement. Using proper transfer techniques and a draw sheet can prevent friction injuries. Lubricants, topical barrier creams, film or hydrocolloid dressings, or protective padding may be used to reduce damage when skin moves across a coarse or hard surface. Shearing results when the body shifts and slides downward; therefore, most shearing injuries can be eliminated with proper placement. For example, not elevating the head of the bed more than 30 degrees and elevating the knees slightly when the head is elevated prevent slipping down in bed. When the patient is sitting in a chair, placing the feet on a stool prevents sliding downward (AHRQ, 2019).

Nutritional status must be closely monitored by assessing food intake, weight, muscle mass, SQ fat stores, localized or generalized fluid accumulation, and hand grip strength (Keller, 2019). Accurate food intake should be monitored routinely to identify both the need for changes before a compromised state develops and nutritionally at-risk patients. Hydration status is another important nutritional component because dehydration may contribute to the development of a pressure injury. The amount of fluid that an older adult should consume each day is determined by their body weight. Current resources suggest that older adults take one-third of their body weight and drink that number of ounces of water per day (National Council on Aging, 2021). For example, an older adult who weighs 100 pounds should drink 33 ounces, or 4 cups, of water per day. This general guideline may need to be changed based on the person's medical comorbidities. A diagnosis such as HF may mandate less fluid intake per day, while a diagnosis of cystic fibrosis may require that the person drink more fluids. The use of an air-fluidized or low-air-loss bed increases daily fluid needs because insensible loss is increased. When the professional nurse recognizes a pattern of decreased food or water intake, a full assessment addressing food preferences, dentition, and swallowing difficulties is warranted. The patient should also be evaluated for constipation or fecal impaction, which decreases appetite. A more comprehensive nutritional assessment may be necessary, which may include a registered dietician consultation, occupational therapy, and a dental appointment; nutritional supplements may be needed. A person's weight typically changes slowly; therefore, weighing the patient monthly is sufficient and is needed more frequently only when assessing cardiovascular status. A weight loss of 5%–10% is significant; weight loss is associated with an increased risk of mortality (Gaddey and Holder, 2021).

Recent evidence suggests that serum protein abnormalities are late indicators of malnutrition in older adults (Keller, 2019). US nutritional societies suggest using the following markers to assess for malnutrition in adults: for the diagnosis to be made, the individual must show at least two or more of the following (Keller, 2019):

- Insufficient energy intake
- Weight loss
- Loss of muscle mass
- Loss of SQ fat
- Localized or generalized fluid accumulation that may sometimes mask weight loss
- Diminished functional status as measured by hand grip strength
- Prealbumin is low

Because of multiple risk factors and their synergistic effect on pressure injury development, prevention is a nursing challenge, offering an opportunity to demonstrate the effect of nursing by recognizing at-risk patients, immediately implementing preventive strategies, and preventing a costly health care problem. Most of all, preventive measures promote high-quality patient care, which is the primary goal of nursing.

Pressure Injury Management

Nurses play a key role in pressure injury management because they are the professionals responsible for wound care and are often the first team members to identify wound changes. In addition, physicians perceive the nurse, especially in long-term care, as an expert in pressure injury management. It is not uncommon for physicians to say, "Do whatever treatment you think is best." Often, the health care provider, when assessing medical management, asks the nurse to describe and evaluate the treatment. Therefore, it is important for the nurse to comprehend the healing process, to understand treatment strategies, and to maintain a current knowledge base. The following discussion reviews the healing trajectory and treatment options, which include nutritional management. It is hoped that the professional nurse will become empowered, promote a positive image for nursing, and, most importantly, be able to deliver more successful patient care by comprehending the physiology of the healing process and the logic for treatment strategies.

Physiology of Wound Healing

An understanding of the healing process is necessary for critically analyzing pressure injury care and determining the best management strategy. Pressure injury research has expanded our understanding of the etiology of pressure injuries and the healing process. The three major stages of wound healing are as follows: (1) the inflammatory stage; (2) the proliferative, or granulation, stage; and (3) the maturation, or matrix formation, stage.

The *inflammatory stage,* characterized by redness, heat, pain, and swelling, lasts approximately 4–5 days. The inflammatory stage initiates the healing process by stabilizing the wound through platelet activity, which stops bleeding and triggers the immune system. Neutrophils, monocytes, and macrophages arrive within 24 hours of the insult to control bacteria, remove dead tissue, and secrete angiogenesis factor (AGF) and other growth factors, which stimulate the development of granulation tissue. Bradykinin and histamine, released from injured cells, cause vasodilation, which leads to swelling. This creates the red, swollen, tender clinical presentation often seen in wounds (Rodrigues et al, 2019). The inflammatory stage is crucial for successful healing, and a delayed or altered response may possibly contribute to the development of chronic, stagnant wounds if appropriate growth factors and responses were not mobilized when the patient was first injured. Medications (e.g., steroids), decreased tissue oxygenation, poor nutritional status, and age-related changes (e.g., decreased response of the immune system) may impede this stage.

The *proliferative,* or *granulation, stage* begins 24 hours after injury and continues for up to 22 days. Three significant events occur: (1) epithelialization, (2) granulation, and (3) collagen synthesis. Epithelialization, via a microscopic epithelial layer, seals and protects the wound from bacteria and fluid loss. This microscopic layer, which is fostered by a moist environment, is extremely fragile and may easily be washed away with aggressive wound irrigation or harsh wiping of the involved area. Granulation, also known as *neovascularization,* is the formation of new capillaries that generate and feed new tissue, creating a beefy-red tissue bed that bleeds easily. Collagen synthesis creates a support matrix that provides strength to the new tissue. Oxygen, iron, vitamin C, zinc, magnesium, and amino acids are necessary for collagen synthesis. Fibroblasts, stimulated in the first phase by AGF, are necessary for collagen production. This phase rebuilds the injured area and can be easily influenced by the effectiveness of the inflammation stage and wound environment.

The *maturation stage,* also known as the *differentiation* or *remodeling phase,* is the final stage. It does not begin until 21 days after the injury and may take years to heal. During this stage, maximum tensile strength is generated through collagen deposits that make the wound thicker and more compact. These collagen deposits contract until closure is attained. Initially, the scarred area is a dark, scarlet red that fades over time to a silvery white. Tensile strength reaches only 80% of preinjury capacity; therefore, the "scarred" area is more vulnerable to breakdown or injury (Rodrigues et al, 2019).

Definition of Terms and Staging Criteria

A *pressure injury* is localized damage to the skin and underlying soft tissue, usually over the bony prominence or related to a medical or other device. The injury can present as intact skin or an open ulcer and may be painful. The injury occurs as a result of intense and/or prolonged pressure, or pressure in combination with shear. The tolerance of soft tissue for pressure and shear may also be affected by microclimate, nutrition, perfusion, comorbidities, and the condition of the soft tissue (Box 15.2; NPIAP, 2021). Box 15.3 provides more definitions of relevant terms.

BOX 15.2 Staging Criteria

Deep Tissue Pressure Injury: Persistent Nonblanchable Deep Red, Maroon, or Purple Discoloration

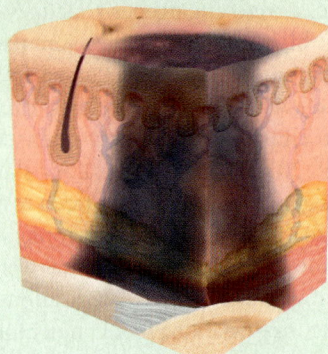

Intact or nonintact skin with a localized area of persistent, nonblanchable deep red, maroon, or purple discoloration, or epidermal separation revealing a dark wound bed or blood-filled blister. Pain and temperature changes often precede skin color changes. Discoloration may appear differently on darkly pigmented skin. This injury results from intense and/or prolonged pressure and shear forces at the bone–muscle interface. The wound may evolve rapidly to reveal the actual extent of tissue injury or may resolve without tissue loss. If necrotic tissue, SQ tissue, granulation tissue, fascia, muscle, or other underlying structures are visible, this indicates a full-thickness pressure injury (Unstageable, Stage 3, or Stage 4). Do not use DTPI to describe vascular, traumatic, neuropathic, or dermatologic conditions.

Stage 1: Nonblanchable Erythema of Intact Skin

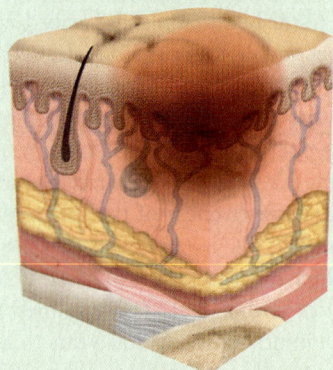

Intact skin has a localized area of nonblanchable erythema, which may appear differently in darkly pigmented skin. The presence of blanchable erythema or changes in sensation, temperature, or firmness may precede visual changes. Color changes do not include purple or maroon discoloration; these may indicate a deep tissue pressure injury.

Stage 2: Partial-Thickness Skin Loss With Exposed Dermis

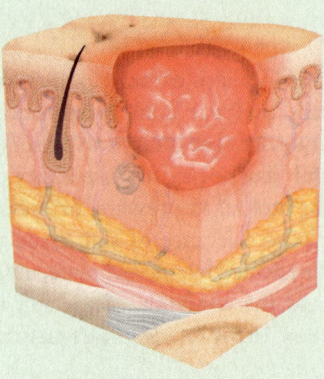

Partial-thickness loss of skin with exposed dermis. The wound bed is viable, pink or red, moist, and may also present as an intact or ruptured serum-filled blister. Adipose (fat) is not visible, and deeper tissues are not visible. Granulation tissue, slough, and eschar are not present. These injuries commonly result from adverse microclimate, shear in the skin over the pelvis, and shear in the heel. This stage should not be used to describe moisture-associated skin damage (MASD), including incontinence-associated dermatitis (IAD), intertriginous dermatitis (ITD), medical adhesive-related skin injury (MARSI), or traumatic wounds (skin tears, burns, and abrasions).

Stage 3: Full-Thickness Skin Loss

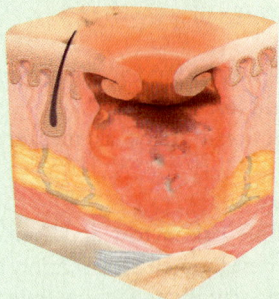

Full-thickness loss of skin, in which adipose (fat) is visible in the ulcer and granulation tissue and epibole (rolled wound edges) are often present. Slough and/or eschar may be visible. The depth of tissue damage varies by anatomic location; areas of significant adiposity can develop deep wounds. Undermining and tunneling may occur. Fascia, muscle, tendon, ligament, cartilage, and/or bone are not exposed. If slough or eschar obscures the extent of tissue loss, this is an Unstageable Pressure Injury.

Stage 4: Full-Thickness Skin and Tissue Loss

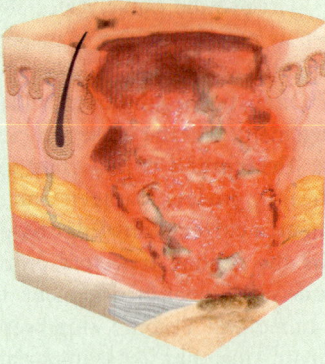

Full-thickness skin and tissue loss, with exposed or directly palpable fascia, muscle, tendon, ligament, cartilage, or bone in the ulcer. Slough and/or eschar may be visible. Epibole (rolled edges), undermining, and/or tunneling often occur. Depth varies by anatomic location. If slough or eschar obscures the extent of tissue loss, this is an Unstageable Pressure Injury.

BOX 15.2 Staging Criteria—cont'd

Unstageable Pressure Injury: Obscured Full-Thickness Skin and Tissue Loss

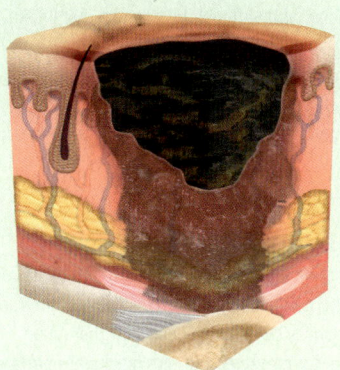

Full-thickness skin and tissue loss, in which the extent of tissue damage within the ulcer cannot be confirmed because it is obscured by slough or eschar. If slough or eschar is removed, a Stage 3 or Stage 4 pressure injury will be revealed. Stable eschar (i.e., dry, adherent, and intact without erythema or fluctuance) on the heel or ischemic limb should not be softened or removed.

From the National Pressure Injury Advisory Panel (2016). Reprinted with permission.

BOX 15.3 Definitions of Terms

Autolysis: Self-debridement of necrotic tissue by WBCs, which is fostered by a dressing that retains moisture (e.g., transparent film); a yellowish-brown fluid is generated from the WBCs and breakdown of tissue.
Debridement: Removal of dead, damaged tissue.
Epithelialization: The growth of a microscopic layer that covers an open wound, which creates a barrier that protects from fluid loss and bacterial assault and that is highly fragile and easily destroyed.
Eschar: Thick, necrotic, devitalized tissue; often black but may be yellowish.
Exudate: Wound discharge that may be serosanguinous, serous, or purulent.
Friction: Rubbing of skin against another surface (e.g., sheets, bed, or chair).
Granulation tissue: New capillary growth that creates a beefy-red color and tissue that bleeds easily (friable).
Interface pressure: Force exerted between body and support surface (e.g., mattress).
Pressure injury: Lesions caused by unrelieved pressure that cause tissue damage and death; usually occur over bony prominences or other pressure points (e.g., tubing, foreign material in bed).

Reactive hyperemia: Transient, blanching erythema from tissue anoxia, which generates a compensatory mechanism resulting in dilated vessels.
Shearing force: Sliding of parallel surfaces when the skeletal frame and deep fascia slide downward; the superficial fascia remains attached to the dermis, thus stretching or occluding the arterial supply to fascia and muscle, which may lead to tissue anoxia and damage; the most common position for this occurrence is when the head of the bed is elevated and the body slides downward.
Sinus tract: A vertical tunnel connecting one anatomic compartment with another.
Tissue tolerance: The skin's (i.e., blood vessels, interstitial fluid, collagen, and other structures) ability to endure the effects of pressure without adverse consequences.
Undermining: Separation of tissue under the dermis creates a horizontal tunnel; length can be measured by inserting a cotton-tipped applicator into the tunnel, marking the length on the applicator, and then placing it next to a tape measure.

Modified from Bryant, R. A., Shannon, M. L., Pieper, B., Braden, B. J. & Morris, D. J. (1992). Pressure ulcers. In R. A. Bryant (Ed.), *Acute and chronic wounds: Nursing management.* St. Louis, MO: Mosby; Agency for Health Care Policy and Research. (1992). *Pressure ulcers in adults: Prediction and prevention,* Clinical Practice Guideline No 3, Rockville, MD: U.S. Department of Health and Human Services; Sanders, S. L. (1992). Pressure ulcers, part II: Management strategies. *Journal of the American Academy of Nurse Practitioners, 4*(3), 101.

Basic Principles of Pressure Injury Management

Three basic principles guide successful pressure injury management:
1. Eliminate or minimize precipitating factors such as pressure, friction, shearing, and poor nutrition.
2. Provide nutritional support and monitor nutritional status.
3. Create and maintain a clean, moist wound environment with adequate circulation and oxygenation.

Pressure injury preventive strategies must be implemented, or wound care efforts are futile (Box 15.4). Through institutional policy and protocol, the nurse should apply an appropriate mattress overlay. The nurse ensures that all staff members use proper technique when repositioning a patient to minimize shearing and friction forces. As leader of the care team, the nurse is responsible for observing nursing aides and other support team members who deliver hands-on care to identify specific learning needs so that pressure, shearing, and friction are minimized. Teaching the logic behind such techniques may motivate staff members to exercise more diligence in performing proper preventive actions. The nurse must rely on teaching principles such as the repetition of key information in a nonthreatening manner. They should reinforce appropriate activity with positive feedback.

Nutritional status should be monitored; specifically, the health care provider should monitor weight and food consumption so that needs can be identified immediately. This also promotes a

BOX 15.4 Pressure Injury Prevention Strategies

Risk Assessment
1. Consider bedfast and chairfast individuals to be at risk for the development of pressure injuries.
2. Use a structured risk assessment, such as the Braden Scale, to identify individuals at risk for pressure injury as soon as possible (but within 8 hours after admission).
3. Refine the assessment by including these additional risk factors:
   a. Fragile skin
   b. Existing pressure injury of any stage, including those ulcers that have healed or are closed
   c. Impairments in blood flow to the extremities from vascular disease, diabetes, or tobacco use
   d. Pain in areas of the body exposed to pressure
4. Repeat the risk assessment at regular intervals and with any change in condition. Base the frequency of regular assessments on acuity levels:
   a. Acute care . . . . Every shift
   b. Long-term care . . . . Weekly for 4 weeks, then quarterly
   c. Home care . . . . At every nurse visit
5. Develop a plan of care based on the areas of risk, rather than on the total risk assessment score. For example, if the risk stems from immobility, address turning, repositioning, and the support surface. If the risk is from malnutrition, address those problems

Skin Care
1. Inspect all of the skin upon admission as soon as possible (but within 8 hours).
2. Inspect the skin at least daily for signs of pressure injury, especially non-blanchable erythema.
3. Assess pressure points, such as the sacrum, coccyx, buttocks, heels, ischium, trochanters, elbows, and beneath medical devices.
4. When inspecting darkly pigmented skin, look for changes in skin tone, skin temperature, and tissue consistency compared with adjacent skin. Moistening the skin assists in identifying changes in color.
5. Cleanse the skin promptly after episodes of incontinence.
6. Use skin cleansers that are pH-balanced for the skin.
7. Use skin moisturizers daily on dry skin.
8. Avoid positioning an individual on an area of erythema or pressure injury.

Nutrition
1. Consider hospitalized individuals to be at risk for undernutrition and malnutrition from their illness or being nothing by mouth (NPO) for diagnostic testing.
2. Use a valid and reliable screening tool to determine the risk of malnutrition, such as the Mini Nutritional Assessment.
3. Refer all individuals at risk for pressure injury from malnutrition to a registered dietitian/nutritionist.
4. Assist the individual at mealtimes to increase oral intake.
5. Encourage all individuals at risk for pressure injury to consume adequate fluids and a balanced diet.
6. Assess weight changes over time.
7. Assess the adequacy of oral, enteral, and parenteral intake.
8. Provide nutritional supplements between meals and with oral medications, unless contraindicated.

Repositioning and Mobilization
1. Turn and reposition all individuals at risk for pressure injury, unless contraindicated due to a medical condition or medical treatments.
2. Choose a frequency for turning based on the support surface in use, the skin's tolerance for pressure, and the individual's preferences.
3. Consider lengthening the turning schedule during the night to allow for uninterrupted sleep.
4. Turn the individual into a 30-degree side-lying position and use your hand to determine whether the sacrum is off the bed.
5. Avoid positioning the individual on body areas with pressure injuries.
6. Ensure that the heels are free from the bed.
7. Consider the level of immobility, exposure to shear, skin moisture, perfusion, body size, and weight of the individual when choosing a support surface.
8. Continue to reposition an individual when placed on any support surface.
9. Use a breathable incontinence pad when using microclimate management surfaces.
10. Use a pressure-redistributing chair cushion for individuals sitting in chairs or wheelchairs.
11. Reposition weak or immobile individuals in chairs hourly.
12. If the individual cannot be moved or is positioned with the head of the bed elevated over 30 degrees, place a polyurethane foam dressing on the sacrum.
13. Use heel-offloading devices or polyurethane foam dressings on individuals at high risk for heel ulcers.
14. Place thin foam or breathable dressings under medical devices.

Education
1. Teach the individual and family about the risk of pressure injury.
2. Engage individuals and families in risk reduction interventions.

From National Pressure Injury Advisory Panel. (2016). *Pressure injury prevention points.* Retrieved from https://npiap.com/page/PreventionPoints.

---

collaborative effort among health care providers. When food intake is first noted to decrease, the nurse should identify reasons, such as not meeting food preferences, a sore mouth, the patient being rushed to eat, conflict with staff, depression, or pain.

For closure of the wound, a clean, moist environment must be created and maintained. This principle is the key to successful healing and should guide the professional nurse and practitioner. Consequently, necrotic tissue must be removed, and any infectious process (as evidenced by erythema, induration, and tenderness in the periwound skin; pus; or a pale wound bed) must be resolved to implement a dressing strategy that fosters rapid epithelialization and granulation.

It is important to know when to culture a wound because of the expense to the patient and the health care system. Also, inappropriate antibiotic use is decreased when wounds are cultured appropriately. All wounds are contaminated; therefore, all cultures grow surface bacteria, and the true pathogen may not be identified. A culture is warranted only when cellulitis (e.g., erythema, induration, and tenderness) or a wound infection (evidenced by a pale wound bed, pus, increased tenderness, persistent exudate, or no new growth) exists. An accurate culture includes both anaerobic and aerobic species. To obtain the culture, the nurse should use the most accurate method, considered the gold standard for wound cultures, which is a deep-tissue or punch biopsy (Spear, 2014). According to the AHRQ treatment guidelines, an ulcer is *not* to be cultured with the use of a culturette because colonized bacteria may be obtained instead of the offending pathogen. The NPIAP treatment guidelines recommend obtaining a tissue biopsy or quantitative swab technique (10-point swab culture). An infected wound is managed topically with antiseptics or systemically, depending on the severity and risk of osteomyelitis.

NPIAP guidelines recommend the use of nontoxic topical antiseptics for a limited time to control bacterial colonization. The following antiseptics are commonly used (NPIAP, 2021; Kramer et al, 2018):

- Iodine compounds (povidone iodine and slow-release cadexomer iodine)
- Silver compounds (including silver sulfadiazine)
- Polyhexanide and betaine (PHMB)
- Chlorhexidine
- Sodium hypochlorite
- Acetic acid

Antiseptic solutions are used with wet-to-dry dressings, which also provide some mechanical debridement. At times, a wound may be irrigated with the antiseptic; however, a rinse with normal saline should follow. If the nurse notices that antiseptic use has continued for longer than 1 week, a reminder or question should be posed to the health care provider.

The first step in pressure injury care is to thoroughly assess the wound to determine the most effective strategy and dressing. The nurse is usually the first person to identify a need for change; therefore, this assessment should be an ongoing process. The nurse should examine the wound, noting its color; any discharge, bleeding, or odor; the degree of undermining or presence of a sinus tract (which may be measured using a cotton-tipped applicator); any necrotic tissue; pain or tenderness; and the amount of erythema surrounding the wound edges. Limited erythema around the wound is a normal phenomenon that signifies increased circulation to provide nutrients; however, if the erythema extends, infection or candidiasis should be suspected and the wound closely monitored. Ideally, the wound base should be a beefy-red color, which is indicative of granulation. However, some hydrogel and hydrocolloid dressings generate a pale pink wound bed, which ordinarily would mean an "ill" wound bed. If the bed is pale pink and not associated with a purulent discharge or cellulitis, the wound environment is most likely clean and should just be observed. Note that granulation tissue has a rich capillary supply and bleeds easily and profusely when disturbed (e.g., when it is irrigated or during a dressing change). Thus, if a tunneling wound bleeds, it can be deduced that granulation tissue exists, although it is not visible because of the tunneling.

The wound assessment should be ongoing and supported with documentation (Fig. 15.19). All new wounds should be described, including location, color, discharge, tenderness, amount of necrotic tissue or undermining, dimensions, and stage. The wound measurements should include length, width, and depth. When measuring undermining, the nurse should use a cotton-tipped applicator, marking depth on the applicator and placing it next to a tape measure to obtain dimension and to note position (e.g., 4 cm at 2 o'clock). It is not imperative that all dimensions or locations of undermining be documented. The nurse should record only the greatest length because the wound cannot be deemed healed until closed. It is recommended that facilities develop a written procedure stating how dimensions should be obtained and documented (e.g., length by width by depth and undermining) to establish continuity and minimize confusion regarding the procedure.

Debridement

Necrotic tissue provides the ideal environment for bacterial growth, which may cause inflammation and impair the body's ability to fight infection. Therefore, necrotic tissue must be debrided as soon as possible, and measures (such as wet-to-dry dressings or topical antimicrobials) should be taken to resolve bacterial insults until purulent discharge has dissipated. If necrotic tissue is not debrided, the nurse's efforts are futile, and the patient's comfort and quality of life are affected.

The removal of dry, hard eschar should be considered because its presence slows the migration of epithelial cells and delays healing, except for stable heel ulcers, in which case dry eschar should be left intact (AHRQ, 2019). At times, this dry eschar may serve as an efficient and comfortable dressing, but the area must be watched for the development of infection. If the patient has diabetes or has an ischemic wound with a dry, hard, intact eschar, it may be more prudent to leave the eschar in place. It serves as a barrier and does not place the patient at risk for any possible problems from frequent dressing changes (e.g., infection, skin tears, and candidiasis). However, the eschar and periwound skin must be monitored. If the eschar becomes soft and boggy, tissue liquefaction is most likely accumulating and must be removed. This is especially true if the wound is tender or has periwound erythema, indicating infection.

Various methods of debridement include mechanical, autolytic, enzymatic, conservative sharp, and surgical sharp. Mechanical debridement (continuously moist gauze or pulsed lavage) is effective for removing slough that cannot be removed surgically or chemically (because of damage to viable tissue). If mechanical debridement using continually moist gauze dressings is employed, the nurse should protect wound borders from maceration with zinc oxide or stoma adhesive. Using pulsed lavage once or twice daily may mechanically debride and should be reserved for large, exuding wounds; this should be discontinued after the wound is clean or demonstrates stability. Mechanical debridement requires more nursing time, is more uncomfortable for the patient, and may destroy fragile epithelial cells. For these reasons, a more efficient method should be sought first (NPIAP, 2021).

Autolytic debridement is effective for removing eschar and slough when less than 50% of the wound bed is involved and no evidence of infection exists in the periwound skin. Autolytic debridement involves using the body's own enzymes to provide additional debriding and cleansing. Hydrocolloid or hydrogel dressings may soften and facilitate the removal of eschar and slough if the wound is not infected. It should be noted that autolysis creates a larger appearing wound because debris is being removed. Autolysis generates a brownish-yellow fluid that may have some pus in it because of dead cells and neutrophils. The nurse should not become alarmed unless clinical evidence of infection exists (e.g., erythema, tenderness, heat, and swelling).

Patient name _____ Patient ID# _____
Ulcer location _____ Date _____

Directions: Observe and measure the pressure ulcer. Categorize the ulcer with respect to surface area, exudate, and type of wound tissue. Record a subscore for each of these ulcer characteristics. Add the subscores to obtain the total score. A comparison of total scores measured over time provides an indication of the improvement or deterioration in pressure ulcer healing.

Length × width	0 0 cm²	1 <0.3 cm²	2 0.3–0.6 cm²	3 0.7–1.0 cm²	4 1.1–2.0 cm²	5 2.1–3.0 cm²	Subscore
		6 3.1–4.0 cm²	7 4.1–8.0 cm²	8 8.1–12.0 cm²	9 12.1–24.0 cm²	10 >24.0 cm²	
Exudate amount	0 None	1 Light	2 Moderate	3 Heavy			Subscore
Tissue type	0 Closed	1 Epithelial tissue	2 Granulation tissue	3 Slough	4 Necrotic tissue		Subscore
							Total score

Length × Width: Measure the greatest length (head to toe) and the greatest width (side to side) using a centimeter ruler. Multiply these two measurements (length × width) to obtain an estimate of surface area in square centimeters (cm²). *Caveat:* Do not guess! Always use a centimeter ruler and always use the same method each time the ulcer is measured.

Exudate Amount: Estimate the amount of exudate (drainage) present after removal of the dressing and before applying any topical agent to the ulcer. Estimate the exudate (drainage) as none, light, moderate, or heavy.

Tissue Type: This refers to the types of tissue that are present in the wound (ulcer) bed. Score as a "4" if there is any necrotic tissue present. Score as a "3" if there is any amount of slough present and necrotic tissue is absent. Score as a "2" if the wound is clean and contains granulation tissue. A superficial wound that is reepithelializing is scored as a "1." When the wound is closed, score as a "0."

- 4 **Necrotic tissue (eschar):** black, brown, or tan tissue that adheres firmly to the wound bed or ulcer edges and may be either firmer or softer than surrounding skin
- 3 **Slough:** yellow or white tissue that adheres to the ulcer bed in strings or thick clumps, or is mucinous
- 2 **Granulation tissue:** pink or beefy red tissue with a shiny, moist, granular appearance
- 1 **Epithelial tissue:** for superficial ulcers, new pink or shiny tissue (skin) that grows in from the edges or as islands on the ulcer surface
- 0 **Closed/resurfaced:** the wound is completely covered with epithelium (new skin)

Directions: Observe and measure the pressure ulcers at regular intervals using the PUSH Tool. Date and record PUSH subscale and total scores on the Pressure Ulcer Healing Record below.

Pressure Ulcer Healing Record										
Date										
Length × width										
Exudate amount										
Tissue type										
Total score										

Version 3.0: 9/15/98
© National Pressure Ulcer Advisory Panel

Fig. 15.19 The Pressure Ulcer Scale for Healing (PUSH) Tool. (From National Pressure Ulcer Advisory Panel. [1998]. Pressure Ulcer Scale for Healing [PUSH]: PUSH Tool 3.0.)

Autolytic debridement may be used in conjunction with mechanical methods to further shorten the time to wound cleansing.

Enzymatic debridement is costly and time-consuming; however, it may be effective on small, necrotic areas or for removing yellow, tender eschar that is difficult to remove surgically. Enzymatic debridement is primarily used in a home setting or nursing facility where appropriately educated or certified professionals are not readily accessible for conservative sharp debridement at the bedside. Enzymatic debridement may save the patient from hospital admission. If used, the enzymatic agent must *not* be applied to healthy, viable tissue because the enzyme will destroy granulation tissue and epithelial cells.

If the wound has a dry, rubbery eschar, conservative, sharp debridement is recommended over enzymatic debridement because enzymatic debridement takes much longer. The main principle that guides conservative sharp debridement is to stop when bleeding occurs, which indicates that viable, healthy tissue has been reached. Because the wound is dirty, an aseptic technique is appropriate. To prevent "showering" of bacteria from conservative sharp debridement and to assist in cleaning up the wound, nurses should apply wet-to-dry dressings moistened with an acceptable antiseptic every shift for 1–3 days, depending on the wound condition.

Surgical sharp debridement is reserved for cases of suspected sepsis, for wounds with tunneling or undermining, if necrotic tissue cannot be removed by other means, or for stage III or IV wounds not healing with conservative treatment.

Wound Care Principles and Dressing Types

The wound care market is a multibillion-dollar business and has created many dressing options. Therefore, the nurse must understand the healing trajectory to select the best treatment option. The major goal is to create an environment that supports healing—a clean, moist (hydrated, not wet) wound bed. If no growth is evident in weekly measurements after 2–4 weeks, consideration should be given to changing the dressing strategy. Table 15.2 provides a brief overview of commonly used dressing types and general treatment principles.

With each dressing change, all open wounds should be *gently* irrigated with approximately 20–50 mL of normal saline with the use of a catheter-tip syringe. After irrigation, the wound can be assessed.

It is prudent to always write the date and time of the dressing change on the outside of the dressing itself. This practice reflects professional accountability and assists in problem-solving. For example, a wound may have more discharge or a significant change because the dressing was not changed soon enough or, inadvertently, not changed at all.

If the wound border has candidiasis, evidenced by a fire-red erythema, usually with satellite lesions and denuded skin, a zinc oxide–nystatin (50/50) mixture may be applied to the affected areas, and then the dressing may be applied. Because candidiasis flourishes in a moist environment, a thorough assessment should be performed to identify the reason for excess moisture. Is a moist dressing overlapping the wound edges? Is the film dressing generating so much fluid retention and maceration that candidiasis is occurring? If so, the zinc oxide–nystatin cream could be applied, and the wound should be monitored. It may be that the dressing type must be changed. After the candidiasis has resolved, a stoma adhesive wafer may be placed around the wound to protect the skin from future problems. Stoma adhesive is recommended over a hydrocolloid dressing because tape and film dressings do not stick to the stoma adhesive barrier as they do to a hydrocolloid wafer. If no infection exists, another alternative that decreases maceration is to apply petroleum jelly or zinc oxide around the wound borders and then apply the dressing.

Gauze dressings have been used for many years with success; however, a large amount of scientific information regarding pressure injuries and wound care has been accumulating since 1962, when moisture was first identified as a facilitator of healing. This discovery has generated many other effective, efficient, and comfortable options. Thus, gauze is primarily used for debriding and cleaning up the wound bed, except when used for protecting closed surgical wounds or when the newer, more expensive dressings are not on the formulary. However, when a wound has tunneling or undermining, saline-moistened gauze, *loosely* packed into the wound, may maintain a moist environment. Caution should be exercised not to pack tightly or have the moistened gauze touching the healing surface surrounding the ulcer to avoid additional damage and maceration. If gauze is being used on a clean wound, the strategy should be wet-to-moist dressing to prevent the drying of epithelial cells. The nurse should slightly moisten the gauze, touching the wound bed with normal saline, and place dry gauze or an abdominal pad over the moist gauze and secure with tape; this should keep the wound moist at all times.

Some gauze is impregnated with materials such as povidone-iodine or petroleum jelly. Gauze ribbons impregnated with povidone-iodine (iodoform gauze) are effective for cleaning up a tunneling wound that has a purulent or foul exudate. However, the povidone-iodine gauze should be stopped when the purulent, foul exudate has resolved so that healthy tissue is not destroyed. Petroleum jelly gauze is a good, inexpensive method for keeping a wound from drying out and protecting the wound and surrounding tissue. Petroleum jelly gauze secured with Kerlix wrapped around the extremity, changed every 2–4 days, and as needed, is an effective strategy for healing skin tears. The petroleum jelly keeps the wound moist and protects it from further insults.

Nonadherent dressings are used when the wound bed must be protected and epithelial cells left undisturbed. Nonadherent dressings are suitable for skin tears, skin grafts, or other wounds that require a minimum insult. Often, an antibiotic ointment is applied to the wound bed (which keeps it moist), and then the bed is covered with a nonadherent dressing, which is changed once or twice a day.

Foam dressings, which are nonadherent, absorbent dressings, protect the wound and assist in minimizing maceration of the wound edges. Consider the use of foam dressings for stage II and shallow stage III pressure injuries, exudating cavity ulcers, painful ulcers, and on body areas and pressure injuries at risk for shear injury (NPIAP, 2021). Foam dressings have also been used around tracheal tubes; they are beneficial when candidiasis exists around tracheal stomas, acting to absorb moisture. Foam dressings are secured with tape or film and may be used in combination with other topical agents or primary dressings.

Transparent films are used for stage I or II pressure injuries (superficial wounds) to secure dressings, to protect vulnerable areas (e.g., elbows) from friction, and to facilitate autolysis. Transparent films are semipermeable, thus allowing the exchange of air. However, they should not be used to cover enzymatic debriding agents, gels, or ointments. Film dressings may be left on for 3–7 days but should be checked a minimum of once a day. Film dressings facilitate autolysis, which causes fluid buildup and may consequently lead to maceration of good tissue and dressing leakage. Petroleum jelly or zinc oxide applied around the wound edges before placement of the film may prevent maceration. A nonadherent dressing or alginate may also be used under the film to assist with exudate management.

Hydrocolloids are sticky, nonpermeable wafers containing a hydrocolloid material that eventually melts, combines with natural body fluids, and keeps the wound bed moist. The nonpermeable wafer also serves as a barrier and creates a

TABLE 15.2 Commonly Used Types of Dressings

Advantages	Drawbacks	Contraindications
Gauze Allows for mechanical debridement via the continually moist gauze dressing method Protects dry, healing wounds Serves as filler dressing for dead space Absorbs exudate Assists with cleaning up wounds; manages exudates	Requires more frequent dressing changes Requires securing with tape or film Requires loose packing, or it may create pressure and possibly enlarge the wound Destroys fragile epithelial cells and slows down healing, especially if gauze dries out	Do not use on a healthy, granulating wound unless moistened with saline or another noncytotoxic solution; even then, fragile epithelial cells may be destroyed. Do not use on dry, necrotic tissue unless you keep eschar in place for protection (appropriate only when no signs of infection exist).
Foam Dressings Decreases trauma to the wound base and fragile epithelial cells because it does not adhere to tissue or the wound base Protects healing wound Has minimum to moderate absorption ability, which can prevent or decrease maceration Insulates wounds and provides comfort Protects "at-risk" tissue	Requires securing with tape or film Usually requires daily to every-shift dressing changes	Not appropriate for mechanical debridement because it does not adhere. Do not use on a healthy, granulating wound unless a topical agent (e.g., bacitracin) is used. Do not use on dry, necrotic tissue, unless keeping eschar in place for protection (appropriate only when no signs of infection exist).
Transparent Film Dressing Retains moisture and is semipermeable and comfortable Is water resistant, thus allowing it to seal and secure other dressings Allows easy inspection to monitor for complications Fosters autolysis because of moisture retention Minimizes friction injury when applied to vulnerable areas (e.g., elbows, coccyx, heels)	May be difficult to apply May leak Should not be used over enzymatic debriding agents, gels, or ointments	Do not use on infected wounds or wounds with cellulitis. Do not use on thin, friable skin surrounding wound edges that cannot be protected with stoma adhesive (risk of creating other open wounds or skin tear). Do not use on exuding wounds.
Hydrocolloid Dressing Retains moisture, which facilitates granulation and is comfortable Provides a water and bacteria barrier, which protects wound Requires fewer frequent dressing changes, which promotes efficient use of nursing time and comfort for patients Promotes the removal of dry necrotic eschar when left in place for several days	Melt-out occurs, creating a foul odor and possible leakage Prevents visibly monitoring wounds May cause hypergranulation tissue (leafy, friable, beefy-red granulation tissue), which impedes healing and usually requires debridement or removal with a sharp instrument or silver nitrate Is expensive but requires fewer dressing changes	Do not use on infected wounds or wounds with cellulitis. Do not use on thin, friable skin surrounding wound edges (more damage may be created when wafer removed). Do not use on heavy, exuding wounds.
Hydrogel Provides moisture, which facilitates granulation Facilitates some debridement for wounds with thin, stringy yellow eschar Promotes removal of dry necrotic eschar when dressing left in place for several days Nonadherent surface, which provides comfort to patient Requires less frequent dressing changes, which promotes efficient use of nursing time and comfort to patient	Must use another product to keep in place and secure with tape or film May cause hypergranulation tissue (leafy, friable, beefy-red granulation tissue), which impedes healing and usually requires debridement or removal with sharp instrument or silver nitrate Is expensive but requires fewer dressing changes	Do not use on heavy, exuding wounds. Do not use on wounds with cellulitis. Do not use on wounds with purulent discharge.

hypoxic wound environment that stimulates granulation if peripheral circulation provides enough oxygen. Consider the use of hydrocolloid dressings on noninfected, shallow stage III pressure injuries and to protect body areas at risk for friction injuries or at risk of injury from tape (NPIAP, 2021). Hydrocolloid dressings should not be used if candidiasis exists. Hydrocolloid wafers are usually changed every 3–7 days. It should be noted that the foul, sour odor generated by hydrocolloid dressings is considered normal. Infection is present when erythema, warmth, tenderness, or purulent discharge exist. Hydrocolloid dressings should *never* be applied to ulcers that are infected, have purulent discharge, or have a suspected infection. The occlusive, moist environment provides a perfect medium for bacterial growth and may worsen the infection.

Hydrogels consist primarily of water and are effective in maintaining a moist ulcer bed, which fosters healing. Hydrogel dressings may be obtained in a sheet form suitable for superficial wounds or as an amorphous gel that can be applied and spread into deep cavity wounds. Hydrogel dressings should not be used on infected wounds because they retain humidity, thus facilitating autolytic debridement. The cover dressing should be chosen based on the health of the surrounding skin and the degree of wound exudate. Examples of cover dressings include gauze, foam, and transparent films. Dressings using a hydrogel may be left in place for 1 day or up to 5–7 days, depending on the setting, product, and ulcer state (see Table 15.3 and Nursing Care Plan: Pressure Injury).

NURSING CARE PLAN

Pressure Injury

Clinical Situation

Mrs. M. is an 80-year-old female who developed a stage IV pressure injury on her sacral area and right ischium while recently hospitalized for pneumonia. Her decreased appetite and poor food intake, a 10-pound weight loss, and her not being initially placed on an egg-crate mattress led to the development of the pressure injury. Mrs. M. was discharged home with home health care.

The sacral and ischial pressure injuries are clean, beginning to granulate, managed with a hydrogel, covered with a foam dressing to lessen maceration, and sealed with a transparent dressing changed every other day. It is estimated that complete healing will take 6–8 months as long as nutritional status and other preventive strategies are maintained.

Analyze Cues and Prioritize Hypotheses (Patient Problems)

- Reduced skin integrity resulting from altered nutrition, altered circulation, and immobilization

Generate Solutions (Planning)

- The patient will have intact skin, as evidenced by clean, healing wounds, maintenance of circulation to the skin, and laboratory values within normal limits.

Take Actions (Nursing Interventions)

- Implement pressure injury preventive strategies to create an environment that will foster healing and prevent further development of ulcers.
- Place the mattress overlay on the bed and obtain an appropriate pressure-relieving chair cushion to decrease ischial pressure.
- Teach the patient and family to position the patient at a 30-degree angle and support extremities with pillows when lying in bed to lessen trochanter pressure.
- Teach the patient, family, and nurse's aide to avoid the use of hot baths and harsh soaps, to use moisturizers for dry skin, and not to massage over bony prominences.
- Teach the patient not to sit at a 45- to 90-degree angle when in bed or on the couch to minimize shearing forces.
- Assess and treat incontinence by cleansing the skin at the time of soiling; use a topical moisture barrier and (if necessary) absorbent undergarments to maintain a dry surface and decrease the risk of additional skin breakdown.
- Inspect the skin during home visits, observing for any pressure points as seen by erythema or skin breakdown. If a stage I or II injury is present but the site is not infected, apply the film or hydrocolloidal dressing to protect from further breakdown.
- Assess the pressure injury when changing the dressing, noting the wound bed and border color, discharge, and general condition.
- Document each assessment and measure weekly. If the wound bed is infected or has developed cellulitis as seen by erythema, tenderness, pale granulation tissue, or purulent discharge, change the dressing to wet-to-dry with an appropriate antiseptic, but only until the wound is improved and no longer than 5–7 days to minimize damage to viable tissue.
- If the wound is stagnant, as documented by serial dimensions over 3–6 weeks, consider changing to another dressing strategy.
- Monitor nutritional status because it may influence skin integrity and the healing process.
- Monitor weight gains or losses monthly.
- Take a 24-hour diet recall with each visit to assess eating habits and nutritional intake.
- Teach the patient and family the role nutrition plays in healing and general health status.
- If weight loss is experienced, interview the patient to determine the reason (e.g., food preferences are not met, or food is cold or esthetically unappealing).
- Examine the oral cavity and, if appropriate, fit for dentures.
- Maintain a clean, moist wound environment to foster healing.
- If necrotic tissue is present, facilitate debridement by arranging for a physician, nurse practitioner, or certified enterostomal therapist to perform bedside debridement.
- If only a small amount of necrotic tissue is present, attempt chemical or mechanical debridement.
- Select the most comfortable and efficient dressing, such as a hydrogel or hydrocolloidal dressing, with the intent of maintaining a moist wound environment, which fosters granulation and thus healing.
- Use clean technique for dressing care; sterile technique is not necessary because the wound is dirty.
- Gently irrigate the wound with normal saline to clean the wound, make an appropriate assessment, and measure the wound dimensions weekly.
- Teach the patient and family dressing care and changing techniques to involve them in the care and to promote self-care.

TABLE 15.3 General Pressure Injury Care Guidelines

Stage	Actions	Dressing Options
1	Implement preventive strategies (e.g., mattress overlay; nutritional assessment; reinforcement of the value of turning, keeping dry, and minimizing friction)	May protect with film or hydrocolloid
2 and 3	Implement preventive strategies, assess for infection, debride necrotic tissue, conduct nutritional assessment, and provide appropriate nutritional support	May use film, if clean, depending on depth; hydrocolloid; hydrogel; foam, honey-impregnated, collagen matrix, continually moist gauze dressing. If infected, manage topically with appropriate antiseptics and continually moisten gauze dressings until the infection is resolved
4	Same as 2 and 3; a specialized bed may be considered	If clean, use hydrogel, hydrocolloid paste and wafer, collagen matrix, or a continually moist gauze dressing; if infected, manage topically with an antiseptic and a continually moist gauze dressing until infection is resolved (but no longer than 5 days)

Alginates are a category of exudate management dressings. The alginate dressings are manufactured from seaweed and are applied to wounds that are moderately to heavily exudative. In most cases, the alginates are safe to use on infected wounds. These dressings have excellent exudate handling properties and are useful in wounds and around drainage tubes when the wound fluid is causing periwound skin maceration.

In addition, some types of dressings are impregnated with various substances, for example, silver-impregnated dressings, which are used for infected or heavily colonized ulcers and stage II and shallow state III pressure injuries; honey-impregnated dressings, which are impregnated with medical-grade honey and are used for stage II and III pressure injuries; and cadexomer iodine dressings, which are used for highly exudating wounds.

Biophysical Agents in Pressure Injury Management

Research has been conducted on the use of different energy forms in the management of pressure injuries. These include acoustic energy (ultrasound) for debridement and treatment of infected wounds, and UV light therapy as adjunctive therapy to reduce bacterial colonization. Negative-pressure wound therapy may be considered an early adjuvant for deep stage III and IV exudative pressure injuries without necrotic tissue. Lastly, hydrotherapy (pulsed lavage with or without suction) can be used as an adjunct for wound cleaning and to facilitate healing (NPIAP, 2021).

SUMMARY

Pressure injuries are a costly health care problem, in terms of not only dollars but also nursing time and human lives. Prevention is the first line of defense against pressure injury development. Nurses have an opportunity to demonstrate the profession's power and accountability by implementing preventive strategies, thereby having a positive effect on a patient's quality of life while preventing a costly health care problem. It is imperative that the nurse conduct pressure injury risk assessments, use mattress overlays, teach support staff prevention and management techniques, monitor the patient's nutritional status, and serve as a role model by focusing on prevention. With expanded pressure injury knowledge and the publication of the AHRQ and NPIAP clinical guidelines, preventive measures are a nurse's responsibility.

The collaborative relationship that the nurse establishes with the health care provider to utilize the most efficient and effective strategies is vital to successful healing. Collaboration develops trust and professional maturity and is necessary for growth.

Successful pressure injury management requires the application of the principles of healing, which should guide the selection of treatment strategies. Frequent review of the healing trajectory, when reinforced with clinical examples, facilitates comprehension of this complex process. Pressure injury management is both a science and an art that requires experience.

HOME CARE

1. Regularly assess for signs and symptoms of skin breakdown in homebound older adults who are at high risk for the development of a pressure injury.
2. Assess for and instruct caregivers and homebound older adults on factors that predispose patients to the development of a pressure injury.
3. Use the services of a wound care advanced practice nurse in assessing, planning, and recommending appropriate wound care management techniques.
4. Prevention is the first-line strategy for pressure injury care. Teach caregivers of at-risk homebound older adults the techniques for preventing a pressure injury—focusing on preventing moisture, avoiding friction and shearing, changing position frequently, and ensuring excellent nutritional intake.

KEY POINTS

- Because of normal, age-related changes in the skin, older adults are more susceptible to skin tears and bruising caused by thinning of the skin.
- Older adults are at greater risk for hypothermia, shearing, pressure damage, and blunt trauma because of decreased SQ tissue.
- Older adults may experience altered medication absorption because of an age-related decrease in fatty tissue and dermal blood supply.
- Older adults are at increased risk of heatstroke because of the compromised cooling mechanism from decreased sweating.
- The typical pattern of spreading for seborrheic dermatitis starts at the scalp margins, progresses downward to the eyebrows, the base of the eyelashes, and around the nose in a butterfly pattern, and continues to the ears and sternum.
- Psoriasis is a common disorder affecting the epidermis and the dermis. It is recognized by the presence of erythematous, scaly, and itchy patches on various parts of the body. Many triggers exacerbate the condition.
- Pruritus warrants a full skin assessment because it may be indicative of many diseases, drug reactions, and possibly cancer. The nurse should determine the location, intensity, alleviating and aggravating events, onset, and what the patient is doing to control it.
- Candidiasis, recognized by fire-red, denuded skin with satellite macules or pustules, develops in moist intertriginous areas.
- Herpes zoster is characterized by prodromal symptoms of itching or burning along a dermatome, followed by a unilateral, bandlike maculopapular rash and vesicles, which rarely cross the midline.
- The nurse should notify the health care provider if the following suspected lesions are found on assessment: actinic keratosis; BCC, SCC, or melanoma.

- Arterial ulcers are usually located on toes or feet and are associated with pain during activity, nighttime, and rest. The cause of decreased arterial blood flow must be corrected for these ulcers to heal.
- Venous hypertension leads to the formation of a capillary fibrin cuff, which causes chronic edema, decreased circulation, and recurring medial lower leg ulcers.
- Diabetic foot lesions are usually located on the plantar foot and result from a loss of protective sensation in the foot, which leads to an abnormal gait and increased pressure on the foot. Bony deformities may develop and further change foot pressure, increasing the likelihood of trauma and subsequent ulceration.
- Pressure injuries are a costly health care problem in terms of not only dollars but also nursing time and human lives. Prevention is the first-line strategy for pressure injury care.
- The nurse should assess the nutritional status of patients with pressure injuries with a determination of monthly weight and laboratory variables.
- To minimize friction, the nurse should use sheets to lift and pull the patient up in bed and apply a film dressing or lotion to vulnerable areas such as the elbows, coccyx, and heels.
- To minimize shearing forces, the nurse should not elevate the head of the bed more than 30–45 degrees.
- Antiseptic solutions should be used only when the wound is infected; they should never be used on a clean, healthy wound because they are cytotoxic and destructive to tissue.
- Surface cultures have been shown to grow different organisms than those in underlying tissues and blood cultures; thus, routine wound cultures are not appropriate.

CLINICAL JUDGMENT EXERCISES

1. Outline major teaching points that would be beneficial to maintaining the integumentary health of older individuals.
2. A 78-year-old Hispanic male has a history of SCC. After having a lesion removed from his upper back 3 years ago, he has been extremely anxious about other skin lesions and skin changes. What approach would you take to help your patient reduce his anxiety and yet remain active in the prevention and early recognition of skin cancer?
3. Your 79-year-old female patient suffered a stroke 6 months ago and is cared for at her sister's home. The patient is dependent on position changes, is unable to communicate the need to be turned, must be fed, and has a stage II pressure injury on her sacral area. Develop a teaching plan for the family to ensure that the patient's needs are met.

REFERENCES

Agency for Healthcare Research and Quality (AHRQ). (2019). *AHRQ National Scorecard on Hospital-Acquired Conditions: Updated baseline rates and preliminary results 2014–2017*. Retrieved from https://www.ahrq.gov/sites/default/files/wysiwyg/professionals/quality-patient-safety/pfp/hacreport-2019.pdf. Accessed July 28, 2023.

American Academy of Dermatology Association (AAD). (2023a). *Dermatologists' top tips for relieving dry skin*. Retrieved from https://www.aad.org/public/everyday-care/skin-care-basics/dry/dermatologists-tips-relieve-dry-skin. Accessed July 28, 2023.

American Academy of Dermatology Association (AAD). (2023b). *What to look for—ABCDEs of melanoma*. Retrieved from https://www.aad.org/public/diseases/skin-cancer/find/at-risk/abcdes. Accessed July 28, 2023.

American Cancer Society. (2022). *Cancer facts & figures 2022*. Atlanta, GA: American Cancer Society.

Armstrong, A. W., Mehta, M. D., Schupp, C. W., Gondo, G. C., Bell, S. J, & Griffiths, C. E. M. (2021). Psoriasis prevalence in adults in the United States. *JAMA Dermatology*, 157(8), 940–946. doi:10.1001/jamadermatol.2021.2007.

Bader, R. S., & Granick, M. S. (2022). *Basal cell carcinoma*. Medscape [website]. Retrieved from https://emedicine.medscape.com/article/276624-overview#a6. Accessed July 28, 2023.

Baraz, S., Zarea, K., Shahbazian, H. B., & Latifi, S. M. (2014). Comparison of the accuracy of monofilament testing at various points of feet in peripheral diabetic neuropathy screening. *Journal of Diabetes and Metabolic Disorders*, 13(1), 19. doi:10.1186/2251-6581-13-19.

Berlowitz, D., Lukas, C. V., Parker, V., Niederhauser, A., Silver, J., & Logan, C. (2014). *Preventing pressure ulcers in hospitals*. Agency for Healthcare Research and Quality, U.S. Department of Health and Human Services. Retrieved from https://www.ahrq.gov/sites/default/files/publications/files/putoolkit.pdf. Accessed July 28, 2023.

Beroukhim, K., Pourang, A., & Eisen, D. B. (2020). Risk of second primary cutaneous and noncutaneous melanoma after cutaneous melanoma diagnosis: A population-based study. *Journal of the American Academy of Dermatology*, 82(3), 683–689. doi:10.1016/j.jaad.2019.10.024.

Bholah, N. G., Oakley, A., & Gomez, J. (2022). *Seborrhoeic dermatitis*. DermNet [website]. Retrieved from https://dermnetnz.org/topics/seborrhoeic-dermatitis. Accessed July 28, 2023.

Blume-Peytavi, U., Kottner, J., Sterry, W., Hodin, M. W., Griffiths, T. W., Watson, R. E. B., et al. (2016). Age-associated skin conditions and diseases: Current perspectives and future options. *The Gerontologist*, 56(Suppl. 2), S230–S242. doi:10.1093/geront/gnw003.

Braden, B. J., & Bergstrom, N. (1989). Clinical utility of the Braden scale for predicting pressure sore risk. *Decubitus*, 2(3), 44–46, 50–51.

Brazen, B. C., Gray, T., Farsi, M., & Miller, R. (2020). Acral lentiginous melanoma: A rare variant with unique diagnostic challenges. *Cureus*, 12(6), e8424. doi:10.7759/cureus.8424.

Brizzi, K. T., & Lyons, J. L. (2014). Peripheral nervous system manifestations of infectious diseases. *The Neurohospitalist*, 4(4), 230–240. doi:10.1177/1941874414535215.

Burden-Teh, E., Thomas, K. S., Ratib, S., Grindlay, D., Adaji, E., & Murphy, R. (2016). The epidemiology of childhood psoriasis: A scoping review. *The British Journal of Dermatology*, 174(6), 1242–1257. doi:10.1111/bjd.14507.

Caesar, J., & Coulson, I. (2020). *Venous insufficiency.* DermNet [website]. Retrieved from https://dermnetnz.org/topics/venous-insufficiency. Accessed July 28, 2023.

Centers for Disease Control and Prevention (CDC). (2023). *About shingles (herpes zoster).* Retrieved from https://www.cdc.gov/shingles/about/index.html. Accessed July 28, 2023.

Clark, G. W., Pope, S. M., & Jaboori, K. A. (2015). Diagnosis and treatment of seborrheic dermatitis. *American Family Physician, 91*(3), 185–190.

Coleman, S., Nixon, J., Keen, J., Wilson, L., McGinnis, E., Dealey, C., et al. (2014). A new pressure ulcer conceptual framework. *Journal of Advanced Nursing, 70*(10), 2222–2234. doi:10.1111/jan.12405.

Coleman, S., Gorecki, C., Nelson, E. A., Closs, S. J., Defloor, T., Halfens, R., et al. (2013). Patient risk factors for pressure ulcer development: Systematic review. *International Journal of Nursing Studies, 50*(7), 974–1003. doi:10.1016/j.ijnurstu.2012.11.019.

Cox, J. (2017). Pressure injury risk factors in adult critical care patients: A review of the literature. *Ostomy/Wound Management, 63*(11), 30–43. doi:10.25270/owm.201.

Dharmarajan, T. S., & Ahmed, S. (2003). The growing problem of pressure ulcers. Evaluation and management for an aging population. *Postgraduate Medicine, 113*(5), 77–90. doi:10.3810/pgm.2003.05.1409.

Dinulos, J. G. H. (2021). *Habif's clinical dermatology: A color guide to diagnosis and therapy* (7th ed.). Philadelphia: Elsevier.

Dissemond, J., Assenheimer, B., Bültemann, A., Gerber, V., Gretener, S., Kohler-von Siebenthal, E., et al. (2016). Compression therapy in patients with venous leg ulcers. *Journal of the German Society of Dermatology, 14*(11), 1072–1087. doi:10.1111/ddg.13091.

Dyer, J. M., & Miller, R. A. (2018). Chronic skin fragility of aging: Current concepts in the pathogenesis, recognition, and management of dermatoporosis. *The Journal of Clinical and Aesthetic Dermatology, 11*(1), 13–18.

Elgash, M., Dlova, N., Ogunleye, T., & Taylor, S. C. (2019). Seborrheic dermatitis in skin of color: Clinical considerations. *Journal of Drugs in Dermatology, 18*(1), 24–27.

European Pressure Ulcer Advisory Panel, & National Pressure Injury Advisory Panel and Pan Pacific Pressure Injury Alliance (EPUAP/NPIAP/PPPIA). (2019). *Prevention and treatment of pressure ulcers/injuries: Quick reference guide.* Haesler, E. (Ed.). EPUAP/NPIAP/PPPIA.

Flowers, R. H., & Elston, D. M. (2020). *Cutaneous candidiasis.* Medscape [website]. Retrieved from https://emedicine.medscape.com/article/1090632-print. Accessed July 28, 2023.

Gaddey, H. L., & Holder, K. K. (2021). Unintentional weight loss in older adults. *American Family Physician, 104*(1), 34–40.

Gillespie, B. M., Chaboyer, W. P., McInnes, E., Kent, B., Whitty, J. A., & Thalib, L. (2014). Repositioning to prevent pressure ulcers. *Cochrane database of systematic reviews, 2014*(4), CD009958. doi:10.1002/14651858.CD009958.pub2.

Jaul, E., Barron, J., Rosenzweig, J. P., & Menczel, J. (2018). An overview of co-morbidities and the development of pressure ulcers among older adults. *BMC Geriatrics, 18*(1), 305. doi:10.1186/s12877-018-0997-7.

Keller, U. (2019). Nutritional laboratory markers in malnutrition. *Journal of Clinical Medicine, 8*(6), 775. doi:10.3390/jcm8060775.

Khan, T., & Khardori, R. (2020). *Diabetic foot ulcers.* Medscape [website]. Retrieved from https://emedicine.medscape.com/article/460282-print. Accessed July 28, 2023.

Kirman, C. N., & Geibel, J. (2022). *Pressure injuries (pressure ulcers) and wound care.* Medscape [website]. Retrieved from https://emedicine.medscape.com/article/190115-print. Accessed July 28, 2023.

Kolluri, R., Lugli, M., Villalba, L., Varcoe, R., Maleti, O., Gallardo, F., et al. (2022). An estimate of the economic burden of venous leg ulcers associated with deep venous disease. *Vascular Medicine, 27*(1), 63–72. doi:10.1177/1358863X211028298.

Kosiak, M. (1958). Etiology and pathology of ischemic ulcers. *Archives of Physical Medicine and Rehabilitation, 40*(2), 62–69.

Kramer, A., Dissemond, J., Kim, S., Willy, C., Mayer, D., Papke, R., et al. (2018). Consensus on wound antisepsis: Update 2018. *Skin Pharmacology and Physiology, 31*(1), 28–58. doi:10.1159/000481545.

Krasner, D. (1991). Resolving the dressing dilemma: selecting wound dressings by category. *Ostomy/Wound Management, 35*, 62, 64–70.

Labropoulos, N. (2019). How does chronic venous disease progress from the first symptoms to the advanced stages? A review. *Advances in Therapy, 36*(Suppl. 1), 13–19. doi:10.1007/s12325-019-0885-3.

Lawton, S. (2019). Skin 1: The structure and functions of the skin. *Nursing Times* [online], *115*(12), 30–33. Retrieved from https://www.nursingtimes.net/clinical-archive/dermatology/skin-1-the-structure-and-functions-of-the-skin-25-11-2019/. Accessed July 28, 2023.

Levine, J. M. (1992). Historical notes on pressure ulcers: The cure of Ambrose Paré. *Decubitus, 5*(2), 23–26.

Meade, R. D., Notley, S. R., Rutherford, M. M., Boulay, P., & Kenny, G. P. (2020). Ageing attenuates the effect of extracellular hyperosmolality on whole-body heat exchange during exercise-heat stress. *The Journal of Physiology, 598*(22), 5133–5148. doi:10.1113/JP280132.

Mercy, K., Kwasny, M., Cordoro, K. M., Menter, A., Tom, W. L., Korman, N., et al. (2013). Clinical manifestations of pediatric psoriasis: Results of a multicenter study in the United States. *Pediatric Dermatology, 30*(4), 424–428. doi:10.1111/pde.12072.

National Council on Aging. (2021). *Hydration for older adults. How to stay hydrated for better health.* Retrieved from https://www.ncoa.org/article/how-to-stay-hydrated-for-better-health. Accessed July 28, 2023.

National Pressure Injury Advisory Panel (NPIAP). (2021). *2021 Fact Sheet: About Pressure Injuries in US Healthcare.* Retrieved from https://cdn.ymaws.com/npiap.com/resource/resmgr/public_policy_files/npiap_word_fact_sheet_08mar2.pdf. Accessed July 28, 2023.

Norton, D. (1989). Calculating the risk: Reflections on the Norton scale. *Decubitus, 2*(3), 24–31.

Oakley, A. (2015a). *Actinic keratosis.* DermNet [website]. Retrieved from https://dermnetnz.org/topics/actinic-keratosis. Accessed July 28, 2023.

Oakley, A. (2015b). *Basal cell carcinoma.* DermNet [website]. Retrieved from https://dermnetnz.org/topics/basal-cell-carcinoma. Accessed July 28, 2023.

Oakley, A. (2015c). *Cutaneous squamous cell carcinoma.* DermNet [website]. Retrieved from https://dermnetnz.org/topics/cutaneous-squamous-cell-carcinoma. Accessed July 28, 2023.

Oakley, A., Dennis, J., & Luther, M. E. (2018). *Intertrigo.* DermNet [website]. Retrieved from https://dermnetnz.org/topics/intertrigo. Accessed July 28, 2023.

Oakley, A., & de Menezes, S. (2016). *Pruritus.* DermNet [website]. Retrieved from https://dermnetnz.org/topics/pruritus. Accessed July 28, 2023.

Oomens, C. W. J, Loerakker, S., & Bader, D. L. (2010). The importance of internal strain as opposed to interface pressure in the prevention of pressure related deep tissue injury. *Journal of Tissue Viability, 19*(2), 35–42. doi:10.1016/j.jtv.2009.11.002.

Padula, W. V., & Delarmente, B. A. (2019). The national cost of hospital-acquired pressure injuries in the United States. *International Wound Journal, 16*(3), 634–640. doi:10.1111/iwj.13071.

Ramji, R., & Oakley, A. (2017). *Cutaneous squamous cell carcinoma in skin of colour*. DermNet [website]. Retrieved from https://dermnetnz.org/topics/cutaneous-squamous-cell-carcinoma-in-skin-of-colour. Accessed July 28, 2023.

Rodrigues, M., Kosaric, N., Bonham, C. A., & Gurtner, G. C. (2019). Wound healing: A cellular perspective. *Physiological Reviews, 99*(1), 665–706. doi:10.1152/physrev.00067.2017.

Scherer, R., Maroto-Sánchez, B., Palacios, G., & González-Gross, M. (2016). Fluid intake and recommendations in older adults: More data are needed. *Nutrition Bulletin, 41*(2), 167–174. doi:10.1111/nbu.12206.

Seebacher, N. A. (2022). *Melanoma*. DermNet [website]. Retrieved from https://dermnetnz.org/topics/melanoma. Accessed July 28, 2023.

Serpa, L. F., Conceição de Gouveia Santos, V. L., Gomboski, G., & Rosado, S. M. (2009). Predictive validity of Waterlow Scale for pressure ulcer development risk in hospitalized patients. *Journal of Wound, Ostomy, and Continence Nursing, 36*(6), 640–646. doi:10.1097/WON.0b013e3181bd86c9.

Siegel, R. L., Miller, K. D., Fuchs, H. E., & Jemal, A. (2022). Cancer statistics, 2022. *CA: A Cancer Journal for Clinicians, 72*(1), 7–33. doi:10.3322/caac.21708.

Spear, M. (2014). *When and how to culture a chronic wound*. Wound Care Advisor [website]. Retrieved from https://woundcareadvisor.com/when-and-how-to-culture-a-chronic-wound-vol3-no1/. Accessed July 28, 2023.

Ständer, S., Zeidler, C., Magnolo, N., Raap, U., Mettang, T., Kremer, A. E., et al. (2015). Clinical management of pruritus. *Journal of the German Society of Dermatology, 13*(2), 101–116. doi:10.1111/ddg.12522.

Stone, A. (2020). Preventing pressure injuries in nursing home residents using a low-profile alternating pressure overlay: A point-of-care trial. *Advances in Skin & Wound Care, 33*(10), 533–539. doi:10.1097/01.ASW.0000695756.80461.64.

Volmer-Thole, M., & Lobmann, R. (2016). Neuropathy and diabetic foot syndrome. *International Journal of Molecular Sciences, 17*(6), 917. doi:10.3390/ijms17060917.

Wells, J. W., & Meyers, A. D. (2021). *Cutaneous squamous cell carcinoma*. Medscape [website]. Retrieved from https://emedicine.medscape.com/article/1965430-overview#a5. Accessed July 28, 2023.

16

Sensory Function

Mary B. Winton, PhD, MSN, RN

http://evolve.elsevier.com/Yeager/gerontologic/

LEARNING OBJECTIVES

On completion of this chapter, the reader will be able to:
1. Describe age-related changes in the senses.
2. Distinguish between cataracts and glaucoma, including the associated nursing interventions.
3. Distinguish between retinal disorders, including the medical and nursing management of each disorder.
4. Identify nursing interventions for older adults with low vision.
5. Describe the proper method for instilling eye medications.
6. Describe common changes in the ear that affect hearing.
7. Identify nursing interventions for hearing impairment.
8. Identify nursing interventions for older patients with xerostomia.
9. Describe safety issues for older adults with diminished vision, hearing, and touch senses.
10. Conduct a sensory system assessment and describe the normal findings.

WHAT WOULD YOU DO?

What would you do if you were faced with the following situations?
- You are caring for a 75-year-old widow who lives independently. You start noticing she is having increased difficulty in reading, she is stumbling into things, and she has told you about a recent fall. What do you do?
- The spouse of your patient states that her husband of 50 years has become withdrawn and complains that everyone mumbles when talking and can't be understood. She complains that she can't stand to be in the room when the television is on because it is so loud. What do you do?
- When assessing a 90-year-old male, you notice he is underweight. He states that family and friends are concerned about his eating habits. He does not enjoy eating because nothing seems to taste the same as he remembers, and his mouth is dry most of the time. What do you do?

The senses connect the human body to the environment. They allow individuals to be aware of and interpret various stimuli, thus enabling interaction with the environment. Sensory changes may dramatically affect the quality of life (QoL) of older adults. Visual and hearing impairments may interfere with communication, social interactions, and mobility, leading to social isolation. Olfactory, gustatory, and tactile deprivations may lead to nutritional problems and safety hazards. Understanding the sensory changes associated with aging is important to help older adults adapt and function independently. An emphasis on maintaining healthy senses is part of Healthy People 2030 (Office of Disease Prevention and Health Promotion, n.d.). This is especially important because impaired senses can be linked to increased mortality (Ehrlich et al, 2021).

The five primary sensory categories include sight, hearing, taste, smell, and touch. Two additional sensory categories that are recognized are general and special. General senses include touch, pressure, pain, temperature, vibration, and proprioception (position sense). These have relatively simple receptors, which are located all over the body. These senses are further classified as somatic (providing sensory information about the body and the environment) or visceral (supplying information about the internal organs). Special senses are produced by highly localized organs and specialized sensory cells. These include the senses of sight, hearing, taste, smell, and balance.

Sensation is a conscious or unconscious awareness of external and internal stimuli, and perception is the interpretation of conscious sensations. The brain receives stimuli from both inside and outside the body. Conscious sensation occurs via action potentials generated by receptors that reach the cerebral cortex.

VISION

Vision is integral to a person's ability to function in the environment. Visual acuity (the ability to see clearly) is an important part of performing activities of daily living (ADLs); dressing, grooming, cooking, sewing, driving, and reading are all tasks that involve the use of eyesight (Fig. 16.1). Poor vision can also

---

Previous authors: Beth Culross, PhD, RN, GCNS-BC, CRRN, FNGNA; Cindy R. Morgan, RN, MSN, CHC, CHPN; and Ramesh C. Upadhyaya, RN, CRRN, MSN, MBA, PhD-C.

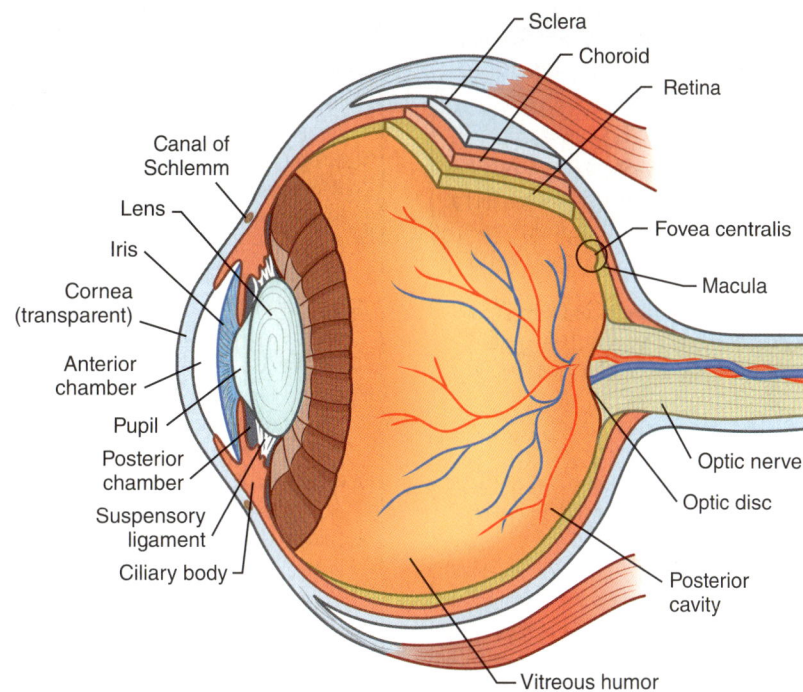

Fig. 16.1 Anatomy of the eye. (From Lewis, S. M., Bucher, L., Heitkemper, M. M., & Harding, M. M. [Eds.]. [2017]. *Medical-surgical nursing: Assessment and management of clinical problems* [10th ed.]. St. Louis, MO: Elsevier. Modified from Patton K. T., & Thibodeau G. A. [2013]. *Anatomy and physiology* [8th ed.]. St. Louis, MO: Mosby.)

increase social isolation among older adults and possibly is linked to dementia (National Institute on Aging [NIA], 2023a). Almost 100,000 cases of dementia could have been avoided by treating vision impairments.

Age-Related Changes in Structure and Function

Normal age-related changes in the external and internal eye have been well documented. The eyelids lose tone and become lax, which may result in ptosis of the eyelids, redundancy of the skin of the eyelids, and malposition of the eyelids. Eyebrows may turn gray and become coarser in males, with outer thinning in all older adults. The conjunctiva thins and yellows in appearance. Additionally, this membrane may become dry because of diminished quantity and quality of tear production. The sclera may develop brown spots. The outer region of the cornea develops a noticeable surrounding ring made up of fat deposits called the *arcus senilis*. The pupil decreases in size and loses some of its ability to constrict. Changes resulting from aging that decrease the size of the pupil and limit the amount of light entering the eye also occur in the iris. The lens increases in density and rigidity, affecting the eye's ability to transmit and focus light. Peripheral vision decreases, night vision diminishes, and sensitivity to glare increases (Boltz et al, 2016; Garrity, 2022). There may be a gradual reduction in the ability to see colors in aging and color deficits due to multiple disease processes, including diabetes, glaucoma, macular degeneration (MD), Alzheimer disease, and Parkinson disease (American Optometric Association, n.d.).

Ophthalmoscopic examination of the retina may reveal the following changes: Blood vessels have narrowed and straightened; arteries seem opaque and gray; and *drusen*, localized areas of hyaline degeneration, may be noted as gray or yellow spots near the macula (Porter, 2023). Two common complaints of older adults, floaters and dry eyes, are discussed in the following section.

Common Complaints
Floaters and Flashers

Floaters appear as dots, wiggly lines, or clouds that a person may see moving in the field of vision. They become more pronounced when a person is looking at a plain background. Floaters occur more often after age 50, as tiny gel or cellular debris clumps float in the vitreous humor in front of the retina. They are caused by degeneration of the vitreous gel and are more common in older adults who have undergone cataract operations or yttrium–aluminum–garnet laser surgery.

In general, floaters are normal and harmless. However, they may be a warning sign of a more serious condition, especially if they increase in number and if changes in the type of floater, light flashes, or visual hallucinations are noted. These symptoms may indicate a vitreous or retinal tear, which could lead to detachment. Additionally, visual hallucinations have been associated with a brain tumor or cortical ischemia. Therefore, any of these symptoms warrants a complete eye examination by an ophthalmologist.

Flashers occur when the vitreous fluid inside the eye rubs or pulls on the retina, producing the illusion of flashing lights or lightning streaks. Flashers that appear as jagged lines, last 10 to 20 minutes, and are present in both eyes are likely caused by a spasm of blood vessels in the brain called a *migraine*. These

EVIDENCE-BASED PRACTICE
Effects of Sensory Impairments in Older Adults

Sample/Setting
The sample for this study consisted of 3005 older adults living in the community. Females represented 1551 and males 1454 of the sample. The age range was 57 to 84. Respondents were from Wave 1 of the study with some additional respondents who refused Wave 1.

Methods
Interviewers from the National Opinion Research Center conducted in-home interviews to collect the following data: demographic, social, psychological, and biological measures. Sensory function was detailed and is discussed in this article.

Findings
Findings included alterations in all sensory function as follows:
- *Vision:* Difficulties were found in driving during the day (14%), driving at night (40%), and an overall 16% stated vision as poor or fair.
- *Hearing:* Poor or fair corrected hearing was reported by 22%; 20% stated they experienced frustration when having conversations with family and 18% stated frustrations when visiting with others. Only 12% reported limitations on personal or social life although 42% had difficulty hearing whispered words. Hearing loss was found to be a significant burden.
- *Touch:* Results indicated a general difference in perception of touch and how appealing it is for the older adult. The indication is that changes in this perception can affect relationships between partners and activities such as exercise.
- *Olfaction:* This was one area that had potential alterations due to 8% of respondents having a cold at the time of the interview. The decline in olfaction may reflect the inability to detect malodor and potentially provide insights into other aspects of health.

Implications
Vision and hearing impairments are highly prevalent in older adults and are related to important functional changes that include personal interactions. The effect is on relationships with family and friends and critical activities that the older adult may participate in such as driving.

Other affected areas include access to health care, personal safety, alterations in communication, and decreased social function and QoL. This can lead to social isolation, depression, and anxiety.

Data from Pinto, J. M., Kern, D. W., Wroblewski, K. E., Chen, R. C., Schumm, L. P., & McClintock, M. K. (2014). Sensory function: Insights from wave 2 of the national social life, health, and aging project. *Journals of Gerontology, Series B: Psychological Sciences and Social Sciences, 69*(8), S144–S153.

BOX 16.1 Aging and Your Eyes: Health Promotion and Illness Prevention

1. Have an eye examination with eyes dilated annually. This will help to detect common eye diseases before the onset of signs or symptoms.
2. Be sure to use adequate lighting for the task you are completing.
3. Wear sunglasses to protect your eyes from ultraviolet (UV) radiation. Wearing a wide-brimmed hat will help as well.
4. Choose eye-healthy foods including fruits, vegetables, and whole grains. Vitamins C and E, zinc, and zeaxanthin have been shown to help eye health.
5. Quit smoking and avoid second-hand smoke to reduce the risk for eye diseases such as cataract and age-related macular degeneration. Smoking also worsens dry eye.
6. Be active and keep a healthy weight. Thirty minutes of daily exercise can help reduce the risk of eye disease that have been linked to other health issues (diabetes, hypertension, and hyperlipidemia).
7. For chronic disease maintenance, maintain normal blood pressure, blood glucose, and cholesterol levels will help reduce the risk for eye disease.
8. Prevent eyestrain by blinking and looking away from computer screens or other electronic devices every 20 minutes. Looking approximately 20 feet away for 20 seconds will help.
9. Know the symptoms of low vision. These include finding lights are not bright enough, can't see well enough for everyday tasks, having difficulty recognizing faces known to you, and having trouble reading street signs.

Data from National Institute on Aging, & National Institutes of Health. (2021). *Aging and your eyes.* Retrieved from https://www.nia.nih.gov/health/vision-and-vision-loss/aging-and-your-eyes; and Rauch, D. (2020). *Perfect vision? 20 tips to keep it that way.* American Academy of Ophthalmology. Retrieved from https://www.aao.org/eye-health/tips-prevention/seven-sight-saving-habits.

---

flashers commonly occur with advancing age. However, they warrant prompt medical attention if they increase in number, if many new flashers appear, or if partial loss of side vision is noted (Boyd, 2023a).

The nurse should refer a patient who experiences any of these symptoms to an ophthalmologist for a comprehensive eye examination. If no cause is found for floaters and flashers, the nurse should teach the patient about the condition and how to live with it. Patients should be taught to look up and down to get the floaters out of the field of vision. Additionally, the nurse should provide the patient with the printed information instruction sheet (Box 16.1).

Dry Eyes

Dry eyes result as the quantity and quality of tear production diminish with aging. Stinging, burning, or a scratchy sensation are common complaints of individuals with dry eyes. Episodes of excess tearing may occur following a period of discomfort, dryness, pain, redness, and possibly discharge in the eyes. Blurred vision and a heavy feel to eyelids may also be experienced (National Eye Institute [NEI], 2023a).

Treatment consists of tear replacement or conservation. Tears may be replaced by an over-the-counter artificial tear preparation to lubricate the eye and replace missing moisture. This type of preparation may be used as often as necessary, especially before activities that require significant eye movement. Solid inserts that gradually release lubricants throughout the day are also available. An ophthalmologist can help conserve the naturally produced tears by temporarily or permanently closing the lacrimal drainage system. Other conservation methods include using a humidifier when the heat is on, wraparound glasses to reduce evaporation of eye moisture caused by wind, and avoiding smoke (NEI, 2023a).

Common Problems and Conditions

Common problems resulting from the aging eye include presbyopia, ectropion and entropion, blepharitis, glaucoma, cataracts, retinal disorders, eye injuries, and visual impairment. Presbyopia is a normal change that occurs with aging. The other problems are eye diseases, which are more prominent in older adults.

Presbyopia

The most common complaint of adults older than 40 is a diminished ability to focus clearly on close objects (arm's length) such as a newspaper. In presbyopia, the lens loses its ability to focus on close objects. Accommodation is impaired as the lens thickens and loses its elasticity. The ciliary muscles weaken the lens's ability to contract. Treatment involves wearing reading glasses or bifocals (two-part lenses that correct near and distant vision); the prognosis for corrected vision is excellent.

Nursing care aims to encourage the patient to adjust to the glasses by wearing them and following up with a visit to the ophthalmologist every 2 years. Information for patient education on vision and aging is available through the National Institute on Aging (see Box 16.1).

Blepharitis

Blepharitis is a chronic inflammation of the eyelid margins commonly found in older adults. It may be caused by seborrheic dermatitis or infection. The use of antihistamines, anticholinergics, antidepressants, and diuretics may exacerbate this condition because of the drying effects of these medications. In addition, the deficiency in tear production with aging may lead to infection. The symptoms include red, swollen eyelids, matting and crusting along the base of the eyelash at the margins, small ulcerations along the lid margins, and complaints of irritation, itching, burning, tearing, and photophobia (NEI, 2023b). Treatment is aimed at removing the causative bacteria and healing the affected areas. Physicians may prescribe topical antibiotics or steroids. However, the nurse can play a significant role in treating this condition by teaching patients certain interventions described later.

The patient must be taught scrupulous eye hygiene, including good hand-washing habits (NEI, 2023b). Mild soap without fragrance or antibacterial ingredients should be used. Contact lens wearers must be taught proper cleaning and storage techniques to prevent eye contamination, as well as lens, lens solution, and lens case contamination. Because cosmetics are a common source of bacterial contamination, eye makeup products should be replaced every 3 to 6 months to avoid bacterial growth. Patients also need to know how to apply makeup with cotton balls and cotton-tipped applicators and understand the importance of discarding the applicators after each use. Mascara should be water resistant, free of lash-extending fibers, and not applied to the base of the lashes. Eyeliner should be a medium-hard pencil and not be applied to the inner margin of the eyelid. Patients should avoid the use of aerosol hairsprays because these may irritate the eyes. Inflammation caused by blepharitis will be resolved, and the patient's comfort level will improve after a week of these hygiene measures.

Glaucoma

Glaucoma is the second leading cause of blindness in the United States and the first cause of blindness among African Americans (especially those over the age of 40). Although glaucoma may occur at any age, those most at risk are adults older than age 60, especially Hispanics (NEI, 2023c; Lewis et al, 2017). Glaucoma is a group of diseases that can result in vision loss and lead to blindness due to damage to the optic nerve. The most common form, open-angle, has few, if any, symptoms and may cause partial vision loss before it is detected. This major public health problem affects approximately 3 million Americans and is associated with more than 2.7 million people affected with the most common form of glaucoma, open-angle glaucoma (Glaucoma Research Foundation [GRF], 2022; National Glaucoma Research [NGR], 2022).

Glaucoma results from a blockage in the drainage of the fluid (the aqueous humor) in the eye's anterior chamber. Normally, this fluid drains through the Schlemm canal and is transported to the venous circulation system. If the fluid forms in the eye faster than it can be eliminated, intraocular pressure (IOP) increases. Pressure is then transferred to the optic nerve, where irreparable damage, possibly even total blindness, may result. In older adults, three types of glaucoma are chronic open-angle glaucoma, acute angle-closure glaucoma, and secondary glaucoma.

Chronic open-angle glaucoma. Chronic open-angle glaucoma is the most common form (making up 90% of all primary glaucoma) and develops slowly. Degenerative changes in the Schlemm canal obstruct the escape of aqueous humor, resulting in increased IOP. This type of glaucoma slowly damages the optic nerve until vision loss occurs. Most people do not have early warning signs (GRF, 2022). Visual loss begins with deteriorating peripheral vision, intolerance to glare, loss of contrast perception, and difficulty adapting to the dark (Boltz et al, 2016; GRF, 2022).

Acute angle-closure glaucoma. Acute angle-closure glaucoma (or acute narrow-angle glaucoma) occurs suddenly because of complete blockage of the drainage canals, causing the IOP to rise quickly (GRF, 2022). This is a medical emergency and requires immediate medical attention to avoid severe vision loss or permanent blindness. The symptoms of acute angle-closure glaucoma include the following:

- Severe eye pain
- Redness in the eye
- Clouded or blurred vision
- Nausea and vomiting
- Rainbow halos surrounding lights

Secondary glaucoma. Secondary glaucoma occurs due to complications from other medical conditions or certain drug therapies (GRF, 2022). Examples include uncontrolled diabetes or hypertension, cataracts, some types of eye tumors, uveitis, or other irritation or inflammation. Steroid drugs may trigger glaucoma. Serious eye injuries or surgical procedures may also lead to the onset of glaucoma.

Nursing care guidelines for glaucoma

Recognize cues (assessment). Patients with glaucoma may complain of dull eye pain, or they may experience no early symptoms. Visual field testing reveals a loss of peripheral vision (tunnel vision), and increased IOP is seen on ophthalmologic examination. Patients may also report increased difficulty seeing in low light or darker rooms and increased sensitivity to glare.

Analyze cues and prioritize hypotheses (patient problems). Potential patient problems for glaucoma include the following:

- Need for patient teaching resulting from lack of exposure and inexperience regarding glaucoma causes and treatments

- Pain resulting from increased IOP
- Potential for infection resulting from eye-drop instillation
- Decreased ability to dress self, resulting from visual impairment

Generate solutions (planning). Expected outcomes for the patient with glaucoma include the following:
1. No further loss of vision
2. Follow prescribed glaucoma care guidelines daily
3. Eye pain is decreased
4. Free from eye infection
5. Perform ADLs safely and independently

Take actions (nursing interventions). Nursing management aims to teach the patient that glaucoma is a chronic condition requiring lifelong medical treatment. Any visual loss is permanent, but following the care guidelines outlined in Box 16.2 may prevent further loss. If medication fails to control rising IOP, surgical intervention may be necessary.

Selective laser trabeculoplasty is usually performed on an outpatient basis, frequently in the doctor's office (NEI, 2023c). Follow-up visits after the procedure are required to measure the IOP. A 4- to 6-week wait is necessary to determine whether the procedure was effective. However, continued use of glaucoma medications is often necessary. Laser treatments are temporary, and some patients may need additional treatments.

Trabeculectomy is done in an outpatient surgical center. The additional opening is created in the top of the eye to allow extra fluid from the eye to drain, thereby decreasing IOP (NEI, 2022). Postoperative nursing care for a patient who has had a trabeculectomy includes:
- Proper hygiene to prevent infections
- Protecting the eye by wearing a shield to prevent rubbing the eye and wearing sunglasses to protect from the sun and irritants, like dust

- Instructing the importance of following instructions on proper instillation of eye drops
- Teaching the importance of avoiding activities that increase IOP, such as bending over, lifting heavy objects, or straining for 2 to 4 weeks

Evaluate outcomes (evaluation). Evaluation includes documentation of the achievement of the expected outcomes, no further vision loss, and the independent performance of ADLs. It is imperative that the patient and family understand the chronic nature of this disease and its treatment. The patient must be able to state the name and dosage of the prescribed eye medications and describe their daily use, even during travel or hospitalization. The patient must also be able to identify significant signs and symptoms so that they can be reported to the ophthalmologist.

Cataracts

Cataracts are the most common disorder found in aging adults. Although cataracts are considered an "age-related" condition, they can occur in individuals in their 40s and 50s but typically do not significantly affect vision (Boyd, 2023b). More than half of Americans over 80 have cataracts or have had a surgical procedure for cataracts (NEI, 2023d). Cataracts can occur in one or both eyes. In addition to aging, other risk factors for cataracts include smoking, prolonged exposure to ultraviolet light, and diabetes. Medications, such as steroids, also increase the risk for cataracts.

Changes in the lens lead to cataracts. Over time, protein meant to keep the lens clear and allow light to pass through starts to clump together behind the lens (NEI, 2023d). This creates a cloud in a small area of the lens, which is called a cataract. As the cataract grows, vision becomes more difficult, including reduced sharpness of images reaching the retina. The lens itself becomes discolored over time with a yellow/brown tint.

There are different types of cataracts, not specifically age-related. A secondary cataract may be related to other health problems, such as diabetes or after surgical eye procedures. Some medications, such as steroids, are also linked to this. A traumatic cataract may develop after an eye injury, maybe years later. A radiation cataract may develop after radiation exposure (NEI, 2023d).

The size and location of a cataract determine the amount of interference with clear sight. A cataract located near the center of the lens produces more noticeable symptoms, such as the following:
- Dimmed, blurred, or misty vision
- The need for brighter light to read
- Glare and light sensitivity
- Halo that appears around lights
- Double vision or multiple images in one eye
- Loss of color perception
- Recurrent eyeglass prescription changes

These symptoms develop slowly and at different rates in each eye (NEI, 2023d).

Nursing care guidelines for cataracts

Recognize cues (assessment). Obtain a history of predisposing factors and subjective complaints, such as trouble reading or needing more light to read, recent eye trauma, vision

---

BOX 16.2 The Patient With Glaucoma

1. Medical follow-up and eye medication will be required for the rest of your life.
2. Eye drops *must* be continued as long as prescribed, even in the absence of symptoms.
    a. Blurred vision decreases with prolonged use.
    b. Avoid driving for 1 to 2 hours after administration of miotics.
3. To prevent complications:
    a. Press lacrimal duct for 1 minute after eye-drop insertion to prevent rapid systemic absorption.
    b. Have a reserve bottle of eye drops at home.
    c. Carry eye drops on person (not in luggage) when traveling.
    d. Carry card or wear MedicAlert bracelet identifying glaucoma and the eye-drops solution prescribed.
4. Bright lights and darkness are not harmful.
5. No apparent relationship exists between vascular hypertension and ocular hypertension.
6. Report any reappearance of symptoms immediately to the ophthalmologist.
7. If admitted to the hospital for a different medical condition, alert staff of continued need to use prescribed eye drops.
8. Avoid the use of mydriatic or cycloplegic drugs (e.g., atropine) that dilate the pupils.

Data from National Eye Institute. (2021). *How to put in eye drops*. Retrieved from https://www.nei.nih.gov/Glaucoma/glaucoma-medicines/how-put-eye-drops.

changes despite wearing corrective lenses, and decreased color perceptions (Rebar et al, 2021). Ask the patient about the use of medications, such as corticosteroids or beta blockers. Lens opacity may be visible on external or internal eye examination.

Analyze cues and prioritize hypotheses (patient problems). Patient problems for cataracts include the following:
- Decreased visual sensory perception
- Anxiety
- Eye discomfort
- Possible injury
- Altered activities of daily living

Generate solutions (planning). The priority problem of decreased visual sensory perception is a safety risk. Patients often live with cataracts for many years before cataract surgery (Rebar et al, 2021). The goals for patients with cataracts are to maximize vision and minimize injury while maintaining ADLs:
1. Remain free from injury due to decreased vision.
2. Recognize when surgery is indicated due to cataracts.
3. Remain free from infection.
4. Demonstrate safe administration of eye drops.
5. Verbalize when to contact the surgeon for symptoms of IOP.
6. Verbalize activities to avoid to prevent increasing IOP.
7. Verbalize appropriate home-care activities to avoid and activities to do after cataract surgery.

Take actions (nursing interventions). Nursing management for a patient with cataracts focuses mainly on pre- and postoperative surgical care because surgery is the only method for treating cataracts (Boyd, 2023b). However, asymptomatic patients do not require referral. Most cataract surgery is performed in an outpatient surgery with the administration of a local anesthetic; this makes preoperative teaching difficult because patients arrive just hours before surgery. Many ambulatory centers conduct preoperative assessment and teaching via phone calls 1 week before surgery. Preoperative care involves administering eye drops and a sedative, as ordered. Postoperative care requires teaching the patient and family home-care procedures after cataract surgery (see Patient/Family Teaching box: Home Care after Cataract Surgery). Following the proper method for instilling eye drops (Box 16.3) is essential. The home care instructions need to include special precautions recommended by the ophthalmologist based on the type of surgery performed. Patients must wear contact lenses or cataract glasses if a lens implant has not been inserted. Patients wearing cataract glasses experience loss of depth perception and distorted peripheral and color vision. They need to be taught that objects are magnified by 25% and appear larger and closer than they really are; this requires home safety measures and the modification of dressing and cosmetic application after surgery (see Nursing Care Plan).

Evaluate outcomes (evaluation). Evaluation includes documentation of the achievement of the expected outcomes. Patients who have had successful cataract surgery will be free from complications and have improved vision. Additionally, they will report the performance of their usual ADLs using lens implants, contact lenses, or corrective glasses. The patient and family will arrange for assistance with ADLs for the first 24 to 48 hours after surgery, or they will notify the home-health agency.

BOX 16.3 Administering Eye Drops

The following steps should be followed to properly administer eye drops:
- Wash hands
- Hold the bottle upside down
- Tilt head back
- Hold the bottle in one hand and place as close as possible to the eye without touching the eye
- Use the other hand to pull down the lower eyelid to form a pocket
- Place the prescribed number of drops into the lower eyelid pocket
- Wait at least 5 minutes in between if administering more than one type of eye drop
- To keep the drops in the eye, close the eye or press the lower lid lightly with one finger for at least 1 minute; this also prevents the drops from draining into the tear duct and increasing the risk of side effects

Data from National Eye Institute. (2021). *How to put in eye drops.* Retrieved from https://www.nei.nih.gov/Glaucoma/glaucoma-medicines/how-put-eye-drops.

PATIENT/FAMILY TEACHING
Home Care After Cataract Surgery

What to Expect
- Protective eye shield will be placed over the eye for protection, which should be worn for several nights to prevent accidental rubbing or scratching
- Vision will be blurry until the brain adapts to the new artificial lens
- Affected eye may be bruised or bloodshot for few days
- Mild discomfort or scratchy feeling in the affected eye for several days
- Eyelid may be slightly swollen

Activity Level and Care
- Avoid driving until vision is clear
- Avoid activities that increase IOP (i.e., biking, running, bending at waist, blowing nose, lifting heavy objects, and sex) for 1 week
- Avoid swimming for 2 weeks to prevent infection
- Light housekeeping is permitted but avoid vacuuming for several weeks
- Shower the next day, but avoid water getting into the affected eye for up to 7 days
- Cool compress to the affected eye to decrease swelling and reduce discomfort may be beneficial
- Avoid alcohol for at least 24 hours
- Do not rub or press on the eye
- Sleep on back or nonoperative side for 2 nights
- Wear the bandage or eye pad as instructed
- Perform regular hand hygiene before attending to any bandage or eye pad
- Instill eye drops using a sterile technique (see Box 16.3)
- May use lubricant drops immediately after surgery
- If instilling multiple eye medications, wait 5 minutes between each medication
- Monitor pain and report if unrelieved with medication
- Recognize signs and symptoms of infection and when to report
- Adhere to eyedrop regimen after surgery
- Follow up with provider as recommended

Data from Mukamal, R. (2022). *Cataract surgery recovery: Exercising, driving, and other activities.* American Academy of Ophthalmology [website]. Retrieved from https://www.aao.org/eye-health/tips-prevention/safe-exercise-driving-cataract-surgery-recovery; and Rebar, C. R., Borchers, S. A., & Borchers, A. A. (2021). Assessment and concepts of care for patients with eye and vision problems. In D. Ignatavicius, M. L. Workman, C. R. Rebar, & N. M. Heimgartner (Eds.). *Medical-surgical nursing: Concepts for interprofessional collaborative care.* (10th ed.). St. Louis: Elsevier.

NURSING CARE PLAN

Cataracts

Clinical Situation

Mrs. D, a 78-year-old retired nurse accompanied by her daughter, was referred to the ophthalmologist for bilateral cataracts. She was recently admitted to the skilled nursing unit of a local hospital for rehabilitation therapy after repair of a right hip fracture after a fall. Mrs. D has no other significant medical history. The patient states she fell down the stairs because of impaired vision that is "getting worse." Since her admission to the hospital, a vision screening detected cataracts in both eyes, and surgery is recommended once she recovers from the hip surgery. Mrs. D requires assistance with all ADLs except eating. She is unable to bear weight on her right leg, so assistance is needed to transfer to the toilet, chair, or bed. She also needs help bathing and dressing the lower half of her body because she cannot reach her legs or feet. Mrs. D states that her biggest concern is fear of falling again.

Analyze Cues and Prioritize Hypotheses (Patient Problems)

- Potential for falls
- Poor vision
- Anxiety related to decreased vision
- Decreased functional ADLs
- Inadequate knowledge about cataracts
- Potential for infection

Generate Solutions (Planning)

- The patient will verbalize questions and concerns regarding cataracts and the recommended surgical treatment.
- The patient will have cataract surgery, when appropriate.
- The patient will not fall.
- The patient will maintain a safe environment.
- The patient will assist with self-care as much as possible, as evidenced by fulfilling needs for cleanliness, grooming, and toileting.
- The patient will report reduced anxiety, as evidenced by a relaxed state and learning about cataract surgery.

Take Actions (Nursing Interventions)

- Provide the patient with the printed information sheet, "Aging and Your Eyes: Promotion and Illness Prevention" (see Box 16.1).
- Encourage the patient and family member to speak with an ophthalmologist about the recommended surgery.
- Explain preoperative and postoperative procedures resulting from the recommended surgery.
- Provide a safe environment (e.g., bed in low position, side rails as needed, and call light and personal items in reach).
- Teach patient about healthy diet and weight.
- Educate about safe instillation of eye drops to prevent infection.
- Assist with transfers until the patient demonstrates safe transfer while unassisted.
- Assess the patient's home for factors that hinder or support vision changes.
- Encourage the patient to perform as much of her own care as possible to help restore independence.
- Provide assistance, supervision, and teaching with the use of assistive devices, as needed, to perform self-care. Assess factors in the patient's home that support or hinder self-care.
- Encourage expression of fears of falling.
- Use therapeutic communication to gain insight into the patient's fears and give realistic feedback.
- Increase attention to the patient when she is feeling anxious.

Evaluate Outcomes (Evaluation)

- The patient will verbalize questions and concerns regarding cataracts and the recommended surgical treatment.
- The patient will have cataract surgery, when appropriate.
- The patient will not fall.
- The patient will maintain a safe environment.
- The patient will assist with self-care as much as possible, as evidenced by fulfilling needs for cleanliness, grooming, and toileting.
- The patient will report reduced anxiety, as evidenced by a relaxed state and learning about cataract surgery.
- The patient will demonstrate safe instillation of eye drops.

Data from Nizami, A. A., Gulani, A. C., & Redmond, S. B. (2022). *Cataract (Nursing)*. StatPearls [Internet]. Treasure Island, FL: StatPearls Publishing. Available at: https://ncbi.nlm.nih.gov/books/NBK568765/.

Retinal Disorders

Three common disorders affecting an older adult's retina are MD, diabetic retinopathy (DR), and retinal detachment.

Age-related macular degeneration. Age-related MD (AMD) is the leading cause of blindness among people over the age of 50 in the United States. It does not cause total blindness but results in loss of central vision. AMD causes damage to the macula, leading to changes in the center of the field of vision. Peripheral vision is unchanged by AMD. The cells within the macula diminish in functional ability with age, and replacement of the damaged cells is decreased, causing irreversible damage to the macula (NEI, 2021). As a result, central visual acuity declines, which makes the performance of ADLs requiring close vision nearly impossible.

Types of AMD include the following:

- **Dry MD.** Also known as *atrophic* AMD, this condition is caused by the breakdown or thinning of macular tissue resulting from the aging process. Vision loss is gradual.
- **Wet MD.** Also known as *neovascular* AMD, this type of AMD results when abnormal blood vessels form and hemorrhage on the retina. Vision loss may be rapid and severe.

AMD is more common among Whites than other races (Boyd, 2023c). There is also an increased risk in those with a family history. Although there are no recommended genetic tests for AMD, nearly 20 genes have been identified that may affect the risk for developing this eye disorder. Smoking has been shown to double the risk for developing AMD. Lifestyle choices can help reduce the risk of developing AMD, such as avoiding smoking, exercising regularly, eating a healthy diet rich in green leafy vegetables and fish, and maintaining BP and cholesterol within a normal range.

Symptoms of MD include the following:

- Difficulty performing tasks that require close central vision, such as reading and sewing
- Decreased color vision (i.e., colors look dim)
- Dark or empty area in the center of vision

- Straight lines appearing wavy or crooked
- Words on a page looking blurred

Diabetic retinopathy. Loss of visual function is one of the most common complications of diabetes (NEI, 2023e). Altered circulation to the eye may result in retinal edema, degeneration, or detachment. This condition is a complication of diabetes that affects the retinal capillary circulation. Ballooning of these tiny vessels leads to hemorrhaging, scarring, and blindness. These vascular changes in and around the retina lead to macular edema, which causes the retina to swell. No symptoms of early retinal changes exist, and no symptoms may be apparent even when the retinopathy is advanced. Early detection requires a complete ophthalmoscopic examination; therefore, patients with diabetes should have yearly examinations by an ophthalmologist.

Hypertension retinopathy. Another form of retinopathy can be caused by untreated chronic hypertension. In this form of retinopathy, chronic hypertension will cause progressive damage to the retina with few or even no symptoms until the late advancement of symptoms. Abnormalities found include permanent arterial narrowing, arteriosclerosis, and vascular wall hyperplasia. The primary treatment is controlling BP with angiotensin-converting enzyme inhibitors, calcium channel blockers, and/or diuretics. Laser procedures or intravitreal injections of corticosteroids or monoclonal antibodies may also be used for vision loss (Mehta, 2022).

Retinal detachment. Retinal detachment occurs when the retina's sensory layer separates from the pigmented layer (NEI, 2023f). Tears or holes occur in the retina because of trauma, aging (degeneration), hemorrhaging, or the presence of a tumor. When a tear occurs, fluid seeps between the layers, which causes detachment. The usual symptoms include the following:

- Light flashes
- A shower of floaters that resembles spots, bugs, or spider webs
- Loss of vision
- Veil or curtain obstructing vision

Nursing care guidelines for retinal disorders

Recognize cues (assessment). There are no early symptoms of DR or hypertensive retinopathy; sometimes, no symptoms are observed even with advanced retinopathy. Patients with MD may complain that they cannot thread a needle or that the words on a page look blurred, making reading difficult. Patients with retinal detachment notice flashes of light followed by floating spots before the eye with progressive vision loss. The specific area of vision loss depends on where the detachment is located. When detachment occurs quickly and is extensive, the patient may feel that a curtain has been drawn before the eyes.

Ongoing nursing assessment involves monitoring the patient's subjective statements about changes in vision and observing for signs of anxiety. All three retinal disorders are diagnosed with ophthalmoscopy.

Analyze cues and prioritize hypotheses (patient problems). Patient problems are determined by analysis of the patient assessment. Possible patient problems for a patient with a retinal disorder include the following:

- Need for patient teaching resulting from lack of exposure to accurate information about the effect of diabetes on the eyes
- Need for patient teaching resulting from retinal detachment condition, surgery, preoperative and postoperative care, and home care after surgery
- Anxiety resulting from fear of blindness

Generate solutions (planning). Expected outcomes for an older person with a retinal disorder include the following:

1. The patient will adjust successfully to vision loss by using low-vision aids.
2. The patient will state in his or her own words the effect of diabetes on the eyes.
3. The patient will see an ophthalmologist yearly.
4. The patient will ask questions about preoperative and postoperative retinal surgery care and report satisfaction with the information.
5. The patient's affected eye will be free from further retinal detachment, infection, or hemorrhaging.
6. The patient will verbalize appropriate home-care activities to participate in after retinal surgery.
7. The patient will demonstrate correct administration of eye drops.
8. The patient will report reduced anxiety.

Take actions (nursing interventions). Patients with MD and DR must learn to cope with chronic, gradual vision loss. Patients with MD are often taught to self-monitor their central vision using an Amsler Grid, which is a small printed grid. The appearance of an increase in waves or curves on the grid may indicate worsening disease. Patients must be taught how to obtain and use low-vision aids (Box 16.4). Teaching about the condition and encouraging yearly follow-up visits with an ophthalmologist help patients understand the disease and how it affects their eyes.

Patients with retinal detachment require the immediate care of bed rest in the proper position (i.e., retinal hole in most dependent position) and eye patches (may be prescribed for one or both eyes) until surgery is performed. Safety precautions and means of communicating are essential for the patient at this point. Postoperative care includes administration of eye

---

BOX 16.4 Low-Vision Aids

- Magnifying devices: glasses, stand or hand magnifier, telescope, video magnifier. Some have built-in lighting
- Audio books or electronic books
- Apps for smartphones, computers, and tablets (e.g., AMagnify, DAISY Talk, TapTapSee, Seeing AI)
- Devices with speech capability: watches, timers, blood glucose monitors, blood pressure cuffs, prescription bottles
- Large-print reading material and items with large-sized numbers/letters and high-contrast colors
- Increased light: higher-watt light bulbs and number of lights indoors, adjust light to reduce glare inside and wear sunglasses or wide-brimmed hat outdoors, use color to create contrast in the house, use a bold felt tip marker to makes lists or notes
- Request a referral early to access the many low-vision aids and devices to help with daily activities; many people will need vision rehabilitation to achieve the best possible QoL. Examples: Light House for the Blind and Visually Impaired (http://lighthouse-sf.org/programs/skills/) or Lions Club International (https://www.lionsclubs.org/en/start-our-global-causes/vision).

medication, pain medication, antiemetics (as needed), and cough medication (as needed). Cold compresses are applied to reduce swelling and promote comfort. Patients must be instructed to avoid jerking movements of the head, as with coughing, sneezing, and vomiting. If the eyes are patched, safety precautions such as keeping call lights, side rails, and necessary items within reach must be instituted. Finally, assistance must be provided with ADLs and walking, as needed, to promote comfort and safety. Home-care instructions to teach the patient and family include the following: (1) report increases in floaters or flashes of light, decreased vision, drainage, or increased pain to an ophthalmologist; (2) administer eye drops; (3) limit physical activity for 1 to 2 weeks, and resume active sports and heavy lifting as indicated by a physician; and (4) make follow-up appointments with the ophthalmologist.

Patients with any retinal disorder may experience anxiety about the loss of vision and possible blindness. Patients must be given the opportunity to discuss their concerns, and nurses must also be knowledgeable about available resources.

Evaluate outcomes (evaluation). Evaluation includes documentation of the achievement of the expected outcomes. Patients with MD and DR will describe the condition and report the use of low-vision aids. These patients will also follow up with annual visits to the ophthalmologist. Patients who have had surgery for retinal detachment will experience no complications and gradual improvement in vision. Patients will limit their physical activity for 1 to 2 weeks with the help of significant others or home healthcare. Patients with MD will monitor their central vision with an Amsler Grid and report changes to the ophthalmologist. Patients with any retinal disorder will report reduced anxiety, as evidenced by their ability to learn about and cope with their disease.

Visual Impairment

Visual impairment is the most common sensory problem faced by older adults. The visually impaired population includes those with low vision (20/50 to 20/200) and those who are legally blind (visual acuity of 20/200 or worse in the better eye with the aid of the best possible correction with the use of spectacles or contact lens) (Lewis et al, 2017). Blindness in older adults results from DR, glaucoma, cataracts, and MD, and its incidence has increased as the number of adults age 65 or older grows.

Sudden vision loss is considered a medical emergency and should be evaluated immediately. It may be caused by retinal detachment or an eye injury. A trained provider must evaluate this as soon as possible. The medical management of vision loss depends on the type, cause, and amount experienced. In the case of a traumatic eye injury, treatment depends on the type of injury (see Emergency Treatment box).

Any patient with a visual disability that cannot be improved by corrective lenses or surgery should be referred to a low-vision specialist or center. Assistive devices for low vision, including talking glucose monitoring instruments, large-print books, talking clocks, talking scales, and computer accessories, are available and continue to be developed for many health issues (Kaur and Gurnani, 2023).

✚ EMERGENCY TREATMENT
Eye Injuries

Determine Etiology
- Trauma: blunt or penetrating
- Burn: chemical (acid or alkaline), thermal (direct or indirect burn)
- Foreign body penetration (glass, metal, wood, plastic, ceramic)

Common Assessment Findings
- Pain
- Photophobia
- Localized or diffuse redness
- Swelling, ecchymosis, tearing
- Absent eye movement
- Fluid drainage
- Visible foreign body
- Visual loss, decreased vision, or visual field defect

Interventions
Initial:
- Determine cause of injury (etiology)
- Ensure airway, breathing, circulation
- Assess for the following: other injuries considering type of exposure, visual acuity, pain, changes around and in the eye
- Do not put pressure on the eye; instruct patient to not blow the nose
- In case of chemical exposure, irrigate the eye immediately and continue until emergency personnel arrive; if no chemical exposure, do not attempt to treat
- Stabilize foreign objects, but do not attempt to remove
- Cover eye with dry, sterile patch and protective shield
- Elevate the head of the patient to 45 degrees
- Do not provide food or drink to patient
- Administer medications/analgesia only as ordered by a provider

Ongoing monitoring:
- Provide reassurance to the patient
- Monitor pain, changes in visual acuity, changes in or around the eye
- Prepare patient for potential surgical repair when appropriate

Modified from Lewis, S. M., Bucher, L., Heitkemper, M. M., & Harding, M. M. et al. (2017). *Medical-surgical nursing: Assessment and management of clinical problems* (10th ed.). St. Louis, MO: Elsevier.

Nursing care guidelines for vision impairment

Recognize cues (assessment). Nursing assessment of the patient with impaired vision requires an understanding of the patient's response to the vision loss. The older adult who becomes suddenly blind usually has a harder time adjusting to the disability than a person who was born blind. Loss of vision may result in a self-esteem disturbance, leading to social isolation. A self-esteem disturbance leads to decreased self-confidence, which may affect interactions with others, the ability to carry out normal daily activities, job performance, and the desire to engage in familiar hobbies. Grief and mourning occur over the loss of vision and result in reactions like those experienced with death, for example, denial, anger, guilt, hopelessness, and depression. The patient's ability to cope with the loss depends on the type, amount, and duration of the vision loss and the patient's support system and coping style. Over time, people with vision loss can compensate by increasing sensitivity in other senses, such as hearing, taste, touch, and balance.

Analyze cues and prioritize hypotheses (patient problems). Potential patient problems for patients with visual impairment include the following:

- Decreased self-esteem resulting from sudden loss of vision
- Social disengagement resulting from impaired communication
- Inadequate coping resulting from sudden loss of vision
- Decreased ability to feed/bathe/dress/toilet self, resulting from visual impairment
- Decreased mobility resulting from visual impairment
- Potential for injury resulting from impaired vision

Generate solutions (planning). Expected outcomes for a patient with visual impairment include the following:

1. The patient will perceive himself or herself positively by making positive statements about self.
2. The patient will participate successfully in activities with others.
3. The patient will demonstrate increased objectivity and ability to solve problems, make decisions, and communicate needs.
4. The patient will safely provide self-care using low-vision aids and environmental strategies.
5. The patient will demonstrate the safe and correct use of adaptive devices.

Take actions (nursing interventions). Counseling allows persons who have become visually impaired to talk about their feelings, concerns, and anxieties. Once these emotions have been identified, patients may be given assistance in identifying their strengths and resources. Problem-solving may lead to alternative ways to complete the tasks of everyday living and participate in recreational activities.

The nurse interacting with a visually impaired patient must rely heavily on various techniques and methods when communicating with that person. See Boxes 16.5 and 16.6 for tips and aids that facilitate communicating and caring for the visually impaired. Remember that these tips can be used in home care, acute care, or long-term care.

Strategies to increase adaptation to daily living include (1) organizing the environment, (2) encouraging the use of the clock method of eating, and (3) using a sighted guide to assist in ambulation (Box 16.7). Organizing the environment means placing clothing items in specific drawers or closets to facilitate selection and placing furniture in specific locations to facilitate mobility. Additionally, using color contrast and color-coding

---

BOX 16.6 Communicating With and Caring for Visually Impaired Nursing Facility Residents

- Always identify yourself clearly.
- Always make it clear when you are leaving the room.
- Make sure you have the resident's attention before you start to talk.
- Try to minimize the number of distractions.
- Whenever possible, choose bright clothes with bold contrasts.
- Check to see that the best possible lighting is available.
- Assess your position in relation to the resident. One of the resident's eye or ear may be better than the other.
- Try not to move items in the resident's room. Narrate your actions.
- Try to keep the resident between you and the window or you will appear as a dark shadow.
- Use some means to identify residents who are known to be visually impaired.
- Use the analogy of clock hands to help the resident locate objects.
- Keep color and texture in mind when buying clothes.
- *Be careful about labeling residents as confused! They may be making mistakes because of poor vision.*
- Obtain and encourage the use of low-vision aids.

Modified from McNeely, E., Griffin-Shirley, M., & Hubbard, A. (1992). Teaching caregivers to recognize diminished vision among nursing home residents. *Geriatric Nursing, 13*(6), 332–335; and Adams-Wendling, L., Pimple, C., Adams, S., & Titler, M. G. (2008). Nursing management of hearing impairment in nursing facility residents. *Journal of Gerontological Nursing, 34*(11), 9–17.

BOX 16.5 Signs and Behaviors That May Indicate Vision Problems

Patient May Report[a]
- Pain in eyes
- Difficulty seeing in darkened area
- Double or distorted vision
- Sudden loss of vision or blurred vision
- Flashes of light
- Halos surrounding lights

Others May Notice the Patient:
- Getting lost
- Bumping into objects
- Straining to read or not reading
- Spilling food on clothing
- Withdrawing socially
- Making less eye contact
- Displaying placid facial expressions
- Viewing the television at close range
- Suffering from a decreased sense of balance
- Mismatching clothes

[a]These issues should be addressed right away.
Modified from McNeely, E., Griffin-Shirley, M., & Hubbard, A. (1992). Teaching caregivers to recognize diminished vision among nursing home residents. *Geriatric Nursing, 13*(6), 332–335.

BOX 16.7 The Sighted Guide

1. Ask the older adult for permission to provide assistance.
2. If assistance is accepted, offer your elbow or arm. The older adult should grasp your arm just above the elbow. If necessary, physically assist the older adult by guiding his or her hand to your arm or elbow.
3. You will then go a half-step ahead and slightly to the side of the older adult. The older adult's shoulder should be directly behind your shoulder (*Note:* If the older adult is frail, locate the hand on your forearm. When this modified grasp is used, the older adult will be positioned laterally to your body.)
4. You and the older adult should be relaxed and walk at a comfortable pace. When approaching doorways or a narrow space, tell the older adult. The older adult should then go directly behind you. Some modifications may be needed for frail older adults; be sure the modifications are safe and comfortable.
5. Describe the surroundings to the older adult as you walk to augment mobility and enrich the experience.

Modified from McNeely, E., Griffin-Shirley, M., & Hubbard, A. (1992). Teaching caregivers to recognize diminished vision among nursing home residents. *Geriatric Nursing, 13*(6), 332–335.

schemes helps the patient locate items; bright, sharply contrasting colors make furniture and personal items visually distinct. For example, a bright-red toothbrush shows up well against a white sink. Coding schemes that facilitate independent living include applying fluorescent tape around light switches, thermostats, and keyholes. Coding with colored paper, textured paper such as sandpaper, or rubber bands may help the patient differentiate among medication containers. The clock method assists the patient at meals because the location of food on the plate is described in terms of a clock face (e.g., beans at the top of the plate are at the 12 o'clock position; potatoes at the bottom of the plate are at the 6 o'clock position). In addition, the patient may use a piece of bread or roll to push food onto the fork. Sighted guides, who lead persons with visual impairments from place to place, can help patients walk confidently (see Box 16.7). Using a cane or a seeing-eye dog also promotes independence in mobility, especially when the patient is in an unfamiliar environment.

The home-health or community health nurse can assist with referral to a social worker who has information on local, state, and federal services available. Services for persons with visual impairments include counseling, mobility training, vocational rehabilitation, self-care skills training, special education, and financial assistance. Low-vision aids such as "talking books," tapes, and tape players are available from public libraries, the National Federation of the Blind, the American Foundation for the Blind, the National Association for Visually Handicapped, the National Braille Association, and the U.S. Library of Congress. Legal blindness entitles a person to some federal assistance based on need. Blind persons can claim an additional tax deduction on their federal income tax returns. The American Council of the Blind (ACB) also has resources for the blind and visually impaired, such as a directory of banks with talking ATMs, a voting access guide for blind voters, and music resources (ACB, n.d.).

Evaluate outcomes (evaluation). Evaluation includes documentation of the achievement of the expected outcomes, demonstrated by the patient actively participating in self-care and social activities. Patients who display signs and symptoms of depression or social isolation require further counseling to talk about their feelings, strengths, and resources. Additionally, alternative visual aids and strategies will need to be identified to increase communication and promote self-care.

HEARING AND BALANCE

The organs of hearing and balance can be divided into three parts: the external ear, the middle ear, and the inner ear. The external and middle ears are involved only in hearing; the inner ear is involved in both hearing and balance. The external ear consists of the auricle and the external auditory canal, a passageway from the outside to the eardrum. The middle ear is an air-filled space that contains the tympanic membrane, the eardrum, and the auditory ossicles. The inner ear contains the sensory organs for hearing and balance. It comprises interconnecting, fluid-filled tunnels and chambers in the petrous portion of the temporal bone (Fig. 16.2).

The organs of balance are located within the inner ear and are divided into two parts. The *vestibule* contains the membranous labyrinth, which consists of the utricle and saccule. This portion evaluates the position of the head relative to gravity or linear acceleration and deceleration. The second part is in the semicircular canals called the *kinetic labyrinth*. This labyrinth evaluates the movements of the head.

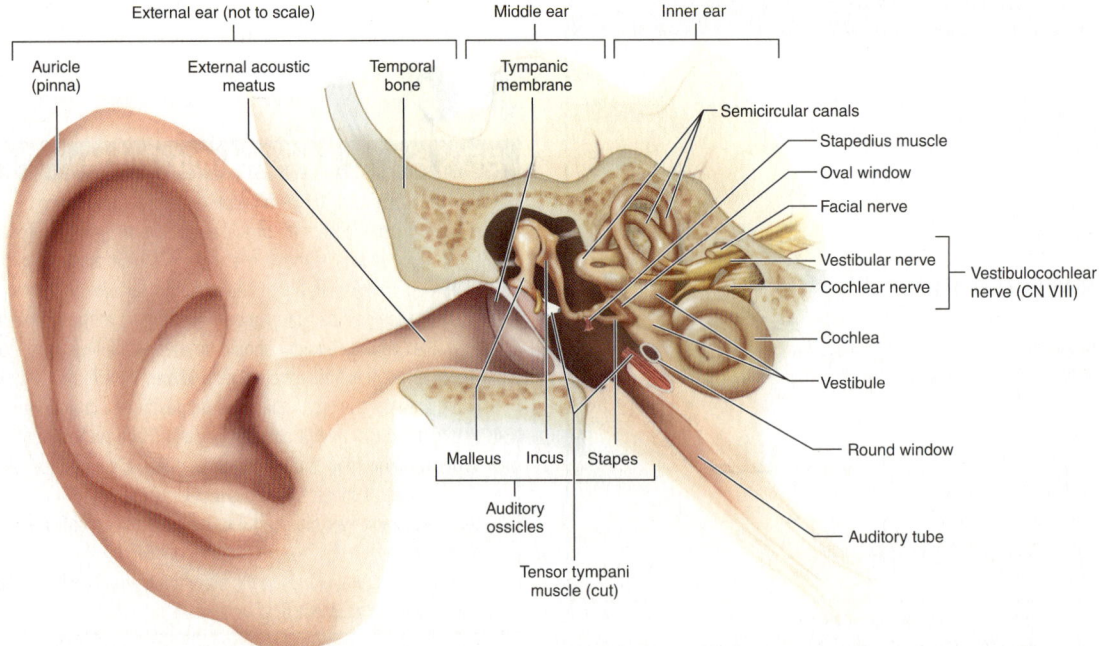

Fig. 16.2 Anatomy of the ear. (From Patton K. T., & Thibodeau G. A. [2013]. *Anatomy and physiology* [8th ed.]. St. Louis, MO: Mosby.)

Age-Related Changes in Structure and Function

Age-related changes in the external ear may be seen in the auricle, which appears larger because of continued cartilage formation and loss of skin elasticity. The lobule of the auricle becomes elongated, with a wrinkled appearance. The periphery of the auricle becomes covered with coarse, wirelike hairs. Compared with females, males have larger tragi, which are laterally situated in the external canal. These tragi become larger and coarser with age. The auditory canal narrows because of inward collapsing. The hairs lining the canal become coarser and stiffer. Additionally, cerumen glands atrophy, causing the cerumen to be much drier. In the middle ear, age-related changes in the tympanic membrane cause a dull, retracted, and gray appearance. Degeneration and calcification of ossicular joints in the middle ear have also been noted. Finally, changes within the inner ear result in decreased vestibular sensitivity.

Age-related balance decline is caused by decreased sensory input, slowing of motor responses, and musculoskeletal limitations. Numerous studies comparing healthy younger and older adults have reported increased postural sway in older adults. Despite this increase, most healthy older adults have enough sensory function reserve to maintain postural control. However, deprivation in multiple systems is likely to lower the balance threshold. Additionally, maintaining balance becomes more difficult under conditions in which balance is maximally stressed, for example, climbing up or down steps or curbs and getting in and out of a bathtub.

Common Problems and Conditions

Pruritus

Pruritus, itching within the external auditory canal, results from age-related atrophic changes in the skin. Atrophy of the epithelium and epidermal sebaceous glands results in dryness. Often, chronic pruritus of the ear canal results from an itch–scratch–itch cycle initiated by dry skin. The problem may be exacerbated by efforts to retard and remove dry earwax buildup. Several drops of glycerin or mineral oil instilled in the ear canal daily will add moisture to the external ear. Instilling steroid-containing medications in the external canal may treat more resistant conditions.

Cerumen Impaction

Cerumen impaction is a reversible, often overlooked, cause of conductive hearing loss. With increasing age, atrophic changes in the sebaceous and apocrine glands lead to drier cerumen. These changes in the cerumen, coupled with a narrowed auditory canal and stiffer, coarser hairs lining the canal, lead to cerumen impaction. The cerumen blockage may interfere with sound vibrations through the external auditory canal to the middle and inner ear, affecting a person's ability to hear and communicate. This impaired communication may then lead to social isolation and depression.

Common symptoms of cerumen impaction include hearing loss, a feeling of fullness in the ear, itching, and tinnitus (ringing in the ears). Identification and removal of the impaction may restore hearing acuity and relieve symptoms associated with impaction. Older adults produce less cerumen and have a drier consistency, creating more risk of impaction in the ear canal (Schwartz et al., 2017).

Nursing care guidelines for cerumen impaction

Recognize cues (assessment). Patients with cerumen buildup may complain of ear fullness, itching, and difficulty hearing. An otoscopic examination will show whether the cerumen obstructs the external ear canal and whether the tympanic membrane is visible.

Analyze cues and prioritize hypotheses (patient problems). Potential problems for a patient with the aforementioned assessment findings includes social disengagement resulting from difficulty communicating with family and friends.

Generate solutions (planning). Expected outcomes for a patient with cerumen impaction include the following:
1. The patient will be free from cerumen impaction.
2. The patient will follow proper instillation of softening agents.
3. The patient will report satisfactory involvement with family and friends.

Take actions (nursing interventions). The nurse must assess patients for signs of hearing impairment that may indicate cerumen impaction, including (1) difficulty understanding the spoken word (patients may ask why others are mumbling or deliberately excluding them from conversation), (2) loud radio and television volume, (3) withdrawal from social activities and accompanying depression, and (4) possible confusion and paranoia. Once an otoscopic examination reveals an impaction, the nurse should follow the protocol for cerumen removal. For patients living in the community, both patients and their families should be taught how to instill the softening agent. Additionally, patients should be instructed to notify their healthcare provider if they experience decreased hearing, any pain, or a ringing or crackling in their ear.

Management of cerumen impaction (modified from Schwartz et al, 2017):

- Before removing cerumen, verify any history of the ruptured tympanic membrane, tympanostomy tubes, or recent ear surgery. These may be contraindications for cerumen removal and must be verified with a provider.
- Impaction may be resolved by instilling fluid into the ear canal. This can be an over-the-counter cerumenolytic agent (carbamide peroxide is the only approved treatment). Other options are two to three drops of baby oil or mineral oil, liquid docusate sodium, or hydrogen peroxide. Avoid hydrogen peroxide if the patient has pruritus or dry skin. The liquid should be instilled daily for 3 to 5 days to resolve the impaction. To instill, have the patient tilt the head to the side not being treated and hold the auricle as straight as possible. Follow the directions on the packaging for the length of time the solution should stay in the ear. The ear may be irrigated to remove the loosened cerumen.
- Water or normal saline warmed to body temperature may be used with an ear syringe to irrigate the ear. This is used when the cerumen is deeper in the ear canal or not cleared with other previously listed methods. For irrigation, the patient should tilt the head to the side being treated with a towel or small basin to catch what is discharged from the ear. Holding the auricle as upright as possible, the irrigating solution

should be administered upward in the ear to avoid pressure on the tympanic membrane.
- In cases where a liquid is contraindicated or does not resolve the problem, a cerumen spoon or curette may be appropriate. For this method of removal, the patient must be able to remain still during the procedure. The cerumen should be visualized in the lateral third of the external ear canal. A physician or advanced practice nurse performs this procedure.

Evaluate outcomes (evaluation). The patient will be free from cerumen impaction and verbalize a decrease in ear fullness and an increase in the ability to hear. The cerumen removal should be documented, noting the irrigation method, the amount and type of debris removed, and the patient's response. The patient will demonstrate the proper method to instill the softening agent. The patient will also state the ear symptoms to report to his or her health-care provider.

Tinnitus

Tinnitus is a chronic combination of both conductive and sensorineural hearing loss. It is a subjective sensation of noise in the ear, defined as a ringing, buzzing, or hissing. Tinnitus occurs more frequently in Whites, and the prevalence of tinnitus is almost twice as frequent in the South as in the Northeast. Individuals at any age may experience tinnitus, but its prevalence increases with advancing age. For most, it is an annoying and bothersome condition; for others, it indicates a permanent hearing loss or a tumor (Benson et al, 2022).

The most common causes of tinnitus are noise or toxin damage to the hair receptors of the cochlear nerve and age-related changes in the organs of hearing and balance. Tinnitus is not a disease but a symptom associated with many diseases, conditions, medications, and medical treatments. Tinnitus is classified as subjective or objective. Subjective tinnitus is audible only to the patient. It is characterized as ringing, buzzing, or humming. Objective tinnitus, although rare, is audible to both the patient and the examiner. It is more likely to be low-pitched and is often associated with an identifiable cause, such as muscle spasms or vascular and musculoskeletal cranial disorders. An additional important classification of tinnitus is whether it is bilateral or unilateral. Unilateral tinnitus is associated with more serious diseases, such as Ménière's disease, tumors, or vascular problems, and requires an extensive workup (Benson et al, 2022; National Institute on Deafness and Other Communication Disorders [NIDCD], 2023).

Nursing care guidelines for tinnitus

Recognize cues (assessment). The Tinnitus Screener can be used to assess the patient for the presence and level of tinnitus (Box 16.8). In addition, the patient should answer questions about the effect of tinnitus on daily living. Tools such as the Tinnitus and Hearing Survey (Henry et al, 2015) can identify the effects of tinnitus, hearing loss, and sound tolerance.

Analyze cues and prioritize hypotheses (patient problems). Potential problems for the patient with tinnitus include the following:
- Inadequate health maintenance resulting from a lack of knowledge about tinnitus prevention practices

---

BOX 16.8 Tinnitus Screener: Interview-by-Clinician Version

During the past year:
1. Have you experienced tinnitus lasting more that 2 to 3 minutes?
   No—stop here—no tinnitus
   Yes—go to #2
2. Have you experienced tinnitus for at least 6 months?
   No—acute tinnitus
   Yes—chronic tinnitus
3. In a quiet room, can you hear tinnitus?
   Always—stop here—constant tinnitus
   Usually—stop here—constant tinnitus
   Sometimes/occasionally—go to #4
4. When you heard tinnitus this past year, was it caused by a recent event? (e.g., loud concert, head cold, allergies, drugs)
   No—go to #6
   Yes, sometimes—go to #5
   Yes, always—stop here—temporary tinnitus
5. Does your tinnitus seem to "come and go" on its own, in addition to being caused by a recent event(s)?
   No—stop here—temporary tinnitus
   Yes—go to #6
6. Do you experience tinnitus on a
   Daily or weekly basis—stop here—intermittent tinnitus
   Monthly or yearly basis—stop here—occasional tinnitus

From National Center for Rehabilitative Auditory Research. (2017). *Tinnitus Screener: Interview-by-clinician version.* Retrieved from https://www.ncrar.research.va.gov/Education/Documents/TinnitusDocuments/TinnitusScreener-Clinician.pdf.

- Anxiety resulting from coping with the chronic condition of ringing in the ears

Generate solutions (planning). Expected outcomes for the patient with tinnitus include the following:
1. The patient will follow tinnitus prevention practices.
2. The patient will use home-masking measures and a hearing aid or tinnitus masker to relieve tinnitus.
3. The patient will cope with anxiety independently by using relaxation techniques.

Take actions (nursing interventions). One primary nursing intervention for tinnitus is reassuring the patient that tinnitus is usually a benign symptom. Determine if the tinnitus is a primary or secondary tinnitus. Removing the underlying cause of secondary tinnitus can reduce or eliminate it (NIA, 2023b). Patients should be taught prevention practices, including (1) treating correctable problems (e.g., cerumen impaction and ear infections) that cause tinnitus, (2) softening loud sounds through improved acoustics, (3) using protective ear plugs, and (4) avoiding foods, drinks, and drugs that contain ototoxic substances. Teach patients about the variety of treatments that can help minimize tinnitus, such as:
- Phone, television, computer, or table-top sound generator
- Wearable sound generators that fit in the ear (similar to hearing aid) that emits soft, pleasant sounds
- Hearing aids for those with hearing loss due to tinnitus
- Tinnitus retraining therapy using counseling and sound therapy to "retrain" the brain

- Behavioral therapy
- Medications, such as antidepressants to improve mood

Patients with tinnitus and age-related hearing loss (sensorineural hearing loss [SNHL]) may benefit from a low-carbohydrate, low-cholesterol diet (Wu et al, 2018). Other conservative management includes reducing stress, caffeine, and alcohol.

Evaluate outcomes (evaluation). Patients following recommended tinnitus interventions and strategies to cope with the chronic ringing in their ears will achieve the expected outcomes. The Tinnitus Handicap Inventory was published in 1996 to identify the problems that individuals have with tinnitus. The 25-question inventory delves into feelings and interference with living issues (American Tinnitus Association, n.d.). Some areas of interference in daily living include the ability to concentrate, frustration, stress, and problems with sleep, among others. Patients noting no improvement or increase in symptoms should be referred to a multidisciplinary team (specializing in tinnitus) composed of an otolaryngologist, audiologist, and psychiatrist for evaluation and counseling. Patients taking medications should be free from side effects. Those displaying adverse side effects should report to their health-care provider for dosage modification, alternative drug therapy, or discontinuation of the medication.

Hearing Loss

Approximately 20% (48 million) of American adults report some degree of hearing loss, and about 28.8 million adults could benefit from hearing aids (Hearing Loss Association of America [HLAA], n.d.[a]). The risk for hearing loss increases with age. About 33% of older adults have hearing loss (NIA, 2023b). Although a strong correlation exists between age and hearing loss, hearing loss does not have to be a normal part of the aging process and should be further evaluated for proper treatment.

Hearing impairment is classified as conductive, sensorineural, or mixed (HLAA, n.d.[a]). Conductive hearing loss results from interruption of the transmission of sound through the external auditory canal and middle ear. Conditions that may result in conductive hearing loss are cerumen impaction, otitis media, and otosclerosis (fixation of auditory ossicles).

SNHL results when the inner ear, auditory nerve, brainstem, or cortical auditory pathways do not function properly, so sound waves are not interpreted correctly. Mixed hearing loss is a conductive loss superimposed on SNHL.

Older adults with SNHL are increasingly selecting cochlear implants. These implants are surgically placed in the mastoid bone (behind the ear), where they transmit electrical signals through the auditory nerve to the brain's hearing center (Ham et al, 2014; NIDCD, 2021).

Presbycusis

Presbycusis, an SNHL due to aging, is the most common form of hearing loss in older adults. Approximately 33% of adults aged 65 to 74 have presbycusis, and nearly 50% of those older than 75 have hearing loss (HLAA, n.d.[b]). Typically, the loss is bilateral, resulting in difficulty hearing high-pitched tones and conversational speech. It affects males more than females. The cause of presbycusis remains unclear. Studies designed to identify a direct cause have proven no clear correlation. Therefore, the diagnosis is one of exclusion, which involves ruling out other causes of hearing loss:

- Noise-induced hearing loss (i.e., prolonged exposure to loud noise)
- Infection
- Head injury
- Metabolic diseases, such as diabetes and kidney disease
- Vascular disease, such as high BP
- Heart disease
- Genetic factors

Signs and symptoms displayed by the patient include the following:

- Increasing the volume on the television or the radio
- Tilting the head toward the person speaking
- Cupping the hand around one ear
- Watching the speaker's lips
- Speaking loudly
- Not responding when spoken to

Nursing care guidelines for hearing loss

Recognize cues (assessment). Subjective data that should be obtained from an older patient with hearing loss include onset, type, and progression of hearing loss, including differences in either ear; a family history of hearing loss; the presence of other symptoms such as pressure or pain in the ears, ringing in the ear, or dizziness; a history of head injury or noise exposure; and current medications with known ototoxic effects. Objectively, the patient may display some behavioral symptoms of hearing loss (Box 16.9). A complete hearing evaluation should be conducted.

Analyze cues and prioritize hypotheses (patient problems). Patent problems based on analysis of the patient's hearing loss include the following:

- Social disengagement resulting from difficulty with communication
- Potential for chronic low self-esteem resulting from hearing loss

---

BOX 16.9 Behavioral Clues Indicating Difficulty Hearing

- Difficulty hearing over the telephone
- Finding it hard to follow conversation when two or more persons are talking at the same time
- Turning up the volume on the television so loud that others complain
- Presence of background noise interferes with ability to hear
- Complaining about people mumbling
- Difficulty understanding women and children talking
- Asking for frequent repetition of what others are saying

Data from National Institutes of Health, & National Institute on Aging (2023). *Hearing loss: A common problem for older adults.* Retrieved from https://www.nia.nih.gov/health/hearing-and-hearing-loss/hearing-loss-common-problem-older-adults.

Generate solutions (planning). Expected outcomes for a patient with a hearing loss include the following:
1. The patient will effectively use aural rehabilitative techniques.
2. The patient will maintain satisfactory social contacts and activities with others.
3. The patient will perceive himself or herself positively, as evidenced by positive self-talk and behaviors.

Take actions (nursing interventions). Interventions for the patient with a hearing impairment focus on aural rehabilitation and facilitation of communication. Patients often deny their hearing loss and need much encouragement and support to explore the various methods to improve hearing. The nurse should provide patients with a printed information sheet on hearing loss (Box 16.10).

Aural rehabilitation includes auditory training, speech and reading training, and hearing aids. Auditory training helps the person with a hearing impairment listen to a speaker by differentiating among gross sounds. Speech and reading training includes lip reading and speech skills. Lip reading requires understanding verbal communication by integrating lip movements, facial expressions, gestures, and environmental clues. This process is extremely difficult without auditory clues. Speech skills must be conserved with the reduced auditory feedback experienced by the patient with impaired hearing. Older adults with hearing impairments must learn to work intelligently with inefficient communication and decreased speech (see Patient/Family Teaching: Communicating with the Hearing Impaired). Hearing aids amplify sound but do not improve the ability to hear. The advancement in technology currently offers patients various amplification options to suit their changing environmental needs (i.e., quiet to noisy). Patients and their families should be instructed on hearing aid use and care (see Patient/Family Teaching: Assisted-Listening Devices). All nurses and nursing assistants should have a basic understanding of how to work with a hearing aid to assist the patient unable to care for the aid. Patients and their families should be taught where to obtain and how to use ALDs (see Patient/Family Teaching: Hearing Aid Assessment Tool for Cleaning, Inserting, and Troubleshooting and Health Promotion/Illness Prevention: The Ear).

PATIENT/FAMILY TEACHING
Communicating with the Hearing Impaired

- Look at the hearing-impaired individual directly, at eye level, and in adequate light.
- Say the individual's name before starting to speak to them, giving them a chance to focus their attention on you.
- Speak slowly and distinctly, but naturally. Do not shout or embellish mouth movements. Use simple, uncomplicated sentences.
- Take your time when speaking, and pause to ensure they have understood you before proceeding.
- When speaking to the listener, observe them closely. Their expression may indicate understanding or misunderstanding. If there is any doubt, tactfully ask them if they understood you, or ask additional leading questions to ensure their understanding.
- Avoid hands near your face while speaking. Actions such as eating, chewing, or smoking while speaking makes speech more challenging for the listener to comprehend.
- Limit unnecessary background noise when speaking.
- When the listener cannot understand a particular word or phrase, try an alternative word or phrase instead of repeatedly saying the original words.
- Provide information that is significant in writing, such as instructions, schedules, directions, etc.
- Be aware that all people have difficulty with hearing and comprehension when ill or tired, not just individuals who are hearing-impaired.

Data from UCSF Health. (n.d.). Communicating with people with hearing loss. University of California San Francisco. Available at: https://www.ucsfhealth.org/education/communicating-with-people-with-hearing-loss. Accessed May 1, 2024.

BOX 16.10 Hearing and Older Adults

1. Presbycusis is the normal hearing loss associated with aging. This is also called age-related hearing loss and comes on gradually. It occurs due to changes in the inner ear and auditory nerve and seems to run in families. It creates difficulty with hearing what others are saying and tolerating loud sounds. Presbycusis may most often affect both ears equally. Due to gradual onset, the individual may not recognize the hearing loss.
2. Tinnitus or ringing in the ears is another common problem for older adults. This is typically described as ringing in the ears and is a symptom, not a disease. It can be as simple as earwax causing a blockage in the ear canal or the result of numerous health conditions (such as high blood pressure or allergies), or can be a medication side effect. Tinnitus may be in one ear or bilateral and described as ringing, roaring, clicking, hissing, or buzzing. It may be constant or intermittent and can accompany other forms of hearing loss.

Data from National Institutes of Health. National Institute on Aging (2023). *Hearing loss: A common problem for older adults.* Available at: https://www.nia.nih.gov/health/hearing-and-hearing-loss/hearing-loss-common-problem-older-adults.

PATIENT/FAMILY TEACHING
Assisted-Listening Devices

Assistive devices or assistive technology has become more accessible and available with advancing technology. These systems allow a hearing-impaired person to communicate more effectively and function more independently.

Assisted listening devices help to improve sound transmission and include:
- Hearing loop systems
- Frequency-modulated (FM) systems
- Infrared systems
- Personal amplifiers

Alerting devices may connect with a sound device such as a doorbell, telephone, or smoke detectors or other alarms and add blinking lights and louder sound.

Augmentative and alternative communication devices include:
- Closed-captioned television and telephones
- Text messaging on mobile phones

Data from National Institute on Deafness and Other Communication Disorders. (2019). *Assistive devices for people with hearing, voice, speech, or language disorders.* National Institutes of Health. Retrieved from https://www.nidcd.nih.gov/health/assistive-devices-people-hearing-voice-speech-or-language-disorders.

PATIENT/FAMILY TEACHING
Hearing Aids Care and Troubleshooting

General care:
- Perform listening checks daily
- Perform battery checks and keep spare batteries on hand
- Clean hearing aids regularly using a soft, dry cloth
- Minimize exposure to moisture; store in a hearing aid drying container with batteries removed
- Avoid feedback; hearing aid should be securely seated in the ear and fitted to proper size

If hearing aid has weak sound or is not working:
- Be sure it is switched on
- Check battery for correct placement
- Check for any blockage in the receiver opening or vent opening with cerumen or other debris
- Check all tubing for proper connections, no bends or twists
- Check microphone for blockage

If sound is distorted or intermittent:
- Check for moisture and remove with an air blower
- Check tubing and any cords that connect the hearing aid or other assistive devices for cracks and holes; notify audiologist if these are present
- Replace battery

Data from Nance, S. (2022). Daily care and troubleshooting tips for hearing aids. *Audiology Information Series*. Rockville, MD: American Speech Language Hearing Association. Available at: https://www.asha.org/siteassets/ais/ais-hearing-aids-troubleshooting.pdf.

HEALTH PROMOTION/ILLNESS PREVENTION
The Ear

Health Promotion
- Notify health-care provider of any pain, discharge, redness, swelling, dizziness, ringing in ears, or loss of hearing.
- See health-care provider for early detection and appropriate treatment of hearing difficulties and ear disease (e.g., cerumen impaction, tinnitus, presbycusis, and vertigo).
- Maintain prescribed hearing aids, ALDs, and medications.

Prevention of Disease
- Have a periodic ear examination and screening for ear disease and hearing problems.
- Avoid exposure to hazardous noise.
- Use protective earplugs in high-risk occupations and activities.

Evaluate outcomes (evaluation). Evaluation is based on documentation of the achievement of expected patient outcomes, as evidenced by the patient using aural rehabilitation techniques and devices to enhance communication. The patient and family should demonstrate the hearing aid's proper use, cleaning, and troubleshooting aid. The older patient should remain actively involved with others and the environment. Those older patients displaying signs and symptoms of depression and social isolation will require further encouragement and support to explore other methods to improve hearing.

Vertigo

Dizziness and disequilibrium are common complaints of older adults. Approximately 30% of those over 60 years and nearly 50% of those over 85 years have balance issues (McKinnon, 2020). Although a general decrease occurs in vestibular sensitivity with aging, the symptoms of dizziness or imbalance should not be considered a normal part of aging. Balance disorders contribute to deficits in ambulation that may interfere with an older person's ability to carry out normal ADLs. Disequilibrium is a major risk factor for unintentional falls, often associated with traumatic brain injury. The five age-related conditions of disequilibrium that have been documented in older adults are as follows:

1. **Benign paroxysmal positional vertigo:** severe episodes of vertigo precipitated by a particular change in head position
2. **Ampullary disequilibrium:** vertigo or disequilibrium associated with rotational head movements
3. **Macular disequilibrium:** vertigo precipitated by a change of head position in relation to the direction of gravitational force (e.g., severe dizziness when rising from bed)
4. **Vestibular ataxia of aging:** a feeling of unbalance when ambulating
5. **Ménière's disease:** an uncommon disease seen most often in older women, characterized by severe vertigo accompanied and usually preceded by tinnitus and progressive low-frequency SNHL

Although the vestibular system of the inner ear is the most common source of dizziness and balance disorders, the following causes must also be considered:

- Visual disturbances
- Musculoskeletal disorders
- Neurologic dysfunctions
- Metabolic abnormalities
- Cardiovascular disease
- Polypharmacy
- Tinnitus

Signs and symptoms vary for each disorder but may include any of the following (NIA, 2022):

- Whirling dizziness when the head is moved in a certain position
- Dizziness or imbalance when the head is moved quickly to the right, left, up, or down
- Constant feeling of imbalance when walking
- Staggered gait
- Lightheadedness or faintness
- Blurred vision

Ménière's Disease

Ménière's disease is one of the most common causes of dizziness caused by pressure within the inner ear's labyrinth due to excessive fluid (American Academy of Otolaryngology-Head and Neck Surgery, 2020). What causes the excessive fluid is unclear. The three major characteristics are vertigo, tinnitus, and hearing loss. Other associated symptoms include loss of balance, nausea and vomiting, and spasmodic eye movements. Roughly 615,000 people have been diagnosed with Ménière's disease in the United States, and another 45,500 are newly diagnosed each year (Haybach and Vestibular Disorders Association, 2013).

Nursing care guidelines for vertigo and ménière's disease
Recognize Cues (Assessment). Subjective data include a description of vertigo episodes (including frequency and duration),

a list of accompanying symptoms, such as nausea and vomiting, hearing loss, or tinnitus, a history of balance problems, and a drug history. Objective data include a complete assessment of hearing and balance, including lower extremity strength, proprioception, and the condition of the patient's feet and shoes.

Analyze cues and prioritize hypotheses (patient problems). Potential problems for the patient with vertigo and Ménière disease include the following:

- Potential for injury resulting from acute onset of vertigo
- Need for patient teaching resulting from lack of exposure and inexperience about the cause of vertigo and its treatment
- Need for patient teaching resulting from lack of exposure to preoperative and postoperative surgical care for Ménière disease
- Anxiety resulting from uncertainty of future vertigo attacks

Generate solutions (planning). Expected outcomes for the patient include the following:

1. The patient will follow the prescribed medication regimen and exercise protocol accurately.
2. The patient will safely follow measures to reduce dizziness and prevent falls.
3. The patient will state the causes and treatment of vertigo.
4. The patient will ask questions about the surgical care for Ménière disease.
5. The patient will meet his or her self-care needs, as evidenced by reports of normal appetite, sleep, and activity.

Take actions (nursing interventions). Pharmacologic treatment includes antivertiginous drugs such as meclizine or diphenhydramine. Meclizine may cause drowsiness; patients should be instructed to avoid alcoholic beverages while taking this drug. Patients with a history of asthma, glaucoma, or enlargement of the prostate gland must be monitored carefully while taking meclizine because of its anticholinergic action. Diphenhydramine, an antihistamine, is likely to cause dizziness, sedation, and hypotension in older patients. Diuretics such as hydrochlorothiazide (HCTZ) and a low-sodium diet help remove excess endolymphatic fluid. Older patients undergoing diuretic therapy need to be monitored for evidence of fluid or electrolyte imbalances.

Vestibular rehabilitation therapy is conducted by a physical therapist who designs an exercise program to help train the brain to use other senses that can substitute for the deficiencies created by a vestibular disturbance (Haybach and Vestibular Disorders Association, 2013).

Surgery may be performed for Ménière disease to prevent further damage and SNHL. An older patient undergoing ear surgery is given a local anesthetic. Preoperative care includes giving instructions for postoperative care and sedating the patient. Postoperative care includes (1) positioning the operative ear up for 4 hours after surgery; (2) medicating for pain and vertigo; (3) following safety precautions (e.g., side rails up, call light in reach, and assistance with ambulation); (4) monitoring the patient for changes in hearing, vertigo, neurologic symptoms (e.g., headache), or facial paralysis; and (5) instructing the patient to keep his or her mouth open when sneezing or coughing.

No complete cure for vertigo exists. Therefore, patients must be taught the following measures to reduce dizziness: (1) move slowly; (2) avoid bright, glaring lights (a quiet, darkened room is best); and (3) if vertigo occurs during ambulation, lie down immediately and hold the head still. The patient with vertigo must be taught the causes of vertigo, pharmacologic treatment, vestibular exercises, and measures to reduce vertigo and promote safety during an acute attack.

Evaluate outcomes (evaluation). Evaluation includes achievement of the expected outcomes, as evidenced by patients accurately following the prescribed medication regimen and exercise protocol. Patients displaying adverse side effects should report these to their health-care provider for a modification in their medication regimen. Patients should be free from falls by following measures to reduce dizziness. Those with reported falls should be evaluated with a fall assessment tool and taught alternative safety measures.

TASTE AND SMELL

The senses of taste and smell detect the esthetics and safety of the environment. Some evidence suggests that the senses of smell and taste diminish with aging. Loss of smell and taste may affect an older person's food choices and intake and subsequently impair nutritional and immune status, which may exacerbate disease states. A decreased sensitivity to odors puts the older person at potential risk for noxious chemicals and poisonings (e.g., a person may fail to detect the odor of smoke or leaking gas).

Age-Related Changes in Structure and Function

Age-related changes in the senses of smell and taste result from alterations in the oral mucosa, tongue, and the pathologic state of the nasal cavity. Anatomic and physiologic changes occur with aging (e.g., reductions in cell number, damage to cells, and diminished levels of neurotransmitters). In healthy older adults, olfactory losses result from normal aging, medications, viral infections, long-term exposure to toxic fumes, and head trauma. Most studies indicate a dramatic decline in sensitivity to airborne chemical stimuli with aging. Additionally, recognition of odors declines dramatically with age.

The cause of taste changes in normal aging is not fully understood. Studies of anatomic losses in the structures of the taste system in older adults report conflicting findings. Taste losses result from disease states of the nervous and endocrine systems, nutritional and upper respiratory conditions, viral infections, and medications. The most common cause of change in the sense of taste is thought to be xerostomia, which is discussed next (Boltz et al, 2016).

Common Problems and Conditions
Xerostomia

Xerostomia, commonly called *dry mouth,* is a subjective sensation of abnormal oral dryness. Reduced salivary flow is a common complaint of older adults. Longitudinal studies have established that salivary flow from the parotid gland is unchanged with advancing age. Factors leading to a dry mouth include disease states (e.g., Alzheimer disease, depression, Sjögren syndrome), conditions (e.g., radiotherapy of the head and neck or mouth breathing), and medications (e.g., sedatives, antihistamines, antidepressants, diuretics, chemotherapy, or anticholinergics).

Dry mouth in older adults may lead to an increased risk for serious respiratory infection, impaired nutritional status, and reduced ability to communicate. Complaints of abnormal taste sensations, burning of the oral tissues and tongue, and cracking of the lips are common. The oral mucosa is dry, thin, and smooth, and the tongue may have a thick, white, foul-smelling coating. The decrease in salivary flow interferes with chewing and swallowing. Patients with dentures may complain of sore gums and tissues and denture slippage from the loss of salivary flow, which forms a mechanical barrier.

Nursing care guidelines for xerostomia

Recognize cues (assessment). Subjective assessment should include a health history of factors leading to decreased salivary flow and the patient's oral complaints. Objective assessment of a patient's lips with xerostomia reveals red, inflamed, cracked, and dry lips, which may bleed. The tongue has red areas and a coated base; it appears thicker, with a prominent lingual groove and papillae. The mucous membranes of the palate and the lining of the mouth and gums appear dry, red, and edematous. The saliva is scant, ropy, and viscid. The amount of moisture in the oral cavity is assessed by running a gloved finger over the oral mucosa to evaluate stickiness, which indicates dry mucous membranes. The patient's voice may be dry and raspy, and he or she may complain of difficulty articulating words. Taste testing is performed to evaluate taste sensation, which may be diminished.

Analyze cues and prioritize hypotheses (patient problems). Potential problems for the patient with xerostomia include the following:
- Inadequate oral mucous membrane resulting from changes induced by xerostomia
- Inadequate nutrition resulting from changes induced by xerostomia

Generate solutions (planning). Expected outcomes for the patient with xerostomia include the following:
1. The patient will verbalize an increase in taste sensation.
2. The patient will exhibit unimpaired oral mucosa tissue integrity, as evidenced by moist, pink, smooth mucosal surfaces.
3. The patient will verbalize no oral discomfort.
4. The patient will state the contributing factors, symptoms, and treatment of xerostomia.
5. The patient will demonstrate a correct oral hygiene regimen.

Take actions (nursing interventions). Nursing interventions for the patient with xerostomia focus on attaining intact oral mucosa tissue integrity. Teaching patients about the factors leading to a decrease in salivary flow and the associated symptoms is key to the prevention and treatment of xerostomia. The treatment regimen focuses on increasing salivary flow. Patients need to be taught the basic oral hygiene of brushing their teeth twice daily with a soft toothbrush, a nonabrasive fluoride toothpaste, and daily flossing. Fluid balance is vital for maintaining moisture in the oral cavity. Patients must take in 2 to 3 liters (L) of fluid per day if not contraindicated. Also, foods prepared with gravy or sauces contain moisture and should be included in the diet if not contraindicated. Additional methods to teach patients to increase salivary flow include the use of artificial saliva, sugar-free hard candy, and gum.

Evaluate outcomes (evaluation). Evaluation of the interventions is based on the appearance of the oral mucous membranes, the patient's relief of symptoms, and an increased level of comfort through effective daily treatment practices.

HOME CARE

1. Sensory changes may lead to social isolation in homebound older adults (e.g., not being able to interact effectively with family members because of visual or hearing deficits).
2. Sensory changes increase safety hazards (e.g., burning or falling) for homebound older adults.
3. Instruct caregivers and homebound older adults about signs and symptoms of age-related sensory changes. Instruct them to report to their physician or home-care nurse any signs and symptoms that interfere with independent function or present safety hazards.
4. Instruct caregivers and homebound older adults about prescribed treatments or surgical procedures (e.g., preoperative and postoperative care of cataract surgery, eye drops, eardrops, and antibiotics).
5. Assist caregivers and homebound older adults in organizing the environment to accommodate any decreased sensory function (e.g., use of color contrast, bold print books, hearing aid on the telephone).

TOUCH

At birth, touch is the most developed sense. Touch involves tactile information on pressure, vibration, and temperature. Although touch, pressure, and vibration are commonly classified as separate sensations, the same types of receptors detect them. The only differences among these three are that (1) touch sensation usually results from stimulation of receptors in the skin or tissues immediately beneath the skin; (2) pressure sensation generally results from deformation of deeper tissues; and (3) vibration sensation results from rapidly repetitive sensory signals.

Sensitivity to light touch diminishes in older adults and may result from a decreased density of cutaneous receptors for touch sensation. Tactile vibratory thresholds progressively increase with age, most likely because of changes in Pacinian corpuscle receptor sensitivity. Studies to evaluate the influence of age on thermal perception report conflicting findings. The warm–cold difference threshold increases with age.

The most common disorders affecting tactile information include cerebrovascular accident (CVA), peripheral vascular disease (PVD), and diabetic neuropathy. All three conditions involve changes in the vascular system that result in decreased blood flow to various body parts. Signs and symptoms of a CVA depend on the cerebral artery affected and the portion of the brain supplied by that artery. In PVD and diabetic neuropathy, the impaired blood flow manifests as a loss of sensation, most commonly noted in the lower extremities.

The common thread among these disorders is the alteration of peripheral tissue perfusion. Nursing interventions are directed toward preventing accidental trauma and injury in the affected limbs. Patient education focuses on skin, leg, and foot care. The effectiveness of nursing interventions is determined by the absence of trauma, especially in the lower extremities.

SUMMARY

The senses of older adults are the key to their interaction with the environment. As these senses decline because of normal age-related changes or pathologic conditions, nurses in every setting must adapt interventions to promote the highest level of independent functioning.

KEY POINTS

- Studies have documented age-related changes in the senses of vision and hearing.
- Age-related changes in the senses of taste and smell remain questionable.
- A cataract is the opacity of the lens and requires surgery for successful treatment.
- Glaucoma is caused by increased IOP and requires lifelong treatment with medications to lower the pressure.
- Retinal detachment requires immediate medical attention and can be repaired only by surgical intervention.
- Wet MD and DR can be treated successfully with laser surgery.
- Creating a safe environment with the appropriate level of assistance is important for an older adult who is visually impaired to maintain independence and prevent injury.
- Hearing loss affects an older person's ability to communicate effectively and may lead to depression, social isolation, and loss of self-esteem.
- Prevention and treatment of cerumen impaction is an important nursing function in caring for older adults to minimize hearing loss.
- Vertigo and tinnitus may be chronic and annoying conditions. Each must be treated in ways to assist the older adult with management and maintaining safety.
- Xerostomia may cause pain in the oral mucosa, gums, and tongue, leading to alterations in taste. Treatment includes a daily oral care regimen and methods to increase salivary production.
- Older adults with a diminished sense of touch are at the potential for injury, especially in the affected limbs.

CLINICAL JUDGMENT EXERCISES

1. A 69-year-old female has tinnitus and episodes of imbalance. Her son and daughter-in-law are concerned about having to leave her alone during the day while they are at work. What strategies could you suggest to the family regarding safety measures in the home?

2. Discuss how loss of sensory function in older adults affects their self-esteem, performance of ADLs, safety, independence, and interactions with others.

REFERENCES

American Academy of Otolaryngology-Head and Neck Surgery. (2020). *Meniere's disease*. ENThealth [website]. Retrieved from https://www.enthealth.org/conditions/menieres-disease/. Accessed January 3, 2024.

American Council of the Blind (ACB). (n.d.). *Resources*. Retrieved from https://www.acb.org/resources. Accessed January 3, 2024.

American Optometric Association. (n.d.). *Color vision deficiency*. Retrieved from https://www.aoa.org/healthy-eyes/eye-and-vision-conditions/color-vision-deficiency?sso=y. Accessed January 3, 2024.

American Tinnitus Association. (n.d.). *Tinnitus handicap inventory (THI)*. Retrieved from https://ata.org/wp-content/uploads/2022/08/Tinnitus_Handicap_Inventory.pdf. Accessed January 3, 2024.

Benson, A. G., McGuire, J. F., 3rd, Djalilian, H. R., Hanks, K. M., & Robbins, W. K. (2022). *Tinnitus*. Medscape [website]. Retrieved from https://emedicine.medscape.com/article/856916-overview?form=fpf. Accessed January 3, 2024.

Boltz, M., Capezuti, E., Fulmer, T., & Zwicker, D. (Eds.). (2016). *Evidenced-based geriatric nursing protocols for best practice* (5th ed.). New York, NY: Springer Publishing.

Boyd, K. (2023a). *What are floaters and flashes?* American Academy of Ophthalmology [website]. Retrieved from https://www.aao.org/eye-health/diseases/what-are-floaters-flashes. Accessed January 3, 2024.

Boyd, K. (2023b). *What are cataracts?* American Academy of Ophthalmology [website]. Retrieved from https://www.aao.org/eye-health/diseases/what-are-cataracts. Accessed January 3, 2024.

Boyd, K. (2023c). *What is macular degeneration?* American Academy of Ophthalmology [website]. Retrieved from https://www.aao.org/eye-health/diseases/amd-macular-degeneration. Accessed January 3, 2024.

Ehrlich, J. R., Ramke, J., Macleod, D., Burn, H., Lee, C. N., Zhang, J. H., et al. (2021). Association between vision impairment and mortality: A systematic review and meta-analysis. *The Lancet Global Health*, 9(4), e418–e430. doi:10.1016/S2214-109X(20)30549-0.

Garrity, J. (2022). Effects of aging on the eyes. In *Merck manual consumer version*. Merck & Co., Inc. Retrieved from https://www.merckmanuals.com/home/eye-disorders/biology-of-the-eyes/effects-of-aging-on-the-eyes. Accessed January 3, 2024.

Glaucoma Research Foundation (GRF). (2022). *Understanding and living with glaucoma: A complete guide for patients and families*. San Francisco: GRF. Retrieved from https://glaucoma.org/wp-content/uploads/2023/12/ug-booklet-09-14-22a-alcon-update.pdf. Accessed August 25, 2024.

Ham, R. J., Sloane, P. D., Warshaw, G. A., Potter, J. F., & Flaherty, E. (2014). *Ham's primary care geriatrics: A case-based approach* (6th ed.). St. Louis: Elsevier.

Haybach, P. J., & Vestibular Disorders Association. (2013). *Meniere's disease*. VeDA [website]. Retrieved from https://vestibular.org/

article/diagnosis-treatment/types-of-vestibular-disorders/menieres-disease/. Accessed January 3, 2024.

Hearing Loss Association of America (HLAA). (n.d.[a]). *Hearing loss basics*. Retrieved from https://www.hearingloss.org/hearing-help/hearing-loss-basics/. Accessed January 3, 2024.

Hearing Loss Association of America (HLAA). (n.d.[b]). *Age-related hearing loss*. Retrieved from https://www.hearingloss.org/hearing-help/hearing-loss-basics/age-related/. Accessed January 3, 2024.

Henry, J. A., Griest, S., Zaugg, T. L., Thielman, E., Kaelin, C., Galvez, G., et al. (2015). Tinnitus and hearing survey: A screening tool to differentiate bothersome tinnitus from hearing difficulties. *American Journal of Audiology, 24*(1), 66–77. doi:10.1044/2014_AJA-14-0042.

Kaur, K., & Gurnani, B. (2023). Low vision aids. In *StatPearls* [Internet]. Treasure Island, FL: StatPearls Publishing. Retrieved from https://www.ncbi.nlm.nih.gov/books/NBK585124/. Accessed February 2, 2024.

Lewis, S. L., Bucher, L., Heitkemper, M. M., & Harding, M. M. (Eds.). (2017). *Medical-surgical nursing: Assessment and management of clinical problems* (10th ed.). St. Louis, MO: Elsevier.

McKinnon, B. J. (2020). *Disequilibrium of aging*. Bulletin [website]. American Academy of Otolaryngology-Head and Neck Surgery. Retrieved from https://bulletin.entnet.org/home/article/21247861/disequilibrium-of-aging. Accessed January 3, 2024.

Mehta, S. (2022). Hypertensive retinopathy. In *Merck manual professional version*. Merck & Co., Inc. Retrieved from https://www.merckmanuals.com/professional/eye-disorders/retinal-disorders/hypertensive-retinopathy. Accessed February 2, 2024.

National Eye Institute (NEI). (2023a). *Dry eye*. National Institutes of Health. Retrieved from https://www.nei.nih.gov/learn-about-eye-health/eye-conditions-and-diseases/dry-eye. Accessed January 3, 2024.

National Eye Institute (NEI). (2023b). *Blepharitis*. National Institutes of Health. Retrieved from https://www.nei.nih.gov/learn-about-eye-health/eye-conditions-and-diseases/blepharitis. Accessed January 3, 2024.

National Eye Institute (NEI). (2023c). *Glaucoma*. National Institutes of Health. Retrieved from https://www.nei.nih.gov/learn-about-eye-health/eye-conditions-and-diseases/glaucoma. Accessed January 3, 2024.

National Eye Institute (NEI). (2023d). *Cataracts*. National Institutes of Health. Retrieved from https://www.nei.nih.gov/learn-about-eye-health/eye-conditions-and-diseases/cataracts. Accessed January 3, 2024.

National Eye Institute (NEI). (2023e). *Diabetic retinopathy*. National Institutes of Health. Retrieved from https://www.nei.nih.gov/learn-about-eye-health/eye-conditions-and-diseases/diabetic-retinopathy. Accessed January 3, 2024.

National Eye Institute (NEI). (2023f). *Retinal detachment*. National Institutes of Health. Retrieved from https://www.nei.nih.gov/learn-about-eye-health/eye-conditions-and-diseases/retinal-detachment. Accessed January 3, 2024.

National Eye Institute (NEI). (2022). *Glaucoma surgery*. National Institutes of Health. Retrieved from https://www.nei.nih.gov/learn-about-eye-health/eye-conditions-and-diseases/glaucoma/glaucoma-surgery. Accessed January 3, 2024.

National Eye Institute (NEI). (2021). *Age-related macular degeneration (AMD)*. National Institutes of Health. Retrieved from https://www.nei.nih.gov/learn-about-eye-health/eye-conditions-and-diseases/age-related-macular-degeneration. Accessed January 3, 2024.

National Glaucoma Research (NGR). (2022). *Glaucoma: Facts & figures. Glaucoma fact sheet*. BrightFocus Foundation. Retrieved from https://www.brightfocus.org/glaucoma/article/glaucoma-facts-figures. Accessed January 3, 2024.

National Institute on Aging (NIA). (2023a). *Take care of your senses: The science behind sensory loss and dementia risk*. National Institutes of Health. Retrieved from https://www.nia.nih.gov/news/take-care-your-senses-science-behind-sensory-loss-and-dementia-risk. Accessed January 3, 2024.

National Institute on Aging (NIA). (2023b). *Hearing loss: A common problem for older adults*. National Institutes of Health. Retrieved from https://www.nia.nih.gov/health/hearing-and-hearing-loss/hearing-loss-common-problem-older-adults. Accessed January 3, 2024.

National Institute on Aging (NIA). (2022). *Older adults and balance problems*. National Institutes of Health. Retrieved from https://www.nia.nih.gov/health/falls-and-falls-prevention/older-adults-and-balance-problems. Accessed January 3, 2024.

National Institute on Deafness and Other Communication Disorders (NIDCD). (2023). *Tinnitus*. National Institutes of Health. Retrieved from https://www.nidcd.nih.gov/health/tinnitus. Accessed January 3, 2024.

National Institute on Deafness and Other Communication Disorders (NIDCD). (2021). *Cochlear implants*. National Institutes of Health. Retrieved from https://www.nidcd.nih.gov/health/cochlear-implants. Accessed January 29, 2024.

Office of Disease Prevention and Health Promotion. (n.d.). *Sensory or communication disorders*. Retrieved from https://health.gov/healthypeople/objectives-and-data/browse-objectives/sensory-or-communication-disorders. Accessed February 2, 2024.

Porter, D. (2023). *What are drusen?* American Academy of Ophthalmology. Retrieved from https://www.aao.org/eye-health/diseases/what-are-drusen. Accessed January 3, 2024.

Rebar, C. R., Borchers, S. A., & Borchers, A. A. (2021). Assessment and concepts of care for patients with eye and vision problems. In D. Ignatavicius, M. L. Workman, C. R. Rebar, & N. M. Heimgartner (Eds.), *Medical-surgical nursing: Concepts for interprofessional collaborative care* (10th ed.). St. Louis: Elsevier.

Schwartz, S. R., Magit, A. E., Rosenfeld, R. M., Ballachanda, B. B., Hackell, J. M., Krouse, H. J., et al. (2017). Clinical practice guideline (update): Earwax (cerumen impaction). *Otolaryngology—Head and Neck Surgery, 156*(Suppl. 1), S1–29. doi:10.1177/0194599816671491.

Wu, V., Cooke, B., Eitutis, S., Simpson, M. T. W., & Beyea, J. A. (2018). Approach to tinnitus management. *Canadian Family Physician, 64*(7), 491–495.

17

Cardiovascular Function

Mary B. Winton, PhD, MSN, RN

http://evolve.elsevier.com/Yeager/gerontologic/

LEARNING OBJECTIVES

On completion of this chapter, the reader will be able to:
1. Explain the age-related changes in the structure and function of the cardiovascular system.
2. Identify contributing risk factors for cardiovascular disease (CVD).
3. Explain the pathophysiology and treatment regimen for common cardiovascular conditions.
4. List nursing interventions for cardiovascular conditions.
5. Implement the nursing process for cardiovascular conditions.

WHAT WOULD YOU DO?

What would you do if you were faced with the following situations?
- An older adult neighbor comes to you with a blood pressure (BP) of 154/89 mm Hg. The BP was taken at a local supermarket. You know the neighbor also has type 2 diabetes mellitus (T2DM) and does not manage their glucose. What would you do?
- You live with an older adult who consumes 64 ounces of beer and smokes 1.5 packs of cigarettes daily. You have also noticed that, with moderate activity, they have difficulty breathing, and their feet have been swelling in the last 15 days. What would you do?

Heart disease is the leading cause of death in the United States and is a major cause of disability. Coronary heart disease (CHD) is the principal type of heart disease. According to the Centers for Disease Control and Prevention (CDC), more than 650,000 people die of heart disease in the United States each year, which is about 25% of all U.S. deaths (CDC, 2023a). Direct and indirect costs for the years 2016–2017 for cardiovascular-related health care were over $350 billion, including health care services, pharmacotherapies, and lost productivity. Risk factors for cardiovascular disease (CVD) include elevated cholesterol, hypertension (HTN), DM, tobacco use, physical inactivity, obesity, alcohol use, advancing age, and heredity. As individuals age, the chances of comorbid conditions increase. The reality is that atherosclerosis, the underlying cause of most clinical cardiovascular problems, is typically present for years before the onset of a clinical event such as a heart attack or symptoms such as angina manifest (Benjamin et al, 2017).

AGE-RELATED CHANGES IN STRUCTURE AND FUNCTION

Aging alters the cardiovascular system both structurally and physiologically. However, increasing evidence suggests that lifestyle and diet may modify some of these age-related changes (Yancy et al, 2017). As people age, changes occur within the heart. For example, the heart rate (HR) decreases, the left ventricular wall thickens, resulting in an overall increase in oxygen demand, and there is increased collagen and decreased elastin in the heart muscle and vessel walls (Huether et al, 2017). The size of the left atrium increases, and aortic distensibility and vascular tone decrease. These changes decrease myocardial muscle contraction, resulting in decreased cardiac output and cardiac reserve. Decreases occur in diastolic pressure, diastolic filling, and beta-adrenergic stimulation; increases occur in arterial pressure, systolic pressure, wave velocity, and left ventricular end diastolic pressure (LVEDP); and the muscle contraction, muscle relaxation, and ventricle relaxation phases are elongated (Banasik, 2013a). An S_4 heart sound commonly occurs in older adults (Huether et al, 2017).

Conduction System

The sinoatrial (SA) node, the atrioventricular (AV) node, and the bundle of His become fibrotic with age (Banasik, 2013a). The number of pacemaker cells located in the SA node decreases with age, which results in less responsiveness of the cells to adrenergic stimulation. Common aging changes reflected by electrocardiography (ECG) include a notched P wave, a prolonged PR interval, decreased amplitude of the QRS complex, and a notched or slurred T wave (Banasik, 2013a).

Vessels

Calcification of vessels occurs, making them tortuous. The elastin in the vessel wall decreases, which causes thickening and rigidity, especially in the coronary arteries (Ball et al, 2014). This increases the risk of atherosclerotic buildup, especially in those individuals with adverse lifestyle practices. Systolic (SBP) is increased in older adults because of a loss of arterial elasticity (Loftsgaarden, 2013). The diastolic blood pressure (DBP) remains the same or may be elevated slightly; thus, the pulse pressure widens. Older adults are less sensitive to the baroreceptor regulation of BP. This causes fluctuations in BP and contributes to increased SBP. Isolated systolic hypertension (ISH) is common in the older adult population.

Response to Stress and Exercise

Decreased cardiac output and cardiac reserve diminish the older adult's response to stress. Reduced stress responses plus changes to the heart and vessels affect the body's reaction to exercise. During stress or stimulation, the HR increases more slowly; however, once elevated, it takes longer to return to the resting rate (Banasik, 2013a). Nonetheless, this does not exclude older adults from participating in exercise programs.

COMMON CARDIOVASCULAR PROBLEMS

Of the CVDs, CHD was the leading cause of death for both males and females in the United States (Tsao et al, 2022). Coronary atherosclerosis, CHF, arrhythmias, acute myocardial infarction (AMI), and stroke were the top 5 causes of cardiovascular-related hospitalizations (Krishnamurthi et al, 2018).

The aging process varies among individuals, which may be attributed to factors of heredity. In addition, the effects of advancing age on cardiovascular structure and function are influenced by the presence of noncardiovascular disease and variations in lifestyle. It may not always be clear which changes in the cardiovascular system are from the normal aging process and which are caused by lifestyle choices (Banasik, 2013b). Many forms of CVD may be accelerated by unhealthy lifestyle choices such as smoking, physical inactivity, high-risk dietary behaviors, obesity, stress, and hormonal use. Chronic diseases such as HTN and DM also play a role in accelerating changes.

Hypertension

HTN continues to be the most prevalent risk factor for ischemic stroke (Rippe, 2018). Approximately 1 in 3 adults in the United States has HTN, and only about 50% are under control (CDC, 2023b). Furthermore, it is estimated that nearly 80% of U.S. older adults will develop HTN by the year 2060 (Patel and Stewart, 2015). HTN contributes to CVD (such as arteriosclerosis and stroke), CHF, and end organ damage (such as kidney disease). HTN is known as the *silent killer*, and many people are unaware of having HTN because they have no warning signs or symptoms (e.g., headache or vomiting; CDC, 2023b). BP is categorized as normal (<120/80 mm Hg), elevated (<120–129/<80 mm Hg), stage 1 HTN (SBP 130–139 mm Hg OR DBP 80–89 mm Hg), stage 2 HTN (SBP ≥140 mm Hg or DBP ≥90 mm Hg), and hypertensive crisis (SBP >180 mm Hg AND/OR DBP 120 mm Hg) (AHA, 2023a). The BP values are based on the average BP taken during office visits for health care.

Among older adults, ISH is more common. Elevated SBP is more predictive of cardiovascular risk than DBP (Patel and Stewart, 2015). However, it is important to note that low DBP (below 65 mm Hg) increases the risk of subtle heart damage and increases the risk of death from all causes (Beddhu et al, 2018). The American College of Cardiology (ACC) and the AHA recently updated the HTN guideline. Older adults age 65 or greater should be treated for HTN with an SBP goal of less than 130 mm Hg and a DBP goal of less than 80 mm Hg. The risk of CVD in older adults has decreased with more intensive treatment. Prevention and proper management of HTN are necessary to reduce the risk of comorbidities such as cardiovascular, renal, and cerebrovascular diseases (Qaseem et al, 2017).

> ### EVIDENCE-BASED PRACTICE
>
> ### *Frailty among In-Hospital Older Adults is Common in Those with Acute Myocardial Infarction (AMI)*
>
> #### Sample / Setting
> Preexisting frailty was assessed among 122,594 in-hospital older adult patients with AMI who participated in the National Cardiovascular Data Registry (NCDR) Acute Coronary Treatment and Intervention Outcomes Network Registry-Get with the Guidelines (ACTION Registry-GWTG) between 2015 and 2016.
>
> #### Methods
> Cognition, ambulation, and functional independence were the 3 domains of preexisting frailty that were included in the ACTION Registry-GWTG. Cognition was defined as normal, mildly impaired, moderate-to-severely impaired, or unknown. Ambulation was defined as unassisted, assisted, use of a wheelchair, nonambulatory, or unknown. Functional independence was defined as the ability to perform activities of daily living (ADLs): independent, partial assist, full assist, or unknown. Patients were categorized as fit / well, mild frailty, moderate frailty, severe frailty, and very severe frailty. Patients were divided according to their score and were compared on their in-hospital mortality and major adverse cardiovascular events (MACE) with the fit / well group. Other metrics, such as pharmacological therapies within 24 hours of hospital presentation, were assessed.
>
> #### Findings
> One (1) in 6 older adult patients was at risk of or had frailty. Older, non-White females were more frail and had a higher risk of not undergoing angiography. Frail patients who presented to the hospital with acute coronary events were less likely to receive intensive acute medical therapy, such as aspirin, beta blockers, and anticoagulants. These patients were at a higher risk of developing in-hospital MACE. Evidence-based practices were less often utilized among frail patients; instead, there was an increased use of comfort care.
>
> #### Implications
> A better understanding of frailty is warranted to improve patient outcomes among older adults with AMI. Clinicians can improve clinical decision-making in the management of cardiac events by evaluating and considering frailty status among their older adult patients.

Data From Udell, J. A., Lu, D., Bagai, A., Dodson, J. A., Desai, N. R., Fonarow, G. C., et al. (2022). Preexisting frailty and outcomes in older patients with acute myocardial infarction. *American Heart Journal*, 249, 34–44.

For primary prevention of CVD in the general public, the ACC and AHA recommend starting drug therapy when the SBP is persistently at or above 140 mm Hg or the DBP of 90 mm Hg or above (Whelton et al, 2018). Treatment for secondary prevention of recurrent CVD events should start if SBP is greater than or equal to 130 mm Hg or DBP is greater than or equal to 80 mm Hg. Other treatments include lifestyle modifications (i.e., smoking cessation, management of glucose intolerance, and hypercholesterolemia), and increased physical activity. The diagnosis of HTN is made with 3 different measurements on more than 2 office visits (Patel and Stewart, 2015). BP should be taken in both arms initially; future BP checks should be performed using the arm with the highest initial BP reading (Whelton et al, 2018).

HTN has been classified into 2 types: primary and secondary. Primary HTN is the most common form. Although the exact cause is unknown, the contributing factors are family history, age, race, diet (e.g., foods high in saturated fats and salt or decreased potassium, magnesium, and calcium intake), smoking, stress, alcohol and drug consumption, lack of physical activity, and hormonal intake.

Secondary HTN refers to elevated BP caused by underlying diseases such as renal artery disease stenosis (RAS), renal parenchymal disorders, endocrine and metabolic disorders, central nervous system (CNS) disorders, coarctation of the aorta, and increased intravascular volume.

In older adults presenting with HTN, the nurse should assess all prescription and over-the-counter (OTC) drugs for possible causes of elevated BP. Drug-induced HTN has occurred with the administration of amphetamines and glucocorticoids. Decongestants, phenobarbital, rifampin, and nonsteroidal antiinflammatory drugs (NSAIDs) may adversely affect the action of some drugs for HTN. NSAIDs have been found to cause elevated BP (Whelton et al, 2018). Many older adults are taking NSAIDs for various musculoskeletal problems. These individuals should have their BP closely monitored.

A positive correlation exists between obesity and HBP. Advancing age is associated with a loss of lean body mass and an increase in adipose tissue. Excess fat in the upper body or a waist circumference of 35 inches or greater in females or 40 inches or greater in males increases the risk for HTN (excess upper body fat correlates with metabolic syndrome, which includes abdominal obesity, glucose intolerance, high triglyceride levels, and low HDL levels). A BP drop of 1 mm Hg for every 1-kg weight reduction is expected with weight loss (Whelton et al, 2018).

Increased sodium intake is closely correlated with HBP. A reduction in sodium to 1000 mg per day may reduce SBP by 2–6 mm Hg. The Dietary Approach to Stop Hypertension (DASH) diet may reduce SBP by 3–11 mm Hg (Whelton et al, 2018).

The pathophysiology of HTN is complex because various environmental, structural, renal, hormonal, and homeostatic mechanisms contribute to BP maintenance, especially in the aging population.

HTN has been associated with arteriolar thickening, vascular smooth muscle (VSM) constriction, and elevated vascular resistance. With age, peripheral vascular resistance increases significantly. The alpha-adrenergic responsiveness of the VSM does not change with age; however, the beta-adrenergic responsiveness declines with age, with a consequent decrease in the relaxation of the VSM. Renal vascular resistance appears to be increased, and renal blood flow appears to be decreased. Left ventricular hypertrophy (LVH) occurs as an adaptation to longstanding HTN and may lead to CHF. Once this occurs, there is a significant increase in cardiovascular risk, particularly for ventricular arrhythmia and sudden death.

In mild-to-moderate HTN, the patient may be asymptomatic. As the disease progresses, the patient may experience fatigue, dizziness, headaches, vertigo, and palpitations. In severe HTN, the patient may experience throbbing headaches, confusion, visual loss, focal deficits, epistaxis, and coma.

It is important that persons with HTN be assessed for end-organ damage and its associated symptoms. HTN may lead to damage to various organs, resulting in the following conditions:

- **Heart:** CHF, ventricular hypertrophy, angina, MI, and sudden death
- **CNS:** transient ischemic attack and stroke
- **Peripheral vessels:** PVD and aneurysm
- **Kidney:** serum creatinine greater than 133 mmol/L (1.5 mg/dL), proteinuria, and microalbuminuria
- **Eye:** hemorrhage or exudates, with or without papilledema

Older adults are likely to have coexisting cardiac, vascular, and renal diseases.

Health-care providers should obtain a history regarding lifestyle factors and conduct an in-depth physical examination. The physical examination should include examination of the neck (to detect carotid bruits, jugular vein distention, or an enlarged thyroid), the heart (to detect abnormalities in rate and rhythm, heaves, lifts, murmurs, and third or fourth heart sounds), the lungs (to detect rales), the abdomen (to detect bruits, masses, and aortic pulsations), and the extremities (to detect peripheral pulses and edema).

Diagnostic tests can be beneficial in determining any effects on end organs due to HTN. The following tests should be included: hemoglobin and hematocrit to exclude anemia or polycythemia vera (PV); urinalysis to investigate for proteinuria or other signs of renal failure; serum sodium, potassium, and creatinine levels; fasting plasma glucose level to determine whether antihypertensive therapy is affecting DM; serum TC and HDL levels to assess for hyperlipidemia; ECG; chest radiograph; and possibly echocardiography to assess left ventricular function and hypertrophy.

Pharmacologic Treatment

One of the most important considerations in drug therapy for older adults is that BP should be lowered gradually, beginning with low doses of a single agent. When treating HTN in older adults, clinicians should consider patient factors such as comorbidities, frailty of patients, and the ability to follow instructions (Oliveros et al, 2020). Other factors to include are:

1. The goal of treatment is a BP less than 130/80 mm Hg.
2. How complex is the regimen?
3. Older adults are more likely to experience an orthostatic drop in BP than younger adults. BP should always be taken with the patient both sitting and standing and in both arms.
4. Isolated HTN should be treated with a calcium antagonist or diuretic.

5. When pharmacologic therapy is used, the dose should be lower than that recommended for younger adults.
6. Both nonpharmacologic interventions and lifestyle modifications should be employed. Older adults respond to modest sodium reduction and weight loss.
7. Select an appropriate drug with consideration for comorbidity. First-line medications include thiazide diuretics, angiotensin-converting enzyme (ACE) inhibitors, calcium channel blockers, and angiotensin II receptor blockers (ARBs).
8. BBs have a high propensity to worsen CVD outcomes and should be avoided if possible.
9. Loop diuretics and alpha blockers should be avoided because of the increased risk of falls.
10. Increase the dose of the first drug, then add a second drug of a different class or substitute a drug from another class.

The use of antihypertensive drugs has been shown to be effective and well tolerated in older adults. The prescription is "to proceed slowly and with caution" and to monitor for adverse reactions. If this principle is adhered to, side effects will be minimal in older adults. Table 17.1 provides the classifications of antihypertensive drugs, their adverse effects, and the nursing implications.

Diuretics. The thiazide diuretics, namely, hydrochlorothiazide and chlorthalidone, continue to be the most commonly prescribed antihypertensive agents for older adults. Initial dosing should start at 12.5 mg – 25 mg/day. Loop diuretics, such as furosemide, are not used unless patients have kidney disease or CHF.

The primary concerns related to diuretic therapy are hypotension, hypokalemia, and hyponatremia. Patients should be aware of the signs and symptoms of hypotension, hypokalemia, and hyponatremia. If hypokalemia continues despite supplementing with potassium, then a potassium-sparing diuretic, such as spironolactone, may be prescribed. With potassium-sparing diuretics, hyperkalemia can occur; therefore, close potassium monitoring is still warranted. Hyponatremia is a common side effect of hydrochlorothiazides. Hypomagnesemia, hyperglycemia, and increased uric acid may also occur. Increases in blood glucose are generally minor with low doses of a thiazide diuretic.

Beta-blockers. Beta-blockers (BBs) are preferred in adults with heart failure with reduced ejection fraction (HFrEF) (Whelton et al., 2018). BBs are effective in lowering morbidity and mortality in older adults. Beta-adrenergic blockage decreases heart rate and contractility. This decreases cardiac workload and is cardioprotective. BBs, such as atenolol and metoprolol, are cardioselective BBs. Noncardioselective BBs include carvedilol. Cardioselective BBs may be better tolerated in older adults with lung disease or PVD. However, carvedilol is the preferred beta-blocker for patients with HFrEF (Whelton et al, 2018).

ACEI. ACEIs inhibit the converting enzyme responsible for the formation of angiotensin II, a potent vasoconstrictor that stimulates the release of aldosterone. These drugs decrease mortality in older adults with decreased left ventricular function and preserve renal function in those with DM. Side effects of these drugs include rash, cough, taste disturbance, neutropenia, and proteinuria. ACEIs should not be used if acute renal failure or bilateral RAS are suspected.

Calcium channel blockers. Calcium channel blockers (CCBs) inhibit the inward movement of calcium across the cell membrane of the VSM, which results in vasodilatation of peripheral, coronary, and renal arteries. They may cause orthostatic hypotension in older adults. These drugs typically have vasodilator effects such as headaches, flushing, dizziness, and weakness. Constipation may also occur. CCBs are useful drugs in treating older adults and may be used when diuretics are not tolerated or are contraindicated.

Prognosis

HTN, if unrecognized and untreated, significantly increases the risk of coronary disease, heart and renal failure, and stroke. Risk increases with smoking, glucose intolerance, hyperlipidemia, left ventricular hypertrophy, male gender, Black race, and increasing age. With an individualized pharmacologic and nonpharmacologic treatment program based on an assessment of total cardiovascular risk, the risk of cardiovascular-related death from stroke and heart attack may be reduced. The degree of end-organ damage affects overall morbidity and mortality (Whelton et al, 2018).

Nursing Care Guidelines for the Older Adult with Hypertension

Recognize cues (assessment). The majority of patients with HTN are asymptomatic. Subjective data are obtained through careful, in-depth history. Symptoms that do occur are variable, depending on the progression of disease in target organs. Vague discomfort, fatigue, headaches, epistaxis, and dizziness may be early indicators. Severe HTN may result in a throbbing headache—particularly prevalent in the morning but disappearing several hours later—as well as confusion, vision loss, focal deficits, and coma. Symptoms of CHF, such as dyspnea, may be present. If the kidneys are affected, hematuria or nocturia may occur.

Objective data are obtained from a thorough assessment of BP on 3 separate occasions. BP readings should be recorded with the patient in both the sitting and standing positions and in both arms. The patient's arms should be bared and supported at heart level. The nurse should instruct the patient not to ingest caffeine or smoke for 30 minutes before the BP reading. The proper cuff size must be used. The bladder of the cuff should surround a minimum of 80% of the arm. Many older individuals will require a large cuff. If these steps are not taken, BP readings may be inaccurate. If BP differs from each arm, then the higher BP should be recorded and used to diagnose HTN.

Analyze cues and prioritize hypotheses (patient problems). Patient problems for an older adult with HTN include the following:

- Potential for injury
- Need for patient teaching resulting from new diagnoses of HTN, self-care management, and interventions
- Poor coping mechanisms resulting from perceived limitations of diagnosis

TABLE 17.1 Classification of Antihypertensive Drugs

Antihypertensive Drug	Adverse Effects	Precautions
Diuretics		
Thiazide Diuretics		
Chlorothiazide	Hyperglycemia	Patients with DM may require an increase in insulin.
Chlorthalidone	Hypokalemia	Encourage patients to restrict their sodium intake and eat foods high in potassium
Hydrochlorothiazide	Hypomagnesemia	
Indapamide	Hyponatremia	Check baseline and later levels of LDL and HDL, cholesterol, and triglycerides
Metolazone	Hyperuricemia	
	Hypercholesterolemia	Report dry mouth, muscle weakness, cramps, drowsiness, and loss of appetite, which may be indicative of an electrolyte imbalance
	Sexual dysfunction	
	Photosensitivity	
	Hypersensitivity to sulfonamides	Be cautious in sunlight
Loop Diuretics		
Bumetanide	Fluid electrolyte imbalance	Observe for signs of dehydration and acid–base imbalance
Furosemide	Diuresis leads to hypovolemia, hypotension, and shock	Monitor BP to detect signs and symptoms of shock
Torsemide	May cause thromboembolism in older patients	Observe for signs and symptoms of thromboembolism
Potassium-Sparing Diuretics		
Amiloride	Hyperkalemia	Monitor serum potassium levels
Triamterene	May cause breast pain and amenorrhea in females	Potassium supplements should be discontinued when these drugs are added to a sulfonamide diuretic regimen
	May cause renal calculi	
	Impotence, sexual dysfunction	Triamterene should be given cautiously to patients taking indomethacin
Aldosterone Receptor Blockers (also potassium-sparing diuretics)		
Eplerenone	Hyperkalemia	Monitor electrolytes, especially potassium
Spironolactone	GI bleeding or ulceration	Use K sparingly
		Do not give NSAIDs
Beta-Blockers		
Atenolol	Cardiac effects, including bradycardia and heart block	Report bradycardia and episodes of dizziness and syncope
Betaxolol	Dizziness and fainting	Do not administer drugs to patients with CHF or advanced degrees of heart block
Bisoprolol	Fatigue, weakness, lethargy, depression, disorientation, and hallucinations	
Metoprolol		Observe the patient for any changes in physical and mental status
Nadolol	Sexual dysfunction	
Propranolol	Nausea, vomiting	Check LDL, HDL, triglyceride, and cholesterol levels.
Timolol	Bronchospasm in patients with asthma	Instruct patients to avoid abrupt discontinuation of the drug
	May mask hypoglycemia	
	May aggravate peripheral vascular insufficiency	
Beta-Blockers with Intrinsic Sympathomimetic Activity		
Acebutolol	Fatigue, dizziness, headache, urinary frequency	Avoid abrupt discontinuation of drug
Penbutolol	May mask hypoglycemia or hyperthyroidism	Monitor weight, blood sugar, and vital signs
Pindolol	Constipation, diarrhea	
	Insomnia	
	Safety concerns	
	Bradycardia, edema, weight gain, hypotension, syncope, and atrioventricular block	
	Diarrhea, nausea, hyperglycemia, abnormal vision, dyspnea	
Combined Alpha- and Beta-Blockers		
Carvedilol	Fatigue, dizziness, postural hypotension, muscle weakness, diarrhea, or constipation	Avoid driving during initial administration
Labetalol		Take it with food
		Report any new cough that continues
		Report any unusual swelling of the extremities

TABLE 17.1 Classification of Antihypertensive Drugs—cont'd

Antihypertensive Drug	Adverse Effects	Precautions
Diuretics		
Angiotensin-Converting Enzyme Inhibitor (ACEIs)		
Benazepril Captopril Enalapril Fosinopril Lisinopril Moexipril Perindopril Quinapril Ramipril Trandolapril	Tickle in the throat or hacking cough Hyperkalemia Rash Reversible renal failure in patients with proteinuria or renal artery stenosis Dizziness, headache, diarrhea, and fatigue Impaired sense of taste and sexual dysfunction are rare	Observe patients for coughs Check the electrolytes for an increase in potassium Observe for rash Check for an increase in BUN or serum creatinine levels Observe for signs of dizziness, headache, and diarrhea
Angiotensin II Blockers		
Azilsartan Candesartan Eprosartan Irbesartan Losartan Olmesartan Telmisartan Valsartan	Dizziness, cough, upper respiratory infection, diarrhea, fatigue, and headache Edema, flushing, and palpitations. Serious reactions include angioedema, anaphylaxis, severe hypotension, hyperkalemia, kidney dysfunction, and rhabdomyolysis.	Monitor renal function Instruct the patient to avoid alcohol, barbiturates, and narcotics Adjust insulin and antidiabetic drugs, which potentiate hydrochlorothiazide, headaches, and dizziness Potentiated by grapefruit juice Avoid BBs, digitalis, and diuretics Do not crush Monitor liver studies in older patients
Calcium Channel Blockers (CCBs)		
Nondihydropyridines		
Diltiazem Verapamil	Headache, dizziness, flushing, and weakness Bradycardia Edema Nausea Constipation (especially with verapamil) Gingival hyperplasia	Monitor HR Monitor BP during dose adjustment Check laboratory results to assess liver and kidney function
Dihydropyridines		
Amlodipine Felodipine Isradipine extended release Nicardipine sustained release Nifedipine long-acting Nisoldipine	Edema, fatigue, palpitations, dizziness, abdominal pain, GI upset, flushing Drowsiness	Monitor for hepatic dysfunction, CVD, and/or aortic stenosis
Alpha₁-Blockers		
Doxazosin Prazosin Terazosin	Syncope with the first dose, dizziness, fatigue, edema, rhinitis, tinnitus, epistaxis, sexual dysfunction, polyuria, urinary incontinence, ataxia, leukopenia, neutropenia, arrhythmia, somnolence, rash, red eyes, dry mouth	Monitor BP Check orthostatic BP Limit ethanol (EtOH)
Central Alpha₂-Agonists and Other Centrally Acting Drugs		
Clonidine Methyldopa Reserpine Guanfacine	Dry mouth, drowsiness, dizziness, weakness, constipation, rash, myalgia, urticaria, nausea, insomnia, agitation, orthostatic hypotension, impotence, and arrhythmias	Monitor BP and supervise ambulation initially due to risk of orthostatic hypotension Monitor fluid and electrolyte status Do not stop abruptly
Direct Vasodilators		
Hydralazine	Headache, tachycardia, angina, palpitations, nausea, vomiting, and diarrhea; serious reactions include MI, severe hypotension, neutropenia, blood dyscrasias, lupus-like syndrome, peripheral neuritis, and hypersensitivity reaction	Monitor BP and HR; monitor for signs and symptoms of lupus with long-term therapy; monitor periodic BUN, creatinine, uric acid, potassium glucose, and ECG

Continued

TABLE 17.1 Classification of Antihypertensive Drugs—cont'd

Antihypertensive Drug	Adverse Effects	Precautions
Diuretics Minoxidil	Hypertrichosis, edema, tachycardia, breast tenderness, weight gain, paresthesia, headache, and ECG abnormalities; serious reactions include pericarditis, pericardial effusion, cardiac tamponade, HF, angina, Stevens-Johnson syndrome, and toxic epidermal necrolysis	Monitor BP and pulse; do not stop drug abruptly, as this could result in MI or CVA; monitor fluid and electrolyte balance periodically; monitor weight and report weight gain of 2 lb in 1 day; monitor for edema and signs, symptoms of HF, and a paradoxical pulse

ACEIs, angiotensin-converting enzyme inhibitors; *BUN,* blood urea nitrogen; *CVA,* cerebrovascular disease; *CVD,* cardiovascular disease; *ETOH,* ethanol; *GI,* gastrointestinal; *HDL,* high-density lipoprotein; *K,* potassium; *LDL,* low-density lipoprotein; *MI,* myocardial infarction; *NSAIDs,* nonsteroidal antiinflammatory drugs.
Data From Whelton, P. K., Carey, R. M., Aronow, W. S., Casey, D. E., Collins, K. J., Himmelfarb, C. D., et al. (2017). 2017 ACC/AHA/AAPA/ABC/ACPM/AGS/APhA/ASH/ASPC/NMA/PCNA guideline for the prevention, detection, evaluation, and management of high blood pressure in adults: A report of the American College of Cardiology/American Heart Association Task Force on Clinical Practice Guidelines. *Hypertension, 71*(6), e13–e115.

- Inadequate nutrition resulting from high fat, caloric, and sodium intake, as well as altered taste

Generate solutions (planning). Expected outcomes for an older patient with HTN include the following:
1. The patient will identify personal risk factors.
2. The patient will explain the disease process and its effects on health and well-being.
3. The patient will incorporate nonpharmacologic treatment measures into their daily lives.
4. The patient will demonstrate the proper use of an automated BP device.
5. The patient will verbalize purpose, dose, action, and significant and reportable side effects of drugs prescribed for HTN.
6. The patient will verbalize the need to increase social interaction.
7. The patient will develop a meal plan that includes a low-fat, low-cholesterol, and reduced-sodium diet.

Take actions (nursing interventions). Knowledge levels vary among older adults with HTN. The teaching plan should incorporate an explanation of the disease process and therapeutic (nonpharmacologic and pharmacologic) interventions. An explanation of the physical examination and appropriate tests should be given to allay anxiety. Anxiety, depression, denial, and fear are often involved in a chronic condition. Although these emotions diminish as the condition is controlled, the patient's ability to absorb this information and make the required changes is initially hampered because the patient may be in denial. For older adults, participation in community-based programs by the AHA or other agencies may be beneficial. It is crucial that any interventions take into account the physiologic changes of aging; for example, using large print and making sure that printed material is appropriate for the patient's culture and educational level.

Patient education includes providing information regarding the disease process, including risk factors for HTN; signs and symptoms of HTN; treatment regimen; drugs and their actions and side effects, including sexual dysfunction; and the need for frequent monitoring of BP. The nurse should explain the importance of a low-sodium, high-potassium, low-fat, and reduced-calorie diet. Weight loss should be encouraged, if indicated. A dietitian may assist with meal planning, preparation, and label reading. Foods are healthier if prepared by baking, broiling, or steaming. The nurse should also discuss the importance of alcohol restriction and smoking cessation; explain the relationships between stress, anxiety, anger, and HTN; identify stressful situations at the patient's home and work; and teach meditation and relaxation techniques. Exercise is beneficial for weight loss and stress reduction. Exercises should include moderate or vigorous aerobic and high-intensity muscle strengthening activities. Older adults should gradually increase their physical activity to a weekly goal of 75 minutes of vigorous or 150 minutes of moderate intensity aerobic exercise and at least 2 days per week of muscle-strengthening activities. Other activities include mall walking and water aerobics. Encourage the patient to reduce or eliminate smoking through a smoking cessation program. Prescription and OTC drugs and other supports are available for smoking cessation. Other alternatives for smoking cessation include hypnotism or behavior modification. Positive reinforcement should be provided whenever possible.

Evaluate outcomes (evaluation). Evaluation consists of determining the patient's achievement of the expected outcomes. The patient's BP should decrease and return to optimal levels. The patient should be able to maintain the treatment plan with minimal side effects or complications. Outcome measures related to QoL are also important because of the chronic nature of HTN. The nurse must determine the patient's perception of any change in QoL resulting from the prescribed therapeutic regimen. Documentation includes accurate records of BP, weight, exercise, and activity patterns; 24-hour dietary intake; cholesterol levels; and any BP monitoring results outside the clinical encounter.

Risk Factors for Heart Disease

Risk factors are classified as nonmodifiable and modifiable (Box 17.1). Age, gender, and family history are risk factors that cannot be modified. Smoking, HBP, a high-fat diet, obesity, physical inactivity, and stress are amenable to change. Research has demonstrated that the adoption of a healthier lifestyle has the potential to reduce or prevent the incidence of morbidity and death from ischemic heart disease and stroke.

Diet

Elevated serum cholesterol levels are a major risk factor for CHD. A total cholesterol (TC) level of 150 milligrams per

> **BOX 17.1   Risk Factors for Cardiovascular Disease**
>
> **Nonmodifiable**
> - Male gender
> - Age (males >45 years, females >55 years)
> - Heredity (including ethnicity)
> - Family history of premature CVD (males <55 years, females <65 years)
>
> **Modifiable**
> - Cigarette smoking / tobacco use
> - HTN or on antihypertensive drugs
> - Physical inactivity
> - Overweight / obesity (body mass index [BMI] 30 kg/m² or higher)
> - DM (HbA1c >6.5%)
> - Atherogenic diet (high intake of sugar, low-calorie sweeteners, high sodium, saturated fats, and cholesterol)
> - Dyslipidemia (high LDL or low HDL cholesterol levels)

BMI, body mass index; CVD, cardiovascular disease; HbA1c, hemoglobin A1c; HDL, high density lipoproteins; kg/m², kilograms per square meter; LDL, low-density lipoproteins; MI, myocardial infarction. Data From Arnett, D. K., Blumenthal, R. S., Albert, M. A., Buroker, A. B., Goldberger, Z. D., Hahn, E. J., et al. (2019). 2019 ACC/AHA guideline on the primary prevention of cardiovascular disease: A report of the American College of Cardiology/American Heart Association Task Force on Clinical Practice Guidelines. *Circulation, 140*(11), e596–646.

deciliter (mg/dL) is the point at which atherosclerosis begins to accelerate. Approximately 28 million adults aged 20 and over have a TC of 240 mg/dL or greater (Benjamin et al, 2017). Females have a higher prevalence of hypercholesterolemia than males. The risk for CHD increases even with modestly elevated cholesterol. The serum levels of LDL and HDL are also important to monitor. LDL (bad cholesterol) carries cholesterol to the walls of the arteries (a positive risk factor), and HDL (good cholesterol) removes LDL from the arterial walls and transports it back to the liver (a negative risk factor). HDL cholesterol levels should be above 60 mg/dL, and LDL cholesterol levels should be below 100 mg/dL (Stone et al, 2014). The levels of cholesterol are taken in context with other risk factors (e.g., diabetes and smoking).

Decreasing fat content in the diet is the first step in reducing TC levels. The American Heart Association (AHA) recommends reducing the risk of CVD by limiting the intake of saturated and *trans* fats to less than 6% of total calories (AHA, 2020). Because of the increased risk of CVD in older adults, even seemingly small improvements in risk factors (i.e., small reductions in BP and LDL cholesterol level through diet and lifestyle changes) are of great benefit. However, because older individuals have decreased energy needs yet their vitamin and mineral requirements remain constant or increase, they should be counseled to select nutrient-dense choices within each food group (Napierkowski and Prado, 2021).

Smoking

Smoking continues to be a major risk factor in the development of heart disease, even though a decline in tobacco use has occurred, largely as a result of health promotion (HP) campaigns, clean air environments, and peer pressure. Cigarette smoking greatly increases an individual's risk of stroke, and smokers are more likely to develop CVD than nonsmokers (Benjamin et al, 2017). Smoking increases platelet aggregation and causes coronary artery spasms. Nicotine increases BP and cardiac demands. Carbon monoxide in tobacco smoke decreases the oxygen-carrying capacity of the blood.

Even smoking a few cigarettes per day greatly increases cardiac risk. Smoking cessation decreases the risk of myocardial infarction (MI). After 10 years of abstinence, an individual's risk is the same as that of a nonsmoker. Smoking cessation should be encouraged at every patient encounter. The Agency for Health care Research and Quality (AHRQ) and Research has established recommendations for smoking cessation (see Chapter 18 for smoking cessation information).

Physical Activity

A sedentary lifestyle is another modifiable cardiac risk factor. The AHA (2021a) recommends moderate to vigorous aerobic activity for a total of 75–150 minutes per week (such as brisk walking) and moderate-to-high-intensity muscle-strengthening activity at least 2 days per week.

Before aerobic exercises, a 10–15-minute warm-up is recommended to allow for a gradual increase in HR and breathing. Walking is the best aerobic exercise for older adults. They may set their own pace, decide the location, and avoid injuries. Health-care professionals should encourage patients to exercise and promote ways to increase activity with daily routines such as parking the car a little farther from the store or using the stairs rather than the elevator.

Obesity

Obesity is another modifiable cardiac risk factor. Obesity is usually associated with a sedentary lifestyle and a high-fat diet, which add to the individual's cardiac risk profile. A healthy body weight is currently defined as a BMI of 18.5–25 kilograms per square meter (kg/m²). Overweight is a BMI between 25 and 29.9 kg/m², and obesity is a BMI of 30 kg/m² or greater (CDC, 2022). Currently, more than one-third of adults are obese (Ogden et al, 2015). The data from the 2011–2014 National Health and Nutrition Examination Survey (NHANES) revealed that 37% of adults aged 60 and over were obese (Ogden et al, 2015). Excess body weight increases cardiovascular risk factors (e.g., by increasing LDL, BP, and blood glucose levels and by reducing HDL levels). Benefits of any physical activity include fewer joint and muscle pains, improved sleep patterns, and a reduction in developing T2DM (AHA, 2014).

Diabetes Mellitus

Hyperglycemia is related to the incidence of CVDs, which include CHD, stroke, peripheral vascular disease (PVD), cardiomyopathy, and CHF (Stone et al, 2014). Individuals with DM are two times more likely to die of cardiovascular causes, and the presence of diabetes is associated with an increased prevalence of HTN and dyslipidemia (AHA, 2021a). Silent MI (asymptomatic MI) is more common in individuals with DM and in older adults. Thus, older adults with DM should be monitored closely for other symptoms of CVD.

Stress

Everyone manages stress differently. Some people respond to stress by overeating, smoking, physical inactivity, or drinking. How a person reacts to stressful situations has a direct effect on their health. Excessive stress can trigger asthma and lead to HTN and irritable bowel syndrome (IBS). Excessive stress has also been linked to CHD. Our bodies respond to stressful events by triggering the *fight or flight* response (adrenaline is released, causing tachypnea, tachycardia, and HTN) (AHA, 2021b).

Stress can be decreased in many ways, and much literature is available on the topic. Yoga, tai chi, meditation, relaxation tapes, visualization, positive self-talk, doing something enjoyable, and physical activity are a few of the methods used. Nurses must help older adults examine environmental issues that cause stress and work with them to find ways to manage the stress (AHA, 2021b; AHA, 2021c).

Menopause

Before menopause, estrogen is believed to have a protective effect by helping to maintain adequate levels of HDL cholesterol and relaxing the smooth muscles of the arteries, which helps maintain normal blood pressure. However, it is believed that these beneficial effects are lost after menopause, and this corresponds to the time when the rate of CHD-related death for females begins to increase (AHA, 2021d).

Coronary Artery Disease

Coronary artery disease (CAD), or ischemic heart disease, refers to a broad group of conditions that partially or completely obstruct blood flow to the heart muscle. Obstruction of coronary arteries may result in ischemia (an imbalance between the oxygen supply and demands of the heart) or infarction (death or necrosis) of the myocardium. Ischemia and infarction occur when the oxygen supply is unable to meet the demands of the heart. Atherosclerosis is the usual cause of CAD; angina, MI, and sudden death may be the final outcomes.

Atherosclerosis usually begins in childhood and is characterized by a local accumulation of lipid and fibrous tissue along the intimal layer of the artery. Lipids accumulate and infiltrate the area, forming a raised fibrous plaque over the site. Eventually, the plaque becomes calcified, which causes the vessel to lose its elasticity and ability to dilate. Progressive narrowing of the artery occurs, resulting in compromised blood flow to the area of the myocardium supplied by that vessel. In the advanced stages of the disease, hemorrhage into the atheromatous plaque, thrombus formation, embolization of a thrombus or plaque fragment, and coronary arterial spasm may cause additional insult to the body. The incidence of atherosclerosis increases with age; the severity of this process may be accelerated by the adverse lifestyle behaviors of smoking, physical inactivity, and obesity, as well as elevated serum cholesterol levels, HTN, and DM. Promoting healthy lifestyles in younger and older individuals is an important aspect of care in the prevention of CAD. The adoption of healthier lifestyles by an older adult may be difficult because of long-term habits; however, healthy behavior changes may slow or halt the progression of the disease (Brodkey, 2022).

CAD is the major cause of morbidity, disability, and mortality in the older adult population. Alterations in cardiac function are likely to cause the older adult to feel afraid or unsure about the future. However, overwhelming fear can interfere with rehabilitation and staying well (AHA, n.d.).

Stable angina is caused by inadequate blood flow to the myocardium. The classic symptom is chest pain during activity that is relieved with rest or nitroglycerin. MI is caused by total disruption of blood flow to an area of the myocardium; it is characterized by more severe, more intense chest pain for a longer time than that associated with stable angina. Other symptoms that may accompany MI include nausea, diaphoresis, shortness of breath, dizziness, and weakness.

But, most often, older adults do not present with classic symptoms. An atypical presentation of MI in an older adult may include vague symptoms such as fatigue, weakness, dizziness, nausea, confusion, and a decline in functional status. More often, older adults report shortness of breath rather than chest pain (Box 17.2). Possible reasons for the atypical presentation include age-related physiologic changes and loss of physiologic reserve, the interaction between acute and chronic conditions, and underreporting of symptoms. Females, especially older females, may not exhibit the classic signs of CAD, and the nurse needs to be aware of this to adequately assess female patients (Garcia et al, 2016). Because symptoms of acute coronary syndrome (ACS) or MI may be vague and atypical of textbook symptoms, older adults may not recognize their seriousness and may not seek medical attention as soon as they should. This may cause a delay in seeking medical attention. Unrecognized ACS or MI may cause permanent cardiac damage and precipitate complications of CHF and pulmonary edema (PE).

Diagnostic Tests and Procedures

Diagnosis is based on patient history, alterations on the ECG, and serum cardiac enzyme levels.

- A 12-lead ECG should be obtained to gather information on rate, rhythm, hypertrophy, and myocardial injury (ischemia or infarction) and to assess for Q waves, ST segment elevation, ST segment depression, and T wave inversion (Zafari and Abdou, 2019).
- Cardiac biomarkers / enzymes: the ACC and AHA recommend cardiac troponin should be obtained when MI is suspected. Troponin (a contractile protein released in the setting of myocardial necrosis) rises when infarction changes cell membrane permeability. Cardiac troponin T increases

---

BOX 17.2 Symptoms Associated with the Atypical Presentation of CAD in Older Adults

- Shortness of breath
- Fatigue
- Weakness
- Nausea
- Dizziness or syncope
- Confusion
- Decrease in functional status
- Abdominal or back pain

3–5 hours after MI and remains elevated for 14–21 days. Cardiac troponin I rises within 3 hours, peaks at 14–18 hours, and remains elevated for 5–7 days (Zafari and Abdou, 2019).
- Complete blood count (CBC) to determine whether angina is caused by anemia (Zafari and Abdou, 2019).
- A comprehensive metabolic panel should be drawn to monitor serum electrolytes, particularly sodium, potassium, and calcium. Elevated or reduced levels of these electrolytes can lead to fluid imbalance or ventricular arrhythmias (Zafari and Abdou, 2019).
- Serum lactate dehydrogenase (LDH) levels rise within 24 hours of an MI, peak in 3–6 days, and return to baseline in 8–12 days (Zafari and Abdou, 2019).
- A chest radiography is used to determine the presence of cardiomegaly, PE, or other indications of CHF (Singh and Aggarwal, 2018).
- A color-flow Doppler transthoracic echocardiography or Doppler echocardiography is used to evaluate wall motion and ventricular performance and detect pericardial effusion and valvular disease (Singh and Agarwal, 2018).
- A Coronary angiography is used to detect the presence, location, and extent of lesions in coronary arteries (Singh and Aggarwal, 2018).
- Exercise stress tests are used to determine activity tolerance. Stress tests may be combined with myocardial imaging to identify changes in myocardial perfusion during exercise. In the absence of an acute cardiac event such as MI, an exercise stress test may be troublesome for older adults with coexisting diseases such as arthritis, PVD, and COPD. Pharmacologic stress tests may be a better choice for these older individuals (Garcia et al, 2016). For older adults who are not able to complete an exercise stress test, dobutamine-stress echocardiography is an option (Singh and Aggarwal, 2018).

Pharmacologic Treatment

Treatment of CAD is directed toward restoring the balance between myocardial oxygen demand and oxygen supply. Pharmacologic therapy plays a major role. Normal changes with aging (e.g., alterations in body mass, water composition, liver size, renal system, and plasma protein concentration) alter the metabolism and excretion of many drugs, so smaller doses are generally prescribed for older adults.

Nitrates. Nitrates are used for the prevention and termination of anginal attacks and for reducing the pain associated with myocardial ischemia. These drugs decrease cardiac preloading and afterload, which reduces the myocardial demand for oxygen. These changes occur due to the vasodilating effects of nitrates on coronary arteries and peripheral vasculature. Intravenous (IV), sublingual, and aerosol preparations have a rapid onset of action (1–3 minutes) and are used to prevent or terminate an anginal attack. Oral and transdermal preparations have a prolonged effect and are used to prevent anginal attacks. Tolerance to oral and transdermal nitrate preparations reduces drug effectiveness; an 8–12-hour nitrate-free interval can reduce tolerance (Fillit et al, 2017). Headache, flushing, dizziness, hypotension, syncope, and tachycardia are side effects attributed to the vasodilating effects. Nitrates are effective in older adults; however, aggressive therapy to reduce preload and afterload may trigger reflex tachycardia and severe orthostatic hypotension. Older adults should take rapid-acting nitrates in the sitting position or supine to prevent falls and should sit up slowly with assistance (Aroesty and Kannam, 2022).

Beta-blockers. Beta-blockers (BBs) are used in patients with stable angina to decrease the frequency of angina or to reduce the size of the infarction and complications of MI. Blockage of beta-adrenergic receptors in the heart decreases sympathetic nervous stimulation, reducing heart rate, stroke volume, and contractility; this leads to decreased myocardial oxygen requirements. Side effects include bradycardia, hypotension, dyspnea, dizziness, syncope, gait difficulties, sexual dysfunction, CHF, heart block, bronchoconstriction, and depression. For patients with lung disease, metoprolol and atenolol are safer drugs, as they are cardioselective. Sudden cessation of therapy may induce myocardial ischemia. Older adults are more sensitive to decreased heart rate, leading to decreased exercise performance and possible syncope (Aroesty and Kannam, 2022).

Calcium channel blockers. Calcium channel blockers (CCBs) are used to treat stable and variant angina and to increase coronary perfusion, reduce BP, and decrease myocardial contractility in individuals with MI. CCBs slow electrical conduction through the heart (to varying degrees), decrease the force of cardiac contraction, and dilate blood vessels by blocking the entry of calcium ions into VSM cells, thereby decreasing myocardial oxygen demand and increasing coronary perfusion. Adverse reactions include bradycardia, constipation, hypotension, flushing, dizziness, syncope, headaches, dyspnea, palpitations, and peripheral edema. Verapamil and diltiazem are not recommended in older adults because they significantly slow electrical conduction through the heart, decreasing HR and increasing the incidence of heart block. Amlodipine, a dihydropyridine CCB, is recommended for older adults because it does not slow cardiac electrical conduction to the extent that nondihydropyridines do (Aroesty and Kannam, 2022; Whelton et al, 2018).

Fibrinolytics, anticoagulants, and antiplatelets. Fibrinolytics, anticoagulants, and antiplatelets are used to prevent, reduce, and dissolve thrombi around atherosclerotic plaques by altering blood-clotting mechanisms. Fibrinolytic or thrombolytic drugs are given intravenously within 6 hours of the onset of symptoms. Patients must be observed for bleeding, arrhythmia, and allergic reactions. Older adults have an increased risk of bleeding with fibrinolytics. Heparin, followed by oral anticoagulation such as warfarin, should be administered after fibrinolytic therapy to prevent secondary clot formation.

Heparin and warfarin are anticoagulants used to prevent the enlargement of existing thrombi and new clot formation after MI. Therapeutic effects of heparin are monitored by PTTs; the antidote is protamine sulfate. Warfarin is monitored by the international normalized ratio (INR); the antidote is vitamin K. Patients who initially receive heparin for anticoagulation and who need oral anticoagulation for maintenance usually take both forms of the drug for 3–5 days to develop therapeutic blood levels. As with thrombolytics, bleeding is a complication. Patients should be educated on signs and symptoms of bleeding, such as unexplained bruising, dark and tarry stools, and bleeding that is not controlled within 15 minutes.

Aspirin, an antiplatelet, decreases the mortality rate of acute MI. It inhibits platelet aggregation and facilitates fibrinolysis. Its effects on platelets occur within 20 minutes of administration. Many aspirin preparations are available. The dose for aspirin can be 81 mg or 325 mg/day.

Lipid-lowering drugs. Lipid-lowering drugs are used to lower serum lipid levels by preventing the absorption of cholesterol and promoting its secretion. Side effects common to all lipid-lowering agents, regardless of class, include diarrhea, constipation, nausea, abdominal pain, and elevation in liver function studies. Lipid-lowering drugs are given to reduce the risk of MI and stroke. They should be prescribed if dietary and activity measures are ineffective in lowering cholesterol, triglycerides, and LDLs. Although some older adults may benefit from lipid-lowering drugs (those with established atherosclerosis), there is debate concerning their benefit for adults over 65. In adults over 75, there is concern that the risk of harm outweighs any benefit (Zoungas, 2017). Older adults and their families should discuss the issue with their health-care providers. When taking lipid-lowering drugs, the benefits related to CAD and stroke prevention should clearly outweigh the potential risk associated with drug therapy (Banach and Serban, 2016; Zoungas, 2017).

Nonpharmacologic Treatment

At each encounter with the health-care system, as appropriate, older adults should be encouraged to quit smoking and avoid second-hand smoke, develop healthy dietary habits, engage in routine exercise, maintain a healthy weight, and manage stress. Improvement in each of these factors has the potential to reduce the progression of CAD.

Surgical Procedures

Percutaneous transluminal coronary angioplasty. Percutaneous transluminal coronary angioplasty (PTCA) is performed to open blocked coronary arteries. In this minimally invasive procedure, a balloon-tipped catheter is inserted through the femoral artery, under fluoroscopy and advanced until it has reached the occluded coronary artery. The balloon is then inflated to compress the obstructing plaque, resulting in a larger vessel lumen and improved blood flow to the myocardium. A *stent* may be placed to keep the vessel open and maintain blood flow through the coronary artery.

Coronary artery bypass graft surgery. Coronary artery bypass graft (CABG) is a surgical procedure to improve blood flow to the ischemic myocardium. During surgery, portions of the saphenous vein or internal mammary artery are grafted to sites above and below the obstructed coronary artery.

Coronary Artery Disease in Females

CAD is the leading cause of death and disability in females older than 55 years. It is estimated that 1 in every 5 females dies of heart disease (CDC, 2023c). Females have smaller coronary arteries that occlude more easily (Duda-Pyszny et al, 2018). Females also have a higher heart rate and stroke volume at rest and lower left ventricular end-diastolic pressure compared with males. Females over the age of 50 have a higher T-cell (TC) level than males. Females experience atypical symptoms associated with CAD, such as diaphoresis, epigastric pain, and shortness of breath.

Differences in treatment between females and males with CAD include the following: Females experience a longer interval between emergency department (ED) admission and the performance of the ECG. Females are less likely to be admitted to an intensive care unit (ICU). Females are less likely to receive thrombolytic therapy. Females have a higher incidence of total occlusion after PTCA. Females have an increased incidence of CABG after PTCA. Females experience more recurrent angina, CHF recurrent infarction, and strokes after MI. Females are referred less often for cardiac rehabilitation. Females have poorer attendance at cardiac rehabilitation if they are referred. Females are typically 10 years older than males when diagnosed with cardiac disease and experience worse outcomes than males (Garcia et al, 2016). The National Coalition for Females with Heart Disease (http://www.womenheart.org) provides information and resource links for both health-care professionals and females diagnosed with heart disease.

Prognosis

Age-related physiologic changes, longstanding unhealthy lifestyles, and chronic conditions in older adults may complicate the progress and treatment of CAD; however, advances in the medical and surgical treatments of CAD and the adoption of healthier lifestyles have the potential to positively influence disease outcomes in older adults.

Nursing Care Guidelines for the Older Adult with CAD

Recognize cues (assessment). Assessment of an older adult with CAD begins with a complete health history and physical examination. Complaints of dyspnea, fatigue, syncope, vertigo, and confusion warrant further investigation. Subjective data may have to be collected when vital signs are stable and discomfort is relieved (Box 17.3).

Specific health questions during the assessment (e.g., "Are you able to shop for groceries?") may elicit more detailed responses than open-ended questions (e.g., "What type of activities at home are difficult for you?"). When gathering objective data on older adults, nurses should keep in mind that slower heart rates, irregular heart rhythms, the presence of a third or fourth heart sound, systolic ejection murmurs, higher systolic BPs (SBPs), and wider pulse pressures may be a result of aging, not the current ischemic episode (Ball et al, 2014).

Analyze cues and prioritize hypotheses (patient problems). Patient problems common for an older patient with CAD include the following:

- Chest discomfort results from an imbalance between oxygen demand and supply
- Ineffective cardiac output results from decreased pumping ability in the heart
- Decreased activity level resulting from decreased cardiac output

> **BOX 17.3 Assessment of Patients with Chest Pain**
>
> **Subjective Data**
> - Chest pain (location, intensity, radiation, onset, and duration)
> - Precipitating factors (activity, emotions, rest, hot or cold exposure, and eating)
> - Associated symptoms (diaphoresis, dyspnea, vomiting, weakness, palpitations, and indigestion)
> - Relieving symptoms (rest and nitrates)
> - Prior hospitalization (for angina, MI, and other disorders)
> - Drugs
> - Family history (parents or siblings with CAD onset before age 50)
> - Modifiable cardiac risk factors (smoking, high cholesterol level, HTN, DM, obesity, and physical inactivity)
> - Psychosocial state (denial, anxiety, fear, or anger)
> - Activity levels
> - Support systems
>
> **Objective Data**
> - Behaviors (nervous, lethargic, rubbing chest, or grimacing)
> - Changes in vital signs
> - Changes in cardiac rhythm
> - Associated symptoms (diaphoresis, pallor, or cold and clammy skin)
> - Peripheral pulses (radial, femoral, and pedal)
> - Heart sounds and murmurs
> - Respiratory rate and breath sounds
> - Jugular vein distention
> - Diagnostic test results (cardiac enzymes, ECG, chest radiography, CBC, and electrolyte levels)

CAD, coronary artery disease; *CBC*, complete blood cell count; *ECG*, electrocardiogram; *MI*, myocardial infarction.

- Potential for nonadherence
- Anxiety resulting from fear of death

Generate solutions (planning). As with all patients, older adults with CAD should be included in the planning of care. Family should also be included in the planning process; however, older adults should be consulted to determine the extent of family involvement. Discharge planning should begin on admission to the hospital, and special attention should be given to the necessary support services in the home.

Expected outcomes for an older patient with CAD include the following:

1. The patient will verbalize pain relief.
2. The patient will maintain adequate perfusion with stable vital signs, mental alertness, urine output greater than 30 milliliters per hour (mL/hr), no ECG changes, and clear breath sounds.
3. The patient will tolerate activity without complaints of chest discomfort or dyspnea.
4. The patient will explain the disease process and therapeutic plan, including causes and risk factors for CAD; precipitating and alleviating factors for angina; and names, dosages, actions, and side effects of drugs.
5. The patient will describe actions to take in the event of chest pain.
6. The patient will express fears and have reduced anxiety.

Take actions (nursing interventions). Interventions for an older adult with CAD focus on relieving pain, improving myocardial blood flow, decreasing myocardial workload, and educating the patient.

Cardiovascular, respiratory, kidney, and neurologic assessments should be conducted on a regular basis to detect progress and prevent complications. Diagnostic testing, especially of potassium levels because older patients are prone to hyperkalemia, should be conducted and evaluated daily, and any adverse changes in patient status should be reported to the physician.

Older adults and their family members may express concern about emergency measures such as resuscitation or life support. Nurses should be sensitive to these needs and initiate discussion with the patient, family, and health-care team to establish a plan of action.

Older adults should be encouraged to participate in cardiac rehabilitation programs to restore their physical and mental health to the highest level of function. Cardiac rehabilitation promotes restoration, diminishes the effects of disease, and encourages optimal physical, psychological, and social functioning. Cardiac rehabilitation consists of 3 phases. Phase 1, or clinical phase, begins in the hospital and includes early ambulation and patient and family education. Phase 2, outpatient cardiac rehabilitation, lasts about 3–12 weeks and takes place in a supervised outpatient setting. Phase 3, post–cardiac rehabilitation, is a maintenance phase that lasts indefinitely; it includes counseling, exercise, education, and socialization (Tessler and Bordoni, 2023).

Exercise should be gradually increased during recovery. Older adults should be taught to monitor their pulse rate to evaluate their tolerance to activity. Walking, with a progressive increase in duration and frequency, is recommended. Heavy lifting should be avoided. Activities should be paced throughout the day. Older adults may benefit from a written plan of progressive activities. Properly designed exercise programs for older adults incorporate longer times for the return to a resting heart rate after exercise. Orthostatic hypotension is more common in the older population because of decreased baroreceptor sensitivity. Thermoregulation among older adults is impaired; thus, caution must be used during exercise in hot and humid environments.

Activities that build endurance, increase the level of self-care, and improve QoL should be encouraged. Activities to suggest include walking, swimming, water aerobics, bowling, and dancing. Older adults with unstable angina should not exercise. Those who require cardiac monitoring during rehabilitation include those who have an ejection fraction of less than 39%, a resting complex ventricular arrhythmia, or decreased BP during exercise. They also include those who escape sudden death, those who experience major complications due to the MI (e.g., CHF or shock), and those who demonstrate an inability to self-monitor their HR because of physical or cognitive impairment.

In spite of the documented benefits of cardiac rehabilitation programs, adherence to rehabilitation remains low. About 14%–35% of patients participate in cardiac rehabilitation (Tessler and Bordoni, 2023). Reasons for low participation include fear of exercise, lack of time, other medical problems, lack of transportation, personal and financial factors, and conflicts with work schedules (Supervía et al, 2017). Females have the poorest adherence to rehabilitation programs. Interdisciplinary teams should recognize these issues and make every effort to assist patients with these problems.

Sexual activity is an important aspect of QoL. The resumption of sexual activity should be discussed with older adults. It is generally safe to resume sexual activity within 4–6 weeks of MI, as long as an older adult is symptom-free during their usual daily activities. The equivalency or expenditure of energy for sexual activity correlates with the same energy expenditure required for climbing a flight of stairs or walking around the block. The pamphlet *Sex and Heart Disease* produced by the AHA may be used to supplement counseling (AHA, 2015).

Visiting nurse programs provide education, support, and supervised activities in the home environment if older patients are unable to attend outpatient services. Home-care services are usually available to assist older patients with ADLs. Both programs typically require physician referrals.

Local heart associations are excellent sources for learning materials and community programs on CAD. Some heart associations offer educational and support programs for patients recovering from CAD or surgery (e.g., Mended Hearts), and they usually provide direction for community programs on risk-factor reduction, cardiopulmonary resuscitation (CPR), and mall walking.

Evaluate outcomes (evaluation). Evaluation and documentation of the progress of an older patient with CAD focus on the achievement of goals outlined in the planning process.

Older adults should demonstrate adequate circulation, the ability to perform ADLs, and control of symptoms. Documentation should focus on the older adult's risk-factor profile and progress, and measures should be aimed at reducing risks because a reduction in behaviors associated with the identified risks will reduce morbidity and mortality (see Nursing Care Plan: Myocardial Infarction).

NURSING CARE PLAN
Myocardial Infarction

Clinical Situation

Mrs. S is an 84-year-old widow who was admitted to the hospital from a nursing facility with complaints of fatigue, weakness, and vertigo. Staff at the nursing facility became concerned after 2 episodes of syncope. Mrs. S suffered a stroke 4 years ago that left her with severe weakness in her left arm and left leg. She was unable to care for herself at home; her daughter encouraged her to enter the nursing facility. She has been following a diet low in saturated fat and cholesterol and takes enteric-coated aspirin daily, as well as levothyroxine for hypothyroidism. Mrs. S is mobile with the use of a walker.

A routine ECG showed pathologic Q waves. Cardiac enzymes were tested. Creatinine phosphokinase (CPK) levels were normal, but LDH was elevated. She was diagnosed with an inferior MI. Because she did not meet the time criteria for fibrinolytic therapy, the physician instituted prophylactic measures with oral anticoagulants (warfarin) on a daily basis. Mrs. S developed occasional premature ventricular contractions and periodic bouts of atrial fibrillation (AFib). Atenolol and nitroglycerin were added to her regimen. She became agitated in the coronary care unit about being a burden to her family and declined invasive treatment procedures. The nurse organized a meeting with the physician, daughter, and patient to discuss her anxiety, and a "no resuscitation" order was written. Lorazepam 1 milligram (mg), as needed 3 times a day, was added to the protocol.

Currently, Mrs. S denies having chest pain and can walk short distances with her walker. She follows a low-cholesterol, low-saturated-fat diet, and she is scheduled for ECG later in the week. Her BP is in the low-to-normal range, and her pulse is irregular at 102 beats per minute (beats/min).

Recognize Cues (Assessment)
- Advanced age with frailty, fatigue, weakness, and vertigo
- History of stroke with left hemiparesis and hypothyroidism
- Two (2) episodes of syncope
- Dependent on daughter for ADLs
- Diagnosis of acute MI
- Dysrhythmias with AFib and occasional premature ventricular contractions (PVCs)
- New medications include warfarin, atenolol, nitroglycerin, and lorazepam
- Agitation and concern about being a burden to family
- Able to ambulate short distances with a walker
- Low-saturated fat and low-cholesterol diet
- Scheduled for ECG

Analyze Cues and Prioritize Hypotheses (Patient Problems)
- Anxiety resulting from the threat of death and a change in health status
- Cardiac tissue injury related to decreased cardiac tissue perfusion as evidenced by pathologic Q waves and elevated cardiac biomarkers
- Dysrhythmia resulting from electrical dysfunction, as evidenced by PVCs and AFib
- Reduced stamina resulting from an imbalance of myocardial oxygen supply and demand and left peripheral limb weakness
- Potential for nonadherence resulting from lack of exposure to disease process and treatment plan

Generate Solutions and Evaluate Outcomes (Planning and Evaluation)
- The patient will verbalize reduced anxiety, as evidenced by a slower HR, reduced apprehension, and participation in self-care.
- The patient will obtain pain relief, as evidenced by verbal statements.
- The patient will maintain adequate circulation, as evidenced by stable vital signs, mental alertness, clear lung sounds, and urine output greater than 30 milliliters per hour (mL/hr).
- The patient will tolerate activity, as evidenced by stable vital signs; absence of pain, weakness, fatigue, and vertigo; and participation in activity.
- The patient will demonstrate knowledge of the disease process, symptoms of ischemia with appropriate responses, and the treatment plan, as evidenced by explanation of and participation in the plan.
- The patient will demonstrate an accurate pulse-taking method.

Take Actions (Nursing Interventions)
- Explain equipment, procedures, and unit routine.
- Encourage verbalization of feelings.
- Teach relaxation techniques and guided imagery to alleviate anxiety.
- Supervise tolerance to visitation.
- Offer lorazepam, as needed.
- Encourage participation in care and emphasize improvements in health status.
- Encourage relaying of pain sensations to the nurse.
- Explain how sensations of fatigue, weakness, and vertigo may be symptoms of ischemia and that these symptoms need to be reported to the nurse.
- Encourage the patient to take nitroglycerin at the onset of chest pain or at sensations of ischemia.

NURSING CARE PLAN—cont'd

- Obtain vital signs during episodes, and contact the physician if the drug is ineffective.
- Offer oxygen, if needed.
- Monitor the therapeutic effects of nitrates and atenolol, observing for hypotensive effects.
- Measure BP, apical pulse, and rhythm every 4 hours. Auscultate the heart and lungs every 8 hours.
- Monitor ECG for reversion to normal sinus rhythm, INR, and digoxin and electrolyte levels.
- Administer and evaluate the effects of warfarin and atenolol.
- Observe for signs of hemorrhage, shock, CHF, and emboli.
- Assist with ADLs, as needed.
- Remind the patient to perform leg exercises every hour and range-of-motion exercises. Apply antiembolic stockings.
- Before the patient ambulates, encourage the patient to do leg exercises and sit at the bedside for 3–5 minutes before standing.
- Gradually increase the distance and frequency of walking.
- Monitor vital signs before and after activity.
- Ensure that the call bell and walker are within reach.
- Encourage the patient to wear shoes with good support and to walk in lighted areas.
- Balance activity with rest.
- Teach the patient to count her own pulse.
- Encourage the patient to recognize sensations of ischemia and cease activity when they occur.
- Include the patient's daughter in teaching sessions.
- Describe the disease and healing process of MI using pictures, models, and large printed material.
- Describe the patient's sensations of ischemia and teach the appropriate use of nitrates and rest.
- Discuss and provide written information for drug dosage, purpose, side effects, and special precautions for warfarin, digoxin, and atenolol.
- Encourage a progressive increase in activity.
- Assess emotions and reassure the patient that depression is common.
- Teach the patient to take a radial pulse and to monitor it before, during, and after activity.

Arrhythmia

Arrhythmia is an abnormal heart rhythm caused by a disturbance in automaticity, conductivity, contractility, or a combination of the three. Arrhythmias can originate in the atria, atrioventricular (AV) junctions, ventricles, bundle of His, or Purkinje fibers and may result in decreased cardiac output and impaired perfusion of coronary arteries.

Older adults may develop any type of arrhythmia; however, AFib, sick sinus syndrome (SSS), and heart block occur more often in the older population due to the loss of cardiac pacemaker cells and the deposition of fat and fibrous tissue in some pathways of the conduction system. Older adults may also have comorbid conditions that damage heart muscle (e.g., HTN or diabetes) and place them at risk for arrhythmias (National Heart, Lung, and Blood Institute, 2022a). The incidence of AFib increases with age and is the most common contributing factor to ischemic stroke in older adults. According to the AHA, the incidence of stroke due to AFib among people aged 50–59 is 1.5%, whereas 23.5% of people aged 80–89 developed stroke due to AFib (Benjamin et al, 2017). In the setting of AFib, stroke is caused by an embolus from the heart that occludes a cerebral vessel. AFib is characterized by chaotic, rapid depolarization within the atria, and an irregular ventricular response. It is a common complication of MI or CABG. Older adults need increased diastolic filling pressures to compensate for structural changes within the heart and to maintain cardiac output, so chaotic or quivering depolarization within the atria diminishes the atrial kick needed for adequate ventricular filling (Ball et al, 2014).

AFib may be triggered or made worse by emotional stress, alcohol use, caffeine, cigarettes, and stimulant drugs. Chronic AFib tends to occur in patients with HTN, CAD, rheumatic heart disease (RHD), valvular heart disease (VHD), CHF, pericarditis, COPD, asthma, cardiomyopathy, hyperthyroidism, obesity, diabetes, sleep apnea, and viral infections (WebMD Editorial Contributors, 2022).

SSS increases the risk of developing AFib. It is characterized by alternating episodes of bradycardia (less than 60 beats/min), normal sinus rhythm (60–100 beats/min), tachycardia (greater than 100 beats/min), and periods of long sinus pauses that fail to stimulate the atria or ventricles. SSS tends to occur in patients with CAD, RHD, and HTN.

Heart block is characterized by delayed or blocked impulses between the atria and ventricles and is classified as first-, second-, or third-degree heart block; each respective classification increases in severity. First-degree block is common in older adults with or without CAD and is a common complication of MI. Digitalis preparations may also cause a first-degree heart block. Second- and third-degree blocks may be caused by degeneration within the conduction system, ischemia, enhanced vagal tone, electrolyte imbalance, and the effects of drugs (e.g., digoxin and BBs).

Symptoms of arrhythmia are related to decreased cardiac output and include weakness, fatigue, palpitations, dizziness, shortness of breath, confusion, chest pain, and syncope, all of which predispose older patients to falls and injuries. Patients with first-degree block and SSS may have no symptoms, whereas patients with AFib may have symptoms associated with rapid ventricular response.

Diagnostic Tests and Procedures

The diagnosis of arrhythmia is made by physical assessment, accompanied by an ECG evaluation, Holter monitor, or patient-activated event recorder. When an arrhythmia is diagnosed, a variety of tests may be performed to determine a causative factor.

Treatment

Treatment should be limited to symptomatic patients with significant arrhythmias.

AFib. The treatment of AFib has 3 objectives: (1) controlling the underlying cause, (2) slowing the heart rate and/or converting the rhythm to a normal sinus rhythm, and (3) preventing stroke with maintenance anticoagulation therapy (Rosenthal et al, 2019). Antiarrhythmic agents, such as calcium channel blockers, cardiac glycosides, and beta blockers, are used for rate or rhythm control (Zathar et al, 2019). CCBs and BBs are first-line agents for new-onset AFib (Rosenthal et al, 2019). Anticoagulants are prescribed to prevent ischemic strokes. Anticoagulant regimen is dependent on the patient's age and comorbidities. Digoxin is recommended if AFib is present along with CHF and reduced left ventricular function. Warfarin is recommended for patients with mechanical heart valves. Otherwise, non–vitamin K oral anticoagulants (NOACs), such as dabigatran and rivaroxaban, are appropriate. Before patients are started on NOACs, renal and hepatic function should be evaluated. Routine aspirin is not recommended for patients with a low risk of blood clots. Elective cardioversion is appropriate for acute AFib if pharmacologic treatment (chemical cardioversion) is not effective and left ventricular hypertrophy (LVH) is NOT present. When the duration of AFib is longer than 48 hours or duration is uncertain, anticoagulants are prescribed to reduce the risk of thromboembolic events.

Sick sinus syndrome. A permanent pacemaker is the treatment of choice for symptomatic patients with bradycardia. If patients have tachycardia, a BB or CCB may be effective. If BBs or CCBs are not tolerated or not effective, patients with tachycardia will require a permanent pacemaker.

Heart block. Treatment for first-degree heart block includes correction of the causative factor (e.g., electrolyte imbalance or drug toxicity). In patients with severe bradycardia or the potential to progress to a higher-degree block, a dual-chamber pacemaker may be used. With symptomatic second- and third-degree blocks, a permanent cardiac pacemaker is the treatment of choice if correction of the underlying cause does not reverse the heart block.

Prognosis

Older adults with arrhythmias have an excellent prognosis when these arrhythmias are corrected. Patients with AFib are at increased risk for complications, such as ischemic stroke.

Nursing Care Guidelines for the Older Adult with Arrhythmia

Recognize cues (assessment). Older adults should be assessed for a history of CAD, CHF, HTN, cardiac valve disease, and current drugs (e.g., cardiac drugs, diuretics, and supplemental electrolytes), which may be causing arrhythmias. Symptoms due to decreased cardiac output include weakness, confusion, palpitations, dizziness, shortness of breath, chest pain, and syncope. They should be assessed for onset, duration, frequency, aggravating and alleviating factors, and home treatment remedies.

Objective data include level of consciousness, orientation, HR and rhythm, BP, peripheral pulses, and urine output. Measuring the apical pulse for 60 seconds yields the most accurate measurement of HR. Apical and radial rates should be compared simultaneously to assess peripheral perfusion. Electrolyte, Hb, and hematocrit values should be assessed for imbalances and anemia.

Analyze cues and prioritize hypotheses (patient problems). Patient problems common for an older patient with arrhythmia include the following:
- Reduced cardiac perfusion resulting from altered HR and rhythm
- Reduced physical stamina resulting from altered heart rate and cardiac output
- Potential for injury resulting from potential thrombus and emboli formation
- Potential for nonadherence resulting from a lack of information about the disease process, drugs, and treatment plan

Generate solutions (planning). The overall goals for a patient with arrhythmia are to maintain ADLs and an adequate HR, sustain cardiac output, and prevent complications. Expected outcomes include the following:
1. The patient will maintain an adequate cardiac output, as evidenced by a HR and rhythm within the normal range, stable BP, adequate peripheral pulses, baseline mental status, a urine output of 30 mL/hr, and clear breath sounds
2. The patient will tolerate activity, as evidenced by stable vital signs and no complaints of dizziness, fatigue, or syncope
3. The patient will remain free from injury
4. The patient will verbalize increased knowledge about his or her diagnosis, treatment plan, and health maintenance behaviors

Take actions (nursing interventions). Vital signs should be monitored every 15–60 minutes if the patient's condition is acute and every 4 hours if it is stable. HR and rhythm should be monitored continuously by telemetry. The patient should be taught to report symptoms of weakness, dizziness, and palpitations to the nurse for correlation to telemetry readings. Cardiovascular, respiratory, and neurologic systems, as well as vital signs, oxygen saturation, and intake / output measurements, should be assessed on a regular basis. The therapeutic response and side effects of prescribed drugs should be determined.

Older patients with slow or rapid ventricular responses to AFib, long periods of sinus arrest with SSS, and second- or third-degree heart blocks are at risk for asystole and sudden cardiac death, so nurses should be prepared to initiate emergency measures.

Sensations of weakness, fatigue, dizziness, or dyspnea affect a patient's activity tolerance. Nurses should assist patients in identifying factors that increase or decrease activity tolerance and developing activity patterns that are spaced with adequate rest. Physiologic responses to activity should be monitored.

Tachycardia, bradycardia, and long periods of sinus pause reduce cardiac output and place patients at a higher risk for fainting and falls. Interventions to prevent injury include (1) having patients sit for 3–5 minutes before activity and (2) protecting patients from objects with sharp or protruding edges by rearranging their living area or padding objects in their environment.

Disease processes and the dosage and side effects of all drugs should be reviewed with the patient. Older patients taking anticoagulants should be taught ways to prevent injury, such as not going barefoot, using a soft toothbrush, shaving with an electric razor, having blood for coagulation studies drawn at the proper times, and taking drugs at the same time every day.

If older patients anticipate difficulty with home recovery, a home-health agency may be consulted. Heart associations are excellent sources for information and community programs. The family or significant others should be encouraged to attend cardiopulmonary resuscitation (CPR) programs. All patients should be encouraged to wear medical-alert bracelets to identify the arrhythmia, the use of a pacemaker, and any drugs they use (see Patient/Family Teaching box: Permanent Pacemakers).

Evaluate outcomes (evaluation). Older adults with arrhythmias or pacemakers should maintain a cardiac rhythm that supports adequate cardiac output. Implantable cardioverter-defibrillators (ICDs) may also be used. If the patient receives a shock from the device, they should sit or lie down immediately to avoid falling (Dechant and Heimgartner, 2018). Encourage patients to maintain a log of the date, time, activity just before the device was discharged, and the number of shocks delivered. The ability to resume ADLs, knowledge of the therapeutic plan, and achievement of expected outcomes define an older adult's readiness for independence in their care. Documentation should focus on the patient's response to the treatment plan, and how well symptoms are controlled. Hemodynamic stability is reflected in the documented trends in the patient's vital signs.

PATIENT / FAMILY TEACHING
Permanent Pacemakers

- Keep handheld cellular phones at least 6 inches away from the pacemaker, and use the ear opposite of the pacemaker.
- Avoid areas with strong electromagnetic fields and electrical appliances, which can cause interference, leading to malfunction, and alter the pacemaker settings.
- Magnetic resonance imaging (MRI) is usually contraindicated, depending on the machine's technology.
- Carry the identification card provided by the manufacturer and wear a medical alert bracelet at all times.
- Inform all health-care providers that you have a pacemaker.
- Report any fever, redness, swelling, or drainage from the incision site.
- Do not manipulate the pacemaker site.
- Take your pulse for 1 full minute at the same time each day and record in the pacemaker diary.
- Know the rate at which your pacemaker is set and the basic functioning of your pacemaker; if the rate changes and/or the pacemaker / battery malfunctions, notify your health-care provider.
- Do not apply pressure over the pacemaker. Avoid restrictive clothing.
- Bathing or showering are permitted without concern for your pacemaker.
- Do not lean over electrical or gasoline engines or motors. Be sure that electrical appliances or motors are properly grounded.
- Avoid all transmitter towers for radio, television, and radar. Radio, television, other home appliances, and antennas do not pose a hazard; avoid using outdated microwave ovens.
- Be aware that antitheft devices in stores may cause temporary pacemakers to malfunction. If symptoms develop, move away from the device.
- Inform airport personnel of your pacemaker before passing through a metal detector and show them your pacemaker identification card. The metal in your pacemaker will trigger the alarm in the metal detector device.
- Stay away from any arc welding equipment.
- If you feel symptoms when near any device, move 5–10 feet away from it and check your pulse. Your pulse rate should return to normal.
- Report any of these symptoms to your primary health-care provider if you experience them: difficulty breathing, dizziness, fainting, chest pain, weight gain, and prolonged hiccupping. If you have any of these symptoms, check your pulse rate and call your primary health-care provider.
- Keep all of your health-care provider and pacemaker clinic appointments.
- Take all medications prescribed.
- Follow your prescribed diet.
- Follow instructions about restrictions on physical activity, such as no sudden, jerky movement, for 8 weeks to allow the pacemaker to settle in place.

Data From Dechant, L. M., & Heimgartner, N. M. (2018). Care of patients with dysrhythmias. In D. D. Ignatavicius, M. L. Workman, C. R. Rebar, & N. M. Heimgartner (Eds.), *Medical surgical nursing: Concepts for interprofessional collaborative care* (9th ed., pp. 664–689). St. Louis, MO: Elsevier.

Orthostatic Hypotension

Orthostatic hypotension is a major risk factor for syncope and falls in older adults. Orthostatic hypotension is defined as a decrease of 20 mm Hg or greater in SBP or a decrease of 10 mm Hg or greater in diastolic BP (DBP) upon standing. The decrease in BP occurs due to blood shifting into the lower extremities. Symptoms associated with the fall in BP include dizziness, light-headedness, confusion, and blurred vision (Thompson and Shea, 2022). Orthostatic hypotension is even more common among persons with certain risk factors, such as autonomic dysfunction, low cardiac output, and hypovolemia. The use of certain drugs, such as sedatives, antihypertensives, vasodilators, and antidepressants, also predisposes older adults to orthostatic hypotension. A drop in SBP is sometimes more pronounced when arising in the morning because of diminished baroreceptor function after prolonged recumbence. Orthostatic hypotension in older adults may be caused by an increase in sedentary activity and the blunting of autonomic reflexes.

Nursing Care Guidelines for the Older Adult with Orthostatic Hypotension

Recognize cues (assessment). Assessment of an older patient begins with taking a complete health history and physical examination. Reports of syncope, falls, and near falls should be thoroughly investigated. Assessment data should reflect drugs (prescription, OTC, herbals, and supplements), environmental factors, and the temporal relationship to meals. Hydration status should be evaluated along with a CBC and serum glucose level; dehydration, anemia, and hypoglycemia can cause syncope and falls.

To assess for orthostatic BP changes, BP and HR should be obtained after the patient has been supine for at least 5 minutes. Then, the nurse should help the patient to a sitting position, with feet dangling or flat on the floor, and repeat the BP and HR after 1 minute and 3 minutes. Then, if the patient can stand, the nurse should obtain a third set of BP and HR readings, noting the differences (Thompson and Shea, 2022); document all measurements in the patient's record. If the patient complains of lightheadedness or dizziness and/or the SBP drops to 20 mm Hg or more or the DBP decreases to 10 mm Hg or more, the findings are considered abnormal (CDC, 2017).

All prescribed and OTC drug and herbal preparations should be reviewed carefully. Special attention should be given to drugs known to induce hypotension in older adults, such as amitriptyline, antidepressants, bromocriptine, antiarrhythmics, antihistamines, diuretics, insulin, monoamine oxidase inhibitors, narcotics, sedatives, nitrates, sympatholytics, sympathomimetics, and vasodilators.

Analyze cues and prioritize hypotheses (patient problems). Patient problems common for an older adult with orthostatic hypotension include the following:
- Potential for reduced cardiac perfusion
- Potential for injury
- Need for health education resulting from positional hemodynamic changes and the risk of falls

Generate solutions (planning). Expected outcomes for an older adult with orthostatic hypotension include the following:
1. The patient will remain free of injury.
2. The patient will verbalize and correctly demonstrate measures to prevent symptoms of orthostatic hypotension.
3. The patient will verbalize their fears and identify coping measures.

Take actions (nursing interventions). The nurse should teach an older adult at risk for or with orthostatic hypotension to move slowly from the recumbent position to the sitting position. The patient should then remain sitting for several minutes before attempting to stand.

Exercising the lower legs and ankles facilitates venous return and raises the BP. Elastic stockings help in the same way. In some instances, a higher salt diet may increase blood volume and ameliorate orthostatic changes. The nurse should work with the patient and physician to eliminate unnecessary drugs that may contribute to orthostatic hypotension; the nurse should also encourage the patient to limit alcohol intake, avoid large meals, and monitor and control DM, which is associated with peripheral autonomic dysfunction.

Environmental safety remains important. Grab bars, nonskid surfaces, and an uncluttered living space minimize injuries. In long-term care settings, low beds are sometimes used for cognitively impaired individuals with orthostatic hypotension and a history of falls.

Fear of falling (also referred to as *postfall syndrome*) produces a fear that frequently causes older adults to limit activity and potentially increases fear for further falls. In addition, caregivers may also fear injury for an older adult and feel compelled to limit the older person's freedom. This leads to a cycle of activity avoidance, increased frailty, and a concomitant increased risk of falling and decreased QoL (Choi et al, 2017; Kapan et al, 2017). Educating patients on the proper technique of standing aids in alleviating this fear. Encouragement and support are also important means of relieving fear.

Evaluate outcomes (evaluation). Evaluation is based on the achievement of the expected outcomes and the safe performance of ADLs. Documentation of the patient's BP trends in the 3 positions aids in evaluating the effectiveness of the recommended treatments.

Syncope with Cardiac Causes

Syncope is a transient loss of consciousness, usually related to decreased cerebral perfusion, with spontaneous recovery (AHA, 2022). Causes of syncope are broadly grouped into the classes of reflex or neurally mediated (e.g., vasovagal), cardiac (e.g., arrhythmias), miscellaneous neurologic (e.g., psychogenic and cerebrovascular), and orthostatic disorders (e.g., dehydration) (Goyal and Maurer, 2016).

Vasovagal syncope occurs when fright, pain, or nausea stimulate the vagus nerve. Signs and symptoms include nausea, diaphoresis, anxiety, and a feeling of warmth. These same manifestations may also be part of the atypical presentation of MI in an older adult. Vasovagal syncope may also be caused by straining during a bowel movement and by pushing up in bed without assistance. Vasovagal attacks usually occur in the upright position, and the patient regains consciousness upon lying down (Goyal and Maurer, 2016).

Cardiac arrhythmias are often first seen as a loss of consciousness that occurs without warning. Ectopic beats, whether supraventricular or ventricular, increase in frequency with age. Specific arrhythmias include supraventricular and ventricular tachycardias and a variety of bradyarrhythmias.

Afib is an atrial arrhythmia recognized by the lack of a clear P wave on the ECG and an irregular ventricular conduction. Because AFib is associated with an increased risk of cerebral embolism, anticoagulation should be considered in any older adult with AFib (Benjamin et al, 2017). AFib may cause syncope if the ventricular rate becomes too fast for adequate ventricular filling during diastole. In addition, the loss of atrial kick, which accounts for 30% of ventricular filling, may be enough to decrease cardiac output and thus cause syncope.

Ventricular tachycardia is a medical emergency. It is a tachycardia without atrial activity, a wide QRS complex, and ventricular rates of 120 beats/min and higher. The problem is inadequate ventricular filling during diastole, leading to significantly diminished cardiac output and syncope if not quickly treated. Ventricular tachycardia associated with hemodynamic instability, such as hypotension, requires immediate electrical cardioversion. Long-term control of this type of arrhythmia is accomplished through drug therapy and implantable automatic defibrillators.

Bradyarrhythmias are more common in older adults because of a dysfunction in the intrinsic conduction system.

Bradyarrhythmias requiring pacemakers are AV blocks, such as Mobitz type II and third-degree heart block, and SSS if the bradycardia is symptomatic (Fillit et al, 2017). Structural problems of the heart, such as aortic stenosis, cardiomyopathy, and acute myocardial cell death, can also cause syncope.

Nursing Care Guidelines for the Older Adult with Syncope

Recognize cues (assessment). The assessment of an older patient with syncope begins with a complete history and physical examination. Family members or other witnesses to the patient's syncopal episode should be asked to describe what the patient was doing just before losing consciousness. The older adult should be examined for evidence of acute infarction and arrhythmias with the use of a 12-lead ECG. The carotid arteries should be auscultated for bruits. Blood work should include CBC and a complete chemistry panel, including glucose levels (Fillit et al, 2017).

Analyze cues and prioritize hypotheses (patient problems). Patient problems for an older adult with syncope include the following:
- Reduced cardiac output resulting from inadequate left ventricular filling, arrhythmia, or orthostasis
- Potential for injury
- Anxiety resulting from a near-or-full loss of consciousness

Generate solutions (planning). Syncope with cardiac causes is often an emergency, requiring intensive care for the older adult. Communication between the medical team and family or other caregivers is very important. It is hoped that a health-care proxy is available if the patient can no longer speak for himself or herself.

Expected outcomes for an older adult with syncope include the following:
1. The patient will regain a normal range of cardiac output as demonstrated by stable vital signs and an alert and oriented sensorium.
2. The older adult and family will verbalize their understanding of the cause of syncope and the therapeutic treatment plan.

Take actions (nursing interventions). Emergency measures such as CPR and defibrillation should be employed, when needed, to correct life-threatening arrhythmias. Oxygen should be administered, and oxygen saturation should be evaluated.

Nurses need to help older adults identify causes of syncope, such as straining during defecation. Constipation is a common complaint among older adults. Measures to avoid constipation include increasing fiber in the diet, adequate fluid intake, and exercise as tolerated. Nurses should instruct the older adult to lie down if they become dizzy or experience other prodromal symptoms.

Evaluate outcomes (evaluation). Evaluation is based on the achievement of the expected outcomes and a positive change in the clinical picture of the older adult. Older adults should be able to identify the cause of their syncope and methods of prevention, including methods of preventing injury if syncope occurs.

Valvular Heart Disease (VHD)

VHD occurs when the cardiac valves do not completely open (stenosis) or close (regurgitation and insufficiency), which prevents the efficient circulation of blood through the heart's chambers and increases the myocardial workload. Mitral and aortic valvular diseases are more common than the tricuspid and pulmonic valves.

Stenosis of the mitral valve impedes blood flow from the left atrium to the ventricle during diastole. With time, the left atrium becomes accustomed to increasing volumes and pressure, which causes dilation and hypertrophy. Stenosis of the aortic valve obstructs blood flow from the left ventricle to the aortic arch during systole. With time, hypertrophy of the left ventricle occurs because of increased pressures and volumes. Both stenotic conditions may eventually lead to hypertrophy of the pulmonary vessels and decreased cardiac output.

Mitral regurgitation allows ejected blood to flow back into the left atrium from the ventricle during systole, resulting in dilation and hypertrophy of the left atrium and ventricle. Aortic regurgitation allows ejected blood to flow back into the left ventricle from the aorta during diastole, leading to volume overload that can cause dilation and hypertrophy of the left ventricle. Mitral valve prolapse (a form of valvular insufficiency) occurs when one or both cusps prolapse into the left atrium during ventricular systole. The prolapse is normally benign but may progress to severe regurgitation with ventricular dilation.

Rheumatic fever is the most common cause of (VHD), although the incidence of rheumatic fever has declined since the introduction of antibiotics. Infective endocarditis (IE), connective tissue disorders (CTDs), and atherosclerosis are other causes of valvular disorders. Mitral regurgitation and aortic stenosis may also be attributed to degeneration or calcification of the valves.

Aortic insufficiency, mitral stenosis, and mitral valve prolapse are more common in younger adults than in older adults. Pulmonary and tricuspid valvular disorders do not often occur in older adults. In older adults, aortic stenosis and mitral regurgitation are more common because of the degeneration or calcification of the valves.

Individuals with VHD may be asymptomatic for many years, but with the deterioration of the valves and hypertrophic changes to the atria or ventricles, symptoms become evident (Box 17.4). Exertional dyspnea is frequently the initial symptom. Other symptoms related to decreased cardiac output include dizziness, fatigue, weakness, and palpitations. AFib is often associated with mitral disorders secondary to distention of the left atria. Symptoms of angina are more common with aortic disorders because of decreased cardiac output. Symptoms of VHD may be difficult to recognize in older adults because symptoms may mimic those of CAD.

Diagnostic Tests and Procedures

Chest radiography and ECG are initial diagnostic tests that may suggest VHD or evaluate damage to the heart from valvular problems. ECG with Doppler and ultrasonography provides the most detailed information on the valve's structure, function (abnormal cusp movement), and any evidence of cardiac hypertrophy. Cardiac catheterization may be performed to assess the severity of the valve disorder (i.e., valve

BOX 17.4 Clinical Manifestations of VHD

Mitral Stenosis
Nocturnal dyspnea and/or on exertion, orthopnea, neck vein distention, fatigue, loud accentuated opening snap, low-pitched rumbling, diastolic murmur heard at apex, and edema

Mitral Regurgitation
Fatigue, dyspnea, palpitations, orthopnea, soft S_3 often present, and high-pitched holosystolic murmur with a harsh and blowing quality that radiates to the axilla

Aortic Stenosis
Angina; syncope; orthopnea; fatigue; nocturnal dyspnea; soft prominent S_4, crescendo–decrescendo, and harsh ejection systolic murmur that radiates to carotids

Aortic Regurgitation
Exertional dyspnea; orthopnea; angina; soft or absent S_2, S_3, or S_4; soft, decrescendo blowing diastolic murmur; widened pulse pressure; and bounding arterial pulse

Data From Dechant, L. M. (2018). Care of patients with cardiac problems. In Ignatavicius, D. D., Workman, M. L., Rebar, C. R., & Heimgartner, N. M. (Eds.) *Medical surgical nursing: Concepts for interprofessional collaborative care* (9th ed., pp. 691–719) (9th ed.). St. Louis, MO: Elsevier, pp 691-719.

size, pressure changes within the chamber, and pressure gradients across valves), and additional effects on the heart. Exercise stress tests may also be conducted to evaluate the patient's exercise capacity and hemodynamic response to exertion and recovery (Garcia et al, 2016).

Treatment

Treatment is directed toward the management of presenting symptoms and the correction of the cause of the valvular disorder. Treatment for symptoms of CHF consists of digoxin, diuretics, vasodilating agents, restricted sodium intake, and oxygen therapy. Symptoms of decreased cardiac output related to AFib are treated with cardioversion, anticoagulants, or antiarrhythmics, such as digoxin, BBs, and CCBs. Symptoms of decreased cardiac output related to ischemia are treated with vasodilating agents. Prophylactic antibiotics before invasive procedures (e.g., surgery, invasive tests, and dental work) are recommended for all patients with valve disorders to prevent infective endocarditis. For patients with valvular disorders resulting from degenerative processes, medical treatment of symptoms tends to be unsuccessful over time, and surgical repair or replacement of diseased valves can become necessary.

Prognosis

Morbidity and mortality are higher for older adults requiring valve surgery. Older adults often have more advanced diseases and multiple coexisting chronic diseases at the time of surgery. Dai and Tan, (2019) report a 75% survival rate at 5 years and a 10-year survival rate greater than 55% for older adults undergoing mitral valve repair. Valvular surgery on older adults has steadily increased during the past decade and has increased the QoL for older adults.

Nursing Care Guidelines for the Older Adult with VHD

Recognize cues (assessment). Assessment should include the history of prior episodes of rheumatic fever, infective endocarditis, staphylococcal and streptococcal infections, and a family history of cardiac disease. Symptoms of VHD (e.g., fatigue, dyspnea, palpitations, dizziness, weakness, syncope, peripheral edema, distended neck veins, periods of memory loss or confusion, and chest pain) or related complications (e.g., arrhythmia, angina, and heart failure) should be noted, as well as the patient's level of fatigue, toleration of activity, and current drugs.

Objective data should be obtained primarily from cardiovascular and respiratory assessments. Cardiovascular data include BP, pulse pressure, HR and rhythm, recent weight loss or gain, peripheral pulses, the presence of peripheral edema, neck vein distention, and heart sounds. Different heart sounds are heard with each valvular disorder, and auscultation should be performed for identification of abnormalities or changes. Respiratory data include rate, depth, and breath sounds.

Aortic stenosis is the most common valvular disorder among older adults because of the calcification of the valve with aging. Stenosis of this valve tends to occur without fusion of the cusps, resulting in a spray of blood through the valve rather than forceful propulsion. Physical examination may reveal softer and more musical heart murmurs that may be associated with the normal aging process rather than with a valvular disorder. Older adults may require diagnostic testing to support a diagnosis of VHD.

Analyze cues and prioritize hypotheses (patient problems). Patient problems common for an older patient with VHD include the following:

- Reduced cardiac output is secondary to altered blood flow through the heart
- Reduced activity level, secondary to decreased cardiac output
- Anxiety, secondary to a new diagnosis, treatment plan, and uncertain outcome
- Need for health education, secondary to a lack of previous exposure to information about the disease process, drugs, and treatment plan

Generate solutions (planning). Expected outcomes for an older patient with VHD depend on the severity and extent of the disease. Outcomes include the following:

1. The patient will maintain adequate cardiac output, as demonstrated by stable vital signs, mental alertness, urine output of 30 mL/hr or greater, and clear breath sounds.
2. The patient will tolerate the usual level of daily activity, as demonstrated by stable vital signs and no dyspnea with activity.
3. The patient will experience reduced anxiety through verbalization of decreased anxiety, the ability to express specific fears.
4. The patient will correctly explain the disease process, therapeutic plan, and preventive precautions.

Take actions (nursing interventions). Cardiovascular and respiratory assessments should be conducted on a regular basis to detect progress and prevent complications. Nurses should monitor patients for therapeutic and adverse reactions to prescribed drugs; monitor BP, HR, respirations, heart sounds, breath sounds, and cardiac rhythm; ensure that the patient maintains an appropriate activity level and performs range-of-motion exercises during bed rest to prevent complications;

elevate the head of the bed to maximize thoracic excursion; and administer oxygen, as prescribed.

Nurses should also assess the older adult's activity level and balance activity with rest periods; organize care to provide rest periods and advance activity according to the patient's tolerance. Because older adults are more prone to dizziness and lightheadedness due to orthostatic hypotension, they should be instructed to rise slowly and stay in the sitting position for a few minutes before standing. Older adults should wear nonslip footwear, and handrails should be available for support and to prevent falls.

Older adults should understand the disease process and treatment plan, recognize the signs and symptoms of CHF, and know when to notify their health-care provider. As appropriate, a low-sodium or other healthy diet should be followed. Bleeding precautions should be reviewed with patients receiving anticoagulant therapy. Patients should be taught the importance of appropriate oral hygiene and its importance in the prevention of trauma and infective endocarditis, as well as the necessity for pretreatment with antibiotics before invasive procedures, including all dental work.

For patients who do not respond to medical treatment, heart valve surgery may be necessary to improve cardiac performance. Older patients benefit more from surgery when their condition is stable, and the procedure is performed on an elective basis. Before heart valve surgery, patients should be informed of the necessity for extensive diagnostic tests and blood studies. The patient and family should also be oriented to the ICU or coronary care unit (CCU) and the equipment that will be used postoperatively. Postoperative assessment activities and treatments should be explained.

After surgery, patients will be monitored closely for complications such as MI, CHF, thromboembolism, hemorrhage, arrhythmia, and infection. Older patients have a greater risk for complications compared with younger adults. Older adults are also prone to the development of delirium after surgery due to multiple factors, including the stress of the procedure, drug therapy and other treatment modalities, and environmental alterations. The presence of family and familiar belongings and the use of personal hearing aids or eyeglasses may help alleviate episodes of delirium.

Recovery from heart valve surgery is generally complete within 6–8 weeks; however, recovery may be delayed in older adults, resulting in a higher incidence of postoperative complications. Exercise and ADLs should be gradually resumed during the first 6 weeks of recovery. Patients should be taught to monitor their pulse and respiratory rate to evaluate their tolerance to activity. Patients should be encouraged to progressively increase the duration and frequency of walking. Patients should avoid lifting heavy objects. Prophylactic use of antibiotics should be explained to the patient. Anticoagulants may be prescribed for patients with prosthetic valves. Signs and symptoms of valve failure should be reviewed with the patient in case deteriorating symptoms develop that necessitate valve replacement following surgical repair of a valve; patients with valve replacements may need new valves after 10–15 years.

Evaluate outcomes (evaluation). The evaluation of an older patient with VHD focuses on the achievement of the expected outcomes. Older adults should demonstrate adequate cardiac output, the ability to perform ADLs within limitations, and control of symptoms. The nurse should also note the patient's and family's ability to manage the care requirements and resolve any problems appropriately. Documentation should accurately reflect the care delivered in the preoperative and postoperative periods and the older adult's response. Assessment of the progress toward self-care and the degree of functional ability must also be documented on an ongoing basis because the older adult's recovery depends in large part on returning to the prior level of functioning.

CHF

Approximately 6.5 million adults in the United States suffer from CHF (Benjamin et al, 2017). More than 900,000 new cases are diagnosed each year. Furthermore, it is estimated that the prevalence of CHF will increase by 46% by the year 2030. Even though mortality rates for CHF have declined over the past years, mortality continues to be high, with approximately 50% of people diagnosed with CHF dying within 5 years.

CHF is a syndrome characterized by poor perfusion of oxygen- and nutrient-rich blood. CHF occurs when the heart does not function as it should, leading to decreased cardiac output (AHA, 2023b). CHF occurs over time and can affect either the right side, the left side, or both. Left-sided CHF can occur with a reduced (systolic failure) or preserved (diastolic failure) ejection fraction (Table 17.2). Right-side CHF prevents oxygen-poor blood from reaching the lungs to obtain oxygen, whereas left-side CHF impedes oxygen-rich blood from leaving the heart and reaching the rest of the body. In systolic CHF, the left ventricle is unable to effectively contract to push enough oxygen-rich blood into circulation; in diastolic CHF, the left ventricle is unable to relax, preventing the heart from filling with oxygen-rich blood. Swelling in the body (e.g., hands, feet, abdomen, neck veins) can occur with right-side CHF, whereas fluid buildup in the lungs can occur with left-side CHF. All types of CHF can cause fatigue and shortness of breath.

CHF is classified according to symptom severity and function status. The ACCF/AHA stages of CHF are used to determine the presence of and severity of failure (Table 17.3), whereas the New York Heart Association (NYHA) functional classification focuses on symptomatology and exercise capability (Heidenreich et al, 2022).

The most common risk factors for CHF include CHD, HTN, DM, obesity, and smoking (AHA, 2023b). The lifetime risk for CHF is higher for males with HTN; among older adults, current and past cigarette smoking increases their risk for CHF. The prevalence of CHF increases as adults age. Hospitalization due to CHF is higher among older adults.

Age-associated cardiovascular and renal changes that affect the clinical course of CHF and responses to treatment include decreased renal and systemic blood flow, increased arterial stiffness and peripheral resistance, reduced ventricular compliance, and reduced maximum aerobic capacity. In the majority of people, the ideal BP is less than 130/80 mm Hg. However, among older adults with CHF or those who are at increased risk of CHF, the optimal goal is an SBP of less than 120 mm Hg (Yancy et al, 2017). But about 50% of older adults

TABLE 17.2 ACC/AHA Definitions of CHF Based on Ejection Fraction

Classification	LVEF (%)	Comments
CHF with reduced ejection fraction (HFrEF) (aka: systolic heart failure)	≤40	Major reduction in systolic function. May also have diastolic dysfunction and variable degrees of LV enlargement.
CHF with preserved ejection fraction (HFpEF) (aka: diastolic heart failure)	Preserved ≥ 50 Mild 41–49 Improved >40	Does not have a major reduction in systolic function. Patients are usually treated for the underlying causes of CHF. Risk factors include DM, obesity, CAD, and AFib.

aka, also known as; *CAD,* coronary artery disease; *LVEF,* left ventricular ejection fraction; *LV,* left ventricle.
Modified From Heidenreich, P. A., Bozkurt, B., Aguilar, D., Allen, L. A., Byun, J. J., Colvin, M. M., et al. (2022). 2022 AHA/ACC/HFSA guideline for the management of heart failure: A report of the American College of Cardiology/American Heart Association Joint Committee on clinical practice guidelines. *Circulation, 145*(18), e895–e1032.

TABLE 17.3 ACCF/AHA Stages of CHF

Stages	Description
A	Asymptomatic. At high risk for CHF. No structural heart disease.
B	Asymptomatic. Pre-CHF. Has structural heart disease.
C	Symptomatic or history of symptoms. Has structural heart disease.
D	Symptomatic. Has refractory CHF, requiring interventions.

Data From Heidenreich, P. A., Bozkurt, B., Aguilar, D., Allen, L. A., Byun, J. J., Colvin, M. M., et al. (2022). 2022 AHA/ACC/HFSA guideline for the management of heart failure: A report of the American College of Cardiology/American Heart Association Joint Committee on clinical practice guidelines. *Circulation, 145*(18), e895–e1032.

with CHF have diastolic dysfunction (Pirmohamed et al, 2016). (See the Evidence-Based Practice box.)

Diagnostic Tests and Procedures

The ACC and AHA guidelines recommend the following diagnostic tests for the initial and serial evaluations of patients with CHF complete laboratory evaluation (e.g., B-type natriuretic peptide, CBC, urinalysis, serum electrolytes, kidney function, thyroid panel, and lipid panel); 12-lead ECG, chest x-ray to assess heart size and to detect other cardiopulmonary diseases; and echocardiogram (ECHO) to assess cardiac function (e.g., LVEF) (Heidenreich et al, 2022). (See the Evidence-Based Practice box.)

EVIDENCE-BASED PRACTICE

CHF in Older Adults

Background
Older adults with acute decompensated CHF who are hospitalized have higher incidences of physical frailty, poorer QoL, slow recovery, and frequent rehospitalizations.

Sample / Setting
Study participants included a total of 349 patients who were hospitalized and randomized, with 175 assigned to rehabilitation intervention (intervention group) and 174 to usual care (control group). Inclusion criteria included persons who were 60 years of age or older, were diagnosed with decompensated CHF, were able to ambulate at least 13 feet, had independent ADLs, and were expected to be discharged home. In both groups at baseline, patients had markedly impaired physical function, 97% were frail or prefrail, and they had a mean of 5 comorbidities.

Method
Study participants were screened at the time of hospital admission and were enrolled in the study before discharge. Participants were randomly assigned to the rehabilitation intervention ($n = 175$) or to usual care ($n = 174$). Randomization was divided according to ejection fraction of less than 45% or greater than 45% and clinical site. The intervention was initiated in the hospital for the control group. They were provided with an early, transitional, tailored, progressive physical rehabilitation focusing on 4 physical-function domains: strength, balance, mobility, and endurance. Types of exercise and exercise intensity were individualized according to the patient's performance level. The goal for the intervention group was to increase the amount of ambulation. Upon discharge, they were transitioned to outpatient treatment for 36 sessions.

Participants in the control group (usual therapy) received a telephone call every 2 weeks and had follow-up clinic visits at 1 month and 3 months after discharge. Information collected from the control group includes the occurrence of symptoms postdischarge and whether rehabilitation therapy was utilized. They did not receive specific postdischarge instructions for exercise, but were encouraged to adhere to postdischarge hospital instructions and follow-up appointments. The main outcome for both groups was the score on the Short Physical Performance Battery (SPPB) at 3 months. The secondary outcome was the rate of rehospitalization at 6 months. Other outcomes included physical function, frailty status, hand-grip strength, and gait speed at 3 months; QoL at 3 months; and depression and cognitive assessments.

Findings
Participants in the intervention group had greater improvement in physical function than in the control group. No significant differences were noted in the rate of rehospitalization between the 2 groups. Results from the analyses of secondary and other outcomes suggested the intervention group had better outcomes than in control group. The rates of rehospitalizations over a 6-month period were high in both groups.

Implications
CHF is one of the most common cardiovascular problems and reasons for hospital admission in older adults. Frailty, physical dysfunction, and depression are often unrecognized in older adults hospitalized for CHF, are usually not addressed in hospital protocols, and most likely contribute to rehospitalization, death, and loss of independence.

Data From Kitzman, D. W., Whellan, D. J., Duncan, P., Pastva, A. M., Mentz, R. J., Reeves, G. R., et al. (2021). Physical rehabilitation for older patients hospitalized for heart failure. *The New England Journal of Medicine, 385*(3), 203–216.

Treatment

Treatment of CHF in older adults requires careful control of precipitating factors, a low-sodium diet, fluid restriction as appropriate, adequate rest, and exercise. Treatment of CHF also includes drug therapy. Table 17.4 lists selected drugs for the treatment of CHF. For adverse effects and nursing implications, see Table 17.1. The American College of Cardiology Foundation (ACCF) and the AHA (Liu and Lampert, 2022) established the guidelines for the treatment of CHF. Depending on the severity of CHF, treatment consists of nonpharmacological and pharmacologic therapy. Nonpharmacological therapies include lifestyle modifications (e.g., regular physical activity, sodium restriction, smoking cessation, and reduced alcohol intake). Pharmacologic therapy for CHF involves several classes of drugs, depending on whether the ejection fraction is preserved or reduced.

Systolic CHF (reduced ejection fraction). Diuretics are important to maintain euvolemia and are prescribed for patients

TABLE 17.4 Selected Drugs for CHF

Drug Classification	Adverse Reactions	Precautions
ACEIs Captopril Enalapril Lisinopril Quinapril Ramipril Trandolapril	Cough (common), skin rash, hypotension, taste disturbance, angioedema	Monitor renal function Avoid sudden changes in position
Aldosterone Antagonist Spironolactone	GI bleeding, sexual dysfunction, fever, urticaria, confusion, and ataxia	Monitor for fluid, electrolyte imbalance, and weight Monitor renal and hepatic levels
Beta-Blockers Bisoprolol Carvedilol Metoprolol Metoprolol extended release	Bradycardia, shortness of breath, fatigue, dizziness, depression, diarrhea, pruritus, rash, arthralgia May mask symptoms of hyperthyroidism and hypoglycemia	Monitor HR Monitor for signs of hyperglycemia
Diuretics		
Thiazide Diuretics Hydrochlorothiazide Metolazone	Electrolyte depletion, hypovolemia, hyperglycemia, gastric irritation	Monitor electrolytes, especially potassium Monitor urine output
Loop Diuretics Furosemide Bumetanide Ethacrynic acid Torsemide	Electrolyte depletion, anorexia, diarrhea, malaise, mental confusion, and ototoxicity A dramatic increase occurs in urine output	Monitor electrolytes, especially potassium Monitor hearing
Cardiac Glycosides Digoxin	Altered color perceptions, visual disturbances, confusion, headache, muscle weakness, nausea, anorexia, arrhythmias, bradycardia	Monitor potassium levels Use with caution in patients with IHSS Half-life may be longer in the elderly, leading to an increased risk of toxicity Monitor vital signs
Sympathomimetics Dopamine Dobutamine Amrinone	Headache, tachycardia, arrhythmias, and HTN Headache, nausea, and hypotension Headache, anorexia, hepatotoxicity, thrombocytopenia, and hypotension	Contraindicated in patients with IHSS or sensitivity to any sulfite Contraindicated in patients with IHSS or hypersensitivity to metabisulfite Use with caution in patients with CAD or recent MI Contraindicated in patients with metabisulfite hypersensitivity

CAD, coronary artery disease; *GI,* gastrointestinal disease; *IHSS,* idiopathic hypertrophic subaortic stenosis; *MI,* myocardial infarction.
Data From Burchum, J. R., & Rosenthal, L. D. (2022). *Lehne's pharmacology for nursing care* (11th ed.). St. Louis, MO: Elsevier; Heidenreich, P. A., Bozkurt, B., Aguilar, D., Allen, L.A., Byun, J. J., Colvin, M. M., et al. (2022). 2022 AHA/ACC/HFSA guideline for the management of heart failure: A report of the American College of Cardiology/American Heart Association Joint Committee on clinical practice guidelines. *Circulation, 145*(18), e895–e1032.

exhibiting evidence of pulmonary or systemic congestion (e.g., furosemide, bumetanide, or torsemide). Kidney function and electrolytes must be closely monitored in older adults because of age-related changes in kidney function. Angiotensin-converting enzyme inhibitors (ACEIs) are first-line therapy in systolic CHF with reduced ejection fraction, as they have been shown to reduce morbidity and mortality. The initial dose should be low; if renal function remains stable, the dose should be titrated up as tolerated. Angiotensin II receptor blocker (ARB) is prescribed if ACEI is not tolerated due to its side effects, such as cough (The Medical Letter, 2015).

BBs (e.g., bisoprolol, carvedilol, and metoprolol succinate) given along with ACEI have been shown to reduce hospitalization and mortality. BBs are started at low doses and increased every 2 weeks to the highest dose tolerated. Patients should be told that symptoms of CHF may worsen slightly the first 2 weeks of treatment and that full therapeutic benefits may not occur for several months (The Medical Letter, 2015).

Aldosterone antagonists (e.g., eplerenone or spironolactone) may be prescribed for patients with systolic CHF with an ejection fraction of 35% or less to reduce hospitalization and mortality. However, life-threatening hyperkalemia can occur with aldosterone antagonists (The Medical Letter, 2015).

Hydralazine and isosorbide dinitrate may be beneficial for some patients, particularly African Americans who have not responded to ACEI and BBs. These 2 drugs in a fixed-dose combination have been shown to reduce mortality. Digoxin has been shown to reduce hospitalizations in patients with advanced CHF and reduced ejection fraction. Digoxin should be prescribed at a low dose (0.125 mg) (The Medical Letter, 2015).

Anticoagulation (e.g., warfarin) is indicated if AFib is present and the older adult has risk factors, such as HTN, DM, or age 75 years or greater, for embolic events. In hospitalized patients, sympathomimetics (e.g., dopamine and dobutamine) may be beneficial to increase the force of myocardial contraction. As with CHF with preserved ejection fraction, exercise is encouraged. Statin drugs and CCBs are not recommended for the treatment of CHF with a reduced ejection fraction.

Diastolic CHF (preserved ejection fraction). The goal is to reduce ventricular filling pressure and control symptoms. The principle goal in treating CHF with preserved ejection fraction is geared toward managing HTN with CCBs, ACEIs, or ARBs; controlling HR with BBs or digoxin; and the use of diuretics to treat pulmonary or systemic congestion. However, overuse of diuretics leading to hypotension and electrolyte imbalance can be problematic for older adults; therefore, close monitoring is warranted.

Prognosis

CHF in older adults is associated with a poor prognosis; 25% of older adults with CHF are readmitted to the hospital within 30 days of discharge, and 70% are readmitted within a year. Mortality is higher for older adults with systolic CHF than for those with diastolic CHF. Mortality rates for older adults discharged to skilled nursing facilities following hospitalization are 50% at 1 year. Mortality rates increase with age; for adults 80 years of age and older, mortality at 5 years is roughly 50% (Benjamin et al, 2017; Dharmarajan and Rich, 2017).

Nursing Care Guidelines for the Older Adult with CHF

Recognize cues (assessment). Older adults should be assessed for a history of CAD, RHD, HTN, arrhythmias, HVD, infection, diabetes, kidney disease, and current drugs. The initial physical evaluation of an older adult suspected of having CHF includes measurement of BP, evaluation for pitting edema of the legs and ankles, assessment of jugular venous distension, heart and lung auscultation, and percussion of the lung for effusions. Assessment for orthopnea, fatigue at rest, paroxysmal nocturnal dyspnea (PND), and nocturnal urination are also important. Nurses should determine how symptoms have affected ADLs in older adults.

Analyze cues and prioritize hypotheses (patient problems). Common diagnoses for an older adult patient with CHF include the following:

- Reduced cardiac output resulting from decreased cardiac contractility
- Altered gas exchange resulting from pulmonary venous congestion
- Increased fluid volume resulting from increased sodium and water reabsorption
- Anxiety resulting from perceived threats to oneself
- Reduced stamina resulting from decreased cardiac output
- Decreased ability to cope resulting from knowledge deficits and fear of uncertain outcomes
- Altered sleep pattern resulting from nocturnal dyspnea and nocturnal urination
- Need for health education resulting from a lack of previous exposure to disease processes, drugs, and treatment plans

Generate solutions (planning). Expected outcomes are aimed at maximizing myocardial function and assisting with the lifestyle modifications and emotional adjustments imposed by the disease. Expected outcomes for an older adult with CHF include the following:

1. Cardiac output will be maximized, as evidenced by vital signs within an acceptable range, no arrhythmia, adequate cardiac output, urine output greater than 30 mL/hr, and an alert mental state.
2. Gas exchange will be improved, as evidenced by decreased or no reported dyspnea, a normal respiratory rate, lungs clear on auscultation, no evidence of central or peripheral cyanosis, and a patient report of improved activity tolerance.
3. Excess fluid volume will be reduced, as evidenced by reductions in water weight, dependent edema, and abdominal girth.
4. The patient will experience less anxiety, as evidenced by communication of fears to the nurse and self-report of the use of coping skills.
5. Activity will be restored to its prior level, as evidenced by fewer or no reports of fatigue with usual activities.
6. The patient will experience adequate coping, as evidenced by the naming of coping skills used in the past and a self-report of feeling positive about the future.

7. The patient will experience an acceptable sleeping pattern, as evidenced by reports of sleep uninterrupted by dyspnea and a feeling of being rested on awakening.
8. The patient will demonstrate an adequate knowledge level, as evidenced by the ability to correctly state information about the disease process, treatment plan, drug indications, dosage, frequency, and side effects.

Take actions (nursing interventions). It is essential for nurses to assess BP, apical pulse, HR, heart and lung sounds, and peripheral edema to detect early signs and symptoms of altered cardiac output. The intake, output, and daily weights should be monitored and recorded. The older adult should be weighed at the same time each day to accurately monitor fluid loss or retention. The older adult's activity should be increased as tolerated, and time for adequate rest should be provided. While in bed, the patient should maintain Fowler's position. Older adults may need more than 1 pillow to sleep with at night. Nurses should instruct patients to take diuretics in the morning so sleep is not disturbed by getting up to void. Nurses should encourage older adults to take slow, deep breaths during dyspneic episodes and maintain a calm environment.

Nurses should instruct the older adult about restricted sodium and fluid intake. A dietitian may be consulted. Older adults should be instructed to avoid canned foods and prepared frozen meals due to their high sodium content and to use salt sparingly. A weight gain of 3 lb in 48 hours and a return of any symptoms should be reported to the health-care provider immediately. Electrolyte levels, especially potassium, and signs and symptoms of electrolyte imbalance should be monitored.

Nurses should give older adults instructions on their condition, procedures, diet, and risk factors in a clear, simple manner, using proper language, an appropriate reading level, and incorporating cultural considerations. When teaching, the environment should be kept relaxed and as quiet as possible; all procedures should be explained and questions answered clearly and concisely. Older adult patients and family members should be given the opportunity to verbalize their concerns.

Referral to a home health agency for assistance with ADLs and referral to Meals-on-Wheels may be necessary for some individuals. Older adults should be encouraged to enter a cardiac rehabilitation program to monitor activity tolerance in a secure environment.

Evaluate outcomes (evaluation). Improved ventricular function is demonstrated by unlabored respirations, decreased or no peripheral edema, improved or no cough or orthopnea, and an increase in urine output. Patients should increase their activity levels as tolerated (i.e., without experiencing dyspnea) and should return to their prior level of ADL function. Documentation of trends is critical for older adults with CHF, especially regarding assessment findings and treatment responses (see Nursing Care Plan: CHF).

NURSING CARE PLAN

CHF

Clinical Situation

Mr. H, an 86-year-old male who is widowed and lives alone, arrives in the ED complaining that he has had difficulty breathing, especially at night, associated with nausea, for the past week. He states that he must sleep with 2 pillows to breathe more easily at night and still does not get a good night's rest. He also complains of a cough that is worse at night and is relieved by nothing. Mr. H is concerned that he has pneumonia. Assessment of Mr. H reveals the following:
- Vital signs: temperature, 98°F; apical HR, 86 beats/min and irregular; respiratory rate, 36 breaths/min and labored; and BP, 170/96 mm Hg
- Skin—pale, cool, and diaphoretic
- Inspiratory bibasilar crackles that do not clear with coughing
- S_3 heart sounds on auscultation
- Visible jugular vein distention
- 3+ bilateral pedal edema

12-lead ECG and a chest radiography (CXR) are ordered. An IV is started at 30 mL/hr. Oxygen via a mask is ordered. IV furosemide is given, and Mr. H is admitted with a diagnosis of CHF.

Recognize Cues (Assessment)
- Advanced age and lives alone
- Nocturnal dyspnea, nausea, and cough
- Vital signs: temperature, 98°F; apical HR, 86 beats/min and irregular; respiratory rate, 36 breaths/min and labored; and BP, 170/96 mm Hg
- Pale, cool skin, and diaphoretic
- Inspiratory bibasilar crackles that do not clear with coughing
- S_3 heart sound on auscultation
- Visible jugular vein distention and 3+ bilateral pedal edema
- Diagnosed with CHF

Analyze Cues and Prioritize Hypotheses (Patient Problems)
- Reduced cardiac perfusion resulting from ineffective myocardial contractility
- Fluid overload resulting from decreased cardiac contractility
- Decreased gas exchange resulting from increased fluid in pulmonary vasculature
- Need for patient teaching resulting from new diagnosis of CHF, disease process, and treatment

Generate Solutions and Evaluate Outcomes (Planning and Evaluation)
- Cardiac output is maximized, as evidenced by vital signs within acceptable limits, controlled arrhythmias, clear breath sounds, fewer dyspneic episodes, decreasing edema, and alert mental status.
- The patient will demonstrate normal fluid balance, as evidenced by reduced pedal and pretibial edema and a loss of water weight with a stable dry weight.
- The patient will correctly verbalize prescribed sodium and fluid restrictions.
- The patient will have improved gas exchange, as evidenced by increased activity tolerance, decreased episodes of shortness of breath and nocturnal dyspnea, and clearer breath sounds.
- The patient will describe CHF and reasons for limitations, identify his own risk factors, and explain techniques to initiate lifestyle changes.
- The patient will participate in the treatment plan.

Take Actions (Nursing Interventions)
- Monitor and document HR, rhythm, BP, respirations, and lung and heart sounds hourly and as needed.
- Assess for edema and jugular vein distention every 2–4 hours.
- Monitor intake and output hourly.
- Assess skin temperature and color, and assess for the presence of diaphoresis at regular intervals.

Continued

NURSING CARE PLAN—cont'd

- Provide a restful environment.
- Administer cardiac drugs as ordered; document the patient's response.
- Monitor intake and output hourly.
- Weigh daily, using the same scale at the same time of day.
- Administer diuretics as ordered; document the patient's response.
- Assess levels of electrolytes, BUN, and creatinine, as well as symptoms of any imbalance.
- Instruct the patient to elevate extremities when sitting.
- Instruct the patient on sodium and fluid restrictions.
- Assess respiratory status hourly and as needed (rate, rhythm, use of accessory muscles, and lung sounds).
- Maintain the patient in Fowler's position to aid breathing.
- Administer oxygen as ordered and monitor oxygen saturation.
- Discuss the benefits of increased activity (e.g., a walking program); instruct the patient to avoid strenuous and taxing activities and to take advantage of peak energy periods.
- Discuss the normal function of the heart and how CHF alters heart function.
- Discuss drug therapy, including indications, side effects, and specific monitoring.
- Discuss specific risk factors and the patient's role in modifying them.
- Review signs and symptoms that need to be immediately reported to a health-care provider.
- Provide an environment that allows the patient to verbalize feelings and ask questions.
- Refer the patient to community resources and support groups.
- Encourage the patient to obtain an annual flu immunization.

Next-Generation NCLEX® Examination-Style Case Study

Scenario: The nurse on the medical-surgical unit is caring for an 86-year-old male patient who was admitted for pulmonary edema. The nurse documents the current assessment findings after reviewing the existing health history, nurses' notes, vital signs, and medication administration record (MAR).

Health History | Flow Sheet | Nurses' Notes | MAR
PH
CAD
T2DM

Health History | **Flow Sheet** | Nurses' Notes | MAR

	0538	0700	1130
Temperature (°F)	97.3°	98.1°	97.9°
Pulse (bpm)	118	109	123
Respirations (bpm)	24	26	22
BP (mm Hg)	142/94	136/90	108/64
Oxygen saturation	84% RA/92% on 2L/NC	94% 2L/NC	94% 2L/NC

Health History | Flow Sheet | **Nurses' Notes** | MAR

0538: Admitted with pulmonary edema. Reported dyspnea on any exertion, coughing up frothy sputum, pressure on the chest, and having to sleep in a recliner. Vital signs were noted. Awake and alert, oriented x 4. He was able to speak 3 words before needing to take a breath. O_2 saturation is 84% on room air. As prescribed, O_2 at 2 L nasal cannula was applied—O_2 saturation is 92%. Lungs with bilateral course crackles. Frequent spitting of frothy white sputum. Head of bed was elevated to 45 degrees, and jugular vein distention was present. Heart with S_3 at the apex. The abdomen was soft, nontender, and active bowel sounds were x 4 quad. Lower extremities were with 2+ pitting edema up to mid-calf. Upper extremities were with 1+ edema. Pulses were 2+ in all areas. IV to right arm patent with 20-gauge angiocath without redness, edema, or discomfort; saline was locked.

Health History | Flow Sheet | **Nurses' Notes** | MAR

0730: Reviewed vital signs. Patient continues with crackles bilaterally and a productive cough. O_2 sat stable on 2 L nasal cannula. Jugular vein distention is still present. Edema is unchanged in the upper and lower extremities. Output of 130 mL since 0600 of dark-colored urine. Notified health care provider of patient's status; new orders received. Administered extra furosemide 40 mg IV piggyback now per orders.

0845: 1400 mL of yellow urine in the urinal. Crackles in the lung field minimizing. Less sputum produced. Edema in the extremities unchanged. Jugular vein distention decreasing.

1000: 2150 mL of yellow urine since 0845. No new concerns were voiced.

1125: Reports chest pain, lightheadedness, weakness, and leg cramps. Vital signs were taken and recorded. 1800 mL of clear urine in the urinal. The health care provider was notified about changes in vital signs and the patient's concerns.

Health History | Flow Sheet | Nurses' Notes | **MAR**

Medications	0500	0600	0700	0800
Metoprolol 50 mg PO now and daily	ID: given at 0515 in ER			
Furosemide 40 mg IVP now and q12 hrs	Now dose given at 0515			
Furosemide 40 mg IVP additional dose—0730				Additional dose given at 0745
Lisinopril 5 mg PO now and daily	Now dose given at 0515			

Which nursing interventions will be implemented at this time? (Select all that apply.)

☐ Administer IV fluids of 500 mL of 0.9% sodium chloride.
☐ Request an order for a 12-lead ECG.
☐ Increase oxygen to 4 L/NC.
☐ Obtain daily weights.
☐ Prepare to administer nebulizer treatment.
☐ Request an order for laboratory tests (CMP and magnesium level).
☐ Place patient on complete bed rest.
☐ Request an order for an additional diuretic dose.
☐ Maintain strict intake and output.
☐ Anticipate administering nitroglycerin sublingually.

Peripheral Artery Disease

PAD is a narrowing of the systemic arteries that impairs tissue perfusion. PAD is associated with significant morbidity and mortality and, if left untreated, can be life-threatening (Gerhard-Herman et al, 2017). The most common causes of PAD are arteriosclerosis and atherosclerosis. Although the exact cause of atherosclerosis is unclear, several risk factors have been identified. These include advanced age, smoking, elevated serum cholesterol levels, HTN, DM, physical inactivity, obesity, and family history.

Atherosclerosis involves the development of atheromatous plaques on the intimal layer of arterial vessels. These lesions progressively narrow the artery lumen and lead to the formation of thrombi, emboli, and aneurysms.

As the lumen narrows, partial or complete obstruction occurs, leading to inadequate tissue perfusion beyond the lesion and ischemia. Common sites for plaque formation are the aortoiliac vessels, femoropopliteal vessels, and popliteal–tibial arteries. Symptoms appear when the artery is unable to supply the tissues with adequate oxygenated blood flow.

Plaques may rupture or break loose and circulate through the arterial system, causing MI or stroke. The emboli also tend to block arteries at bifurcation points of the femoral and popliteal arteries. Impaired blood flow and ischemia occur at sites distal to the occlusion.

As the atheromatous plaque progresses, the medial layer of the wall calcifies and loses elasticity, which weakens the arterial wall. As the vessel wall weakens, pouches, or aneurysms form. Pressure within the arteries, especially in the presence of HTN, may further dilate the aneurysm until it ruptures. Aneurysms commonly occur in large arteries, such as the abdominal aorta. Multiple aneurysms may develop in the popliteal artery. Thrombi may form within the aneurysm and circulate to smaller distal vessels in the arterial system.

Signs and symptoms of arterial insufficiency depend on the site, extent of occlusion, and degree of collateral circulation. Collateral circulation often develops in the setting of gradual occlusion caused by plaque formation.

Intermittent claudication (exercise-induced reversible muscle ischemia) is one of the initial symptoms of atherosclerosis obliterans. Pain in the foot or calf is experienced with exercise and subsides with rest (Stephens and Peak, 2022). As the disease progresses, the distance walked becomes shorter before pain is felt. Burning pain in the foot at rest or during sleep indicates a severe form of the disease. Cold, numbness, and tingling may accompany the pain. The foot appears pale when elevated and dusky red in dependent positions (dependent rubor). Dry skin, thickened toenails, loss of pedal hair, and cool skin may result from poor circulation. Painful arterial ulcers may be noticed on the toes, between the toes, or on the upper aspect of the foot. Cold extremities with mottling, delayed filling of capillaries, and absent pedal pulses are indicative of acute arterial insufficiency and should be treated immediately. Care should be taken to examine both extremities for comparison. Advanced stages of ischemia lead to necrosis, ulceration, and gangrene of the toes.

The pain with arterial emboli is sudden and severe. The affected extremity appears pale and cool, and distal pulses are absent. Impaired motor and sensory function is evident. Shock may develop if large arteries are occluded.

Diagnostic Tests and Procedures

Screening all patients for asymptomatic PAD is not recommended. Patients who have increased risk for PAD should have a comprehensive history and physical assessment for clinical manifestations (Gerhard-Herman et al, 2017). SBPs should be obtained in both arms and ankles in patients with PAD, and the ankle–brachial index should be calculated. A low (≤ 0.90) ankle–brachial index indicates PAD:

- Mild (0.71–0.90)
- Moderate (0.41–0.70)
- Severe (≤ 0.40)

Other diagnostics for patients with PAD include imaging studies. Doppler ultrasound (Duplex) imaging detects and measures the velocity of blood flow through arterial segments. Angiography is performed to determine the exact location and extent of arterial occlusion. Contrast material is injected into the arterial system through a specialized catheter inserted into the brachial or femoral artery, and a series of radiographic studies trace the dye through the arterial system.

Treatment

Treatment of PAD includes lifestyle modifications, such as adopting a structured exercise regimen of swimming or biking and smoking cessation, which is crucial for patients with PAD. Pharmacotherapy should be guideline-based to reduce cardiovascular and limb-related events. Antiplatelet therapy with aspirin alone or combined with clopidogrel is highly recommended for symptomatic patients to reduce cardiovascular events, such as MI and stroke. Antiplatelet drugs inhibit the adherence and aggregation of platelets along damaged vessels. Dipyridamole and cilostazol are other antiplatelet drugs that inhibit platelet aggregation (Gerhard-Herman et al, 2017).

Statin drugs, such as simvastatin, are also indicated for patients with symptomatic PAD to improve blood flow, reduce cardiovascular events, and decrease loss of limbs. Control of BP with antihypertensive drugs is necessary to decrease cardiovascular events.

Surgical Procedures

Percutaneous transluminal angioplasty involves gaining access to the arterial system with a specialized balloon-tipped catheter. The catheter is advanced under fluoroscopy to the atherosclerotic lesion and inflated over the site to compress the plaque and improve blood flow. Intravascular stents keep the vessel open. A thromboendarterectomy is the opening of the artery and the removal of plaque. Revascularization (arterial bypass and reconstruction) may be performed to increase blood flow. Advanced cases of atherosclerosis and gangrene of the extremities necessitate amputation of the limb.

Prognosis

The key to preventing or halting the progression of PAD and subsequent complications appears to be controlling the risk factors for atherosclerosis through adherence to a healthy diet, a program of exercise, weight loss if needed, and smoking cessation. If lifestyle changes are ineffective, pharmacologic therapy or surgical intervention may be necessary (see Patient / Family Teaching box: PAD).

PATIENT / FAMILY TEACHING
Peripheral Artery Disease (PAD)

- Prevention is the key to the management of PAD.
- Control risk factors: stop smoking; lose weight; control HTN and DM; eat a low-fat, low-cholesterol diet; and exercise daily by walking.
- Do not cross legs while sitting; do not stand or sit for long periods.
- Do not wear constricting garments.
- Foot care is essential. Inspect the feet daily, and keep them clean and dry. Do not soak feet. Use mild soap and a washcloth to clean. Check the water temperature with a thermometer or elbow, but do not use your toes. After bathing, dry well between toes; lubricate feet with lotion daily. Avoid walking barefoot, and wear proper-fitting footwear that is flexible yet protective.
- Immediately notify the health-care provider of changes in color, temperature, or sensation of the affected area or damage to skin integrity.

Data From Heimgartner, N. M. (2018). Care of patients with vascular problems. In D. D. Ignativicius, M. L. Workman, C. R. Rebar, & N. M. Heimgartner (Eds.), *Medical surgical nursing: Concepts for interprofessional collaborative care* (9th ed., pp. 720–750). Philadelphia, PA: Elsevier.

Nursing Care Guidelines for the Older Adult with PAD

Recognize cues (assessment). Assessment of an older adult with PAD begins with a complete history and physical examination. Assessment data should reflect the presence of acute or chronic arterial insufficiency.

Subjective and objective assessment of a patient with PAD is outlined in Box 17.5.

Analyze cues and prioritize hypotheses (patient problems). Patient problems for older adults with PAD include the following:

- Decreased peripheral tissue perfusion resulting from decreased arterial blood flow
- Decreased ADLs resulting from an imbalance between tissue needs and blood supply

BOX 17.5 Assessment of Older Adults with Peripheral Artery Occlusive Disease

Subjective Data
- Pain in extremities (onset, duration, intensity, location)
- Precipitating factors (activity or rest)
- Relieving factors (activity or rest and position)
- Presence of intermittent claudication (frequency and distance)
- Modifiable risk factors (smoking, high cholesterol levels, HTN, DM, obesity, and physical inactivity)
- Personal and family history (of CAD and PAD)
- Psychosocial state (anxiety, fear, or depression)

Objective Data
- Skin changes (color, temperature, appearance, and sensations)
- Condition of nails
- Circulation (peripheral pulses, bruits, and capillary filling)
- Muscle tone

CAD, coronary artery disease; *PAD*, peripheral artery occlusive disease.

- Potential for skin integrity issues
- Need for health education resulting from a lack of previous exposure to disease processes, drugs, and treatment plans

Generate solutions (planning). Older patients with PAD and their family members should be included in the planning of care. Discharge planning should begin as soon as an older adult is admitted to the hospital. Additional support services may be necessary during home recovery.

Expected outcomes for an older adult patient with PAD include the following:

1. The patient will manifest reduced signs and symptoms of arterial insufficiency, as evidenced by a warm skin temperature over the affected area, the presence of pedal pulses, and decreased claudication in the affected extremities.
2. The patient will successfully participate in activities within the limits imposed by the disease.
3. The patient will demonstrate protective behavior and self-care measures to prevent injury to the skin.
4. The patient will correctly describe the disease process and treatment plan, including drug actions, dosage, and side effects.
5. The patient will identify personal risk factors and methods to reduce these factors.

Take actions (nursing interventions). Nursing interventions include the initiation of a graduated, regular exercise program. Patients should be encouraged to balance activities with rest and may need assistance to develop a schedule of paced activities. Patient education is also important for preventing injuries.

Evaluate outcomes (evaluation). The evaluation of an older adult patient with PAD focuses on the achievement of expected outcomes. Short-term evaluation focuses on those interventions aimed at reducing risk factors. Long-term evaluation is based on trends in progress toward improving tissue perfusion and viability. Involvement of the older adult and their family in planning care is a crucial factor in achieving a successful outcome over time (see Nursing Care Plan: PAD).

Chronic Venous Insufficiency

Chronic venous insufficiency (CVI) is any disturbance that impairs tissue perfusion. The most common disorders due to CVI are (1) varicose veins, (2) venous ulcerations, and (3) venous thrombosis.

Varicose veins of the leg occur, particularly in females, and may be divided into primary and secondary varicose veins. Primary varicose veins are more common, and the varicosity, which occurs in the wall of the vein, may be related to weakness of the wall, incompetent valves of the saphenofemoral junction, or perforating veins. Underlying causes include obesity, estrogenic hormones, and, in older adults, a previous occupation that required long periods of standing. Varicose veins are unattractive but generally do not lead to other serious vascular diseases. Complications of primary varicose veins due to CVI are venous ulcers. The superficial system is subjected to high pressure, which results in poor tissue oxygenation of the lower limbs. Venous ulcers occur on the medial side of the lower half of the leg. The ulcer is usually painful, may easily be infected,

NURSING CARE PLAN

PAD

Clinical Situation

A 72-year-old female is complaining of a decreased activity level because of pain in her right leg when walking. This has been getting worse over the past few months, and it is now difficult for her to walk to the mailbox without pain. She states that sometimes her toes tingle at night. She does not complain of chest pain or shortness of breath. She denies smoking and takes amlodipine for HBP and aspirin as needed for arthritis.

Assessment of Mrs. A reveals the following:

- Vital signs: temperature, 98.4°F; HR, 84 beats/min and regular; respiratory rate, 16 breaths/min and not labored; BP, 160/84 mm Hg at the left arm and 143/80 mm Hg at the right arm
- Height: 5 ft, 6 in; weight: 164 lb
- Skin: warm and dry
- Right foot pale and cooler than left
- Pedal pulse: right foot 1+ and left foot 2+
- Femoral pulse: 2+ bilateral
- Able to move toes equally

Pentoxifylline is ordered, and an exercise program is prescribed. Doppler studies are scheduled.

Recognize Cues (Assessment)

- Advanced age with decreased activity
- Worsening pain to right leg with ambulation and occasional tingling to toes
- History of HTN and arthritis
- Right foot pale and cooler than left
- Pedal pulse: right foot 1+ and left foot 2+
- Femoral pulse: 2+ bilateral
- Able to move toes equally

Analyze Cues and Prioritize Hypotheses (Patient Problems)

- Decreased activity resulting from pain when walking
- Altered tissue perfusion resulting from decreased circulation
- Risk of skin breakdown
- Need for health teaching resulting from lack of knowledge of the disease and the treatment plan

Generate Solutions and Evaluate Outcomes (Planning and Evaluation)

- The patient will identify factors that cause pain.
- The patient will participate in a plan to increase activity and decrease claudication.
- The patient will demonstrate no signs of skin breakdown or impairment in skin integrity.
- The patient will identify the risk factors for the disease, describe lifestyle changes, and participate in the treatment plan.

Take Actions (Nursing Interventions)

- Plan activities to include a walking program.
- Encourage the patient to increase their walking regimen daily, up to 30 minutes per day, with intermittent rest periods if experiencing pain.
- Encourage the patient and give reassurance that activity does not harm painful tissue.
- Assist the patient in identifying, reducing, and eliminating risk factors (e.g., reducing weight and controlling HTN).
- Assess for ischemic ulcers.
- Have the patient report ulcers or darkened areas on her skin to the health-care provider.
- Teach foot care measures, including daily inspection, daily washing using mild soap, and drying well; the patient may use lotion but should avoid use between the toes.
- Teach the patient proper nail care and to wear proper-fitting closed-toe shoes.
- Explain drug therapy, including side effects and when to call the health-care provider.
- Identify available community resources.

---

and, if left untreated, may involve the circumference of the leg. The management of venous ulceration depends on relieving the HTN occurring in the superficial system through bed rest, elevation of the limb, and single or multi-layer compression dressings. A characteristic brownish discoloration of the skin develops from deposits of melanin and hemosiderin. Older adults often complain of heaviness in their legs. The signs and symptoms of varicose veins are protrusion of veins on the legs, aching, ankle swelling, night cramps, skin changes such as itching, varicose eczema, and (in extreme cases) hemorrhage. Most varicose veins may be treated with conservative therapy, including the use of compression dressings or stockings, elevation of the lower extremities when sleeping or relaxing, regular exercise, and weight reduction. In more severe cases, surgical interventions such as sclerotherapy, ligation, ablation, or phlebectomy (vein stripping) may be required.

Secondary varicose veins are the result of thrombosis in the deep system, which may subsequently occur with obstruction of the valves. Deep vein thrombosis (DVT) due to the Virchow Triad (venous stasis, hypercoagulability, and intimal changes to the vessels) is a common and serious disorder. The CDC estimates an annual occurrence of DVT at 300,000–600,000, with 34% being fatal pulmonary embolism (PE). Immobility, advancing age, obesity, hormonal usage, and cigarette smoking are contributing factors. Medical conditions predisposing individuals to DVT include blood dyscrasias, cancer, systemic infection, dehydration, heart disease, stroke, IBD, and incompetent venous valves. Incidences greatly increase with age for both males and females (Benjamin et al, 2017).

Diagnostic Tests and Procedures

Indirect methods to detect obstruction include Doppler ultrasonography, plethysmography, venous duplex ultrasonography, and contrast venography. Doppler ultrasonography measures venous obstruction and reflux of blood by changes in the frequency of sound waves. Laboratory work includes a CBC, prothrombin time, PPT and activated PPT, INR, highly-sensitive D-dimer, and chemistry panel.

Treatment

The therapeutic aim of treatment for more serious CVI is to preserve not only the extremity but also its function. Interventions range from palliative measures to ease symptoms to the use of pharmacologic and surgical strategies to enhance blood flow and prevent clot formation.

Palliative measures are important for maintaining comfort. Preservation of skin integrity is of prime importance in maintaining the overall health of the extremity. Pharmacologic intervention is directed at increasing blood flow and preventing clot formation. For prophylaxis, rather than treatment during the acute phase, low-molecular-weight heparins (LMWHs), such as enoxaparin sodium, are used for their antithrombotic action. This class of drug has a lower risk of bleeding and does not require laboratory monitoring for therapeutic doses. Typically, LMWHs are given subcutaneously once or twice a day. Anticoagulation therapy, such as heparin and warfarin, is used to prevent further clot formation. A variety of surgical procedures may be performed to reduce the effects of CVI.

Nursing Care Guidelines for the Older Adult with CVI

Recognize cues (assessment). Assessment of an older adult with CVI begins with a complete history and physical examination. Subjective data include pain in the extremity, precipitating factors, relieving factors, modifiable risk factors, and personal and family history. Objective data include skin color, hair distribution, atrophy, edema, varicosities, petechiae, lesions, and ulcerations. Table 17.5 provides more information for the assessment of PAD and PVD.

Analyze cues and prioritize hypotheses (patient problems). Patient problems for an older adult with CVI include the following:
- Potential for skin integrity issues resulting from venous stasis
- Decreased peripheral tissue perfusion resulting from an interruption of venous flow
- Pain resulting from inflammatory processes

Generate solutions (planning). Expected outcomes for an older patient with CVI include the following:
1. Skin integrity will be maintained or improved.
2. The patient will exhibit no ulceration or signs of the inflammatory process.
3. Tissue perfusion will be improved, as evidenced by decreased edema and fewer complaints of discomfort.

Take actions (nursing interventions). Nursing interventions for an older patient with venous disease include assessment of skin integrity (e.g., skin texture, skin temperature, pain, color, edema, and pulses). The nurse should use a Doppler sensor if pulses are absent. The affected extremity should be elevated to facilitate venous circulation, and the size of the affected limb should be measured and recorded at least daily. Elastic compression stockings may also be ordered; it is helpful to demonstrate their application and removal and require a return demonstration to assess the patient's ability to correctly apply them. Devices are available through medical supply companies for assistance with application, if necessary. Stockings should be replaced every 3–6 months in the absence of any evidence of excess wear.

Bed rest versus early ambulation in patients with DVT has not been associated with an increased risk of PE (Liu et al, 2015). Early ambulation has also been shown to decrease pain. Instruct older adults to apply their elastic compression stockings before walking and to avoid standing or immobility for prolonged periods. Instruction on foot care is an important part of the prevention plan for venous ulcers. The skin should be inspected daily, washed gently in tepid water with a neutral soap, and patted dry with special attention paid to adequately drying between the toes. A foot cream or moisturizer, then cotton socks, should be applied after washing to aid in retaining moisture. A professional should perform nail care. Shoes should fit well and provide good support.

Evaluate outcomes (evaluation). Evaluation focuses on the patient's progress in maintaining skin integrity, improving venous circulation, and reducing pain and discomfort. Documentation should include accurate recording of the skin assessment, including measurements of the affected extremity, as well as the older adult's response to other nursing interventions.

Anemia

Anemia is defined as a reduction in red blood cell (RBC) mass, a decreased quantity of Hb, and a decreased hematocrit (HCT). The National Heart, Lung, and Blood Institute (NHLBI) indicates the normal range for Hb is adults is 14–17 gm/dL in males and 12–15 gm/dL in females (NHLBI, 2022b). Approximately 15% of adults over the age of 60 are anemic (Guralnik et al,

TABLE 17.5 Differentiating Arterial and Venous Insufficiency

Assessment	PAD	PVD
Pain	Achy to sharp cramps; activity aggravates and is relieved by rest	Little or no pain; achy to cramps; relieved by activity or elevating extremity
Skin texture	Thin, dry, shiny; hairless	Stasis dermatitis; veins may be visible; darkened pigmentation
Skin color	Pallor or reactive hyperemia (pallor when the limb is elevated; rubor when limb is dependent)	Brawny (reddish brown); cyanotic, if dependent
Skin temperature	Cool or cold	Warm
Skin breakdown (ulcers)	Severely painful; usually on or between toes or on upper surface of foot over metatarsal heads or other bony prominence	Mildly painful, with pain relieved by leg elevation; usually in ankle area
Edema	None or mild, usually unilateral	Typically present (usually foot to calf); may be unilateral or bilateral; increases throughout day and with dependent position
Pulses	Diminished, weak, or absent	Normal

Modified From Cooper, K., & Gosnell, K. (2023). Care of the patient with a cardiovascular or a peripheral vascular disorder. In K. Cooper, & K. Gosnell (Eds.), *Adult health nursing* (9th ed., pp. 299–374) St. Louis, MO: Elsevier.

2022). The number of older adults with anemia increases with age and is common among the most frail. Anemia in older adult typically has a different etiology from anemia in younger adults; it is usually insidious in nature and an incidental finding on hematological studies. When anemia is discovered, it is important for reversible causes to be identified, as anemia in older adults is correlated with increased hospitalizations, morbidity, and mortality.

The most common causes of anemia in older adults are iron deficiency anemia (IDA), anemia of chronic disease, and anemia related to CKD (Guralnik et al, 2022). Other causes of anemia include deficiency in vitamin B_{12} or folate, and myelodysplastic syndromes (MDS). However, many cases of anemia go unexplained.

Symptoms vary in frequency and severity. Fatigue and weakness are frequent complaints of older adults with anemia. Pallor is another common sign. Skin color is not a good indicator of pallor because of varying pigmentation. Oral mucous membranes, as well as conjunctivae and nail beds, are better indicators. Headaches, dyspnea on exertion, palpitations, poor concentration, and dizziness are other common symptoms of anemia. Older adults may exhibit symptoms of anemia (e.g., fatigue and dizziness) but attribute these to the aging process or to other chronic diseases. The nurse should be aware of the nonspecific nature of symptoms so that detection and treatment can be initiated as soon as possible (Guralnik et al, 2022).

Diagnostic Tests, Procedures, and Treatment

In addition to a thorough history and physical examination, the following laboratory tests should be obtained:
- CBC with differential and peripheral smears
- Reticulocyte count
- LDH level
- Serum ferritin
- Serum iron
- Total iron-binding capacity
- Vitamin B_{12}, folate, and thyroid-stimulating hormone (TSH).
- Serum chemistry with an estimated glomerular filtration rate (eGFR)

In IDA, in addition to the serum iron level, serum ferritin is the most useful test (a ferritin level <12 ng/mL is specific for IDA; levels between 18 and 44 ng/mL are suggestive of IDA; levels over 100 mg/dL indicate adequate iron stores). Although a low mean corpuscular volume (MCV) is suggestive of IDA, the MCV should not be completely relied on, as microcytosis is a late finding and other factors may influence changes in RBC size (Olmedo and Pakbaz, 2022). Stools should be tested for occult blood, and if positive, the patient should be evaluated for anemia caused by gastrointestinal (GI) blood loss. Treatment includes dietary sources of iron and supplemental intake of iron (i.e., ferrous sulfate, 325 mg, 3 times a day). Iron therapy should continue until ferritin levels normalize. If there is no response to oral replacement, IV iron should be tried.

Anemia from chronic disease is related to inflammatory processes; inflammation inhibits erythropoiesis. In this form of anemia, iron levels are decreased, but ferritin levels are normal or increased (Olmedo and Pakbaz, 2022). Additional laboratory testing that may be useful includes C-reactive protein, fibrinogen, erythrocyte sedimentation rate, IL6, and hepcidin levels. The treatment focuses on treating the underlying disease along with administration of an erythropoiesis-stimulating agent (e.g., epoetin alfa or darbepoetin alfa) if necessary (Goodnough and Schrier, 2014).

Folate deficiency is usually the result of inadequate dietary intake or malabsorption; it also occurs in the setting of alcoholism and the use of methotrexate, phenytoin, and trimethoprim. In addition to decreased folic acid levels in folate deficiency, serum homocysteine levels are elevated; folate deficiency is a macrocytic anemia (MCV >100 fL). In addition to the common symptoms associated with anemia, patients with folate deficiency also experience mouth sores and tongue swelling (glossitis). Treatment includes increased dietary intake (e.g., citrus fruits and dark green vegetables) of folic acid; older adults with alcoholism usually require exogenous folic acid (Waterbury, 2021).

Older adults frequently experience low vitamin B_{12} levels. A level <200 pg/mL may be indicative of malabsorption or pernicious anemia. If the B_{12} level is between 200 and 350 pg/mL, a methylmalonic acid level should be drawn; an elevated methylmalonic acid level is indicative of B_{12} deficiency (please note, methylmalonic acid levels are elevated in CKD) (Olmedo and Pakbaz, 2022). Patients with B_{12} deficiency may experience paresthesia and exhibit ataxia, decreased proprioception, and decreased vibratory sensation on examination, in addition to the more common symptoms of anemia. Lifelong treatment with cyanocobalamin (vitamin B_{12}) is necessary; dosing may be oral, nasal, or by subcutaneous (subcut) or intramuscular (IM) injections.

Prognosis

The prognosis for anemia depends on the cause. With drugs and dietary changes, the prognosis is usually good.

Nursing Care Guidelines for the Older Adult with Anemia

Recognize cues (assessment). The assessment of an older adult with anemia focuses on identifying the underlying cause and its effects on functional ability (Box 17.6).

Analyze cues and prioritize hypotheses (patient problems). Patient problems for an older adult with anemia include the following:
- Decreased activity resulting from an imbalance between oxygen supply and demand
- Inadequate nutrition resulting from malabsorption or decreased intake of vitamins, minerals, and nutritious foods
- Need for patient teaching resulting from a lack of exposure to information about the condition and treatment plan

Generate solutions (planning). Expected outcomes for the older adult include the following:
1. The patient will experience increases in activity without dyspnea or other previous symptoms over a period of 3–6 weeks.
2. The patient will consume a well-balanced diet with foods high in minerals and vitamins, as evidenced by a food diary or planned weight gain.
3. The patient will verbalize an understanding of the cause of anemia and an understanding of the treatment plan.

> **BOX 17.6 Assessment of Older Adults with Anemia**
>
> **Subjective Data**
> - History (e.g., gastric surgery, liver or kidney disease, recent blood loss, or trauma)
> - Current drugs (e.g., prescription, OTC, vitamins and minerals, and NSAIDs)
> - Nutritional habits (i.e., ask the older adult to give a 24-hour diet recall)
> - Alcohol intake
> - Change in bowel habits (e.g., color and consistency)
> - Weight loss
> - Complaints (e.g., fatigue, palpitations, dyspnea, paresthesia, painful tongue, dizziness, headache, or tinnitus)
>
> **Objective Data**
> - Pallor (e.g., nail beds, conjunctivae, or oral mucous membranes)
> - Physical appearance
> - Tachycardia
> - Tachypnea
> - Crackles on pulmonary auscultation
> - Edema
> - Syncope
> - Systolic murmur
> - Confusion
> - Unsteady gait
> - Stomatitis
> - Vital signs (including orthostatic BP/P)
> - Laboratory values

NSAIDs, nonsteroidal antiinflammatory drugs; *BP,* blood pressure; *P,* pulse.

In addition to dietary recommendations, the gerontologic nurse should ensure that the older adult patient has adequate income to purchase necessary foods, the functional ability to acquire and prepare foods, and adequate oral health, including properly fitting dentures. The nurse should also be alert to the presence of other variables that may adversely affect the older adult's ability to eat, such as loneliness, grief, depression, or alcoholism.

Older patients and their families should also be instructed to balance rest and activity. It is helpful for older adults to identify peak energy periods during waking hours and carry out desired or important activities during those times. However, patients should not carry out activities to the point of fatigue or dyspnea; rather, they should rest at intervals until activities are completed.

Evaluate outcomes (evaluation). Evaluation focuses on the patient's progress toward meeting the expected outcomes. Specifically, the older patient should have fewer complaints of dyspnea, fatigue, and dizziness, and their weight should be within the established norm. Normal values of the older adult's Hb, HCT, and RBC count indicate the success of interventions. The older patient's symptoms, weight trends, and activity levels should be documented, along with any patient and family teaching.

NUTRITIONAL CONSIDERATIONS

DASH Diet

Daily Food Group	Servings	Significance of Each Food
Grains	6–8	Energy and fiber
Vegetables	4–5	Potassium, magnesium, and fiber
Fruits	4–5	Potassium, magnesium, and fiber
Low-fat or nonfat dairy foods	2–3	Calcium and protein
Lean meats, poultry, and fish	6 or less	Protein and magnesium
Nuts, seeds, and legumes	4–5 per week	Energy, magnesium, potassium, protein, and fiber
Fats and oils	2–3	The DASH study had 27% of calories as fat, including fat in or added to foods
Sweets and added sugars	5 or less per week	Sweets should be low in fat

DASH, Dietary Approaches to Stopping Hypertension.
Modified From National Institutes of Health, National Heart, Lung, and Blood Institute. (2021). *Description of the DASH eating plan.* Retrieved from https://www.nhlbi.nih.gov/education/dash-eating-plan.

Take actions (nursing interventions). Nursing interventions for an older adult with anemia focus on dietary management, a balance of rest and activity to support functional ability, and education about the condition. Environmental safety issues are also important for an older patient experiencing symptoms that increase the risk of injury.

The patient and family should be instructed about appropriate food selection and meal preparation to promote RBC formation. The nurse should provide a list of foods high in iron, folic acid, and vitamin B_{12} to incorporate into the daily meal plan. The health-care provider may order supplemental iron preparations, and if so, the nurse should assess the patient's tolerance of the preparation. Side effects of oral iron preparations include GI upset, constipation or diarrhea, and green or black stools. It may be helpful to recommend taking the iron preparation after meals to minimize GI upset.

SUMMARY

CVD remains the leading cause of death in the United States. In the older adult population, it is often difficult to clearly distinguish between CVD and normal aging. The presentation and effects of CVD may vary widely from person to person. Older adults often display atypical symptoms of CVD, enabling the disease process to advance before discovery and treatment are initiated. The challenge for the nurse is to obtain an accurate and complete assessment of the older adult patient that allows the planning and initiation of appropriate physical and psychosocial care. The nurse should focus on assisting older patients in modifying risk factors and optimizing their health status.

HOME CARE

1. Homebound older adult patients, spouses, family, significant others, and caregivers should be included in all aspects of the care-planning process in the home-care setting.
2. Older patients value education in the home-care setting, and this should continue to be an important focus of care after hospitalization.
3. Older adult patients dealing with chronic disease management in the home setting often experience anxiety, frustration, and depression. This factor should be taken into consideration when providing home-care services, and appropriate interagency referrals should be initiated.
4. The fear of dying is often a major factor for homebound older adults with CVD, particularly those with CHF. Counseling and referrals to agencies should be provided.
5. Homebound older adults have a high-anxiety level about needing help and not being able to obtain it. Establishing a link with an emergency community service, such as a lifeline program, may alleviate some anxiety.
6. The nurse should direct the teaching of homebound older adults about the anatomy and physiology of the heart, modifiable risk factors for CVD, drug regimens (especially regarding dosage and side effects), exercise tolerance, daily weight monitoring, and dietary modification (e.g., low-sodium and low-fat diets and fluid restriction).
7. Caregivers need to be educated about signs that suggest deterioration in status.
8. Assistance with ADLs may be required, especially for those homebound older adults who live alone or are responsible for household tasks. Often, these older adult patients do not request assistance, so the nurse should offer these services where appropriate.
9. Participation in a cardiac rehabilitation program or activities such as walking or swimming should be encouraged by the home-care nurse.
10. Homebound older adult patients should be encouraged to wear medical alert bracelets that identify the patients' conditions and drugs.

KEY POINTS

- CVD is the leading cause of death among both males and females.
- For those older than age 65, mortality rates for CVD rise sharply, and it is anticipated that the actual number of deaths resulting from CVD will escalate as the proportion of the older adult population increases.
- Older adults who stay physically fit have twice the work capacity and a lower amount of body fat than older adults who are sedentary.
- Smoking cessation in older adults significantly reduces the risks of coronary events and cardiac death within 1 year of quitting. The risk continues to decline gradually for many years thereafter.
- Smokers have twice the chance of developing CAD and 4 times the chance of sudden death compared with nonsmokers.
- It is estimated that more than 45% to 50% of the population older than age 65 has HBP, and the consequences are the most common causes of morbidity and mortality, including MI, CHF, and CVI.
- Older adults may have difficulty adopting healthier lifestyles because of long-term habits; however, healthy behavior changes may slow or halt the progression of disease.
- Older adults have more atypical signs of CAD.
- Older adults may not recognize the onset of ischemia. Initial symptoms may consist of sudden dyspnea, confusion, fatigue, weakness, vertigo, syncope, vomiting, and an exacerbation of CHF.
- The incidence of AFib increases with age and is the most common contributing factor to ischemic stroke in older adults.
- AFib, SSS, and heart block appear more often in the older adult population because of fewer pacemaker cells and extensive deposits of fat and fibrous tissue throughout the conduction system.
- Orthostatic hypotension is a major risk factor for syncope and falls in older adults.
- Older adults are prone to dizziness with position changes, resulting from decreased sensitivity of baroreceptors.
- CHF is the leading cause of hospitalization in the older adult population.
- Older adults may exhibit symptoms of anemia that are attributed to the aging process or to a variety of chronic diseases.
- Nursing interventions (e.g., education on the role of cardiovascular risk factors, preventive measures, and treatment regimens) may enhance the QoL of older patients, reduce hospitalization, and positively affect the cost-effectiveness and efficiency of cardiovascular programs.

CLINICAL JUDGMENT EXERCISES

1. You are preparing to teach an 85-year-old female about the actions and side effects of nitroglycerin for the treatment of angina. What aspects of teaching would you emphasize, given the patient's age?
2. A 78-year-old female has a long-standing history of AFib. She takes digoxin 0.125 mg and warfarin 2.0 mg daily. She recently read about the advantages of taking aspirin and started taking 4 tablets daily. How would you intervene in this situation, and why?
3. What specific assessment findings indicate that an older adult patient being treated for CHF is not responding to digoxin, furosemide, and vasodilator therapy? How would you differentiate among expected, adverse, and toxic side effects?

REFERENCES

American Heart Association (AHA). (2023a). *Understanding blood pressure readings*. Retrieved from https://www.heart.org/en/health-topics/high-blood-pressure/understanding-blood-pressure-readings. Accessed April 29, 2024.

American Heart Association (AHA). (2023b). *Types of heart failure*. Retrieved from https://www.heart.org/en/health-topics/heart-failure/what-is-heart-failure/types-of-heart-failure. Accessed July 28, 2023.

American Heart Association (AHA). (2022). *Syncope (fainting)*. Retrieved from https://www.heart.org/en/health-topics/arrhythmia/symptoms-diagnosis—monitoring-of-arrhythmia/syncope-fainting. Accessed July 28, 2023.

American Heart Association (AHA). (2021a). *Cardiovascular disease and diabetes*. Retrieved from https://www.heart.org/en/health-topics/diabetes/diabetes-complications-and-risks/cardiovascular-disease--diabetes. Accessed July 28, 2023.

American Heart Association (AHA). (2021b). *Stress and heart health*. Retrieved from https://www.heart.org/en/healthy-living/healthy-lifestyle/stress-management/stress-and-heart-health. Accessed July 28, 2023.

American Heart Association (AHA). (2021c). *3 tips to manage stress*. Retrieved from https://www.heart.org/en/healthy-living/healthy-lifestyle/stress-management/3-tips-to-manage-stress. Accessed July 28, 2023.

American Heart Association (AHA). (2021d). *Menopause and heart health infographic*. Retrieved from https://www.goredforwomen.org/en/know-your-risk/menopause/menopause-and-heart-health-infographic. Accessed July 28, 2023.

American Heart Association (AHA). (2020). *The skinny on fats*. Retrieved from https://www.heart.org/en/health-topics/cholesterol/prevention-and-treatment-of-high-cholesterol-hyperlipidemia/the-skinny-on-fats. Accessed July 28, 2023.

American Heart Association (AHA). (2015). *Sexual activity and heart disease*. Retrieved from https://www.goredforwomen.org/en/health-topics/consumer-healthcare/what-is-cardiovascular-disease/sex-and-heart-disease. Accessed July 28, 2023.

American Heart Association (AHA). (2014). *Body mass index (BMI) in adults (BMI calculator for adults)*. Retrieved from https://www.heart.org/en/healthy-living/healthy-eating/losing-weight/bmi-in-adults. Accessed July 28, 2023.

American Heart Association (AHA). (n.d.). *Coping with feelings*. Retrieved from https://www.heart.org/en/health-topics/cardiac-rehab/taking-care-of-yourself/coping-with-feelings. Accessed July 28, 2023.

Aroesty, J. M., & Kannam, J. P. (2022). Patient education: Medications for angina (beyond the basics). In B. J. Gersh, J. Givens, & N. Parikh (Eds.), *UpToDate*. Waltham, MA: UpToDate. Retrieved from https://www.uptodate.com/contents/medications-for-angina-beyond-the-basics. Accessed July 28, 2023.

Ball, J. W., Dains, J. E., Flynn, J. A., Solomon, B. S., & Stewart, R. W. (2014). *Seidel's guide to physical examination* (8th ed.). St. Louis: Elsevier.

Banach, M., & Serban, M. C. (2016). Discussion around statin discontinuation in older adults and patients with wasting diseases. *Journal of Cachexia, Sarcopenia and Muscle, 7*(4), 396–399. doi:10.1002/jcsm.12109.

Banasik, J. L. (2013a). Cardiac function. In L. E. Copstead & J. L. Banasik (Eds.), *Pathophysiology* (5th ed., pp. 378–407). St. Louis: Elsevier.

Banasik, J. L. (2013b). Alterations in cardiac function. In L. E. Copstead & J. L. Banasik (Eds.), *Pathophysiology* (5th ed., pp. 349–377). St. Louis: Elsevier.

Beddhu, S., Chertow, G. M., Cheung, A. K., Cushman, W. C., Rahman, M., Greene, T., et al. (2018). Influence of baseline diastolic blood pressure on effects of intensive compared with standard blood pressure control. *Circulation, 137*(2), 134–143. doi:10.1161/CIRCULATIONAHA.117.030848.

Benjamin, E. J., Blaha, M. J., Chiuve, S. E., Cushman, M., Das, S. R., Deo, R., et al. (2017). Heart disease and stroke statistics—2017 update. *Circulation, 135*(10), e146–e603. doi:10.1161/CIR.0000000000000485.

Brodkey, F. D. (2022). *Aging changes in the heart and blood vessels*. MedlinePlus [website]. Retrieved from https://medlineplus.gov/ency/article/004006.htm. Accessed July 28, 2023.

Centers for Disease Control and Prevention (CDC). (2023a). *Heart disease facts*. Retrieved from https://www.cdc.gov/heartdisease/facts.htm. Accessed July 28, 2023.

Centers for Disease Control and Prevention (CDC). (2023b). *High blood pressure*. Retrieved from https://www.cdc.gov/bloodpressure/index.htm. Accessed July 28, 2023.

Centers for Disease Control and Prevention (CDC). (2023c). *Lower your risk for the number 1 killer of women*. Retrieved from https://www.cdc.gov/healthequity/features/heartdisease/index.html. Accessed July 28, 2023.

Centers for Disease Control and Prevention (CDC). (2022). *Overweight & obesity*. Retrieved from https://www.cdc.gov/obesity/index.html. Accessed July 28, 2023.

Centers for Disease Control and Prevention (CDC). (2017). *Assessment: Measuring orthostatic blood pressure*. Retrieved from https://www.cdc.gov/steadi/pdf/Measuring_Orthostatic_Blood_Pressure-print.pdf. Accessed July 28, 2023.

Choi, K., Jeon, G. S., & Cho, S. I. (2017). Prospective study on the impact of fear of falling on functional decline among community dwelling elderly women. *International Journal of Environmental Research and Public Health, 14*(5), 469. doi:10.3390/ijerph14050469.

Dai, X., & Tan, W. A. (2019). Cardiovascular disease in the elderly. In G.A. Stouffer, M. S. Runge, C. Patterson, & J. S. Rossi (Eds.), *Netter's cardiology* (3rd ed., pp. 517–523). Philadelphia, PA: Elsevier.

Dechant, L. M., & Heimgartner, N. M. (2018). Care of patients with dysrhythmias. In D. D. Ignatavicius, M. L. Workman, C. R. Rebar, & N. M. Heimgartner (Eds.), *Medical surgical nursing: Concepts for interprofessional collaborative care* (9th ed., pp. 664–690). St. Louis, MO: Elsevier.

Dharmarajan, K., & Rich, M. W. (2017). Epidemiology, pathophysiology, and prognosis of heart failure in older adults. *Heart Failure Clinics, 13*(3), 417–426. doi:10.1016/j.hfc.2017.02.001.

Duda-Pyszny, D., Trzeciak, P., & Gąsior, M. (2018). Coronary artery disease in women. *Polish Journal of Cardio-Thoracic Surgery, 15*(1), 44–48. doi:10.5114/kitp.2018.74675.

Fillit, H. M., Rockwood, K., & Young, J. (2017). *Brocklehurst's textbook of geriatric medicine and gerontology* (8th ed.). Philadelphia, PA: Elsevier.

Garcia, M., Mulvagh, S. L., Merz, C. N. B., Buring, J. E., & Manson, J. E. (2016). Cardiovascular disease in women: Clinical perspectives. *Circulation Research, 188*(8), 1273–1293. doi:10.1161/CIRCRESAHA.116.307547.

Gerhard-Herman, M. D., Gornik, H. L., Barrett, C., Barshes, N. R., Corriere, M. A., Drachman, D. E., et al. (2017). 2016 AHA/ACC guideline on the management of patients with lower extremity peripheral artery disease: A report of the American College of Cardiology/American Heart Association Task Force on Clinical Practice Guidelines. *Circulation, 135*(12), e726–e779. doi:10.1161/CIR.0000000000000471.

Goodnough, L. T., & Schrier, S. L. (2014). Evaluation and management of anemia in the elderly. *American Journal of Hematology*, 89(1), 88–96. doi:10.1002/ajh.23598.

Goyal, P., & Maurer, M. S. (2016). Syncope in older adults. *Journal of Geriatric Cardiology*, 13(5), 380–386. doi:10.11909/j.issn.1671-5411.2016.05.002.

Guralnik, J., Ershler, W., Artz, A., Lazo-Langner, A, Walston, J., Pahor, M., et al. (2022). Unexplained anemia of aging: Etiology, health consequences, and diagnostic criteria. *Journal of the American Geriatrics Society*, 70(3), 891–899. doi:10.1111/jgs.17565.

Heidenreich, P. A., Bozkurt, B., Aguilar, D., Allen, L. A., Byun, J. J., Colvin, M. M., et al. (2022). 2022 AHA/ACC/HFSA guideline for the management of heart failure: A report of the American College of Cardiology/American Heart Association Joint Committee on Clinical Practice Guidelines. *Circulation*, 145(18), e895–e1032. doi:10.1161/CIR.0000000000001063.

Huether, S. E., McCance, K. L., Brashers, V. L., & Rote, N. S. (2017). *Understanding pathophysiology* (6th ed.). St. Louis, MO: Elsevier.

Kapan, A., Luger, E., Haider, S., Titze, S., Schindler, K., Lackinger, C., et al. (2017). Fear of falling reduced by a lay led home-based program in frail community-dwelling older adults: A randomised controlled trial. *Archives of Gerontology and Geriatrics*, 68, 25–32. doi:10.1016/j.archger.2016.08.009.

Krishnamurthi, N., Francis, J., Fihn, S. D., Meyer, C. S., & Whooley, M. A. (2018). Leading causes of cardiovascular hospitalization in 8.45 million US veterans. *PLoS One*, 13(3), e0193996. doi:10.1371/journal.pone.0193996.

Liu, E., & Lampert, B. C. (2022). Heart failure in older adults: Medical management and advanced therapies. *Geriatrics (Basel)*, 7(2), 36. doi:10.3390/geriatrics7020036.

Liu, Z., Tao, X., Chen, Y., Fan, Z., & Li, Y. (2015). Bed rest versus early ambulation with standard anticoagulation in the management of deep vein thrombosis: A meta-analysis. *PLoS One*, 10(4), e0121388. doi:10.1371/journal.pone.0121388.

Loftsgaarden, T. G. (2013). Alterations in blood flow. In L. E. Copstead & J. L. Banasik (Eds.), *Pathophysiology* (5th ed., pp. 309–331). St Louis: Elsevier.

Napierkowski, D. B., & Prado, K. B. (2021). Nutritional needs in the older adult, guidelines and prevention strategies to optimize health and avoid chronic disease. *Geriatrics, Gerontology and Aging*, 15, e0210027. doi:10.5327/Z2447-212320212100010.

National Heart, Lung, and Blood Institute. (2022a). *What is an arrhythmia?* Retrieved from https://www.nhlbi.nih.gov/health/arrhythmias. Accessed July 28, 2023.

National Heart, Lung, and Blood Institute. (2022b). *What is anemia?* Retrieved from https://www.nhlbi.nih.gov/health/anemia. Accessed July 28, 2023.

Ogden, C. L., Carroll, M. D., Fryar, C. D., & Flegal, K. M. (2015). Prevalence of obesity among adults and youth: United States, 2011–2014. *NCHS Data Brief*, (219), 1–8.

Oliveros, E., Patel, H., Kyung, S., Fugar, S., Goldberg, A., Madan, N., et al. (2020). Hypertension in older adults: Assessment, management, and challenges. *Clinical Cardiology*, 43(2), 99–107. doi:10.1002/clc.23303.

Olmedo, K., & Pakbaz, Z. (2022). *Anemia in elderly persons*. Medscape [website]. Retrieved from https://emedicine.medscape.com/article/1339998-overview. Accessed July 28, 2023.

Patel, A., & Stewart, B. F. (2015). *On hypertension in the elderly: An epidemiologic shift*. American College of Cardiology. Retrieved from http://www.acc.org/latest-in-cardiology/articles/2015/02/19/14/55/on-hypertension-in-the-elderly. Accessed July 28, 2023.

Pirmohamed, A., Kitzman, D. W., & Maurer, M. S. (2016). Heart failure in older adults: Embracing complexity. *Journal of Geriatric Cardiology*, 13(1), 8–14. doi:10.11909/j.issn.1671-5411.2016.01.020.

Qaseem, A., Wilt, T. J., Rich, R., Humphrey, L. L., Frost, J., & Forciea, M. A. (2017). Pharmacologic treatment of hypertension in adults aged 60 years or older to higher versus lower blood pressure targets: A clinical practice guideline from the American College of Physicians and the American Academy of Family Physicians. *Annals of Internal Medicine*, 166(6), 430–437. doi:10.7326/M16-1785.

Rippe, J. M. (2018). Lifestyle medicine: The health promoting power of daily habits and practices. *American Journal of Lifestyle Medicine*, 12(6) 499–512. doi:10.1177/1559827618785554.

Rosenthal, L., McManus, D. D., & Sardana, M. (2019). *Atrial fibrillation treatment and management*. Medscape [website]. Retrieved from https://emedicine.medscape.com/article/151066-treatment. Accessed July 28, 2023.

Singh, V. N., & Aggarwal, K. (2018). *Acute myocardial infarction imaging*. Medscape [website]. Retrieved from https://emedicine.medscape.com/article/350175-overview#a1. Accessed July 28, 2023.

Stephens, E., & Peak, D. A. (2022). *Peripheral vascular disease clinical presentation*. eMedicine [website]. Retrieved from https://emedicine.medscape.com/article/761556-clinical. Accessed July 28, 2023.

Stone, N. J., Robinson, J. G., Lichtenstein, A. H., Merz, C. N. B., Blum, C. B., Eckel, R. H., et al. (2014). 2013 ACC/AHA guideline on the treatment of blood cholesterol to reduce atherosclerotic cardiovascular risk in adults: a report of the American College of Cardiology/American Heart Association Task Force on Practice Guidelines. *Circulation*, 129(25 Suppl. 2), S1–S45. doi:10.1161/01.cir.0000437738.63853.7a.

Supervía, M., Medina-Inojosa, J. R., Yeung, C., Lopez-Jimenez, F., Squires, R. W., Pérez-Terzic, C. M., et al. (2017). Cardiac rehabilitation for women: A systematic review of barriers and solutions. *Mayo Clinic Proceedings*, S0025-6196(17)30026-5. doi:10.1016/j.mayocp.2017.01.002.

Tessler, J., & Bordoni, B. (2023). *Cardiac rehabilitation*. StatPearls [Internet]. Retrieved from https://www.ncbi.nlm.nih.gov/books/NBK537196/. Accessed July 28, 2023.

The Medical Letter. (2015). Drugs for chronic heart failure. *The Medical Letter on Drugs and Therapeutics*, 57(1460), 9–13.

Thompson, A. D., & Shea, M. J. (2022). Orthostatic hypotension. In *merck manual professional version*. Merck & Co., Inc. Retrieved from http://www.merckmanuals.com/professional/cardiovascular-disorders/symptoms-of-cardiovascular-disorders/orthostatic-hypotension. Accessed July 28, 2023.

Tsao, C. W., Aday, A. W., Almarzooq, Z. I., Alonso, A., Beaton, A. Z., Bittencourt, M. S., et al. (2022). Heart disease and stroke statistics – 2022 update: A report from the American Heart Association. *Circulation*, 145(8), e153–e639. doi:10.1161/CIR.0000000000001052.

Waterbury, S. (2021). *Anemia in the elderly*. NetCE [website]. Retrieved from http://www.netce.com/coursecontent.php?courseid=1145. Accessed July 28, 2023.

WebMD Editorial Contributors. (2022). *Atrial fibrillation: Causes, risk factors, and triggers*. WebMD [website]. Retrieved from https://www.webmd.com/heart-disease/atrial-fibrillation/causes-risks-triggers-afib. Accessed July 28, 2023.

Whelton, P. K., Carey, R. M., Aronow, W. S., Casey, Jr., D. E., Collins, K. J., Himmelfarb, C. D., et al. (2018). 2017 ACC/AHA/AAPA/ABC/ACPM/AGS/APhA/ASH/ASPC/NMA/PCNA Guideline for the prevention, detection, evaluation, and management of high blood pressure in adults: A report of the American College of Cardiology/American Heart Association Task Force on Clinical Practice Guidelines. *Hypertension, 71*(6), e13–e115. doi:10.1161/HYP.0000000000000065.

Yancy, W. C., Jessup, M., Bozkurt, B., Butler, J., Casey, Jr., D. E., Colvin, M. M., et al. (2017). 2017 ACC/AHA/HFSA focused update of the 2013 ACCF/AHA guideline for the management of heart failure: A report of the American College of Cardiology/American Heart Association Task Force on Clinical Practice Guidelines and the Heart Failure Society of America. *Journal of the American College of Cardiology, 70*(6), 776–803. doi:10.1016/j.jacc.2017.04.025.

Zafari, A. M., & Abdou, M. H. (2019). *Myocardial infarction workup*. Medscape [website]. Retrieved from https://emedicine.medscape.com/article/155919-workup#c14. Accessed July 28, 2023.

Zathar, Z., Karunatilleke, A., Fawzy, A. M., & Lip, G. Y. H. (2019). Atrial fibrillation in older people: Concepts and controversies. *Frontiers in Medicine, 6*, 175. doi:10.3389/fmed.2019.00175.

Zoungas, S. (2017). *How old is too old for cholesterol lowering medications?* TheConversation.com [website]. Retrieved from http://theconversation.com/how-old-is-too-old-for-cholesterol-lowering-medications-78102. Accessed July 28, 2023.

18

Respiratory Function

Jennifer Mundine, EdD, MSN, RN, CNE

http://evolve.elsevier.com/Yeager/gerontologic/

LEARNING OBJECTIVES

On completion of this chapter, the reader will be able to:
1. Describe anatomic changes in the lungs resulting from the normal aging process.
2. Describe age-related changes in ventilation.
3. Identify nursing interventions and outcomes for older adults with various respiratory alterations.
4. Discuss smoking cessation methods and interventions.
5. Identify risk factors for the development of tuberculosis in older adults.
6. List the benefits of pulmonary rehabilitation for older adults with chronic obstructive pulmonary disease (COPD).

WHAT WOULD YOU DO?

What would you do if you were faced with the following situations?
- Your 72-year-old patient comes to the clinic for their annual physical examination. During the history, your patient notes that they continue to smoke one pack per day. A chart review indicates that they have received smoking cessation counseling on their last three visits. What should you do?
- Your 68-year-old patient, newly diagnosed with sleep apnea, is struggling to wear their continuous positive airway pressure (CPAP) when sleeping. What additional measures can they take to help with nocturnal oxygenation?

The respiratory system is responsible for gas exchange between the environment and the blood and involves two processes: ventilation and oxygenation. *Ventilation* is the movement of air into and out of the lungs and consists of inhalation and exhalation. During inhalation, oxygen-rich air is moved into the lungs, and then during exhalation, carbon dioxide (CO_2)-rich air is moved out. During *oxygenation*, CO_2 is transferred from the vasculature to the pulmonary side of the lungs, and oxygen is transferred from the pulmonary side to the vasculature, where it is loaded onto hemoglobin. The processes of respiration, including rate and depth, are controlled by chemoreceptors in the medulla oblongata, the arch of the aorta, and the carotid artery and are sensitive to oxygen levels and pH. Respiration depends on adequate structures for moving air during ventilation, an environment where oxygen and CO_2 can transfer, and chemoreceptors sensitive to the maintenance of oxygenation and pH levels.

AGE-RELATED CHANGES IN STRUCTURE AND FUNCTION

Normal aging results in changes to the ribs and vertebrae. The ribs become less mobile, and chest wall compliance decreases. Osteoporosis and calcification of the costal cartilage lead to increased rigidity and stiffness of the thoracic cage. If kyphosis or scoliosis is present, degeneration of the intervertebral disks occurs, resulting in a shorter thorax with an increased anteroposterior diameter. Advanced cases may result in a marked limitation of thoracic movement because the rib cage rests on the pelvic bones. Such changes in the chest wall can impair respiratory compliance, leading to increased breathing.

Progressive loss of elastic recoil of the lung parenchyma and conducting airways, reduced elastic recoil of the lung, and the opposing forces of the chest wall are also present. The lung becomes less elastic as collagenic substances surrounding the alveoli and alveolar ducts stiffen and form cross-linkages that interfere with the elastic properties of the lungs. Any and all of these structural changes make it more difficult for the older person to ventilate, leading to increased work of breathing and heightened energy expenditure. Table 18.1 summarizes various

Previous author: Debra L. Sanders, PhD, RN, GCNS-BC

TABLE 18.1 Age-Related Changes in the Respiratory System

Functions	Pathophysiologic Changes	Clinical Presentation
Structures	Chest wall stiffening Costal cartilage calcification	Barrel chest Kyphotic posture Decreased chest wall movement Decreased deep breathing Decreased cough effectiveness Decreased breath sounds Decreased vital capacity Increased residual capacity Decreased PaO_2 and SaO_2
Defense mechanisms	Decreased cell mediated immunity and antibodies Decreased cilia function Decreased cough force Decreased alveolar macrophage function Decreases sensation in the pharynx	Decrease secretion clearance Thickened mucous Decreased cough effectiveness Increased risk for aspiration and infection Infections may be more severe and last longer
Respiratory control	Decreased response to hypoxemia Decreased response to hypercapnia	A slight decrease in PaO_2 and an increase in $PaCO_2$ Decreased ability to maintain acid–base balance Significant hypoxemia or hypercapnia may develop Retained secretion, excessive sedation, or positioning that impairs chest wall expansion
Sleep and breathing	Decreased ventilatory drive Decreased upper airway muscle tone Decreased arousal	Increased frequency of apnea, hypopnea, and arterial oxygen desaturation during sleep Increased risk of aspiration Snoring Obstructive sleep apnea
Exercise capacity	Muscle deconditioning Decreased muscle mass Decreased efficiency of respiratory muscles Decreased reserves	Decreased maximum oxygen consumption Breathlessness at low exercise levels
Breathing pattern	Decreased responsiveness to hypoxemia and hypercapnia Change in respiratory mechanics	Increased respiratory rate Decreased V_T Increased minute ventilation

PaO_2, partial pressure of arterial oxygen; $PaCO_2$, partial pressure of arterial carbon dioxide; SaO_2, saturation arterial oxygen; V_T, tidal volume.
Modified From Pierson, D. J., & Kacmarek, R. M. (Eds.). (1992). *Foundations of respiratory care*. New York: Churchill Livingstone.

changes in the aging respiratory system (McCance and Huether, 2019).

As muscle strength declines with age and as respiratory muscles weaken, it becomes increasingly difficult to exert inspiratory and expiratory forces. A functional decline with age affects respiratory muscles, decreasing maximum inspiratory pressure (Morisawa et al, 2021). The combination of an increasingly stiffer skeletal structure and weaker muscles results in additional effort and energy to breathe. The diaphragm, a major respiratory muscle, flattens and becomes less efficient in patients with advancing COPD. Because of this, older adults use the less efficient accessory muscles of respiration, such as the abdominal, sternocleidomastoid, and trapezius muscles. As the abdominal muscles become more important to older adults, their breathing patterns may become more affected by positioning and increased abdominal pressure.

Respiratory rates generally are faster and shallower in older adults; a normal rate is 16–25 breaths per minute. This combination results in a relatively unchanged arterial CO_2 pressure ($PaCO_2$). However, shallow breathing patterns may result in hypoxemia and hypercapnia as the alveoli at the base of the lungs are underventilated, which, in turn, results in a decreased ventilation–perfusion ratio and less effective alveolar gas exchange. Age-related reductions in cardiac output and mixed venous oxygen content compound the effect of the ventilation–perfusion imbalance in older adults. In healthy older adults, the number of alveoli remains relatively unchanged, but their structure may be altered. As a result, the number of functioning alveoli decreases. With age, alveolar supporting structures deteriorate, which leads to a progressive loss of the intraalveolar septum. As the alveolar septal walls become thinner, the alveoli enlarge because of the dilation of the proximal bronchioles, but fewer capillaries are available for gas exchange. The increase in physiologic dead space is seen as the capillary structures surrounding the alveoli diminish. The result is a decrease in the surface area available for gas exchange, which can mimic those with emphysema or lung disease (Staheli and Rondeau, 2022).

Older adults may also have a decrease in the number and effectiveness of cilia in the tracheobronchial tree, which results in increasing difficulty clearing secretions. As immunoglobulin A (IgA), which is found on the nasal respiratory mucosal surface, decreases with aging, the older adult's ability to neutralize viruses becomes hindered. This combination of decreased IgA and an increase in pooling secretions from impaired mucociliary transport makes infections more likely. With repeated respiratory tract infections or smoking, the effectiveness of the ciliary action and the number of cilia are significantly decreased, resulting in difficulty in managing mucus (SmokeFree.gov, n.d.).

One of the primary functions of the respiratory system is gas exchange. For a healthy adult, the normal partial pressure of oxygen in alveolar air (PaO_2) is 80–100 mm Hg. However, after the age of 60, the PaO_2 drops by 1 mm Hg per year. Therefore, a PaO_2 of 70 mm Hg for a 70-year-old is relatively normal, which is how the phrase "70 at 70" originated. The expected decrease in PaO_2 is most likely caused by some of the factors previously discussed—reduced tidal volume (V_T), less alveolar surface area, and increased residual volume (RV) (Sorenson, 2006).

The oxygen-carrying capacity of blood is also reduced with age. Hemoglobin is the molecule most responsible for oxygen transport to peripheral tissues, but its levels are diminished in older adults. The alveolar–arterial (A-a) oxygen gradient, a measure of the efficiency of oxygen transfer from the lungs to the blood, compares the PAO_2 with the PaO_2. With rapid diffusion in a healthy adult, the net difference is close to zero. This gradient normally increases in older adults, most likely because of the ventilation–perfusion mismatch (Brashers and Huether, 2020).

The arterial pH of the older person remains within the normal adult range of 7.35–7.45 unless influenced by an acute illness or comorbidity. Despite an increase in RV, $PaCO_2$ does not normally rise, primarily because of increased ventilation. However, older adults do not react as quickly to changes in either hypoxemia or hypercapnia. The normal clinical response to hypoxemia is an increase in the rate and depth of respiration and an increase in heart rate and blood pressure. Older patients show a lower increase in heart rate and a lower response to increasing CO_2. In fact, their ventilatory responses to hypoxia and hypercapnia may be diminished by as much as 50% in comparison with adults in their 20s, largely as a result of a reduced sympathetic nervous system response. Therefore, careful assessment is crucial. The most sensitive clinical indicator for hypoxia and hypercapnia in older adults is mental status changes and complaints of occipital headaches or forgetfulness that are not otherwise explained. Finally, dyspnea on exertion is an increasing problem because any increased oxygen demand may lead quickly to symptomatic hypoxia (Brashers and Huether, 2020; McCance and Huether, 2019).

As previously described, many of the changes in pulmonary functions in older adults are related to the changes in elastic recoil and musculoskeletal changes of the chest wall. Table 18.2 lists the lung volumes measured, the normal findings, and alterations related to aging. The ability to determine accurate pulmonary function by testing requires patience on the part of the healthcare provider, as an older patient may not be able to perform quickly. Ensure adequate time for this assessment of the older adult patient.

Although the total lung capacity (TLC) remains relatively unchanged, the individual volumes that comprise TLC change dramatically. V_T is decreased in older adults. Vital capacity (VC) is also decreased as a result of decreased mobility of the chest wall and altered inspiratory and expiratory capabilities. The rate of reduction in VC is greater in older males than in older females. The inspiratory capacity of older adults is affected by their decreased ability to take deep breaths. Decreased compliance of the thorax accounts for the increase in RV and expiratory reserve volume (ERV). RV is also reduced because of decreased muscle strength and a shallow breathing pattern. As a result, functional dead space ventilation is increased from one-third to as much as one-half of each breath, which results

TABLE 18.2 Pulmonary Function Changes in Older Adults

		AVERAGE VALUE	
	Description	Adult Male	Older Patient
Lung Volume			
Tidal volume (V_T)	Volume of air inhaled or exhaled per breath	5–10 (mL/kg)	Decreased
Inspiratory reserve volume (IRV)	Volume of air inhaled in addition to normal V_T	3000 mL	Decreased
Expiratory reserve volume (ERV)	Maximum volume of air that can be exhaled in addition to normal V_T	1200 mL	Decreased
Residual volume (RV)	Volume of air left in the lungs after maximum exhalation	1200 mL	Increased by as much as 25%
Lung Capacity			
Functional residual capacity (FRC)	Volume of air left in the lung after a normal exhalation (RV + ERV)	2400 mL	Increased
Residual volume/total lung capacity (RV/TLC)	The ratio of RV to TLC is expressed as percentage	33%	Increased
Vital capacity (VC)	Volume of air exhaled after maximal inhalation (IRV + V_T + ERV)	4800 mL	Decreased by as much as 25%
Total lung capacity (TLC)	Total volume of air in the lungs after maximum inhalation (IRV + V_T + ERV + RV)	6000 mL	Unchanged

in a decrease in the volume of air that can participate in gas exchange (Brashers and Huether, 2020; McCance and Huether, 2019).

Airflow in the tracheobronchial tree is affected by the size of the airway, resistance in the airway, muscle strength, and elastic recoil. When measured in the older patient, all of these indices decreased. Forced expiratory volume in 1 second (FEV_1) is reported to drop between 25 and 30 milliliters (mL) per year after age 30. Changes in the airflow measures are related to the stiffness of the chest wall and the loss of elastic recoil in the lungs. The decrease in thoracic muscular strength contributes to the decreased force of the air moved, and as much as a 50% reduction may occur in the maximum voluntary ventilation and FEV between ages 30 and 90.

At low V_Ts, small airways tend to close early because of the loss of elastic recoil and decreased flow rates caused by increased airway resistance, trapping air in the alveoli. Closing capacity (CC), the volume at which the smallest airways close, increases with age, and by the age of 65, it exceeds the functional residual capacity (FRC) when in the upright position. This contributes to early airway closure. Other factors contributing to early airway closure include increased time in a supine position and shallow breathing.

In younger adults, pulmonary vascular circulation is a relatively low pressure system with high distensibility and low resistance. As adults age, these vessels become less distensible and more fibrous, which results in increased pulmonary artery diameter and greater thickness of the vessel wall; in turn, these increases result in increased pulmonary vascular resistance and increased pulmonary artery pressure. The alveolar capillary membrane also thickens, which further reduces the surface area available for gas exchange. The number of functional capillaries declines, which results in decreased alveolar vascularity; this, in combination with a diminished cardiac output, causes a decrease in pulmonary capillary blood flow (Brashers and Huether, 2020).

FACTORS AFFECTING LUNG FUNCTION

Exercise and Immobility

Exercise has a positive effect on the respiratory and cardiovascular systems. However, the ability of older patients to perform exercise is affected by changes in cardiac output, skeletal muscle function, joint function, and overall coordination.

Increased oxygen demands during exercise periods may well exceed the abilities of older patients, and for those with COPD, activity intolerance is exacerbated. In addition, older patients are more likely to have comorbidities involving the cardiovascular and respiratory systems that may deter exercise ability. Strength and endurance may also be reduced, which leads to increased immobility and increased breathlessness when activity is attempted. Older patients with COPD and immobility may benefit from a program of regular exercise to increase strength and endurance and decrease breathlessness as the respiratory muscles become trained (see Health Promotion/Illness Prevention box).

> **HEALTH PROMOTION/ILLNESS PREVENTION**
> **The Respiratory System**
>
> - Avoid cigarettes and secondhand smoke
> - Avoid environmental and air pollutants
> - Avoid allergens
> - Maintain a healthy diet
> - Exercise
> - Keep immunizations up to date
> - Use masks, scarves, and filters to protect against community-acquired illnesses
> - Incorporate stress management activities into daily life
> - Ensure early diagnosis and treatment of respiratory tract infections
> - Adhere to a medical regimen for chronic respiratory illnesses
> - Maintain a clean environment (i.e., dust regularly, change air filters in the furnace and air conditioner every 3 months, and change toothbrushes every 3–4 months and after an illness)
> - Maintain adequate hydration (at least 64 ounces of water daily)

Smoking

Smoking damages the lungs. Prolonged exposure to secondhand smoke has also been shown to damage the lungs of nonsmokers. Heavy smokers may demonstrate a nine-times increase in the reduction in FEV_1 over normal expected reductions. Cilia, which are paralyzed by nicotine, are unable to protect and clean the lungs, and, when coupled with the increased mucus production of goblet cells induced by tobacco, respiratory infections become more likely. Cigarette smoke also causes bronchoconstriction, increased airway resistance, and increased closing volumes and interferes with gas exchange because carbon monoxide, a byproduct of tobacco, competes with oxygen for the hemoglobin molecule. Many medications are also affected by smoking, which decreases clearance and increases serum drug levels. Some drugs altered by the chemicals present in smoking include antidepressants, propranolol, theophylline, insulin, clopidogrel, methadone, warfarin, erythromycin, and lidocaine (Fiore et al, 2008; Sarna and Bialous, 2010; Lucas and Martin, 2013).

During an assessment of social behaviors, a smoking history needs to include pack-years, that is, the number of packs smoked per day multiplied by the number of years the patient has smoked. An example is someone who smoked two packs per day from age 15 through age 40 but increased to three packs until quitting smoking at age 62. Subtract 15 from 40 and multiply by 2; then, subtract 40 from 62 and multiply by 3. Add the two numbers, and the total is 106 pack-years (Masters, 2020).

Smoking Cessation

Smoking cessation is imperative to prevent a decline in lung function with aging and comorbid disease. The five components of smoking cessation, known as the "Five A's", consist of asking, advising, assessing, assisting, and arranging (Agency for Healthcare Research and Quality [AHRQ], 2012). At each encounter, the patient is asked about tobacco use. This gives the healthcare worker an opportunity to advise, discuss the health benefits, and promote smoking cessation. When speaking to older adults, the nurse should use strong, clear, and personalized language. The nurse should assess older adults for their willingness to give up smoking and determine how soon they are ready to start the process. Then, the nurse assists older adults with smoking cessation by encouraging them to set a quit date, reviewing preparations for quitting (e.g., removing associated objects such as ashtrays), recommending nicotine replacement therapy, providing advice on successful quitting (e.g., avoid constant exposure to other smokers), providing supplemental educational materials, and offering appropriate skills training and support. Finally, the nurse arranges for follow-up (U.S. Preventive Services Task Force, 2022).

Many new treatments are available for older smokers to assist with quitting. These include the use of bupropion hydrochloride, varenicline, nicotine gum, nicotine patches, and nicotine inhalation systems. Bupropion hydrochloride is given for 3 days at 150 milligrams (mg) per day and then increased to 150 mg twice a day, with doses 8 hours apart and the first dose in the morning. Older patients can smoke during the first week of treatment and are encouraged to set a quit-smoking date before the end of the first 14 days of treatment. Varenicline, a nicotinic receptor partial agonist, is initiated 1 week before the quit date with a dosing of 0.5 mg daily, increasing to 0.5 mg twice daily on the fourth day. On the actual quit date, the dose is increased to 1 mg twice daily for 12 weeks. Varenicline has shown efficacy in dampening cravings for smoking, particularly when used in tandem with behavioral approaches. Nicotine inhalation systems, gums, and patches are used to replace the patient's need for nicotine. While vaping can be used, it still causes inflammation of the lungs and a potentially fatal lung injury (Shmerling, 2021). While using these nicotine substitutes, the older adult patient should not smoke. Gradually, over a 6–8-week period, the frequency of usage decreases (Woo and Robinson, 2020).

Obesity

The effect of obesity on respiratory function results in a decrease in chest wall compliance and a reduction in FRC, VC, and ERV because the additional weight of the relatively stiffer chest and larger abdomen creates a mechanical disadvantage to breathing and impedance to overall body movement. As a result, pulmonary functions are reduced and breathlessness increases. The combination of decreased ability to take a deep breath, early airway closure, and the increased likelihood of immobility puts the older patient at high risk of developing atelectasis and upper and lower respiratory tract infections.

Moreover, excessive weight can lead to hypoventilation with or without hypercapnia, further interfering with adequate respiratory ventilation and perfusion. Obesity is a well-recognized precursor to obstructive sleep apnea (OSA), a periodic reduction or cessation of breathing during sleep that causes narrowing or occlusion of the upper airway. OSA is increasing in prevalence due to escalating obesity rates. The World Health Organization (WHO, n.d.) defines overweight as a body mass index (BMI) equal to or greater than 25 kg/m^2 and obesity as a BMI equal to or greater than 30 kg/m^2. Even a 10% reduction in body weight can significantly improve VC and respiratory mechanics in older adults. Nurses can play an integral role in educating older adults about obesity and the modifiable risk factors associated with weight gain and concomitant disease (Cash and Glass, 2019).

Anesthesia and Surgery

Because aging can decrease overall pulmonary reserves, older adults are more susceptible to respiratory compromise during the perioperative and postoperative periods. An older patient undergoing surgery has an increased risk of aspiration as a result of a loss of laryngeal reflexes. If surgery is an emergency, this risk is increased because of the older patient's delayed gastric emptying and the potential for a full stomach. Even younger, healthier adults have the risk of postoperative atelectasis because of general anesthesia and the inability or unwillingness to cough and deep breathe because of incisions, pain, and drowsiness. In the older adult, these risks are amplified because of decreased muscle strength, a decreased cough reflex, and a greater likelihood of alterations in consciousness. Postoperative immobility decreases ventilation and increases the risk of airway clearance problems. Because a healthy adult patient can tend to be slightly "dry" after surgery in combination with a reduced thirst sensation, the older adult has an increased risk of hypovolemia and resultant thickened secretions that are difficult to clear. Promotion of deep breathing for effective pain management, adequate hydration, frequent position changes, and early mobility will decrease the risk of developing atelectasis. Furthermore, anesthetic agents used during surgical procedures can increase the risk of perioperative hypercapnia, hypoxemia, and postoperative complications such as respiratory failure. This risk is compounded in older adults who have cardiovascular or respiratory comorbid diseases (Barnett, 2022).

RESPIRATORY FINDINGS COMMON IN OLDER PATIENTS

Respiratory symptoms common in older patients include alterations in breathing patterns, dyspnea, and coughing. Abnormal breathing patterns in older patients may also be indicative of other metabolic and respiratory illnesses. An early sign of respiratory problems is a change in mental status. Because the physiologic responses to hypoxemia and hypercapnia are blunted in older patients, compensatory changes in heart rate, respiratory rate, and blood pressure may be delayed and cerebral perfusion may suffer. Mental status changes may include subtle increases in forgetfulness and irritability. Older patients may also complain of an occipital headache or confusion when awakening from sleep. If these signs persist, a more in-depth evaluation of the older patient's respiratory status is indicated.

Complaints of dyspnea or breathlessness in older patients are often associated with underlying respiratory and cardiac disease. Dyspnea is a subjective perception of breathlessness that is difficult for the older patient to quantify; dyspnea may therefore be dismissed, especially when no clinical evidence can be attributed to the complaint. Older patients most often describe their breathlessness as a sensation of an inability to get enough air, difficulty taking a deep breath, breathing rapidly, or a choking or smothering feeling. Dyspnea at rest is most often associated with an acute respiratory or cardiac illness, whereas dyspnea on exertion may be related to immobility, obesity, respiratory muscle deconditioning, or an overall deconditioned state. Older patients with COPD may experience dyspnea on exertion initially and dyspnea at rest as the disease progresses. Dyspnea is a common complaint in older patients with pulmonary disease. However, older patients usually do not complain of dyspnea until it begins to interfere with their activities of daily living (ADLs), and then only if those activities are important to them. For example, it may become difficult to use the stairs; therefore, an older patient may simply choose the elevator or escalator and not consider reporting the shortness of breath associated with stair climbing. It is important to determine which ADLs an older patient no longer participates in and why.

The cough mechanism in older patients is altered because of the loss of elastic recoil and decreased respiratory muscle strength. Causes of coughing in older patients include postnasal drip, chronic bronchitis, acute respiratory tract infections, aspiration, gastroesophageal reflux disease (GERD), congestive heart failure (CHF), interstitial lung disease, cancer, and angiotensin-converting enzyme inhibitor (ACEI) medications for hypertension and CHF. Because of the age-related changes that affect an older patient's coughing mechanism, it is important to recommend cough suppressants with caution. Suppression of the cough and depression of any respiratory function could lead to retention of pulmonary secretions, plugged airways, atelectasis, and aspiration.

RESPIRATORY ALTERATIONS IN OLDER PATIENTS

Chronic respiratory disease affects not only older patients but also their families (Cruz et al, 2017). Many patients with respiratory illnesses feel a loss of control over their lives because of breathlessness during exertion and at rest. They may become demanding and controlling in dealing with their families and friends. The quality of older patients' lives depends on their feelings about and control of the disease. Support groups sponsored by the American Lung Association and local hospitals are available to help patients and families deal with anger, loss of control, and hopelessness. The family, or a significant other, needs to be included in all aspects of planning and caring for an older patient with a respiratory illness. The patient's success in complying with the medical recommendations may depend on the assistance they receive in getting to the physician's office, getting to the pharmacy for medications, administering medications, and performing ADLs. Older patients with respiratory disease need a good family support system and a healthcare team to support both them and their families (see Evidence-Based Practice: COPD Self-Management in Ethno-Cultural Communities).

Respiratory disease is divided into two categories: (1) obstructive pulmonary disease and (2) restrictive pulmonary disease. Obstructive lung diseases are characterized by changes in expiratory airflow rates and obstruction of the airway. The lumen of the airway may be decreased by mucus, edema of the airway lining, or constriction of the muscles surrounding the airway, causing bronchoconstriction. Restrictive lung disease is characterized by a decreased ability to expand the chest, impaired inhalation, and decreased lung volumes. Changes in the chest wall, lung parenchyma, pleural space, and extrapulmonary factors, such as body mass, may result in restrictive lung disease. Examples of these diseases include bronchogenic carcinoma and tuberculosis (TB). Other respiratory diseases seen in older patients include bronchopulmonary infections, pulmonary edema, and pulmonary emboli (PE).

OBSTRUCTIVE PULMONARY DISEASE
Asthma

Asthma is a chronic inflammatory disease that affects the airways and is characterized by reversible airway obstruction, airway inflammation, and increased airway responsiveness to a variety of stimuli. Asthma has higher morbidity and mortality rates in older adults than in other age groups. Older patients diagnosed with asthma have lower expiratory flow rates and fewer symptom-free periods. Because of other comorbidities, the provider may delay a diagnosis of asthma. Asthma occurs in about 8.3% of older adults after age 65, and many of these older adults have asthma as a continuing chronic disorder (Global Initiative for Asthma [GINA], 2022a).

Airway inflammation contributes to airway hyperresponsiveness; airflow limitations, including acute bronchoconstriction, airway edema, and mucous plug formation; airway wall remodeling; respiratory symptoms; and disease chronicity (GINA, 2022a; McCance and Huether, 2019). Inflammation causes recurrent episodes of wheezing, breathlessness, chest tightness,

---

> **EVIDENCE-BASED PRACTICE**
>
> **COPD Self-Management in Ethno-Cultural Communities**
>
> **Sample/Setting**
> The study included 30 patients with COPD and 16 family members.
>
> **Methods**
> Qualitative data were collected via interviews.
>
> **Findings**
> Five themes emerged: current knowledge and practice of COPD self-management; trusted sources of health information; insufficient care from medical doctors; information they wish to receive; and barriers to accessing health information.
>
> **Implications**
> Consider diverse cultural beliefs and practices when developing educational materials; engage patients and families in the development of educational materials; and ensure that education is appropriate and relevant to the patient's and family's ethnic and cultural beliefs and practices to facilitate adherence.

Data From Shum, J., Poureslami, I., Cheng, N., & FitzGerald, J. M. (2014). Responsibility for COPD self-management in ethno-cultural communities: The role of patient, family member, care provider, and system. *Diversity and Equality in Health and Care, 11*, 201–213.

and coughing, often at night or early in the morning. Blood vessel dilation and capillary leakage are caused by inflammation of the airway mucous membranes. This leads to tissue swelling and increased secretions associated with mucus production (Brashers and Huether, 2020).

Recent evidence suggests that persistent abnormalities in lung function are associated with subbasement membrane fibrosis in some patients. Patients with asthma, especially older patients who may not have had this disease through most of their lives, require careful education to include self-management, how to adjust medications during exacerbations, and the correct way to prepare themselves for exposure to known triggers.

An asthma attack may be precipitated by exposure to allergens or irritants such as changes in weather, odors, or stress. In older patients, asthma is often associated with viral respiratory infections. Signs and symptoms include dyspnea, audible wheezing, cough, palpitations, tachypnea, tachycardia, use of accessory muscles of respiration, pulsus paradoxus, diaphoresis, and hypoxemia. Initially, a patient may hyperventilate and effectively blow off increased CO_2. However, falling PaO_2 levels and pH, along with rising $PaCO_2$, are indicative of imminent respiratory failure. The increasing $PaCO_2$ is a result of the patient's exhaustion and inability to hyperventilate as a result of increased breathing work.

Prognosis

The prognosis for older adults with asthma is relatively good. Success is based on a partnership between the patient and the healthcare provider to properly use prescribed medications, avoid asthma triggers, identify early signs of exacerbation, and maintain a healthy lifestyle.

Treatment

The goals of asthma therapy are to control asthma by reduction in impairment and risk, which may be achieved by (1) preventing chronic and troublesome symptoms such as coughing or breathlessness during the day, at night, or after exercise, (2) maintaining (near) normal pulmonary function, (3) maintaining normal activity levels, including exercise and attendance at work or school, (4) requiring infrequent use (≤ 2 days a week) of inhaled short-acting beta$_2$-agonists (SABAs) and satisfying the patient's and family's expectations of asthma care, (5) preventing recurrent exacerbations and minimizing emergency department visits, and (6) providing optimal pharmacologic treatment with minimal or no adverse effects (GINA, 2022a). A stepwise approach to pharmacologic management is recommended by the GINA (2022a) clinical practice guidelines. The specific drug, dose, and frequency are dictated by the severity of the asthma attack at the time that therapy is initiated, and subsequently, the drug should be stepped down to maintain long-term control with the minimum medication necessary. Medications are classified into two categories: (1) long-term control medications and (2) quick-relief medications.

Long-term control medications. Long-term control medications are taken daily and include antiinflammatory agents, long-acting bronchodilators, and leukotriene modifiers. Corticosteroids are the most potent and effective long-term control medications in the treatment of mild, moderate, or severe persistent asthma. They are well tolerated and safe when used at the recommended dosage. Most of the benefit is achieved with relatively low doses, and the potential for side effects increases with the dose. However, for asthma not controlled with maintenance doses of corticosteroids, two options are now available. The first is to combine the corticosteroids with long-acting beta$_2$-agonists (LABAs), and the second, most recent recommendation is to increase the dose of corticosteroids (GINA, 2022b). The clinical response to corticosteroids is a reduction in airway inflammation, improvement in peak expiratory flow rate (PEFR), diminished airway hyperresponsiveness, prevention of exacerbations, and possible prevention of airway wall remodeling. Corticosteroids are generally inhaled twice a day.

LABAs act by relaxing the smooth muscle of the airways and stimulating beta$_2$-receptors to increase cyclic adenosine monophosphate (cAMP). They are not recommended as a monotherapy for long-term control but, rather, are often prescribed in combination with corticosteroids. The duration of action is 12 hours for a single dose. These medications are also not indicated for acute exacerbations, although they may be used to prevent exercise-induced exacerbations; however, when beta$_2$-agonists are used on a long-term basis before exercise, their effects last only 5 hours. An example of these medications is inhaled salmeterol or formoterol.

Leukotriene modifiers are potent biochemical mediators released from mast cells, eosinophils, and basophils. They act on the lungs, causing airway smooth muscle contraction and increased mucous secretion; they also attract and activate inflammatory cells in the airways. Leukotriene antagonists improve lung function, diminish symptoms, and reduce the need for SABAs. They are an alternative, although not preferred, therapy for the treatment of mild, persistent asthma. They may also be used with corticosteroids, although LABAs are the preferred adjunct. An example of a leukotriene antagonist is montelukast or zafirlukast. These drugs block the leukotriene receptors, whereas zileuton prevents leukotriene synthesis. These drugs do not reverse symptoms during an asthma attack, should not be used as rescue medication, and have decreased exacerbations in patients with obstructive lung disease (Koarai et al, 2020).

Cromolyn and nedocromil stabilize mast cells. Although they are not the preferred method of treatment, they are also an alternative therapy for mild persistent asthma and may also be used before exercise or before a known exposure to a trigger.

The immunomodulators are monoclonal antibodies that prevent the binding of IgE to the receptor cells of basophils and mast cells. They are used for the treatment of severe, persistent asthma, especially if allergies are the primary trigger. The nurse should always be prepared and equipped to treat any anaphylaxis that may occur.

Quick-relief medications. Quick-relief medications are used to treat acute symptoms and exacerbations such as chest tightness, coughing, and wheezing. This group of medications includes SABAs, anticholinergics, and systemic corticosteroids. SABAs are bronchodilators that provide smooth muscle relaxation within 30 minutes and are the drug of choice for treating acute asthma symptoms and preventing exercise-induced exacerbations (GINA, 2022a). Older patients who use more than one canister per month do not have adequate control and need additional antiinflammatory therapy. Daily use of SABAs is not recommended. Those with symptoms of COVID-19 should not use nebulizer treatments but rather inhalers to decrease the spread of infected aerosols (GINA, 2022a).

Anticholinergics such as ipratropium bromide may provide an additive benefit to inhaled beta$_2$-agonists in the treatment of severe exacerbations. They may also be used as an alternative to SABAs in patients who do not tolerate them well. Finally, systemic corticosteroids, although not short-acting, may be used in the treatment of moderate to severe asthma exacerbations as an adjunct to the SABAs. Their onset of action is more than 4 hours, and they act by preventing progression of the exacerbation, speeding recovery, and preventing early relapse (GINA, 2022a).

Asthma medications administered through a stepwise approach

Step 1: No daily medication is indicated. SABAs are used as required (PRN). If they are used more than two times a week, consider long-term control therapy.

Step 2: A daily low-dose of inhaled corticosteroid is indicated.

Step 3: A daily low-dose of inhaled corticosteroid is used in conjunction with a long-acting bronchodilator. An alternative is to increase the corticosteroid dose to a medium level without the addition of a long-acting bronchodilator. If ineffective, a leukotriene modifier may be added to a low-dose corticosteroid. SABAs are used prn. With daily or increased usage, an additional long-term control therapy is added.

Step 4: A daily antiinflammatory, inhaled corticosteroid (medium dose), and a long-acting bronchodilator are recommended. If ineffective, a leukotriene modifier may be substituted for the long-acting bronchodilator. SABAs are used prn. An additional long-term control therapy is added if SABAs are used daily or if there is an increase in use.

Step 5: A daily inhaled corticosteroid (high dose) and a long-acting bronchodilator are recommended. An immunomodulator is considered for patients with allergies. SABAs are used prn. Add additional long-term control therapy with daily or increased usage.

Step 6: A daily inhaled corticosteroid, a long-acting bronchodilator, and an oral corticosteroid are suggested. Consider an immunomodulator for patients with allergies.

(GINA, 2022b; Cash and Glass, 2019).

Patient education, environmental control, and quick management of comorbidities are required at each step. An asthma specialist should be considered at Step 3 and implemented at Step 4.

In older adults, asthma management may occur alongside the management of chronic bronchitis or emphysema. A trial of systemic corticosteroids is useful in determining the presence of reversible airflow obstruction (GINA, 2022a). An older adult may have medical conditions, such as cardiac disease and osteoporosis, that are aggravated by asthma medications. Older adults with ischemic heart disease may be more sensitive to beta$_2$-agonist side effects, such as tremors and tachycardia; the dosage may need to be adjusted, or different medications may need to be added as an adjunct.

Corticosteroids may cause confusion, agitation, and changes in glucose metabolism in older adults. The use of inhaled corticosteroids in older adults may predispose them to a reduction in bone mineral content, especially in the presence of preexisting osteoporosis, changes in estrogen levels affecting calcium utilization, and a sedentary lifestyle. The GINA (2022a) guidelines recommend calcium and vitamin D supplements as well as estrogen replacement therapy when appropriate. An increased risk for adverse drug and disease interactions exists, such as asthma, which may be exacerbated using nonsteroidal antiinflammatory drugs (NSAIDs) for arthritis, aspirin for circulation, nonselective beta-blockers for hypertension, or glaucoma eye drops that contain beta-blockers. Finally, it is imperative that older adults are carefully assessed for their ability to use prescribed medications appropriately and devices correctly, as the increased risk of physical (arthritis and visual) or cognitive impairments could be challenging for them (Cash and Glass, 2019).

Nursing Care Guidelines for Asthma

Recognize cues (assessment). Evaluation of respiratory symptoms includes effects on ADL's and breathlessness, the hallmark symptom of COPD (Miravitlles and Ribera, 2017), the presence of asthma triggers, and the frequency of the need for bronchodilator therapy. Physical assessment includes inspection of the chest for shape and symmetry, determination of respiratory rate and pattern, body position, use of accessory muscles of respiration, and amount and color of sputum production. Palpation and percussion of the chest are indicated so that increased tactile fremitus, chest wall movement, and diaphragmatic excursion can be assessed. When the chest wall is auscultated, the older adult should be given enough time to take deep breaths comfortably without becoming dizzy. Determine the presence of any wheezing, the phase of respiration in which it occurs, and whether it is present during a forced expiratory maneuver. Determination of the PEFR with a peak expiratory flow meter (PEFM) is important in determining trends of airway resistance (Fig. 18.1).

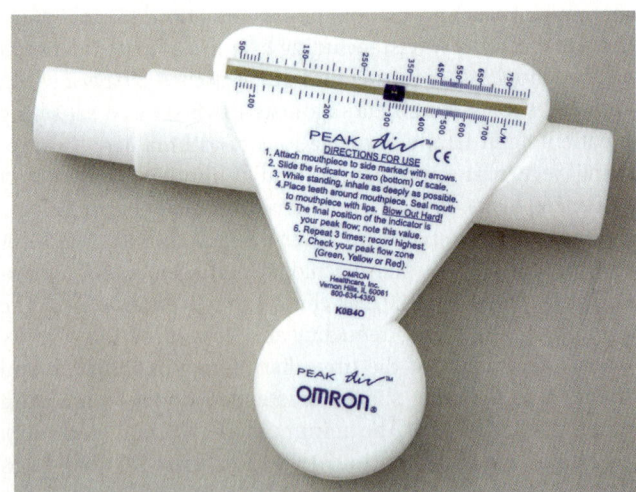

Fig. 18.1 A sample of a peak expiratory flow meter. This model displays results in colored areas: faster exhalation rates are in green, reduced exhalation rates in yellow, and seriously reduced exhalation rates in red. (From Aehlert, B. [2011]. *Paramedic practice today: Above and beyond.* St. Louis, MO: Elsevier.)

Analyze cues and prioritize hypotheses (patient problems). Patient problems common for an older patient with asthma include the following (Mondor, 2020):
- Airway obstruction resulting from bronchospasm, excessive mucus production, tenacious secretions, adventitious breath sounds, or a combination of all of these
- Reduced gas exchange resulting from alveolar–capillary membrane changes
- Need for health teaching about asthma

The diagnosis of asthma is based on episodic symptoms of partially reversible airflow obstruction. Key indicators for the diagnosis of asthma include (1) wheezing, (2) a history of a cough that is worse at night, (3) recurrent difficulty breathing and chest tightness, (4) variation in PEFR of 20% or more, and (5) symptoms that worsen during exercise, with viral infection in the presence of environmental irritants, such as animal fur, dust mites, mold, smoke, pollen, changes in weather, airborne chemicals, or dust, during menses, or with strong emotional expression (GINA, 2022a; Cash and Glass, 2019).

Pulmonary function tests (PFTs) are used to measure the presence and amount of airway obstruction. An FEV_1–forced vital capacity (FVC) ratio of less than 65% indicates obstruction of airflow. Measurements of FEV_1, FVC, and the FEV_1–FVC ratio before and after inhaled short-acting bronchodilators are recommended. Other diagnostic procedures include methacholine, histamine, or exercise challenge; chest radiography; allergy testing; ear, nose, and throat evaluation for nasal polyps and sinus disease; evaluation for gastroesophageal reflux; a 1–2-week evaluation of diurnal variation in PEFR; and evaluation for vocal cord dysfunction (GINA, 2022a).

The diagnosis and management of asthma in older patients is more difficult than in younger patients. The symptoms of asthma mimic those of other conditions, such as myocardial ischemia or pulmonary embolus. Asthma may appear as late as the eighth or ninth decade of life. Older adults with asthma may not show allergic skin sensitivity; therefore, serum IgE and eosinophil levels may be more predictive. Incomplete reversibility of airflow obstruction is increasingly common. Older adult patients with asthma may achieve only a 12% improvement in their FEV_1, even with optimally prescribed inhaled bronchodilators. In older patients with heartburn, coughing, nocturnal symptoms occurring early in the night, and resistance to routine therapy, gastroesophageal reflux disease should be considered (GINA, 2022a; Cash and Glass, 2019).

Asthma is classified into three categories according to (1) severity of symptoms, (2) frequency of nighttime symptoms, and (3) lung function (Table 18.3). Asthma also occurs as seasonal asthma, cough variant asthma, and exercise-induced asthma.

Generate solutions (planning). Older patients with asthma and their families should be included in care planning (GINA, 2022a; Cash and Glass, 2019). It is important to incorporate the changes in ADLs required for the ongoing monitoring and maintenance of patients with asthma. Expected outcomes include the following:
1. The patient will maintain a patent airway.
2. The patient will maintain arterial blood gas (ABG) values at baseline.
3. The patient will be able to demonstrate proper use of the PEFM.
4. The patient will be able to demonstrate relaxation techniques to control breathing.
5. The patient will be able to list the significant and reportable signs and symptoms.

Well-controlled asthma results in temporary and reversible airway changes. Poorly controlled asthma leads to chronic inflammation, which may cause damage and hyperplasia of the bronchial epithelial cells and bronchial smooth muscle (GINA, 2022a).

Take actions (nursing interventions). Interventions for patients with asthma include health maintenance, lifestyle changes, administration of medications at designated time intervals, exercise, and promotion of hydration and good nutrition.

TABLE 18.3 Classification of Asthma by Severity of Disease Before Treatment[a]

Characteristic	Mild	Moderate	Severe
Frequency of exacerbations	≤ 2 times/week; lasting less than 1 hour	> 2 times/week; may last days; not frequently severe	Frequent exacerbations, often severe
Frequency of symptoms	Minimal	Often	Continuous
Exercise tolerance	Minimal	Diminished	Poor; activity limited
Frequency of nocturnal asthma	≤ 2 times/month	> 2 times/week	Almost nightly, chest tight in the morning
School or work attendance	Good	Fair	Poor
Pulmonary function: peak expiratory flow rate (PEFR)	> 80%	60%–80%	< 60%
PEFR variability	< 20%	20%–30%	> 30%
Spirometry	Minimal airway obstruction	Airway obstruction is evident with reduced expiratory flow at low lung volumes	Substantial airway obstruction with increased lung volumes and marked unevenness of ventilation

[a]After treatment, severity is measured by the minimum medications needed to maintain good health.
From National Heart, Lung, and Blood Institute, National Institutes of Health (NIH). (2007). *Expert Panel Report 3: Guidelines for the diagnosis and management of asthma*. Retrieved from https://www.nhlbi.nih.gov/sites/default/files/media/docs/EPR-3_Asthma_Full_Report_2007.pdf. Accessed July 28, 2024.

Education is started at the time of diagnosis and is integrated into every aspect of care. Emphasis is placed on asthma self-management; basic facts about asthma; roles of medications; environmental control measures; the use of inhalers, spacers, and PEFMs; and a daily written action plan for management of exacerbations (Cash and Glass, 2019). Additional topics include smoking cessation, weight gain or loss, exercise requirements, and breathing retraining.

In addition to the basic interventions already described, older patients may require special considerations. The nurse should be accommodating to any neurologic changes such as altered senses, decreased fine motor movements, and memory loss. These expected changes may be managed with a number of strategies (GINA, 2022a) as follows:
- Make treatment plans simple.
- Use short explanations and easily explained graphs.
- Make sure instructional materials are in large type and use color-coded PEFM diaries.
- Increase lighting, and speak in a low-pitched, clear voice.
- Have the patient read and then repeat the instructions.
- Allow sufficient time for instruction, demonstrations, and return demonstrations.

Evaluate outcomes (evaluation). Physical evaluation is based on normal breath sounds and the ability to clear secretions and maintain airways with a normal respiratory rate. The evaluation of self-management is based on the patient's success in following through with the plan. Determine the frequency of rescue inhaler use, success at avoiding triggers, and the patient's ability to monitor and address lifestyle changes. Making permanent changes rather than temporary adjustments, although initially difficult for older adults, will be more likely to be achieved after thorough education. Continue to stress the need for regular follow-up with the primary care provider. Pictures and instructions on the use of multiple inhaler devices are available for download at the Ginasthma.org website.

Chronic Bronchitis

Chronic bronchitis is a clinical syndrome characterized by excessive mucous production with a chronic or recurrent cough on most days for a minimum of 3 months of the year for at least 2 consecutive years in a patient in whom other causes have been ruled out. Hypertrophy of the bronchial mucous glands, an increase in the number of goblet cells, and a decrease in the effectiveness of the mucociliary escalator all occur, usually as a result of repeated infections. Cigarette smoking is the single most important factor that exacerbates chronic bronchitis. Chronic bronchitis is associated with right-sided heart failure, cor pulmonale, polycythemia, hypoxemia, and respiratory insufficiency. Clinical symptoms often include a persistent cough, dyspnea on exertion, purulent sputum, cyanosis, crackles on auscultation, tachycardia, pedal edema, unexplained weight gain, and a decreased PaO_2 with a normal or elevated $PaCO_2$ (McCance and Huether, 2019).

Emphysema

Emphysema usually occurs between ages 60 and 70 and is characterized by progressive destruction of the alveoli and their supporting structures. The alveoli distal to the terminal bronchioles become enlarged, and loss of elastic recoil leads to chronic airflow limitation. Loss of connective tissue supporting the alveoli leads to permanent obliteration of the peripheral airways. Physical signs include the classic barrel chest appearance and the use of accessory muscles for respiration. Emphysema is often associated with a history of smoking. The clinical presentation includes dyspnea on exertion or at rest, decreased weight, a chronic cough with little sputum production, digital clubbing, hyperresonance of the chest on percussion, an elevated hemoglobin level, markedly decreased breath sounds or, at times, crackles and wheezes on auscultation, and abnormal PFTs with decreased VC, increased TLC, increased FRC, increased RV, and decreased FEV_1 (McCance and Huether, 2019).

Chronic Obstructive Pulmonary Disease

COPD is characterized by progressive airflow limitation that is not fully reversible and, during the course of the disease, lung tissue that becomes abnormally inflamed. The changes manifested include peripheral airway inflammation, airway fibrosis, hypertrophy of smooth muscles, hyperplasia of goblet cells and resultant mucus hypersecretion, and, eventually, the destruction of the lung parenchyma (McCance and Huether, 2019). The two reversible components in COPD are airway diameter and expiratory flow rate. COPD is a broad term that describes two obstructive airway diseases: chronic bronchitis and emphysema. Asthma may also be included in COPD, especially if a component of airway hyperreactivity exists; however, it may be difficult to differentiate between the two, especially if a history of cigarette smoking is present.

COPD is a progressive and ultimately fatal disease. The fatality rate for COPD is more than two times higher in males than in females between the ages of 65 and 74 and three times higher between the ages of 75 and 84. The number of females with COPD has been increasing since 1991 (GOLD, 2021), likely a result of the increase in the number of females who smoke. Risk factors for COPD include age, male gender, reduced lung function, air pollution, exposure to secondhand smoke, familial allergies, poor nutrition, and alcohol intake. COPD is often a comorbid factor in deaths from pneumonia and influenza; it accounts for increased physician visits and is preventable and treatable (GOLD, 2021).

Signs and Symptoms

The characteristic symptoms of COPD are chronic and progressive dyspnea, coughing, and sputum production. Chronic coughing and sputum production may precede limits on airflow by many years, which provides a real opportunity for intervention before it becomes a major health problem. It is also possible that airflow limitations may develop without either a chronic cough or excess sputum production (GOLD, 2021).

Diagnostic Tests and Procedures

A diagnosis of COPD should be considered based on a history of exposure to tobacco smoke or other occupational irritants and progressive dyspnea, a chronic cough, and chronic sputum production; the diagnosis should then be confirmed with spirometry testing. COPD is staged based on the percent of the predicted value of FEV_1 (Table 18.4).

TABLE 18.4 Staging Chronic Obstructive Pulmonary Disease by Level of Airflow

Stage	% Predicted FEV$_1$	Description
I: Mild	≥ 80%	Mild airflow limitation. Possibly cough and sputum, but possibly not. The patient may be unaware of altered lung function
II: Moderate	≥ 50% and < 80%	Worsening airflow Shortness of breath, especially on exertion Cough and sputum may be present, but not always Usually, this is the stage where people seek medical help
III: Severe	≥ 30% and < 50%	Further worsening of airflow Increased shortness of breath and dyspnea on exertion Fatigue Repeated exacerbations that affect quality of life
IV: Very severe	< 30% or < 50% plus the presence of chronic respiratory failure	Severe airflow limitation Respiratory failure is defined as PaO$_2$ < 60 mm Hg at sea level Cardiac complications may occur (e.g., cor pulmonale) Quality of life is appreciably affected, and exacerbations are frequent and life threatening

FEV1, forced expiratory volume in 1 second; *PaO2*, partial pressure of arterial oxygen.
Modified From Rabe, K. F., Hurd, S., Anzueto, A., Barnes, P. J., Buist, S. A., Calverley, P., et al. (2007). Global strategy for the diagnosis, management, and prevention of chronic obstructive pulmonary disease: GOLD executive summary. *American Journal of Respiratory and Critical Care Medicine, 176*(6), 532–555.

Most patients seek medical treatment because of progressive dyspnea leading to breathlessness and anxiety. Chronic coughing is often the first sign of COPD, but the absence of coughing does not rule it out. Initially, chronic coughing is intermittent, and patients may describe "good days and bad days." As the disease progresses, the cough is present every day. Wheezing and "chest tightness" may vary from day to day and may vary throughout a single day. Once again, an absence of tightness or wheezing does not rule out COPD. Weight loss, anorexia, depression, and anxiety often accompany the pulmonary signs of COPD (GOLD, 2021).

Treatment

Managing COPD focuses on increasing treatment, depending on the disease severity; the clinical status of the patient with airflow limitations provides a general guide. Treatment is focused on symptom management through education about the disease and the active engagement of the older patient in care management. Aspects of management include smoking cessation, a stepwise approach to pharmacotherapy, limited occupational exposure to toxins and air pollution, and a healthy lifestyle, including regular exercise and weight control. Proper nutrition is essential for promoting efficient respiratory muscle work, as COPD patients use a lot of calories and energy to breathe. Shielding measures, such as wearing a mask, social distancing, and hand washing, are important for the prevention of exacerbations (GOLD, 2021). Pneumococcal, COVID-19, Tdap, shingles, and annual influenza vaccinations are recommended for older patients (GOLD, 2021). During peak influenza season, older patients with COPD should avoid crowds to decrease the risk of contracting influenza.

The single most important and cost-effective intervention is smoking cessation. Smoking cessation improves FEV$_1$ and helps relieve symptoms. Benefits of smoking cessation include a reduction in the number of respiratory infections, an improvement in the function of the mucociliary clearance of the lungs, decreased coughing and dyspnea, increased appetite, and decreased sputum production. Older patients with COPD should also avoid secondhand smoke, as it may also cause bronchospasm and coughing. Many pharmacotherapies are now available to help older patients quit smoking. Nicotine replacement drugs, some antidepressants (bupropion and nortriptyline), and varenicline may increase smoking abstinence rates but should be used as part of an overall program of abstinence (GOLD, 2021; Cash and Glass, 2019).

Pulmonary pharmacotherapy is recommended in a stepwise manner based on the severity of airway obstruction and patient symptoms. None of the medications modify the long-term decline of the patient and are thus only used to reduce symptoms and complications. Bronchodilators are key in managing the symptoms of COPD and are given for both long-term therapy and during acute exacerbations; they include beta-adrenergic drugs, anticholinergics, and methylxanthines. Once a patient reaches stage 3, the addition of inhaled glucocorticosteroids is appropriate. However, chronic treatment with systemic glucocorticosteroids is not recommended unless patients are thought to have a significant asthmatic component.

Bronchodilators. Bronchodilators are the central pharmacologic tool used in managing the symptoms of COPD. They may be prescribed for long-term maintenance or short-term exacerbations. Inhaled medications are preferred because the systemic complications they cause are both less severe and more rapidly reversed. However, with inhalation therapy, proper training is essential. The primary bronchodilators used are beta$_2$-agonists, anticholinergics, and methylxanthines. The choice of drug will depend on the patient's response.

Beta$_2$-agonists. These sympathomimetic drugs work by stimulating the beta$_2$-receptors in the lungs, which results in bronchial dilation, increased mucociliary clearance, and possibly increased diaphragmatic function. The drugs may be administered by metered-dose inhaler (MDI) with a spacer, dry powder inhalation, or aerosolized therapy. Beta$_2$-agonists should be used with caution in older patients with ischemic heart disease. Examples of beta$_2$-agonists include albuterol, metaproterenol sulfate, and pirbuterol acetate.

Anticholinergics. Inhaled anticholinergics—ipratropium bromide or oxitropium bromide—are used to treat chronic bronchitis. They work by inhibiting vagal stimulation of the lungs, preventing contraction of the smooth muscle, and decreasing mucous production. A combination of an SABA and an anticholinergic results in a greater and more sustained improvement than with either drug alone (GOLD, 2021). Tiotropium, a long-acting antimuscarinic antagonist (LAMA), which blocks the bronchoconstrictor effect of acetylcholine, has been shown to have a greater effect on exacerbations rates compared with LABA alone.

Glucocorticosteroids. Inhaled glucocorticosteroids do not reduce the decline of the older adult with COPD, but for those patients with advanced disease (stage 3 or 4), they have been shown to reduce the frequency of exacerbations and improve overall health status. Chronic oral steroid use is no longer recommended as it may lead to steroid myopathy, which is associated with muscle weakness and respiratory failure. Steroid therapy may not be well tolerated in older patients (GOLD, 2021).

Vaccines. Influenza vaccines reduce serious illness and death in patients with COPD (GOLD, 2021). Pneumococcal vaccines are effective in reducing the incidences of community-acquired pneumonia among older adults. The COVID-19 vaccine (m-RNA) is effective in reducing hospitalization and death (Centers for Disease Control and Prevention [CDC], 2023a). Vaccines containing killed or live inactivated viruses are recommended for older adults, and the pneumococcal polysaccharide vaccine is recommended for those older than 65 years.

Oxygen therapy. Long-term oxygen therapy increases survival rates, improves hemodynamics, exercise and lung capacity, and mental status, and can decrease the long-term effects of a heart stressed by chronic hypoxemia. Supplemental oxygen therapy is indicated for patients with resting PaO$_2$ of 55 mm Hg or less or saturation of arterial oxygen (SaO$_2$) of 88% or less with or without hypercapnia. Oxygen therapy may also be indicated if the patient's PaO$_2$ is between 55 and 60 mm Hg, the SaO$_2$ is 88% or less, or evidence of pulmonary hypertension, peripheral edema, or polycythemia (hematocrit level > 55%) exists. The primary goal of oxygen therapy is to increase baseline PaO$_2$ to at least 80 mm Hg and SaO$_2$ to at least 90% (GOLD, 2021).

Pulse oximetry recognizes hemoglobin saturation, which normally is between 95% and 100%. The pulse oximeter uses infrared light waves and a sensor placed on the finger of the patient. However, the oximeter probe may be placed on toes, earlobes, or even the nose if circumstances do not permit a finger to be used. Pulse oximetry can detect desaturation before the physical appearance of dusky skin, pale mucosa, or pale nail beds is noted.

Antibiotics. No evidence suggests that the prophylactic long-term use of antibiotics has any beneficial effect. Antibiotics should be used only when a concomitant bacterial infection is present.

Surgical options. Surgical options consist of a bullectomy, which reduces dyspnea and improves lung function by allowing previously compressed lung tissue to expand. Another option is a lung volume reduction surgery, which, thus far, shows some promise for those with upper lobe emphysema and low exercise capacity. Lung transplantation is the final surgical option and does improve quality of life. All three procedures are extremely expensive and somewhat controversial because all are essentially palliative by nature (GOLD, 2021).

Nursing Care Guidelines for COPD

Recognize cues (assessment). Dyspnea is the hallmark symptom of COPD. It is the primary reason that patients seek treatment and the major cause of disability and anxiety. As such, spirometry remains the primary tool for determining the severity and staging of COPD. Evaluation of respiratory symptoms also includes assessing their effect on ADLs, quantifying breathlessness on a scale of 1–10, and identifying environmental and social factors that may contribute to the symptoms. The nurse also identifies the type of onset of the symptoms—whether sudden or insidious—and any precipitating factors such as exercise, temperature changes, and stress. Physical assessment includes assessment of the shape and symmetry of the chest, respiratory rate and pattern, pulse oximetry, body position, use of accessory muscles of respiration, color, temperature, appearance of extremities, and the color, amount, consistency, and odor of sputum.

To assess cyanosis in darkly pigmented older adults, the nurse should examine the patient with favorable lighting conditions (e.g., use overbed light or natural sunlight). The nurse should be attentive to factors that may mask cyanosis by causing vasoconstriction, which may include environmental conditions (e.g., air conditioning and mist tents) and patient behaviors (e.g., smoking and taking medications causing vasoconstriction). Examine the usual places in which cyanosis is found, namely, the lips, nail beds, around the mouth, cheek bones, and earlobes. Be aware that the darker skin may mask the underlying cyanosis, and the region around the mouth is often darker in people of Mediterranean descent. When cyanosis is questionable, apply light pressure to create pallor. In cyanosis, tissue color returns slowly from the periphery to the center. Normally, color returns in 1 second, from below the pallid spot as well as from the periphery. Cyanosis of an extremity may become more recognizable if the elevation of an extremity is changed.

The nurse should observe for other clinical manifestations of decreased oxygenation of the brain. These include changes in the level of consciousness, increased respiratory rate, the use of accessory muscles for respiration, nasal flaring, positional changes, and other manifestations of respiratory distress.

The nurse should use palpation and percussion of the chest to assess for increased tactile fremitus, chest wall movement, and diaphragmatic excursion. When auscultating the chest wall, the nurse must give an older adult enough time to take deep breaths comfortably without becoming dizzy.

Analyze cues and prioritize hypotheses (patient problems). The primary patient problems common for an older patient with COPD include the following (Mondor, 2020):

- Airway obstruction resulting from retained secretions
- Decreased gas exchange resulting from an altered oxygen supply
- Impaired nutritional status

- Insomnia resulting from anxiety, dyspnea, depression, and hypoxemia, hypercapnia, or both, paroxysmal nocturnal dyspnea, and orthopnea
- Potential for infection resulting from inadequate primary and secondary defenses and chronic disease

Generate solutions (planning). As with all patients, older patients with COPD should be included in the care planning. It is important to include the spouse or significant other, family, and any other caregivers in the planning process. Discharge planning should begin as soon as an older patient is admitted to the hospital. If an older patient requires special equipment for home care, such as supplemental oxygen therapy or aerosolized therapy, the patient and his or her family will benefit from learning the new skills in the acute care setting. Expected outcomes for the older patient with COPD include the following (Moorhead et al, 2018):

1. The patient will maintain a patent airway.
2. The patient will maintain a stable weight.
3. The patient will maintain ABG values at baseline.
4. The patient will maintain a balanced intake and output.
5. The patient will be able to effectively clear secretions.
6. The patient will be able to demonstrate diaphragmatic and pursed-lip breathing.
7. The patient will be able to demonstrate relaxation techniques to control breathing.
8. The patient will maintain a respiratory rate between 16 and 25 breaths per minute.
9. The patient will be able to list significant and reportable signs and symptoms.

Take actions (nursing interventions). Interventions for patients with COPD include maximizing the effects of bronchodilator therapy, administering medications at designated intervals, and promoting hydration, good nutrition, and increased mobility (Cash and Glass, 2019). The majority of nursing care for patient with COPD involves extensive education. Topics include normal respiratory anatomy and changes associated with the disease; medical intervention, including tests and medications; and lifestyle changes such as smoking cessation, weight gain or loss, exercise, and breathing retraining (see Nursing Care Plan: Chronic Obstructive Pulmonary Disease).

NURSING CARE PLAN

Chronic Obstructive Pulmonary Disease

Clinical Situation

Mr. W is an 80-year-old retired truck driver admitted to the medical intensive care unit (ICU) for exacerbation of his COPD. He lives with his wife, who is 78 years old. Mr. W continues to smoke one to two packs of cigarettes per day, as he has done since the age of 15.

Over the past week, Mrs. W has noticed a decrease in Mr. W's activity level and attention span. He has a productive cough of thick, tenacious sputum, averaging 1 cup per day. Over the past week, the sputum has become yellow. His appetite has decreased, and he has difficulty sleeping at night, often awakening and gasping for breath. Mr. W is having increasing difficulty bathing and dressing.

A physical examination reveals a thin male with a weight of 138 pounds (lb). He has a barrel chest and uses his accessory muscles of respiration to breathe. Auscultation of the chest reveals diminished breath sounds with scattered coarse crackles bilaterally and no wheezes. Mr. W's blood pressure is 138/68 mm Hg, his pulse is 92 beats per minute, and his respiratory rate is 35 breaths per minute. His oral temperature is 101°F (38.3°C).

Laboratory tests show ABG measurements as follows: pH, 7.40; $PaCO_2$, 68 mm Hg; PaO_2, 58 mm Hg; SaO_2, 80%; and bicarbonate (HCO_3), 28. Mr. W has a white cell count of 12,000. Sputum cultures reveal the presence of *Haemophilus influenzae*. A diagnosis of *H. influenzae* pneumonia is made.

Because of increasing shortness of breath and decreasing oxygenation, Mr. W is intubated and begins receiving mechanical ventilation according to the couple's wishes. Intravenous antibiotic therapy is started, and bronchodilator therapy is initiated to reduce airway resistance and promote pulmonary hygiene. Mr. W receives mechanical ventilation for 6 days until he is successfully weaned off the ventilation and then transferred to the medical division.

He remains in the medical division for 10 additional days. Mr. W is sent home, with home oxygen therapy and bronchodilators, and he is told absolutely not to smoke.

Analyze Cues and Prioritize Hypotheses (Patient Problems)
- Reduced stamina resulting from decreased strength and endurance
- Airway obstruction resulting from retained secretions
- Decreased gas exchange resulting from alveolar hypoventilation
- Reduced spontaneous ventilation resulting from infection and decreased respiratory muscle endurance
- Inability to communicate resulting from endotracheal intubation
- Need for patient teaching about home oxygen therapy and smoking cessation resulting from inexperience with concepts

Generate Solutions (Planning)
- The patient will be able to safely and comfortably perform ADLs.
- The patient will be able to effectively clear secretions with coughing or suctioning.
- The patient will be able to maintain spontaneous ventilation without mechanical assistance.
- The patient will be able to effectively communicate with caregivers and family.
- The patient and family will be able to demonstrate the use of the home oxygen equipment.
- The patient and family will be able to verbalize oxygen safety measures.
- The patient and family will be able to verbalize the need to quit smoking and techniques for achieving success.

Take Actions (Nursing Interventions)
- Provide active and passive range-of-motion exercises and early mobilization to maintain mobility.
- Assess the need for supplemental oxygen to enhance activity tolerance.
- Arrange for physical and occupational therapy consultation.
- Pace activities to provide rest and decrease episodes of breathlessness and fatigue.
- Provide chest physiotherapy (CPT) to promote secretion removal and chest expansion, as tolerated.
- Provide hydration to maintain fluid volume status and to decrease the viscosity of secretions.
- Turn every 2 hours to promote ventilation and to help drain pulmonary secretions.
- Monitor ABGs, as ordered.
- Monitor pulse oximetry continuously.

Continued

> **NURSING CARE PLAN—cont'd**
>
> - Provide mechanical ventilation during an acute phase if indicated for acute respiratory failure.
> - Suction as needed based on assessment findings; maintain a patent airway.
> - Monitor ventilator settings every 2 hours.
> - Provide reassurance for the patient and family.
> - Provide oral care every 2 hours.
> - Provide rest periods.
> - Schedule care activities based on the patient's energy level.
> - Provide an alternative method of communication, such as a picture board, talking board, or alphabet board.
> - Speak in clear, short sentences, and ask questions that require only a short response.
> - Provide the patient and family with information about home oxygen therapy, liter flow, and equipment for home use. Provide instructions about oxygen safety.
> - Instruct the patient and family in smoking cessation techniques and how this relates to oxygen safety.
> - Provide information about local smoking cessation programs.
> - Refer to the outpatient pulmonary rehabilitation program for COPD education and exercise training.

Pulmonary rehabilitation. Patients with COPD at all stages benefit from COPD education for self-management and exercise training. Pulmonary rehabilitation programs are designed to provide the patient with exercise training, breathing retraining, education, smoking cessation, medications, ADL retraining, nutrition counseling, and group support. The exercise component should include 20–30 minutes of moderate-intensity exercise three to five times a week, as well as strength training, and should result in increased exercise tolerance and decreased dyspnea and fatigue. It may also reduce cardiovascular disease risks, improve musculoskeletal functioning, help control weight or promote weight loss, and may help prevent bone loss in older patients (GOLD, 2021; Garvey et al, 2016). One of the best exercises is walking or using a treadmill. It strengthens both the legs and the upper body, especially if the arms are used. Exercise on a stationary bicycle is also useful, but it does not have the benefit of overall body conditioning that can be achieved with walking. Older patients with COPD may start a program in small increments, for example, walking or biking for 3–5 minutes daily. It is important to develop an exercise program that is achievable for an older patient. Targets are based on desired outcomes. The appropriate exercise intensity for health benefit is maintaining a heart rate of at least 55% of the maximum rate for a patient's age (i.e., a rate of 88 beats per minute [beats/min] for a 60-year-old and 80 beats/min for a 75-year-old). Adding strength training to a comprehensive exercise program can help to improve overall muscle mass, enhance muscle efficiency, and complement conditioning. Strength training can also help to reduce oxygen consumption and minimize dyspnea (Garvey et al, 2016).

Another benefit of a formal pulmonary rehabilitation program is the social aspect. Pulmonary rehabilitation classes and exercise times usually allow many patients to participate in a group setting. This group setting helps motivate older patients, provides emotional support, and offers them an opportunity for socialization and interaction. The pulmonary class sessions are often mini-support groups. Pulmonary rehabilitation may help reduce healthcare costs by reducing the frequency of hospitalizations and helping older patients and their families learn to cope with the disease process (GOLD, 2021; Garvey et al, 2016).

Smoking cessation. Smoking cessation is the best and most cost-effective way to reduce exposure to risk factors. Older patients with COPD who continue to smoke increase their risk of repeated respiratory infections and the progression of the underlying disease process. Older patients should be offered an opportunity for smoking cessation, and it should be offered at every opportunity. It is important to provide support for older patients attempting to quit smoking. Success depends, in part, on the support of family and friends. Many older patients find it impossible to stop smoking completely. They should be encouraged to reduce the amount and frequency of their smoking and perhaps consider nicotine replacement therapy to facilitate total cessation. Although smoking reduction is not ideal, it may help decrease some of the symptoms associated with respiratory illness. Programs are available through the American Lung Association, the American Cancer Society, and many community hospitals. The U.S. Public Health Service provides a framework for cessation (CDC, 2022a; U.S. Department of Health and Human Services, 2020) (Table 18.5).

Nutrition. Older patients should be instructed on the benefits of eating nutritious meals. Adequate nutrition is often difficult to maintain in older patients, and those with COPD have the additional problem of breathlessness. The patient should be instructed to eat frequent small meals, avoid gas-producing foods, reduce carbohydrates to only 50% of the diet (the breakdown of carbohydrates has been shown to increase the CO_2 load, thereby increasing the work of breathing, especially in those with CO_2 retention), eat high-protein foods, and reduce the intake of fat (see Nutritional Considerations box).

TABLE 18.5 How to Help the Patient Who Is Willing to Quit Smoking

Ask	Identify all tobacco users at every visit. For every patient, regardless of setting, tobacco usage is queried and documented.
Advie	Strongly urge them to quit. Be clear. Be caring. Be personable.
Assess	Determine the patient's readiness to quit. Ask every patient at every opportunity if they is willing to try to quit.
Assist	Help patients with a quit plan. Provide counsel. Provide support. Help the patient obtain treatment. Help patients with approved pharmacotherapy.
Arrange	Schedule follow-up contact either in person or by phone.

Modified From Fiore, M. C., Bailey, W. C., Cohen, S. J., Dorfman, S. F., Goldstein, M. G., Gritz, E. R., et al. (2000). The Tobacco Use and Dependence Clinical Practice Guidelines Panel, Staff, and Consortium Representatives. A clinical practice guideline for treating tobacco use and dependence: A U.S. Public Health Service report. *JAMA, 283*(24), 3244–3254.

NUTRITIONAL CONSIDERATIONS
Respiratory System

The nutrient requirements for patients with respiratory disease are as follows:
- Calories—25–35 kilocalories per kilogram (kcal/kg) of body weight for maintenance; 35–40 kcal/kg for replacement and building
- Protein—1–1.5 grams (g)/kg of body weight for maintenance; 1.5–2 g/kg for replacement and building; and 25%–50% of caloric intake
- Carbohydrates—50% of caloric intake; the breakdown of carbohydrates increases the CO_2 load and may increase the work of breathing, especially in older patients with CO_2 retention
- Fats—20%–25% nonprotein calories

Breathing retraining. The goals of breathing retraining include decreasing the work of breathing, improving oxygenation, increasing the efficiency of breathing patterns, and promoting patient control of breathing. Two of the most commonly taught techniques are diaphragmatic breathing and pursed-lip breathing (Boxes 18.1 and 18.2; Figs. 18.2 and 18.3).

Diaphragmatic breathing increases the patient's awareness of breathing patterns and improves the efficiency of breathing. Pursed-lip breathing increases expiratory pressure, improves

BOX 18.1 Diaphragmatic Breathing
1. Lie in the supine or semi-Fowler position.
2. Place one hand in the middle of the stomach, below the sternum.
3. Place the other hand on the upper chest.
4. Inhale slowly through the nose. The stomach should expand. (Note the movement of the hand over the stomach.)
5. Exhale slowly through pursed lips. The stomach should contract.
6. Rest.
7. Repeat.

BOX 18.2 Pursed-Lip Breathing
1. Assume a comfortable position.
2. Inhale slowly through the nose, keeping the mouth closed.
3. Remember to use the diaphragmatic breathing technique.
4. Pucker the lips as if blowing out a candle, kissing, or whistling.
5. Exhale slowly, blowing through pursed lips (exhalation should be at least twice as long as inhalation).
6. Rest.
7. Repeat.

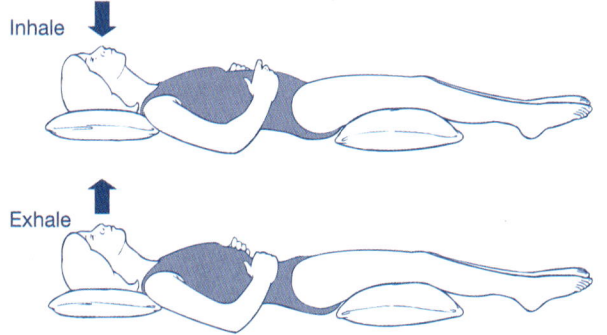

Fig. 18.2 Diaphragmatic breathing.

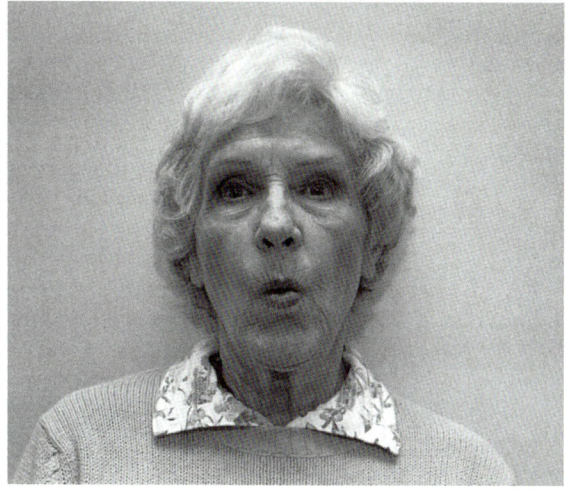

Fig. 18.3 Pursed-lip breathing. (Courtesy of Ursula Ruhl, St. Louis, MO.)

oxygenation, helps prevent early airway closure, increases exhalation time, reduces the respiratory rate, and allows the patient to slow the breathing.

Chest physiotherapy. CPT includes chest percussion, postural drainage (PD), and vibration for patients who have difficulty clearing their own secretions. Contraindications include hemoptysis, pulmonary emboli, osteoporosis, and bleeding disorders. PD consists of positioning the patient in a head-down position after CPT to facilitate drainage of pulmonary secretions. Older patients may not tolerate the head-down position of PD or the percussion of CPT. The nurse should explain to patients that they may experience increased breathlessness as a result of the mobilization of secretions and increased coughing as they try to clear the airway. To help decrease the discomfort associated with chest percussion, the nurse should place a bath towel over the percussed area.

Pulmonary hygiene. Pulmonary hygiene consists of hydration, deep breathing exercises, and coughing techniques (Box 18.3). Older patients are prone to dehydration and therefore are at risk for airway plugging. The nurse should encourage a volume of oral fluids of 4–6 quarts a day, if not contraindicated by cardiovascular disease. The nurse should also instruct older patients to sip fluids all day to decrease the chance of feeling full by drinking a large amount at one time and prevent dyspnea from bloating in the abdomen.

Medications. Patient education regarding medications includes the purpose of the medication, dosage, side effects, and schedule of administration. Medications are administered by mouth, MDI (Box 18.4), dry powder inhaler (DPI), or nebulizer. Inhaled medications are only as effective as the delivery technique. Simple human errors that affect the delivery of inhaled medications include failure to shake the inhaler before use, failure to exhale slowly before inhaling, lack of mechanical coordination of compression of the inhaler and inhaling, rapid inhalation or lack of deep inhalation, not waiting at least 30 seconds between puffs, failure to clean the MDI periodically, holding the MDI upside down, and failure to remove the cap before spraying the medication. A spacer device can help overcome errors in delivery technique and promote better

> **BOX 18.3 Effective Coughing Techniques**
>
> **Cascade Cough**
> 1. Take a deep breath and hold it for 1–3 seconds.
> 2. Cough out forcefully several times until the all air is exhaled (usually two to six coughs).
> 3. Inhale slowly through the nose.
> 4. Repeat once, if necessary.
> 5. Rest.
> 6. Repeat as needed.
>
> **Huff Cough**
> 1. Take a deep breath and hold it for 1–3 seconds.
> 2. Keeping the glottis open, cough out several times until all the air is exhaled (usually two to six coughs). Sometimes, it helps to say the word *huff* while coughing.
> 3. Inhale slowly through the nose.
> 4. Repeat as necessary.
>
> **End-Expiratory Cough**
> 1. Take a deep breath and hold it for 1–3 seconds.
> 2. Exhale slowly.
> 3. At the end of the exhalation, cough once.
> 4. Inhale slowly through the nose.
> 5. Repeat, as necessary.
> 6. Follow with a cascade or huff cough, in which secretions are moved from smaller to larger airways.
>
> **Augmented Cough**
> 1. Take a deep breath and hold it for 1–3 seconds.
> 2. Perform one or more of the following maneuvers:
>   a. Tighten knees and buttocks to increase intraabdominal pressure.
>   b. Bend forward at the waist to increase intraabdominal pressure.
>   c. Place hands flat on the upper abdomen just under the xiphoid process and press in and up abruptly during the cough or exhalation, or place hands on the lateral rib cage and quickly press in and release with each cough (this is called *rib springing*).
>   d. Keep hands on the chest wall and press inward with each cough.
> 3. Inhale slowly through the nose.
> 4. Rest if necessary.
> 5. Repeat, as needed.

> **BOX 18.4 Using a Metered-Dose Inhaler**
> 1. Select the appropriate canister of medication.
> 2. Shake the inhaler 15–20 times.
> 3. Hold the inhaler directly in front of the mouth, about 2–3 inches from the lips. When a spacer is used, place the inhaler in the spacer and place the mouthpiece directly into the mouth.
> 4. Take a deep breath and exhale completely.
> 5. Open the mouth wide. When a spacer is used, seal the lips around the mouthpiece.
> 6. Activate the inhaler.
> 7. Inhale slowly and deeply.
> 8. Hold breath for a count of 10.
> 9. Exhale slowly.
> 10. Wait 1–5 minutes between puffs. Repeat the steps for each puff ordered.

drug deposition into the lung (Woo and Robinson, 2020). The patient's inhaled medication technique should be evaluated and reviewed at every healthcare encounter.

Home oxygen therapy. Oxygen therapy decreases morbidity and mortality rates for patients with COPD when used for more than 18 hours a day. A patient's acceptance of oxygen therapy and attitude about the disease determine the level of compliance with treatment. Oxygen is a medication, and patients and their families need to be taught the correct administration, which includes proper liter flow, the times that oxygen is to be used, and the proper use of the equipment.

Home oxygen therapy is available in E-cylinders, concentrators, and liquid systems. A liquid oxygen system with portability is the most easily transported and may provide older patients with more mobility. However, it is the most expensive option. The concentrator is a machine about the size of a small bedside table. It is stationary and usually accompanied by an E-cylinder for limited portability. The E-cylinder, a small green tank that can be pulled on a cart like a luggage rack, is economical, although it is a little less portable because of its size.

All the persons involved in a patient's care—patient, family, physician, and nurse—should discuss the patient's level of activity and select the right oxygen system to support his or her lifestyle. Social workers may be helpful in determining the amount and type of insurance coverage the patient has available for home oxygen therapy. Many third-party payers do not cover liquid oxygen systems unless the patient is active and spends a good portion of the day out of the home. If an older patient is homebound, only leaving the home for medical appointments, the most economical system is the concentrator with an E-cylinder.

Exacerbations of disease and self-monitoring. It is critical that patients with COPD are taught how to monitor their symptoms for signs of lung infection and what action to take should they suspect they are experiencing an exacerbation of the disease. Knowing the signs/symptoms of infection can enable the patient to seek prompt medical attention, shorten the length of an exacerbation, and hopefully prevent worsening disease and function. Exacerbations can sometimes be managed at home; however, if symptoms are severe, hospitalization may be necessary, as exacerbations can be serious enough to be fatal. Therefore, early detection and treatment are essential.

Patients should discuss with their healthcare providers what steps or actions they should take for exacerbations; this "Action Plan" can outline specific steps and instructions at the first signs of exacerbation (American Lung Association, 2022). Experiencing worsening shortness of breath; a change in the quality, amount, or color of sputum; coughing; wheezing; and the need for increased use of inhaled medication can all be signs of a lung infection. Because an underlying lung infection can often cause exacerbations, antibiotics and oral corticosteroids may be necessary in an acute exacerbation (Woo and Robinson, 2020). Patients can be taught how and when to start these medications as part of their overall "Action Plan."

Although not all exacerbations can be prevented, measures like quitting smoking, getting an annual flu vaccine and updating a vaccination for pneumonia, avoiding close contact with sick individuals, and good hand washing are a few strategies that may help to minimize exacerbations.

A quick reference fact sheet on COPD exacerbations found in the GINA Pocket Guide can be obtained from the Ginasthma.org website's Guidelines and Reports.

Evaluate outcomes (evaluation). Evaluation of an older patient with COPD focuses on airflow as measured by spirometry, the ability to accomplish ADLs, and minimization of exacerbations. Older patients may need additional caregivers in the home because the spouse or significant other is most likely of a similar age and may also have chronic health problems. Older patients may need more time to learn the educational materials; however, once taught, they should have a good understanding and be able to adapt these techniques to their lifestyles.

RESTRICTIVE PULMONARY DISEASE

Restrictive lung disease results in the loss of functioning alveoli, the loss of lung volume, and decreased chest wall compliance. Restrictive lung disease may be the result of extrapulmonary factors such as excessive weight and muscle mass, a chest splint, or a restrictive dressing. Mechanisms of restrictive lung disease include pleural-based diseases, impaired lung expansion, impaired neuromuscular contraction, and thoracic deformities.

Lung Cancer

Lung cancer is the second-leading cause of cancer deaths. Approximately 236,740 new cases of lung cancer are reported annually in the United States. It is rare in patients younger than 45 years of age but increases in incidence between ages 60 and 70, and the average age at diagnosis is 70 years (American Cancer Society [ACS], 2023).

Risk factors for the development of lung cancer include tobacco use; marijuana use; recurring inflammation; or exposure to asbestos, talcum powder, or minerals. Less frequently, radon exposure, heredity, vitamin A deficiency, and exposure to air pollution may be risk factors. The leading cell types of lung cancer are small-cell lung carcinoma (SCLC), which accounts for 13% of cases, and non–small cell lung carcinoma (NSCLC), including squamous cell carcinoma and adenocarcinoma, which accounts for 84%, and other specified and nonspecified types, which account for about 3% of cases (ACS, 2023). The most lethal type of lung cancer is SCLC, which usually has a 5-year survival rate of 6.3%. SCLC is an aggressive cancer that metastasizes to the central nervous system (CNS), bones, and liver. NSCLC is a slower growing and less aggressive cancer that has a 5-year survival rate of 17.5% (National Cancer Institute [NCI], n.d.).

Diagnostic Tests and Procedures

The diagnosis is based on the clinical history and chest radiography. The initial workup includes a complete blood cell (CBC) count, carcinoembryonic antigen (CEA) level, chest radiography, computed tomography (CT), ABG measurements, PFTs, and an electrocardiogram (ECG). Sputum cytology is used to determine the cell type. If metastasis is suspected, additional diagnostic tests include magnetic resonance imaging (MRI) of the brain, bone scintigraphy, exercise PFTs, quantitative ventilation–perfusion scanning, treadmill exercise tests, Doppler echocardiography, and carotid Doppler ultrasonography. Fiberoptic bronchoscopy is used to obtain tissue confirmation of the diagnosis. Surgical diagnosis includes cervical mediastinoscopy, mediastinotomy, and thoracotomy. PFTs are used to determine impairment in ventilation and help predict functionality if surgery is a consideration. On the basis of diagnostic testing, the stage of NSCLC involvement is determined (Table 18.6). SCLC is not staged because it is extremely aggressive and is always assumed to be systemic once diagnosed.

Treatment

Treatment is based on histologic analysis and staging. SCLC has a median survival of 2–4 months from diagnosis and is very aggressive. It is much more responsive to chemotherapy and radiation therapy, but a cure is very difficult. The treatment of NSCLC depends on the staging and is basically divided into three groups of patients. The first group contains those patients with resectable cancer. Generally, this is stage 1 and 2 and some stage 3 cancers. These patients have the best prognosis. The second group of patients includes the remainder of NSCLC patients, except for those with stage 4 cancer. This second group may benefit from a mixed modality of surgery, radiation therapy, and chemotherapy. The final group is those with stage 4 cancer, and they receive palliative treatment that includes chemotherapy, radiation therapy, and endobronchial laser therapy (NCI, n.d.). If an older patient has significant lung disease, resection of the lung or segmental resection may not be possible. The decision to perform a surgical resection depends on the amount of functional lung tissue that would remain after the surgery.

Careful management of pain, nausea, vomiting, and chemotherapy-related side effects is important for providing as much physical comfort as possible for the patient and mental comfort for the family. Older patients may not be able to tolerate a complex medical regimen, especially with other organ involvement or underlying disease processes.

TABLE 18.6 Staging of Non–Small Cell Lung Carcinoma

Stage	Description
1a	Tumor < 3 cm, localized, no lymph node involvement
1b	Tumor > 3 cm, invading local areas, no lymph node involvement
2a	Tumor < 3 cm, lymph node involvement on the same side of the chest
2b	Tumor > 3 cm, lymph node involvement on the same side of the chest, tissue involvement of local organs
3a	Spread nearby (chest wall, pleura, and pericardium) and to regional lymph nodes
3b	Extensive tumor (heart, trachea, esophagus, scalene, and supraclavicular lymph nodes)
4	Distant metastasis

Data From PDQ® Adult Treatment Editorial Board. (2021). *PDQ non-small-cell lung cancer treatment*. Bethesda, MD: National Cancer Institute. Retrieved from https://www.cancer.gov/types/lung/patient/non-small-cell-lung-treatment-pdq.

Nursing Care Guidelines for Lung Cancer

Recognize cues (assessment). Assessment includes the identification of risk factors for lung cancer. The clinical presentation of lung cancer may easily be mistaken for other chronic lung diseases, such as chronic bronchitis. Often, no symptoms are present, or the symptoms are ignored or attributed to smoking or a preexisting lung disease. Common early signs include coughing, chest pain, and hemoptysis. It is also important to assess the patient's and the family's understanding of the numerous diagnostic tests that will be performed shortly. An assessment of the anxiety level is also appropriate.

Analyze cues and prioritize hypotheses (patient problems). Patient problems with lung cancer include the following (Mondor, 2020):

- Decreased gas exchange resulting from altered blood flow and alveolar–capillary membrane changes
- Acute pain and chronic pain resulting from the pressure of the tumor on surrounding structures
- Inadequate nutrition
- Anxiety resulting from a lack of knowledge of the diagnosis or unknown prognosis and treatment
- Hopelessness resulting from failure or deterioration of a physiologic condition and long-term stress

Generate solutions (planning). Planning includes developing interventions and expected outcomes for the patient that focus on improving gas exchange, promoting airway clearance, increasing comfort, and reducing anxiety. Expected outcomes include the following (Moorhead et al, 2018):

1. The patient will be able to maintain ABG values at baseline.
2. The patient will be able to sustain spontaneous respiration.
3. The patient and family will be able to verbalize their feelings related to the diagnosis of lung cancer.
4. The patient's pain will be controlled.
5. The patient will report a decrease in the number of episodes of breathlessness.
6. The patient's lungs will be clear on auscultation.
7. The patient will maintain a stable weight.
8. The patient will report feeling a decrease in fatigue.
9. The patient will maintain a realistic level of activity.

Take actions (nursing interventions). Nursing care for an older patient with lung cancer includes relief of pain, emotional support, counseling, and discussion of options and alternatives. The older patient may have fewer friends and family members for support. Interventions include providing factual information concerning the diagnosis, treatment, and prognosis; encouraging an attitude of realistic hope as a way of dealing with feelings of helplessness; acknowledging the patient's spiritual and cultural background; and encouraging verbalization of feelings, perceptions, and fears (NCI, n.d.). The nurse needs to be sensitive to the values of older patients and how they see the diagnosis affecting their quality of life. Many older patients may be more concerned about immediate survival and quality-of-life issues than the 5-year postoperative survival rate.

Evaluate outcomes (evaluation). Symptom management is evaluated by assessing how often symptoms occur, how the patient has been able to incorporate changes into his or her lifestyle, and how the symptoms alter the patient's ADLs. The nurse should determine the success of pain management and the level of patient comfort. Older adults may not have the same tolerance for pain and discomfort as younger patients. The nurse should help patients quantify their pain on a scale of 1–10. This will help both the nurse and the patient monitor the effectiveness of pain management. The nurse should also evaluate the older adult's use of pain medication. The main goal of pain management is to optimize physiologic, social, and spiritual well-being, improving quality of life (Brant, 2018). Many older adults are concerned about becoming addicted to their pain medication or think pain is a normal part of aging and, therefore, may not use pain medication appropriately as prescribed. Nurses should be astute to pain management protocols for older adults and employ accurate assessment and evaluation in managing the older adult's pain (Brant, 2018). The nurse should ensure that the older patient understands that the dose and frequency of medications will be carefully monitored. In addition, many older adults may become depressed after a diagnosis of cancer and should be monitored for signs of depression; a referral should be made if depression is suspected.

Tuberculosis

TB is caused by the organism *Mycobacterium tuberculosis*. TB is most often seen in populations living in crowded quarters and in those with little or no healthcare or preventive care. It is the number one fatal and communicable disease in the United States. TB is divided into primary and active varieties. TB is transmitted by the inhalation of infected droplets aerosolized in the air from the cough or sneeze of an infected person. The body's immune system responds to the local inflammation by walling off the bacteria. When active, the patient with TB is seen with symptoms of inflammation of the airway that lead to the development of a lesion and necrosis of the tissue. TB may remain inactive in the body for decades. Although TB primarily attacks the lungs, it can travel via the pulmonary lymphatics or enter the vascular system and affect the brain, kidneys, spine, bones, and joints. The bacillus infects a greater number of older adults than causes active TB. However, active TB may be present in any patient admitted with pneumonia, pleural effusion, human immunodeficiency virus (HIV) or acquired immunodeficiency syndrome (AIDS), weight loss, cancer, or alcohol or substance abuse (CDC, 2023b; Cash and Glass, 2019).

In an older patient, the presence of TB may be a reactivation of a dormant organism that has been present in the individual for some time. As patients age, changes in the immune system increase the risk of reactivation of TB. Medical risk factors that substantially increase the risk of TB include silicosis, gastrectomy, jejunal bypass, weight more than 10% *below* ideal body weight, chronic renal failure, diabetes mellitus, and hematologic disorders such as leukemia, lymphomas, and other malignancies. Older residents of nursing homes and other long-term care facilities are at increased risk of developing TB; they have a two to seven times greater incidence of the disease compared with older adults in the general population (CDC, 2023b).

Many older adult patients have underlying lung disease that puts them at higher risk of morbidity and mortality should they become infected. Most nursing home and long-term care facility residents are older adults. These concentrations of older adults, many of whom are infected and some of whom are immunocompromised, create high-risk situations for the transmission of TB. Hispanic Blacks and African Americans are eight times as likely to develop TB (CDC, 2023b). This higher incidence is due to treatment duration, socioeconomic factors, and HIV and other immunologic diseases (CDC, 2023b).

Diagnostic Tests and Procedures

Older patients with any of the following symptoms should alert the practitioner to a high probability of TB: night sweats, atypical pneumonia, low-grade fever, nonproductive coughing, hemoptysis, anorexia, and weight loss. However, tuberculin skin testing in older patients is an unreliable indicator of TB because they are more likely to have false-negative results because of reduced immune system activity. If skin testing is used, it is recommended that the standard 5 tuberculin unit (5 TU) Mantoux test be given and then repeated to create a booster effect. The second test may be a 5 TU or a second strength 250 TU test. If the size of the induration is 10 mm or greater (or ≥ 5 mm in an HIV-positive patient), the purified protein derivative (PPD) is positive. In the event of a positive PPD with symptoms, chest radiography is recommended within 72 hours (CDC, 2023b; Cash and Glass, 2019).

A positive chest radiography result with the following strongly indicates TB: infiltration in the posterior and apical segments of the upper lobes or in the superior segments of the lower lobes, cavitation, nodular infiltrates, atelectasis, fibrotic scarring with retraction of the hilum, and deviation of the trachea. Older adults may show lower lobe nodular infiltrates without cavitation. Diffuse, finely nodular, and uniformly distributed lesions characterize hematogenous TB. Older patients with any persistent infiltrate must be suspected of having TB. Although the previously mentioned radiographic changes are most common, TB may produce almost any form of pulmonary radiographic abnormality. Older patients should be questioned about potential exposure to TB, tested for HIV infection, and screened for other symptoms such as chronic osteomyelitis, chronic urinary tract infections, and any of the previous symptoms not present on initial examination. If a patient has a positive PPD and is asymptomatic, prophylaxis with isoniazid for 4 months is indicated (WHO, 2021; CDC, 2023b; Cash and Glass, 2019).

For older patients with a positive PPD, symptoms, and positive chest radiography, many additional laboratory tests and referrals are indicated. These include the CBC count, erythrocyte sedimentation rate, chemistry panel, sputum test for AFB performed three times, and bone marrow biopsy. A referral to an infectious disease specialist is also recommended, especially if the patient has been determined to have multidrug-resistant TB (MDR-TB) or extensively drug-resistant TB (XDR-TB).

Treatment

Treatment with the standard four-drug anti-TB therapeutic regimen will cause a rapid reduction in the number of viable mycobacteria (WHO, 2021; CDC, 2023b; Cash and Glass, 2019). A reduction in the viable organism load is seen within 2 weeks. Cultures will convert to negative within 3 months in patients compliant with therapy. Medications include a combination of bactericidal drugs. The most common drugs are isoniazid, rifampin, ethambutol, streptomycin, and pyrazinamide (CDC, 2023b). Other drugs used in the treatment of TB include ethionamide, kanamycin, para-aminosalicylic acid, cycloserine, and rifabutin. Fluoroquinolones, such as ciprofloxacin, are also being used to treat TB.

Monitoring of liver function on a monthly basis is recommended because older adults are at greater risk of developing hepatitis. Isoniazid may lead to toxic hepatitis and peripheral neuropathy, especially in malnourished or diabetic older adults.

Because the incidence of MDR-TB has been on the rise, the CDC recommends anti-TB drug-susceptibility testing on the initial *Mycobacterium tuberculosis* isolated from all patients with TB. MDR-TB is more common in patients who have spent time with someone with MDR-TB, in those who do not take their medicine regularly or do not take all their prescribed medication, in those who redevelop TB after having been treated, and in those who come from areas high in MDR-TB incidence, come from countries with high MDR-TB burden, which include Bangladesh, China, DPR Korea, DR Congo, Ethiopia, India, Indonesia, Kazakhstan, Kenya, Mozambique, Myanmar, Nigeria, Pakistan, Philippines, Russian Federation, South Africa, Thailand, Ukraine, Uzbekistan, and Vietnam (WHO, 2021).

Prognosis

The prognosis for an older patient with TB is good if the patient follows the medical regimen and maintains good nutrition. The greater problems are the side effects of isoniazid and the risk of spreading TB to other vulnerable older adults.

Nursing Care Guidelines for Tuberculosis

Recognize cues (assessment). Signs and symptoms include fatigue, weight loss, weakness, night sweats, low-grade fever, purulent sputum, and sputum positive for AFB. Older adults may not always manifest all the classic symptoms of TB, so the nurse should suspect TB when an older patient complains of weight loss and a chronic cough. If the disease has progressed, the patient may have hemoptysis, lung consolidation, crackles and wheezes on auscultation, upper lobe patchy infiltrates, and cavitation on chest radiography.

Analyze cues and prioritize hypotheses (patient problems). Patient problems for an older patient with TB include the following (Mondor, 2020):

- Inadequate breathing pattern resulting from decreased lung capacity
- Need for health education due to a lack of knowledge about the disease process and therapeutic regimen
- Inadequate health behaviors resulting from a lack of knowledge of the disease process, a lack of motivation, and the long-term nature of treatment
- Restricted calorie intake resulting from chronic poor appetite, fatigue, and a productive cough

Generate solutions (planning). Planning for older patients with TB must include the patient and their family. If a patient is a resident of a nursing or extended care facility, the medical and nursing directors need to be included in the planning as well. Expected outcomes include the following (Moorhead et al, 2018):

1. The patient will be able to demonstrate safe coughing techniques.
2. The patient and family will be able to verbalize the medication regimen.
3. The patient and family will be able to verbalize the side effects of the anti-TB medications.
4. The patient will be able to verbalize the need for continued medication.
5. The patient and family will be able to state how TB is transmitted.
6. The patient will be able to verbalize feelings related to social isolation.

Take actions (nursing interventions). Nursing measures for patients with TB include education about TB and how it is transmitted. Patients and their families should be educated about the measures necessary to prevent further TB transmission, the importance of continued medication administration, and good nutrition. Table 18.7 lists the most common drugs used to treat TB, their dosages, adverse reactions, and nursing considerations. The nurse should teach the patient that, if any of the adverse reactions named in Table 18.7 occur, they should call the doctor or nurse immediately. Patients should not drink alcohol while taking isoniazid.

Other TB drug side effects to report to the healthcare practitioner include skin rashes, easy bleeding, aching joints, dizziness, tingling or numbness around the mouth, easy bruising, blurred or changed vision, ringing in the ears, and hearing loss. Nurses should inform older adults that rifampin may cause urine, stool, saliva, sputum, sweat, and tears to turn red or orange and may stain clothes or contact lenses (Vallerand and Sanoski, 2023).

Older adults may view TB as a socially unacceptable disease. They may remember the stigma of TB in the early 1900s, when a person with TB was required to be separated from family and friends and placed in a sanatorium. Finally, the nurse must address the need for psychosocial interaction and support.

Evaluate outcomes (evaluation). Evaluation of an older patient with TB includes assessment of compliance because older adults may find it difficult to adhere to the lengthy medication regimen. The nurse should also evaluate compliance with public health measures, such as wearing a mask in public. Evaluation also includes monitoring of hepatic and renal function and repeated sputum cultures for AFB. The patient's mood should be evaluated for depression because of social isolation.

Pneumonia

Pneumonia is an inflammation of the lung parenchyma, usually associated with the filling of the alveoli with fluid. Pneumonia

TABLE 18.7 Tuberculosis Medications

Medication	Dosage	Adverse Reactions	Nursing Considerations
Isoniazid	Primary therapy: 5 mg/kg, PO/IM, daily up to 300 mg/day	Anemia, hepatitis, hypersensitivity, peripheral neuritis, seizures, and systemic lupus erythematosus	Therapy lasts for 6–9 months and is used in conjunction with other antituberculosis medication. Instruct the patient to avoid alcohol.
Rifampin	10 mg/kg body weight (maximum 600 mg)	Decreased effectiveness of oral contraceptives, hemolysis, hepatic toxicity, increased metabolism of hepatically excreted drugs, induction of methadone withdrawal, renal failure, thrombocytopenia, orange body fluids, and rash	Monitor hepatic, renal, and hemolytic parameters. Give 1 hour before or 2 hours after meals. Monitor hepatic function (urine may become red-orange in color). Instruct the patient to avoid alcohol. Usually used with one other drug.
Pyrazinamide (PZA)	15–30 mg/kg/day up to 2 g/day	Anorexia, arthralgia, gout (rare), hepatitis, hyperuricemia, nausea, renal failure (rare), and vomiting	Monitor the platelet count and complete blood cell count (CBC). Have the patient take medication with meals or snacks to reduce gastric irritation. Instruct patient to report any problems with urination. Monitor liver function tests. Instruct the patient regarding signs of thrombocytopenia, such as unexplained bleeding or bruising, the appearance of petechiae, and nosebleeds.
Ethambutol	15 mg/kg PO daily in adults with no prior anti-TB therapy Increase to 25 mg/kg PO daily if previous therapy	Headache, nausea/vomiting, blurry vision, joint pain, and skin rashes	May take with or without food Refrain from getting immunizations while on ethambutol Monitor renal function, hepatic function, and uric acid

g/day, gram per day; *mg/kg/day*, milligram per kilogram per day; *PO*, by mouth; *IM*, intramuscular.
Data From Centers for Disease Control and Prevention (CDC). (2022). *Tuberculosis (TB)*. Retrieved from https://www.cdc.gov/tb/default.htm; Cash, J. C., & Glass, C. A. (2019). *Adult-gerontology practice guidelines* (2nd ed.). New York: Springer.

may be viral, bacterial, or caused by aspiration, which occurs more frequently in older adults. In fact, for older adults, pneumonia is an extremely serious illness that often results in death. The increased risk of mortality in older adults is related to the normal age-related deterioration of the immune system, an increased likelihood of underlying chronic illnesses, a weakened cough reflex, and decreased mobility. However, the diagnosis of pneumonia in an older adult may be missed because the symptoms may be obscured by a coexisting disease or the chronic use of corticosteroids or antiinflammatory drugs. In addition to the typical pneumonia signs and symptoms, an older patient may also manifest more atypical symptoms such as altered mental status, dehydration, and a failure to thrive. The patient may require hospitalization and admission to the ICU, with subsequent intubation and mechanical ventilation. The incidence of pneumonia in older adults in long-term care institutions is particularly higher than it is among older adults in the community (Henig and Kaye, 2017; Cash and Glass, 2019). The Pneumonia Severity Index Calculator (Fine, n.d.) can be used to estimate the risk of pneumonia mortality and help decide if the patient should be treated on an inpatient or outpatient basis.

Community-Acquired Pneumonia

Community-acquired pneumonia (CAP) is a lower respiratory tract infection that has an onset in the community or emerges within the first 2 days of hospitalization. Classic symptoms of community-acquired or bacterial pneumonia include fever, cough, sputum production, general feelings of fatigue and malaise, and shortness of breath. Older patients do not always exhibit fever and coughing but often have symptoms of dehydration, confusion, and a respiratory rate greater than 26 breaths per minute. Other signs may include tachycardia, chest discomfort, dyspnea, headache, nausea, vomiting, myalgia, arthralgia, fatigue, weakness, abdominal pain, diarrhea, and anorexia (Cash and Glass, 2019). In multiple-lobe pneumonia, chest radiography may show incomplete consolidation of the lung. Some older patients manifest dramatic symptoms, resembling septic shock or adult respiratory distress syndrome (ARDS). *Streptococcus pneumoniae* is the leading cause of CAP in older adults, accounting for approximately 25% of pneumonia cases; its associated death rate is 30%–40% among older adults (CDC, 2022b). The 2019 novel coronavirus (COVID-19) is now associated with categories of CAP (CDC, 2023c). COVID-19-viral associated pneumonia will be discussed further in the viral pneumonia section. About 5%–15% of cases are caused by *Haemophilus influenzae, Moraxella (Branhamella) catarrhalis,* and *Legionella pneumophila* (Table 18.8).

Healthcare-Associated Pneumonia, Hospital-Acquired Pneumonia, and Ventilator-Associated Pneumonia

Healthcare-associated pneumonia (HCAP) is new-onset pneumonia. It is seen in a patient who (1) was hospitalized in an acute care facility after 2 days or longer within 90 days of the infection; (2) resided in a long-term care facility; (3) received recent intravenous antibiotic therapy, chemotherapy, or wound care within a month of the current infection; or (4) was seen in a hemodialysis facility. Hospital-acquired pneumonia (HAP) occurs within 48 hours or longer after hospital admission but is not found to be incubating at the time of admission. Ventilator-associated pneumonia (VAP) occurs more than 48 hours after endotracheal intubation. These infections increase the incidence of death from pneumonia. The costs associated with these diagnoses and longer hospital stays are significantly higher than a direct admission for pneumonia treatment alone. A major problem with treatment for any of these diagnoses is MDR. The virulence of the organisms may significantly reduce the availability and appropriateness of antimicrobial therapy (McCance and Huether, 2019).

Nosocomial Pneumonia

Staphylococcus aureus, Klebsiella pneumoniae, Pseudomonas aeruginosa, and *Escherichia coli* most often cause nosocomial pneumonia. Older patients have an incidence of nosocomial pneumonia three times higher than younger patients, probably because of the age-related decline in the immune system and a high incidence of comorbidities. In addition, older adults are more likely to be in high-risk areas such as residential centers, hospitals, and extended care facilities for other coexisting diseases.

Viral Pneumonia

Viral pneumonia in older patients is most often associated with a history of the influenza A virus and severe acute respiratory syndrome (SARS) COVID-19 (CDC, 2023c). Most infected with COVID-19 have mild to moderate symptoms, such as coughing and fever, but others may experience serious symptoms, such as acute respiratory distress syndrome. With COVID-19 infections, about 5% develop serious symptoms, leading to ventilator

TABLE 18.8 Criteria for Severe Community-Acquired Pneumonia (CAP)

Minor Criteria			Major Criteria
Respiratory rate (RR) ≥ 30	Uremia (BUN ≥ 20)	Hypothermia Core temperature < 96.8°F	Invasive mechanical ventilation
Multilobar infiltrate	Leukopenia (WBC < 4000)	Hypotension requiring fluid resuscitation	Septic shock with a need for vasopressors
Confusion/disorientation	Thrombocytopenia Platelets < 100,000		

Note: either one major criteria or three minor criteria qualify for intensive care unit admission. *BUN,* blood urea nitrogen; *WBC,* white blood cell.
From Mandell, L. A., Wunderink, R. G., Anzueto, A., Bartlett, J. G., Campbell, G. D., Dean, N. C., et al. (2007). Infectious Diseases Society of America/American Thoracic Society consensus guidelines on the management of community-acquired pneumonia in adults. *Clinical Infectious Diseases, 44*(Suppl. 2), S27–S72.

use and management (Bernstein, 2022). Older adults are especially susceptible to secondary bacterial infections from *S. aureus* and *H. influenzae*.

Older adults are more likely to develop the long-term effects of COVID-19 because they have underlying health conditions and maintain a multisystem inflammatory response (MIS) (CDC, 2023d). Long COVID-19 effects can cause scarring of the lung tissue, inflammation of the heart muscle, kidney damage, loss of smell and taste, and neurologic and cognitive issues. With long COVID-19, older adults have increased barriers because of additional ongoing multisystem organ issues, activities of daily living, and increased complexities in treatments (Chung et al, 2022). Clinical trials are underway to determine medications and treatments that may be helpful in long COVID-19. Additional support includes therapies for breathing, mobility, strength, and nutrition.

Severe Acute Respiratory Syndrome

The first outbreak of SARS initially occurred in China in 2003 (Hodgens & Gupta, 2023), with the latest SARS viral strain being in 2019 (COVID-19) and, within months, spreading across the world, becoming a pandemic. The patient's history of potential exposure to other known positive cases or exposure to someone with COVID-19 symptoms makes it imperative to determine if exposure to or close contact within 10 days of symptoms with a person known to have or suspected of having SARS. Generally, a patient may be asymptomatic or have a mild respiratory illness. The signs and symptoms often include a temperature over 100.4°F, coughing, shortness of breath, headache, malaise, or myalgias.

Severe illness, including death, is at higher incidence in those over the age of 65 (CDC, 2023c). Viral lung damage as a result of the COVID-19 condition is a result of rapid onset, and 84% of cases affect both lungs. Additionally, with severe infection, a phenomenon of disseminated intravascular coagulation (DIC) can increase the risk of mortality and multisystem organ failure. Especially in those studies over the age of 65, leukocytosis was also noted (Essetova et al, 2022). Long COVID-19 is especially apparent in older adults who experience severe illness from the infection.

The detection of antibodies to SARS coronavirus (CoV) drawn during the acute illness or 21 days after the onset of the illness confirms the diagnosis. Other diagnostic tests include the COVID-19 nasal swab, chest radiography, CBC, ABG analysis, clotting profile, respiratory viral panel for influenza and syncytial viruses, lactic dehydrogenase, metabolic profile, cross-reactive protein (CRP) test, and *Legionella* and pneumococcal urinary antigen testing. The patient should wear a mask and wash their hands, and universal precautions should be observed as the illness is thought to be spread by person-to-person contact and respiratory droplets. Care is usually supportive. COVID-19 is ongoing throughout the world, with the identification of further strains, diagnostics, vaccinations, and treatment recommendations being updated.

Aspiration Pneumonia

Aspiration pneumonia is commonly associated with clinical situations such as stupor, coma, cardiopulmonary resuscitation, alcohol or drug intoxication, neurologic illness, nasogastric feeding, and general anesthesia. Aspiration is a misdirection of oropharyngeal secretions or gastric contents into the larynx and lungs (Metheny, 2018). Aspiration may result in obstruction, chemical pneumonitis, or infection. Older adults are especially prone to aspiration pneumonia because of dysphagia, decreased coughing, and gagging reflexes. In addition, positioning, feeding, and the use of a feeding tube place older patients at increased risk for aspiration pneumonia. The use of narcotic medications, alcohol, and sedatives increases the risk of aspiration.

Older adults may have atypical symptoms of aspiration, such as delirium or coughing. Since aspiration can occur in small incidents, symptoms such as fever, chest pain, and crackles on auscultation may not manifest for many days. Other diagnostics include chest X-rays and a white blood cell (WBC) count to determine the presence of an infection. Swallow tests performed by a speech pathologist can assist in determining the risk of aspiration and needed nutritional modifications to prevent or as a result of aspiration (Metheny, 2018; Chen et al, 2021).

The best practice to prevent aspiration pneumonia is to modify food and drink consistency, engage in swallowing exercises, use of a chin tuck, and sit upright to help control secretions (Metheny, 2018). Small bites, assisted feeding, and coaching can help patients manage their food and secretions. For older adults who may receive nutrition through supplemental gastrointestinal tube feedings, the use of prevention measures is important. Ensuring the patient does not have excessive gastrointestinal contents already in the stomach (check residual) is the first step. Sitting the patient upright and giving the feeding slowly will prevent gastric contents from aspirating into the lungs. If coughing, nausea, vomiting, or abdominal pain occur, stop the feeding, as these may be signs of gastric overfill, putting the patient at risk for aspiration.

Diagnostic Tests and Procedures

The diagnosis of pneumonia is made based on a *history* of colds, influenza, and exposure to COVID-19 and the *clinical presentation*. Signs and symptoms include fever, chills, pleuritic chest pain, crackles on auscultation, and a productive cough with purulent sputum. Atypical pneumonia is first seen with a fever, constitutional symptoms, a dry cough, and a headache. Laboratory sampling includes total WBC count, blood cultures, Gram stain, and sputum culture. Of older patients, 20%–25% fail to demonstrate leukocytosis, and about one-third are unable to produce a sputum sample. *Chest radiography* (posterior, anterior, and lateral) is performed to identify infiltrates and assess for complications such as effusions or lung abscesses. Chest radiography is the gold standard for diagnosis. If the patient is dehydrated, infiltrates may not be evident even if they are present (Ramirez, 2023; CDC, 2022b; Cash and Glass, 2019).

Treatment

Treatment consists of the administration of the appropriate antibiotics, hydration, good nutrition, and rest. The length of treatment with antibiotics may range from 10 to 14 days, depending on the causative organism. The initial management of immunocompetent patients with CAP emphasizes empiric treatment instead of extensive testing because of the difficulty in determining the etiologic pathogen in the disease.

The severity of the illness, site of acquisition (e.g., community or nursing facility), age, and presence of comorbid illnesses are all considerations in determining initial antibiotic therapy. Therapy is aimed at pneumococcal and atypical pneumonia. Antibiotics used include macrolides such as azithromycin and clarithromycin for outpatients. For patients with advanced age and comorbidity, a second-generation cephalosporin such as cefuroxime or a combination agent such as trimethoprim–sulfamethoxazole is added. If an older patient is hospitalized, a second-generation or third-generation cephalosporin or a beta-lactam or beta-lactamase inhibitor is used in combination, with or without a macrolide. Patients with resistant or severe CAP may need an aminoglycoside, an antipseudomonal agent, or quinolone (CDC, 2022b; Woo and Robinson, 2020).

The American Thoracic Society Criteria for Assessing Pneumonia Severity established guidelines for ICU admission of older patients. To qualify for admission, the patient must meet either one major or at least three minor criteria (see Table 18.8), including a respiratory rate of 30 beats/min or more, PaO_2, or fractional concentration of oxygen in inspired gas (FiO_2) of 250 mm Hg or less, multilobe infiltrates on chest radiography, and hypotension requiring fluid resuscitation (Ramirez, 2023). Healthcare providers may use various guidelines that attempt to quantify the risk factors of individual patients when determining whether the patients should be hospitalized (Table 18.9). Some of the factors in these indexes include age greater than 65 years, presence of coexisting illness, altered mental status, chronic alcohol abuse, dehydration, malnutrition, nursing facility residency, aspiration, history of cigarette smoking, recent upper respiratory tract infection or influenza, and previous hospitalization within 1 year (Singanayagam et al, 2009) (see Table 18.9). Clinical signs include unstable vital signs, extrapulmonary involvement, leukopenia, hypoxemia, and PaO_2 of 60 mm Hg or less.

Prognosis

Clinical improvement usually occurs between 3 and 5 days after the initiation of treatment. Patients failing to respond to therapy will require aggressive evaluation to assess for noninfectious causes, complications, or MDR causes. Pneumonia remains the most common cause of death in older adults because of the altered immune response related to aging, underlying chronic disease, and a diminished cough reflex.

Nursing Care Guidelines for the Older Adult with Pneumonia

Recognize cues (assessment). A history of generalized fatigue, malaise, decreased appetite and fluid intake, or a recent viral infection may indicate a bronchopulmonary infection in an older adult. Fever, chills, shortness of breath, sputum production, and an abnormal chest examination suggest pneumonia. The nurse should assess the chest for decreased breath sounds, wheezing, dullness to percussion, egophony, and increased vocal and tactile fremitus. The nurse should also assess for symptoms of dehydration and confusion and other signs and symptoms such as tachycardia, tachypnea, chest discomfort, dyspnea, headache, nausea, vomiting, myalgia, arthralgia, fatigue, weakness, abdominal pain, diarrhea, and anorexia.

The nurse must be alert to signs and symptoms suggestive of an increasing severity of illness and a potential need for intensive care. These include tachypnea (30–35 breaths per minute or more); severe respiratory failure (PaO_2 or FiO_2 of 250 mm Hg or less); shock (diastolic hypotension of 60 mm Hg or systolic hypotension of 90 mm Hg or less); fever (temperature over 102.6°F [39.3°C]); decreased urine output (20 milliliters per hour [mL/hr]); and abnormal laboratory values for blood urea nitrogen (BUN over 20 milligrams per deciliter [mg/dL]), creatinine (over 1.2 mg/dL), WBCs (4000 or over 30,000), hemoglobin (9 grams per deciliter [g/dL]), PaO_2 (60 mm Hg), or $PaCO_2$ (over 50 mm Hg) (Ramirez, 2023; CDC, 2022b). Another sign that may indicate more intensive care is needed is a rapid change in chest radiography that consists of spreading infiltrates and extrapulmonary sites of infection. An older patient with such indications needs close monitoring, ongoing nursing care, and possibly even short-term mechanical ventilation for respiratory support.

TABLE 18.9 Variables Used to Calculate Pneumonia Risk and to Determine Hospitalization

Demographics	Comorbidity	Vitals	Diagnostics	Other
Age ≥ 65	Neoplastic	Respiratory rate > 30	pH < 7.35	Altered mental status
Male	Cerebrovascular	SBP < 90	BUN > 10.7 mmol/L	New-onset mental confusion
Nursing home resident	CHF	Temp either < 95°F or > 104°F	Sodium < 130 mEq/L	
	Chronic renal	Pulse > 125	Hematocrit < 30%	
	Chronic liver		PaO_2 < 60 mm Hg	
			Glucose > 13.9 mm Hg	
			Radiography shows effusion	

BUN, blood urea nitrogen; *CHF*, congestive heart failure; *mEq/L*, milliequivalents per liter; *mm Hg*, millimeters per mercury; *mmol/L*, millimoles per liter; *PaO₂*, partial pressure arterial oxygen; *SBP*, systolic blood pressure.
Modified from Singanayagam, A., Chalmers, J. D., & Hill, A. T. (2009). Severity assessment in community-acquired pneumonia: A review. *QJM, 102*(6), 379–388.

Analyze cues and prioritize hypotheses (patient problems). Patient problems for a patient with a bronchopulmonary infection include the following (Mondor, 2020):
- Airway obstruction resulting from decreased energy and tracheobronchial infection, obstruction, and secretions
- Decreased gas exchange resulting from altered oxygen supply and alveolar–capillary membrane changes
- Impaired breathing pattern resulting from respiratory muscle fatigue
- Fluid imbalance resulting from altered intake and factors influencing fluid needs
- Acute pain resulting from inflammation as well as ineffective pain management, comfort measures, or both, as evidenced by the patient's report of pleuritic chest pain and the presence of pleural friction rubbing and shallow respirations
- Activity intolerance resulting from altered oxygen supply to promote activity function

Generate solutions (planning). Planning for an older adult with pneumonia should include the patient and their family. It is important to focus on supporting respiratory function, promoting good pulmonary hygiene, and maintaining adequate oxygenation. Expected outcomes for an older patient with a bronchopulmonary infection include the following (Moorhead et al, 2018; Cash and Glass, 2019):

1. The patient will maintain a patent airway.
2. The patient will maintain a PaO_2 of 80 mm Hg by ABG analysis or an arterial oxygen saturation (SaO_2) greater than 90% by pulse oximetry.
3. The patient will have fewer complaints of fatigue.
4. The patient will have clear lungs on auscultation.
5. The patient will be able to clear secretions effectively.
6. The patient will be able to sleep through the night without episodes of breathlessness or coughing.
7. The patient will maintain baseline vital signs and weight.

Take actions (nursing interventions). Nursing care guidelines for an older patient with a bronchopulmonary infection include maintenance of hydration, promotion of effective airway clearance, and proper positioning. Other interventions include monitoring fluid, monitoring vital signs and oxygenation parameters, maintaining a clean environment, and assisting the patient with airway clearance by encouraging coughing or by suctioning (CDC, 2022b; Cash and Glass, 2019). Because of the ventilation–perfusion imbalance in the lung, it is important to position the patient with the "good lung down." This technique promotes the drainage of secretions from the lung with pneumonia and increases the perfusion of the healthy lung, which results in improved oxygenation. It may be a challenge to keep the older patient positioned on the appropriate side.

The key to pneumonia prevention is early vaccination. Antibodies to most pneumococcal vaccine antigens remain elevated in healthy adults for at least 5 years. Antibody declines have been shown in older adults after 5–10 years (CDC, 2022b). Therefore, all persons aged 65 or older should receive the pneumococcal vaccine, including all persons who have not previously been vaccinated and those who have not received the vaccination within 5 years and were 65 or younger at the time of their last vaccination. Vaccination is recommended for all persons with unknown vaccination status (CDC, 2022b). Revaccination is recommended for immunocompromised patients aged 65 or older, including those with HIV infection, leukemia, lymphoma, Hodgkin's disease, generalized malignancy, chronic renal failure, organ or bone marrow transplantation, and those taking long-term systemic corticosteroids or undergoing immunosuppressive chemotherapy (CDC, 2022b). Older adults should also receive the COVID-19 vaccination in accordance with the recommendations of the vaccine manufacturer (CDC, 2023a).

Nurses should assess older patients for their potential for aspiration. Nursing care planned to prevent aspiration focuses on careful assessment of the RVs of feedings and proper positioning of the older patient during and after eating. Minimize the use of sedatives and hypnotics if a meal will follow afterward. Provide a 30-minute rest period before eating. If assisting the older patient with meals, nurses should alternate between solid and liquid boluses. Determine the food viscosity that is best tolerated for each patient. Be aware of which patients have aspirated previously. Clinical signs of aspiration include a sudden appearance of coughing, cyanosis, or voice changes. Notify the provider if suspicion of aspiration exists.

Evaluate outcomes (evaluation). Evaluation includes the achievement of the expected outcomes, the return of sputum to preinfection color and consistency, and the return to baseline respiratory status. The nurse should monitor the patient for adequate hydration by assessing vital signs, body weight, and tissue turgor. Dehydration contributes to secretion retention and an inability to clear the airways. The effectiveness of an older adult's cough should be monitored because a weaker cough is common in older adults, and ineffective coughing may contribute to fatigue and result in aspirated secretions. The nurse should also monitor the patient's lungs for adventitious lung sounds and monitor the respiratory pattern for effective breathing and the use of accessory muscles of respiration.

OTHER RESPIRATORY ALTERATIONS

Cardiogenic and Noncardiogenic Pulmonary Edema

Pulmonary edema is an abnormal increase in the amount of fluid in the alveoli and interstitial spaces of the lungs and may be a complication of many cardiac and lung diseases. The most common form of pulmonary edema is a result of left ventricular failure. Left ventricular failure commonly occurs in older adults, especially in persons age 85 or older, because of coronary artery disease, mitral stenosis and insufficiency, and aortic stenosis. Cardiogenic pulmonary edema is the most common form of pulmonary edema and is caused by the increased capillary hydrostatic pressure that results from myocardial infarction, mitral stenosis, decreased myocardial contractility, left ventricular failure, or a fluid overload. Other predisposing factors include CHF, infusion of excessive volumes or an overly rapid infusion of intravenous fluids, impaired pulmonary lymphatic drainage from Hodgkin's disease or obliterative lymphangitis after radiation, inhalation of irritating gases, left atrial myxoma, pneumonia, and pulmonary venoocclusive disease. A rise in pulmonary capillary pressure occurs because of elevated left ventricular end-diastolic filling pressure, elevated left atrial pressure, and elevated pulmonary venous pressure.

The clinical presentation of acute cardiogenic pulmonary edema includes acute shortness of breath; orthopnea; frothy, blood-tinged sputum; cyanosis; diaphoresis; and tachycardia. Physical findings include crackles in the bases on auscultation, fremitus, and dullness on percussion.

Noncardiogenic pulmonary edema results from a variety of noncardiac causes. Examples of noncardiogenic pulmonary edema include ARDS, reexpansion pulmonary edema, neurogenic pulmonary edema, posttraumatic head injury, salicylate toxicity, pulmonary embolus, and opioid overdose (Givertz, 2022).

Cardiogenic Pulmonary Edema

Diagnostic tests and procedures. Diagnosis is based on clinical presentation and diagnostic testing. ABG measurements are drawn to determine arterial PO_2, arterial PO_2 saturation, and pH. A reduced oxygen tension and saturation and a resultant acidity related to retained CO_2 would be expected with pulmonary edema. The biomarker B-type natriuretic peptide (pro-BNP) may be drawn to help provide additional data for cardiogenic versus noncardiogenic pulmonary edema. Because underlying conditions that may predispose to heart failure may be etiologic factors for cardiogenic pulmonary edema, other cardiac-specific markers may be included in the workup (Garan, 2022). Hemodynamic measurements often reveal decreased cardiac output, increased pulmonary artery pressure, and right-sided heart pressure in biventricular failure. Because older patients have difficulty maintaining normal hemoglobin levels, it is important to take blood samples judiciously.

Treatment. The nurse must help reduce preload and afterload and correct the underlying process if possible. The first step is supplemental oxygen administration; mechanical ventilation should not be used unless necessary (Mayo Clinic Staff, 2022). Myocardial function is improved by reducing preload, which is the quantity of blood returned to the heart. This is accomplished through diuresis (furosemide) and pulmonary or cardiac dilation (nitroglycerin). Morphine is also a mainstay of treatment; it reduces anxiety and therefore reduces oxygen demand. Afterload (the force the heart pumps against) is reduced through peripheral vasodilation (nitroprusside and enalapril). Inotropic support may involve the use of drugs like dobutamine or catecholamines (dopamine and norepinephrine) (Sovari et al, 2020). Pulmonary edema is extensive; an older patient may require transfer to the ICU, initiation of mechanical ventilation, and insertion of a pulmonary artery catheter.

Prognosis. The prognosis for a patient with cardiogenic pulmonary edema is good when symptoms are easily reversed and cardiac complications are controlled. However, older adults usually have one or more comorbidities, such as underlying cardiac or lung disease, which increases their risk for complications. With extensive rehabilitation and physical therapy, older adults may be able to return to independent living and baseline ADLs.

Noncardiogenic Pulmonary Edema: ARDS

Diagnostic tests and procedures. The most commonly used test is the ABG, which determines the degree of hypoxia. Other tests include chest radiography, CT, CBC, and hemodynamic measurements (Mayo Clinic Staff, 2022). Older patients may need intubation and mechanical ventilation. In addition, the placement of an arterial line and a pulmonary artery catheter may be indicated so that oxygenation and cardiopulmonary hemodynamics can be monitored.

Treatment. Treatment consists of supplemental oxygen therapy, ventilation support, and maintenance of hemodynamics. Neuromuscular blocking agents, sedatives, and narcotics may be used to reduce anxiety, decrease the work of breathing, decrease oxygen consumption, and increase oxygen delivery. Positive end-expiratory pressure may be added to mechanical ventilation to improve oxygenation.

A pulmonary artery catheter may be used to monitor fluid volume status. Fluids and vasopressors may be indicated for the maintenance of adequate blood pressure. If a bacterial infection is evident, antibiotic therapy may be added. Corticosteroids are reserved for ARDS caused by a chemical injury or fatty emboli.

Prognosis. Overall, the prognosis is fair to poor, and the mortality rate is approximately 30%–60%. Comorbidity, frailty, and nosocomial infections put older adults at increased risk for complications. If an older adult does not require mechanical ventilation, the prognosis is good to fair, depending on underlying disease states and complications. Extensive rehabilitation, physical therapy, and retraining of ADLs may be necessary to return the older adult to independent living (Farley et al, 2009).

Nursing Care Guidelines for the Older Adult with Pulmonary Edema

Recognize cues (assessment). The nurse should determine through the patient's health history whether the patient has risk factors for the development of pulmonary edema. Assessment begins with the evaluation of respiratory and cardiac status. The nurse should observe the older patient for signs and symptoms of pulmonary edema. Nonspecific signs may include insomnia, wandering, anorexia, nausea, delirium, weakness, and weight gain.

Assessment for noncardiogenic pulmonary edema involves identifying predisposing factors, which include aspiration of gastric contents, pneumonia, thoracic injury, pulmonary contusions, smoke inhalation, multiple blood transfusions, uremia, cardiopulmonary bypass surgery, fracture of long bones, and sepsis. The clinical presentation of noncardiogenic pulmonary edema includes refractory hypoxemia, crackles on auscultation, hypotension, cyanosis, tachypnea, hyperventilation, and increased tracheobronchial secretions.

Analyze cues and prioritize hypotheses (patient problems). Patient problems for an older patient with pulmonary edema include the following (Mondor, 2020):

- Inadequate breathing patterns resulting from decreased energy
- Decreased gas exchange resulting from alveolar–capillary membrane changes and altered blood flow
- Airway obstruction resulting from decreased energy and tracheobronchial obstruction
- Fluid overload resulting from a compromised regulatory mechanism
- Reduced spontaneous ventilation resulting from metabolic factors and respiratory muscle fatigue

- Potential for infection resulting from inadequate primary and secondary defenses
- Need for health education resulting from a lack of previous experience with cardiogenic or noncardiogenic pulmonary edema

Generate solutions (planning). Planning includes developing interventions and expected outcomes for older patients that focus on the restoration of the oxygen supply and demand balance. The patient and family must be included to help the patient achieve the expected outcomes. It is important that both the patient and the family know about expected outcomes and necessary interventions such as oxygen administration or mechanical ventilation. Expected outcomes include the following (Moorhead et al, 2018):

1. The patient will maintain ABG values within normal limits.
2. The patient will maintain oxygenation within normal values.
3. The patient will have a cardiac output within normal values.
4. The patient will be able to verbalize feelings related to the illness.
5. The patient will maintain a patent airway.
6. The patient will maintain a balanced intake and output.
7. The patient will have an alternative method of communication if receiving mechanical ventilation.
8. The patient will maintain skin integrity.
9. The patient will be able to sustain spontaneous ventilation without mechanical ventilation.
10. The patient will have stable hemodynamics.

Take actions (nursing interventions). The effect of pulmonary edema may be severe in older adults because of its associated functional disability secondary to activity intolerance, drug therapy, and frequent rehospitalizations. The nurse should be alert to these factors and plan interventions that include daily weight assessments, energy-conserving ADLs, elevation of the feet and legs, a reduction in or elimination of sodium intake, and the use of diuretics. The nurse should assess the patient for adventitious lung sounds, respiratory muscle fatigue and the use of accessory muscles of respiration, and airway patency. The patient should be positioned to facilitate ventilation–perfusion matching and to minimize respiratory efforts. This can be accomplished by adding pillows at the back and under the arms and encouraging the patient to sit up straight with legs and feet elevated. The patient should be encouraged to cough effectively, which may require splinting and analgesic interventions; the patient should also be encouraged to change positions frequently and practice slow, deep breathing.

Inpatient interventions for pulmonary edema include positioning the patient to improve ventilation by elevating the head of the bed by 30 degrees. If the patient is producing large amounts of frothy sputum, they should be turned to the side to facilitate drainage; frequent suctioning then becomes appropriate. The nurse should reassure the patient and family or significant other and, if necessary, prepare them for intubation and mechanical ventilation, which may be particularly frightening for an older patient. An integral part of planning nursing care for older patients requiring intensive care is a discussion about the patient's wishes with regard to high-technology medical care. The patient and family should be asked if they have any advance medical directives (AMDs) or durable powers of attorney in case the older patient becomes unable to speak. If the patient is unaware of AMDs but expresses an interest, a family conference including the physician, nurse, social worker, and pastoral caregiver should be planned to help the older patient express his or her wishes. If the older patient has an AMD or a durable power of attorney, a copy should be filed in the medical record and reviewed with the older patient, family, physician, and any other caregivers. It is important to understand and respect the wishes of older patients and their families before initiating high-technology medical care.

Interventions include supplemental oxygen, mechanical ventilation, and nursing measures to promote oxygen balance. Monitoring PaO_2 saturation helps the nurse determine which activities deplete oxygen saturation. Interventions such as suctioning, turning, and positioning have been well documented as increasing oxygen consumption and decreasing arterial and mixed venous oxygen levels. The nurse should plan care to decrease the number of interventions performed at one time so as to minimize oxygen consumption and stress. It is important to provide an alternative means of communication for older patients receiving mechanical ventilation. If a patient has a hearing aid, it may be difficult for them to hear over the noise of the technology in the intensive care setting.

Older patients in the ICU need astute assessment, monitoring, and interventions to help prevent ICU delirium (DiSabatino Smith and Grami, 2016). The ICU provides no cues as to day and night; therefore, patients need to be continually oriented to time. Furthermore, older patients are particularly sensitive to continuous stimuli in the unit—sound, sights, smells, and textures—and may become confused and combative. The nurse should try to establish a regular nighttime routine with older patients, for example, vital sign assessment, oral care, and toileting. The lighting should then be reduced as much as possible to promote rest and sleep while allowing for safe care. This helps older patients establish a routine or pattern that they can recognize as "time to sleep." Such nursing measures can help reduce the incidence of ICU delirium, which will only prolong hospital days and potentially lead to additional complications for the patient.

Evaluate outcomes (evaluation). Evaluation is based on improvement in the clinical picture, resolution of symptoms, and prevention of further complications. The nurse should monitor the patient's vital signs, cardiac function, and oxygenation status for stability and improvement. The nurse should also monitor the older adult's reaction to frightening therapies and invasive interventions. Older adults need continual reassurance and information to reduce their anxiety. The nurse should constantly monitor the airway for effective clearance of secretions. A careful evaluation of daily weight and the patient's intake and output will help determine whether the patient is retaining additional fluids. The nurse should monitor the patient's subjective measure of dyspnea using the dyspnea scale.

Pulmonary Emboli

A pulmonary embolus (PE) is an occlusion of pulmonary arteries by a thrombus, fat, or air. Often, in the older patient, the occlusion is a result of a deep vein thrombosis. The thrombosis breaks loose, becoming an embolus, and travels to the lungs through the venous system, where it is trapped in a small vessel of pulmonary circulation. Occlusion of the lung with a large embolus causes pulmonary infarction, which results in necrosis of the lung tissue. The embolus, which is composed of platelets, red blood cells (RBCs), and WBCs, releases vasoactive substances that cause bronchial constriction, ventilation–perfusion mismatch, and hypoxia. The amount of physiologic dead space—ventilation in excess of perfusion—is increased, which leads to an increase in intrapulmonary shunting and hypoxia.

Risk factors for the development of PE include an age older than 40 years, immobility, recent surgery, recent trauma, history of hospital or nursing home confinement, central venous catheter placement, neurologic disease with extremity paresis, a history of vascular disease, COPD, heart disease, diabetes mellitus, malignancy, and previous PE. Thromboembolism is more difficult to establish with nonspecific symptoms, some of which may be already present in older adults (Vyas and Goyal, 2022).

The clinical presentation includes coughing, dyspnea at rest, hypotension, hypoxia, hemoptysis, tachycardia, anginal or pleuritic chest pain, decreased PaO_2, and S_3 or S_4 gallop (Thompson et al, 2023).

Diagnostic Tests and Procedures

Diagnosis is based on ventilation–perfusion lung scanning (VQ scan) or pulmonary angiography. ABG measurements may reveal hypoxemia with a PaO_2 between 60 and 80 mm Hg. ECG may show a right axis deviation, right bundle branch block, tall peaked P waves, a depressed ST segment, and supraventricular tachycardia if the emboli are extensive. Massive PE may result in electromechanical dissociation, in which electrical conduction continues without heart muscle response or cardiac output. Chest radiography may reveal an elevated hemidiaphragm; atelectasis, consolidation, or both; and pleural effusion. Additionally, the workup may include a D-dimer used in conjunction with probability assessment. The Wells score for PE may be helpful in classifying patients regarding the predetermination of a low, moderate, or high probability of a PE, along with other diagnostic tests and symptomatology (Thompson et al, 2023).

Treatment

The patient with suspected PE should initially be resuscitated and stabilized, focusing on hemodynamics and oxygenation. Unless contraindicated, anticoagulation should be started. Heparin is usually the anticoagulant of choice in the inpatient setting, and unfractionated heparin levels should be monitored. Heparin can be administered subcutaneously or intravenously to achieve a prothrombin time of 1.5–2.5 times control. Thrombolytic therapy, such as the use of streptokinase, urokinase, or tissue plasminogen activator (TPA), is used in patients with extensive PE who exhibit unstable hemodynamic situations. Patients with a likelihood of recurring PE are treated on a long-term basis with warfarin (Coumadin) and monitoring of their international normalized ratio (INR). The goal range of the INR is 2.5–3.0. Patients with recurrent PE or in whom anticoagulation is contraindicated may be good candidates for Greenfield vena cava filters.

Prognosis

The prognosis for PE is variable. The incidence increases with aging, and older adults treated for PE are more at risk for complications of the disease and anticoagulation. Furthermore, the ability to predict mortality in older adults seems to be lower than with younger populations (Polo Friz et al, 2015).

Nursing Care Guidelines for the Older Adult with Pulmonary Embolus

Recognize cues (assessment). Assessment begins with the identification of risk factors for the development of PE. In older adults, dehydration and immobility are the leading causes. If an older patient has a history of a recent fracture of a long bone or a pelvic fracture secondary to falling, fat emboli should be suspected. Clinical signs and symptoms may include sudden dyspnea, chest pain, restlessness, a weak and rapid pulse, tachypnea, and tachycardia.

Analyze cues and prioritize hypotheses (patient problems). Diagnoses for an older patient with pulmonary emboli include the following (Mondor, 2020):

- Decreased gas exchange resulting from altered blood flow and oxygen supply
- Decreased perfusion resulting from an interruption of arterial flow
- Reduced spontaneous ventilation resulting from metabolic factors

Generate solutions (planning). Planning includes developing interventions and expected outcomes for the older patient that are aimed primarily at improving oxygenation and reducing pain. Expected outcomes include the following (Moorhead et al, 2018):

1. The patient will maintain ABG values within normal limits.
2. The patient will maintain adequate respiratory muscle function.
3. The patient will be able to sustain spontaneous ventilation without mechanical ventilation.
4. The patient will maintain adequate oxygenation.
5. The patient will have adequate pain control.
6. The patient will maintain adequate cardiac output.
7. The patient will maintain adequate vital signs.

Take actions (nursing interventions). The primary goals of treatment are to stop the clot from getting bigger and to prevent new clots from forming. Although treatment is focused on these goals, maintaining effective oxygenation and ventilation is paramount. The nurse should monitor tissue oxygen delivery, signs and symptoms of respiratory failure, laboratory values for changes in oxygenation or acid–base balance, and hemodynamic parameters and respiratory pattern for symptoms of respiratory difficulty. Oxygen therapy is administered to improve oxygenation and decrease breathlessness. Heparin therapy is initiated to prevent the formation of future clots. Older patients need reassurance and careful monitoring of their vital signs. Sedation relieves pain and anxiety, and reduces oxygen demand. If an older patient is dehydrated or has hypotension, intravenous fluids are administered. The nurse may use vasopressors if hypotension cannot be reversed with fluids.

The patient needs to be monitored for bleeding complications from anticoagulant therapy. The nurse should observe the urine for color changes, check the stool for occult blood, and monitor for other complications, including bruising, gastric bleeding, hemorrhaging, and stroke.

Because immobility is a risk factor for the development of PE, it is important to promote mobility as soon as medically possible. The nurse should use an antiembolic compression hose and passive and active range-of-motion exercises during the acute phase. The older patient should be encouraged to move about as soon as is medically feasible.

Education topics for the older patient and his or her family include signs and symptoms of pulmonary emboli, long-term anticoagulant therapy (warfarin), and the importance of exercise and mobility. Education on anticoagulant therapy includes the elimination of aspirin or NSAIDs, the elimination of green leafy vegetables, cautionary use of over-the-counter medications that potentiate the anticoagulation effect, and prompt reporting of any bleeding. An electric razor is recommended for male patients. The nurse must also help the patient understand the importance of regular monitoring of the INR and the importance of taking anticoagulation medication at the same time every day.

Evaluate outcomes (evaluation). Evaluation is based on the successful achievement of the expected outcomes. The nurse should monitor the older patient's response to oxygen therapy, respiratory support, and effective pain management and relief by using a pain scale. The nurse should also monitor the patient for follow-up care with INR blood draws, dietary restrictions, and medication compliance. With older adults, it is especially important to evaluate the patient's ability to recall the signs of excessive anticoagulation.

Obstructive Sleep Apnea

Obstructive sleep apnea syndrome (OSAS) is a disorder of breathing during sleep due to a periodic reduction (hypopnea) or cessation (apnea) of breathing due to an obstruction of the upper airway (Cash and Glass, 2019; McCance and Huether, 2019). This upper airway obstruction can be associated with oxygen desaturation and hypercapnia. Pathogenic factors include intermittent hypoxemia or hypercapnia, mechanoreceptor activation during obstructed efforts, chemoreflex activation through chronic body and CNS excitability, and arousal that results from abnormal breathing (McCance and Huether, 2019). These changes result in partial awakening of the patient with a startle response of snorts and gasps, which move the tongue and soft palate and relieve the obstruction. Chronic effects on the cardiovascular system are a result of increased sympathetic nervous system activity. During obstructive apnea, large fluctuations in intrathoracic pressure occur, causing changes in venous return, left ventricular filling, cardiac output, baroreflex, and the release of volume-regulatory peptides (McCance and Huether, 2019).

Obesity is the dominant risk factor for OSAS in both males and females. OSAS is twice as common in males as in females, and the risk increases with age. Because obesity is a strong predictive factor, even a 10% reduction in weight can lead to a substantial decrease in the respiratory disturbance index (RDI) (Wickramasinghe et al, 2020). Other risk factors for OSAS include family history, increased neck circumference, genetic syndrome, smoking, alcohol use, employment requiring shift rotation or sleep restrictions, tonsillar hypertrophy, craniofacial abnormalities, medications, and ethnicity (African Americans, Hispanics, and Pacific Islanders have a higher incidence of OSAS compared with Whites) (Cash and Glass, 2019).

Diagnostic Tests and Procedures

The diagnosis of OSAS is made based on the patient's history and the objective measurement in tandem with polysomnography (PSG) in the sleep laboratory. PSG is the gold standard diagnostic test for OSA and is particularly important in patients with underlying cardiovascular disease, hypoventilation syndrome, stroke, and insomnia (Kapur et al, 2017). Diagnostic criteria include complaints of excessive daytime sleepiness, frequent episodes of obstructed breathing during sleep, loud snoring, morning headaches, dry mouth on awakening, and falling asleep during normal awake-time activities or driving. Sleep study criteria include more than five episodes of obstructive apnea longer than 10 seconds in duration per hour of sleep and one or more of the following: frequent arousal from sleep, bradycardia, tachycardia, and arterial oxygen desaturation associated with apneic episodes. Clinical practice guidelines for OSA identify other tools such as the Epworth Sleepiness Scale (ESS), a self-report scale for evaluating inclination toward daytime sleepiness or dozing, and the STOP-BANG questionnaire as an OSA screening tool, which can be used to provide additional information and supplement PSG.

Treatment

Treatment starts conservatively and involves teaching the older patient to avoid alcohol or sedatives at bedtime, humidify the air, and wear a dental device to keep the jaw forward. Weight loss should also be encouraged, as overweight and obesity can be associated with an increased incidence of OSAS. These interventions may be enough to relieve sleep apnea problems in some individuals. The next line of treatment for patients with OSAS is nasal CPAP therapy. CPAP provides immediate prevention of upper airway collapse and can lead to correction of ABG derangements, improved sleep continuity, improved cognition, and a reduction in sleepless symptoms. The most critical factor in the use of nasal CPAP is the patient's level of adherence to the treatment modality. It is estimated that 29%–83% of patients are nonadherent to CPAP therapy (< 4 hrs/nightly) (Weaver, 2022). Alternatives to nasal CPAP may include weight reduction, sleep position training, and the avoidance of alcohol, sedative-hypnotic and narcotic medications, cigarette smoking, and sleep deprivation.

Surgical interventions include tracheotomy or uvulopalatopharyngoplasty (UVPP or UPPP). The goal of UVPP or UPPP is to remove redundant or obstructing tissue of the soft palate, uvula, and posterolateral pharynx, thereby eliminating obstruction. The procedure may eliminate snoring but may not reduce the apneic episodes (Adil and Meyers, 2020).

Prognosis

The prognosis for a patient with OSAS is good. Patient commitment to medical management, such as weight loss and daily use of nasal CPAP, is essential for a good outcome. Older adults may have difficulty with weight reduction. Patients may also find the nasal CPAP machine annoying and disruptive to their sleep and therefore not wear it consistently at night. Although surgery may be an option, comorbidity may preclude its use in some older adults.

Nursing Care Guidelines for the Older Adult with OSA

Recognize cues (assessment). The nurse should assess the patient for the presence of chronic loud snoring, gasping, or choking episodes during sleep, excessive daytime sleepiness (especially when driving), automobile or work-related accidents attributed to fatigue, and personality changes or cognitive difficulties. Clinical signs include obesity, systemic hypertension, nasopharyngeal narrowing, and, in rare cases, pulmonary hypertension and cor pulmonale.

Analyze cues and prioritize hypotheses (patient problems). Patient problems for a patient with OSAS include the following:
- Fatigue resulting from the increased energy required for ADLs
- Disrupted sleep patterns resulting from sensory alterations.
- Inadequate breathing patterns resulting from decreased energy or fatigue.

Generate solutions (planning). Expected outcomes for an older patient with OSAS include the following (Moorhead et al, 2018):
1. The patient will verbalize a feeling of rest and well-being
2. The patient will verbalize an improvement in quality of life.
3. The patient will report an absence of sleepy episodes during the day
4. The patient will have an increased ability to concentrate
5. The patient will have increased endurance, as evidenced by their ability to participate in ADLs
6. The patient will maintain adequate vital signs
7. The patient will maintain adequate oxygenation and ventilation during sleep, as evidenced by continuous pulse oximetry monitoring

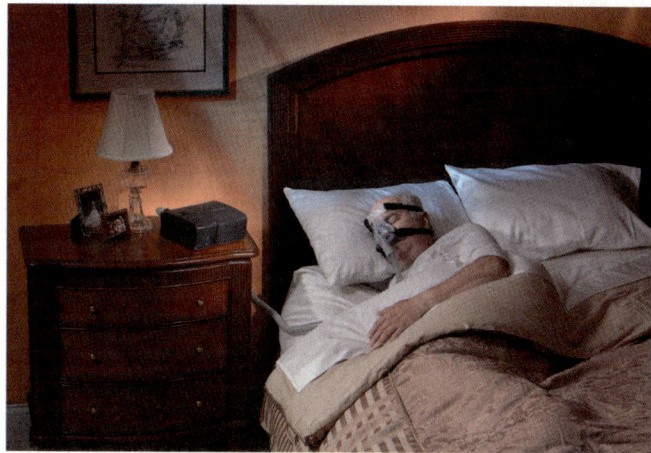

Fig. 18.4 The management of sleep apnea often involves sleeping with a nasal mask in place. The pressure supplied by air coming from the compressor opens the oropharynx and nasopharynx. (From Lewis, S. M., Dirksen, S., Heitkemper, M. M., Bucher, L., & Camera, I. [2011]. *Medical-surgical nursing: Assessment and management of clinical problems* [8th ed.]. St. Louis, MO: Elsevier.)

8. The patient will achieve or maintain an appropriate body weight.

Take actions (nursing interventions). Interventions for a patient with OSAS include monitoring the patient's sleep pattern; noting physiologic and psychologic circumstances that interrupt sleep; implementing sleep-promoting therapies and bedtime routines conducive to sleep, lifestyle modifications, and the use of CPAP (Fig. 18.4). The nurse should assist the patient with nutrition counseling, weight reduction, and exercise plans (Cash and Glass, 2019). Exercise may be especially difficult for older adults with underlying orthopedic problems and decreased activity. Exercise programs that incorporate water aerobics may be helpful for older adults with joint problems. The nurse should encourage healthy food choices such as fresh fruits and vegetables and less processed and prepackaged foods, which may be challenging for older adults who live alone and do not cook regularly.

Evaluate outcomes (evaluation). Evaluation is based on the achievement of the expected outcomes and an improvement in the patient's perception of sleep. The nurse should evaluate the patient's daytime somnolence and ability to complete ADLs, noting the frequency of napping and monitoring for lower extremity edema, fluid retention, and weight gain.

HOME CARE

1. Encourage homebound older adult patients with respiratory disease to drink 8–10 glasses of water a day, if not contraindicated.
2. Encourage homebound older adult patients with respiratory disease to exercise within their capacity to promote thoracic muscle conditioning.
3. Monitor homebound older adult patients for smoking and exposure to secondhand smoke. Encourage family members to refrain from smoking in the presence of the patient.
4. Encourage homebound older adult patients to use pursed-lip breathing to control breathlessness and improve oxygenation.
5. Monitor pulse oximetry to assess oxygenation.
6. Encourage frequent small meals to reduce the breathlessness associated with eating.
7. If a patient is using home oxygen, assess the home environment for potential safety hazards, including the possibility of the patient tripping over oxygen tubing.
8. Assess patients for confusion, occipital headaches, and forgetfulness. These symptoms may be indicative of CO_2 retention. Teach family caregivers these signs as well.

SUMMARY

Neurochemical control and the respiratory muscles are involved in the process of respiration. The structures of the lungs include upper and lower airways and extrapulmonary and intrapulmonary structures. Age-related changes in pulmonary structure and function include elastic recoil, musculoskeletal changes of the chest wall, and decreased compliance of the thorax. Asthma, chronic bronchitis, emphysema, and pneumonia are respiratory conditions common in older adults. Chronologic age and tobacco use put older patients at risk for bronchogenic carcinoma. Nursing care guidelines for older patients with respiratory alterations focus on a complete and accurate physical assessment, minimization of risk factors for disease development, development of partnerships with the patient to successfully implement lifestyle changes and treatment regimens, and, most importantly, pulmonary hygiene and airway patency.

KEY POINTS

- Changes in lung functions associated with the aging process, in the absence of primary pulmonary disease, are not associated with decreased activity or increased breathlessness.
- Older adults with chronic lung disease can lead active lives with proper medical and nursing care guidelines.
- Breathing retraining (e.g., pursed-lip breathing and diaphragmatic breathing) may result in decreased breathlessness and increased oxygenation.
- It is important to include the family in planning care for an older adult with chronic lung disease.
- An older patient with chronic lung disease may demonstrate unacceptable behavioral patterns because of the loss of control experienced with chronic illness.
- Smoking cessation may not be achievable for some older patients; interventions for these patients should focus on reducing the number of cigarettes smoked.
- Exercise plays an important part in overall lung function and has been shown to improve breathing in older patients.
- Care planning that includes the use of mechanical ventilation or other technology should include the patient and family.
- Primary patient problems for the older patient with respiratory disease focus on increasing airway clearance, decreasing breathlessness, and improving oxygenation.

CLINICAL JUDGMENT EXERCISES

1. How might pulmonary hygiene measures be revised for a frail older adult with a history of CHF and osteoporosis?
2. You are caring for a 71-year-old male who has a history of smoking for 75 pack-years. He has COPD but continues to smoke, stating that it would be impossible to quit now and, besides, "It's too late." How would you assist this patient?
3. Think about your own personal views regarding advanced life-support measures for the older adult population. What are the ethical implications of placing (or not placing) an 80-year-old person on mechanical ventilation for acute respiratory failure? How would you assist patients and/or family members faced with decisions of this nature?

REFERENCES

Adil, E. A., & Meyers, A. D. (2020). *Uvulopalatopharyngoplasty*. Medscape [website]. Retrieved from https://emedicine.medscape.com/article/1942134-overview. Accessed July 28, 2023.

Agency for Healthcare Research and Quality (AHRQ). (2012). *Five major steps to intervention (the 5 A's)*. Retrieved from https://www.ahrq.gov/prevention/guidelines/tobacco/5steps.html. Accessed July 28, 2023.

American Cancer Society (ACS). (2023). *Key statistics for lung cancer*. Retrieved from https://www.cancer.org/cancer/lung-cancer/about/key-statistics.html. Accessed July 28, 2023.

American Lung Association. (2022). *My COPD action plan*. Retrieved from https://www.lung.org/getmedia/c7657648-a30f-4465-af92-fc762411922e/fy20-ala-copd-action-plan.pdf. Accessed July 28, 2023.

Barnett, S. (2022). Anesthesia for the older adult. In G. P. Joshi & N. A. Nussmeier (Eds.), *UpToDate*. Waltham, MA: UpToDate. Retrieved from https://www.uptodate.com/contents/anesthesia-for-the-older-adult. Accessed July 28, 2023.

Bernstein, S. (2022). *Coronavirus and pneumonia*. WebMD [website]. Retrieved from https://www.webmd.com/lung/covid-and-pneumonia#1. Accessed July 28, 2023.

Brant, J. M. (2018). Assessment and management of cancer pain in older adults: Strategies for success. *Asia-Pacific Journal of Oncology Nursing, 5*(3), 248–253. doi:10.4103/apjon.apjon_11_18.

Brashers, V. L., & Huether, S. E. (2020). Alterations of pulmonary function. In S. E. Huether, K. L. McCance, & V. L. Brashers (Eds.), *Understanding pathophysiology* (7th ed., pp. 670–696). St. Louis, MO: Elsevier.

Cash, J. C., & Glass, C. A. (2019). *Adult-gerontology practice guidelines* (2nd ed.). New York: Springer.

Centers for Disease Control and Prevention (CDC). (2022a). *Cessation materials for tobacco control programs*. Retrieved from https://www.cdc.gov/tobacco/quit_smoking/cessation/index.htm. Accessed July 28, 2023.

Centers for Disease Control and Prevention (CDC). (2022b). *Pneumococcal disease*. Retrieved from https://www.cdc.gov/pneumococcal/index.html. Accessed July 28, 2023.

Centers for Disease Control and Prevention (CDC). (2023a). *About COVID-19*. Retrieved from https://www.cdc.gov/coronavirus/2019-ncov/your-health/about-covid-19.html. Accessed July 28, 2023.

Centers for Disease Control and Prevention (CDC). (2023b). *Tuberculosis*. Retrieved from https://www.cdc.gov/tb/default.htm. Accessed July 28, 2023.

Centers for Disease Control and Prevention (CDC). (2023c). *COVID-19 risks and information for older adults*. Retrieved from https://stacks.cdc.gov/view/cdc/119720. Accessed July 28, 2023.

Centers for Disease Control and Prevention (CDC). (2023d). *Long COVID or post-COVID conditions*. Retrieved from https://www.cdc.gov/coronavirus/2019-ncov/long-term-effects/index.html. Accessed July 28, 2023.

Chen, S., Kent, B., & Cui, Y. (2021). Interventions to prevent aspiration in older adults with dysphagia living in nursing homes: A scoping review. *BMC Geriatrics*, 21(1), 429. doi:10.1186/s12877-021-02366-9.

Chung, T., Mastalerz, M. H., Morrow, A. K., Venkatesan, A., & Parker, A. (2022). *Long COVID: Long-term effects of COVID-19*. Johns Hopkins Medicine [website]. Retrieved from https://www.hopkinsmedicine.org/health/conditions-and-diseases/coronavirus/covid-long-haulers-long-term-effects-of-covid19. Accessed July 28, 2023.

Cruz, J., Marques, A., & Figueiredo, D. (2017). Impacts of COPD on family carers and supportive interventions: A narrative review. *Health & Social Care in the Community*, 25(1), 11–25. doi:10.1111/hsc.12292.

DiSabatino Smith, C., & Grami, P. (2016). Feasibility and effectiveness of a delirium prevention bundle in critically ill patients. *American Journal of Critical Care*, 26(1), 19–27. doi:10.4037/ajcc2017374.

Essetova, G. U., Idrissova, L. R., & Muminov, T. A. (2022). Outpatient COVID-19 pneumonia in elderly patients in Kazakhstan. *Fortune Journal of Health Sciences*, 5, 446–453.

Farley, A., McLafferty, E., & Hendry, C. (2009). Pulmonary embolism: Identification, clinical features and management. *Nursing Standard*, 23(28), 49–56. doi:10.7748/ns2009.03.23.28.49.c6924.

Fine, M. J. (n.d.). *PSI/PORT Score: Pneumonia severity index for CAP*. MDCalc.com [website]. Retrieved from https://www.mdcalc.com/psi-port-score-pneumonia-severity-index-cap. Accessed July 28, 2023.

Fiore, M. C., Jaén, C. R., Baker, T. B., Bailey, W. C., Benowitz, N. L., Curry, S. J., et al. (2008). *Treating tobacco use and dependence: 2008 update*. Clinical Practice Guideline. Rockville, MD: U.S. Department of Health and Human Services. Public Health Service. Retrieved from https://www.ncbi.nlm.nih.gov/books/NBK63952/. Accessed July 28, 2023.

Garan, A. R. (2022). Pathophysiology of cardiogenic pulmonary edema. In W. S. Colucci & T. F. Dardas (Eds.), *UpTodate*. Waltham, MA: UpToDate. Retrieved from https://www.uptodate.com/contents/pathophysiology-of-cardiogenic-pulmonary-edema. Accessed July 28, 2023.

Garvey, C., Bayles, M. P., Hamm, L. F., Hill, K., Holland, A., Limberg, T. M., et al. (2016). Pulmonary rehabilitation exercise prescription in chronic obstructive pulmonary disease: Review of selected guidelines: An official statement from the American Association of Cardiovascular & Pulmonary Rehabilitation. *Journal of Cardiopulmonary Rehabilitation and Prevention*, 36(2), 75–83. doi:10.1097/HCR.0000000000000171.

Givertz, M. M. (2022). Noncardiogenic pulmonary edema. In S. S. Gottlieb & G. Finlay (Eds.), *UpToDate*. Waltham, MA: UpToDate. Retrieved from https://www.uptodate.com/contents/noncardiogenic-pulmonary-edema. Accessed July 28, 2023.

Global Initiative for Asthma (GINA). (2022a). *Global strategy for asthma management and prevention, 2022*. Retrieved from https://ginasthma.org/gina-reports/. Accessed July 28, 2023.

Global Initiative for Asthma (GINA). (2022b). *Pocket guide for asthma management and prevention (for adults and children older than 5 years)*. Retrieved from https://ginasthma.org/pocket-guide-for-asthma-management-and-prevention/. Accessed September 30, 2022.

Global Initiative for Chronic Obstructive Lung Disease (GOLD). (2021). *Global strategy for the diagnosis, management, and prevention of chronic obstructive pulmonary disease: 2022 report*. Retrieved from https://goldcopd.org/wp-content/uploads/2021/12/GOLD-REPORT-2022-v1.1-22Nov2021_WMV.pdf. Accessed July 28, 2023.

Henig, O., & Kaye, K. S. (2017). Bacterial pneumonia in older adults. *Infectious Disease Clinics of North America*, 31(4), 689–713. doi:10.1016/j.idc.2017.07.015.

Hodgens, A., & Gupta, V. (2023). Severe acute respiratory syndrome. *StatPearls* (Internet). Retrieved from https://www.ncbi.nlm.nih.gov/books/NBK558977/. Accessed October 7, 2024.

Kapur, V. K., Auckley, D. H., Chowdhuri, S., Kuhlmann, D. C., Mehra, R., Ramar, K., et al. (2017). Clinical practice guideline for diagnostic testing for adult obstructive sleep apnea: An American Academy of Sleep Medicine clinical practice guideline. *Journal of Clinical Sleep Medicine*, 13(3), 479–504. doi:10.5664/jcsm.6506.

Koarai, A., Sugiura, H., Yamada, M., Ichikawa, T., Fujino, N., Kawayama, T., et al. (2020). Treatment with LABA versus LAMA for stable COPD: A systematic review and meta-analysis. *BMC Pulmonary Medicine*, 20(1), 111. doi:10.1186/s12890-020-1152-8.

Lucas, C., & Martin, J. (2013). Smoking and drug interactions. *Australian Prescriber*, 36, 102–104. doi:10.18773/austprescr.2013.037.

Masters, N. J. (2020). Smoking pack years calculator. *The British Journal of General Practice*, 70(694), 230. doi:10.3399/bjgp20X709553.

Mayo Clinic Staff. (2022). *Pulmonary edema: Diagnosis and treatment*. MayoClinic.org [website]. Retrieved from https://www.mayoclinic.org/diseases-conditions/pulmonary-edema/diagnosis-treatment/drc-20377014. Accessed July 28, 2023.

McCance, K. L., & Huether, S. E. (Eds.). (2019). *Pathophysiology: The biologic basis for disease in adults and children* (8th ed.). St. Louis, MO: Elsevier.

Metheny, N. A. (2018). Preventing aspiration in older adults with dysphagia. *Try This: Best Practices in Nursing Care to Older Adults. Hartford Institute for Geriatric Nursing*, Issue number 20. Retrieved from https://hign.org/sites/default/files/2020-06/Try_This_General_Assessment_20.pdf. Accessed July 28, 2023.

Miravitlles, M., & Ribera, A. (2017). Understanding the impact of symptoms on the burden of COPD. *Respiratory Research*, 18(1), 67. doi:10.1186/s12931-017-0548-3.

Mondor, E. (2020). Lower respiratory problems. In M. M. Harding, J. Kwong, D. Roberts, D. Hagler, & C. Reinisch (Eds.), *Lewis's medical-surgical nursing: Assessment and management of clinical problems* (11th ed., pp. 502–540). St. Louis, MO: Elsevier.

Moorhead, S., Swanson, E., Johnson, M., & Maas, M. L. (2018). *Nursing outcomes classification (NOC): Measurement of health outcomes* (6th ed.). St. Louis: Elsevier.

Morisawa, T., Kunieda, Y., Koyama, S., Suzuki, M., Takahashi, Y., Takakura, T., et al. (2021). The relationship between sarcopenia and respiratory muscle weakness in community-dwelling older adults. *International Journal of Environmental Research and Public Health, 18*(24), 13257. doi:10.3390/ijerph182413257.

National Cancer Institute (NCI). (n.d.). *Lung cancer—Patient version.* Retrieved from https://www.cancer.gov/types/lung. Accessed July 28, 2023.

Polo Friz, H., Molteni, M., Del Sorbo, D., Pasciuti, L., Crippa, M., Villa, G., et al. (2015). Mortality at 30 and 90 days in elderly patients with pulmonary embolism: A retrospective cohort study. *Internal and Emergency Medicine, 10*(4), 431–436. doi:10.1007/s11739-014-1179-z.

Ramirez, J. A. (2023). Overview of community-acquired pneumonia in adults. In T. M. Jr. File, S. Bond, & P. Dieffenbach (Eds.), *UpToDate.* Waltham, MA: UpToDate. Retrieved from https://www.uptodate.com/contents/overview-of-community-acquired-pneumonia-in-adults. Accessed July 28, 2023.

Sarna, L., & Bialous, S. A. (2010). Using evidence-based guidelines to help patients stop smoking. *American Nurse Today, 5*(1), 44–47.

Shmerling, R. H. (2021). *Can vaping help you quit smoking?* Harvard Health Publishing [website]. Retrieved from https://www.health.harvard.edu/blog/can-vaping-help-you-quit-smoking-2019022716086. Accessed September 30, 2022.

Singanayagam, A., Chalmers, J. D., & Hill, A. T. (2009). Severity assessment in community-acquired pneumonia: A review. *QJM, 102*(6), 379–388. doi:10.1093/qjmed/hcp027.

SmokeFree.gov. (n.d.). *Health effects.* SmokeFree.gov [website]. Retrieved from https://smokefree.gov/quit-smoking/why-you-should-quit/health-effects. Accessed July 28, 2023.

Sorenson, H. M. (2006). Arterial oxygenation in the elderly. *19*(2), 17. Elite Learning [website]. Retrieved from https://www.elitelearning.com/resource-center/respiratory-care-sleep-medicine/arterial-oxygenation-in-the-elderly/. Accessed July 28, 2023.

Sovari, A. A., Kocheril, A. G., & Baas, A. S. (2020). *Cardiogenic pulmonary edema treatment & management.* Medscape [website]. Retrieved from https://emedicine.medscape.com/article/157452-treatment. Accessed July 28, 2023.

Staheli, B., & Rondeau, B. (2022). *Anesthetic considerations in the geriatric population.* Treasure Island, FL: StatPearls Publishing.

Thompson, B. T., Kabrhel, C., & Pena, C. (2023). Clinical presentation, evaluation, and diagnosis of the nonpregnant adult with suspected acute pulmonary embolism. In J. Mandel, K. S. Zachrison, & G. Finlay (Eds.), *UpToDate.* Waltham, MA: UpToDate. Retrieved from https://www.uptodate.com/contents/clinical-presentation-evaluation-and-diagnosis-of-the-nonpregnant-adult-with-suspected-acute-pulmonary-embolism. Accessed July 28, 2023.

U.S. Department of Health and Human Services. (2020). *Smoking cessation: A report of the Surgeon General.* Retrieved from https://www.hhs.gov/sites/default/files/2020-cessation-sgr-full-report.pdf. Accessed July 28, 2023.

U.S. Preventive Services Task Force. (2021). *Tobacco smoking cessation in adults, including pregnant persons: Interventions.* Retrieved from https://www.uspreventiveservicestaskforce.org/uspstf/recommendation/tobacco-use-in-adults-and-pregnant-women-counseling-and-interventions. Accessed July 28, 2023.

Vallerand, A. H., & Sanoski, C. A. (2023). *Davis' drug guide for nurses* (18th ed.). Philadelphia, PA: F.A. Davis Company.

Vyas, V., & Goyal, A. (2022). *Acute pulmonary embolism.* Treasure Island, FL: StatPearls Publishing.

Weaver, T. E. (2022). Assessing and managing nonadherence with continuous positive airway pressure (CPAP) for adults with obstructive sleep apnea. In N. Collop & G. Finlay (Eds.), *UpToDate.* Waltham, MA: UpToDate. Retrieved from https://www.uptodate.com/contents/assessing-and-managing-nonadherence-with-continuous-positive-airway-pressure-cpap-for-adults-with-obstructive-sleep-apnea. Accessed July 28, 2023.

Wickramasinghe, H., Rowley, J. A., Downey, R., 3rd, Sharma, S., & Gold, P. M. (2020). *Obstructive sleep apnea (OSA).* Medscape [website]. Retrieved from https://emedicine.medscape.com/article/295807-overview. Accessed July 28, 2023.

Woo, T. M., & Robinson, M. V. (2020). *Pharmacotherapeutics for advanced practice nurse prescribers* (5th ed.). Philadelphia, PA: F. A. Davis Company.

World Health Organization (WHO). (n.d.). *Obesity.* Retrieved from https://www.who.int/health-topics/obesity#tab=tab_1. Accessed July 28, 2023.

World Health Organization (WHO). (2021). *WHO TB guidelines: recent updates. Global Tuberculosis Report 2021.* Retrieved from https://www.who.int/publications/digital/global-tuberculosis-report-2021/featured-topics/tb-guidelines. Accessed July 28, 2023.

19

Gastrointestinal Function

Renae Authement, DNP, MSN, RN

http://evolve.elsevier.com/Yeager/gerontologic/

LEARNING OBJECTIVES

On completion of this chapter, the reader will be able to:
1. Describe the age-related physiologic and functional changes in the gastrointestinal (GI) system.
2. Explain primary and secondary preventive care related to the GI tract for older adults and the rationales for such care.
3. Discuss the alterations in normal structure and function accompanying common GI diseases in older adults.
4. Describe an appropriate evaluation of older patients with symptoms related to a GI disorder.
5. Describe the cause, incidence, and pathophysiology of the various types of GI disorders, including cancer and liver disease.
6. Discuss the nursing management of GI disorders in older adults.
7. Write an appropriate care plan for an older adult with a GI disorder.

WHAT WOULD YOU DO?

What would you do if you were faced with the following situations?
- While rounding on your patient, they ask for "something for constipation." Records indicate a bowel movement yesterday. What should you do?
- Your patient reports nausea, trouble eating, lack of appetite, vague abdominal pain, decreased peripheral sensation, and edema. What additional assessment data should you gather? Which interventions should you plan?

The GI system functions in the ingestion, digestion, and absorption of nutrients as well as in the excretion of solid wastes from the body. The accessory organs of digestion—salivary glands, liver, pancreas, and gallbladder—aid in the absorption of nutrients by secreting enzymes involved in the digestive process. GI system–related symptoms and complaints are common with advancing age, and the nurse is often the first healthcare provider to identify and acknowledge them. Therefore, knowledge of normal and age-related changes in the GI system is essential to providing appropriate nursing care.

AGE-RELATED CHANGES IN STRUCTURE AND FUNCTION

Although many health-related complaints from older adults pertain to the GI system, these complaints are rarely responsible for death. Older adults are usually aware of alterations in GI function, and many of these changes can be alleviated through appropriate self-care practices. Normal aging causes some changes in the GI tract (Table 19.1); however, multiple factors such as polypharmacy, stress, poor nutrition, multiple comorbidities, and poor hygiene may all contribute to alterations in GI function. Misinformation about changes in GI function may lead to more complex problems because of a failure to seek healthcare or engage in appropriate preventive and treatment measures. The nurse has the responsibility of teaching health promotion and disease prevention strategies to these patients.

Many of the systemic changes in the digestion and absorption of nutrients from the GI tract result from changes in older adults' cardiovascular and neurologic systems rather than their GI systems. For example, atherosclerosis and other cardiovascular problems may cause a decrease in mesenteric blood flow, leading to a decrease in absorption in the small intestine. Additionally, the central and peripheral nervous systems affect the motility of the entire GI system, and any change may alter peristalsis, thereby altering transit time. A decrease in mobility, often seen in older adults, may also affect GI function.

Oral Cavity and Pharynx

Changes in the oral cavity have an effect not only on an older person's well-being, comfort, and health but also on overall nutrition and digestion. The most obvious change in the mouth is the loss of teeth. In five adults 65 or older, one is edentulous (without teeth), and the prevalence of tooth loss doubles by age 75 or older. Periodontal gum disease, caused by bacterial infection and inflammation under the gum line, damages bone and connective tissue. Smoking also increases the risk of developing gum disease. In addition, persons with chronic diseases such as

TABLE 19.1 Alterations in Assessment Findings: Gastrointestinal System

Expected Aging Changes	Alterations in Assessment Findings
Gingival retraction	Loss of teeth, presence of dentures, and difficulty chewing
Decreased taste buds, decreased sense of smell	Diminished sense of taste (especially salty and sweet)
Decreased volume of saliva	Dry oral mucosa
Atrophy of gingival tissue	Poor-fitting dentures
Esophagus Lower esophageal sphincter pressure decreased; motility decreased	Epigastric distress, dysphagia, potential for hiatal hernia, and aspiration
Abdominal Wall Thinner and less taut	More visible peristalsis and easier palpation of organs
Decrease in the number and sensitivity of sensory receptors	Less sensitivity to surface pain
Stomach Atrophy of the gastric mucosa, decrease in blood flow	Food intolerances, signs of anemia as a result of cobalamin malabsorption, and decreased gastric emptying
Small Intestines Slight decreases in the secretion of most digestive enzymes and motility	Complaints of indigestion, slowed intestinal transit, and delayed absorption of fat-soluble vitamins
Liver Decreased size and lower position	Easier palpation because of the lower border extending past the costal margin
A decrease in protein synthesis and an ability to regenerate decreased	Decrease in drug metabolism
Large Intestine, Anus, and Rectum Decreased anal sphincter tone and nerve supply to the rectal area	Fecal incontinence
Decreased muscular tone and decreased motility	Flatulence, abdominal distention, and relaxed perineal musculature
Increase in transit time and decrease in the sensation of defecation	Constipation and fecal impaction
Pancreas Pancreatic ducts distended, lipase production decreased, and pancreatic reserve impaired	Impaired fat absorption and decreased glucose tolerance

Modified from Harding, M. M., Kwong, J., Roberts, D., Hagler, D., & Reinisch, C. (2020). *Lewis's medical-surgical nursing: Assessment and management of clinical problems,* (11th ed). St. Louis, MO: Elsevier.

heart disease, COPD, and diabetes are more likely to develop periodontal gum disease (Centers for Disease Control and Prevention [CDC], 2021).

Taste buds both decrease in number and atrophy beginning at age 60, resulting in a decreased ability to discriminate between salty and sweet, followed by bitter and sour. This may contribute to decreased enjoyment of food, resulting in poor eating habits and nutritional deficiencies. Drugs such as diuretics, anticholinergics, certain antidepressants, and antipsychotics reduce saliva production, leading to xerostomia (dry mouth). A reduction in saliva increases the risk for tooth decay and gum disease. Saliva normally protects the oral tissues by cleaning teeth and neutralizing acids (Harding et al, 2020).

Healthy People 2030 reflects on the importance of oral health as an integral component of health and well-being. Poor oral health and periodontal disease lead to pain and disability. One of the goals of *Healthy People 2030* is to improve oral health by increasing access to oral healthcare and to reduce the proportion of adults over the age of 45 with moderate and severe periodontitis (U.S. Department of Health and Human Services, 2022) (see Evidence-Based Practice box).

EVIDENCE-BASED PRACTICE

Effectiveness of a Mouth Care Program Provided by Nursing Home Staff

Background
Strategies to reduce pneumonia in nursing homes are needed, as pneumonia affects over 250,000 residents annually. One strategy is daily oral care. The objective of this study was to determine the effectiveness of Mouth Care Without a Battle, a program designed to increase staff knowledge and attitudes about oral hygiene.

Sample/Setting
In total, 2152 nursing home residents from 14 nursing homes in New Hampshire (NHs) participated in a pragmatic cluster randomized trial lasting 2 years. The nursing homes were selected due to the high proportion of resident rehospitalizations due to pneumonia. Each home was pair-matched and randomly assigned to either the intervention or control groups.

> **EVIDENCE-BASED PRACTICE—cont'd**
>
> The overall mean age was 79.4; participants were 66.2% females and 62.2% Caucasian.
>
> **Methods**
> The intervention, Mouth Care Without a Battle, teaches that oral care is healthcare. The program teaches staff about individualized techniques and products for oral care for residents who are resistant to care or who have special situations. The control group utilized standard oral care.
>
> **Findings**
> Over the two years, there was no statistical difference in the incidence of pneumonia between the two groups. In the second year, the rate of pneumonia was nonsignificantly higher in the intervention group versus the control group. Adjusted post hoc analyses limited to the first year found a significant reduction in pneumonia incidence in intervention nursing homes "[Incident rat ratio (IRR)], 0.69; upper bound of 1-sided 95% Confidence interval (CI), 0.94; $p = .03$" (p. 1).
>
> **Implications**
> Although a reduction was found during the first year of Mouth Care Without a Battle compared with standard care, there was no significant reduction in pneumonia incidence at 2 years. "The lack of significant results in the second year may be associated with sustainability. Improving mouth care in US NHs may require the presence and support of dedicated oral care aides" (p. 1).

Data From Zimmerman, S., Sloane, P. D., Ward, K., Wretman, C. J., Stearns, S. C., Poole, P., et al. (2020). Effectiveness of a mouth care program provided by nursing home staff vs standard care on reducing pneumonia incidence: A cluster randomized trial. *JAMA Network Open, 3*(6), e204321.

Esophagus

Age-related changes in the smooth muscle lining the esophagus contribute to a decrease in the strength of esophageal contractions and lower esophageal sphincter weakness, leading to decreased food transit time. The highest incidence of gastroesophageal reflux disease (GERD) diagnosis occurs between the ages of 60 and 69. In addition, GERD symptoms are increased and have more severe comorbidities, and polypharmacy can also exacerbate GERD symptoms (Commisso and Lim, 2019). Neurogenic, hormonal, and vascular changes secondary to comorbidities may also contribute to a decrease in esophageal motility. These changes may lead to complaints of dysphagia, heartburn, or vomiting of undigested foods. Subsequently, poor nutrition, dehydration, and decreased food intake result.

Stomach

Age-related changes in the stomach include decreased production of gastric acid, pepsin, bicarbonate, prostaglandins, and mucus. By the age of 60, gastric secretions decrease to 70%–80% of those of the average adult. In older adults, intrinsic and HCL acid secretions are decreased (Harding et al, 2020). A decrease in pepsin may hinder protein digestion, whereas a decrease in hydrochloric acid and intrinsic factor may lead to malabsorption of iron, vitamin B_{12}, calcium, and folic acid. Altered absorption and decreased gastric acid production, combined with altered gastric defense mechanisms, increase the incidence of pernicious anemia, peptic ulcer disease (PUD), and stomach cancer. Gastric emptying time has decreased, mainly due to diabetes. However, amyloidosis, neurologic diseases, and medication side effects can also contribute (Shane and Moshiree, 2021). The stomach of an older adult is not able to accommodate large amounts of food, resulting in a feeling of fullness or early satiation.

Small Intestine

Age-related changes in the small intestine include broadening of the villi and a reduction in mucosal surface areas (Dumic et al, 2019). Over time, the gastric mucosa atrophies, which leads to a decrease in the absorption of iron and vitamin B_{12} and a rapid increase in bacteria. In turn, persons with an overgrowth of bacteria may experience atrophic gastritis (Ignatavicius et al, 2021).

Large Intestine

The main function of the large intestine is the storage, propulsion, and evacuation of feces. Age-related changes in the large intestine motility reduction may be caused by a lessening of enteric smooth muscle contractility and relaxation or by changes in the enteric nervous system and a lightening in the concentration of neurotransmitters (Dumic et al, 2019). As nerve impulses and peristalsis lessen, a person's sensation to defecate decreases, which leads to constipation and impaction (Ignatavicius et al, 2021).

Gallbladder

The gallbladder and bile ducts are unaffected by aging. However, the incidence of gallstones does increase with age and is seen more in females than men (Shanmugam et al, 2020). Bile may become more lithogenic with advancing age, possibly because of an increase in biliary cholesterol related to diet and hormonal changes that affect cholesterol metabolism. The bile salt pool also decreases because of a decrease in bile salt synthesis. These predispositions for stone development, along with a tendency for dehydration in older adults, explain the increased incidence of cholelithiasis and cholecystitis in older adults. In addition, obesity, insulin resistance, metabolic syndrome, hormone replacement, and a sedentary lifestyle may contribute to gallstone production (Shanmugam et al, 2020). The complications of cholelithiasis in older adults include empyema, perforation, and choledocholithiasis (calculi in the common bile duct). These complications are often seen in persons older than the age of 65 and those with diabetes.

Pancreas

The pancreas shows some age-related changes such as fibrosis, fatty acid deposits, and atrophy; weight, but not size, is affected (Harding et al, 2020). Evidence suggests that the volume of pancreatic secretions (chymotrypsin and pancreatic lipase) declines with age. This decrease in enzyme activity affects the digestion of fats and may account for a vague intolerance of fatty foods in older adults. The decrease in fat absorption may cause steatorrhea (Ignatavicius et al, 2021). The incidence of pancreatic cancer and pancreatitis increases in older adults.

Liver

The liver is a sturdy organ and retains most of its functions throughout the life span. Although liver size decreases after age 50, liver function tests may remain within normal limits. A decline in cardiac output associated with aging contributes to a decrease in hepatic blood flow. As hepatic blood flow slows, drug metabolism is reduced, which leaves the aging liver more susceptible to drugs and toxins (Harding et al, 2020). As enzyme activity lessens, drug metabolism decreases (Ignatavicius et al, 2021). Older adults have a decreased ability to compensate for infectious, immunologic, and metabolic disorders. Some evidence suggests that normal aging may adversely affect liver tissue regeneration (Harding et al, 2020). The mechanism of this effect is not fully known, but it may be a result of a generalized slowing of repair or an inadequate response to regeneration of liver tissue.

PREVENTION

Although some changes in the GI system are associated with aging, screening recommendations for both primary and secondary prevention of problems arising from these changes are outlined by the American Cancer Society (ACS) (Wolf et al, 2018). Nurses caring for older adults should educate their patients concerning these recommendations.

COMMON GI SYMPTOMS

No clear-cut GI disease can be attributed directly to the aging process. However, many conditions show a higher incidence in older adults and have a greater effect on their physical and social well-being. These complaints may be related to normal physiologic changes associated with aging but must be distinguished from pathologic problems that increase in frequency with aging.

Older adults may report GI symptoms not related to a specific diagnosis. Any symptom reported by an older patient needs a thorough assessment by the nurse. What follows are the most frequently reported GI symptoms experienced by older adults. The sections include information on their definitions, assessments, nursing interventions, and self-care measures.

Nausea and Vomiting

Vomiting is controlled through a central vomiting center in the medulla. This center is close to the pain and respiratory centers; it is also near the centers that control vestibular and vasomotor function. Occasionally, stimuli from one center spill over to another, and symptoms may become mixed (Fig. 19.1).

Nausea may be difficult for patients to describe; many use the phrase "I feel sick" to convey the symptom of nausea. It is important to keep in mind that, although nausea usually precedes vomiting, it may also be an isolated symptom. In general,

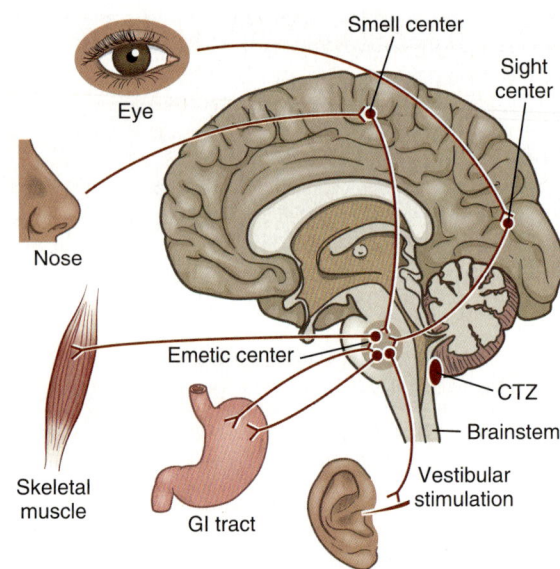

Fig. 19.1 Stimuli involved in the act of vomiting. *CTZ*, chemoreceptor trigger zone; *GI*, gastrointestinal. (Modified from McKenry, L., Tessier, E., & Hogan, M. [2006]. *Mosby's pharmacology in nursing* [22nd ed.]. St. Louis, MO: Elsevier.)

nausea in the absence of vomiting is of central, rather than peripheral, origin (i.e., the symptom is initiated centrally in the brain rather than peripherally in the GI tract). Central nausea is usually a response to a metabolic disorder.

It is important to obtain a detailed description of the events surrounding reports of nausea and vomiting. Data should be elicited about precipitating factors (e.g., the relationship of nausea and vomiting to food intake, drugs, and activity). The patient should be questioned about the presence of nausea and vomiting, as well as diarrhea or constipation. It is important to obtain information about the amount and characteristics of the emesis and whether the vomitus contained food particles, bile, or blood (bright red or the color of coffee grounds). Other symptoms, such as fever, sweating, pallor, dizziness, and pain, should be determined. Because older adults are at risk for dehydration and electrolyte imbalances, it is essential to establish the frequency and amount of vomiting and to examine patients for signs and symptoms of fluid and electrolyte imbalances.

Nursing interventions include establishing many self-help measures, including dietary changes such as drinking clear liquids, progressing from eating bland foods to solid foods, and small, frequent meals. If vomiting occurs, fluid replacement should be a priority. Sips of fluids every 15 minutes until more can be tolerated may decrease episodes of dehydration. Older adults are at high risk for aspiration, and they should be placed in the semi-Fowler or side-lying position when drinking liquids. It is important that older adults be made aware of the signs and symptoms of dehydration and electrolyte imbalances, as well as when to seek medical care. Any episodes of prolonged nausea or vomiting require careful evaluation by a healthcare provider. In addition, it should be made clear that pharmacologic therapy used to treat nausea and vomiting may cause sedation, confusion, and delirium in older adults.

Anorexia

Anorexia as a symptom should not be confused with anorexia nervosa, which is an eating disorder of psychiatric significance. The term *anorexia* literally means "lack of appetite." Hunger and appetite are not synonymous; hunger is related to the physiologic need for food. It is important for the nurse to ascertain whether food intake is truly decreased because of a loss of appetite. Once that is determined, the nurse must ask questions regarding other symptoms, including weight loss, nausea, vomiting, abdominal pain, diarrhea, and constipation. In addition, psychosocial factors such as stress, grief, pain, and concomitant illnesses may need to be assessed. Food insecurity, due to limited financial resources, is also a contributing factor (Keith-Jennings et al, 2019).

Nursing interventions for older patients with anorexia include monitoring of intake, output, and weight. It is important to acknowledge a patient's symptoms and provide gentle encouragement to eat for nutritional purposes. Small, frequent meals may be helpful. Encouraging older patients to seek medical attention for anorexia is also important because patients may not be aware of the problem.

Abdominal Pain

Abdominal pain as a symptom is often difficult to assess in a complete manner. With older adults, it may be even more difficult, even for a skilled clinician. The assessment of pain may be made easier by thinking in terms of the three pathways for pain impulses. The first are the *visceral pain pathways,* which are activated by receptors in the wall of the abdominal viscera and develop from stretching or distending the abdominal wall or from inflammation. This type of pain is often diffuse, is poorly localized, and has a gnawing, burning, or cramping quality. The second are *somatic* or *parietal pathways,* which are activated by receptors in the parietal peritoneum and other supporting tissues. This type of pain is usually sharp, more intense, constant, and better localized than visceral pain. The third are *referral pathways,* which account for referred pain (i.e., pain felt at a different site than the source of the pain but sharing the same dermatome). This type of pain is usually sharp and well localized; it may resemble somatic pain (Fig. 19.2).

In assessing any type of pain, the nurse should elicit information about its duration, location, mode of onset (sudden or gradual), intensity, quality, rhythm, relationship to food, alleviating and aggravating factors, and radiation (e.g., back, neck, or groin), as well as the older patient's ability to pass stool and gas. Older persons may complain of vague symptoms and wait much longer than their younger counterparts to seek medical care. Older adults with infections are less likely to exhibit fever or abnormal laboratory values (Penner and Fishman, 2021).

Nursing care includes measures to increase comfort and pain relief. The nurse should encourage older patients to see their healthcare provider for a complete evaluation of the abdominal pain. Abdominal pain that is severe is often referred to as an *acute abdomen.* Nursing procedures for acute abdomen include (1) starting intravenous fluids, as ordered; (2) placing a nasogastric tube for decompression of the stomach; (3) monitoring and recording vital signs and reporting abnormal findings; (4) monitoring intake and output accurately every hour; and (5) completing an assessment on the onset of pain, the presence of vomiting or diarrhea, and the presence of fever, and taking an accurate medical and surgical history.

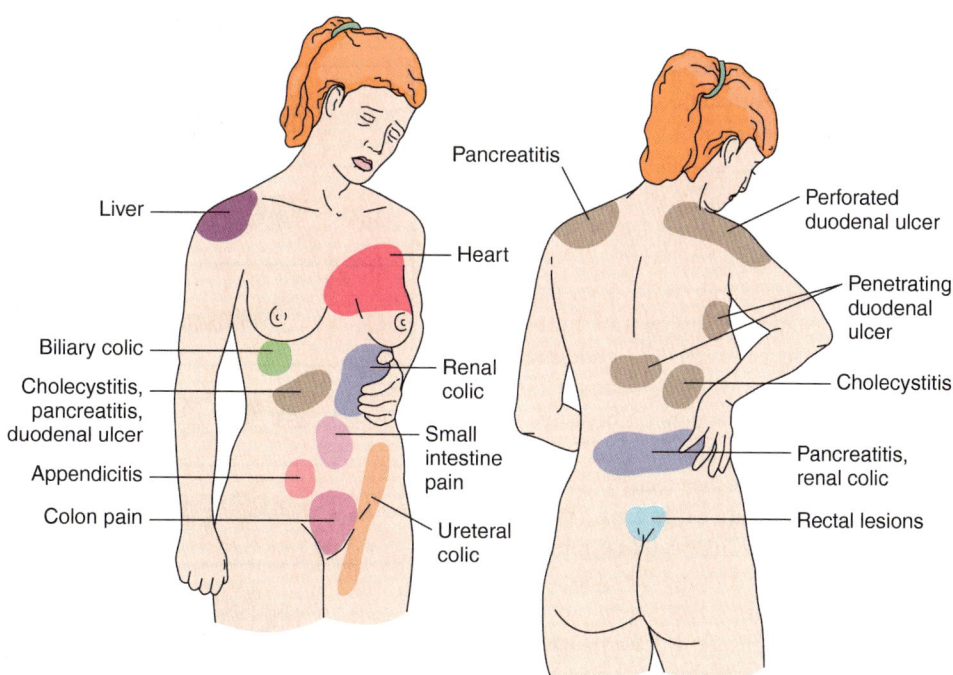

Fig. 19.2 Common sites of referred abdominal pain. (Modified from Saxton, D. F., Nugent, P. M., & Pelikan, P. K. [2009]. *Mosby's comprehensive review of nursing for the NCLEX-RN® Examination* [19th ed.]. Elsevier.)

Gas

Belching, bloating, fullness, and flatus are some of the complaints associated with gas. About 99% of the gas present in the GI tract of adults comprises five gases: nitrogen, oxygen, hydrogen, carbon dioxide, and methane. The percentage of each individual gas depends on the source; these sources include swallowing, diffusion of gas from the bloodstream to the intestinal lumen, and processing of food. All these gases are odorless; the unpleasant odor associated with flatus is probably a result of hydrogen sulfide metabolized from sulfur-containing foods. A frequency of 7–20 expulsions of gas a day is considered normal. Intestinal gas is frequently accompanied by intense abdominal pain, which may be relieved by repositioning or walking.

Although belching primarily comes from the unconscious swallowing of air, it is important to assess patients for other symptoms suggestive of gastritis or PUD. Many complaints of bloating and fullness are related to a motility disorder or malabsorption; however, in older adults, the complaints must be taken seriously. Further assessment through questioning about changes in bowel function, pain, and other GI tract symptoms is required.

Although the expulsion of flatus is a normal event, excessive flatus may have several causes. Some patients form more gas within the gut, some swallow more air, and others may have excessive flatus because of the nature of the foods consumed. Common culprits include beans, cabbage, legumes, raisins, and artificial sweeteners. In addition, patients who are lactose-intolerant may produce more gas. Careful questioning may reveal one or a combination of these causes.

Nursing interventions focus on patient education about the cause and nature of intestinal gas. The keys to treatment are changes in dietary factors (e.g., focusing on eating more slowly and avoiding gas-producing foods) and a routine exercise plan.

Diarrhea

Diarrhea is an increase in the frequency of defecation, but many definitions also include a change in the consistency of feces (e.g., watery stools). Diarrhea may be caused by increased bowel motility or interference in the normal absorption of water and nutrients from the GI tract. When an older adult reports diarrhea, it is important to ascertain exactly what is meant. Keep in mind that the description of diarrhea is useless unless a patient's normal bowel habits are known.

The nurse should ask about precipitating events (e.g., travel out of the country or eating at a restaurant), timing (intermittent or continuous), associated factors (fever, weight loss, abdominal pain, vomiting, dietary or drug changes, and any systemic diseases), characteristics of the diarrhea (frequency, consistency, volume, foul smell, presence of mucus or blood, incontinence, awakening from sleep [e.g., nocturnal diarrhea usually points to an organic cause rather than a functional or infectious cause]), and whether the onset was sudden. All these questions help assess the diarrhea further to aid in determining the cause.

Nursing care focuses on maintaining adequate fluid and electrolyte balance, assessing for complications, and providing emotional support as necessary. Usual water loss accompanying bowel movements is 150 milliliters per day (mL/day); severe diarrhea can account for up to 5 to 10 liters (L) of water loss daily. Therefore, assessing for signs and symptoms of dehydration and volume depletion in older patients is important. Patients and their families need to be taught to report complications such as increased thirst, weakness, dizziness, palpitations, and fatigue. If fluid and electrolyte imbalances occur, either oral or parenteral therapy may be required because diarrhea in older adults may be life-threatening. Nursing interventions should also be aimed at identifying and correcting the cause. The administration of antibiotics may be necessary for infectious diarrhea. Depending on the causative factor, antispasmodic and antidiarrheal drugs may also be used. The education of patients and their families should include instruction on dietary changes. Older patients with chronic diarrhea should avoid gas-forming foods, vegetables, spices, and milk products; patients with acute diarrhea should consume bland foods, such as the BRAT (bananas, rice, applesauce, and toast) diet, and clear liquids.

Constipation

Constipation is a common problem among older adults secondary to physiologic changes and is often a complication of polypharmacy. Over 65% of individuals over the age of 65 experience constipation (Kernisan, 2018). Females are affected more often compared with males. It is also more common in African Americans and individuals of lower socioeconomic status. The older adult often associates constipation with straining to have a bowel movement (Dumic et al, 2019). Typical definitions of constipation also include hard, dry stools that are difficult to pass. Bowel movements less than three times a week are often associated with constipation. However, normal bowel patterns differ greatly among individuals. The Bristol Stool Chart (Fig. 19.3)

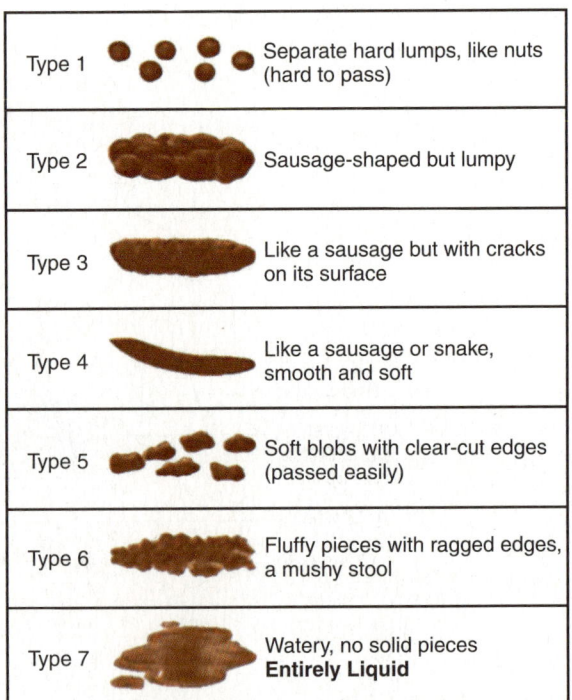

Fig. 19.3 Bristol stool chart. (From Kliegman, R. M., Stanton, B. F., St. Geme, J. W., & Schor, N. F. [2016]. *Nelson textbook of pediatrics* [20th ed.]. Philadelphia, PA: Elsevier.)

is a useful tool that may help individuals identify impending constipation by fecal consistency (Çevik et al, 2018). Common causes of constipation in older adults are related to genetic factors (family history), lifestyle factors (diet and exercise), and psychologic factors (like depression) (Vriesman et al, 2020). However, decreased mobility, cognitive impairment, comorbid medical problems, polypharmacy, and dietary changes (decreased fiber) are all contributing factors (Dumic et al, 2019). Other risk factors include foods, medications, and diseases (Ignatavicius et al, 2021).

Perhaps the most widespread cause of constipation in older adults is diet. It is usually a lack of certain foods, rather than the addition of certain foods, that leads to the problem. For example, many foods, such as fresh fruits and vegetables, contain natural laxatives, although older adults may have difficulty eating these foods because of dental problems. A second dietary cause of constipation is a lack of fiber or bulk and a decrease in fluid intake. In general, unrefined foods have more fiber than the refined foods popular in American society.

Limitations on mobility may greatly affect the ability of an older person to feed themselves and reach the toilet. They may feel awkward about depending on others for these functions. Subsequently, they may ignore the urge to defecate rather than ask for help to get to the toilet. They may also decrease fluid intake to prevent urinary incontinence. These factors may greatly influence regular bowel patterns (Ignatavicius et al, 2021; Harding et al, 2020).

Constipation is treated through dietary measures such as increasing fluid intake and increasing fiber, combined with light exercise and the development of a regular toileting routine that includes responding to the urge to defecate. In teaching older adults about dietary changes, the nurse should educate them about fiber being a "food" rather than a "medicine."

It is, however, important to understand that certain medications may cause or worsen constipation in older adults (Box 19.1) (Pont et al, 2019). Laxatives may be helpful in managing constipation. In the past, the overuse of laxatives was believed to be a contributing factor in constipation; however, there is no scientific evidence to support this concern (Kernisan, 2018).

Multiple drugs are available to treat constipation, and many of them are available over the counter (OTC). Laxatives are defined as drugs used to facilitate or stimulate the passage of feces and are classified as bulking agents (bran and psyllium), surfactants (stool softeners), emollients (mineral oil), contact stimulants (cascara, castor oil, and bisacodyl), saline cathartics (magnesium hydroxide [Milk of Magnesia], citrate, sodium, or potassium phosphate), osmotic agents (lactulose, sorbitol), and prokinetic agents (prucalopride). Laxatives may also be categorized by speed of action: (1) group I drugs (castor oil and saline laxatives in high doses) act in 2–6 hours and produce watery stool, (2) group II drugs (other contact stimulants and low-dose saline laxatives) act in 6–12 hours and produce a semiformed stool, and (3) group III drugs (bulking agents, surfactants, and lactulose) produce soft stools in 1–3 days.

In addition to oral laxatives, several rectal agents are available. Enemas provide immediate relief but should be limited in their use for long-term treatment. Soap-suds enemas should

> **BOX 19.1 Medications and Constipation**
>
> **Overview**
> *Medications* have a direct effect on constipation in older adults. Some medications can cause or worsen constipation, while others help treat or prevent it.
>
> **Medications Associated with Constipation**
> - Anticholinergics
> - Antacids
> - Opiates
> - Diuretics
> - Antihistamines
> - Antipsychotics
> - Calcium channel blockers
> - Calcium supplements
> - Nonsteroidal antiinflammatory drugs
> - Sympathomimetics
> - Iron supplements
> - Antidiarrheal medications
>
> **Medications Used to Treat Constipation**
> - Stool softeners and emollients
> - Laxatives:
>   - Osmotic agents
>   - Stimulant agents
>   - Bulking agents
>   - Prokinetic agents
>   - Secretory agents
>
> Data from Pont, L. G., Fisher, M., & Williams, K. (2019). Appropriate use of laxatives in the older person. *Drugs & Aging, 36*(11), 999–1005.

never be used because they lead to mucosal irritation. Small-volume enemas such as Fleets are the easiest to use. Rectal suppositories (bisacodyl and glycerin) may also be used, but they must be retained for 20–30 minutes for optimal results and so may be more difficult for older patients to use.

The management of constipation in older adults should be individualized. Comorbid conditions, drug interactions, and potential side effects should be considered when developing a treatment plan (Pont et al, 2019).

Fecal Incontinence

Fecal incontinence, the involuntary passing of feces, may be acute or chronic, and it demands evaluation. For older adults, the loss of bowel control is devastating and may significantly alter their quality of life. Fecal incontinence may lead to skin breakdown, which increases the risk for infection and discomfort. Loss of bowel control can lead to depression and anxiety as well. (Ignatavicius et al, 2021). Fecal incontinence may be a result of trauma (childbirth and anorectal surgery) and neurologic conditions (including stroke and multiple sclerosis) (Harding et al, 2020). In addition, comorbidities, such as stroke, dementia, and diabetes can be associated with fecal incontinence (Shaw and Wagg, 2021).

Nursing interventions focus on education concerning the prevention and treatment of incontinence in older adults. Examining the cause of the incontinence is important for the nurse, patient, and family. Laxative abuse is completely preventable and treatable with education and reassurance to the patient that being "regular" does not necessarily mean one or two bowel movements a day.

Management strategies should focus on the cause and may include lifestyle, behavioral, pharmacologic, and surgical interventions (Shaw and Wagg, 2021). However, regardless of the cause, a program of bowel control (see Patient/Family Teaching box) may usually help an older patient who is aware of and distressed by incontinence. It is important to reassure older patients that control and retraining are achievable because many older adults believe that fecal incontinence is the first step on the road to permanent institutionalization. Interventions may include avoiding artificial sweeteners, caffeine, and fatty foods. In addition, performing pelvic floor exercises and avoiding constipation are recommended (Shaw and Wagg, 2021). Other nursing interventions include methods to deal with the embarrassment caused by the incontinence, ways to decrease fecal odor, the use of adult diapers, and skin care.

PATIENT/FAMILY TEACHING
Bowel Training for the Patient with Incontinence

Overview
Fecal incontinence refers to the inability to voluntarily control defecation. It may result from decreased anal muscle tone, disturbances in the neural innervations of the rectum, loss of cortical control, rectal prolapse, diarrhea, constipation with overflow related to impaction, or altered cognition.

Contributing Factors
Factors that contribute to fecal incontinence include altered bowel habits, weakness in the internal or external anal sphincter, nerve damage that innervates the anorectum, and anal tissue damage.

Goal
Control of bowel elimination

Take Actions (Nursing Interventions)
- Assess the patient's bowel status, including patterns prior to the development of incontinence.
- Assess current bowel habits.
- Assess the consistency, frequency, and volume of the stool.
- Assess symptoms, including pain during defecation.
- Assess for a sensation of urgency to evacuate the bowel or to pass flatus.
- Ask the patient about lifestyle activities, including diet, activities, and degree that incontinence interferes.
- Assess for skin irritation or breakdown.
- Implement bowel training based on pattern.
- If necessary, stimulate the anorectal reflex with a glycerin suppository, or a small phosphate enema 15–30 minutes after the usual evacuation time.

Data from Harding, M. M., Kwong, J., Roberts, D., Hagler, D., & Reinisch, C. (2020). *Lewis's medical-surgical nursing: Assessment and management of clinical problems* (11th ed.). St. Louis, MO: Elsevier.

COMMON DISEASES OF THE GI TRACT

The following is an overview of common GI disorders seen in older patients, including related nursing care.

Gingivitis and Periodontitis

The gingivae, or gums, are subject to localized and systemic diseases, problems caused by drug therapy, poor oral hygiene, and poor nutrition. Diseases such as dementia, Parkinson disease, and osteoarthritis can negatively affect oral health in older adults (Hazara, 2020).

Gingivitis, an inflammation of the gums surrounding the teeth, may result in pain and bleeding; it may lead to *periodontitis,* a spreading of inflammation to the underlying tissues, bones, or roots of teeth. This is the most common reason for tooth loss with advancing age.

Candida albicans, or thrush, is an infection causing white lesions on the oral mucosa. It is often seen in persons with compromised immune systems and in those with suppressed immunity, such as individuals taking immunosuppressant drugs and antibiotics. *Candida albicans* is the most common cause of denture stomatitis (Gad and Fouda, 2020).

Nursing Care Guidelines for the Patient with Gingivitis and Periodontitis

Recognize cues (assessment). Assessment begins with a good history of dental care and dental hygiene practices. A complete health history focusing on other illnesses and concomitant drugs, as well as a physical assessment of the mouth, is necessary.

Analyze cues and prioritize hypotheses (patient problems). The most common patient problems for an older patient with gingivitis or periodontitis include the following:
- Inadequate oral mucous membrane
- Inadequate dentition
- Inadequate health maintenance
- Inadequate nutrition resulting in pain

Generate solutions (planning). An older adult must understand the relationship between oral health and overall health and well-being. The nurse must determine a patient's feelings and attitude about performing the self-care necessary to achieve the desired goals.

Expected outcomes for an older patient with gingivitis or periodontitis include the following:
1. The patient will maintain a comfortable and functional oral cavity.
2. The patient will establish and maintain a mouth care routine, including regular professional dental care.
3. The patient will maintain a normal body weight and nutritional status.

Take actions (nursing interventions). Nursing management of an older patient with gingivitis or periodontitis includes promotion of regular oral hygiene, regular preventive dental care, and maintenance of nutritional status. In addition, assessing the patient's knowledge of the importance of oral hygiene and frequently reinforcing oral hygiene practices are important roles for the nurse. Oral hygiene includes flossing regularly, brushing teeth or dentures, and using saline mouth rinses, as needed. Professional dental care should be sought routinely every 6 months or more often, as needed. Proper fit of dentures initially and at all subsequent visits to both the dentist and the primary healthcare provider is also encouraged. Pain relief, which will facilitate adequate nutrition, may be managed with nonnarcotics (e.g., acetaminophen), frequent mouth rinses, and a liquid or soft diet.

The key to the treatment of gingivitis and periodontitis is prevention. Although good oral hygiene needs to begin early in life, it is never too late for an older patient to begin routine dental care and oral hygiene. The nurse should discuss with the patient the use of nutritional foods that are nonirritating, for example, soft foods such as pudding or custard, and the use of nutritional supplements such as Ensure.

Evaluate outcomes (evaluation). Evaluation includes documentation of the achievement of the expected outcomes, the establishment and maintenance of regular dental care and oral hygiene practices, and the prevention of infection. Evaluation focuses on an older adult's ability to carry out the recommendations and whether any changes in self-care have occurred as a result. Findings of an oral cavity inspection should be noted, as should any instructions or explanations provided to the patient. The patient's response to recommended treatment measures should also be documented.

Dysphagia

Dysphagia (difficult swallowing) is a common problem in the older adult population. Weakened esophageal smooth muscle and incompetent sphincter function are contributory factors in older adults who develop dysphagia. Dysphagia is a symptom with many underlying causes, including stroke, neurologic disease (e.g., Alzheimer disease and Parkinson disease), local trauma or tissue damage, and tumors that may obstruct the flow of food and liquids in the esophagus. Symptoms may range from mild to severe to a complete inability to swallow (Harding et al, 2020). Dysphagia may compromise the nutritional status of an older adult, increase the risk of aspiration pneumonia, and lead to a decreased quality of life (Box 19.2).

Nursing care is aimed at ensuring the patient receives adequate evaluation, nutrition, hydration, and safe positioning during meals to prevent aspiration. Dietary modification may be recommended following a speech–language pathologist evaluation and a modified barium swallow.

Nursing Care Guidelines for the Patient with Dysphagia

Recognize cues (assessment). Assessment begins with an accurate and precise history that focuses on whether dysphagia occurs with liquids, solids, or both, as well as the time frame for the progression of the dysphagia. A thorough physical examination includes (1) neurologic assessment, (2) assessment of the oral cavity and salivary glands, (3) observation of swallowing capability for both liquid and solid substances, and (4) examination of the neck and thyroid glands.

Analyze cues and prioritize hypotheses (patient problems). Patient problems for an older patient with dysphagia include the following:
- Inadequate nutrition
- Potential for aspiration resulting from abnormal swallowing
- Acute pain resulting from odynophagia (painful swallowing in the mouth or esophagus)
- Fear resulting from the diagnosis and prognosis

BOX 19.2 Feeding Tubes in Advanced Dementia

The American Geriatrics Society recommends careful hand feeding over tube feedings in older adults with advanced dementia (American Geriatrics Society Ethics Committee and Clinical Practice Models of Care Committee, 2014). Persons with advanced dementia are at risk of tube-related complications, such as aspiration pneumonia related to gravitational backflow and pressure sores due to increased urine and fecal incontinence (Lee et al, 2021).

"Tube feeding is linked with recurrent and new-onset aspiration, aspiration-related infection, oral secretions, poor oral hygiene, anxiety, tube malfunction, use of physical and chemical restraints, and development of pressure ulcers" (Siniora et al, 2022).

Therefore, careful hand feeding may be a better first option prior to tube placement.

Data from American Geriatrics Society Ethics Committee and Clinical Practice and Models of Care Committee. (2014). American Geriatrics Society feeding tubes in advanced dementia position statement. *Journal of the American Geriatrics Society*, 62(8), 1590–1593; Lee, Y. F., Hsu, T. W., Liang, C. S., Yeh, T. C., Chen, T. Y., Chen, N. C., et al. (2021). The efficacy and safety of tube feeding in advanced dementia patients: A systemic review and meta-analysis study. *Journal of the American Medical Directors Association*, 22(2), 357–363; Siniora, D. N., Timms, O., & Ewuoso, C. (2022). Managing feeding needs in advanced dementia: Perspectives from ethics of care and ubuntu philosophy. *Medicine, Health Care, and Philosophy*, 25(2), 259–268.

Generate solutions (planning). It is essential to determine whether an older patient is ready and able to learn the self-care measures necessary to reduce the symptoms associated with dysphagia. Determining the extent of a patient's specific fears created by learning about the nature of interventions is important because the type and degree of fear affect the nurse's specificity in intervention strategies.

Expected outcomes for an older patient with dysphagia include the following:
1. The patient will maintain a weight within 10% of their ideal body weight.
2. The patient will remain free from aspiration.
3. The patient will learn techniques to swallow that minimize aspiration and pain.
4. The patient will be free from epigastric discomfort.
5. The patient will be able to verbalize fears related to the diagnosis and prognosis.

Take actions (nursing interventions). Nursing management of an older patient with dysphagia includes maintenance of hydration and nutritional status, prevention of aspiration, and the provision of emotional support and information regarding the diagnosis and prognosis. Additionally, the nurse provides support and reassurance directed at a patient's fear of eating related to pain, difficulty swallowing, and frequent regurgitation. Optimizing nutritional status and preventing weight loss are important because fear of eating may lead to chronic weight loss. Instructions regarding eating habits and swallowing techniques, as well as maintaining weight and nutrition, are important. For example, eating small, frequent meals consisting of pureed or soft high-protein, high-calorie foods; taking only small sips of fluid or using thickened liquids; and turning head to the side are helpful. The nurse should instruct the patient to elevate the head of the bed to prevent nocturnal aspiration.

Evaluate outcomes (evaluation). Evaluation includes documentation of achievement of the expected outcomes, prevention of aspiration, and maintenance of nutrition. Evaluation of how the patient is coping with the diagnosis may be assessed through the patient's resumption of activities and ability to verbalize feelings. Additionally, evaluation focuses on a patient's ability to satisfactorily incorporate and adhere to the dietary recommendations and modify behaviors and lifestyle to reduce symptoms.

Gastroesophageal Reflux and Esophagitis

GERD is a prevalent condition found in 23% of the older adult population. Atypical symptoms include dysphagia, cough, wheezing, hoarseness, and vomiting (Kurin and Fass, 2019). Causes are lower esophageal sphincter dysfunction, delayed gastric emptying, hiatal hernia, and increased intraabdominal pressure. Older adults also take drugs that increase the symptoms of GERD. Examples of such drugs include theophylline anticholinergics, B-adrenergic blockers, diazepam, morphine sulfate, nitrates, progesterone, and theophylline. In addition, alcohol, chocolate, fatty foods, nicotine, peppermint, and caffeine may increase symptoms (Harding et al, 2020).

Esophagitis refers to inflammation of the esophagus. Most often, these result from gastroesophageal reflux caused by either prolonged vomiting or an incompetent lower esophageal sphincter. The amount of mucosal damage is related to the contact time between the esophageal mucosa and the gastric contents, as well as the acidity and quantity of gastric secretions. Additional causes of esophagitis include viral, fungal, or bacterial infections.

Symptoms of GERD and esophagitis include heartburn, retrosternal discomfort, and the regurgitation of sour, bitter material. Symptoms are often precipitated by the ingestion of a large amount of fatty or spicy foods or alcohol. Strictures, caused by esophageal scarring, may develop and make food passage difficult. Dysphagia for both liquids and solids occurs as scar tissue builds and the esophageal lining stiffens, leading to esophageal narrowing. If regurgitation occurs often, substernal pain may result, occasionally mimicking a heart attack. Reflux may be aggravated by postural changes, such as sleeping in the supine position, but may occur in any position. Pulmonary aspiration because of reflux is common; when severe, it may lead to pneumonia.

Hiatal Hernia

In hiatal hernia (diaphragmatic or esophageal hernia), a major cause of reflux and esophagitis, part of the stomach protrudes through an opening of the diaphragm (Fig. 19.4). The condition may be intermittent or continuous. The continuous type is the least common, accounting for only about 10% of cases. Either part or all of the stomach, and even the intestines, may herniate, causing dyspepsia, severe pain, and often a gastric ulcer. The intermittent type, or sliding hernia, occurs with changes in position or with increased peristalsis. The stomach is forced through the opening of the diaphragm when the person is prone, and it moves back to its normal position when the person stands up. Most hiatal hernias are asymptomatic and

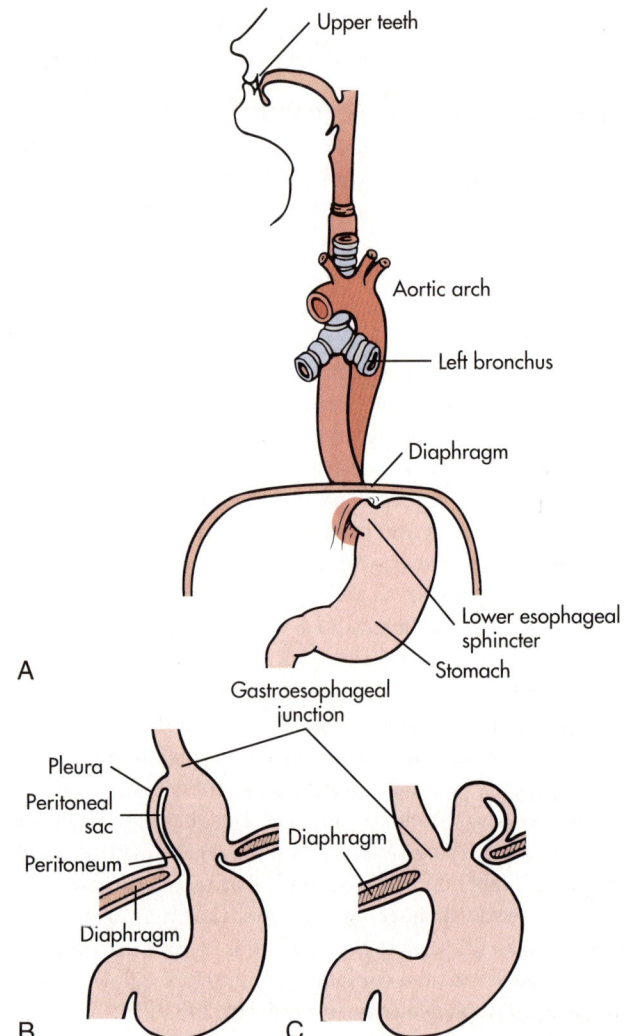

Fig. 19.4 Hiatal hernias. **A,** Normal esophagus. **B,** Sliding hiatal hernia. **C,** Rolling or paraesophageal hernia. (From Salvo, S. G. [2009]. *Mosby's pathology for massage therapists* [2nd ed.]. St. Louis, MO: Elsevier.)

require no treatment. Symptoms, when they arise, include heartburn, gastric regurgitation, dysphagia, and indigestion (Harding et al, 2019). These symptoms are accentuated (1) when assuming the supine position after meals, (2) after overeating, (3) after physical exertion, or (4) with a sudden change in posture.

Nursing Care Guidelines for the Patient with Gastroesophageal Reflux

Recognize cues (assessment). Assessment begins with a history of symptoms and possible aggravating factors. Older patients may use terms such as *indigestion* or *heartburn* rather than *pain*, and these terms need to be clearly defined. Patients may also not understand what *regurgitation* means, especially in relation to vomiting. Older adults may have atypical symptoms, including hoarseness, chest pain, postprandial fullness, respiratory symptoms, and belching. Alcohol and drug use must also be determined, as these are contributing factors. Drug and diet histories are also important components of the assessment.

Analyze cues and prioritize hypotheses (patient problems). Patient problems for an older patient with gastroesophageal reflux include the following:
- Potential for aspiration resulting from regurgitation
- Inadequate nutrition resulting from pain or dysphagia
- Need for health education resulting from a lack of exposure to disease processes and treatment modalities

Generate solutions (planning). It is essential to determine whether a patient is ready to learn the preventive measures necessary for reducing symptoms. The presence of additional health problems may affect an older patient's ability to participate in an educational plan or carry out interventions.

Expected outcomes for an older patient with gastroesophageal reflux include the following:
1. The patient will remain free from aspiration.
2. The patient will maintain a weight within 10% of their ideal body weight.
3. The patient will verbalize an understanding of the disease process and treatment approaches.

Take actions (nursing interventions). Nursing management of older patients with GERD includes maintenance of adequate nutrition, prevention of aspiration, and instruction to patients and their families about the disease process and treatment approach. Nonpharmacologic treatment includes avoiding foods that increase symptoms, maintaining health, and quitting smoking. Support from caregivers, spouses, or significant others is key to success.

Evaluate outcomes (evaluation). Evaluation includes documentation of the achievement of expected outcomes, the prevention of complications, and appropriate dietary and lifestyle changes. Because most patients improve after 1 month of conservative management with antacids and lifestyle changes, it is important for the nurse to ascertain whether symptoms have subsided. If they have not, a referral for further medical management is warranted.

Vitamin B_{12} Deficiency

Vitamin B_{12} deficiency is a condition present in more than 20% of older adults. Malabsorption causes most cases; however, pernicious anemia accounts for about one-fifth of known cases. Contributing factors to malabsorption include socioeconomic factors, physical illness, drug-nutrient interactions, and inadequate diets (Harding et al, 2020). Conditions that increase the risk of malabsorption include chronic alcohol abuse, drugs with antinutrient or catabolic properties, gastritis, gastric surgery, dementia, and nutrient losses from malabsorption, dialysis, and diarrhea (Harding et al, 2020). In pernicious anemia, degeneration of the parietal cells in the gastric mucosa leads to a decrease in the production of the intrinsic factor, resulting in a reduced absorption of vitamin B_{12}. Persons with vitamin B_{12} deficiency can develop severe neurologic impairment. Persons with pernicious anemia are typically treated with injections of vitamin B_{12}, as oral vitamin B_{12} is not well absorbed. Oral supplementation is recommended for individuals who cannot take IM injections (Rodriquez and Shackelford, 2022).

Gastritis

Gastritis refers to inflammation of the gastric mucosa and occurs in acute or chronic forms. The amount of gastric acid secretion might not be excessive in cases of gastritis.

Acute gastritis causes transient inflammation, hemorrhages, and erosion into the gastric mucosal lining. Although the cause may be undetermined, it is frequently associated with alcoholism, aspirin or NSAID ingestion, smoking, and severely stressful conditions such as burns, trauma, central nervous system (CNS) damage, chemotherapy, and radiotherapy.

Chronic gastritis involves inflammation of the stomach lining that may occur repeatedly or continue over time. Among its possible causes are ulcers, hiatal hernias, vitamin deficiencies, chronic alcohol use, gastric mucosal atrophy, achlorhydria, and peptic ulceration. The continual loss of gastric mucosa eventually decreases gastric secretion and may lead to pernicious anemia, PUD, or gastric cancer.

The major symptom of gastritis is abdominal pain. Other symptoms include indigestion, distention, decreased appetite, nausea, and vomiting. Many patients with chronic gastritis are asymptomatic.

Stress-Induced Gastritis

Stress-induced gastritis or erosion may occur in critically ill patients, such as those with burns, sepsis, multiorgan failure, major surgery, or head injuries. These erosions are superficial defects of the stomach mucosa that usually do not penetrate the muscularis layer; however, they may result in significant blood loss.

Two mechanisms are thought to produce stress ulcers: (1) mucosal ischemia resulting from a lack of blood supply to the gastric mucosa during the poststress period and (2) a decrease in mucosal bicarbonate concentration leading to increased sensitivity of the gastric mucosa to hydrochloric acid and pepsin.

The major clinical manifestation of stress ulcers is painless, gastric bleeding. Because of the danger of bleeding after acute stress and the difficulty of stopping it once it has started, preventive measures are routinely used to decrease hydrogen ion secretion and neutralize gastric acid. These include the administration of antacids, as well as histamine blockers, sucralfate, or both.

Nursing Care Guidelines for the Patient with Gastritis

Recognize cues (assessment). Assessment begins with a history and review of systems, which may include complaints of indigestion, abdominal, or epigastric discomfort; nausea; vomiting; or anorexia. Questioning patients about possible GI blood loss (e.g., hematemesis or melena) is also important. With acute gastritis, signs of dehydration may be present.

Analyze cues and prioritize hypotheses (patient problems). Patient problems for an older patient with gastritis include the following:
- Acute pain resulting from epigastric discomfort, cramping secondary to acidity, or both
- Dehydration resulting from decreased intake, vomiting and blood loss, or both
- Need for health education resulting from the disease process

Generate solutions (planning). Because most patients receive treatment on an outpatient basis, the nurse must determine an older patient's ability to adhere to the recommended treatment

strategies. Expected outcomes for an older patient with gastritis include the following:
1. The patient will experience relief from epigastric symptoms.
2. The patient will maintain adequate fluid and electrolyte balance.
3. The patient will verbalize their understanding of the disease and the factors that contribute to it.

Take actions (nursing interventions). Nursing management of an older patient with gastritis includes acid-suppressant drugs, as ordered; small, frequent, easily digested meals; maintenance of a calm environment to decrease the effects of stress; monitoring of fluid and electrolyte status; and teaching the older patient about precipitating and contributory factors. GI bleeding is a possible complication of gastritis, and prevention and early diagnosis are important. An older patient must understand the necessity of limiting or eliminating alcohol and tobacco use, avoiding aspirin and other NSAIDs, and seeking prompt medical attention for symptoms of indigestion and epigastric pain.

Evaluate outcomes (evaluation). Evaluation includes documentation of achieved expected outcomes, a decrease in symptoms, and no evidence of GI hemorrhaging or other complications. The nurse should note an older patient's adherence to necessary lifestyle changes.

Peptic Ulcer Disease

PUD is an ulcerative condition caused by the erosion of the GI mucosa resulting from the digestive action of hydrochloric acid and pepsin. Although PUD refers to injury anywhere in the GI tract, the most common occurrence is in the stomach and duodenum (Fig. 19.5). The exact cause of peptic ulcers is unclear, but research has identified conditions that predispose individuals to their development. *Helicobacter pylori* infection plays a central role in the development of PUD in nearly 80% of gastric and 90% of duodenal ulcers (DUs). The infection leads to bacterial gastritis and subsequent gastric atrophy. The long-term effects of gastric mucosal atrophy include decreased gastric acid production, intestinal metaplasia, and gastric carcinoma. The organism secretes urease, which generates free ammonia, and a protease that breaks down the gastric mucus. These substances mediate inflammation in the gastric mucosa, which makes it more vulnerable. Non-*H. pylori* gastric ulcers and DUs are typically associated with NSAID use. Other drugs associated with PUD include corticosteroids and anticoagulants (Harding et al, 2020).

Both genetic and environmental factors have been proposed as the cause of peptic ulcers because both gastric ulcers and DUs tend to occur in families. At present, no direct evidence exists that indicates dietary or occupational factors as causes of ulcer disease. In addition, although psychologic factors such as anxiety or stress play a role in the response of peptic ulcers to treatment, little evidence supports the common belief that only a person with the type A personality, who is constantly striving for perfection, develops ulcers. However, prolonged stress may produce a stress ulcer in anyone.

Gastric Ulcers

The risk of gastric ulcers increases in those over the age of 50 and is more prevalent in females. In gastric ulcers, the level of hydrochloric acid secretion is usually normal or reduced. The problem lies in the increased rate of diffusion of gastric acid back into the tissue. Patients with benign gastric ulcers should be encouraged to receive frequent follow-up and monitoring because these ulcers can become malignant. Risk factors for the formation of gastric ulcers include *H. pylori* infection, NSAID use, cigarette smoking, and alcohol use disorder. Caffeine and excessive stress may aggravate symptoms.

The most common symptom with gastric ulcers is gnawing or burning pain in the epigastric region that comes and goes; eating may lead to pain relief. Pain may be worse on an empty stomach. If the ulcer has eroded through the mucosa, food aggravates symptoms rather than alleviating them (Harding et al, 2020). Nausea, vomiting, and weight loss are common. Perforation may lead to hemorrhage and peritonitis. Healings and recurrences are common. A lack of healing or failure to decrease in size suggests malignancy.

Duodenal Ulcers

Duodenal ulcers (DUs) account for around 80% of peptic ulcers. In contrast to gastric ulcers, people with DUs have normal back diffusion of gastric acid but an increased rate of gastric acid secretion. They also have an increased emptying rate of acid from the stomach to the duodenum. If the increase in acid is not buffered in the stomach, the acid is propelled into the duodenum, which leads to irritation of the duodenal mucosa. Most of these ulcerations occur in the first part of the duodenum, close to the pylorus. It is believed that the bacterium *H. pylori* migrates from the stomach to the duodenum in the presence of dysplastic changes in the duodenal mucosa.

Typically, the symptoms of DUs are patterned by periods of exacerbation and remission and follow a pain–food–relief pattern. The pain begins 1–2 hours after meals and is immediately relieved by food or antacids. The pain is in the mid-epigastrium and may be described as a burning or cramp-like pain (Harding et al, 2020). The pain may manifest as back pain. Other GI symptoms include heartburn and the regurgitation of sour, acidic juice into the back of the throat. Anorexia and weight loss are rare because the patient usually seeks food to relieve the

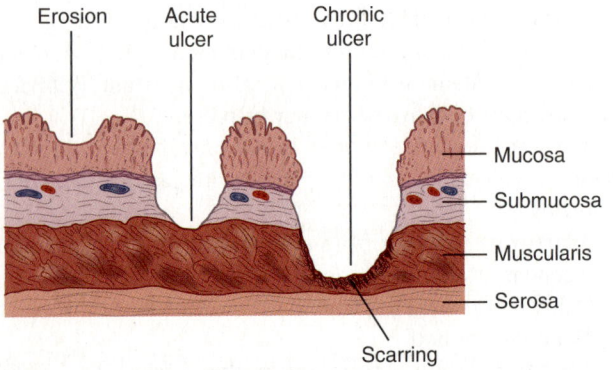

Fig. 19.5 Peptic ulcers, including an erosion, an acute ulcer, and a chronic ulcer. (From Harding, M. M., Kwong, J., Roberts, D., Hagler, D., & Reinisch, C. [2020]. *Lewis's medical-surgical nursing: Assessment and management of clinical problems* [11th ed.]. St. Louis, MO: Elsevier.)

pain. A DU may rupture because of erosion through the duodenal wall, and this leads to contamination of the peritoneal cavity (peritonitis). A slowly bleeding ulcer may reveal guaiac-positive stools. On physical examination, the only abnormality observed is possibly a tender epigastrium.

Nursing Care Guidelines for the Patient with PUD

Recognize cues (assessment). Assessment begins with an evaluation of a patient's complaint of abdominal or epigastric pain, the most common symptom of peptic ulcers. Pain should be assessed for presence, location, character, and especially alleviating and precipitating factors. Peptic ulcer pain is usually described as gnawing, burning, or aching, usually in the epigastric area, and may radiate around to the back. The pain usually begins when the stomach is empty and may disappear with the ingestion of food or an antacid. Because of this, pain often occurs at night when the stomach is empty, especially with DUs. A patient may also exhibit signs of complications from the peptic ulcer. Hemorrhaging may manifest as either melena or hematemesis. Older adults typically have a blunt presentation.

Analyze cues and prioritize hypotheses (patient problems). The most frequently used patient problems for an older patient with PUD include the following:

- Acute pain resulting from mucosal lesions
- Need for health education resulting from a lack of exposure to disease processes and treatments
- Inadequate family therapeutic management resulting from the complexity of the healthcare regimen

Generate solutions (planning). Because not all older patients with PUD have the same set of symptoms, the nurse must determine individual patient needs regarding education and other interventions. Expected outcomes for an older patient with PUD include the following:

1. The patient will report a decrease in abdominal or epigastric pain.
2. The patient will adhere to the prescribed dietary, activity, and drug regimen.
3. The patient will acknowledge aggravating factors such as smoking, alcohol use, stress, or frequent use of aspirin or NSAIDs.

Take actions (nursing interventions). Nursing management for an older patient with PUD includes education of the patient on lifestyle changes, dietary modifications, and drugs that may be used in the treatment plan. Lifestyle changes include cessation of smoking, cessation of alcohol consumption, and avoidance of other irritants such as aspirin-containing products and NSAIDs. In addition, stress reduction techniques such as exercise, relaxation training, biofeedback, and other appropriate outlets should be explored and individualized, depending on patient needs and wishes. Dietary changes include avoiding foods that irritate the mucosa of the stomach, for example, caffeine and foods that cause pain.

Drugs need to be taken as prescribed. An older patient needs to be instructed that antacids work quickly to neutralize acid in the stomach and are only to be used intermittently for heartburn and acid indigestion. Drugs to reduce or prevent acid production (H_2 receptor antagonists and PPIs) should be taken exactly as ordered, but these agents take longer to provide relief. The patient should also understand that antacids last only 20–30 minutes, whereas drugs to reduce or prevent acid production have a long-term effect. Another important point to discuss with the older patient is the effect of the ulcer drug on other drugs. For example, cimetidine, an H_2 receptor antagonist, interferes with the metabolism of warfarin, theophylline, and phenytoin.

If surgery is performed, more dietary modifications may be necessary because of a reduction in the size of the stomach. A response known as *dumping syndrome* is common after gastric resection; it is manifested by dizziness, nausea, and diaphoresis after meals. The institution of small, frequent meals that are low in carbohydrates will diminish the incidence of these symptoms. Resting after eating and drinking fluids between (rather than during) meals will also help alleviate these symptoms. Maintaining adequate nutrition and fluid and electrolyte balance is especially important for older patients and may be achieved by making these dietary modifications.

Evaluate outcomes (evaluation). Evaluation includes documentation of the achievement of the expected outcomes, the prevention of complications, the elimination of symptoms, and an increased knowledge base regarding PUD. Any complications from recommended medical treatments should be noted.

Enteritis

Enteritis, or *gastroenteritis,* refers to an inflammatory process of the stomach or small intestine. Bacteria, viruses, drugs, radiation, ingestion of foods that irritate the gastric mucosa, or allergic reactions may cause it. Bacterial enteritis, commonly known as "food poisoning," is often caused by the ingestion of food contaminated by bacteria containing toxins. Examples of these bacteria include *Staphylococcus aureus, Salmonella,* and *Clostridium botulinum.*

In addition, enteritis may result from parasitic infections such as amebiasis and trichinosis. Amebiasis is caused by a protozoal parasite that primarily invades the large intestine. The inactive form, a cyst, is ingested through food or water contaminated by feces and passes into the intestines. There, the active form is released and enters the intestinal wall, causing ulceration of the intestinal mucosa. Amebiasis is prevalent primarily in tropical countries and in places with poor sanitation.

Trichinosis is transmitted through improperly cooked pork and is caused by the larvae of a roundworm that became imbedded in the striated muscles. When the contaminated pork is eaten, gastric acid releases the larvae from cysts; they develop into adults in the host's intestine. The adult females release larvae, which move toward the host's muscles, where they may remain for many years. Acute enteritis is a result of a direct bacterial or viral infection or the effect of the toxins produced by bacteria. This results in either an increased secretion of water into the intestinal lumen or an increase in motility, causing large amounts of food and fluid to be excreted. In general, enteritis causes inflammatory changes in the intestinal mucosa, which return to normal when the offending agent is removed.

The pathologic process has varying manifestations, resulting in symptoms of abdominal cramping, profuse diarrhea, and vomiting. With profuse diarrhea, large amounts of fluid and electrolytes may be lost, which leads to dehydration and electrolyte imbalances such as hyponatremia and hypokalemia. Older adults are particularly at risk for dehydration and electrolyte imbalance. Prompt treatment is required.

Nursing Care Guidelines for the Patient with Enteritis

Recognize cues (assessment). Assessment begins with a history of recent food intake, nausea, vomiting, and diarrhea, including amount, duration, frequency, and stool characteristics. The nurse should inquire about recent drug use, especially antibiotics, and recent travel. If food poisoning is suspected, the nurse should also question the patient regarding possible sources of contamination. Physical examination includes inspection of mucous membranes and assessment of orthostatic blood pressure, temperature, and abdominal tenderness. A urine specimen for specific gravity may be helpful in assessing hydration.

Analyze cues and prioritize hypotheses (patient problems). The most common patient problems for an older patient with enteritis include the following:
- Dehydration resulting from vomiting and diarrhea
- Diarrhea resulting from intestinal inflammation

Generate solutions (planning). Expected outcomes for an older patient with enteritis include the following:
1. The patient will maintain adequate fluid volume and electrolyte balance.
2. The patient will have a continual decline in the number of liquid, nonformed stools until baseline is achieved.

Take actions (nursing interventions). Nursing management of an older patient with enteritis includes maintenance of hydration and monitoring of fluid and electrolyte status. With severe vomiting and diarrhea, intravenous hydration and hospitalization are required. With milder forms of enteritis, clear liquids may be offered at home. In all cases, monitoring for signs and symptoms of dehydration is imperative. In addition, it is important for the nurse to determine whether an older patient has someone nearby to assist them or summon for help if the condition worsens. Older patients need to be educated about the signs and symptoms of dehydration and when to seek further medical care. Prevention of bacterial and parasitic enteritis should also be discussed, and the need for thorough hand washing, especially before meals and food preparation, should be stressed.

Evaluate outcomes (evaluation). Evaluation includes documentation of the achievement of the expected outcomes, the prevention of complications, and the return to baseline status. The nurse should monitor the older patient for a reduction in symptoms as the problem resolves. Careful monitoring of oral intake and tolerance for an advancing diet is also documented.

Intestinal Obstruction

Intestinal obstruction occurs whenever partial or complete blockage of the GI tract occurs in either the small intestine or the large intestine. This may be the result of several conditions, which are usually classified as mechanical or paralytic ileus.

Mechanical obstructions are the most common and are primarily caused by tumors, adhesions, or hernias (Fig. 19.6). Another mechanical cause of intestinal obstruction is volvulus, or the twisting of a part of the intestine. Although this is a rare

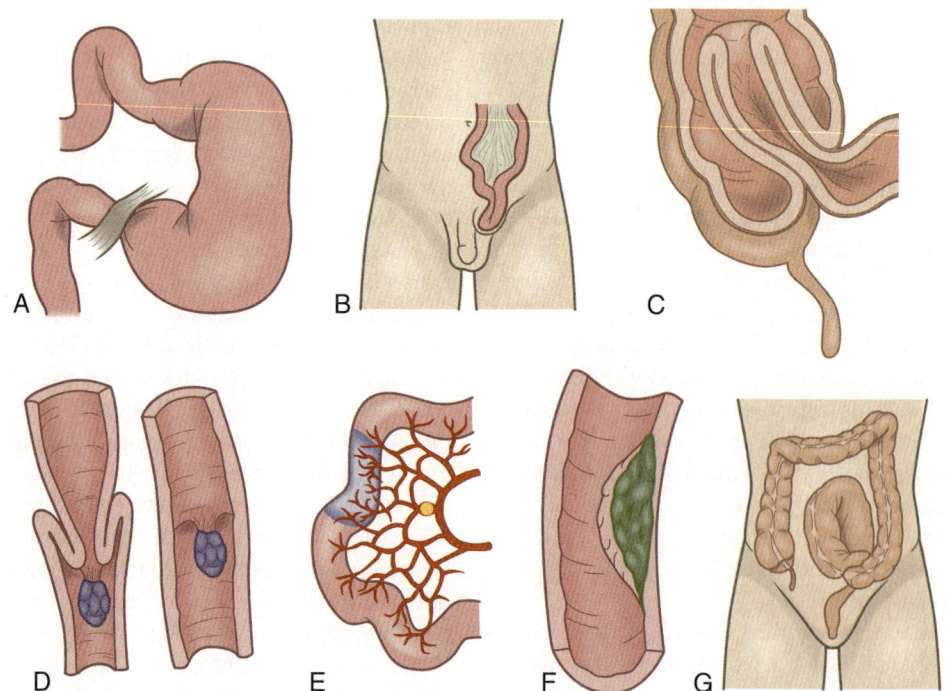

Fig. 19.6 Bowel obstructions. **A,** Adhesions. **B,** Strangulated inguinal hernia. **C,** Ileocecal intussusception. **D,** Intussusception from polyps. **E,** Mesenteric occlusion. **F,** Neoplasm. **G,** Volvulus of the sigmoid colon. (Modified from Harding, M. M., Kwong, J., Roberts, D., Hagler, D., & Reinisch, C. [2020]. *Lewis's medical-surgical nursing: Assessment and management of clinical problems* [11th ed.]. St. Louis, MO: Elsevier.)

cause of obstruction overall, it is more common in older adults because the mesenteric ligaments weaken over time.

Paralytic ileus involves decreased or absent peristalsis resulting from neurologic or vascular disorders. Peristalsis becomes diminished or absent because of a triggering of the inhibitory reflex by noxious stimuli such as anesthesia, peritoneal injury, interruption of the nerve supply, abdominal injury or surgical manipulation, intestinal ischemia, electrolyte imbalances, or side effects of certain drugs such as antidepressants or drugs to control pain. Neurologic causes, which may be overlooked, include diabetes-related neuropathy, multiple sclerosis, stroke, or Parkinson disease. It is a common postoperative problem, especially after abdominal surgery.

Vascular disorders may cause intestinal or mesenteric ischemia, resulting in obstruction. Prolonged ischemia results in the death of the surface of the villi and epithelial cells, which, in turn, impairs the absorption of nutrients. In addition, the mucosal layer becomes necrotic, and peristalsis diminishes. Although intestinal or mesenteric ischemia is relatively rare, its high mortality rate and predominance in older adults make it important for nurses caring for older adults. Some degree of intestinal ischemia is present in all patients who have a history of other forms of ischemia, thrombosis, or infarction, or in patients who have chronic ischemia, for example, those with atherosclerosis. Most of these patients have a history of cerebrovascular disease, peripheral vascular disease, coronary heart disease, or all these conditions. Ischemic bowel disease comprises a spectrum of acute and chronic syndromes that usually affect older adults. The major syndromes of ischemic intestinal disease include acute embolic ischemia, acute thrombotic occlusion (ischemic colitis), nonocclusive ischemia, chronic intestinal ischemia (abdominal angina), and venous occlusive disease.

Whatever the cause of intestinal obstruction, after the blockage occurs, the bowel becomes distended by gas and air proximal to the area of blockage. If the process continues, gastric, biliary, and pancreatic secretions, along with water, electrolytes, and serum proteins, begin to accumulate in the area, causing an increase in intraluminal pressure. A third space shift may occur when the circulating blood volume decreases because of the movement of water into the intestinal lumen, which may lead to dehydration, electrolyte imbalances, and hypovolemia.

Clinical findings with an obstruction include the acute onset of severe cramping pain that correlates roughly to the area or level of obstruction. The pain may decrease in severity as the distention of the bowel increases. In mesenteric ischemia, the clinical presentation is initially nonspecific and may mimic other, more common abdominal problems such as diverticulitis, appendicitis, and cholecystitis. Although the major symptom is abdominal pain, the clue to mesenteric ischemia is that the pain is out of proportion to what is found on physical examination. Atherosclerotic ischemia may create angina-like cramping abdominal pain that becomes worse after meals and then dissipates. In colonic ischemia, the pain is worse in the left lower quadrant. Vasospasm and emboli produce acute, severe abdominal pain with associated vomiting and diarrhea.

Abdominal distention will be present, especially if the obstruction is in the lower small intestine or colon. Percussion will elicit a tympanic sound because of the accumulation of gas and air in the bowel. Hyperactive bowel sounds are present above the site of a mechanical obstruction as the intestine attempts to push the contents downward. The increase in the rate and force of peristalsis may cause *borborygmi* (loud and high-pitched bowel sounds); these may progress to an absence of bowel sounds as the condition persists. Bowel sounds below the obstruction will be absent. Vomiting is almost always present and may (rarely) be bilious or feculent, depending on the level of the obstruction. Diarrhea may occur if the obstruction is not complete, allowing watery contents to pass. The patient may develop signs of dehydration and shock.

Complications of intestinal obstruction include perforation of the bowel, chemical or bacterial peritonitis, hypovolemic shock, and septic shock. The increased pressure on the mucosa of the affected bowel segment may lead to bowel necrosis, resulting in changes in the permeability of the bowel wall. Normal bacteria of the intestine may then escape into the peritoneal cavity, causing peritonitis that may escalate to bacteremia. Perforation of the thinned intestinal wall results in the loss of fluid into the abdominal space, chemical peritonitis, and possible abscess formation. Infection and the loss of fluid and electrolytes are major problems. Hypovolemic shock may result when there is a shift of fluid greater than 10% of body weight. Septic shock may also occur because of the contamination of the bloodstream when the bowel ruptures or becomes gangrenous. Sepsis and hypovolemic shock are life-threatening and must be treated aggressively.

Nursing Care Guidelines for the Patient with Bowel Obstruction

Recognize cues (assessment). Assessment begins with a thorough history of the precipitating event; the nurse should focus on the type and frequency of vomiting and diarrhea (e.g., profuse or fecal) and the location and character of pain (e.g., cramping, constant, or diffuse). A sudden change in a patient's description of abdominal pain from generalized and dull to localized and sharp must be taken seriously; this is a characteristic presentation of peritonitis. A physical examination should focus on the presence and character of bowel sounds (e.g., loud, frequent, absent, or weak), the presence of abdominal distention, vital signs, and urinary output. A sudden elevation of temperature is another classic sign of peritonitis.

Analyze cues and prioritize hypotheses (patient problems). Patient problems for an older patient with bowel obstruction or ileus include the following:

- Dehydration resulting from the loss of body fluids and inadequate fluid volume intake
- Inadequate nutrition resulting from vomiting and obstruction
- Nausea resulting from GI irritation
- Constipation resulting from decreased motility or obstruction

Generate solutions (planning). Expected outcomes for an older patient with an ileus or intestinal obstruction include the following:

1. The patient will maintain adequate fluid volume and electrolyte balance.

2. The patient will verbalize a tolerable level of discomfort.
3. The patient will regain and maintain adequate nutrition, as evidenced by the achievement of preillness body weight.
4. The patient will report relief from nausea.
5. The patient will maintain passage of soft, formed stool.

The older adult with bowel obstruction requires careful and close observation because the classic signs of pain and fluid loss may be blunted.

Take actions (nursing interventions). Nursing management of an older patient with intestinal obstruction or ileus includes maintenance of hydration and promotion of comfort. Dehydration may be prevented through the provision of intravenous fluids and electrolytes, as ordered. Monitoring intake and output and the specific gravity of urine, as well as monitoring for signs of fluid overloading or dehydration, is important. Nasogastric or nasointestinal tubes are usually required for decompression, and maintenance of their patency and placement is imperative. Pain relief measures may include drug therapy; however, narcotics are sometimes not allowed because of their effects on the bowel and their masking of important symptoms. Other comfort measures include repositioning, mouth care, skin care, and music or meditation. If surgery is required, the preparation of the patient and family concerning what should be expected is also important.

Evaluate outcomes (evaluation). Evaluation includes documentation of the achievement of expected outcomes and the prevention of complications (see Nursing Care Plan: Ileus). Vital signs, intake and output, bowel sounds, and bowel elimination patterns should also be recorded. If surgery was performed, monitoring of the incision site and wound healing status is necessary.

NURSING CARE PLAN

Ileus: Obstruction Resulting from Diverticulitis

Clinical Situation

Mrs. M is a 78-year-old retired seamstress who was recently admitted to the emergency department with abdominal pain. Her son and daughter-in-law, with whom she lives, brought her in. Her son reported that his mother had been complaining of abdominal pain for the past 24 hours, and because it did not subside, he encouraged her to seek medical attention. Over the past 24 hours, Mrs. M reported left-sided lower abdominal pain, nausea, and, more recently, vomiting. She was unsure whether she had a fever. Her daughter-in-law added that her mother-in-law had had a lot of constipation recently, for which Mrs. M had taken various types of laxatives.

Her medical history included hypertension (for which she takes extended-release nifedipine and hydrochlorothiazide) and hypercholesterolemia (for which she takes lovastatin daily). Her son also remembered the doctor telling his mother a few years ago that she had diverticulosis, which was diagnosed from an incidental finding on radiography. Her only past surgery was an uncomplicated cholecystectomy about 20 years ago for cholecystitis. Mrs. M stated that she ate a regular diet without restrictions and did not have much weight fluctuation over the past few years.

Physical examination revealed a thin female, weighing 128 pounds (lb), with a temperature of 100.9°F (38.3°C) (orally), a pulse of 98 beats per minute (beats/min), a respiratory rate of 24 breaths/min, and a blood pressure of 140/84 mm Hg. She was lying on the stretcher, curled in a semifetal position. Her abdomen was not obviously distended, and her only scar was a midline incisional scar from her previous cholecystectomy. She had loud, high-pitched bowel sounds but no audible bruits. Her abdomen was tender, and a firm mass was palpable in the lower left quadrant. She had no elicitable rebound tenderness. She had tenderness on rectal examination and was thought to have stools high up in her rectal vault. Her stool occult test was guaiac negative.

Laboratory tests revealed a white blood cell (WBC) count of 90,000 microliters (µL) and a normal hemoglobin count. Urinalysis was normal, as were serum electrolyte levels. Serum amylase was 500 units per deciliter (units/dL). Plain abdominal radiography revealed air–fluid levels but no free air in the abdomen. She was given the diagnosis of ileus, or obstruction resulting from diverticulitis.

Mrs. M was admitted to a general medical unit and had a surgical consultation. She was started on intravenous fluids, restricted to nothing by mouth (NPO) status, and had a nasogastric tube placed on high intermittent suction. Intravenous antibiotic therapy was begun and continued for the remainder of her hospitalization. She was monitored closely and managed medically. She was found to have only an ileus and never required surgery for a small bowel obstruction or perforation. She was discharged home on the eighth day after admission. She resumed her previous drugs.

Analyze Cues and Prioritize Hypotheses (Patient Problems)
- Dehydration resulting from active loss of body fluid secondary to nasogastric tube output
- Inadequate nutrition resulting from prolonged NPO status
- Constipation resulting from decreased mobility, daily ingestion of constipating drugs, and a lack of dietary fiber
- Need for health education resulting from a lack of exposure to knowledge about the prevention and complications of diverticular disease
- Pain (abdominal) resulting from reluctance to take drugs to control pain

Generate Solutions (Planning)
- The patient will maintain adequate fluid volume and electrolyte balance.
- The patient will maintain preadmission weight.
- The patient will establish a regular pattern of fecal elimination.
- The patient and family will be able to verbalize dietary changes and be able to prevent constipation and further complications.
- The patient will obtain pain relief.

Take Actions (Nursing Interventions)
- Monitor vital signs every 4 hours or as ordered.
- Maintain intravenous therapy as ordered.
- Monitor intake and output (hourly); skin moisture, color, and turgor; specific gravity of urine (every 4 hours); serum electrolyte levels; and level of consciousness.
- Weigh the patient every day or as ordered.
- Monitor serum albumin and protein levels.
- Administer intravenous total perineal nutrition, as ordered.
- When the patient is no longer NPO, encourage high-protein, high-calorie foods.
- Administer stool-softening drugs, if ordered.
- When the patient is no longer NPO, encourage a daily fluid intake of 2 liters (L) and the consumption of high-fiber foods. Teach the patient about fiber-rich foods to be included in the diet.
- When the patient is able, encourage her to increase her activity level.
- Teach about constipating side effects of drugs.
- Provide the patient and family with written and verbal information concerning the importance of a high-fiber diet, the need to maintain an adequate fluid intake, and the need for light exercise.
- Provide the patient and family with written and verbal information concerning complications of diverticulosis, such as diverticulitis.
- Assess and monitor the degree of pain every 4 hours.
- Provide the patient with verbal and written instructions about analgesics.
- Provide other measures of pain relief, such as guided imagery, repositioning, and diversional activities.
- Provide encouragement by informing the patient that the pain will decrease as the ileus improves.

Diverticula

Diverticula are saclike protrusions of the mucosa along the GI tract. These small sacs are formed by herniation of the mucous membrane outward through a separation in the circular muscle fibers of the intestine, where blood vessels penetrate the muscle layer.

Diverticula are a result of increased intraluminal pressure and can develop in any part of the digestive tract. They occur most often in the descending and sigmoid colons. Colonic diverticula are usually multiple.

The exact cause of diverticula is unknown. Because of the frequency of diverticula in older adults, it is thought that they are related to the blood supply or nutrition of the bowel. Lack of dietary fiber, or roughage, and decreased fecal bulk have also been correlated with this process. With an increase in food bulk (as with consumption of dietary fiber), the pressure in the colon decreases. In contrast, when little waste is present in the colon, stronger muscle contractions are necessary to excrete it, and the pressure increases. This increase in pressure leads to muscle hypertrophy and the development of diverticula. In this manner, diverticula have also been linked to chronic constipation and obesity in older adults. Atrophy of the musculature of the bowel wall may weaken the intestine and be another factor in the development of diverticula in older adults. The presence of multiple diverticula that are not inflamed is termed *diverticulosis*. Diverticulosis may be symptom-free and is often diagnosed as an incidental finding on radiography or sigmoidoscopy. When symptoms are present, they may be associated with vague abdominal discomfort, constipation, or diarrhea. More than 50% of Americans over the age of 60 have diverticulosis; therefore, the prevalence of diverticulitis is high (Strate and Morris, 2019).

Diverticulitis is an inflammation of or around a diverticular sac, usually caused by the retention of undigested food, stool, and bacteria. In diverticulitis, stasis leads to inflammation, infection, or both. The mucous membranes may erode or perforate blood vessels, causing bleeding. Obstruction of the large intestine, fistulae, and abscesses may result. The rupture of the infected material into the peritoneal cavity may result in peritonitis. Approximately 5% of those with diverticulosis develop diverticulitis (Strate and Morris, 2019).

Clinical manifestations of symptomatic diverticular disease include constipation or diarrhea, left-sided lower abdominal pain, and fever. More than half of patients with diverticulitis experience some change in bowel habits; most complain of constipation. Other symptoms include flatulence, nausea, and vomiting. Older adults with diverticulitis may be afebrile and have little abdominal discomfort. Complications include perforation and peritonitis, ureteral obstruction, and significant lower GI bleeding. Surgery may be necessary if an obstruction or perforation is suspected.

Nursing Care Guidelines for the Patient with Diverticula

Recognize cues (assessment). Assessment begins with an older patient's history of elimination patterns and changes in these patterns, such as frequency of defecation, stool characteristics (e.g., color, size, and consistency), toileting habits, and course (e.g., improving or worsening and recurrent or chronic changes in bowel habits). Exercise patterns, pain, bloating, nausea, vomiting, medical history (e.g., hemorrhoids or bowel surgery), and family history of bowel problems such as polyps or colon cancer are also important. With diverticulitis, the patient may have a fever and chills. A physical examination may be unremarkable, but it may also reveal left lower quadrant tenderness or a guaiac-positive stool.

Analyze cues and prioritize hypotheses (patient problems). The most common patient problems for an older patient with diverticulosis or diverticulitis include the following:

- Potential for constipation resulting from decreased fluid, bulk in the diet, or both
- Acute pain resulting from bowel obstruction
- Need for health education resulting from the lack of exposure to disease processes, prevention, and treatment

Generate solutions (planning). Expected outcomes for an older patient with diverticulosis or diverticulitis include the following:

1. The patient will experience fewer episodes of constipation, as evidenced by the establishment of a regular pattern of bowel activity.
2. The patient will verbalize pain relief and remain free from abdominal pain.
3. The patient will verbalize self-care practices to minimize symptoms of diverticulosis and prevent complications of diverticulitis.

Take actions (nursing interventions). Nursing management of an older patient with diverticulosis or diverticulitis includes the prevention and elimination of constipation and the initiation of dietary changes. This includes teaching the patient and family about the development of diverticula and the escalation to diverticulitis. In addition, teaching should include the importance of eating high-fiber foods, which include beans, whole grains, brown rice, fruits (e.g., apples, bananas, and pears), and vegetables (e.g., broccoli, carrots, corn, and squash). Patients should be encouraged to drink eight cups of fluids each day, unless contraindicated by cardiac status.

An older patient with diverticulitis needs pain management (with antispasmodics, analgesics, or other measures such as a heating pad), bowel rest (intravenous fluids if given NPO status), and hospitalization if acutely ill. The nurse should teach self-care practices that promote bowel regularity and the administration of stool softeners (such as docusate) as necessary. Preventing constipation is of the utmost importance.

Evaluate outcomes (evaluation). Evaluation includes documentation of the achievement of the expected outcomes, the prevention of complications, and the maintenance of regular bowel patterns and habits. Asking an older adult to verbalize how they have incorporated self-care practices into their daily lives is an effective way to ascertain whether the patient understands the disease and is able to take measures to prevent complications.

Colon Polyps

Colon polyps are growths on the mucous membranes of the GI tract. A polyp may be sessile (flat, broad, and attached directly to the intestinal wall) or pedunculated (attached to the wall by a thin stem). The most common type of polyp is termed an *adenomatous polyp* or *adenoma*. Adenomatous polyps may become cancerous. The larger the polyp, the more likely it is to be malignant (greater than 1 millimeter [mm]). Having numerous polyps increases the likelihood of developing cancer.

The most common nonmalignant polyps are of the hyperplastic type. These rarely grow large and never cause clinical symptoms. Many patients with polyps are asymptomatic. These growths are often discovered incidentally by sigmoidoscopy, colonoscopy, or barium enema. Occasionally, they may bleed, causing bright red blood in the feces.

Nursing Care Guidelines for the Patient with Polyps

Recognize cues (assessment). Assessment begins with a thorough history of any changes in an older adult's routine pattern of elimination and any symptoms such as blood in the stools or on the toilet paper. A detailed family history should be taken, and specific questions should be asked regarding polyps in family members. A physical examination may be unremarkable; however, guaiac-positive stools may be found on a rectal examination.

Analyze cues and prioritize hypotheses (patient problems). The most common patient problems for an older patient with polyps include the following:
- Need for health education resulting from a lack of exposure to the disease process, the importance of treatment, and follow-up
- Anxiety resulting from a threat to health status

Generate solutions (planning). Expected outcomes for an older patient with polyps include the following:
1. The patient will verbalize knowledge of the disease process and potential outcomes.
2. The patient will obtain medical follow-up as suggested by the ACS or a healthcare provider.

Take actions (nursing interventions). Nursing management of an older patient with polyps includes education and reinforcement of the guidelines suggested by the ACS for the prevention and early detection of colorectal cancer. The teaching of a patient who is to undergo colonoscopy may need to include reinforcement of the importance of having the polyps removed. Reminders should be given to older patients regarding the time for a repeated screening sigmoidoscopy (according to their healthcare provider or ACS guidelines). Patients may also need to be reminded that, although polyps are often asymptomatic, they may bleed. The presence of any blood in the stool may indicate the need for a repeated sigmoidoscopy or colonoscopy.

Evaluate outcomes (evaluation). Evaluation includes documentation of the achievement of the expected outcomes and the prevention of complications such as invasive colorectal cancer.

Hemorrhoids

Hemorrhoids are dilations of the veins in the mucous membrane inside the rectum or near the anal opening. These dilations are common and develop in susceptible people because of the increased pressure on the veins in the pelvic and rectal areas. Patients may be predisposed because of diarrhea or constipation, obesity, pregnancy, liver disease, prolonged sitting, pelvic tumors, and anal intercourse.

Internal hemorrhoids may cause bleeding with defecation. The dilated venous sacs may protrude into the anal canal, where they become exposed and result in pain; thrombus, ulcerations, and bleeding then develop. External hemorrhoids produce varying degrees of pain, as well as pressure, itching, irritation, and a palpable mass. Bleeding occurs only if the external hemorrhoid is injured or ulcerated. Usually, blood loss is insignificant; however, with persistent bleeding, anemia from a chronic disease may develop.

Nursing Care Guidelines for the Patient with Hemorrhoids

Recognize cues (assessment). Assessment begins with an older patient's history of constipation and symptoms of rectal pain or blood in the stools or on toilet paper. The physical examination may be unremarkable except for a painful anus and rectum—painful to the point where a thorough examination may be difficult. However, a prolapsed hemorrhoid may be detected and should be assessed for swelling, thrombosis, and ischemia. Guaiac-positive stools may be found.

Analyze cues and prioritize hypotheses (patient problems). The most common patient problems for an older patient with hemorrhoids include the following:
- Potential for constipation resulting from pain during defecation
- Acute pain in the anal and rectal areas resulting from swelling and inflammation
- Need for health education resulting from a lack of previous exposure to treatment and prevention

Generate solutions (planning). Expected outcomes for an older patient with hemorrhoids include the following:
1. The patient will experience fewer episodes of constipation.
2. The patient will establish a regular pattern of fecal elimination.
3. The patient will report a decrease in anal and rectal pain.
4. The patient will verbalize knowledge of self-care practices to minimize the occurrence of hemorrhoids.

Take actions (nursing interventions). Nursing management of an older patient with hemorrhoids includes the prevention and elimination of constipation. This includes a review of high-fiber, high-roughage foods, including indigestible fibers such as whole grains, legumes, and fresh fruits. Older patients should be encouraged to increase their fluid intake daily, particularly water. The nurse should encourage light exercise on a regular basis and review the importance of a regular toileting routine. OTC anesthetic ointments, creams, and sitz baths may be used for pain relief. Patients should be encouraged not to strain when defecating; this may worsen the hemorrhoids (Pullen, 2022). The nurse should emphasize that it is important to report any rectal bleeding to rule out the possibility of a more serious disorder.

Evaluate outcomes (evaluation). Evaluation includes documentation of achievement of the expected outcomes, prevention of complications, and maintenance of regular bowel patterns and habits.

DISORDERS OF THE ACCESSORY ORGANS

Cholelithiasis and Cholecystitis

Cholelithiasis is the presence or formation of gallstones in the gallbladder. When the gallbladder empties slowly or incorrectly, stasis occurs and encourages the aggregation of cholesterol crystals, eventually leading to stone formation. Gallstones are primarily composed of two main substances: cholesterol and calcium bilirubinate. The incidence of gallstones varies among racial groups (i.e., higher incidence in Hispanic and Native Americans) and countries; however, it is not known whether this is a result of environmental or genetic factors. Risk factors include obesity, female sex, multiparity, sedentary lifestyle, diabetes, drugs (e.g., cholesterol-lowering agents, estrogen, and antibiotics), and advancing age (Harding et al, 2020). Additionally, persons who have undergone bariatric surgery are at increased risk of developing gallstones.

Gallstones may be present for many years without signs and symptoms. The classic symptom is right upper quadrant pain, which may radiate to the right scapular area. The pain may be sharp, crampy, or dull and begins suddenly, often directly after a meal. The pain may last from 15 minutes to 6 hours, and nausea and vomiting may occur. These attacks of pain may occur as infrequently as once every few years or as often as every few days. Often, these episodes are precipitated by the ingestion of fatty foods. The symptoms of biliary pain are caused by an obstruction of the cystic or common bile duct, causing increased pressure and distention of the gallbladder. Often, the pain is so severe that it is mistaken for a heart attack. When the stones lodge along the biliary tract, they obstruct the flow of bile. This may result in jaundice because of the blockage of the flow of bilirubin. When the common bile duct becomes blocked, the bile cannot enter the duodenum, and the stool is clay colored because the fecal matter lacks pigment. In addition, obstruction of the common bile duct may cause biliary pain, jaundice, pancreatitis, or cholangitis (inflammation of the bile ducts).

Cholecystitis may be acute or chronic and is usually associated with gallstones or other obstructions of the biliary system. The inflammation in cholecystitis results in a thickening of the wall of the gallbladder. This can lead to ischemia, necrosis, gangrene, and possible perforation of the gallbladder itself, leading to peritonitis. In chronic cholecystitis, the walls become thickened and inefficient at emptying. This is a result of chronic chemical or mechanical irritation from stones exerting pressure on the mucosa or from biliary stasis.

Nursing Care Guidelines for the Patient with Cholelithiasis or Cholecystitis

Recognize cues (assessment). Assessment begins with a history of episodes of pain; the nurse should identify its location, quality, and duration. Associated symptoms include nausea and vomiting. Precipitating factors (e.g., large, fatty meals) and alleviating factors (e.g., pain relievers or changes of position) need to be documented. A physical examination may reveal a tender right upper quadrant and possibly jaundice.

Analyze cues and prioritize hypotheses (patient problems). The most common patient problems for an older patient with cholelithiasis or cholecystitis include the following:
- Acute pain resulting from gallbladder inflammation
- Need for health education resulting from a lack of previous exposure to the condition and treatment options
- Altered sleep pattern resulting from pain

Generate solutions (planning). Expected outcomes for an older patient with cholelithiasis or cholecystitis include the following:
1. The patient will experience pain relief.
2. The patient will verbalize knowledge of the disease process, prevention of complications, and treatment options available.
3. The patient will verbalize feeling rested after nighttime sleeping.

Take actions (nursing intervention). Nursing management of an older patient with cholelithiasis or cholecystitis includes providing pain relief and instructing the patient and family about the disease process, treatment options, and potential complications. Older patients with cholelithiasis need to know that foods high in fat may precipitate an attack of pain. They need to be aware of treatment options, including types of surgery, medical dissolution, and lithotripsy, as well as the advantages and disadvantages of each. The patient with cholecystitis may require hospitalization and may receive intravenous fluids and antibiotics. If managed at home, patients need to be on a clear liquid diet until pain is resolved and then slowly advance to a regular diet, avoiding fatty foods. Signs and symptoms of complications need to be reviewed with both patients and their families. Additional nursing care is based on an older patient's response to the initial treatment.

Evaluate outcomes (evaluation). Evaluation includes documentation of the achievement of expected outcomes, the prevention of complications, the prevention of infection, and the assessment of a patient's knowledge of the disease process. The nurse also evaluates the patient's response to food intake and monitors the patient's food choices to ensure dietary adherence.

Pancreatitis

Pancreatitis is an inflammation of the pancreas and often has no known cause. The disorder may be acute or chronic. In acute pancreatitis, the organ returns to normal after treatment. In chronic pancreatitis (CP), permanent and progressive destruction of the pancreas occurs, whereby the normal tissue is replaced by fibrous tissue.

Acute pancreatitis may be alcohol-induced or related to biliary tract disease; however, in nearly a third of cases, the cause is unknown. In older adults, acute pancreatitis is most often related to biliary tract disease. Other causes of acute pancreatitis include drugs, surgery, trauma, and metabolic disorders.

Acute pancreatitis is believed to be caused by the activation of pancreatic enzymes, which may cause autodigestion of the pancreas; activation of the enzymes is thought to result from reflux of bile into the pancreatic duct, obstruction of the pancreatic duct, ischemia, anorexia, trauma, and toxins.

The most common cause of CP in the United States is alcohol consumption. However, CP in the elderly is less frequently caused by alcohol (Hirth et al, 2019). Other causes include obstruction caused by gallstones, tumors, trauma, and systemic diseases such as lupus erythematosus, autoimmune pancreatitis, and cystic fibrosis (Harding et al, 2020). Additional factors in the development of CP include hereditary pancreatitis, cystic fibrosis, elevated triglycerides, cholelithiasis, and drugs.

Symptoms include severe abdominal pain in the epigastric to the right upper quadrant area, occasionally radiating through to the back. Pain is usually more intense in the supine position, and the patient often remains in a flexed position to relieve pain. Nausea, vomiting, abdominal distention, and fever are common. In CP, the pain may be continuous and accompanied by weakness and jaundice. In addition, in CP, the stools often become bulky, fatty, and foul-smelling; weight loss may occur because of malabsorption. Glucose intolerance is a late sign of CP. The development of easily identifiable CP may take years. Clinical occurrences, such as pseudocysts, pain, endocrine insufficiency, and other complications, are more prevalent in individuals over the age of 60 (Hirth et al, 2019). Calcification of the pancreas may take decades to develop, and diabetes (glucose intolerance) and steatorrhea may only develop after 10–20 years of disease progression (Forsmark, 2008).

Nursing Care Guidelines for the Patient with Pancreatitis

Recognize cues (assessment). Assessment begins with an older patient's history of precipitating factors such as alcohol use disorder or the presence of gallstones. Symptoms of abdominal pain, anorexia, nausea, and vomiting need to be assessed in detail. The patient may be in tremendous pain and unable to answer, so reliance on information from a family member may be necessary. Depending on the patient's pain, a physical examination may be difficult.

Analyze cues and prioritize hypotheses (patient problems). The most common patient problems for an older patient with pancreatitis include the following:
- Dehydration resulting from nausea or vomiting; restricted oral intake
- Acute pain resulting from obstruction of the pancreatic tract
- Inadequate nutrition resulting from anorexia and vomiting

Generate solutions (planning). Expected outcomes for an older patient with pancreatitis include the following:
1. The patient will maintain adequate fluid volume and electrolyte balance.
2. The patient will obtain pain relief.
3. The patient will stabilize and maintain weight.
4. The patient will not experience complications.

Take actions (nursing interventions). Nursing management of an older patient with pancreatitis includes maintenance of fluid and electrolyte balance, establishment of pain relief measures, and prevention of complications. This includes monitoring intravenous therapy, vital signs, intake and output, serum electrolyte values, and weight. Pain management may be extremely difficult, especially for patients with CP. Often, the expertise of a pain consultant is necessary.

An important consideration in acute pancreatitis is the prevention of recurrence. When pancreatitis results from an alcohol use disorder, teaching should focus on the need to avoid alcohol consumption to prevent future acute episodes. Referrals and counseling may be needed. For the patient with pancreatitis resulting from biliary tract disease, information on maintaining a low-fat diet is important. Providing information and emotional support is important for patients who may need surgery.

Evaluate outcomes (evaluation). Evaluation includes documentation of achievement of expected outcomes, prevention of complications, prevention of recurrence (for acute pancreatitis), and maintenance of adequate nutrition and hydration. Older adults addicted to alcohol may go through withdrawal, requiring the nurse to carefully monitor and record patient responses to treatment for this secondary problem.

Hepatitis

Hepatitis is a general term referring to inflammation of the liver. It may be caused by a variety of factors, such as drugs, chemicals, and alcohol, but the most common cause is a viral infection. Although five major viruses (and possibly a sixth), as well as mononucleosis and cytomegalovirus, may act as the causative agents for hepatitis, hepatitis A, B, and C viruses are the most common causative agents in the United States.

Hepatitis A virus (HAV), a ribonucleic acid (RNA) virus, causes hepatitis A. The primary mode of transmission of this organism is the fecal–oral route, commonly through the ingestion of contaminated food or water. Risk groups for hepatitis A include institutional populations such as patients in daycare centers and travelers to endemic areas. The clinical disease tends to be mild and of short duration. There is no residual liver disease after recovery, and no indications of a chronic state are present. The rate of hepatitis A is decreasing in the United States, as routine vaccination is now given to all children, travelers to certain countries, and persons at risk for the disease (Harding et al, 2020).

Hepatitis B virus (HBV), a deoxyribonucleic acid (DNA) virus, causes hepatitis B. This virus is transmitted through blood and body fluids, and risk factors include intravenous drug use and sexual contact. It is considered a sexually transmitted disease (STD) by the CDC. Hepatitis B follows a more severe course compared with hepatitis A and has an increased risk for liver disease (e.g., cirrhosis and cancer). A 5%–10% incidence of a chronic state, defined as continuing to test positive for the viral antigen for 6 months or longer, is present. Affected individuals may be asymptomatic or have subclinical symptoms; however, they remain contagious as long as the antigen is present. Hepatitis D virus (HDV) is an obligate virus of HBV; this virus is spread by the same mechanisms as HBV and results in severe acute illness and life-threatening chronic liver disease.

Hepatitis C (HCV) is a virus that causes both acute and chronic infections, ranging in severity from mild to a serious life-long illness (World Health Organization [WHO], 2022). It is estimated that 2.4 million people in the United States have the virus, and most do not know they have it (U.S. Department of Health and Human Services, 2016). The clinical course of HCV is usually milder than that of hepatitis B, and the affected person may even be asymptomatic. Around 30% of infected individuals spontaneously clear the virus within 6 months without treatment. The remaining 70% will develop an HCV infection and will require treatment. Fifteen to thirty percent of individuals infected with HCV are at risk of developing cirrhosis within 20 years (WHO, 2022).

The pathophysiologic events leading to the liver inflammation seen in hepatitis are similar for all the viruses. Once the virus is introduced into the individual by its specific mode of transmission, it enters the circulation and seeks out hepatic tissue. The virus enters the cell and uses the host cell's DNA to

TABLE 19.2 Viral Hepatitis

	Hepatitis A Virus (HAV)	Hepatitis B Virus (HBV)	Hepatitis C Virus (HCV)
Transmission	Person-to-person through the fecal–oral route or consumption of contaminated food or water	Via blood, semen, or another body fluid; can happen through sexual contact; sharing needles, syringes, or other drug–injection equipment; or from mother to baby at birth	Most people become infected with the Hepatitis C virus by sharing needles or other equipment to inject drugs
Incubation period	May be spread without symptoms, 2–6 weeks after exposure	Spread: blood, semen, or other body fluid 6 weeks–6 months	20–90 days
Risk groups	Institutional populations, including daycare centers, and travelers to endemic areas	Intravenous drug use and sexual contact are considered by the CDC to be sexually transmitted disease	Recipients of blood or blood product transfusions, invasive medical procedures (e.g., injections and hemodialysis), injecting drug users, high-risk behaviors (e.g., anal sex without using a condom), and persons with HIV
Course of disease	Self-limited disease that does not result in chronic infection	The course is more severe than with hepatitis A	Either asymptomatic or have a mild clinical illness
	Symptomatic usually less than 2 months	70% of adults and children older than 5 years will develop symptoms	
Chronic state	No	Approximately 90% of infected infants become chronically infected, compared with 2%–6% of adults	Data suggests that spontaneous clearance might be as high as 46%. Chronic infection occurs in persons who do not spontaneously clear the virus. Approximately 5% to 25% of persons with chronic hepatitis C will develop cirrhosis over 10–20 years.
Prevention/vaccination	Yes	Yes	No
	2 injections, 6 months apart	3–4 shots over a 6-month period	
Liver cancer risk	None	Yes (and also other liver diseases like cirrhosis)	Yes

NOTE: HDV is uncommon in the United States. Hepatitis D occurs only among people infected with the hepatitis B virus because HDV is an incomplete virus that requires the helper function of HBV to replicate. HDV can be an acute, short-term infection or a long-term, chronic infection. Hepatitis D is transmitted through percutaneous or mucosal contact with infectious blood and can be acquired either as a coinfection with HBV or as a superinfection in people with HBV infection. There is no vaccine for hepatitis D, but it can be prevented in persons who are not already HBV-infected by hepatitis B vaccination. Hepatitis E virus (HEV) is a self-limited disease that does not result in chronic infection. Although rare in the United States, hepatitis E is common in many parts of the world. It is transmitted through the ingestion of fecal matter, even in microscopic amounts, and is usually associated with contaminated water supplies in countries with poor sanitation. There is currently no FDA-approved vaccine for hepatitis E.

Data from Schillie, S., Wester, C., Osborne, M., Wesolowski, L., & Ryerson, A. B. (2020). CDC recommendations for Hepatitis C screening among adults-United States, 2020. *MMWR Recommendations and Reports*, *69*(2), 1–17; American Cancer Society. (2020). *American Cancer Society Guidelines for Colorectal Cancer Screening*. Retrieved from https://www.cancer.org/cancer/colon-rectal-cancer/detection-diagnosis-staging/acs-recommendations.html.

reproduce itself. This may directly injure or kill the hepatocyte, which is believed to be the primary cause of cell damage in hepatitis A, or the responding immunologic cells may harm the liver cell in the process of destroying the virus, which is the probable pathologic cause in hepatitis B and C (Table 19.2).

There are also viral hepatitis types D, E, and G. HDV is a small virus that requires concomitant infection with HBV to survive. HDV cannot survive on its own because it requires HBV to make a surface antigen to enable it to infect liver cells. HDV is spread by shared needles among persons with substance use disorders, contaminated blood, and sexual contact. Individuals who already have chronic HBV infection can acquire HDV infection at the same time as they acquire the HBV infection or later. Those with chronic hepatitis due to HBV and HDV develop cirrhosis rapidly. The combination of HDV and HBV is very difficult to treat (Davis, 2022).

Hepatitis E virus (HEV) is like HAV in terms of disease and occurs mainly in Asia, where it is transmitted by contaminated water. Hepatitis G virus (HGV, also termed GBV-C) was recently discovered and resembles HCV, but, more closely, the flaviviruses; the virus and its effects are under investigation, and its role in causing disease in humans is unclear (Davis, 2022).

The clinical picture of hepatitis is essentially the same for diseases caused by all the viruses, but the overall course is shorter for hepatitis A. Typically, the illness is divided into three phases. In the *prodromal phase*, patients have generalized symptoms of malaise, fatigue, possible right upper quadrant pain, nausea and vomiting, anorexia, and a low-grade fever. Patients often think they have the flu, or the infected individuals do not recall experiencing the symptoms as they are very mild. The second phase, in which jaundice and dark urine appear, is termed the *icteric phase*. Sometimes, jaundice does not occur. Patients may start to feel better during this phase. Finally, in the *convalescent phase*, jaundice and other symptoms disappear, and patients feel fully recovered. It is important that patients understand that it will take 3–6 months for the liver to return to its normal functioning status. Care should be taken regarding rest and drug and alcohol consumption during this phase; a relapse is possible.

Nursing Care Guidelines for the Patient with Hepatitis

Recognize cues (assessment). Assessment begins by reviewing with the patient any possible exposure to a hepatitis virus. The nurse should ask questions about recent travel, food intake, blood transfusions, and close contact with persons who may have had hepatitis in the past. Assess clinical manifestations such as jaundice, right-upper-quadrant tenderness, fatigue, and malaise. The nurse should question the patient about changes in functional status; for example, whether the patient's activity level and ability to perform activities of daily living (ADLs) have decreased from baseline levels. The nurse should also review nutritional intake and assess for anorexia, as well as question changes in the way clothes fit and ask if family and friends have noticed weight loss in the patient. Palpation of the abdomen may reveal an enlarged liver.

Analyze cues and prioritize hypotheses (patient problems). Patient problems for an older patient with hepatitis include the following:
- Inadequate health maintenance resulting from deficient knowledge about hepatitis, the treatment regimen, and the prevention of spreading the virus
- Reduced stamina resulting from generalized weakness and fatigue
- Inadequate nutrition resulting from anorexia, nausea, and liver dysfunction
- Inadequate family therapeutic management resulting from a lack of knowledge

Generate solutions (planning). Expected outcomes for an older patient with hepatitis include the following:
1. The patient will verbalize the causes of hepatitis, the treatment plan, and mechanisms to prevent spreading the virus to others.
2. The patient will participate in ADLs without experiencing fatigue.
3. The patient will consume a well-balanced, high-calorie diet, as evidenced by a food diary.
4. The patient will demonstrate self-care activities as much as possible within their physical limitations.

Take actions (nursing interventions). The nurse must teach patients and their significant others about the spread of hepatitis and mechanisms for prevention. Depending on the specific mode of transmission of the virus, the nurse should also discuss hygiene practices in the home, especially with regard to feces; instruct males and females on condom use; discuss proper disposal of needles; instruct the patient and family on the purchase and preparation of certain foods, such as shellfish (i.e., eating raw shellfish should be avoided); and instruct the patient to avoid alcohol and drugs containing acetaminophen.

Frequent rest periods are necessary. The nurse should explain that rest is an important treatment for hepatitis, and activities such as visiting, cooking, and housework need to be curtailed. A patient with hepatitis best tolerates a high-carbohydrate, low-fat diet. Several small feedings throughout the day will help alleviate the effects of anorexia. Fluid intake should increase to 2,000–3,000 mL/day unless contraindicated by cardiovascular status.

The cause of jaundice should be explained, and the patient should be warned that changes in the colors of urine, skin, and sclera may be seen; this is a temporary condition that will resolve once the acute phase of illness has run its course.

If the jaundice causes pruritus (common in chronic HCV), the nurse should discuss the use of nonalcohol-based lotions, soft clothes and linens, and tepid baths using as little mild soap as possible. The nurse should instruct patients and caregivers about keeping patients' fingernails short to avoid injury from scratching.

Evaluate outcomes (evaluation). Evaluation includes documentation of the achievement of the expected outcomes, coupled with the patient's successful self-management of the disease. Careful attention to an older adult's food intake, weight trends, and activity tolerance is crucial.

Cirrhosis Secondary to Alcohol Use Disorder

Cirrhosis is a general term referring to a chronic disorder of the liver in which permanent, irreversible destruction of the hepatocytes and the normal architecture of the organ occurs. The causes of this disease are many and include fatty liver, hepatitis, cystic fibrosis, and primary biliary cirrhosis; however, about 80% of cases in the United States are attributed to alcohol use disorder.

The progressive loss of functioning liver tissue is manifested by the appearance of general signs and symptoms of liver failure; over time, other manifestations of declining liver function appear (Fig. 19.7). Early signs and symptoms of liver failure from cirrhosis are like those of hepatitis. The patient experiences fatigue, malaise, anorexia, changes in fecal elimination pattern (either diarrhea or constipation), nausea and vomiting, and dull, heavy pain in the right upper quadrant. Later symptoms include jaundice and edema in peripheral sites. Ultimately, serious complications such as bleeding, portal hypertension, ascites, and encephalopathy develop. Bleeding tendencies are the result of declining clotting and coagulation factors. One of the many functions of the liver is the production of clotting factors V, VII, IX, and X, as well as the production of fibrinogen and prothrombin. Decreased amounts of these proteins result in a bleeding diathesis in any patient with advanced liver disease, regardless of the cause.

Ascites is the accumulation of serous fluid in the abdominal cavity. It is the result of several factors relating to poor liver function, but the most important of these is the decreased production of albumin by the liver. Insufficient amounts of this major plasma protein in the blood cause the escape of plasma fluid into the abdominal space. Another factor is the increased venous pressure from portal hypertension, which forces the fluid out of the vessel. The most serious effect of ascites is respiratory compromise, which occurs when the diaphragm is pushed upward by increasing abdominal fluid, thus decreasing thoracic space for pulmonary excursion.

Portal hypertension is an increase in pressure in the portal vein and its feeders because of liver congestion or obstruction.

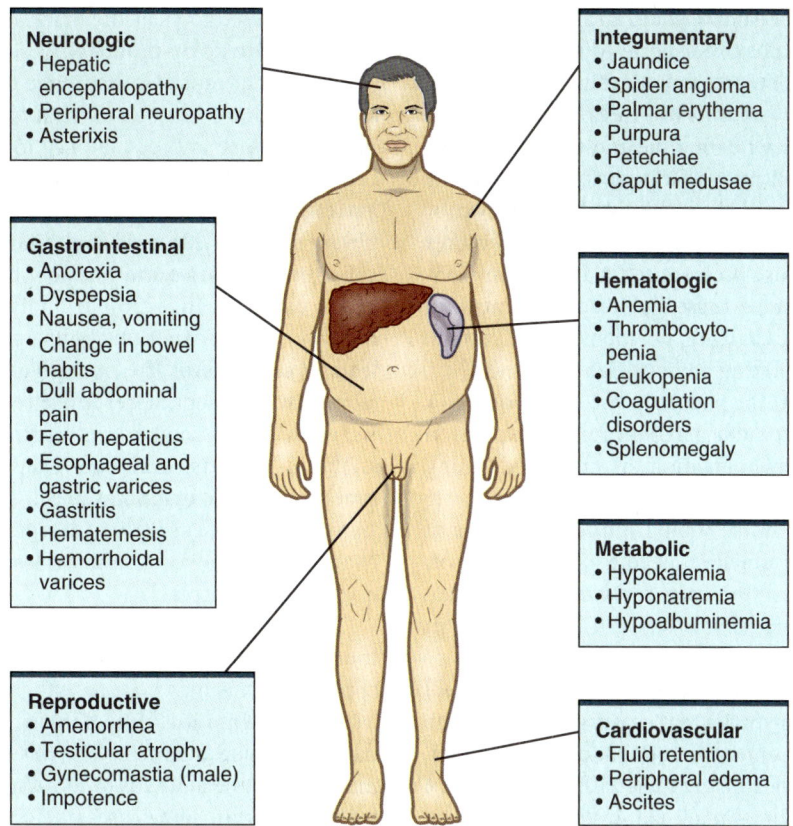

Fig. 19.7 Systemic clinical manifestations of liver cirrhosis. (Modified from Harding, M. M., Kwong, J., Roberts, D., Hagler, D., & Reinisch, C. [2020]. *Lewis's medical-surgical nursing: Assessment and management of clinical problems* [11th ed.]. St. Louis, MO: Elsevier.)

In addition to contributing to the development of ascites, portal hypertension and the backflow of venous blood cause severe problems with hemorrhoids, splenomegaly, and esophageal varices. The effect of portal hypertension on the esophageal veins is the most dangerous because these vessels are fragile and susceptible to rupture with any increase in intraabdominal pressure. Patients who bleed from esophageal varices are gravely ill. One-third of deaths from cirrhosis are from esophageal varices.

A late-stage event in long-term liver disease is the development of *encephalopathy*, which is caused by the diseased liver's inability to carry out its function of detoxifying metabolic by-products. One of the most critical of these is ammonia, an end-product of protein metabolism. Although it is not clear whether the ammonia is directly toxic to the brain or interferes with glucose uptake, decreasing blood ammonia levels is correlated with successful treatment. A patient with high ammonia levels will begin to exhibit changes in behavior, irrationality, agitation, combativeness, and muscle tremors (asterixis). If the condition remains untreated, hepatic coma ensues and has a mortality rate of 90%.

Nursing Care Guidelines for the Patient with Cirrhosis

Recognize cues (assessment). Assessment of the patient with cirrhosis involves a careful history of the onset and duration of symptoms. The nurse should question the patient about changes in the color of the stool, rectal bleeding, and bloody emesis. A thorough physical assessment of all body systems, especially the skin and abdomen, and respiratory and mental status are indicated. Assessment of nutritional status is also important.

Analyze cues and prioritize hypotheses (patient problems). Patient problems for an older patient with cirrhosis include the following:

- Potential for reduced skin integrity resulting from pruritus, edema, and ascites
- Inadequate breathing pattern resulting from increased pressure on the diaphragm secondary to ascites
- Potential for injury resulting from decreased clotting factors
- Acute confusion resulting from increased serum ammonia levels
- Inadequate nutrition resulting from anorexia, nausea, and vomiting
- Potential for decreased self-esteem resulting from guilt about damage done to oneself and significant others

Generate solutions (planning). Expected outcomes for an older patient with alcoholic cirrhosis include the following:

1. The patient will be free from skin breakdown.
2. The patient will demonstrate the ability to pace activity and ADLs within current ventilatory function.
3. The patient will remain free from injuries and bleeding.
4. The patient will demonstrate resolution of cerebral dysfunction, as evidenced by no injury to self or others; achieve an appropriate sleep-wake pattern; communicate meaningfully with others; and be oriented to time, person, and place.

5. The patient will maintain or gain weight to an appropriate level.
6. The patient will identify positive aspects of themselves and express an optimistic outlook regarding relationships.

Take actions (nursing interventions). Interventions for an older adult with cirrhosis may be multiple and complex; a major focus is preventing complications. Skin care is a priority. The nurse should inspect the skin daily for signs of breakdown or redness. The skin should be kept clean and dry, especially after toileting. The nurse should use pressure relief devices on a patient's bed and chair. The nurse must also teach patients and caregivers the importance of changing positions every 2 hours. A bed trapeze may facilitate lifting and position changes.

The nurse should position the patient in the semi-Fowler or high-Fowler positions to promote maximum chest expansion and maintain oxygen supplementation as indicated. Lung sounds must be assessed at least daily.

To prevent bleeding, the nurse should limit the number of venipunctures and use the smallest needle possible. A soft toothbrush or oral swabs may be used for mouth care. Male patients should use an electric razor to shave. The environment should be kept free of clutter.

Orientation and psychomotor function should be assessed. The nurse should reorient the patient on a consistent basis. The number of new people who enter the room should be limited. Mouth care should be provided before meals. The environment should be conducive to eating. Small, bland feedings may be given, especially if the patient complains of nausea. The nurse should consider the patient's food preferences and remember that a high-carbohydrate, no-protein, or low-protein, low-fat diet will be ordered. The nurse should also remember that fruit juices are often well tolerated by individuals with anorexia.

The nurse should encourage the patient to discuss feelings about self-esteem while always maintaining a judgment-free environment. The nurse should also reinforce positive abilities and traits and help the patient identify negative automatic behaviors. Resources such as pastoral care may be used, as indicated.

Evaluate outcomes (evaluation). Evaluation includes documentation of the achievement of the expected outcomes and the prevention or early detection of complications. Given the long-term nature of the condition, the nursing care plan should be reviewed and updated on a regular basis.

Drug-Induced Hepatitis

Throughout the world, the older population has increased over the years, and as a result, the rate of polypharmacy and drug-induced liver injury (DILI) has increased as well (Pedraza et al, 2021). Because one of the major functions of the liver is the metabolism and detoxification of chemicals, including drugs, this organ is subject to potential damage from these substances. Hepatic injury may result from direct toxicity, the conversion of a drug to a toxic metabolite, or immune mechanisms responding to the presence of a "foreign" invader.

Some agents cause liver cell damage in all individuals at a predictable dose level. A common example of a dose-related toxic drug is acetaminophen. With an overdose of these agents, the normal metabolic pathway is exhausted, and alternative means are used to clear the drug from the body. These mechanisms yield toxic by-products.

Drugs that cause liver damage in an unpredictable manner are said to have *idiosyncratic toxicity*. These reactions are unrelated to dose and occur only in a small percentage of susceptible individuals. Idiosyncratic toxicity is manifested in a variety of ways. A massive hepatocellular injury may occur. Drugs such as isoniazid, halothane, and benoxaprofen may cause liver necrosis and possibly hepatic failure, especially in older patients. Ingestion of poisonous mushrooms causes massive cell destruction. Substances such as vinyl chloride lead to sclerosis of the portal venules and portal hypertension. Another hepatic response to toxic exposure is *cholestasis*, an arrest or cessation of normal bile flow. Drugs such as anabolic steroids, oral contraceptives, phenothiazines, and oral antidiabetic drugs cause this response. Other manifestations of liver disease from idiosyncratic toxicity include fatty changes in the liver and mass lesions such as liver cell adenoma and hyperplasia.

The clinical manifestations of drug-induced hepatitis are like those of viral hepatitis. At first, GI and influenza-like symptoms appear. Patients may be seen with jaundice, especially with cholestatic presentation. Hepatomegaly and other signs of liver damage may also appear. The onset of symptoms may be immediate or several weeks to months after exposure to the hepatotoxic agent. In some cases, the onset of liver failure is abrupt, and the clinical course lasts only a few days, with outcomes ranging from resolution to organ transplantation to death.

Nursing Care Guidelines for the Patient with Drug-Induced Hepatitis

Recognize cues (assessment). In addition to the previously discussed assessments related to liver disease, it is essential that information be obtained regarding the exact name of the ingested substance, the dosage and amount taken, and the length of time since ingestion occurred. A history of emesis after ingestion is also pertinent.

Analyze cues and prioritize hypotheses (patient problems). The most common patient problems for an older patient with drug-induced hepatitis include the following:
- Need for health education resulting from a lack of exposure to disease causes, treatment regimens, and outcomes
- Potential for injury resulting from end-stage liver failure
- Need for health education resulting from drugs and interactions

Generate solutions (planning). Expected outcomes for an older patient with drug-induced hepatitis include the following:
1. The patient will verbalize their understanding of the disease process and interventions.
2. The patient will not experience life-threatening complications from liver failure.
3. The patient will verbalize their understanding of current drugs and their interactions.

Take actions (nursing interventions). Nasogastric suction, if required, needs to be explained and performed in a calm manner. The nurse should also discuss the adverse effects of certain drugs with the patient and provide written material as a reminder to avoid these drugs. The nurse must monitor the patient carefully for signs and symptoms of liver failure, percuss liver size, assess the skin and sclera of the eyes, and monitor the level of consciousness.

Interventions for older adults presenting with complications of liver failure are discussed in the section on alcoholic cirrhosis.

Evaluate outcomes (evaluation). Evaluation includes documentation of the achievement of the expected outcomes and the prevention of complications.

GI CANCERS

Cancers of the GI system account for more than 25% of cancer deaths in the United States each year. Cancers of the GI tract are one of the top three causes of cancer deaths in both males and females. Most tumors of the GI tract are adenocarcinomas, except for tumors of the esophagus and anus, where squamous cell malignancies predominate. Although the GI tract begins at the oral cavity and ends at the anus, oral cancer is considered along with head and neck cancers. Discussion of GI cancer will begin with cancer of the esophagus.

Esophageal Cancer

Early esophageal cancer usually remains asymptomatic. Medical evaluation is typically sought when symptoms such as dysphagia, choking when eating, hoarseness, heartburn, unintentional weight loss, and fatigue develop. Many people with esophageal cancer attribute these signs and symptoms to some of the more common disorders that affect older adults and fail to seek treatment. Because of this fact, patients with esophageal cancer have a 5-year survival rate of about 20%.

Risk factors for the development of adenocarcinoma include obesity, GERD, and a history of Barrett esophagus; for squamous cell carcinoma, risk factors include heavy alcohol consumption, cigarette smoking, a diet low in fruits and vegetables, and infection with the human papilloma virus (HPV). Additionally, those older than 55, males, and African Americans are at a higher risk of developing esophageal cancer.

The two main forms of esophageal cancer are adenocarcinoma and squamous cell carcinoma. Adenocarcinoma is the most prevalent form in the United States, most often affecting older White males. It typically develops at the distal portion of the esophagus. Worldwide, squamous cell carcinoma is the most common, affecting the middle of the esophagus. The tumor often metastasizes to the lungs, the liver, and the CNS.

Persons with a known Barrett esophagus are urged to seek screening for esophageal cancer. The proximity of the tumor to the aorta and the trachea, in addition to the potential for metastasis, results in a generally poor prognosis. The natural history of the disease includes esophageal obstruction, coughing, hiccups, bleeding, malnutrition, cachexia, pneumonia, and death.

Nursing Care Guidelines for the Patient with Esophageal Cancer

Recognize cues (assessment). Assessment begins with an accurate history that focuses on risk factors for esophageal cancer. A review of the systems may reveal symptoms of dysphagia, eating difficulties, and aspiration. A physical examination will probably reveal a few findings definitive of the diagnosis. However, in advanced disease, the nurse may find palpable lymph nodes and perhaps organ enlargement resulting from metastasis. Other findings include significant and recent weight loss and substernal epigastric pain radiating to the neck, jaws, ears, and shoulder (Harding et al, 2020).

Analyze cues and prioritize hypotheses (patient problems). Patient problems for an older patient with esophageal cancer include the following:

- Inadequate nutrition resulting from inadequate intake of nutrients in the diet because of dysphagia
- Potential for aspiration
- Fear resulting from an uncertain prognosis, possible disfigurement, and loss of ability to eat

Generate solutions (planning). Expected outcomes for an older patient with esophageal cancer include the following:

1. The patient will initially stabilize their weight and then achieve an individually determined weight gain.
2. The patient will remain free from aspiration.
3. The patient will verbalize fears related to the diagnosis and prognosis.

The medical treatments of radiotherapy, chemotherapy, and surgery will require additional, specific nursing interventions. The nurse should include the older adult and family in planning all aspects of nursing care related to anyone or a combination of these modalities.

Take actions (nursing interventions). Nursing management of an older patient with esophageal cancer includes maintenance of hydration and nutritional status, prevention of aspiration, maintenance of comfort, and provision of emotional support. Optimizing nutritional status and preventing further weight loss is accomplished with small, frequent feedings; high-protein, high-calorie foods; supplements such as Ensure; and tube feedings, if necessary. Nursing care to prevent aspiration focuses on the assessment of respiratory status, the assessment of difficulty with eating and drinking, and proper positioning during and after eating. The risk of aspiration increases in older adults when the bed is kept in a horizontal position.

The nurse's role in the prevention and early detection of esophageal cancer may lead to early identification and perhaps an improved prognosis for older patients. Persons with risk factors for esophageal cancer should be instructed on means to reduce or eliminate these factors. Counseling on the need for frequent medical follow-up, proper nutrition, and the elimination of smoking and alcohol consumption is important for prevention. Older patients with frequent upper GI complaints should be advised to seek medical attention immediately.

Evaluate outcomes (evaluation). Evaluation includes documentation of achievement of the expected outcomes, prevention of aspiration, and maintenance of adequate nutrition (see Nursing Care Plan: Esophageal Cancer).

NURSING CARE PLAN

Esophageal Cancer

Clinical Situation

Mr. B, a 66-year-old retired salesman, has come to the outpatient clinic with a complaint of dysphagia. Within the past 4 months, he has had pain and difficulty swallowing solid food; he therefore proceeded to eat soft, then liquid foods. However, within the past month, the problem has progressed to difficulty swallowing even liquids. He reported one episode of nocturnal regurgitation this past week. Other symptoms include a loss of 20 pounds (lb) over the past 6 months, fatigue, and a dull backache. Mr. B admits that he still smokes but has cut down from two packs to one pack a day. In addition, he admits to ingestion of beer and hard liquor, although he has cut down in amount and frequency over the past few years since his retirement.

His medical history is otherwise unremarkable. He lives alone but near his daughter, who convinced him to come to the clinic when he did not eat anything at her recent Easter dinner.

Physical examination reveals a thin, older male with a weight of 140 lb, a temperature of 98°F (36.6°C), a pulse of 80 beats per minute (beats/min), a respiratory rate of 18 breaths/min, and a blood pressure of 120/82 mm Hg. Inspection of his oropharynx reveals no abnormalities except for poor dentition. The examination of his abdomen and rectal area was also unremarkable. Laboratory values reveal iron deficiency anemia, but initial screening is otherwise unremarkable. He is scheduled for an endoscopy the next day. He returns to the clinic 1 week later to get his results, and his diagnosis is esophageal cancer. He is scheduled for radiotherapy and possibly surgery once the tumor has shrunk in size.

Analyze Cues and Prioritize Hypotheses (Patient Problems)

- Inadequate nutrition resulting from inadequate intake of nutrients secondary to dysphagia
- Decreased ability to swallow resulting from mechanical obstruction secondary to the tumor
- Fear resulting from uncertain prognosis, possible disfigurement, and loss of ability to eat
- Potential for aspiration resulting from dysphagia

Generate Solutions (Planning)

- The patient will stabilize his weight.
- The patient will swallow safely without gagging or aspirating.
- The patient will maintain adequate nutrition and hydration.
- The patient and family will identify sources of fear and acquire knowledge to deal with them.

Take Actions (Nursing Interventions)

- Encourage small, frequent meals. Encourage the use of high-protein, high-calorie foods and the use of supplements such as Ensure. Refer to a dietitian, if necessary, for specific recommendations.
- Discuss the possibility of using tube feedings with the patient to supplement nutrients or as the sole means of delivering necessary nutrients.
- Arrange for a speech therapist consultation to provide instructions regarding swallowing.
- Instruct the patient and family regarding the need for upright positioning during and after eating.
- Instruct the patient and family to rotate the patient's head toward the affected side to facilitate swallowing.
- Provide rest periods before, during, and after feedings.
- Provide thick liquids first, adding thin liquids last; begin with cold liquids and progress to hotter ones.
- Instruct the patient to begin with pureed foods, progressing to soft ones, while taking small bites.
- Encourage the patient and family to verbalize their fears.
- Provide information to reduce distortions in perceptions.
- Encourage the patient and family to attend cancer support groups.
- Instruct the patient and family about impending treatments such as surgery and radiotherapy.
- Assess the patient's ability to eat and drink.
- Assess respiratory status before, during, and after eating.
- Monitor for signs of aspiration: dyspnea, coughing, wheezing, tachycardia, and an elevated temperature.
- Observe and record the color and character of the sputum.
- Instruct the patient and family to keep the patient's head elevated during and after eating or feeding.

Gastric Cancer

As with other forms of GI cancer, gastric cancer is insidious. Symptoms may be vague until the cancer has infiltrated and spread throughout the body, when the overt signs of cancer become evident. In addition, stomach cancer mimics other diseases, such as ulcers and gastritis, so misdiagnosis and self-medication for chronic "stomach problems" are common and may delay the diagnosis and treatment of stomach cancer.

Gastric cancer accounts for around 10,800 deaths in the United States each year. Asian Americans, Pacific Islanders, Hispanics, and Blacks have a higher incidence than non-Hispanic Whites. It occurs twice as often among males than females and mostly affects older people (Harding et al, 2020).

The cause is unknown, although the incidence is higher when gastric acid is low, as with chronic gastritis and pernicious anemia. Gastric cancer is also associated with environmental and genetic factors, including diet (e.g., diets high in salt, nitrate-preserved foods, and smoked foods, and diets low in fruits and vegetables), smoking, and heavy alcohol consumption. It may also be precipitated by polyps or degenerative changes in gastric ulcers, previous stomach surgery, or achlorhydria. Finally, occupational risks such as those faced by rubber and coal workers and those working in nickel refineries also play a role. A relationship exists between gastric cancer and infection with *H. pylori*.

Adenocarcinomas account for more than 90% of stomach cancers. Adenocarcinomas arise from the mucosal lining of the stomach. Additional types of stomach cancer are (1) lymphomas, (2) GI stromal tumors, (3) carcinoid tumors, and (4) rarely squamous cell carcinomas or small cell carcinomas. Adenocarcinomas may metastasize by extension and infiltration along the mucosa into the stomach wall and lymph nodes. The tumor may metastasize to the lung, bone, liver, spleen, pancreas, peritoneum, and esophagus. Once the tumor has spread outside of the stomach, a cure is not possible.

Because of its elusive nature, gastric cancer is usually well advanced when symptoms begin to appear. When they do manifest, they are vague and of variable duration. Because of this, people usually delay seeking medical attention for a few months after the initial onset of symptoms. Initially, the patient may complain of a vague, uneasy sense of fullness, indigestion, and distention after meals, which may be passed off as stomach upset. As the disease progresses, anorexia, nausea, and vomiting may develop and lead to weight loss. Other symptoms include dysphagia, back pain, weakness, fatigue, hematemesis, and a change in fecal elimination patterns. Unfortunately, definitive clinical signs occur mostly with advanced disease and include weight loss, pain, vomiting, anorexia, dysphagia, and a palpable abdominal mass. Prognosis is best for tumors in the lower stomach (antrum) and worse for tumors that occur higher in the stomach (fundus).

Nursing Care Guidelines for the Patient with Gastric Cancer

Recognize cues (assessment). Assessment begins with a thorough history and review of symptoms pertaining to the GI system, particularly symptoms that an older patient may not report unless asked. These include indigestion, discomfort after eating, nausea, anorexia, vomiting, or any chronic "stomach problem." In addition, the nurse should question older adults regarding changes in dietary or bowel patterns and habits, the use of prescription and OTC drugs, and the use of home remedies. A physical examination may reveal no obvious abnormalities except that, when advanced, the tumor may be palpable, especially through the thin skin and musculature of an older patient's abdomen. In addition, lymph nodes may be palpable when metastases have occurred.

Analyze cues and prioritize hypotheses (patient problems). The most common patient problems for an older patient with gastric cancer include the following:
- Anticipatory grieving resulting from a poor prognosis
- Inadequate nutrition resulting from gastric distress
- Acute pain resulting from gastric distress and discomfort

Generate solutions (planning). Expected outcomes for an older patient with gastric cancer include the following:
1. The patient will discuss thoughts and feelings related to the diagnosis with appropriate people.
2. The patient will use appropriate resources for support counseling.
3. The patient will maintain adequate nutrition, as evidenced by the stabilization and maintenance of weight and the consumption of a well-balanced, high-calorie diet.
4. The patient will effectively manage pain, as evidenced by the verbalization of comfort and pain relief after analgesic use.

Take actions (nursing interventions). Nursing management of an older patient with gastric cancer includes maintenance of hydration, nutrition, fluid and electrolyte balance, and the provision of emotional support to the individual and family. Many patients and their families feel guilty and negligent about the delay in seeking medical attention for the vague symptoms of gastric cancer. The nurse may support patients and families by dispelling misconceptions and offering a realistic sense of hope.

Nursing care should also focus on the prevention and early diagnosis of gastric cancer, including encouragement for all older patients with GI symptoms, however trivial, to seek medical attention. In addition, identifying those at risk and encouraging them to seek medical care for evaluation on a regular basis is also important.

Evaluate outcomes (evaluation). Evaluation includes documentation of achievement of the expected outcomes, prevention of malnutrition, maintenance of comfort, and continued family support. As the disease advances and the older patient becomes more debilitated, the focus of care will change, requiring the nurse to collaborate and coordinate with other healthcare team members regarding alternative care arrangements.

Colorectal Carcinoma

Cancer of the colon and rectum is the fourth leading cause of cancer in the United States and the second leading cause of cancer death. Forty-two percent of new diagnoses are in persons over the age of 65, and the probability of developing them increases with age. Females are at greater risk of developing the disease than males (Nee et al, 2020).

Although the cause of colorectal cancer is unknown, research has indicated that diet, environment, smoking, heavy alcohol use, obesity, sedentary lifestyle, and genetics all play important roles in the development of the disease, as does a personal history of colon polyps and inflammatory disease of the bowel. Colon cancer is more prevalent in the United States, probably because the typical American diet is low in fruits and vegetables and high in red meat. A diet high in fat and refined carbohydrates and low in roughage is considered a risk factor for colorectal cancer. Genetic studies also suggest an inheritable susceptibility to colorectal cancer. Individuals with first-degree relatives diagnosed with colorectal cancer have double the risk for the development of adenomatous polyps, which are considered precursors of carcinoma.

Adenocarcinoma accounts for 95% of the carcinomas of the colon. The tumors tend to grow slowly and may remain asymptomatic for a long time. Cancer of the rectum is manifested as bright red bleeding from the rectum, along with changes in the characteristics of the stool. Carcinomas in the sigmoid and descending colon tend to grow around the bowel, encircling it and leading to an obstruction. For these patients, a change in fecal elimination pattern is a common symptom. On the right side, a few symptoms are seen. If present, crampy abdominal pain may be difficult to pinpoint. Anemia may also be present.

The clinical manifestations of colorectal cancer depend on the location and extent of the tumor. Left-sided lesions often cause melena, diarrhea, constipation, and a feeling of retained stool. Right-sided tumors often cause weakness, malaise, and weight loss. Abdominal pain is rare with either type and may result from obstructions or nerve involvement. Obstruction is often the first sign of the disease. Often, if a mass is palpated on a physical examination or a routine rectal examination, the stool is guaiac positive. Although the duration of symptoms is not effective in predicting the degree of tumor advancement, the early diagnosis of cancer in asymptomatic persons has been shown to be related to improved chances of survival. Colorectal cancer in stages I, II, and III is considered curable; if the cancer does not return in 5 years after treatment, it is considered cured. Stage VI cancer is not considered curable. Should metastases occur, they are primarily to the liver and lymphatic system, although other sites include the brain, lungs, bones, and adrenal glands.

Colorectal cancers produce a wide variety of tumor antigens; the carcinoembryonic antigen (CEA) is the most well-known. The CEA level is used to gauge the effectiveness of therapy and may be useful at the time of diagnosis for prognostic value. In addition, it is used to monitor for recurrence. The current use of the CEA level in mass screening and detection is limited.

Nursing Care Guidelines for the Patient with Colorectal Cancer

Recognize cues (assessment). Assessment begins with an older patient's history of symptoms such as diarrhea, constipation, abdominal pain, blood in stools, or melena. Generalized symptoms may have been overlooked by an older patient; these include malaise, weight loss, weakness, and fatigue. Eliciting a family history of colorectal cancer, polyps, and any previous bowel surgeries is also important. Because of the potential for multiple losses with colorectal cancer, the nurse must also assess an older patient's coping skills and abilities. A physical examination may reveal a mass in the abdomen or guaiac-positive stools, or it may be unremarkable.

Analyze cues and prioritize hypotheses (patient problems). The most common patient problems for an older patient with colorectal cancer include the following:
- Inadequate nutrition resulting from anorexia
- Acute pain resulting from GI distress
- Distorted body image resulting from a colostomy

Generate solutions (planning). Expected outcomes for an older patient with colorectal cancer include the following:
1. The patient will maintain the recommended weight and adequate nutrition.
2. The patient will verbalize comfort after taking an analgesic.
3. The patient will verbalize acceptance of permanent or temporary body changes resulting from a colostomy.

Take actions (nursing interventions). The nursing management of an older patient with colorectal cancer depends on the stage of the disease and the treatment modalities necessary. In general, older patients are at risk for weight loss and malnutrition because of cancer and symptoms of vomiting or diarrhea. Eating small, frequent, high-calorie, high-protein meals should be encouraged. Allowing patients to eat some of their favorite foods on a regular basis may help maintain the recommended weight. The use of supplements such as Ensure or nighttime tube feedings may be necessary to maintain adequate nutrition. Not every patient with colorectal cancer complains of pain, but if present, pain can be managed with both pharmacologic and nonpharmacologic relief measures. If an older patient requires a colostomy either for treatment or as a palliative measure, the patient should be encouraged to verbalize and express feelings on a regular basis. Referral to a support group or counseling may be necessary. Having an older patient speak with or visit someone with a colostomy may help reduce the anxiety, concerns, and fears associated with it. If the colorectal cancer is completely resected, reminding and encouraging the older patient to have follow-up examinations and procedures to check for recurrence is of the utmost importance.

Nursing care should also focus on the prevention and early diagnosis of colorectal cancer. Nearly all colorectal cancers begin as polyps. Colonoscopy screening should begin at the age of 45 and is no longer recommended after the age of 85. When caught in the early stages, colorectal cancer is nearly always curable. Older adults with identified risk factors should be taught the importance of dietary changes (e.g., low-fat and high-fiber diets) and lifestyle changes (e.g., weight loss and increased physical activity).

Evaluate outcomes (evaluation). Evaluation includes documentation of the achievement of the expected outcomes and the prevention of complications. In addition, documentation of the patient's methods of coping with the lifestyle changes imposed by the various treatment modalities is essential.

Pancreatic Cancer

Pancreatic cancer accounts for approximately 3% of all cancers in the United States. Slightly more than 20% of affected individuals survive for 1 year after diagnosis, and the 5-year survival rate is less than 5%. Pancreatic cancer is lethal. The disease usually affects older adults; the incidence of pancreatic cancer is slightly higher in men than in females and higher in Blacks than in Whites. Additional risk factors include smoking, obesity, diabetes, cirrhosis, and a family history of pancreatic cancer. An increased risk attributable to environmental factors has been suggested because the incidence is higher in those exposed to industrial pollutants or who live in urban areas.

Cancer of the pancreas is primarily an adenocarcinoma. Although the head, body, or tail of the pancreas may be involved, it is primarily a disease of the exocrine portion of the gland. It arises in the head of the organ in 60%–70% of cases.

As tumor growth advances within the pancreas or on lymph nodes along the biliary tree, obstruction and compression of the common bile duct result. Eventually, the carcinoma may infiltrate the duodenum, stomach, transverse colon, spleen, kidney, and surrounding blood vessels. Invasion by the celiac nerve plexus accounts for the severe pain associated with cancer of the body or tail of the pancreas. Cancer of the pancreas grows rapidly, so at the time of diagnosis, the cancer has invaded locally or metastasized in 90% of individuals. Metastasis occurs through the bloodstream and by peritoneal seeding, frequently causing cancers in the lungs and bones.

Symptoms generally occur late in the course of the disease and are vague and insidious at onset. Manifestations of the disease differ according to the location of the tumor within the pancreas: pain and weight loss (tail of the pancreas), steatorrhea, weight loss, and jaundice (head of the pancreas). Nonspecific findings include anorexia, fatigue, digestive problems, blood clots, and diarrhea.

Nursing Care Guidelines for the Patient with Pancreatic Cancer

Recognize cues (assessment). Assessment begins with a history of symptoms and a review of possible risk factors for pancreatic cancer. An accurate assessment of the pain pattern is also important. The nurse should obtain a symptom analysis for any of the usual symptoms of nausea, vomiting, weight loss, weakness, and stool changes. A physical examination may be unremarkable.

Analyze cues and prioritize hypotheses (patient problems). Patient problems for an older patient with pancreatic cancer include the following:
- Acute pain resulting from abdominal discomfort
- Decreased ability to cope resulting from the diagnosis of terminal stage
- Decreased family's ability to cope resulting from the diagnosis of terminal stage

Generate solutions (planning). Expected outcomes for an older patient with pancreatic cancer include the following:
1. The patient will verbalize adequate relief of pain or the ability to cope with incompletely relieved pain.
2. The patient and family will verbalize concerns and feelings related to the diagnosis and prognosis.
3. The patient and family will demonstrate improved coping strategies, as evidenced by the incorporation of alternative coping behaviors and techniques in their interactions.

Take actions (nursing interventions). Nursing management for an older patient with pancreatic cancer focuses on the provision of pain relief and encouragement to verbalize feelings. Pain relief may require narcotics, and the patient and family may require teaching concerning their prolonged use. Other nonpharmacologic measures of pain relief (e.g., diversional activities, repositioning, meditation, and massage) need to be offered. The patient and their family may benefit from attending a support group for cancer patients. However, because of the poor prognosis, encouraging families to spend time with the older patient is also important. Assisting the patient and family in dealing with an imminent death may also be necessary.

Evaluate outcomes (evaluation). Evaluation includes documentation of the achievement of expected outcomes, prevention of complications, and provision of a comfortable environment.

Liver Cancer

The incidence of primary liver cancer (hepatocellular carcinoma) is less than 5% in the United States; however, in countries where hepatitis is endemic, the incidence of primary liver cancer is as high as almost 50%. In addition to hepatitis, risk factors for the development of hepatocellular carcinoma include alcoholic cirrhosis, hemochromatosis, fatty liver disease, obesity, diabetes, anabolic steroid use, and exposure to aflatoxins (poisons produced by molds). Additionally, hepatocellular carcinoma is more common in males, Asian Americans, and Pacific Islanders.

Metastatic cancer in the liver is named after the organ in which it began (e.g., metastatic breast cancer). In the case of metastatic disease, the common original sites are the lungs, breasts, kidneys, and other organs in the GI tract. Most often, multiple masses are present in the liver and spread throughout the organ via its vascular system. The diagnosis of liver metastasis is usually an indicator that the primary cancer is incurable. Weight loss is a common early finding in cases of metastatic liver disease. Signs and symptoms of liver involvement are the late signs of organ failure (e.g., ascites and portal hypertension); by the time of the diagnosis of metastasis, the overall prognosis is poor. The 5-year survival rate is 5%; if untreated, death will occur in 6–8 weeks after diagnosis. The cause of death is most often pneumonia, malnutrition, emboli, hepatic failure, or hemorrhage.

Nursing management for older patients with metastatic liver disease is similar to that for patients with alcoholic cirrhosis.

HOME CARE

1. Regularly monitor and assess the diagnosed GI disease or disorder for signs and symptoms indicating exacerbation or instability.
2. Weigh at regular intervals to monitor weight loss or gain; encourage homebound older adults to use nutritional supplements, if indicated.
3. Teach caregivers and homebound older adults appropriate dental hygiene practices.
4. Instruct caregivers and homebound older adults on reportable signs and symptoms related to the GI problem or disorder and when to report these symptoms to the home care nurse or healthcare provider.
5. Instruct caregivers and homebound older adults on the name, dose, frequency, side effects, and indications of both prescribed and OTC drugs used to treat the identified GI problem.
6. Instruct caregivers and homebound older adults about laboratory indices used to evaluate GI disturbances. Inform them of the results of any tests after the healthcare provider has been notified.
7. Assess and instruct older adults on the importance of maintaining hydration in the presence of GI disturbances.
8. Instruct caregivers and homebound older adults on all aspects of any treatments used to provide nutritional support in the absence of a functioning GI system (e.g., enteral nutrition, total parenteral nutrition, and formula supplements).

SUMMARY

Many older adults' health concerns are related to the GI system. Because these problems are often amenable to appropriate self-care practices, the nurse is responsible for teaching prevention and self-management strategies to these patients. However, the nurse must also teach older adults that GI-related symptoms should not be dismissed as part of the normal aging process; they should be reported so that an accurate determination can be made and timely interventions can be instituted.

KEY POINTS

- A decline in the normal function of the GI tract may occur with aging without any effect on physiologic processes.
- A significant decrease in liver function is not an inevitable outcome of aging, but because the incidence of chronic disease increases with advancing age, liver disorders are more common in older adults.
- Any weight loss or complaint of dysphagia, indigestion, heartburn, vomiting, change in appetite, or change in stool in an older patient warrants prompt evaluation by the healthcare provider.
- Primary and secondary prevention of problems in the GI tract should be part of the care of all older patients (e.g., colonoscopy and dental examination).
- Smoking, alcohol, obesity, and dietary factors are important risk factors for the development of GI cancer in older patients.
- Gastric ulcers have a higher incidence of becoming malignant compared with DUs.
- Intestinal ischemia should be included in the differential diagnosis of an older patient who has a history of cardiovascular disease and complains of abdominal pain.
- Guaiac-positive stools in an older adult should be considered pathologic until proven otherwise.
- Intestinal polyps and a positive family history of polyps are the main risk factors for the development of colorectal cancer.
- Although 60% of polyps and cancers are visualized with flexible sigmoidoscopy, a colonoscopy is necessary to detect any suspected cancers in the right colon.
- Although treatment of asymptomatic gallstones is not currently recommended, the rise in new therapeutic treatment options for cholecystitis should lead to a decline in morbidity and mortality previously associated with cholecystectomies in older adults.
- GI cancers present a common concern in that the symptoms are often overlooked or self-treated until the disease has become well established.
- Although the incidence of pancreatic cancer is increasing in the United States, treatment remains palliative.
- The high correlation between polypharmacy, increased drug consumption, and age makes the older person more prone to drug-induced liver disorders.

CLINICAL JUDGMENT EXERCISES

1. Your patient has smoked at least a pack of cigarettes a day for the past 33 years. At present, they are being treated for gastric ulcers. What relationship, if any, exists between age, smoking history, and a GI disorder?
2. Your 83-year-old neighbor confides in you that they have recently had bright red blood in their stools but think it is because of hemorrhoids. They are reluctant to see their healthcare provider because they do not want to be admitted to the hospital. What advice should you give? Why are bloody stools of particular importance to older adults? What would the plan of care be because they are older than 80 years?
3. A 65-year-old is admitted to the hospital with a diagnosis of cirrhosis of the liver. During the shift report, the primary care nurse states that the patient has been agitated and anxious but has not exhibited any manifestations of alcohol withdrawal. What assumptions did the nurse make? Are these assumptions valid? Explain.
4. Discuss the nursing care measures that would be similar for an older adult patient with cirrhosis and one with hepatitis.

REFERENCES

Centers for Disease Control and Prevention (CDC). (2021). *Older adult oral health*. Retrieved from https://www.cdc.gov/oralhealth/basics/adult-oral-health/adult_older.htm. Accessed October 3, 2022.

Çevik, K., Çetinkaya, A., Gökbel, K. Y., Menekse, B., Saza, S., & Tikiz, C. (2018). The effect of abdominal massage on constipation in the elderly residing in rest homes. *Gastroenterology Nursing, 41*(5), 396–402. doi:10.1097/SGA.0000000000000343.

Commisso, A., & Lim, F. (2019). Lifestyle modifications in adults and older adults with chronic gastroesophageal reflux disease (GERD). *Critical Care Nursing Quarterly, 42*(1), 64–74. doi:10.1097/CNQ.0000000000000239.

Davis, C. P. (2022). *Hepatitis (viral hepatitis, A, B, C, D, E, G)*. MedicineNet.com [website]. Retrieved from https://www.medicinenet.com/viral_hepatitis/article.htm. Accessed October 3, 2022.

Dumic, I., Nordin, T., Jecmenica, M., Stojkovic Lalosevic, M., Milosavljevic, T., & Milovanovic, T. (2019). Gastrointestinal tract disorders in older age. *Canadian Journal of Gastroenterology & Hepatology, 2019*, 6757524. doi:10.1155/2019/6757524.

Forsmark, C. E. (2008). The early diagnosis of chronic pancreatitis. *Clinical Gastroenterology and Hepatology, 6*(12), 1291–1293. doi:10.1016/j.cgh.2008.08.008.

Gad, M. M., & Fouda, S. M. (2020). Current perspectives and the future of Candida albicans-associated denture stomatitis treatment. *Dental and Medical Problems, 57*(1), 95–102. doi:10.17219/dmp/112861.

Harding, M. M., Kwong, J., Roberts, D., Hagler, D., & Reinisch, C. (2020). *Lewis's medical-surgical nursing: Assessment and management of clinical problems* (11th ed.). St. Louis, MO: Elsevier.

Hazara, R. (2020). Oral health in older adults. *British Journal of Community Nursing, 25*(8), 396–401. doi:10.12968/bjcn.2020.25.8.396.

Hirth, M., Härtel, N., Weiss, C., Hardt, P., Gubergrits, N., Ebert, M. P., & Schneider, A. (2019). Clinical course of chronic pancreatitis in elderly patients. *Digestion, 100*(3), 152–159. doi:10.1159/000494349.

Ignatavicius, D., Workman, L., Rebar, C., & Heimgartner, N. (2021). *Medical-surgical nursing: Concepts for interprofessional collaborative care* (10th ed.). St. Louis, MO: Elsevier.

Keith-Jennings, B., Llobrera, J., & Dean, S. (2019). Links of the Supplemental Nutrition Assistance Program with food insecurity, poverty, and health: Evidence and potential. *American Journal of Public Health, 109*(12), 1636–1640. doi:10.2105/AJPH.2019.305325.

Kernisan, L. (2018). *How to evaluate, prevent & manage constipation in aging*. Better Health While Aging [website]. Retrieved from https://betterhealthwhileaging.net/how-to-prevent-and-treat-constipation-aging/. Accessed October 3, 2022.

Kurin, M., & Fass, R. (2019). Management of gastroesophageal reflux disease in the elderly patient. *Drugs & Aging, 36*(12), 1073–1081. doi:10.1007/s40266-019-00708-2.

Nee, J., Chippendale, R. Z., & Feuerstein, J. D. (2020). Screening for colon cancer in older adults: Risks, benefits, and when to stop. *Mayo Clinic Proceedings, 95*(1), 184–196. doi:10.1016/j.mayocp.2019.02.021.

Pedraza, L., Laosa, O., Rodríguez-Mañas, L., Gutiérrez-Romero, D. F., Frías, J., Carnicero, J. A., et al. (2021). Drug induced liver injury in geriatric patients detected by a two-hospital prospective pharmacovigilance program: A comprehensive analysis using the Roussel Uclaf Causality Assessment Method. *Frontiers in Pharmacology, 11*, 600255. doi:10.3389/fphar.2020.600255.

Penner, R. M., & Fishman, M. B. (2021). Evaluation of the adult with abdominal pain. In A. D. Auerbach, M. D. Aronson, & J. Givens (Eds.), *UpToDate*. Waltham, MA: UpToDate. Retrieved from https://www.uptodate.com/contents/evaluation-of-the-adult-with-abdominal-pain. Accessed December 8, 2022.

Pont, L. G., Fisher, M., & Williams, K. (2019). Appropriate use of laxatives in the older person. *Drugs & Aging, 36*(11), 999–1005. doi:10.1007/s40266-019-00701-9.

Pullen, R., Jr. (2022). Hemorrhoidal disease: What nurses need to know. *Nursing, 52*(5), 19–24. doi:10.1097/01.NURSE.0000827128.26047.32.

Rodriguez, N. M., & Shackelford, K. (2022). Pernicious anemia. In *StatPearls* [Internet]. Treasure Island, FL: StatPearls Publishing.

Shane, M. A. S., & Moshiree, B. (2021). Esophageal and gastric motility disorders in the elderly. *Clinics in Geriatric Medicine, 37*(1), 1–16. doi:10.1016/j.cger.2020.08.002.

Shanmugam, H., Molina Molina, E., Di Palo, D. M., Faienza, M. F., Di Ciaula, A., Garruti, G., et al. (2020). Physical activity modulating lipid metabolism in gallbladder diseases. *Journal of Gastrointestinal and Liver Diseases, 29*(1), 99–110. doi:10.15403/jgld-544.

Shaw, C., & Wagg, A. (2021). Urinary and faecal incontinence in older adults. *Medicine, 49*(1), 44–50. doi:10.1016/j.mpmed.2020.10.012.

Strate, L. L., & Morris, A. M. (2019). Epidemiology, pathophysiology, and treatment of diverticulitis. *Gastroenterology, 156*(5), 1282–1298. doi:10.1053/j.gastro.2018.12.033.

U.S. Department of Health and Human Services. (2022). *Healthy People 2030*. Retrieved from https://health.gov/healthypeople. Accessed October 3, 2022.

U.S. Department of Health and Human Services. (2016). *Viral hepatitis in the United States: Data and trends*. Retrieved from https://www.hhs.gov/hepatitis/learn-about-viral-hepatitis/data-and-trends/index.html. Accessed October 3, 2022.

Vriesman, M. H., Koppen, I. J. N., Camilleri, M., Di Lorenzo, C., & Benninga, M. A. (2020). Management of functional constipation in children and adults. *Nature Reviews Gastroenterology & Hepatology, 17*(1), 21–39. doi:10.1038/s41575-019-0222-y.

Wolf, A. M. D., Fontham, E. T. H., Church, T. R., Flowers, C. R., Guerra, C. E., LaMonte, S. J., et al. (2018). Colorectal cancer screening for average-risk adults: 2018 guideline update from the American Cancer Society. *CA: A Cancer Journal for Clinicians, 68*(4), 250–281. Retrieved from https://acsjournals.onlinelibrary.wiley.com/doi/full/10.3322/caac.21457#caac21457-tbl-0001. Accessed July 27, 2023. doi:10.3322/caac.21457.

World Health Organization (WHO). (2022). *Hepatitis C*. Retrieved from https://www.who.int/news-room/fact-sheets/detail/hepatitis-c. Accessed October 3, 2022.

20

Urinary Function

Linda Bub, MSN, RN, GCNS-BC, NPD-BC

http://evolve.elsevier.com/Yeager/gerontologic/

LEARNING OBJECTIVES

On completion of this chapter, the reader will be able to:
1. Describe how aging affects normal bladder function.
2. List multiple causes of transient incontinence.
3. List multiple causes of established incontinence.
4. Discuss the role of functional and environmental assessment in the evaluation of urinary incontinence (UI).
5. Describe the behavioral interventions used to treat UI in cognitively intact patients.
6. Develop a patient teaching plan for a patient with incontinence.
7. Develop a caregiver teaching plan for a patient with functional UI resulting from dementia.
8. Describe the effects of normal aging on renal function.
9. Identify the possible causes of acute and chronic kidney disease (CKD).
10. Identify the treatment options for patients with bladder cancer.
11. List supportive services for the individual who has undergone a cystectomy.
12. Differentiate between benign prostatic hyperplasia (BPH) and prostate cancer.
13. Identify the treatment options for patients with prostate cancer.
14. Apply the nursing process to the care of older adults with select urinary system conditions.

WHAT WOULD YOU DO?

What would you do if you were faced with the following situations?
- Your 75-year-old patient denies any UI during their admission history, but you can smell a strong scent of urine. What do you do?
- Your patient, who is one day postoperation open reduction and internal fixation (ORIF) left femur, tells you and their doctor that they have too much pain when they get up. The doctor tells you to put a catheter in. What do you do?

UI is one of the most common health problems affecting older adults. UI is an involuntary loss of bladder control sufficient to interfere with daily and social activities. It is a significant cause of disability and dependency. Physical health, psychologic well-being, interpersonal relationships, and social functioning are adversely affected by incontinence. Individuals with UI are at increased risk for urinary tract infection (UTI), skin problems (e.g., infections and pressure injuries), sleep disturbances, sexual dysfunction, and falls; additionally, incontinence may also result in anxiety and depression (Batmani et al, 2022). Incontinence contributes to psychologic distress and social isolation. It is a cause of caregiver burden and plays a significant role in the decision to place older adults in long-term care facilities. The cost of UI is staggering; the combined estimate of direct and indirect costs is upward of $82.6 billion per year (projected) (Coyne et al, 2014).

AGE-RELATED CHANGES IN STRUCTURE AND FUNCTION

UI is not a normal part of aging. Normal age-related changes in the lower urinary tract (Fig. 20.1) increase an older adult's susceptibility to other insults in the lower urinary tract. As a result, these insults (e.g., drug side effects, UTIs, and conditions impairing mobility) are more likely to produce incontinence in older patients than in younger ones.

With age, bladder capacity decreases, the prevalence of involuntary bladder contractions increases, and more urine is produced at night. The reduction in bladder capacity and increased involuntary bladder contractions may lead to urgency and frequency. Many older adults find that they must empty their bladders more often than they did when they were younger. Increased urine formation at night leads to nocturia,

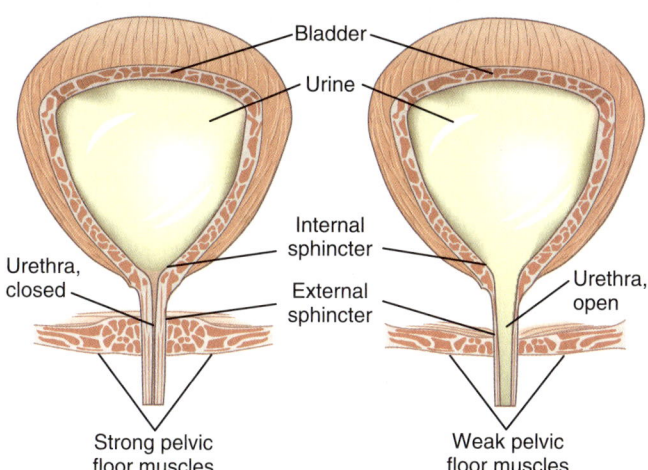

Fig. 20.1 Female urinary bladder with strong pelvic floor muscles *(left)* and weak pelvic floor muscles *(right)*. (From National Institute of Diabetes and Digestive and Kidney Diseases. [2016]. *Bladder control problems in women [urinary incontinence]*. Retrieved March 28, 2018, from https://www.niddk.nih.gov/health-information/urologic-diseases/bladder-control-problems-women.)

defined as the need to void one or more times during the sleeping period of the night (Oelke et al, 2017). Nocturia occurs frequently in older adults and is a major contributor to disruptions in normal sleep patterns and falls.

Changes occur in the urethra because of the aging process and decreased levels of estrogen after menopause. Thinning and increased friability of the urethral mucosa may contribute to urgency and frequency. A decrease in muscle tone and bulk may decrease urethral resistance. In addition to changes in the urethra, declining estrogen levels affect pelvic floor muscle tone and function.

As males age, the prevalence of BPH increases, with more than 50% experiencing BPH by the time they are over the age of 65. Enlargement of the prostate may interfere with bladder emptying and precipitate involuntary bladder contractions, resulting in incontinence or urinary retention.

PREVALENCE OF UI

UI is common in older adults, affecting approximately 60% of females in the United States (Patel et al, 2022). UI is more common among nursing facility residents, affecting 43%–80% of all nursing facility residents (John et al, 2016). UI is considered one of the geriatric syndromes, along with delirium, cognitive impairment, geriatric depression, fecal incontinence, and decreased mobility. UI is considered a geriatric syndrome that is associated with admissions to skilled nursing facilities (SNFs), with admission rates for UI ranging from 80%–95% (Bell et al, 2016).

Even though awareness of UI has increased in recent years due to commercials for incontinence products and drugs to treat UI (Milsom and Gyhagen, 2019), the number of older adult females who speak to their healthcare providers remains low, at just over 30%, and the older the female, the less likely they are to report it (Lane et al, 2021). Research studies have indicated that common beliefs about UI may lead older adults, particularly older females, to think that incontinence is not worth reporting to health care providers. Many health care providers do not ask patients about incontinence. And, when patients inform them about incontinence, many providers do not provide adequate diagnosis and treatment.

COMMON INCONTINENCE PROBLEMS AND CONDITIONS

Transient Incontinence

Transient incontinence has a sudden onset and is often associated with gastrointestinal, genitourinary, neuropsychiatric, and systemic disorders, as well as restricted mobility and various drugs. Transient incontinence generally resolves when the underlying cause is corrected (Table 20.1). The mnemonic DIAPPERS is useful for remembering the transient causes of incontinence (Shenot, 2021):

- **D**elirium
- **I**nfection (commonly, symptomatic UTIs)
- **A**trophic urethritis and vaginitis
- **P**harmaceuticals (i.e., those with alpha-adrenergic, cholinergic, or anticholinergic properties; diuretics; sedatives)
- **P**sychiatric disorders (particularly depression)
- **E**xcess urine output (polyuria)
- **R**estricted mobility
- **S**tool impaction

Established Incontinence

Established incontinence is caused by a persistent problem affecting nerves or muscles. Specific issues include bladder outlet incompetence or obstruction, detrusor overactivity or underactivity, detrusor-sphincter dyssynergia, or a combination of problems. Major types of established incontinence include urge, stress, overflow, functional, and mixed incontinence (Shenot, 2021).

Urge Incontinence

Urge incontinence is the most common type of incontinence in the older adult population. Urge incontinence may be associated with an overactive bladder. Common causes of urge incontinence include local genitourinary conditions, such as UTI, drugs, bladder irritants (e.g., caffeine and carbonated drinks), bowel issues, dementia, stroke, Parkinson disease, and cancers of the uterus and the urinary system. Individuals with urge incontinence typically have a history of involuntary urine loss after a sudden urge to void. Urgency and involuntary urine loss may be precipitated by the sound of running water, cold weather, or the sight of a toilet. Urinary accidents are sometimes large. Urge incontinence is often accompanied by nocturia and complaints of daytime frequency, with individuals often needing to void more than seven times per day (Shenot, 2021).

Stress Incontinence

Stress incontinence is the second most common form of incontinence in females. Involuntary loss of urine follows a sudden increase in intraabdominal pressure. Stress incontinence occurs when pressure in the bladder (intravesical pressure) exceeds

TABLE 20.1 Causes of Transient Urinary Incontinence

Cause	Comments
Gastrointestinal disorders	
Fecal impaction	Impaction may cause mechanical disruption of the bladder or urethra
	May experience urges and overflow incontinence
Genitourinary disorders	
Atrophic urethritis	Thinning of the urethral and vaginal epithelium and submucosa may cause local irritation
Atrophic vaginitis	Persons may experience urgency, and scalding dysuria
Urinary calculi	Bladder irritation precipitates spasms
Foreign bodies	
Urinary tract infections	Only symptomatic UTIs cause incontinence
	Dysuria and urgency can prevent persons from reaching the toilet before voiding
Neuropsychiatric disorders	
Delirium	Awareness of the need or ability to void is impaired
Depression	
Psychosis	
Restricted mobility	
Weakness	Access to the toilet is impaired
Injury	
Use of physical restraints	
Systemic disorders	
Excess urine output due to various disorders (i.e., diabetes insipidus, and diabetes mellitus)	Frequency, urgency, and nocturia can result
Drugs	
Alcohol	Alcohol has a diuretic effect and can cause sedation, delirium, or immobility, which can result in functional incontinence
Caffeine (i.e., coffee, tea, cola and other soft drinks, cocoa, chocolate, and energy drinks)	Urine production and output are increased, causing polyuria, frequency, urgency, and nocturia
Alpha-adrenergic antagonists (i.e., alfuzosin, doxazosin, prazosin, tamsulosin, terazosin)	Bladder neck muscle in females or prostate smooth muscle in males is lax and may result in stress incontinence
Anticholinergics (i.e., antihistamines, antipsychotics, benztropine, tricyclic antidepressants)	Bladder contractility can be impaired, sometimes causing urinary retention and overflow incontinence
	These drugs can also cause delirium, constipation, and fecal impaction.
Calcium channel blockers (i.e., diltiazem, nifedipine, verapamil)	Detrusor contractility is decreased, sometimes causing urinary retention and overflow incontinence, nocturia due to peripheral edema, constipation, and fecal impaction
Diuretics (i.e., bumetanide, furosemide [not thiazides])	Urine production and output are increased, causing polyuria, frequency, urgency, and nocturia
Hormone therapy (systemic estrogen/progestin therapy)	Collagen in the paraurethral connective tissues is degraded, causing ineffective urethral closure
Misoprostol	It relaxes the urethra and may result in stress incontinence
Opioids	Cause urinary retention, constipation, fecal impaction, sedation, and delirium
Psychoactive drugs (i.e., antipsychotics, benzodiazepines, sedative-hypnotics, tricyclic antidepressants)	Awareness of the need to void is heightened, and dexterity and mobility are decreased
	These drugs can cause delirium

From the MSD Manual Professional Version, edited by Sandy Falk. Copyright © 2024 Merck & Co., Inc., Rahway, NJ, USA and its affiliates. All rights reserved. Available at https://www.msdmanuals.com/professional. Accessed May 2024.

urethral resistance. This may be caused by a lack of estrogen, obesity, previous vaginal deliveries, surgeries, or all these factors. Individuals with stress incontinence often leak urine with physical exertion, such as coughing, sneezing, laughing, lifting, and exercise. Older females may report leakage when they change positions (e.g., get out of a chair) or lift small weights, such as a small child. These activities increase intraabdominal pressure, which increases bladder pressure. If the urethra, supporting tissues, and bladder neck are abnormal, urethral resistance may be too low to withstand the increased pressure on the bladder, which results in involuntary urine loss. Stress incontinence is unusual in males, and it mainly occurs after radical prostatectomy, when the anatomic sphincters are damaged (Shenot, 2021).

Overflow Incontinence

Overflow incontinence occurs when bladder pressure in a chronically full bladder rises to a level higher than urethral resistance, causing involuntary loss of urine. Based on history alone, overflow incontinence may be difficult to differentiate from stress or urge incontinence. It is the second most common form of incontinence in males. Typically, individuals with overflow incontinence complain of constant dribbling. They may have had both daytime and nighttime accidents. Overflow incontinence may result from urethral blockage (e.g., BPH, scar tissue, stones), weakened bladder muscles, nerve injury or damage (e.g., diabetes, Parkinson disease, and multiple sclerosis), constipation, or drugs (Shenot, 2021).

Functional Incontinence

In functional incontinence, incontinence results from physical, mental, psychologic, or environmental factors interfering with the ability to make it to the toilet on time. Individuals with physical disabilities affecting their gait or their ability to undress may have difficulty reaching the bathroom on time and unbuttoning or unzipping clothes in a timely manner; individuals with cognitive impairment may not recognize their need to void or may have difficulty finding the toilet and preparing to void. Those with psychologic problems such as severe depression may lack the motivation to toilet appropriately. Environmental factors may play a role in causing incontinence, especially in acute and long-term care settings. Residents confined to beds and wheelchairs, or restrained, are dependent on caregiver assistance for toileting. If that assistance is not available in a timely manner, the resident often becomes incontinent. This is especially true in the case of urgency (Shenot, 2021). Functional incontinence should be a diagnosis of exclusion.

Mixed Incontinence

Mixed incontinence is described as a combination of two or more other types: stress, urge, overflow, or functional incontinence. Among community-dwelling older adults, mixed urge incontinence and stress incontinence are common. Urge incontinence with functional incontinence is most common in residential facilities (Shenot, 2021).

Diagnosis of the UI

The basic evaluation for all persons with UI includes a history, physical examination (to include pelvic examination for females and rectal examination), postvoid residual (PVR) measurement via bladder scan, blood chemistry, and urinalysis. Urodynamic testing or cystoscopy may also be necessary (Shenot, 2021).

Incontinence can be cured, or the problem can be significantly alleviated, if treatable factors contributing to the incontinence are identified and appropriate medical and nursing interventions are implemented. As quality of life is significantly affected by UI, efforts to restore urinary continence should be based on an older person's satisfaction and tolerance of the interventions and strategies to achieve the outcome.

NURSING CARE GUIDELINES FOR INCONTINENCE

Recognize Cues (Assessment)

The purpose of the nursing assessment is to determine the type of incontinence and contributing factors so appropriate nursing interventions can be planned and implemented. In addition, nursing assessment enables the nurse to identify patients who need referral to a healthcare provider for a more complete evaluation. Assessment consists of a history assessment, functional assessment, environmental assessment, psychosocial assessment, physical examination, tests of provocation, and evaluation of bladder habits.

History

During the history assessment, information is collected about the patient's incontinence symptoms and bladder habits, general health and functional status, medical problems, current drugs, and past medical, surgical, and obstetric histories. If patients can provide a history, they are the most accurate source of data. In situations in which a patient has cognitive impairment, the nurse may need to rely on secondary sources such as family caregivers or medical records.

When taking the incontinence history, the following information should be collected (Sharma and Chakrabarti, 2018; Stewart, 2018):

- How long has the UI been going on, and if it has been worsening?
- Triggering events (cough, sneezing, etc.)
- Constant or intermittent loss of urine and what prompts it
- What other symptoms is the patient experiencing, such as frequency, urgency, and dysuria
- Fecal incontinence
- Other medical history, such as diabetes
- Obstetrical history, including difficult births
- History of pelvic surgeries
- History of spinal surgeries
- Lifestyles such as smoking and alcohol use
- Existing pelvic organ prolapse
- Cancers
- Medication (prescription and over-the-counter [OTC])
- Mobility
- Quality of life impact

Functional Assessment

Because functional problems often contribute to UI, functional assessment is one of the most important parts of the evaluation. Information should be collected about the patient's ability to perform normal activities of daily living (ADLs), including grooming, dressing, getting in and out of bed, and walking. Patients who have difficulty performing these ADLs often have difficulty toileting. Functional status may be assessed by using unstructured questioning or by using a structured questionnaire such as the Katz Index of ADLs (Katz et al, 1963).

Mental status should also be assessed during the functional assessment. Cognitive ability may affect the patient's ability to recognize the need to urinate, locate the toilet, and undress for toileting. In addition, knowledge of a patient's cognitive status is essential in planning nursing interventions for incontinence. The Montreal Cognitive Assessment (MoCA) is useful for general screening as it assesses multiple cognitive functions (Newman, 2020).

Environmental Assessment

Environmental barriers may contribute to UI. For example, the bathroom may be too far away or inaccessible to the patient, or the toilet may be too low or difficult for the patient to get on and

off. The patient may need assistance with toileting, which may not be readily available. For these reasons, environmental assessment is an important component of the evaluation of UI. It is necessary to note the following:
- Proximity of the toilet
- Any barriers between the patient's usual location and the toilet, for example, poor lighting, steps, furniture, or other objects
- The size of the bathroom: Is it large enough to accommodate the patient and any assistive devices (wheelchair or walker) that must be used?
- Toilet height: Is it adequate, too high, or low?
- Presence of grab bars, if needed
- Availability of caregiver or nursing staff assistance, if needed
- Availability of a call bell, if needed

Psychosocial Assessment

Psychosocial assessment focuses on the effect of incontinence on the patient's life and on the availability and quality of caregiver assistance. The nurse should ask the patient how incontinence has affected social activities (e.g., visiting family and friends and attending social functions and church), self esteem, mood, sexual activity, and family relationships; the nurse should also assess the patient's desire and willingness to participate in a treatment program for incontinence. Effective nursing interventions for UI require active patient involvement, so motivation is an essential component of success. If a patient does not want treatment for incontinence, the reasons should be explored. What is the reason? For example, is it a knowledge deficit, depression, or an overwhelming physical, social, or psychologic problem?

If the patient depends on another person's assistance in toileting, caregiver assessment is an essential component of the psychosocial assessment. Is the caregiver (1) physically able to assist the patient, (2) available on a consistent basis, and (3) willing to assist the patient? What is the caregiver's attitude toward the patient and toward incontinence? Does the caregiver have an adequate understanding of the problem and its management?

Physical Examination

The physical examination should include the following:
- Inspection of gait, balance, and body mass index (BMI)
- Neurologic assessment of any weakness, paralysis, or sensory deficit in the lower extremities
- Abdominal examination for bladder distention, suprapubic tenderness (occurs in bladder infections), and costovertebral angle tenderness (occurs in kidney infections)
- Rectal examination for fecal impaction; rectal sensation and tone; and, in males, the size, shape, and consistency of the prostate gland
- Measurements of sitting and standing blood pressure to detect orthostatic hypotension and dizziness
- Pelvic examination, including inspection of the vagina for atrophic changes, vaginitis, cystocele, rectocele, or uterine prolapse
- Urinary stress testing: With a full bladder, the patient sits upright on the examination table with legs spread, relaxes the perineal area, and coughs vigorously once

- Immediate leakage that starts and stops with a cough confirms stress incontinence
- Delayed or persistent leakage suggests detrusor overactivity triggered by the cough

Bladder Habits

One of the most effective ways to assess bladder habits is to ask the patient or caregiver to keep a diary of the frequency of urination and any incontinent episodes, their relative volume, and the circumstances that precipitated their occurrence (e.g., coughing, sneezing, urgency, and changing position). Fig. 20.2 shows a sample bladder diary. Bladder diaries may be used in the home, hospital, or nursing facility and may be kept by the patient or caregiver. They provide a more objective and accurate measure of a patient's bladder habits than can be obtained by recall alone. They may be especially useful for a patient who has short-term memory problems. For bladder diaries to be accurate, patients and caregivers need careful instructions on their maintenance.

Collecting bladder diaries during assessment helps establish the type of UI and aids in planning nursing interventions.

Analyze Cues and Prioritize Hypotheses (Patient Problems)

The data collected during assessment and the nurse's knowledge of UI often permit a diagnosis of the type of incontinence. Sometimes, a more complex evaluation is needed to determine the cause and most appropriate treatment for UI. In any new case of incontinence, the nurse should consider acute and potentially reversible causes. If transient incontinence is ruled out or treated and involuntary urine loss persists, a diagnosis of chronic incontinence must be considered.

The following patient problems are appropriate for patients with established incontinence: stress UI, urge UI, overflow UI, and functional UI.

Stress UI

History: The patient reports leaking urine with activities that increase intraabdominal pressure (e.g., coughing, sneezing, laughing, lifting, position changes, walking, climbing steps, or exercise).

Objective observations: Leaking urine with stress provocation; signs of pelvic floor relaxation (e.g., cystocele, rectocele, or uterine prolapse) are observed on pelvic examination.

Bladder records: Documentation of urine loss during physical activities that increase intraabdominal pressure.

Urge UI

History: The patient reports a sudden urge to void, followed by involuntary urine loss; the patient may also report that running water or cold weather precipitates involuntary urine loss.

Objective observations: Leaking urine with urge provocation.

Bladder records: Documentation of urine loss associated with urgency; frequent urination and nocturia are also frequently recorded.

Your Daily Bladder Diary

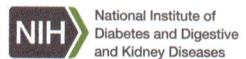

This diary will help you and your health care team figure out the causes of your bladder control trouble. The "sample" line shows you how to use the diary.

Time	Drinks — What kind?	Drinks — How much? oz, mL, cups	Trips to the Bathroom — How many times?	Trips to the Bathroom — How much urine? (sm/med/lg)	Accidental Leaks — How much urine? (sm/med/lg)	Did you feel a strong urge to go?	What were you doing at the time? Sneezing, lifting, arriving home, sleeping, etc.
Sample	Juice	8 ounces	✓✓	(sm circled)	(sm circled)	Yes (circled) / No	Running
6–7 a.m.						Yes / No	
7–8 a.m.						Yes / No	
8–9 a.m.						Yes / No	
9–10 a.m.						Yes / No	
10–11 a.m.						Yes / No	
11–12 noon						Yes / No	
12–1 p.m.						Yes / No	
1–2 p.m.						Yes / No	
2–3 p.m.						Yes / No	
3–4 p.m.						Yes / No	
4–5 p.m.						Yes / No	
5–6 p.m.						Yes / No	
6–7 p.m.						Yes / No	
7–8 p.m.						Yes / No	
8–9 p.m.						Yes / No	
9–10 p.m.						Yes / No	
10–11 p.m.						Yes / No	
11–12 mid.						Yes / No	
12–1 a.m.						Yes / No	
1–2 a.m.						Yes / No	
2–3 a.m.						Yes / No	
3–4 a.m.						Yes / No	
4–5 a.m.						Yes / No	
5–6 a.m.						Yes / No	

Use this sheet as a master for making copies that you can use as a bladder diary for as many days as you need.

I used _____ pads today. I used _____ diapers today (write number).

Questions to ask my health care team: _____

Fig. 20.2 Sample bladder diary. (From National Institute of Diabetes and Digestive and Kidney Diseases. [n.d.]. *Your daily bladder diary.* Retrieved from https://www.niddk.nih.gov/-/media/Files/Urologic-Diseases/diary_508.pdf.)

Overflow UI

History: Patient histories vary, but they often show frequent involuntary urine loss of small amounts. Urine loss may be associated with physical exertion. Complaints may include decreased force of the urine stream, hesitancy, a feeling of incomplete bladder emptying, and frequent urination of small amounts of urine. Patients may also have risk factors for urinary retention, such as diabetes or the use of anticholinergic drugs.

Objective observations: An elevated PVR (> 100 mL) is the hallmark of overflow incontinence (Shenot, 2021). This should be part of the initial evaluation of patients with UI. On abdominal examination, a distended bladder may be detected on percussion. When overflow incontinence is associated with prostatic hyperplasia, an enlarged prostate can be detected on rectal examination. In females, a large cystocele observed during pelvic examination may suggest the cause of overflow incontinence.

Bladder records: Documentation of frequent small-volume urinary accidents.

Functional UI

History: The patient or caregiver reports large-volume urine loss in places other than the toilet, commode, bedpan, or urinal in the absence of symptoms of stress, urge, or overflow incontinence. The patient may be unaware of the need to void or have a significant mobility impairment.

Objective observations: In pure functional incontinence, leaking is not seen with stress or urge provocation, and the PVR result is normal. A mental status examination may reveal cognitive impairment. Functional assessment may reveal impaired mobility and toileting skills.

Bladder records: Documentation of involuntary urine loss (often large accidents) without symptoms of urge or stress incontinence.

Generate Solutions (Planning)

For all types of UI, the nurse must determine the patient's and caregiver's desire for treatment and willingness to carry out the recommended self-care practices and interventions.

Stress UI

The long-term goal is that the patient will reduce or eliminate the number of stressful accidents. Short-term goals include the following:
1. The patient will master interventions (e.g., pelvic floor muscle exercises) designed to increase pelvic muscle tone.
2. The patient will recognize factors that precipitate stress accidents and use behavioral interventions to prevent accidents.

Urge UI

The long-term goal is that the patient will reduce or eliminate urge accidents. Short-term goals include the following:
1. The patient will master interventions (e.g., pelvic floor muscle exercises and bladder retraining) designed to increase pelvic muscle tone and decrease urge accidents.
2. The patient will recognize factors that precipitate accidents and use behavioral interventions to prevent accidents.

Overflow UI

The long-term goal is that the patient reduces or eliminates incontinence caused by urinary retention and overflow. Short-term goals for the patient vary depending on the underlying mechanism responsible for the incontinence, but they might include the following:
1. The patient will seek a urologic evaluation of incontinence.
2. If the patient has an atonic bladder, the patient will master in-and-out self-catheterization.

Functional UI

The long-term goal is that, with caregiver assistance, the patient will reduce or eliminate urinary accidents. Short-term goals for the caregiver include the following:
1. The caregiver will provide timely assistance with toileting.
2. The caregiver will remove environmental barriers to proper toileting.

Take Actions (Nursing Interventions)

First-line nursing interventions for UI focus on lifestyle modifications and behavioral therapies. These therapies are effective for all types of UI and have limited to no side effects. Pharmacologic options are offered to patients with urge incontinence or mixed incontinence who have failed a trial lasting up to 3 months of lifestyle and behavioral therapies (Davis et al, 2020; Dufour and Wu, 2020). Nursing needs to improve its skills in managing and implementing incontinence interventions. The most appropriate behavioral intervention depends on the type of incontinence, the patient's cognitive status, and the level of family assistance (Davis et al, 2020).

Lifestyle Modifications

Individuals with UI may decrease fluid intake to prevent accidents. This is not an effective method of managing incontinence and may lead to UTIs, constipation, and dehydration. Patients and caregivers should be cautioned not to decrease fluid intake to less than six glasses a day.

Individuals with incontinence, particularly those with urge accidents, should be advised to eliminate or restrict caffeine intake. Products containing caffeine include coffee, tea, caffeinated colas, and chocolate. Caffeine has been shown to increase the occurrence of abnormal detrusor contractions, which are the cause of urge incontinence. Additionally, alcohol should be discouraged, as it is a bladder stimulant and causes increased urgency and frequency, sedation, and altered mobility.

Weight loss is another important lifestyle modification. Excessive weight increases pressure on the pelvic floor muscles and the bladder. Although studies have not shown resolution of UI symptoms, significant decreases in frequency of episodes and cost of UI management have been demonstrated with a decrease in weight (Patel et al, 2022).

Some older adults, even those who are continents, complain of frequent nocturia that disrupts their sleep. Getting up at night is probably a normal effect of aging. For patients who get up more often and think that the quality of their sleep is disrupted, some measures, such as restricting fluid intake in the evening, may be helpful. Although it is important for patients to

> **BOX 20.1 Nonpharmacologic Management of Nocturia**
>
> - Restrict fluids 2–4 hours before going to sleep. It is important to drink enough fluids (usually 2 liters a day), but the bulk of fluids should be ingested during the day.
> - Limit caffeine containing beverages (e.g., caffeinated cola and tea, chocolate) and alcohol, especially in the evening.
> - Reduce dietary salt and protein intake late in the day.
> - Ensure diuretics are not taken within 6 hours of bedtime.
> - Take an afternoon nap; naps allow fluid to be absorbed back into the bloodstream. Avoid long naps to avoid nighttime sleep disruption. Do not nap after 3 pm.
> - Elevate the legs in the afternoon so the feet and ankles are not swollen when going to bed.
> - Wear compression socks to reduce peripheral edema.
> - Optimize treatment of underlying medical conditions, such as diabetes and heart failure.
> - Pelvic floor exercises (Kegel exercises)
>
> Data From Leslie, S. W., Sajjad, H., & Singh, S. (2023). *Nocturia*. StatPearls [website]. Retrieved from https://www.statpearls.com/ArticleLibrary/viewarticle/25914; Urology Care Foundation. (n.d.). *What is nocturia?* Retrieved from https://www.urologyhealth.org/urology-a-z/n/nocturia.

have adequate fluid intake, individuals with frequent nocturia should drink the bulk of this fluid before dinner. These individuals should be advised to eliminate caffeine in the evening. When an older adult goes to bed with swollen ankles and feet, nocturia frequently increases. Patients with such swelling should be advised to elevate their legs for several hours during the afternoon to limit the amount of edema present at bedtime (Box 20.1).

Frail older adults are at increased risk for constipation and fecal impaction, which may cause transient incontinence and exacerbate persistent incontinence. Nurses should assess bowel habits regularly and institute preventive measures such as increased fiber intake, adequate fluids, and increased activity levels.

UI increases the risk of skin rashes, infections, and skin breakdown. Frequent changes of incontinence pads and scrupulous skin care provide the best protection against these complications. For short-term use in conjunction with other treatment measures, incontinence pads or garments provide convenience and comfort. However, they are expensive for long-term use and may be associated with skin rashes and breakdown if not changed often. They should not be used as a substitute for the evaluation and treatment of incontinence.

Cognitively Intact Patients

Two behavioral interventions useful for cognitively intact individuals are bladder retraining and pelvic floor muscle exercises. These interventions may be used alone or in combination, depending on the type of incontinence.

Bladder retraining. The patient is encouraged to adopt a gradually expanding voiding schedule with the goal of 2–4 hours between toiletings. Retraining is useful for correcting the habit of frequent toileting and for diminishing urgency. A schedule is established for voiding times; voiding because of urgency is discouraged. This procedure is most useful for patients with urge incontinence and frequent urination.

Pelvic floor muscle exercises. Kegel (1948) was the first to report pelvic floor muscle exercises as a treatment for UI. These exercises consist of alternating contractions and relaxations of the levator ani muscles, which are the muscles of the pelvic floor. These muscles, including the pubococcygeal muscle surrounding the midportion of the urethra, contract as a unit. In older adults, these muscles are often weak from disuse atrophy. Performed correctly, pelvic floor muscle exercises strengthen the muscles, increase urethral resistance, and allow the patient to use the muscles voluntarily to prevent urinary accidents (Stewart, 2018); reports vary, but about 75% of females with stress incontinence experience resolution or improvement in symptoms when they perform pelvic floor muscle exercises properly (Vasavada et al, 2023).

However, many older adults need additional help in identifying and learning to use their pelvic floor muscles. These patients can benefit from biofeedback. Biofeedback is an intensive therapy where the patient is given immediate feedback on pelvic floor muscle contractions by attaching sensors that detect electrical signals from the pelvic floor muscles. The electric signals from pelvic floor muscles are visible on a computer screen, providing minute-by-minute feedback (Vasavada et al, 2023).

After training with biofeedback, the patient must practice the pelvic floor muscle exercises at home. The patient should be instructed to practice contracting and relaxing the pelvic floor muscles at least 45 times a day, in three or four practice sessions. The patient should exercise lying down, sitting, and standing. This facilitates the patient's ability to identify and use the muscles in any position. The nurse should remind the patient to relax the abdominal muscles when exercising, as this is essential for the successful performance of exercises. The nurse may ask patients to try occasionally to slow or stop their urine stream while voiding. This allows the patients to monitor their progress in using and strengthening the correct muscles (Box 20.2).

Once patients master the exercises, they should be taught strategies to prevent involuntary urine loss (stress and urge strategies). Patients with stress accidents should be instructed to contract their pelvic floor muscles before and during activities that precipitate leaking, such as coughing, sneezing, lifting, or changing positions. Those with urge incontinence may be taught to contract their pelvic floor muscles to inhibit involuntary bladder contractions. A patient should respond to an urge to void by relaxing and contracting the pelvic floor muscles three or four times quickly. When the urgency subsides, the patient should walk to the toilet at a normal pace (Box 20.3).

Pessaries. Pessaries are an option for older females with stress or mixed UI and those with prolapse. A pessary is a stiff ring or dish-like object inserted into the vagina to compress the urethra against the symphysis pubis, thereby elevating the bladder neck. Once fitted by the healthcare provider, care of the pessary is based on type. A ring pessary is usually removed at least weekly (it may be removed nightly) and cleaned with mild soap and water, rinsed, and reinserted after it dries. A healthcare provider must remove a Gellhorn pessary; it is removed

BOX 20.2 Kegel Exercises

What Are Kegel Exercises?
Pelvic floor muscle exercises, also known as *Kegels* or *Kegel exercises*, are one of the best ways to improve and maintain bowel and bladder functions. They increase the strength of pelvic floors and may improve or even eliminate bladder leakage.

There is a sling of muscles extending from the inside of the pubic bone to the anus and woven around the vagina, urethra, and rectum. This group of muscles helps indirectly control the contractions of the detrusor muscle (bladder muscle) and the urethral pressures. The pelvic floor muscles relax to allow urination and tighten to stop the stream of urine. Contraction of the pelvic floor muscles closes the lower urethra, squeezing any remaining urine back up into the bladder.

Pelvic floor muscle exercises will help restore muscle function before it is permanently lost and will lessen the symptoms of incontinence.

How To Do Kegel Exercises
Like any exercise, it can be difficult at first to know if the Kegel exercises are being done properly. But with a daily commitment, it becomes instinctive. Here are a few tips:

- **Which muscles?** If the urination flow can be stopped midstream, the pelvic floor muscles have been identified. That's the most difficult part of the exercise.
- **Increase the routine over time.** When performing with an empty bladder, the first goal should be to tighten the pelvic floor muscles for 5 seconds. Then relax them for 5 seconds. Try to do 5 reps on the first day. While gaining confidence from the new routine, aim for 10 seconds at a time, relaxing for 10 seconds between contractions.
- **Watch outs.** Be careful not to flex the abdominal muscles, thighs, or buttocks. Also, breathe freely during the exercises to keep from stressing the rest of the body.
- **Repeat 3 times a day.** Aim for at least 3 sets of 10 repetitions per day.
- **Give yourself encouragement.** These exercises will feel foreign in the beginning. But continuing these exercises, the better the bladder health will become. As a bonus, Kegels have been reported to increase sexual pleasure as well.

To give the pelvic floor a full workout, perform the two exercises. The first exercise is called a short contraction, and it works the fast-twitch muscles that quickly shut off the flow of urine to prevent leakage. The muscles are quickly tightened, lifted, and then released. While contracting the muscles, be sure to exhale, then continue to breathe normally while exercising.

The second exercise works on the supportive strength of the muscles and is referred to as a long contraction. The slow-twitch muscles are gradually tightened, lifted, and held for several seconds. At first, it may be difficult to hold the contraction for more than 1 or 2 seconds. Ultimately, the goal is to hold the contraction for 10 seconds, then rest for 10 seconds between each long contraction to avoid taxing the muscles. A solid exercise plan would be to perform 3 sets of 10 short and 10 long contractions twice per day. Doing the exercises right trumps doing a bunch of them incorrectly. Improvements to the strength of the pelvic floor are usually seen in 3 to 6 months.

Use vaginal weights, wands, or other devices as a training aid for Kegels. These provide resistance against muscle contractions. Some of these aids are prescribed by a health professional and used under professional supervision, while others are available without a prescription.

Signs of Pelvic Floor Strength Improvement
Do not be discouraged if the control of the bladder does not occur quickly, but rather look for these signs as proof that the pelvic floor muscle exercises are working towards better bladder health:

- Longer time between bathroom visits
- Fewer "accidents"
- Ability to hold the contractions longer, or to do more repetitions
- Drier underwear, without the feeling of always being wet

Females who have difficulty performing pelvic floor muscle exercises on their own may find biofeedback therapy helpful. With professional instruction from a nurse specialist or physical therapist, many females witness significant improvement in pelvic floor muscle strength. It is crucial to remember that incontinence and pelvic floor symptoms almost always have solutions and should not be shrugged off as normal. Find time each day to squeeze it into a regular exercise routine.

Modified from National Association for Continence. (2022). *Kegel exercises*. Retrieved July 24, 2023 from https://nafc.org/kegel-exercises/.

BOX 20.3 Urge Strategies

The nurse should instruct the patient to do the following when they have the urge to void:

1. Try to "hold it" for longer than normal. Build up longer intervals over a 12-week period. The goal is to urinate every three to four hours.
2. Change the routine. If the patient runs to the bathroom as soon as they get to work or home, stop. The urge to urinate may diminish after 30 to 60 seconds.

Data from WebMD Editorial Contributors. (2021). *Urge incontinence: Tips for daily life*. WebMD [website]. Retrieved July 24, 2023 from https://www.webmd.com/urinary-incontinence-oab/oab-tips.

and cleaned every one to three months (Fig. 20.3) (Dufour and Wu, 2020; WebMD Editorial Contributors, 2021).

Cognitively Impaired Patients

The techniques already described (bladder retraining, pelvic floor muscle exercises, and biofeedback) require active patient involvement. Treating UI in individuals with cognitive impairment requires the use of other behavioral techniques that depend on the caregiver rather than the patient. These include scheduled toileting, habit training, and prompted voiding. The success of these techniques in large part depends on the availability and motivation of the caregiver and the dedication of the nursing staff.

Scheduled toileting. The patient is assisted to the bathroom to void on a fixed schedule. Beginning at the time the patient wakes up, the patient is assisted to the toilet every two hours. The schedule can be adjusted to every two and a half hours to three hours if the patient remains dry when taken every two hours.

Habit training. Habit training creates a schedule based on the patient's usual voiding pattern. After determining the person's normal schedule (either through observation or by checking for soiling), take them to the toilet about 10 minutes before their anticipated need to void.

Prompted voiding. Prompted voiding is most successful with patients who can recognize the need to void. It depends on active caregivers and patient involvement. The goal is to increase a patient's awareness of the need to void and increase the frequency of self-initiated toileting. Patients are approached on a regular schedule, asked if they are wet or dry, and then

CHAPTER 20 Urinary Function

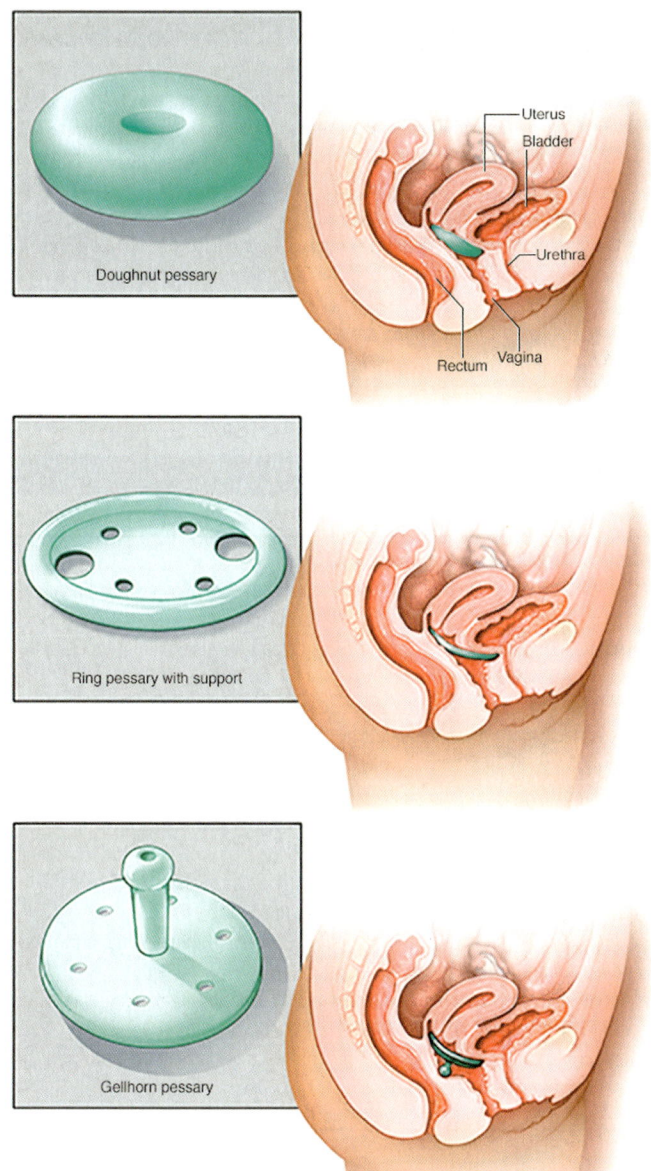

Fig. 20.3 Types of pessaries. (From https://www.mayoclinic.org/diseases-conditions/cystocele/diagnosis-treatment/drc-20369457. Used with permission of Mayo Foundation for Medical Education and Research, all rights reserved.)

> **BOX 20.4 Prompted Voiding Instructions**
>
> 1. Approach the patient at the scheduled times and ask if they are feeling wet or dry.
> 2. Check to see if the patient is wet or dry.
> 3. If the patient correctly identified their present continent status, give positive feedback.
> 4. Ask the patient if they prefer to use the toilet. If the response is yes, toilet the patient; if it is no, encourage the patient. *Never* force the patient to go to the toilet.
> 5. Give positive feedback regarding appropriate toileting. Do not give any negative feedback.
> 6. Inform the patient of the next scheduled voiding time.
> 7. Encourage the patient to hold urine until the next scheduled time.

Data From Newman, D. K., Eason, S., & Specht, J. (2018). *Prompted voiding for persons with urinary incontinence.* Iowa City, IA: The University of Iowa College of Nursing. Retrieved from https://csomaycenter.uiowa.edu/sites/csomaycenter.uiowa.edu/files/2022-05/2018_Prompted%20Voiding_Guideline.pdf.

prompted to toilet (Box 20.4). A patient should never be forced to toilet or reprimanded for failing to toilet appropriately. Self-initiated toileting should not be discouraged. To relieve the stress that may occur because of sleep disruption for both caregiver and patient, toileting protocols may be modified for the nighttime hours.

Once contributing causes have been ruled out or treated, and if trials of scheduled toileting, habit training, and prompted voiding have failed, the use of disposable incontinence pads and other protective garments may be the only feasible method of managing UI in older adults with dementia (Payne, 2020).

Evaluate Outcomes (Evaluation)

Evaluation is an integral ongoing component of the management of UI. Patient goals are the focal point of evaluation. A patient's perception of the effectiveness of and satisfaction with their treatment should be assessed and documented. Many older adults with incontinence may require more than one treatment modality to achieve a satisfactory reduction in incontinence episodes. As a result, the care plan often evolves over time (see Nursing Care Plan: Mixed Incontinence and Nursing Care Plan: Functional Incontinence boxes).

NURSING CARE PLAN

Mixed Incontinence

Clinical Situation

Mrs. W is a 72-year-old retired administrative assistant who was discharged from the hospital after an amputation of a gangrenous toe. The nurse sees her three times a week to change the dressing and assess wound healing. Mrs. W's medical history includes type 2 diabetes mellitus for 26 years, complicated by peripheral neuropathy. She also has coronary artery disease (one myocardial infarction), hypertension, peptic ulcers, and rheumatoid arthritis. She has had a bilateral hip replacement. She walks with a walker, and her gait is slow and sometimes unsteady. Her current drugs include insulin glargine, lansoprazole, acetaminophen, diltiazem extended release, triamterene and hydrochlorothiazide, nitroglycerin, docusate sodium, and oxybutynin. Her OTC drugs include a multivitamin, Metamucil, Citrucel, and Tums. She needs assistance with personal grooming and bathing.

She has had problems with constipation but finds that daily Metamucil and docusate sodium help with regularity. Mrs. W has been incontinent for 2 years. She describes both stress and urge symptoms and states that she has about 14 accidents per week. She also experiences nocturia. She drinks three or four cups of regular coffee or tea a day and drinks a considerable amount of iced tea in the summer. She has seen a urologist, and he prescribed oxybutynin for her. She has been taking it for 2 years. Although it somewhat reduced the number of accidents, she does not think it is very effective. She finds the incontinence disturbing and wishes something more could be done.

Continued

> ### NURSING CARE PLAN—cont'd
>
> **Analyze Cues and Prioritize Hypotheses (Patient Problems)**
> - Inadequate urinary elimination
>
> **Generate Solutions (Planning)**
> - The patient will master pelvic floor muscle exercises.
> - The patient will experience a decrease in the number of urinary accidents.
>
> **Take Actions (Nursing Interventions)**
> - Ask the patient to keep a baseline bladder diary before treatment.
> - Teach the patient pelvic floor muscle exercises using verbal feedback of pelvic floor muscle contractions during rectal examination.
> - Provide written instructions for practicing the exercises.
> - Ask the patient to continue to keep bladder diaries during treatment.
> - Review the diaries and assess the patient's progress during weekly visits.
> - Once the patient has mastered the exercises, teach strategies to manage urge incontinence and then strategies for stress incontinence, if indicated by the diaries.
> - If the patient is unable to identify her pelvic floor muscles using verbal feedback or is not making adequate progress, refer her to the nurse specialist who deals with continence for biofeedback.
> - Advise the patient to substitute decaffeinated coffee and tea for the regular coffee and tea that she now drinks.

> ### NURSING CARE PLAN
> *Functional Incontinence*
>
> **Clinical Situation**
> Mrs. G is a 78-year-old retired teacher who receives visits from a nursing agency for congestive heart failure. Mrs. G was diagnosed with mild Alzheimer disease 3 years ago. She lives with her niece, who is also her primary caregiver. Mrs. G is legally blind. She had a fall and fractured her right hip 1 year ago. She has a moderate amount of bilateral ankle and foot edema. She also suffers frequently from constipation. Her current drugs include furosemide, a calcium channel blocker, and a stool softener. She requires assistance with ambulation and ADLs. She has had UI for 3 years. Mrs. G generally feels the urge to void but has frequent accidents. Mrs. G now requires incontinence undergarments. She also has enuresis, and the pad is usually wet in the morning.
>
> **Analyze Cues and Prioritize Hypotheses (Patient Problems)**
> - Inadequate urinary elimination
>
> **Generate Solutions (Planning)**
> - The patient's caregiver will master a prompted voiding and toileting program with the patient.
> - The patient will experience a reduction in the number of episodes of incontinence.
>
> **Take Actions (Nursing Interventions)**
> - Collect baseline bladder diaries to establish the frequency of UI and precipitating factors.
> - Assess the caregiver's willingness to participate in a behavioral program to treat the patient's incontinence.
> - Teach the caregiver how to implement a prompted voiding program.
> - Assess the patient's understanding by having her conduct a return demonstration of the technique.
> - Visit weekly to assess the implementation and success of the program.
> - Have the caregiver keep the bladder diaries during treatment.
> - Assess the patient's daily fluid intake.
> - If daily fluid intake is less than six to eight glasses of fluid per day, instruct the caregiver to increase the patient's fluid intake.
> - Instruct the caregiver to restrict the patient's fluids in the evening, providing the bulk of her fluids during the day.
> - Instruct the caregiver to restrict the patient's caffeine intake and eliminate caffeine in the evening.
> - Instruct the caregiver to have the patient elevate her legs in the afternoon to reduce the amount of edema.

AGE-RELATED RENAL CHANGES

The process of aging results in anatomic and functional changes in the renal system. Kidneys decrease in size and number of nephrons with aging. In addition, individuals with atherosclerosis experience decreased renal blood flow due to fibrous tissue and calcification-hardening renal vasculature. These factors combine, leading to a decrease in the glomerular filtration rate (GFR). Despite the anatomic and functional changes associated with age, the kidneys remain capable of performing their functions well into the ninth decade of life unless acute illness or comorbidities result in renal dysfunction.

With age, arterial changes and ischemia in the kidney result in the gradual loss of renal tissue and nephrosclerosis. Additionally, the number of nephrons decreases by about 6800 per year. After age 30, the GFR decreases at an average of 1 mL/min/m^2/year; this results in a GFR of 60 mL/min by age 75. This reduction in GFR is independent of comorbidities (Mathew, 2020).

The effect of aging on the renal system has implications for clinical management. Changes in renal function affect all aspects of pharmacokinetics. Drug dosages should be adjusted based on GFR, or creatinine clearance. Older adults lack adaptive mechanisms; therefore, fluid and electrolyte alterations may occur in the setting of acute illness. It is also important for nurses to recognize comorbidities likely to affect renal function in the older adult population, for example, cardiovascular disease and diabetes.

COMMON RENAL PROBLEMS AND CONDITIONS

Acute Kidney Injury

Acute kidney injury (AKI) is the sudden decline in renal function accompanied by fluid and electrolyte alterations and acid–base disturbance. It may or may not be associated with oliguria. Symptoms may include anorexia, nausea, and vomiting. If left untreated, seizures and coma may occur. AKI is classified as

> **BOX 20.5 Causes of Acute Kidney Injury**
>
> **Prerenal**
> Sudden and severe reduction in blood pressure (shock) of interruption of blood flow to the kidneys from severe injury or illness
> - Blood loss
> - Dehydration
> - Heart failure
> - Sepsis
> - Vascular occlusion
>
> **Intrinsic Renal**
> Direct injury to the kidneys by inflammation, drugs, toxins, infection, or reduced blood supply
> - Acute tubular necrosis
>   - Drugs
>   - Toxins
>   - Prolonged hypotension
> - Glomerulonephritis
> - Acute tubular necrosis
>   - Drugs
>   - Toxins
>   - Autoimmune disease
>   - Infection
> - Small-vessel vasculitis
>
> **Postrenal**
> Sudden obstruction of urine flow due to enlarged prostate, kidney stones, bladder injury or tumor
> - Benign prostatic hyperplasia
> - Cervical cancer
> - Meatal stenosis/phimosis
> - Retroperitoneal fibrosis
> - Prostate cancer
> - Urinary calculi

From Thongprayoon, C., Hansrivijit, P., Kovvuru, K., Kanduri, S. R., Torres-Ortiz, A., Acharya, P., et al. (2020). Diagnostics, risk factors, treatment and outcomes of acute kidney injury in a new paradigm. *Journal of Clinical Medicine, 9*(4), 1104. doi: 10.3390/jcm9041104.

prerenal, renal (also referred to as intrinsic), or postrenal based on causative factors (Box 20.5).

Prerenal failure occurs because of inadequate perfusion (e.g., fluid sequestration in liver failure or heart failure). It is not accompanied by parenchymal damage; therefore, restoring perfusion should restore renal function.

Renal causes of AKI occur due to abnormalities within the kidney and may be caused by ischemia, sepsis, inflammation, or injury. Acute tubular necrosis (ATN) is the most common cause of intrarenal failure. The three stages of ATN are as follows:

1. **Initiation:** Blood urea nitrogen (BUN) and creatinine levels rise, and urine output decreases.
2. **Maintenance:** A continued decrease in renal function lasting for 7–21 days during which supportive therapy (e.g., dialysis) may be necessary.
3. **Recovery:** Urine output increases, accompanied by a decrease in BUN and creatinine levels. During this time, regeneration of tubular epithelial cells occurs.

Postrenal failure results from an obstructive or mechanical process in the urinary tract (e.g., renal calculi or BPH) that interferes with the outflow of urine. Removal of the obstructive process usually restores renal function.

In older adult patients who experience AKI, evaluation should begin with an attempt to determine the underlying cause. Once the cause is corrected, renal function is typically recovered. Clinical manifestations of AKI include fluid and electrolyte disturbances, metabolic acidosis, and uremic symptoms (e.g., anorexia, nausea, anemia, fatigue, edema, and crackles). The patient may also have a history of exposure to nephrotoxic substances or a recent infection. Moreover, 90-day mortality is as high as 23% (Wiersema et al, 2019).

The diagnosis of AKI is made based on an elevated BUN level, an elevation in serum creatinine, and a decrease in creatinine clearance accompanied by decrease in urine output. In addition to correcting the underlying cause of AKI, treatment includes the correction of acidosis and hematologic abnormalities, the removal of nephrotoxic agents, and the maintenance of fluid hemostasis.

Chronic Kidney Disease

CKD is the presence of kidney damage for more than 3 months accompanied by a decrease in GFR (Box 20.6). The symptoms manifested depend on the extent of the disease. The five stages of CKD are as follows (Arora, 2023):

- Stage 1: Kidney damage with normal or increased GFR (> 90 mL/min/1.73 m^2).
- Stage 2: Mild reduction in GFR (60–89 mL/min/1.73 m^2).
- Stage 3a: Moderate reduction in GFR (45–59 mL/min/1.73 m^2).
- Stage 3b: Moderate reduction in GFR (30–44 mL/min/1.73 m^2).
- Stage 4: Severe reduction in GFR (15–29 mL/min/1.73 m^2).
- Stage 5: Kidney failure (GFR < 15 mL/min/1.73 m^2 or dialysis).

Typically, patients with CKD stages 1–3 are asymptomatic. On entering stages 4 and 5, patients may develop weakness, edema, fatigue, hypertension, heart failure, impaired cognition and immune function, dry skin and pruritus, anorexia, nausea, malnutrition, increased bleeding, anemia, peripheral neuropathy, and an overall decreased quality of life. Management strategies include treatment of the underlying cause of CKD, aggressive control of blood pressure (systolic blood pressure [SBP] ≤ 130 mm Hg and diastolic blood pressure [DBP] ≤ 80 mm Hg), treatment of hyperlipidemia, blood sugar control in diabetics (glycated

> **BOX 20.6 CKD By the Numbers**
> - Kidney diseases are a leading cause of death in the United States.
> - About 37 million US adults are estimated to have CKD, and most are undiagnosed.
> - 40% of people with severely reduced kidney function (not on dialysis) are not aware of having CKD.
> - Every 24 hours, 360 people begin dialysis treatment for kidney failure.
> - In the United States, diabetes and high blood pressure are the leading causes of kidney failure, accounting for 3 out of 4 new cases.
> - In 2019, treating Medicare beneficiaries with CKD cost $87.2 billion, and treating people with ESRD cost an additional $37.3 billion.

From Centers for Disease Control and Prevention. (2022). *Chronic kidney disease basics*. Chronic Kidney Disease Initiative. Retrieved from https://www.cdc.gov/kidneydisease/basics.html.

hemoglobin [Hb$_{A1c}$] < 7%), avoidance of nephrotoxic drugs (e.g., nonsteroidal antiinflammatory drugs [NSAIDs]), use of angiotensin-converting enzyme inhibitors (ACEIs), and angiotensin receptor blockers (ARBs) in individuals with proteinuria (protein > 300 mg/24 hours). Additional management strategies include restricting sodium, potassium, and phosphorus in the diet; restricting protein in the diet; restricting fluid intake; weight management and promotion of exercise; and use of multivitamins and iron supplements (see Patient/Family Teaching: Chronic Kidney Disease box).

PATIENT/FAMILY TEACHING
Chronic Kidney Disease

The kidneys perform crucial functions that affect all parts of the body. The kidneys, in fact, keep the rest of the body in balance and working properly. When CKD causes the kidneys to fail, the whole body stops functioning correctly, and the person can become extremely ill unless the condition is treated.

How Do the Kidneys Work?
The kidneys are the size of a person's fist and are located on either side of the spine. Each kidney has about a million working units called *nephrons*. Nephrons are the kidney's filters. Once blood is filtered, the waste products are removed from the body as urine.

The kidneys' job is to filter extra water and waste out of your blood to make urine.

The kidneys are also responsible for regulating the body's salts and minerals. Your kidneys also produce hormones that control blood pressure, make red blood cells, and keep your bones strong.

What Causes CKD?
CKD is a common disease in the United States. As many as 37 million people have been diagnosed with it. There are some risk factors for CKD:
- Diabetes can damage the blood vessels in the kidney and is the leading cause of CKD.
- High blood pressure over time can damage the small blood vessels in the kidney and is the second most common cause.
- Heart disease: there is a connection between kidney disease and heart disease. Researchers are working on determining the connection.
- Family history: if your nuclear family has CKD, you are more at risk.

Other factors to consider are age, and African Americans, Hispanics, and American Indians have higher rates of diabetes and high blood pressure, and those put them at higher risk.

What Are the Signs of Kidney Failure?
Because kidney failure sometimes gives no warning signs, it may go undiagnosed until it is well advanced. However, some warning signs may be present:
1. Decreased energy and fatigue
2. Trouble concentrating
3. Puffiness around the eyes
4. Loss of appetite
5. Nighttime muscle cramps
6. Swelling in feet and ankles
7. Dry, itchy skin
8. Urinating more frequently at night
9. Nausea and vomiting

How Is Kidney Failure Treated?
In the early stage of kidney failure, the disease may be slowed by ensuring control of high blood pressure and control of other chronic diseases such as diabetes. Additionally, the patient may be asked to take drugs to treat anemia, reduce swelling, lower cholesterol, and protect bones. The diet may be changed as well, to reduce waste products in the blood. However, as the disease progresses and the kidneys no longer perform their duties of removing bodily waste, other treatments must be used. Blood must be cleansed by using an artificial kidney (hemodialysis) three times a week at a special facility or at home, or by introducing a cleansing solution into the abdomen (peritoneal dialysis), performed daily in the home. Kidney transplantation, in which healthy, donated kidneys replace the failed kidneys, may restore normal kidney function.

Outlook
No cure exists for CKD. Following the program prescribed by the healthcare provider is vitally important as it helps people with kidney failure. Many people with kidney disease manage to live active, productive lives.

Data from The National Institute of Diabetes and Digestive and Kidney Diseases. (2017). What is chronic kidney disease? The National Institutes of Health. Retrieved July 24, 2023, From https://www.niddk.nih.gov/health-information/kidney-disease/chronic-kidney-disease-ckd/what-is-chronic-kidney-disease.

The diagnosis of CKD is usually made based on an increase in creatinine and BUN and a decrease in creatinine clearance. Additionally, tests are performed to evaluate blood sugar levels, parathyroid hormone and calcium levels, hematocrit and hemoglobin levels, other iron studies, and reticulocyte count. Urinalysis is performed to determine the amount of protein in the urine. The remainder of the evaluation is identical to that of a patient with AKI. Treatment of renal failure in an older adult is initially conservative. Older adult patients with kidney failure generally have concomitant diseases such as diabetes, cardiac disease, or cancer.

Nursing Care Guidelines for Kidney Disease

Recognize cues (assessment). Data collection should include a thorough health history and physical examination; special attention should be paid to the drug history. Box 20.7 summarizes the nursing history and physical assessment data to be obtained.

Analyze cues and prioritize hypotheses (patient problems). Appropriate patient problems for a patient with CKD include the following:
- Fluid overload resulting from compromised urinary regulatory mechanisms
- Inadequate nutrition resulting from anorexia
- Potential for infection resulting from a compromised immune system
- Need for health education resulting from a lack of exposure to disease processes, treatment regimens, and follow-up care
- Inadequate coping resulting from an uncertain outcome of illness

BOX 20.7 Recognizing Cues in the Nursing Assessment of the Renal System

History
- Personal or family history of renal disease
- Recent surgeries or illnesses (predisposing to renal dysfunction)
- Symptoms:
  - Urine (e.g., frequency, color, amount, and appearance)
  - Nausea and vomiting
  - Anorexia
  - Weight loss
  - Confusion
  - Fatigue
  - Pruritus
  - Edema
- Drugs (e.g., antibiotics, antineoplastics, and nonsteroidal anti-inflammatory drugs)
- Diet
- Current support systems

Physical Assessment
- Neurologic status: altered mental status and presence of asterixis
- Cardiopulmonary status: rales and pericardial rub
- Gastrointestinal status: nausea and vomiting, abdominal discomfort, and intolerance to diet
- Musculoskeletal status
- Ophthalmoscopic examination and visual inspection

- Reduced stamina resulting from fatigue
- Inadequate toileting self-care resulting from weakness and fatigue
- Potential for reduced skin integrity resulting from pruritus and immobility
- Reduced cardiac output resulting from fluid volume excess
- Alteration of protective mechanisms resulting from nutritional deficiencies (anemia)
- Inadequate sexuality pattern resulting from uremia and the psychologic effects of CKD

Generate solutions (planning). The development of a care plan for an older adult with renal failure must include the patient and family or significant others because of the potential for self-care deficits. Expected outcomes include the following:

1. The patient will achieve a normal level of fluid volume use, as evidenced by the re-establishment of baseline "dry" weight.
2. The patient will consume a well-balanced, appropriately restricted diet on a regular basis.
3. The patient will remain free from infection, as evidenced by an afebrile state during hospitalization.
4. The patient will demonstrate knowledge of the disease process and therapeutic regimen, as evidenced by adherence to prescribed self-care and other treatment measures.
5. The patient will demonstrate the use of effective coping strategies, as evidenced by the verbalization of feelings and seeking support.
6. The patient will demonstrate the ability to carry out ADLs without undue stress or fatigue.
7. The patient will maintain skin integrity, as evidenced by no reddened areas or broken skin.
8. The patient will have adequate cardiac output, as evidenced by the absence of pulmonary crackles.
9. The patient maintains hemoglobin above 10 g/dL.
10. The patient and partner express satisfaction with the expression of intimacy.

Take actions (nursing interventions). Interventions for an older adult with renal failure should focus on maintaining fluid and electrolyte balances; monitoring nephrotic symptoms; educating about treatment regimens (Box 20.8), dietary management, and drug usage; and managing fatigue and low energy levels. Patients and their significant others must be educated on the interventions. The typically prescribed diet is a low-protein, low-sodium, low-potassium, and low-phosphorus diet. At times, the diet is less than palatable, so with the normal age-related changes in the sense of taste and smell, adherence to a renal diet presents a challenge. The use of spices and seasonings to enhance taste may be helpful. For those individuals with CKD who experience nausea resulting from uremic symptoms, it might be beneficial to administer a prescribed antiemetic before meals (Box 20.9 and Patient/Family Teaching: Management of Kidney Disease).

BOX 20.8 Dialysis Therapies

Many factors determine the choice of hemodialysis or peritoneal dialysis (Fig. 20.4).

Hemodialysis is more appropriate for persons with recent abdominal surgery, other abdominal wounds, or defects in the abdominal wall. Hemodialysis is performed three times a week for 3–5 hours. Hemodialysis can take place at a center where dialysis staff manage the treatment. Or, it can be performed at home, where a care partner can help with the treatments. People treated at home typically have longer lives with improved quality of life. Common complications of hemodialysis include hypotension. Additionally, vascular access patients may become infected or develop thrombosis or stenosis. Treatment of stenosis or thrombosis includes angioplasty, stenting, or surgery.

Peritoneal dialysis is better tolerated by people with blood pressure fluctuations. Peritoneal dialysis is performed at home. There are two types of peritoneal dialysis (with several subtypes that are not discussed in this text).

- Continuous ambulator peritoneal dialysis does not require a machine to make the exchanges. The adult infuses 2–3 liters of dialysate into the abdomen four to five times per day. At night, the dialysate remains in the abdomen for 8–12 hours. After the specified dwell time, the dialysate is manually drained.
- Continuous cycle peritoneal dialysis uses a long daytime dwell (12 to 15 hours) and three to six nighttime exchanges performed with an automated cycler.

Peritonitis is the most common complication of peritoneal dialysis. Signs and symptoms include abdominal pain, cloudy peritoneal fluid, fever, and nausea. Peritonitis is treated with antibiotic therapy.

Data from Hechanova, L. A. (2022). Dialysis. In *Merk Manual Consumer Version* [website]. Retrieved From https://www.merckmanuals.com/home/kidney-and-urinary-tract-disorders/dialysis/dialysis.

BOX 20.9 Diet for CKD

The Kidney Foundation has chapters in most states. It is a good place for people with kidney disease and their families to find programs and information. You need to take in enough calories each day to keep you healthy and prevent the breakdown of body tissue. Ask your provider and dietitian what your ideal weight should be. Weigh yourself every morning to make sure you are meeting this goal.

Carbohydrates

If you do not have a problem eating carbohydrates, these foods are a good source of energy. If your provider has recommended a low-protein diet, you may replace the calories from protein with:
- Fruits, bread, grains, and vegetables. These foods provide energy, as well as fiber, minerals, and vitamins.
- Hard candies, sugar, honey, and jelly. If needed, you can even eat high-calorie desserts such as pies, cakes, or cookies, if you limit desserts made with dairy, chocolate, nuts, or bananas.

Fats

Fats can be a good source of calories. Make sure to use monounsaturated and polyunsaturated fats (olive oil, canola oil, and safflower oil) to protect your heart health. Talk to your provider or dietitian about fats and cholesterol that may increase your risk for heart problems.

Protein

Low-protein diets may be helpful before you start dialysis. Your provider or dietitian may advise a lower-protein diet based on your weight, stage of disease, how much muscle you have, and other factors. But you still need enough protein, so work with your provider to find the right diet for you.

Once you start dialysis, you will need to eat more protein. A high-protein diet with fish, poultry, pork, or eggs at every meal may be recommended.

People on dialysis should eat 8–10 ounces (225–280 grams) of high-protein foods each day. Your provider or dietitian may suggest adding egg whites, egg white powder, or protein powder.

Calcium and Phosphorous

The minerals calcium and phosphorous will be checked often. Even in the early stages of CKD, phosphorous levels in the blood can get too high. This can cause:
- Low calcium. This causes the body to pull calcium from your bones, which can make your bones weaker and more likely to break.
- Itching

You will need to limit the number of dairy foods you eat, because they contain large amounts of phosphorus. This includes milk, yogurt, and cheese. Some dairy foods are lower in phosphorous, including:
- Tub margarine
- Butter
- Cream, ricotta, brie cheese
- Heavy cream
- Sherbet
- Nondairy whipped toppings

You may need to take calcium supplements to prevent bone disease and vitamin D to control the balance of calcium and phosphorous in your body. Ask your provider or dietitian about how best to get these nutrients.

Your provider may recommend medicines called "phosphorous binders" if diet changes alone do not work to control the balance of this mineral in your body.

Fluids

In the early stages of kidney failure, you do not need to limit the fluid you drink. But, as your condition gets worse, or when you are on dialysis, you will need to watch the amount of liquid you take in.

In between dialysis sessions, fluid can build up in the body. Too much fluid will lead to shortness of breath, an emergency that needs immediate medical attention.

Your provider and dialysis nurse will let you know how much you should drink every day. Keep a count of foods that contain a lot of water, such as soups, fruit-flavored gelatin, fruit-flavored ice pops, ice cream, grapes, melons, lettuce, tomatoes, and celery.

Use smaller cups or glasses, and turn over your cup after you have finished it. Tips to keep from becoming thirsty include:
- Avoid salty foods
- Freeze some juice in an ice cube tray and eat it like a fruit-flavored ice pop (you must count these ice cubes in your daily amount of fluids)
- Stay cool on hot days

Salt or Sodium

Reducing sodium in your diet helps you control high blood pressure. It also keeps you from being thirsty and prevents your body from holding onto extra fluid. Look for these words on food labels:
- Low-sodium
- No salt added
- Sodium-free
- Sodium-reduced
- Unsalted

Check all labels to see how much salt or sodium foods contain per serving. Also, avoid foods that list salt near the beginning of the ingredients. Look for products with less than 100 milligrams (mg) of salt per serving.

DO NOT use salt when cooking, and take the salt shaker away from the table. Most other herbs are safe, and you can use them to flavor your food instead of salt.

DO NOT use salt substitutes because they contain potassium. People with CKD also need to limit their potassium.

Potassium

Normal blood levels of potassium help keep your heart beating steadily. However, too much potassium can build up when the kidneys no longer function well. Dangerous heart rhythms may result, which can lead to death.

Fruits and vegetables contain large amounts of potassium, and for that reason, they should be avoided to maintain a healthy heart.

Choosing the right item from each food group can help control your potassium levels.

When eating fruits:
- Choose peaches, grapes, pears, apples, berries, pineapple, plums, tangerines, and watermelon.
- Limit or avoid oranges and orange juice, nectarines, kiwis, raisins or other dried fruit, bananas, cantaloupe, honeydew, prunes, and nectarines.

When eating vegetables:
- Choose broccoli, cabbage, carrots, cauliflower, celery, cucumber, eggplant, green and wax beans, lettuce, onion, peppers, watercress, zucchini, and yellow squash.
- Limit or avoid asparagus, avocado, potatoes, tomatoes or tomato sauce, winter squash, pumpkin, and cooked spinach.

Iron

People with advanced kidney failure also have anemia and usually need extra iron.

Many foods contain extra iron (liver, beef, pork, chicken, lima and kidney beans, and iron-fortified cereals). Talk to your provider or dietitian about foods with iron that you can eat because of your kidney disease.

From *MedlinePlus* [Internet]. Bethesda, MD: National Library of Medicine (US). *Diet – chronic kidney disease*. Reviewed 2021. Retrieved July 24, 2023 from https://medlineplus.gov/ency/article/002442.htm.

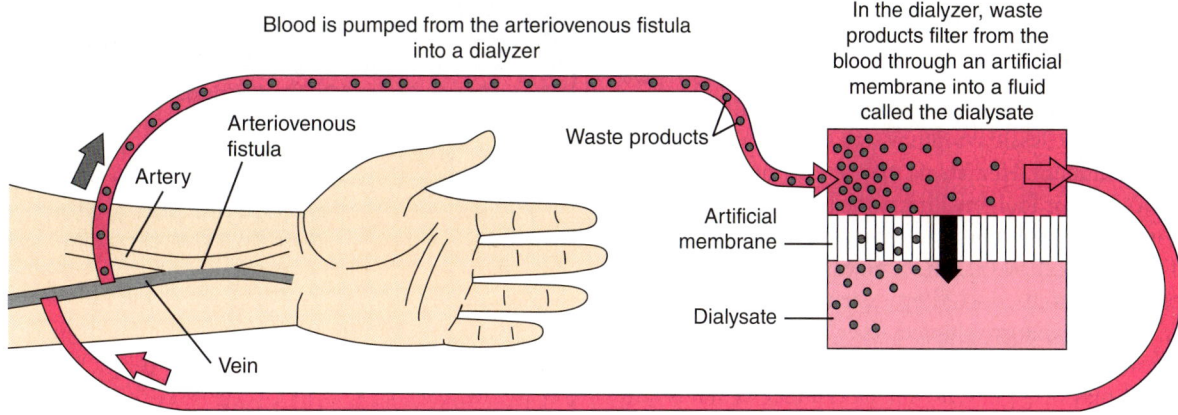

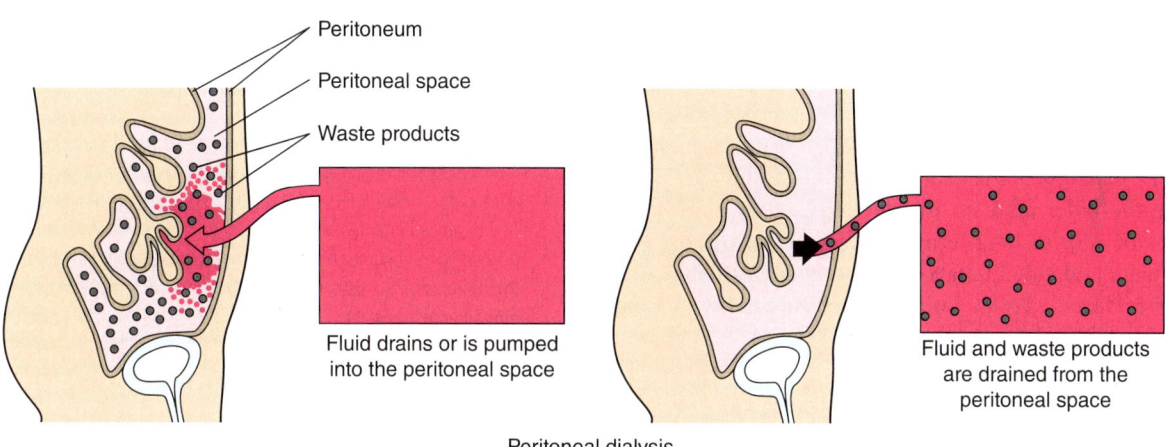

Fig. 20.4 Comparing hemodialysis with peritoneal dialysis. (From the MSD Manual Professional Version, edited by Sandy Falk. Copyright © 2024 Merck & Co., Inc., Rahway, NJ, USA and its affiliates. All rights reserved. Available at https://www.msdmanuals.com/professional. Accessed May 2024.)

PATIENT/FAMILY TEACHING
Management of Kidney Disease

Ten ways to manage kidney disease:
1. Control your blood pressure.
2. Meet your blood glucose goal if you have diabetes.
3. Work with your health care team to monitor your kidney health.
4. Take medicines as prescribed.
5. Work with a dietitian to develop a meal plan.
6. Make physical activity part of your routine.
7. Aim for a healthy weight.
8. Get enough sleep.
9. Stop smoking.
10. Find healthy ways to cope with stress and depression.

From National Institute of Diabetes and Digestive and Kidney Diseases. (2016). *Managing chronic kidney disease*. National Institutes of Health. Retrieved from https://www.niddk.nih.gov/health-information/kidney-disease/chronic-kidney-disease-ckd/managing.

With the varied treatment options available to individuals with renal failure, it is important to educate patients and significant others about prescribed modalities. The National Kidney Foundation provides patient and family resources helpful to persons with CKD.

Evaluate outcomes (evaluation). Evaluation is an important component in the care of older adults with CKD. Subjective data include the patient's reported symptoms and quality of life. Objective data include improved or stable renal function, as evidenced by stable levels of BUN and creatinine, hematocrit, and fluid and electrolytes.

Urinary Tract Infection

UTIs and asymptomatic bacteriuria are common in the older adult population. The prevalence of bacteriuria increases dramatically in females and males older than the age of 80. The incidence of bacteriuria is higher in females than males, partly because of the proximity of the urethral meatus to the rectum. The incidence is also higher for residents of long-term care facilities compared with those living at home. Higher rates of bacteriuria in nursing facilities are likely caused by the increased incidence of bowel and bladder incontinence, functional disability, and dementia. *Escherichia coli* continues to be the most common infectious organism. Other common organisms are *Klebsiella, Proteus, Enterobacter,* and *Pseudomonas* (Rodriguez-Mañas, 2020). Methicillin-resistant *Staphylococcus aureus* (MRSA), vancomycin-resistant *Enterococcus* (VRE), and fluoroquinolone-resistant Gram-negative bacilli are becoming more prevalent as the causative organisms found in UTIs, especially in the long-term care setting.

Symptomatic UTIs in older adults result in over 551,000 hospitalizations per year (U.S. Department of Health and Human Services, n.d.). Classic symptoms of a UTI include dysuria, frequency, and urgency. Hematuria may or may not be present. In isolation, cloudy or foul-smelling urine is not an indicator of UTI, as it is also present in asymptomatic bacteriuria or dehydration (Franks, 2022). A UTI in an older adult often presents with atypical symptoms, including delirium (Krinitski et al, 2021), confusion, lethargy, blunted fever, new-onset incontinence, and anorexia (Rodriguez-Mañas, 2020). Older adults with dementia may also present with altered mental status and agitation (Sabih and Leslie, 2022). Left untreated, UTIs can lead to kidney failure or death in older adults (U.S. Department of Health and Human Services, n.d.)

Asymptomatic Bacteriuria

Asymptomatic bacteriuria (ASB) is defined as ≥100,000 colony-forming units per milliliter (CFU/mL) without the symptoms of UTI. Changes in the urinary tract that occur with aging predispose the older adult to the development of ASB. Incidence rates of ASB in long-term care facilities are as high as 50% in females and 40% in males. For those with catheters, the prevalence is close to 100%. Guidelines advise against treating ASB (Franks, 2022).

Nursing Care Guidelines for UTI

Recognize cues (assessment). Data collection concerning patterns of elimination should be completed, and alterations in normal voiding patterns and symptoms such as burning, urgency, frequency, or atypical symptoms should be determined. The characteristics of the urine should also be noted. In addition, a mental status examination may be indicated, as older adults may experience altered mental status in the presence of a UTI.

Analyze cues and prioritize hypotheses (patient problems). Patient problems for an older adult experiencing a UTI include the following:
- Pain resulting from altered urinary elimination
- Inadequate urinary elimination resulting from the infectious process
- Need for health education related to unfamiliarity with the treatment of UTI

Generate solutions (planning). Expected outcomes for an older adult with a UTI include the following:
1. The patient will experience adequate pain control, as evidenced by reports of no further dysuria or burning with urination.
2. The patient will resume a normal voiding pattern, free from frequency, urgency, and dysuria.
3. The patient or caregiver verbalizes knowledge of the causes and treatment of UTI.

Take actions (nursing interventions). Nursing management should focus on the education of older adults, including appropriate perihygienic measures such as showering, front-to-back wiping techniques, adequate daily fluid intake, frequent bladder emptying, adherence to the prescribed drug regimen, and reportable signs and symptoms of a recurrent infection. The sterile technique should be used with urinary catheterization; the use of indwelling catheters should be minimized (Box 20.10).

Evaluate outcomes (evaluation). Evaluation includes ongoing data collection related to expected outcomes and documentation of findings. Documentation also includes routine vital signs, functional status, and other associated risk factors.

BOX 20.10 Indications for Bladder Catheterization

Examples of *Appropriate* Indications for Indwelling Urethral Catheter Use
- Patients have acute urinary retention or bladder outlet obstruction.
- Need for accurate measurements of urinary output in critically ill patients.
- Perioperative use for selected surgical procedures:
  - Patients undergoing urologic surgery or other surgery on contiguous structures of the genitourinary tract.
  - Anticipated prolonged duration of surgery (catheters inserted for this reason should be removed in PACU).
  - Patients are anticipated to receive large-volume infusions or diuretics during surgery.
  - Need for intraoperative monitoring of urinary output.
- To assist in the healing of open sacral or perineal wounds in incontinent patients.
- Patient requires prolonged immobilization (e.g., potentially unstable thoracic or lumbar spine, multiple traumatic injuries such as pelvic fractures).
- To improve comfort for end-of-life care if needed.

Examples of *Inappropriate* Uses of Indwelling Catheters
- As a substitute for nursing care for the patient or resident with incontinence.
- As a means of obtaining urine for culture or other diagnostic tests when the patient can voluntarily void.
- For prolonged postoperative duration without appropriate indications (e.g., structural repair of urethra or contiguous structures, prolonged effect of epidural anesthesia, etc.).

From Gould, C. V., Umscheid, C. A., Agarwal, R. K., Kuntz, G., Pegues, D. A., & the Healthcare Infection Control Practices Advisory Committee (HICPAC). (2009; updated 2019). *Guideline for prevention of catheter-associated urinary tract infections 2009*. Washington, DC: Centers for Disease Control and Prevention. Retrieved from https://www.cdc.gov/infectioncontrol/guidelines/cauti/.

EVIDENCE-BASED PRACTICE

Deferring Antibiotic Prescribing to Nursing Home Residents With Asymptomatic Bacteriuria: A Pilot Educational Intervention

Background
Overuse of antibiotics in nursing homes leads to multidrug-resistant bacteria, adverse drug events, polypharmacy, and increased costs. The purpose of the study was to determine the effectiveness of an educational intervention for clinical staff covering best practices for the management of asymptomatic bacteriuria. The primary outcome was the percentage of patients with asymptomatic bacteriuria who were treated with antibiotics before and after the educational intervention.

EVIDENCE-BASED PRACTICE—cont'd

Sample/Setting
Residents of long-term care facilities who went to Butler Memorial Hospital emergency department (ED), a rural, nonprofit organization located in Butler, Pennsylvania, between February 1, 2018, and November 10, 2018. Inclusion criteria in retrospective chart review: no urinary symptoms, discharged back to long-term care, bacterial growth in urine culture of at least 10^5 CFU/mL. Exclusion criteria: positive urine culture with more than three organisms. One hundred and five residents met the criteria; 73 in the six months before the educational intervention and 32 in the three months following. Of the 105 residents, 73 were females and 32 were males, with a mean age of 81.8 years.

Methods
A multifaceted educational intervention was provided to the ED staff, which emphasized the importance of not treating older adults with asymptomatic bacteriuria, who resided in long-term care settings. Educational content included current evidence-based information, clarification of misconceptions, and discussion of current cases treated in the ED. The intervention included a self-paced educational module presentation slides, pocket cards highlighting the Infectious Diseases Society of America guidelines for asymptomatic bacteriuria, and educational posters placed on the walls throughout the ED. Retrospective chart data was collected for 6 months before the educational intervention and 3 months after the intervention.

Results
Among the 73 residents with asymptomatic bacteriuria prior to the educational intervention, 16.4% were unnecessarily given antibiotics and discharged back to long-term care with a diagnosis of UTI. Following the educational intervention, 12.5% of the 32 residents seen in the ED were treated with antibiotics and given the inaccurate diagnosis of UTI, a reduction of 3.9%.

Implications
The results of this pilot educational intervention aimed at providers in a rural ED indicate that an educational intervention on asymptomatic bacteriuria may enhance antibiotic stewardship. Although this was a small pilot study at one hospital, further research conducted at multicenter sites may be beneficial for ongoing and future stewardship initiatives.

Data from Kennedy, E. (2020). Deferring antibiotic prescribing in nursing home residents with asymptomatic bacteriuria: A pilot educational intervention. *Journal of Infectious Diseases and Epidemiology, 6*(2).

NEXT-GENERATION NCLEX® EXAMINATION-STYLE CASE STUDY

Phase 1, Question 1

Scenario: A patient is brought to the ED by a squad following a fall and striking their head.

Nurses' Notes

Day 1
0930:
- The patient was admitted to the ED for evaluation after a fall in their bathroom last night. The patient does not remember hitting their head, just that their legs went out from under them, and they were on the floor.
- The patient lives alone and has three adult children who live in neighboring states.
- The patient has a history of heart failure, type 2 diabetes, hypertension, and osteoporosis. They were recently started on furosemide for symptomatic heart failure. The patient states that they missed a dose yesterday and took the medication with dinner when they remembered.
- The patient denies headaches, blurred vision, shortness of breath, or nausea. They are alert to person, place, and times. Hair is clean. Clothes are clean. The patient has a faint odor of urine.
- Lungs have faint crackles in bilateral lower lobes on auscultation, heart regular rate and rhythm with normal S_1S_2; faint S_3 audible. No murmurs. Abdomen with normoactive bowel sounds in all four quadrants. There is 2+ peripheral edema bilateral lower extremities. Extremity pulses are palpable throughout. Skin is warm and dry, with natural coloring.
- Vital signs: blood pressure 132/86 mm Hg, pulse 92 beats per minute, respirations 18 per minute, temperature 99°F (37.2°C), oxygen saturation 94% on room air.

Medications

	0600	0700	0800	0900	1000	1100	1200
Metformin 1000 mg twice daily Scheduled 0800 and 1700							
Glipizide 20 mg twice daily Scheduled 0730							
Sitagliptin 100 mg daily Scheduled 0800							
Furosemide 40 mg daily Scheduled 0900							
Valsartan 160 mg daily Scheduled 0900							
Calcium citrate 200 mg daily Scheduled 0800							
Vitamin D 1000 IU a day Scheduled 0800							
Risedronate 150 mg orally each month First Saturday each month at 0730							
Aspirin 325 mg each night Scheduled 2100							
Acetaminophen 500 mg ii 3 times per day Scheduled 0600, 1400, 2200							
Gemfibrozil 600 mg twice daily Scheduled 0900, 2200							

Continued

NEXT-GENERATION NCLEX® EXAMINATION-STYLE CASE STUDY—cont'd

Health History | Nurses' Notes | Medications | Laboratory Values

	Results	Reference Range
Blood urea nitrogen	24 mg/dL **H**	7–20 mg/dL
Creatinine	1.6 mg/dL **H**	0.7–1.3 mg/dL
Glucose	200 mg/dL **H**	70–100 mg/dL
Sodium	132 mEq/L **L**	136–145 mEq/L
Potassium	3.5 mEq/L **L**	3.7–5.2 mEq/L
White blood cell count	8.0×10^9/L	$4.5\text{–}10 \times 10^9$/L
Hemoglobin	12 g/dL	12–15 g/dL
Hematocrit	36%	36%–48%
Platelets	150×10^9/L	$150\text{–}400 \times 10^9$/L
LDL cholesterol	68 mg/dL	<70 mg/dL
HDL cholesterol	45 mg/dL	>40 mg/dL
Triglycerides	132 mg/dL	<150 mg/dL
Albumin	3.4 g/dL	3.4–5.4 g/dL
Aspartate aminotransferase	15 units/L	8–33 units/L
Alanine transaminase	30 units/L	4–36 units/L
Thyroid-stimulating hormone	5.0 µU/mL	0.5–5.0 µU/mL
C-reactive protein	1.2 mg/L **H**	0.3–1.0 mg dL
Brain natriuretic peptide	250 pg/mL **H**	<100 pg/mL
eGFR	60 mL/min/1.73 m² **H**	90–120 mL/min/1.73 m²
Hgb A1C	8.8 % **H**	<5.7%

Highlight the findings that require follow-up.

Phase 1, Question 2

Which additional information related to the incontinence history would be helpful or significant to the nurse? (Select all that apply.)

a. History of urinary leakage with urgency.
b. How often do they wake up at night to urinate.
c. Associated symptoms, like frequency.
d. Assessment of the home environment.
e. Evaluation of the patient's gait.
f. Determining a history of alcohol use.
g. If female, history of childbirth.
h. Ability to perform self-care.

Phase 2, Question 1

Scenario: The nurse gathers additional data on the patient.

Health History | Nurses' Notes | Medications | Laboratory Values

Day 2
1145:

- Accompanying provider on rounds. The results of the urine analysis are available, along with a preliminary culture.
- The patient requests assistance going to the bathroom. Incontinent × one during the night but remains dry during the day. Denies dizziness while standing. Steady on feet with standby assistance. Up to chair for meals. The nursing assistant helped the patient sponge bathe this morning at sink side.
- Denies pain or other discomfort. Provided with fresh ice water, a call light within reach, as well as a TV remote and cell phone.
- The patient reports mild shortness of breath with exertion and nausea.
- They are alert to person, place, and time. The hair is clean. Sitting on the side of the bed, wearing a hospital gown. The blue pad on the bed is wet and smells of urine.
- Lungs have crackles bilateral lower lobes on auscultation, heart regular rate and rhythm with normal S_1S_2; faint S_3 audible. No murmurs. Abdomen with normoactive bowel sounds in all four quadrants. There is 2+ peripheral edema bilateral lower extremities. Extremity pulses are palpable throughout. Skin is warm and dry, with natural coloring.
- Vital signs: blood pressure 138/86 mm Hg, pulse 98 beats per minute, respirations 18 per minute, temperature 100.0°F (37.22°C), oxygen saturation 94% on room air. Finger-stick blood glucose this morning was 225 mg/dL.

Health History | Nurses' Notes | Medications | Laboratory Values

Test	Results	Usual Range
Urinalysis		
Color	Amber	Yellow
Appearance	Hazy	Clear
Glucose	2+	Negative
Bilirubin	Negative	Negative
Ketone	Negative	Negative
Specific gravity	1.015	1.002–1.030
Blood	Trace	Negative
pH	7.5	5.0–8.0
Protein	1+	Negative
Urobilinogen	1.0	0.1–1.0 mg/dL
Nitrite	Negative	Negative
Leukocyte esterase	1+	Negative
Microscopic		
RBC	Occasional	None seen/hpf
WBC	Trace	None seen/hpf
Epithelial cells	4/hpf	1–5 squamous/hpf
Bacteria	2+	0–1+
Culture Report		
Preliminary: >=10,000 CFU/mL of two organisms	Susceptibility testing pending	Final report: >100,000 CFU/mL Gram-negative bacilli

NEXT-GENERATION NCLEX® EXAMINATION-STYLE CASE STUDY—cont'd

Health History | **Nurses' Notes** | **Medications** | **Laboratory Values**

Antibiotic	MIC	
Amikacin	≤ 1	S
Ampicillin sulbactam	16	I
Cefotaxime	16	I
Ciprofloxacin	≥ 4	R
Gentamicin	≤ 1	S
Nitrofurantoin	≤ 1	S
Trimethoprim/ sulfamethoxazole	≥ 16	R

I = indeterminate; R = resistant; S = sensitive

For each finding, place an "X" to specify if the finding is consistent with the disease process of heart failure, UTI, or incontinence. Each finding may support more than one disease process.

Finding	Heart Failure	UTI	Incontinence
The blue pad on the bed is wet			
Crackles in bilateral lower lung fields			
Audible S_3			
Blood glucose is 225 mg/dL			
Urine protein 1+			
>=10,000 CFU/mL of two organisms			

Phase 2, Question 2
Based on the findings, which two (2) provider orders would the nurse expect at this time?
a. Restrict oral fluids to 1000 mL/day.
b. Foley catheter for gravity drainage.
c. Begin intravenous fluids, D_5 ½ NS at 125 cc/hr.
d. Acetaminophen 325 mg ii every six hours as needed.
e. Clear liquid diet; advance as tolerated.
f. Nitrofurantoin ER 100 mg twice daily for 5 days.
g. Bladder scan for postvoid residual.
h. Begin sliding-scale insulin before meals.

Phase 3, Question 1
Scenario: The nurse gathers additional data on the third day of the patient's admission.

Health History | **Nurses' Notes** | **Medications** | **Laboratory Values**

Day 3
1430:
Orders received to discharge the patient home.
The patient denies shortness of breath with exertion and states that nausea is resolved.
Alert to person, place, time, and situation. The hair is clean. Sitting up in a chair wearing street clothes. No residual odor of urine
Lungs are clear to auscultation, and the heart has a regular rate and rhythm with normal S_1S_2. No murmurs. Abdomen with normoactive bowel sounds in all four quadrants. There is trace peripheral edema bilateral lower extremities; wearing TED hose. Extremity pulses are palpable throughout. Skin is warm and dry, with natural coloring.
Vital signs: blood pressure 124/76 mm Hg, pulse 82 beats per minute, respirations 16 per minute, temperature 98.9°F (37.22°C), oxygen saturation 97% on room air. Finger-stick blood glucose this morning was 175 mg/dL.

Discharged home on:
Nitrofurantoin: 100 mg twice daily for 4 days.
Metformin: 1000 mg twice daily.
Glipizide: 10 mg daily.
Sitagliptin: 100 mg daily.
Furosemide: 60 mg daily.
Valsartan: 160 mg daily.
Calcium citrate: 200 mg daily.
Aspirin: 325 mg each morning with food.
Tylenol: 325 mg ii tabs every 6 hours as needed.
Prescriptions were provided for nitrofurantoin and furosemide.

Which discharge teaching would the nurse provide in preparation for the patient to go home? (Select all that apply.)
a. Call the provider if sclera become yellow.
b. Take furosemide no later than 2 pm daily.
c. Report a weight gain of 2 pounds in 4 days.
d. Use portable oxygen as directed.
e. Drink eight glasses of water a day.
f. Practice double voiding to empty the bladder.
g. Wipe front to back after using the bathroom.
h. Keep a three-day bladder diary.

Phase 3, Question 2
For each body system below, select the current assessment findings that indicate conditions have improved. More than one finding may be selected for each body system/function.

Body System/Function	Current Assessment Finding
Cardiovascular	❏ Oxygen saturation is 97% ❏ S_3 heart sound
Genitourinary	❏ No smell of urine ❏ Urine protein is 1+
Metabolic	❏ Blood sugar is 175 mg/dL ❏ Denies any nausea

Bladder Cancer

Bladder cancer is common and has a high rate of recurrence. The most common type is urothelial carcinoma. Other forms include squamous cell carcinoma and adenocarcinomas. The biggest risk factor for developing bladder cancer is cigarette smoking. Occupational exposures to dyes, diesel exhaust, petroleum products, and solvents increase the risk of developing bladder cancer. Exposure to arsenic may also be a risk factor in the development of bladder cancer. Chronic bladder irritation resulting from stones and chronic UTIs, as well as long-term indwelling catheters, are risk factors for the development of bladder cancer. Bladder cancer occurs more often in males than in females and more often in Whites than in other races (Babaian et al, 2023).

Painless hematuria occurs in up to 90% of patients and is considered the "classic" presentation. It may also be accompanied by dysuria, urgency, and frequency in roughly a third of patients. In more advanced stages, the patient may experience bony pain (particularly in the pelvis), lower-extremity edema, or flank pain (Babaian et al, 2023).

Nursing Care Guidelines for Bladder Cancer

Recognize cues (assessment). Data collection should include a thorough history with attention to changes in urinary elimination patterns, the presence of pain, hematuria, dysuria, urgency, frequency, and voiding of small volumes. Data collection should also include the results of urine studies, cytology, cystoscopy, biomarker testing, and other blood tests.

Analyze cues and prioritize hypotheses (patient problems). Patient problems appropriate for an older patient with bladder cancer include the following:
- Anxiety resulting from an uncertain prognosis
- Inadequate urinary elimination resulting from surgical diversion
- Distorted body image resulting from surgical diversion
- Inadequate coping resulting from an uncertain outcome of treatment
- Reduced sexual expression resulting from anatomic alterations

Generate solutions (planning). Developing a care plan for a patient with bladder cancer involves the patient, family, and significant others. Expected outcomes include the following:
1. The patient will experience reduced anxiety, as evidenced by a decrease in symptoms.
2. The patient will develop a routine for managing urinary diversion.
3. The patient will verbalize acceptance of urinary diversion and associated changes.
4. The patient will demonstrate the use of effective coping strategies, as evidenced by the verbalization of feelings and seeking support.
5. The patient will verbalize concerns about sexuality.
6. The patient will express satisfaction with alternative positions for intercourse.

Take actions (nursing intervention). Nursing interventions for patients with bladder cancer focus on patient education, psychosocial support, management of pain, and maintenance of adequate fluid and nutritional intake. Surgery is performed to remove the cancer; the type of surgery depends on the stage of the cancer. A transurethral resection of the bladder tumor removes noninvasive cancer. A partial or total cystectomy is used to remove invasive tumors. An ileal conduit as a means of urinary diversion is the most frequent means of managing urinary elimination following cystectomy. The social stigma associated with the excretion of body fluids into an external device compounds the patient's fears and concerns regarding the diagnosis of cancer. Because patients may have difficulty coping, it is important to encourage them to verbalize their fears and concerns and to refer them to the appropriate supportive services, if necessary.

If a patient requires chemotherapy, nursing interventions include monitoring for infection, irritative voiding symptoms, allergic reactions, and bone marrow suppression. Patient education should include instructions for follow-up care and the importance of cystoscopy every 3 months for 1 year, then every 6 months to 1 year thereafter. Patients who smoke should be counseled to stop smoking.

Evaluate outcomes (evaluation). The evaluation of nursing interventions is based on the achievement of expected outcomes. Documentation of ongoing biopsychosocial assessment is key to the provision of holistic nursing care.

Benign Prostatic Hyperplasia

BPH is an age-related enlargement of the prostate gland that constricts the urethra and obstructs the outflow of urine. Roughly 50% of males have histopathologic demonstrations of BPH by age 60 and 90% by age 85. The development of BPH is the result of structural, functional, and hormonal (testosterone and dihydrotestosterone) changes. About half of the males with histopathologic BPH experience lower urinary tract symptoms (Deters et al, 2023).

With early prostatic enlargement, the patient may be asymptomatic because the muscles compensate for increased urethral resistance. As the prostate gland enlarges, the patient begins to manifest symptoms of an obstructive process. Symptoms include frequency, urgency, hesitancy, a decrease in the force of the urinary stream, straining to initiate and maintain urination, terminal dribbling, a sensation of a full bladder after voiding, urinary retention, and nocturia (Deters et al, 2023). Urethral obstruction may cause urinary stasis, UTIs, hydronephrosis, and renal calculi.

The purpose of the diagnostic evaluation of BPH is to determine the extent of obstruction. Diagnostic evaluation includes a history and physical examination, digital rectal examination (DRE), urinalysis, and measurement of BUN and serum creatinine levels. Although BPH is not related to prostate cancer, a prostate-specific antigen (PSA) test may be ordered in some cases to rule out prostate cancer. Although not indicated as part of the initial evaluation of BPH, abdominal ultrasonography or cystoscopy may be indicated in persons with urinary retention, renal impairment, or suspected cancer.

Nursing Care Guidelines for BPH

Recognize cues (assessment). The purpose of the data collection for an individual with BPH is to determine the extent of prostate enlargement and its effect on function so that an

> **BOX 20.11 Recognizing Cues in the Nursing Assessment for BPH**
>
> **History**
> - General health
> - Functional status
> - Medical and surgical history
> - Current drugs
> - Voiding habits and patterns:
>   - The initiation and caliber of the urinary stream
>   - Dysuria
>   - Frequency
>   - The presence of obstructive symptoms:
>   - Diurnal frequency
>   - Nocturia
>   - Hesitancy
>   - Urgency
>   - Urge incontinence
>   - Incomplete bladder emptying
>   - Postvoid dribbling
>   - Signs and symptoms of UTI
>
> **Physical Examination**
> The physical examination is usually conducted by the healthcare provider or an advanced practice nurse and includes the following:
> - DRE to evaluate the size, shape, and consistency of the prostate gland
> - Abdominal examination to determine the presence of bladder distention, suprapubic tenderness, and costovertebral angle tenderness

appropriate plan of care can be developed and implemented. Data collection consists of history-taking, physical examination, and evaluation of voiding patterns (Box 20.11).

Analyze cues and prioritize hypotheses (patient problems). Patient problems appropriate for the patient experiencing BPH include the following:

- Inadequate urinary elimination resulting from bladder outlet obstruction
- Potential for infection resulting from stasis
- Reduced sexual expression resulting from erectile dysfunction
- Need for health education resulting from a new diagnosis

Generate solutions (planning). Expected outcomes for a patient with BPH include the following:

1. The patient will maintain a regular schedule of complete bladder emptying.
2. The patient will remain free from UTIs, as evidenced by using measures to prevent infection.
3. The patient will verbalize sexual concerns and describe measures to cope.
4. Patient demonstrates understanding of evaluation and treatment of BPH.

If surgery is indicated, expected outcomes might include the following:

1. The patient will have satisfactory pain control, as indicated by 3 or less on a 0–10 scale.
2. The patient will regain urinary control like that experienced in the premorbid state.

Take actions (nursing interventions). Nursing interventions for BPH focus on patient education regarding the diagnosis and management of the disease. Education regarding the management of alterations in urinary elimination should include the establishment of frequent voiding schedules. The educational plan should also include teaching patients about the sympathomimetic actions of decongestant drugs and diet pills, as they may cause acute urinary retention.

Nursing interventions must also consider the treatment regimen. For patients treated with nonsurgical methods, interventions should focus on education about the signs and symptoms of progressive BPH. As the prostate gland enlarges, the urine stream becomes weaker, hesitancy increases, and it becomes increasingly difficult to completely empty the bladder. Patient education should also focus on the drugs used to relieve symptoms, their side effects, and drug interactions. For patients undergoing surgery, nursing interventions should initially focus on immediate postoperative care. Most surgical procedures require general anesthesia and a short hospital stay. Interventions should focus on maintaining patients' levels of function and preventing postoperative complications related to immobility. Following discharge from the hospital, patients require education related to temporary activity restrictions, signs and symptoms of infection and urinary obstruction, and possible temporary incontinence. Surgical interventions may result in temporary sexual dysfunction; patients should be given the opportunity to verbalize concerns and to be referred to appropriate supportive services, such as a urologist or a certified sex therapist (see Patient/Family Teaching: Benign Prostatic Hyperplasia box).

PATIENT/FAMILY TEACHING

Benign Prostatic Hyperplasia (BPH)

Lifestyle, dietary, and other factors may be included in the treatment of BPH.

- Lifestyle factors: Limit fluid intake in the evening and before bed, empty bladder before going to bed, lose weight, and increase physical activity.
- Dietary factors: Reduce intake of alcohol, coffee, and other foods or fluids that may irritate the bladder. Eat a healthy diet high in fruits and vegetables.
- Avoid using decongestants and antihistamines (over-the-counter cold and allergy medications). Some antidepressants and diuretics may worsen symptoms and require discussion with the provider.
- Kegel exercises can help prevent leaking urine.
- Double void: After emptying the bladder, wait a moment, then try to urinate again.
- Prevent and/or treat constipation.
- Empty bladder when the urge is first felt. Try to urinate at least every 3 hours. Do not strain to empty the bladder.

Mild enlargement of the prostate may not require treatment. After a complete evaluation, the patient, family, and provider decide the need to start treatment.

Treatment includes watchful waiting—only 57% of BPH symptoms progress in 9 years, and only 10% require surgical intervention. Several medications are available that help shrink the prostate and relax muscles around the urethra,

Continued

> **PATIENT/FAMILY TEACHING—cont'd**
>
> making it easier to empty the bladder (alpha-blockers, phosphodiesterase inhibitors, and alpha-reductase inhibitors). Should surgery be necessary, several procedures are available to reduce the size of the middle lobes of the prostate. Newer procedures do not result in erectile dysfunction.
>
> Seek medical care if these symptoms occur:
> - Fever (≥100.4° F; 38° C); chills; back, side, or abdominal pain
> - Pain with urination and blood or pus in urine
> - Inability to urinate

Data from: De Pietro, M. (2019). What is benign prostatic hyperplasia? MedicalNewsToday.com [website]. Available at: https://www.medicalnewstoday.com/articles/314998. Accessed May 1, 2024; University of Rochester Medical Center. (2024). Benign prostatic hyperplasia (BPH). Available at: https://www.urmc.rochester.edu/encyclopedia/content.aspx?ContentTypeID=85&ContentID=P01470. Accessed May 1, 2024; Mason, N., Read, A., & Powley, G. (2019). Patient Fact Sheet: Benign prostatic hyperplasia. Society of Urologic Nurses and Associates. Available at: https://www.suna.org/sites/default/files/download/resources/SUNA_bphFactSheet.pdf. Accessed May 1, 2024; UpToDate. (2023). Patient education: Benign prostatic hyperplasia (enlarged prostate) (The basics). UpToDate, Inc. Available at: https://pro.uptodatefree.ir/Show/15355. Accessed May 1, 2024.

Evaluate outcomes (evaluation). Evaluation of interventions is based on the return of urinary function to the premorbid state, relief of urinary symptoms, avoidance or prompt management of UTIs, and a return to satisfactory sexual activity. Documenting the care of a patient with BPH includes noting the effectiveness of the nursing interventions, including validation that the patient understands the disease process, treatment regimen, and urinary elimination patterns.

Prostate Cancer

The incidence of prostate cancer increases with age; by age 90, it is estimated that 70% of males have some degree of prostate cancer. Prostate cancer is the most common form of cancer in males and the second-leading cause of cancer-related death. The rate of mortality from prostate cancer is higher among Black males than among White males. Risk factors include advancing age, family history of the disease, and Black race (MedlinePlus, 2022).

Most prostatic cancers are adenocarcinomas; other forms include transitional cell carcinomas, small cell carcinomas, and sarcomas. Prostate cancer may metastasize through the lymphatic system and the bloodstream to the lymph nodes, bones, lungs, and liver.

Early prostate cancer is typically asymptomatic. As the tumor enlarges, the patient may experience a urine stream that is hard to start and weak, urgency, frequency, dysuria, and hematuria (MedlinePlus, 2022). If obstruction of the urethra occurs, the patient may manifest symptoms of postrenal failure. Other symptoms may include perineal and rectal discomfort, weakness, nausea, hematuria, and lower extremity edema (with metastasis to pelvic nodes). Skeletal pain and pathologic fractures may indicate an advanced disease with metastases.

It is important for males to follow the recommendations of the American Cancer Society about screening for prostate cancer (American Cancer Society, 2023):

- "Age 50 for males who are at average risk of prostate cancer and are expected to live at least 10 more years.
- Age 45 for males at high risk of developing prostate cancer. This includes African Americans and males who have a first-degree relative (father or brother) diagnosed with prostate cancer at an early age (younger than age 65).
- Age 40 for males at even higher risk (those with more than one first-degree relative who had prostate cancer at an early age)."

Men and their health care provider should discuss individual risk for prostate cancer, the pros and cons of the screening tests, and then decide if prostate screening is right for them (American Cancer Society, 2023).

Nursing Care Guidelines for Prostate Cancer

Recognize cues (assessment). Data collection for a patient with prostate cancer is essentially the same as that for a patient with BPH. The nurse should determine the patient's health beliefs and fears related to a malignant process.

Analyze cues and prioritize hypotheses (patient problems). Appropriate patient problems for a patient with prostate cancer include the following:

- Inadequate urinary elimination resulting from bladder outlet obstruction
- Anxiety resulting from an uncertain prognosis
- Reduced sexual expression resulting from treatment measures
- Need for health education resulting from a lack of previous exposure to treatment modalities and prognosis

Generate solutions (planning). Expected outcomes for a patient with prostate cancer include the following:

1. The patient's urinary elimination patterns will return to their premorbid state.
2. The patient's expressions of anxiety about the diagnosis, treatment, and prognosis will be replaced with an understanding of the prognosis.
3. The patient and partner will have a mutually satisfying sexual relationship.
4. The patient will demonstrate knowledge of treatment methods and prognostic indicators.

Take actions (nursing interventions). Nursing interventions for a patient with prostate cancer include educating the patient on diagnostic tests and treatment options. If surgery is indicated, nursing interventions should include the following:

1. Administration of analgesics for pain control.
2. Suggestion of options for sexual counseling if the patient indicates a need.
3. Education of the patient on the importance of a follow-up check of PSA levels and evaluation for disease progression.

If hormonal therapy is indicated, the nurse should educate the patient on the administration of intramuscular or subcutaneous injections. If bone metastasis has occurred, the nurse should encourage safety measures around the home to decrease the incidence of pathologic fractures. The patient should be educated on when to report symptoms of worsening urethral obstruction, such as increased frequency, urgency, hesitancy, and urinary retention (see Nursing Care Plan: Prostate Cancer box).

Evaluate outcomes (evaluation). Evaluation of interventions is based on a patient's relief of symptoms from the obstruction and his return to the premorbid urinary elimination pattern. The patient should verbalize an understanding of the disease process, the staging of the tumor, and the recommended treatment. The patient and his partner should regain satisfactory sexual relations. Documentation should include all ongoing assessment findings related to expected outcomes.

NURSING CARE PLAN
Prostate Cancer

Clinical Situation

Mr. C is a 68-year-old Black male. He has no major health problems. At his annual physical examination, he was found to have prostatic enlargement; serum PSA testing showed a level of 30 nanograms per milliliter (ng/mL). He then underwent magnetic resonance imaging (MRI) and was found to have a grossly enlarged prostate. A needle-guided biopsy was performed, and it showed adenocarcinoma of the prostate gland. Because of the large size of the prostate mass, evaluation for metastasis, consisting of bone scintigraphy and chest radiography, was performed. The evaluation did not show any metastatic disease.

Mr. C promptly scheduled a consultation with a urologist at a major medical center for the treatment of the prostate tumor. On evaluation, he was found to have stage C prostate cancer. The decision was made to treat the prostate tumor with a radical prostatectomy.

Mr. C, his wife, and children are experiencing anxiety, fear, and anticipatory grief related to the diagnosis. Mr. C lost his father 5 years ago to prostate cancer and has many bad memories of his father's illness and death.

Analyze Cues and Prioritize Hypotheses (Patient Problems)
- Anxiety resulting from the diagnosis of cancer
- Need for health education resulting from a lack of previous exposure to current treatment modalities and prognosis

Generate Solutions (Planning)
- Expressions of anxiety about the diagnosis and prognosis will be replaced by a realistic understanding of the disease and the likely prognosis, as evidenced by satisfactory engagement in activities.
- The patient and family will verbalize understanding of the treatment regimen.
- The patient and family will seek supportive services.

Take Actions (Nursing Interventions)
- Reassure the patient and family that prostate cancers are typically slow growing and treatable.
- Reiterate the explanation of the diagnosis and treatment. Include the family in teaching, whenever possible.
- Refer the patient and family to cancer support group services. Emphasize the importance of continuing present activities. Assist the patient in gaining awareness of anxiety.
- Teach the patient relaxation techniques.
- Provide written information regarding prostate disease and treatment regimens.
- Encourage the patient and family members to attend educational and supportive services provided by the American Cancer Society.

HEALTH PROMOTION/ILLNESS PREVENTION
Urinary Function

Health Promotion
- Follow a healthy diet
- Limit salt and caffeine
- Drink at least eight glasses of water daily, unless contraindicated by other chronic conditions
- Avoid alcohol
- Maintain a healthy weight
- Exercise regularly (at least 30 minutes of moderate activity a day, if able)
- Manage stress
- Avoid constipation
- Adherence to the prescribed bladder training program, exercises, and techniques for UI
- Adherence to a regularly scheduled program monitoring of conditions as appropriate (e.g., PSA, blood pressure, urinalysis, and laboratory tests)
- Prompt treatment of urinary tract symptoms

Disease Prevention
- Establish a routine pattern of urinary elimination
- Use appropriate hygiene measures to avoid urinary tract contamination
- Stop smoking
- Manage comorbid illnesses, such as hypertension and diabetes

HOME CARE

1. Regularly monitor and assess homebound older adults for signs and symptoms of exacerbation of a diagnosed renal or urinary disease or disorder.
2. Instruct caregivers and homebound older adults on reportable signs and symptoms related to the diagnosed renal or urinary system disorder and when to report these symptoms to the home care nurse or health care provider.
3. Instruct caregivers and homebound older adults on the name, dose, frequency, and side effects of drugs prescribed to treat the diagnosed renal or urinary system disease or disorder.
4. Assess functional and environmental factors that contribute to UI in homebound older adults.
5. Instruct caregivers and homebound older adults to keep a voiding diary to help the home care nurse establish the type of UI and plan nursing interventions.
6. Instruct caregivers and homebound older adults on behavioral interventions (e.g., bladder retraining and pelvic floor exercises) to treat UI.
7. If a homebound older adult is cognitively impaired, the success of behavioral techniques (e.g., habit training and prompted voiding) used to treat UI will depend on the caregiver's availability and motivation.
8. Instruct caregivers and homebound older adults on measures to reduce UI and maintain comfort.

SUMMARY

The changes that occur in urologic function with aging may be challenging. Impaired urinary elimination may cause problems that have a significant effect on day-to-day activities, self-concept, and functioning. The nurse's role includes assessment, patient advocacy, emotional support, and appropriate referral. Individualized care plans should be developed that focus on the promotion of self-care and functional ability (see Health Promotion/Illness Prevention box).

KEY POINTS

- UI is one of the most common health problems among older adults.
- Although the aging process does affect lower urinary tract function, aging alone does not cause UI.
- Drugs, including many OTC drugs, may cause transient UI.
- Functional and environmental assessments are important components of the evaluation of UI.
- Bladder diaries provide a more objective measure of the severity and type of incontinence than recall alone and should be part of the evaluation of UI.
- Behavioral interventions are the initial treatment of choice for many patients with UI.
- Cognitively intact patients with urge or stress incontinence often respond well to properly taught pelvic floor muscle exercises.
- Once a patient masters pelvic floor muscle exercises, the nurse may teach urge or stress strategies to prevent involuntary urine loss.
- Scheduled toileting, habit training, and prompted voiding may effectively reduce incontinence in patients with cognitive impairment, but the success of these methods depends on caregiver compliance.
- Aging affects kidney function; however, impaired kidney function is not a normal consequence of aging. Older adult patients must be assessed, and attention must be directed to adequate hydration, adjusted drug dosages, and the existence of comorbidities that may lead to renal dysfunction.
- AKI, which is classified into three types, is a reversible process. The nurse must focus on education regarding proper diet and drugs used to treat renal failure to halt the progression of AKI.
- CKD is not reversible but may be managed with drugs and diet modification unless it has progressed to end-stage renal disease; in this case, dialysis is typically required as a bridge to successful transplantation.
- Alterations in urinary elimination patterns are common in males with BPH. The nurse must be prepared to educate patients about drugs and Kegel exercises after surgery.
- PSA screening is a personal decision made after a discussion of the risks and benefits between the male and his health care provider.

CLINICAL JUDGMENT EXERCISES

1. Your 78-year-old patient complains that they have leakage of urine during the day. What additional information do you need to assess their urinary function?

2. An 82-year-old is admitted to the ED with confusion, nausea, fatigue, and a poor appetite. The healthcare provider orders a urinalysis with culture and sensitivity, BUN, and creatinine. Why does the healthcare provider suspect it is a problem?

REFERENCES

American Cancer Society. (2023). *American cancer society recommendations for prostate cancer early detection*. Retrieved from https://www.cancer.org/cancer/types/prostate-cancer/detection-diagnosis-staging.html. Accessed July 24, 2023.

Arora, P. (2023). *Chronic kidney disease (CKD)*. Medscape [website]. Retrieved from https://emedicine.medscape.com/article/238798-overview. Accessed July 24, 2023.

Babaian, K. N., Adams, P. G., McClure, C., Tompkins, B., & McMurray, M. (2023). *Bladder cancer*. Medscape [website]. Retrieved from https://emedicine.medscape.com/article/438262-overview#a7. Accessed July 24, 2023.

Batmani, S., Jalali, R., Mohammadi, M., & Bokaee, S. (2022). Correction: Prevalence and factors related to urinary incontinence in older adult women worldwide: A comprehensive systematic review and meta-analysis of observational studies. *BMC Geriatrics, 22*(1), 454. doi:10.1186/s12877-022-03111-6.

Bell, S. P., Vasilevskis, E. E., Saraf, A. A., Jacobsen, J. M. L., Kripalani, S., Mixon, A. S., et al. (2016). Geriatric syndromes in hospitalized older adults discharged to skilled nursing facilities. *Journal of the American Geriatrics Society, 64*(4), 715–722. doi:10.1111/jgs.14035.

Coyne, K. S., Wein, A., Nicholson, S., Kvasz, M., Chen, C. I., & Milsom, I. (2014). Economic burden of urgency urinary incontinence in the United States: A systematic review. *Journal of Managed Care Pharmacy, 20*(2), 130–140. doi:10.18553/jmcp.2014.20.2.130.

Davis, N. J., Wyman, J. F., Gubitosa, S., & Pretty, L. (2020). Urinary incontinence in older adults. *The American Journal of Nursing, 120*(1), 57–62. doi:10.1097/01.NAJ.0000652124.58511.24.

Deters, L. A., Costabile, R. A., Leveillee, R. J., Moore, C. R., & Patel, V. R. (2023). *Benign prostatic hyperplasia (BPH)*. Medscape [website]. Retrieved from https://emedicine.medscape.com/article/437359-overview#a1. Accessed July 24, 2023.

Dufour, S., & Wu, M. (2020). No. 397 – Conservative care of urinary incontinence in women. *Journal of Obstetrics and Gynaecology Canada, 42*(4), 510–522. doi:10.1016/j.jogc.2019.04.009.

Franks, S. (2022). Asymptomatic bacteriuria in institutionalized elderly. *American Nurse, 17*(10), 44–46. Retrieved from https://www.myamericannurse.com/asymptomatic-bacteriuria-in-institutionalized-elderly/. Accessed July 24, 2023.

John, G., Bardini, C., Combescure, C., & Dällenbach, P. (2016). Urinary incontinence as a predictor of death: A systematic review and meta-analysis. *PLoS One, 11*(7), e0158992. doi:10.1371/journal.pone.0158992.

Katz, S., Ford, A. B., Moskowitz, R. W., Jackson, B. A., & Jaffe, M. W. (1963). Studies of illness in the aged: The index of ADL—A standardized measure of biological and psychosocial function. *JAMA, 185*, 914–919. doi:10.1001/jama.1963.03060120024016.

Kegel, A. H. (1948). Progressive resistance exercise in the functional restoration of the perineal muscles. *American Journal of Obstetrics and Gynecology, 56*(2), 238–248. doi:10.1016/0002-9378(48)90266-x.

Krinitski, D., Kasina, R., Klöppel, S., & Lenouvel, E. (2021). Associations of delirium with urinary tract infections and asymptomatic bacteriuria in adults aged 65 and older: A systematic review and meta-analysis. *Journal of the American Geriatrics Society, 69*(11), 3312–3323. doi:10.1111/jgs.17418.

Lane, G. I., Hagan, K. Erekson, E., Minassian, V. A., Grodstein, F., & Bynum, J. (2021). Patient–provider discussions about urinary incontinence among older women. *The Journals of Gerontology. Series A, Biological Sciences and Medical Sciences, 76*(3), 463–469. doi:10.1093/gerona/glaa107.

Mathew, T. (2020). The Aging Kidney. *BMH medical journal* - ISSN 2348–392X, 7(Suppl). Retrieved from https://www.babymhospital.org/BMH_MJ/index.php/BMHMJ/article/view/230.

Milsom, I., & Gyhagen, M. (2019). The prevalence of urinary incontinence. *Climacteric, 22*(3), 217–222. doi:10.1080/13697137.2018.1543263.

Newman, G. (2020). How to assess mental status. In: *Merck manual professional version*. Merck & Co., Inc. Retrieved from https://www.merckmanuals.com/professional/neurologic-disorders/neurologic-examination/how-to-assess-mental-status. Accessed July 24, 2023.

Oelke, M., De Wachter, S., Drake, M. J., Giannantoni, A., Kirby, M., Orme, S., et al. (2017). A practical approach to the management of nocturia. *International Journal of Clinical Practice, 71*(11), e13027. doi:10.1111/ijcp.13027.

Patel, U. J., Godecker, A. L., Giles, D. L., & Brown, H. W. (2022). Updated prevalence of urinary incontinence in women: 2015–2018 National Population-Based Survey Data. *Female Pelvic Medicine & Reconstructive Surgery, 28*(4), 181–187. doi:10.1097/SPV.0000000000001127.

Payne, D. (2020). Managing incontinence in people with dementia. *British Journal of Community Nursing, 25*(9), 430–436. doi:10.12968/bjcn.2020.25.9.430.

Prostate cancer. (2022). *MedlinePlus* [Internet]. Bethesda, MD: National Library of Medicine (U.S.). Retrieved from https://medlineplus.gov/prostatecancer.html#. Accessed July 24, 2023.

Rodriguez-Mañas, L. (2020). Urinary tract infections in the elderly: A review of disease characteristics and current treatment options. *Drugs in Context, 9*, 2020-4-13. doi:10.7573/dic.2020-4-13.

Sabih, A., & Leslie, S. W. (2022). Complicated urinary tract infections. In: *StatPearls* [Internet]. Treasure Island, FL: StatPearls Publishing. Retrieved from https://pubmed.ncbi.nlm.nih.gov/28613784/. Accessed July 24, 2023.

Sharma, N., & Chakrabarti, S. (2018). Clinical evaluation of urinary incontinence. *Journal of Mid-life Health, 9*(2), 55–64. doi:10.4103/jmh.JMH_122_17.

Shenot, P. J. (2021). Urinary incontinence in adults. In: *Merck manual professional version*. Merck & Co., Inc. Retrieved from https://www.merckmanuals.com/professional/genitourinary-disorders/voiding-disorders/urinary-incontinence-in-adults. Accessed July 24, 2023.

Stewart, E. (2018). Assessment and management of urinary incontinence in women. *Nursing Standard, 33*(2), 75–81. doi:10.7748/ns.2018.e11148.

U.S. Department of Health and Human Services. (n.d.). *Reduce the rate of hospital admissions for urinary tract infections among older adults — OA-07*. Healthy People 2030 [website]. Retrieved from https://health.gov/healthypeople/objectives-and-data/browse-objectives/infectious-disease/reduce-rate-hospital-admissions-urinary-tract-infections-among-older-adults-oa-07. Accessed July 24, 2023.

Vasavada, S. P., Barat, O., & Leone, G. (2023). *Urinary incontinence*. Medscape [website]. Retrieved from https://emedicine.medscape.com/article/452289-overview. Accessed July 24, 2023.

WebMD Editorial Contributors. (2021). *What are vaginal pessaries?* WebMD [website]. Retrieved from https://www.webmd.com/urinary-incontinence-oab/what-are-vaginal-pessaries. Accessed July 24, 2023.

Wiersema, R., Eck, R. J., Haapio, M., Koeze, J., Poukkanen, M., Keus, F., et al. (2019). Burden of acute kidney injury and 90-day mortality in critically ill patients. *BMC Nephrology, 21*(1), 1. doi:10.1186/s12882-019-1645-y.

21

Musculoskeletal Function

Mary B. Winton, PhD, MSN, RN

http://evolve.elsevier.com/Yeager/gerontologic/

LEARNING OBJECTIVES

On completion of this chapter, the reader will be able to:
1. Describe the normal structure and function of the musculoskeletal system.
2. Discuss the age-related changes in the musculoskeletal system.
3. Discuss the nursing management of patients with fractures of the hip, wrist, clavicle, and vertebra.
4. Distinguish differences among osteoarthritis, rheumatoid arthritis, gout, and polymyalgia rheumatica.
5. Identify the nursing interventions associated with osteoarthritis, rheumatoid arthritis, gout, and polymyalgia rheumatica.
6. Discuss the pathophysiology, treatment, and nursing management of osteoporosis.
7. Describe the indications for amputation in older adults and the nursing management of these patients.
8. Discuss the causes and management of common foot problems in older adults.

WHAT WOULD YOU DO?

What would you do if you were faced with the following situations?
- You are taking care of a 75-year-old female who sustained a fracture of the proximal femur 3 months ago. She reports that she has completed physical therapy following the injury and is scheduled to travel overseas on a 10-day European river cruise in 6 months. She is inquiring about additional measures she can take to enhance her safety while traveling abroad. What do you advise her?
- Your patient is an 85-year-old male who has recently been diagnosed with polymyalgia rheumatica. He is currently prescribed long-term corticosteroids and has been experiencing multiple physical changes, such as increased bruising, weight gain, and an increased incidence of upper respiratory tract infections. He is requesting advice on how to maintain health while recovering from an illness while taking the prescribed long-term corticosteroids. What do you tell him?

Musculoskeletal problems are common among older adults. Recent reports have indicated that one out of five Americans has been diagnosed with arthritis. With the aging of the population, coupled with the high incidence of obesity, it is anticipated that the number of activity limitations attributable to arthritis and the number of people diagnosed with arthritis will continue to rise (Hootman et al, 2016). Complaints in the musculoskeletal system are common because normal aging predisposes people to the development of diseases such as osteoarthritis (OA) and osteoporosis (Browne and Merrill, 2015).

Diseases of the musculoskeletal system are usually not fatal but may lead to chronic pain and disability. Chronic conditions of the musculoskeletal system may contribute to impaired function and disability in older adults in the areas of self-care and mobility. They may suffer impairments in the ability to perform activities of daily living (ADLs) such as bathing, dressing, and eating, and impairments in the ability to perform instrumental activities of daily living (IADLs) such as managing finances, preparing food, managing transportation, and keeping house. Functional impairment of ADLs and IADLs may be devastating to older adults who desire to maintain independence. When dependence occurs, it may result in a loss of self-esteem, the perception of a decreased quality of life, and depression (Allen et al, 2016).

AGE-RELATED CHANGES IN STRUCTURE AND FUNCTION

The musculoskeletal system is affected in numerous ways by the aging process. A pronounced decrease in muscle mass and muscle strength occurs gradually over time. The actual number of muscle cells decreases, and they are replaced by fibrous connective tissue. As a result, muscle mass, tone, and strength decrease. The elasticity of ligaments, tendons, and cartilage decreases, as does bone mass, which results in weaker bones. The intervertebral disks lose

---

Previous authors: Laurie Kennedy-Malone, PhD, GNP-BC, FAANP, FGSA; Ramesh C. Upadhyaya, RN, CRRN, MSN, MBA, PhD-C.

water, causing a narrowing of the vertebral space. This shrinkage may result in a loss of 1.5–3 inches of height. The lordotic or convex curve of the back flattens, and both flexion and extension of the lower back are decreased. Posture and gait change. Posture, as a result of the changes in the spine, assumes a position of flexion. Changes in posture result in a shift in the center of gravity. In males, the gait becomes small-stepped with a wider-based stance. Females become bowlegged (genus varus), have a narrow standing base, and walk with a waddling gait (Manini et al, 2016). The articular cartilage erodes in older adults. It is unknown whether this is a result of the aging process or the result of wear and tear on the joints.

All the changes mentioned may cause pain, impaired mobility, self-care deficits, and an increased risk of falls for older adults. Approximately 25% of those aged 65 or older have falls each year. A recent report from the Centers for Disease Control and Prevention (CDC) found that, in 2018, over 3 million nonfatal falls resulted in emergency room care and more than 800,000 required hospitalization related to the injury sustained (CDC, 2023); moderate to severe injuries included hip fractures, lacerations, and traumatic brain injury (Gray-Miceli, 2017). Furthermore, of the 1.6 million residents in nursing homes, 50% of them fall each year (Agency for Healthcare Research and Quality [AHRQ], 2017).

Falls are the most common cause of traumatic brain injury, and 95% of hip fractures are related to falls (CDC, 2023). When falls result in injury and hospitalization, the risk of iatrogenic illness and immobility may lead to a downward trajectory, which may ultimately result in death. Falls may also cause a cycle of disuse. This pattern of disuse usually occurs after the individual has experienced repeated falls. The fall experience causes a fear of falling. To avoid falls, the individual decreases mobility; with decreased mobility, muscle strength decreases, joints become stiff, and pain develops, resulting in disability, loss of independence, and frailty (Gray-Miceli, 2017; Taylor-Piliae et al, 2017). Current research has documented that some of the diseases and decline in the musculoskeletal system may be reduced or prevented through the use of regular programs of active exercise and resistive muscle strengthening (CDC, 2016).

COMMON PROBLEMS AND CONDITIONS OF THE MUSCULOSKELETAL SYSTEM

Fractures are common among older adults and often result in some loss of function. A *fracture* is a break or disruption in the continuity of the bone. Fractures may occur because of major trauma, or they may be the result of pathologic processes such as osteoporosis or neoplasms (Wedrow, 2022). Osteoporosis makes bones more fragile, which increases the risk of fractures from minor falls or while performing normal activities of daily living (AGS, 2022). Weakened bones due to osteoporosis and falls are the most common causes of fractures in older adults. More than 25% of older adults aged 65 or older fall each year (NIA, 2022). The most frequently occurring fractures among older adults include hip, femur, wrist, and spine fractures. Fractures are classified as open or closed by the location and type of the fracture (AGS, 2022) (Fig. 21.1).

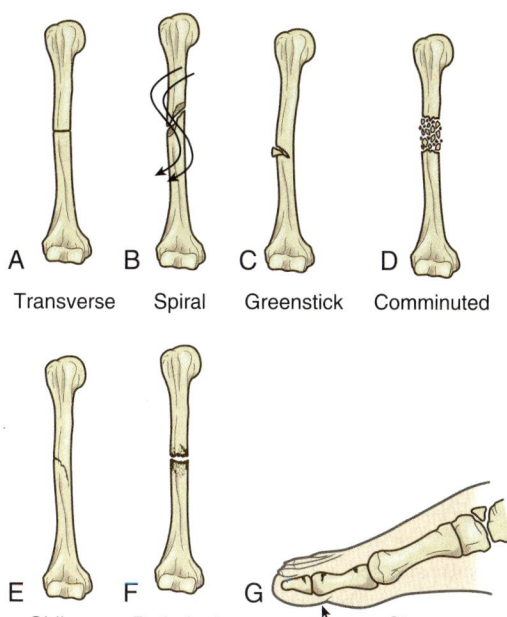

Fig. 21.1 Types of fractures. **A,** Transverse fracture: the line of the fracture extends across the bone shaft at a right angle to the longitudinal axis. **B,** Spiral fracture: the line of the fracture extends in a spiral direction along the bone shaft. **C,** Greenstick fracture: an incomplete fracture with one side splintered and the other side bent. **D,** Comminuted fracture: a fracture with more than two fragments. The smaller fragments appear to be floating. **E,** Oblique fracture: the line of the fracture extends across and down the bone. **F,** Pathologic fracture: a spontaneous fracture at the site of a diseased bone. **G,** Stress fracture: occurs in normal or abnormal bone that is subject to repeated stress, such as from jogging or running. (From Lewis, S. L., Bucher, L., Heitkemper, M. M., Harding, M. M., Kwong, J., & Roberts, D. [2017]. *Medical-surgical nursing: Assessment and management of clinical problems* [10th ed.]. St. Louis, MO: Elsevier.)

The history given by a patient with a fracture usually includes trauma followed by immediate local pain. Tenderness, swelling, muscle spasms, deformity, bleeding, and a loss of function are also seen with fractures (Corrarino, 2015) (see Emergency Treatment box). In addition to physical assessment, it is important for the nurse to carefully evaluate the older adult's perception of mobility and functional ability to determine preceding factors leading up to the fall and individualize care to maximize their function and mobility (Gray-Miceli, 2017).

⊕ EMERGENCY TREATMENT
Fractures

If a fracture is suspected, assess the injured area for the following:
- Movement
- Pain
- Color
- Temperature
- Pulse
- Sensation

If a fracture is open and bleeding is present:
- Apply pressure
- Apply sterile dressing
- Immobilize the fracture site

Hip Fracture

Hip fractures are the most disabling type of fracture for older adults. They are usually caused by falls and result in direct trauma to the hip. Approximately 25% of patients with hip fractures die within 1 year after the injury (AGS, 2022). The complications of hip fractures are generally related to immobility. They include pneumonia, sepsis from urinary tract infections, and pressure ulcers. With the growing number of older adults, especially those older than 75, it is expected that the incidence of hip fractures will increase (CDC, 2016).

Hip fractures are classified according to their locations. *Intracapsular* fractures, or subcapital fractures, occur within the hip capsule. *Extracapsular* fractures occur outside or below the capsule and are referred to as *intertrochanteric* and *subtrochanteric* locations (Fischer and Gray, 2020) (Fig. 21.2). Most common fractures occur at the intertrochanteric and femoral necks.

After the fall or injury that results in the fractured hip, the patient has an affected extremity that is usually externally rotated and shortened. Tenderness and severe pain at the fracture site may be present. Immediately after the injury, the joint should be stabilized until surgery. Controversy exists about the application of traction before surgery (Ikpeze et al, 2017; Ackermann et al, 2021; American Academy of Orthopaedic Surgeons [AAOS], 2021). Surgery within 24 hours of injury and pain management provide a more favorable outcome and decrease the risks of infection and delirium. If traction is needed, a Buck or Russell traction (Fig. 21.3) is used until the patient has surgery. The type of surgical repair depends on the location and type of fracture and may include internal fixation with pins, plates, and screws, or prosthetic replacement of the femoral head (Emmerson et al, 2023) (Fig. 21.4).

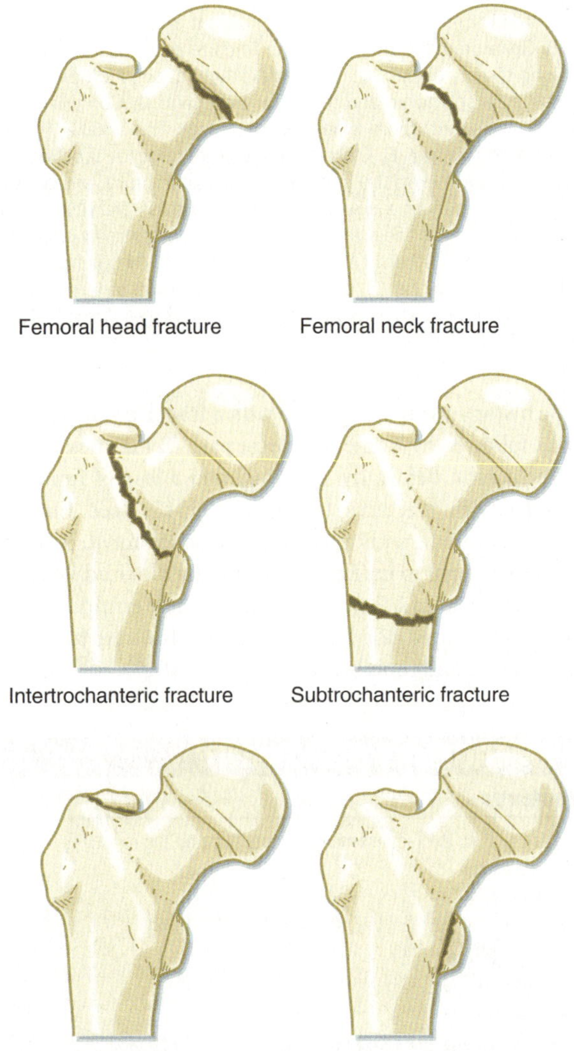

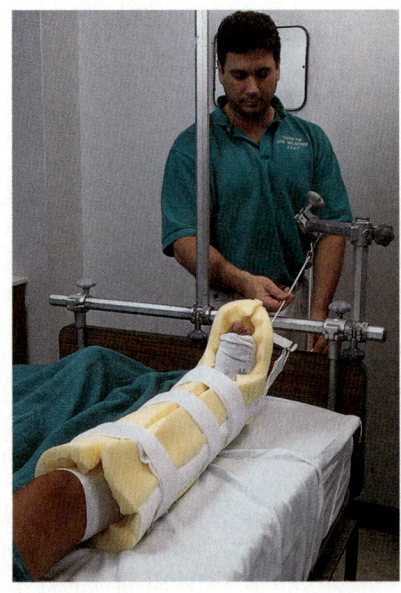

Fig. 21.3 Buck extension. The heel is supported off the bed to prevent pressure on the heel, the weight hangs free of the bed, and the foot is well away from the footboard of the bed. The limb should lie parallel to the bed unless prevented by a slight knee flexion contracture. (From Perry, A. G., Potter, P. A., & Ostendorf, W. R. [2016]. *Nursing interventions and clinical skills* [6th ed.]. St. Louis, MO: Elsevier.)

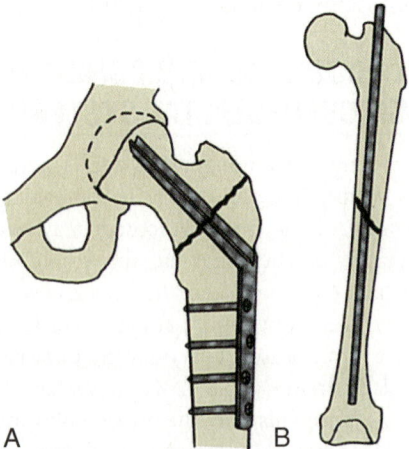

Fig. 21.2 Fractures of the hip. (From Adams, J. G., Barton, E. D., Collings, J. L., DeBlieux, P. C.C., Gisondi, M. A., & Nadel, E. S. [2013]. *Emergency medicine: Clinical essentials* [2nd ed.]. Philadelphia, PA: Elsevier.)

Fig. 21.4 A, Neufeld nails and screws, used in the repair of intertrochanteric fracture. **B,** Küntscher nail (intramedullary rod) used in the repair of the midshaft femoral fracture. (Modified From Monahan, F. D., Sands, J., Neighbors, M., et al. [2007]. *Phipps' medical-surgical nursing: Health and illness perspectives* [8th ed.]. St. Louis, MO: Elsevier.)

Nursing Care Guidelines for the Older Adult with Hip Fracture

Recognize cues (assessment). Hip fractures are most often related to falls. After any fall or other injury that may cause hip trauma, the nurse assesses the hips and lower extremities for evidence of fracture. This includes inspecting the site for direct evidence of fracture, shortening of the extremity, and abnormal rotation. Also assessed is the presence of tenderness, swelling, ecchymosis, or decreased sensation or circulation to the affected extremity (Corrarino, 2015). Note if the patient reports pain with any motion. Given that the injury was severe enough to sustain a fracture, the patient should be assessed for other injuries. On admission and postoperatively, the patient's cognition should be assessed to identify underlying dementia or acute postoperative delirium (Emmerson et al, 2023).

Analyze cues and prioritize hypotheses (patient problems). Patient problems for a patient with a hip fracture include the following:
- Pain resulting from the discomfort from the muscle and bone trauma
- Decreased mobility resulting from the immobilization of the fracture and the healing process
- Potential for reduced skin integrity resulting from immobilization required for healing
- Potential for infection resulting from inadequate wound healing, compromised nutrition, and the effects of immobility
- Inadequate bathing/dressing/feeding/toileting self-care resulting from discomfort and decreased mobility
- Inadequate home maintenance resulting from decreased independence and the recovery period needed for fracture healing

Generate solutions (planning). Nursing care for a patient with a hip fracture involves the perioperative, postoperative, and rehabilitation periods. Each of these stages of treatment and recovery requires specific nursing interventions and includes the following expected outcomes:
1. The patient will report an adequate level of pain control.
2. The patient will remain free from postoperative complications such as altered skin integrity and infection.
3. The patient will adhere to the prescribed physical therapy regimen to regain function in the affected joint.
4. The patient will be able to participate in physical and occupational therapies.
5. The patient will be able to safely demonstrate the use of assistive devices for mobility and ADLs.
6. The patient will be able to return to the preinjury level of independence with appropriate support and assistive devices.

Take actions (nursing interventions). On arrival in the acute care setting, the patient's hip should be stabilized and pain controlled. The patient should be assessed for any comorbidities that may delay surgery. Surgical intervention is usually warranted and is recommended within 24 hours of the injury. During this preoperative period, the nurse's focus is on keeping the patient comfortable and hydrated, and preventing complications of immobility. Preoperatively, hip fractures may produce severe muscle spasms, causing intense pain. Pain medications, traction, or immobilization and proper positioning are used to manage the pain. Preoperative education should include information regarding the surgical procedure, postoperative treatments, potential complications, and expected outcomes for rehabilitation and recovery.

The immediate postoperative period requires monitoring of vital signs, intake, and output. Turning, deep breathing, and coughing are used to prevent respiratory complications. The operative site is monitored for signs of infection and bleeding. Movement, circulation, and sensation of the extremity are assessed to determine impaired circulation. Mental status should be assessed and any changes noted. Postoperative delirium may occur in older patients after a hip fracture; the effects of surgery, anesthesia, analgesic drugs, loss of familiar surroundings, pain, and immobility may increase the potential for delirium. Care planning should include familiarizing the patient with his or her surroundings, providing for safety, instituting comfort measures, decreasing anxiety, and assisting with maintaining a sense of independence and identity.

EVIDENCE-BASED PRACTICE
Fall Prevention Program

Sample/Setting

This quality improvement pilot study examined the effectiveness of a fall prevention program in four assisted living facilities (ALFs) in North Carolina. All residents in the facilities were the intended population for the study. A target sample of 50 residents who met the eligibility criteria of 65 years and older, non-bed bound, or residents of a dementia or hospice unit were invited to participate.

Methods

The researchers collected data via observations, chart reviews, and conversations with the staff at baseline, and 4 months after the implementation of a fall quality improvement (QI) program. After consenting to be a subject in the study, the residents were assessed by trained researchers using the Morse Falls Scale and the Timed Get Up and Go Test. Additional data were extrapolated from the residents' Minimum Data Set scores that pertained to cognition and ADLs. The actual QI program was the Assisted Living Falls and Prevention and Monitoring Program (AL-FPMP). At each site, there was a dedicated team that oversaw all aspects of the program.

Findings

Of the 277 residents who were eligible to participate, 175 consented to participate; after 4 months, 146 residents continued in the program. The mean age of the participants was 85.7. Although there were challenges in each ALF to full implementation of the QI falls program, there was an improvement in participants' Morse Falls Scale, although the results were not statistically significant.

Implications

The need for a fall prevention program in ALFs remains great. To be successful, however, it was recommended that a specific falls team be established, that there be a "champion" who will lead the continued efforts of a program, that staff be trained to assess residents using the Morse Falls Scale, and finally that other programs that increase function and have been shown to reduce falls, such as t'ai chi and walking, be added to the AL-FPMP.

Data from Zimmerman, S., Greene, A., Sloane, P. D., Mitchell, M., Giuliani, C., Nyrop, K., et al. (2017). Preventing falls in assisted living: Results of a quality improvement pilot study. *Geriatric Nursing, 38* (3), 185–191.

Pain is managed through the careful administration of pain drugs. Because of the normal physiologic aging changes that affect pharmacokinetics and pharmacodynamics, older adults are at risk for developing changes in mental status, respiratory depression, and sedative effects with the use of opioid analgesics. These problems are prevented by the use of lower initial doses of opioids. The individual's response to the pain medication and the pain are closely monitored. After determining the patient's level of tolerance, the dose may be carefully increased. Keeping the affected extremity in alignment during turning also decreases pain. This is performed with the use of pillows between the knees or an abduction splint.

Another common problem a patient recovering from hip surgery has is constipation, which often causes fecal impaction because of the side effects of the analgesics and the hazards of immobility. Assess the patient's frequency of bowel movements and determine whether a stool softener and/or laxative are needed to relieve constipation.

Patients who have their fractures repaired with hemiarthroplasty are at risk for dislocation. The nurse should give the patient and family instructions on preventing dislocation. Dislocation may occur when the joint is adducted and internally rotated. Activities to avoid include crossing the legs and feet while seated, sitting on low seats, and adducting the legs when lying on the nonoperated side. The patient is instructed not to put on socks or shoes without the aid of assistive devices, not to cross the legs, not to lie on the affected side, to use a raised toilet seat and a shower chair, and to use a pillow between the legs while in bed. Activities that may cause dislocation should be avoided for 6 weeks until the muscles surrounding the joint are healed and the joint is stabilized. Symptoms of dislocation are sudden, severe pain, and external rotation of the leg.

After hip fracture and surgery, comprehensive interdisciplinary rehabilitation focuses on returning the patient to the prior level of function and preventing disability (Della Rocca et al, 2013). Specific areas of treatment are gait and transfer training, muscle strengthening through active assistive exercises, teaching the use of adaptive techniques for dressing, and teaching the correct use of assistive devices, such as walkers and canes (Fig. 21.5) (see Patient/Family Teaching box: Correct Use of Walkers).

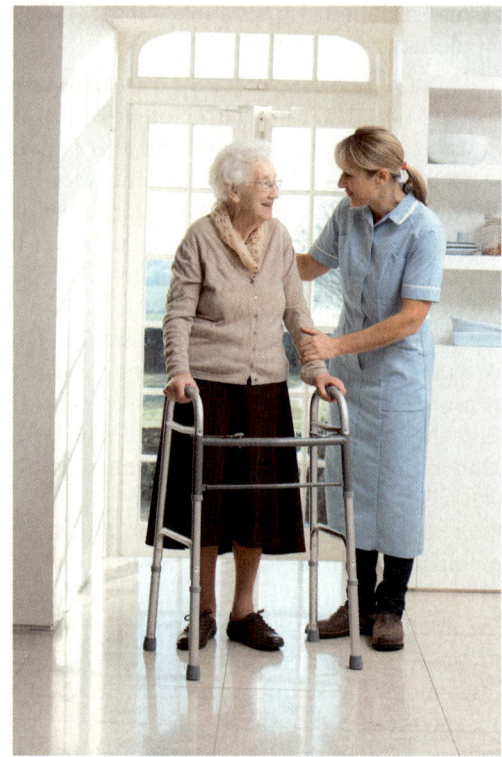

Fig. 21.5 Walking with a walker. The walker is moved about 6 inches in front of the resident. Both feet are moved up to the walker. (© monkeybusinessimages/iStock/Thinkstock.)

> ### PATIENT/FAMILY TEACHING
> **Correct Use of Walkers**
> - A walker should always rest on all four legs.
> - Correct body position should be maintained:
>   - Posture erect
>   - Elbows slightly bent
>   - Wrists extended
>   - Shoulders relaxed
> - Sturdy, comfortable, hard-soled shoes should be worn.
> - Walker first, then the affected leg. While supporting the weight on the walker, move the unaffected leg.
> - Be alert for hazards such as uneven surfaces, wet floors, or area rugs.

The loss of independence and decreased functional ability should also be addressed during rehabilitation. These losses may lead to depression. The nurse's role is to identify the patient's strengths, give positive feedback, and reinforce the progress made in achieving goals. Discharge planning focuses on using family and social support networks and ongoing therapy programs.

Evaluate outcomes (evaluation). Successful achievement of the expected outcomes after a hip fracture will allow the patient to return to a preinjury level of function. Those living independently should be successful in meeting therapy goals and should regain their self-care abilities, which will allow them to return home. Home health agencies may also be useful in successfully returning the patient to independent living.

Patients who were living in other types of health care facilities before the injury should be expected to return to their previous level of activity. Complications will prolong the recovery period and may lead to long-term changes in the level of independence. Patients should report minimum pain at the fracture or surgical site. The skin should remain intact. Muscle strength, joint movement, level of mobility, and degree of safety while performing ADLs should be continually evaluated throughout the recovery period. Continued physical and occupational therapies may be required to achieve goals and expected outcomes (see Nursing Care Plan: Fractured Hip).

NURSING CARE PLAN
Fractured Hip

Clinical Situation

Ms. W, an 86-year-old female who still works as an executive secretary, is admitted to the skilled nursing unit of the local hospital for restorative care after surgery for a fractured left hip. The hip was repaired with a femoral head prosthesis. Ms. W had a fall when getting on the city bus. Before this incident, Ms. W worked 3 days a week. Her general health status is good. She lives alone on the second floor of a two-story building. Her only family is a niece who lives 60 miles away.

On admission, Ms. W is a slender female who looks younger than her stated age. She is in no acute pain. The left hip incision is clean and dry, with the staples intact. Ms. W transfers with the moderate assistance of two people. During the transfer, she becomes tense and tells the nurses that she is afraid of falling and that she has to get on her feet so that she can get back to work. Because the surgical procedure has caused decreased range of motion and weakness in her left leg, Ms. W requires assistance with bathing and clothing for her lower extremities.

Analyze Cues and Prioritize Hypotheses (Patient Problems)

- Reduced mobility resulting from alteration in musculoskeletal function as a result of fracture and surgical repair
- Inadequate bathing and dressing self-care (bathing and dressing lower extremities) resulting from alteration in musculoskeletal function secondary to fracture and surgical repair
- Need for patient teaching resulting from limited exposure to home care programs

Generate Solutions (Planning)

- Patient will be able to transfer with minimal assistance.
- Patient will be knowledgeable about pain relief measures prior to transfer.
- Patient will demonstrate proper use of assistive devices for transfer.
- Patient will implement measures for self-care.
- Patient will familiarize themselves with home care programs prior to discharge.
- Patient will remain free from infection.

Take Actions (Nursing Interventions)

- Consult with a physical therapist for a program of muscle strengthening, transfer training, and gait training.
- Reinforce physical therapy training.
- Give positive feedback for gains made.
- Instruct the patient to take deep breaths and relax before transfers.
- Assist with transfers.
- Give specific instructions before transfers. Instruct on hip precautions.
- Teach the use of a walker.
- Give a pain medication 30–60 minutes before physical therapy.
- Consult with the occupational therapist for specific assistive devices.
- Teach the use of assistive devices.
- Allow adequate time for bathing and dressing.
- Assess support systems and the need for home services.
- Instruct on wound care, home safety, and home exercise programs.
- Plan for discharge with the patient and team members.
- Use community services, a visiting nurse, physical therapy, and a niece for assistance.

Evaluate Outcomes (Evaluation)

With proper interventions, outcomes include the following:
- Ambulate 50 feet with the assistance of a walker.
- Demonstrate the ability to bathe and dress themselves with the use of assistive devices.
- Verbalize knowledge of home care programs.

Colles Fracture

A Colles fracture is a fracture of the distal radius that is usually the result of reaching out with an open hand to break a fall. This fracture is seen most often in perimenopausal females, and although the incidence increases following menopause, the rate of Colles fractures remains relatively stable beginning at age 65 (Ensrud, 2013). Patients with a Colles fracture have pain at the site of the fracture that begins immediately after the traumatic episode, local edema, swelling, and a visible deformity from the displacement of the distal bone fragment. Treatment of a Colles fracture usually consists of closed reduction and immobilization with a forearm splint or cast. Nursing measures include elevating the extremity to decrease edema and neurovascular assessment to monitor for complications. The patient is instructed to actively move the thumb and fingers to improve venous return and decrease edema. Range-of-motion exercises for the elbow and shoulder prevent stiffness of the extremity.

Clavicular Fracture

Fractures of the clavicle, like Colles fractures, may occur after a fall on an outstretched hand or on a fall to the shoulder. Clavicular fractures are one of the most common fractures among older adults who fall (Wedrow, 2022). The majority of these fractures occur in the middle third of the clavicle. The patient with a fractured clavicle has point tenderness, local edema, and crepitus. The shoulder is noticeably deformed, dropping downward, forward, and inward. Treatment of most clavicular fractures includes placing the affected arm and shoulder in a sling while it is healing (Githens and Lowe, 2022). If the bone is significantly out of place or is broken into several pieces, surgery will be required for proper healing. Nursing measures include monitoring for neurovascular complications such as compartment syndrome, elevating the extremity, and instructing the patient to actively move the hand and fingers. Physical therapy will be required to maintain motion of the elbow and shoulder.

Casts and Cast Care

Casts are one type of device used to immobilize an injured body part. At the same time, casts provide a means of providing pain relief, decreasing swelling, and reducing muscle spasms (AAOS, 2020). They maintain proper positioning of the injured area, prevent further deformity, protect realigned bones, and promote healing. Used on the lower extremities, they may also allow for earlier weight bearing.

Casting materials include plaster or fiberglass. Patients are instructed to keep both types of casts dry; plastic or purchased cast protectors may be used during showering or bathing. Synthetic casts are immersed in water only with physician approval and should be dried thoroughly afterward. A hair dryer set at a low temperature may be used for this purpose.

Patients are instructed to keep the extremity elevated above the heart for the first 24–48 hours after cast application to decrease edema (Schweich, 2023). The patient should also be instructed to maintain movement of the extremity to prevent muscle atrophy and joint stiffness above or below the cast (see Patient/Family Teaching box: Cast Care). Ice can be applied to the cast to reduce swelling. Nursing care includes assessment for potential areas of skin irritation or breakdown. The patient should be instructed to report any redness or discomfort along the edges of the cast and any signs of drainage or odor coming from the cast.

> ### PATIENT/FAMILY TEACHING
> #### Cast Care
> Keep the casted extremity elevated for the first 24 hours.
> When the cast is wet, lift it with their palms.
> Observe the extremity for swelling, color changes, movement, and sensation.
> If any changes occur, contact a health care provider.
> Do not put anything inside the cast.
> Do not get plaster cast wet; cover with plastic for bathing.

A neurovascular assessment of the extremity is performed to determine that the cast is not too constrictive. Excessive constriction caused by the cast could result in compartment syndrome, leading to ischemia and tissue destruction of the extremity. Any change in capillary refilling, skin color, skin temperature, or excessive pain not controlled with pain medication or elevating the affected extremity should be immediately reported to the physician.

Casts are generally used to immobilize fractures for 6–8 weeks. A variety of assistive devices may be used for patients with lower extremity casts (Fig. 21.6). The nurse prepares the patient for self-care and the prevention of complications during this treatment period.

Osteoarthritis

Osteoarthritis (OA), also known as *degenerative joint disease,* is a noninflammatory disease of joints characterized by progressive articular cartilage deterioration and the formation of new bone in the joint space. This is the most common type of arthritis seen in older adults and the leading cause of disability in the United States.

The exact cause of OA is not well understood. Aging alone does not cause the degeneration of the joint. Age, trauma, lifestyle, obesity, and genetics have been cited as predisposing factors in the development of OA. The underlying pain associated with OA is related to pressure on the ligaments, bone spur formation, and the stretching of the joint capsule (Ashford and Williard, 2014; Ayhan et al, 2014). In OA, the articular cartilage thins and is lost, particularly in areas of increased stress. As the cartilage deteriorates, bone proliferation occurs at the margins of the joints. When the joint cartilage is lost, the two bone surfaces come into contact with each other. This results in joint pain. The distal interphalangeals, proximal interphalangeals, the carpometacarpal joint, the first metatarsophalangeal joint, the knees, hips, and spine are the joints most commonly affected by OA (Shelton, 2013; Onat et al, 2015).

The most common symptom is a gradual onset of joint pain. The pain occurs with activity and is relieved with rest. Stiffness may occur on awakening or after periods of inactivity that resolve with movement. *Crepitus,* a grating sound and sensation, may be heard and felt with range of motion in affected joints. Affected joints also have a decreased range of motion (Onat et al, 2015). The degeneration of the joint structure may result in muscle spasms, gait changes, and disuse of the joint. Bony

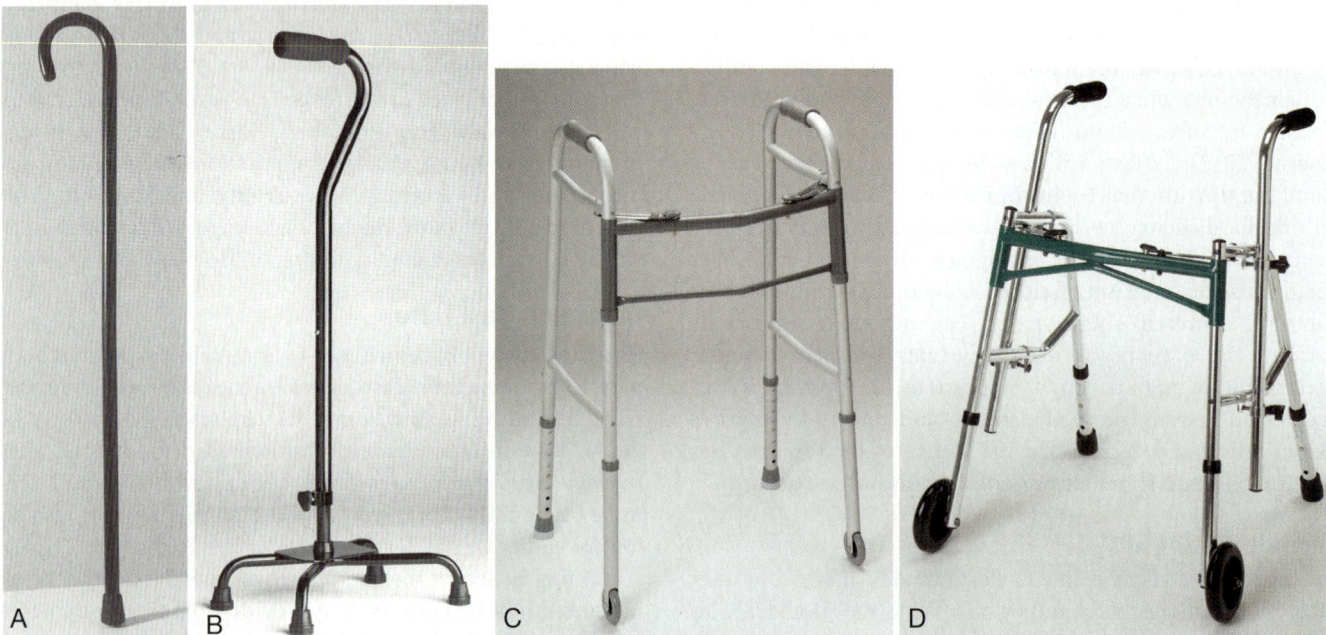

Fig. 21.6 Assistive devices. **A,** Cane. **B,** Quad cane offers more support than a single-stem walker. **C,** Walker with front wheels allow constant contact with the ground. **D,** Walker with adjustable front wheels. (From Cameron, M. H., & Monroe, L. G. [2007]. *Physical rehabilitation: Evidence-based examination, evaluation, and intervention.* St. Louis, MO: Elsevier.)

enlargements, called Heberden nodes, may be seen on the distal interphalangeals, and Bouchard nodes are the nodules of the proximal joints (Fig. 21.7) (LeBlond et al, 2015).

Nursing Care Guidelines for the Older Adult with Osteoarthritis

Recognize cues (assessment). Nursing assessment of a patient with OA begins with taking a thorough history of the problem. The data gathered includes information about the onset, location, quality, and duration of the joint pain. Inquire with the patient about the sensation of joint locking in the knee. Determine whether any associated muscle spasms have occurred (LeBlond et al, 2015). Questions about precipitating factors; medications used to relieve pain, including prescription and over-the-counter (OTC) agents; nonpharmacologic interventions, such as heat or cold therapy and exercise; and their effect on functional abilities should be asked. Affected joints should be inspected for tenderness, swelling, redness, crepitation, and range of motion. Note the presence of muscle atrophy in the surrounding muscles.

Analyze cues and prioritize hypotheses (patient problems). Patient problems for the older adult patient with OA include the following:
- Pain resulting from inflammation and deterioration of the joint cartilage
- Reduced mobility as a result of lower extremity joint stiffness
- Inadequate self-care is a result of limitations in joint movement and strength

Generate solutions (planning). The focus of the nursing care plan is to protect and preserve joint motion and function. Expected outcomes for the patient are individualized and specific to the joints affected. Outcomes include the following:
1. The patient will verbalize an improved level of comfort with activities.
2. The patient will be able to successfully use various adaptive devices to maintain independence in ADLs and IADLs.
3. The patient will demonstrate the safe use of assistive devices for ambulation.
4. The patient will demonstrate an understanding of the use of orthotics.

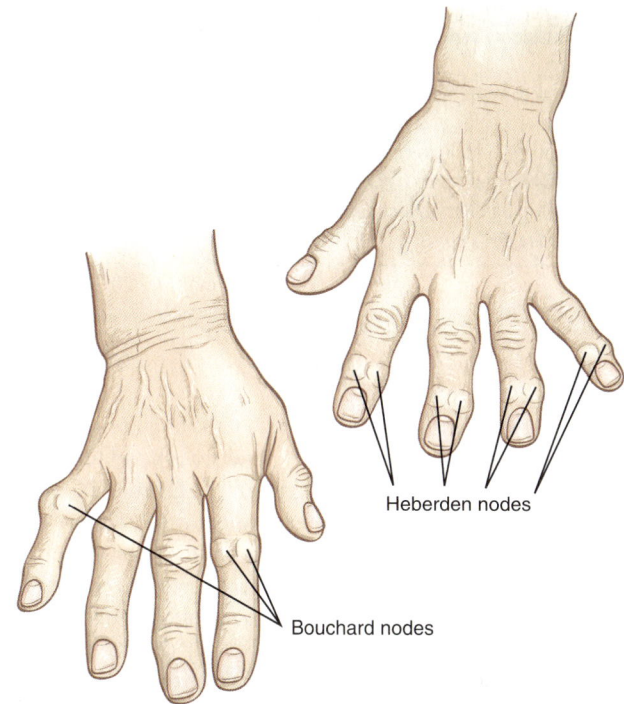

Fig. 21.7 Nodes and arthritis. (From McCance, K. L., & Huether, S. E. [2014]. *Pathophysiology: The biologic basis for disease in adults and children* [7th ed.]. St. Louis, MO: Elsevier.)

Take actions (nursing interventions). Instructions on joint protection and energy conservation are given. For patients with mild pain, a gentle exercise program that improves muscle tone and prevents joint stiffness may be used. Water therapy has been found to be effective in alleviating osteoarthritic pain and improving overall function (Bhatia et al, 2013). Rest periods between activities are recommended. Heat or cold therapy for the joints may also be used to decrease joint pain. Simple measures such as a warm bath or shower in the morning may help reduce the early morning stiffness that may accompany the pain. Other pain relief interventions may be incorporated into the treatment plan (see Evidence-Based Practice box: Osteoarthritis and Benefits of Shared Yoga Intervention for Sleep Disturbances).

EVIDENCE-BASED PRACTICE

Osteoarthritis and Benefits of Shared Yoga Intervention for Sleep Disturbances

Background
Older adults are at cumulative risk for developing OA, with increasing age a leading risk factor. Recent studies have indicated that regular participation in yoga has reduced pain and improved function in patients with OA. This study looked at the effect of a shared yoga intervention on insomnia in older adults with OA.

Sample/Setting
Seventeen community-dwelling older adults who met the inclusion criteria of a designated age range (50–85) diagnosed with OA of the hip, knee, or ankle in pain and reported insomnia directly related to the OA were randomized to a shared yoga or individual yoga program. The age range of the participants was 50–72, with 53% of the sample male and 41% female. Following telephone screenings, a baseline visit was made to obtain consent and provide participants with a sleep diary, Actigraph and yoga equipment, and an audio-guided CD to be used at home.

Methods
Before participating in the yoga classes, participants were instructed to keep a sleep diary and wear the Actigraph. The yoga programs for each group consisted of 12 weeks of classes that consisted of a brief warm-up followed by 30 minutes of yoga. Participants were also asked to practice yoga moves at home on days when no classes were scheduled. If the participant was in the partner group, the partner also practiced yoga.

Continued

> **EVIDENCE-BASED PRACTICE—cont'd**
>
> **Findings**
> No differences were found between the two groups on attendance at classes or at home practicing yoga lessons. Participants who had a partner reported feeling motivated to go to class. The efficacy outcomes of yoga classes were found in both groups to be perceived improvement in sleep rather than actual hours slept or on indicators of depression from the eight item Patient Health Questionnaire (PHQ-8).
>
> **Implications**
> Participating in yoga, whether alone or with a partner, may improve self-reported sleep issues. Although the overall actual quality of sleep was not found to improve, nurses can recommend participation in yoga as a means of improving self-reported sleep issues, which are quite common in older adults with OA.
>
> Data from Buchanan, D. T., Vitiello, M. V., & Bennett, K. (2017). Feasibility and efficacy of a shared yoga intervention for sleep disturbance in older adults with osteoarthritis. *Journal of Gerontological Nursing, 43*(8), 42–52.

The physician may also prescribe various nonsteroidal anti-inflammatory drugs (NSAIDs) and nonopioid analgesics to control the pain. Patients may initially be given OTC drugs, then gradually progress to a prescription anti-inflammatory agent. The use of a topical anti-inflammatory gel on an affected area, such as the knee, has been shown to reduce pain (Derry et al, 2017). Other medical treatment options for more severe pain may include directly injecting the painful joint with steroids. This may be performed two or three times a year for chronic pain. More recent developments in arthritis treatment include the injection of hyaluronic acid into a painful knee joint if more conservative measures have not been effective. The nurse should educate the patient about these conservative measures for treating the symptoms of arthritis. Information regarding the correct dosing of oral drugs, contraindications, side effects, and adverse effects should be provided.

When conservative measures for treating chronic arthritis pain fail and the patient becomes more disabled, surgical procedures may be considered. The main indications for surgery are severe pain and increasing disability. Arthroplasty, a surgical replacement of the affected joint, is one of the most common procedures. Joint replacement surgery is currently successful for many joints that may be involved with arthritis, including the shoulders, elbows, fingers, hips, and knees. Other surgical options include arthroscopic procedures and joint fusion surgery. These procedures do not replace the joint but may result in improved function and reduced pain.

For patients undergoing joint replacement surgery for the hip or knee, the preoperative period focuses on education about the surgical procedure, its risks, any potential complications, and the postoperative course. After surgery, the goals of nursing care are to prevent complications, relieve surgical pain, and assist the patient in achieving higher levels of function and activity. Major complications after joint replacement surgery may include thromboembolism (deep venous thrombosis [DVT]), joint or wound infection, blood loss, nerve injury, joint dislocation, and surgical pain (Forster and Stewart, 2016). The risk of DVT is highest between the first and second weeks after surgery. Various prophylactic measures should be ordered to prevent DVT. These may include various lower extremity compression devices, oral or injectable anticoagulants, and physical therapy to mobilize the patient (O'Connell et al, 2016).

Nursing interventions in the postoperative period include measures to prevent infection, control pain, and assist with daily activities. Aseptic precautions should be taken with surgical wound dressings, urinary catheters, and surgical drains to prevent infection. The patient may be given prophylactic antibiotics for a short time (24 hours) after surgery.

Infection of the site of joint replacement is a serious complication. The incidence of deep infection after joint replacement is 1%–2% and 4%–5% after joint revision (Bullock, 2021). The infection may be a result of contamination during surgery, hematoma formation, or delayed wound healing, or it may be hematogenous from a distant site, as with a urinary tract infection. The most common contaminants are bacteria, such as staphylococci and Gram-positive aerobic streptococci. Because the new joint is a foreign body, pathogens may be introduced and will persist on the metal or plastic surfaces of the prosthesis, leading to chronic, deep infection of the joint.

Patients with rheumatoid arthritis (RA), diabetes mellitus, or poor nutritional status and those receiving long-term corticosteroid therapies are at increased risk for developing joint infections. If infection occurs in a joint replacement, long-term intravenous antibiotic therapy is instituted. In some cases, the infected joint may be replaced. Joint infections may lead to increased disability and prolonged rehabilitation.

Pain control during the first 24–48 hours may be accomplished with intravenous or epidural administration of narcotic analgesics. Patient-controlled analgesia is frequently used to provide adequate pain control. As the patient's pain decreases, oral analgesics should be ordered. Mild analgesics may be required for up to 6 weeks postoperatively as the surgical site heals.

Patients who have total hip replacement surgery are at risk for hip dislocation. The hip should be maintained in a position of abduction and neutral alignment. Some physicians may require the use of pillows or abduction splints while the patient is in bed. Nurses should reinforce hip precautions as described in the Patient/Family Teaching box: Precautions After Total Hip Replacement Surgery.

> **PATIENT/FAMILY TEACHING**
> **Precautions After Total Hip Replacement Surgery**
>
> Sit with your hips at a 90-degree or greater angle (keep your knees below the hip).
> Do *not* bend forward more than 90 degrees.
> Do *not* lift the knee on the operating side higher than your hip.
> Do *not* cross legs at the knees or ankles.
> Keep pillows between your legs when lying on your nonsurgical side or your back.
> Do *not* lie on the surgical side.
> Do *not* bend to put on shoes; use a long shoehorn.
> Do *not* bend down to reach items on the floor.
> Do *not* sit in low chairs.
> Use an elevated toilet seat to keep your knees below your hips.

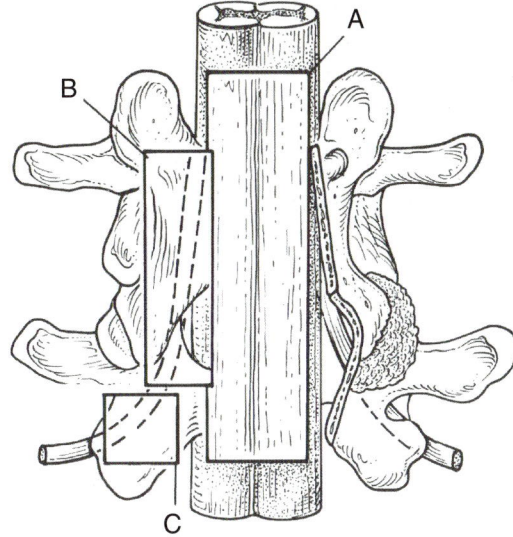

Fig. 21.8 Three-dimensional illustration of segmental stenoses. **A,** Anatomic. **B,** Segmental. **C,** Pathologic. (Redrawn from Ciric, I., Mikhael, M. A., Tarkington, J. A., & Vick, N. A. [1980]. The lateral recess syndrome: A variant of spinal stenosis. *Journal of Neurosurgery*, 53, 433–443.)

The goal of total knee replacement surgery is to restore at least 90 degrees of knee flexion. For patients to achieve this, active and passive physical therapy is instituted. In addition, the physician may order a continuous passive motion device, which continuously moves the knee through a preset range of flexion and extension. Rehabilitation for a patient with a joint replacement begins within 24–48 hours of the surgical procedure and includes muscle strengthening and range-of-motion exercises. The patient is instructed on the use of a cane, walker, or crutches. Occupational therapy provides the patient with instructions for independence in daily activities. A short stay in a rehabilitation facility may follow the acute hospital stay. However, many patients are able to quickly return to their own homes with continued home therapy services.

Evaluate outcomes (evaluation). The goals of caring for a patient with OA are to relieve pain and restore function. Patients should report minimum pain and improved ability to perform ADLs. Conservative measures (as outlined earlier) will improve mobility and increase comfort for many older patients. If surgical intervention is used, the patient needs to understand the expected outcomes as well as the risks associated with the procedure. Patients with OA may benefit from support groups and group exercise programs especially those designed for patients with arthritis. The patient's self-care practices should include regular exercise, the use of adaptive devices, and adherence to prescribed drug regimens. Understanding the disease process and treatment measures will assist an older adult in maintaining function and independence.

Spinal Stenosis

Changes of the spine leading to functional limitation and pain in older adults are becoming more common. Spinal stenosis, or compression of the spinal canal, can pinch the nerve roots and spinal cord, causing pain, weakness, and numbness (Yang, 2023). Spinal stenosis can occur due to age-related degenerative changes, such as OA. Lumbar spinal stenosis is one of the most frequently encountered, clinically important degenerative disorders in the aging population. Approximately 95% of those age 50 and older have degenerative changes to the spine (Park, 2021). Degenerative spinal stenosis is a bony overgrowth of the facet joints of the vertebrae, which leads to narrowing of the spinal canal and possible compression of the nerve roots. Although spinal stenosis may occur at any level of the spine, it is most frequently seen in the lumbar region at levels L3 and L4 (Fig. 21.8). Degeneration of the vertebral joints and disks of the spine, along with nerve compression, leads to progressive back pain and possible weakness of the lower extremities. Patients with spinal stenosis may develop claudication-like symptoms of burning and numbness in their lower extremities (Kalff et al, 2013).

Nursing Care Guidelines for the Older Adult with Spinal Stenosis

Recognize cues (assessment). The goals of nursing assessment focus on the patient's symptoms. The exact location of pain or numbness, the duration of the symptoms, and successful pain relief measures should be identified. Pain caused by degenerative spinal stenosis tends to occur primarily in the back and buttocks, but it may also radiate into the thighs, calves, and feet. The pain may be unilateral or bilateral and generally worsens with prolonged standing or activity. Symptoms are generally relieved with flexion of the spine. Patients may usually report specific positions or activities that aggravate or reduce their symptoms. They may report that activities such as leaning over a grocery cart lessen their pain. Comfort levels during routine ADLs should always be assessed.

Analyze cues and prioritize hypotheses (patient problems). Patient problems for an older patient with spinal stenosis include the following:

- Chronic pain resulting from spinal nerve root narrowing
- Reduced mobility as a result of discomfort with walking and movement
- Potential for reduced stamina as a result of chronic pain
- Potential for injury resulting from pain and difficulty with ambulation

Generate solutions (planning). The focus of the nursing care plan for a patient with spinal stenosis is the management of chronic pain, maintenance of strength and mobility, and promotion of independence with daily activities. The severity of symptoms and assessment of current limitations of activity will determine the individual needs of patients with degenerative spinal stenosis. Expected outcomes include the following:

1. The patient will report a minimum or tolerable level of pain.
2. The patient will demonstrate improved mobility and tolerance for activity.
3. The patient will be able to incorporate a plan for lifestyle modifications that includes activity and rest.
4. The patient will demonstrate safe use of assistive devices and make necessary environmental changes to promote safety.

Take actions (nursing interventions). Nursing care for an older patient with spinal stenosis depends on the severity of spinal cord narrowing, the patient's state of health, and the degree of pain and immobility. For the patient being treated conservatively, the nurse should instruct them to allow sufficient periods of rest and to limit activities that produce pain. Physical therapy for range of motion and muscle strengthening may be ordered by the physician. Pain relief measures should be initiated and then evaluated for their effectiveness. The physician may order NSAIDs, analgesics, and injectable steroid treatments for more severe pain (Lee et al, 2015). The use of pain assessment scales helps determine pain patterns, the severity of pain, and the effectiveness of pain relief measures. Other nursing measures to relieve pain include the use of heat or cold applications to the back, massage therapy, relaxation techniques, and position changes for the patient while in bed. Older patients with unrelieved chronic pain may be considered for pain team consultation and interdisciplinary treatment efforts, such as physical therapy and pain management. In many patients with chronic pain, depression may accompany and increase the intensity of the pain symptoms. A physician consultant may recommend the use of a mild antidepressant drug in addition to the other pain relief measures.

Evaluate outcomes (evaluation). The patient's ability to perform ADLs independently with minimum discomfort is evaluated by self-report and observation. The effectiveness of pain relief measures is discussed with the patient, and changes are made when drugs have lost their effectiveness. For patients undergoing epidural injections or surgical procedures, the nurse would reinforce instructions about precautions and activities. The nurse would also ascertain whether the patient is able to verbalize potential complications and expected outcomes of treatment. Documentation of patient interactions includes the use of an appropriate pain scale and information about current activity levels and restrictions.

Rheumatoid Arthritis

RA is a chronic, systemic, inflammatory disease that causes joint destruction and deformity and results in disability. The onset of the disease most commonly occurs in the third or fourth decade. However, RA may also develop in older adults, known as *elderly-onset rheumatoid arthritis* (EORA). The disease is usually a chronic problem for 1% of the population, and the occurrence of EORA has an equal gender distribution compared with RA in the younger adult population (Yung, 2017).

The cause of RA is not known. The most widely accepted theory is that it is an autoimmune disease that causes inflammation, most often in the joints but sometimes also in connective tissue. Joint involvement most often starts with the proximal interphalangeals, metacarpophalangeals, and wrists; in the later stages of the disease, knees and hips are affected.

In the initial phase of RA, the synovial membrane becomes inflamed and thickens, and production of synovial fluid is increased. The change is called *pannus*. As pannus tissue develops, it causes erosion and destruction of the joint capsule and subchondral bone. These processes result in decreased joint motion, deformity, and finally ankylosis, or joint immobilization.

The course of RA is variable. Generally, the onset is gradual, and the course is one of remissions and exacerbations. The symptoms are painful, stiff joints, decreased range of motion in the joints, joint swelling, and deformity (Fig. 21.9). The joint stiffness is present in the morning or after a prolonged period of inactivity and lasts for more than 30 minutes. On examination, the affected joints are warm and swollen. Deformities of the joints include ulnar deviation of the wrists, boutonnière deformity caused by contractures of the distal and proximal interphalangeal joints, and swan-neck deformity caused by contractures of the distal interphalangeal joint (Fig. 21.10).

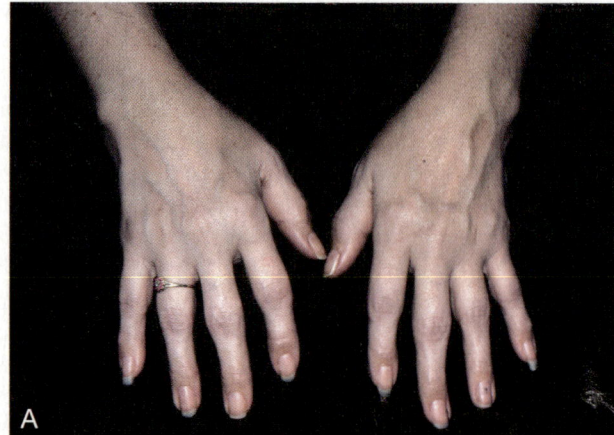

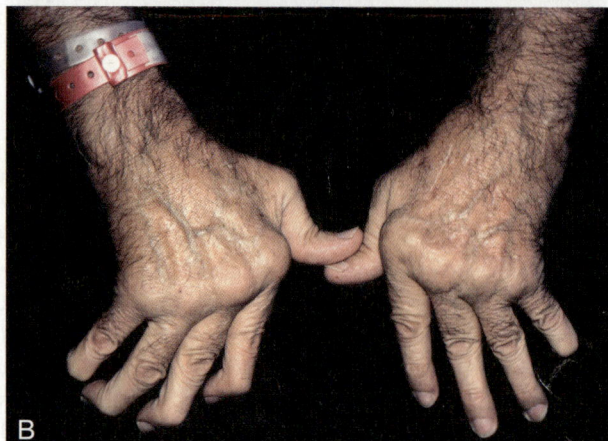

Fig. 21.9 Rheumatoid arthritis of the hand. **A,** Early stage. **B,** Advanced stage. (From Hochberg, M. C., Silman, A. J., Smolen, J. S., et al. [2009]. *Rheumatoid arthritis.* Philadelphia, PA: Elsevier.)

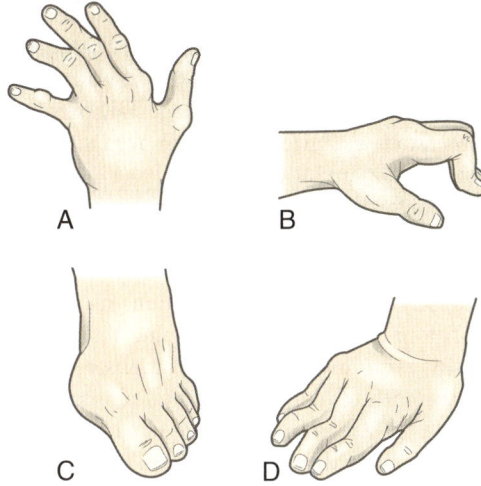

Fig. 21.10 Typical deformities of rheumatoid arthritis. **A,** Ulnar drift. **B,** Boutonnière. **C,** Hallux valgus. **D,** Swan-neck deformity. (From Lewis, S. L., Bucher, L., Heitkemper, M. M., Harding, M. M., Kwong, J., & Roberts, D. [2017]. *Medical-surgical nursing: Assessment and management of clinical problems* [10th ed.]. St. Louis, MO: Elsevier.)

TABLE 21.1 Differentiating Rheumatoid Arthritis From Osteoarthritis

	Rheumatoid Arthritis	Osteoarthritis
Age at onset	Fourth through sixth decades Late-onset RA peaks between 60 and 80 years of age	Fifth and sixth decades
Onset	Gradual	Gradual
Disease course	Exacerbations and remissions	Variable, progressive
Duration of stiffness	1–24 hours	30 minutes or less
Joint pain	Worse in the morning	Worse after activity
Joints involved	Proximal interphalangeal Metacarpophalangeal Metatarsophalangeal Knees, hips, wrists	Distal interphalangeal Knees, hips Lumbar, cervical Spine
Symmetric pattern	Almost always	Occasionally
Constitutional manifestations	Present	Absent
Synovial fluid	Increased cells Decreased viscosity	Few cells Normal viscosity
Radiography findings	Abnormalities present	Abnormalities present
Erythrocyte sedimentation rate	Almost always elevated	Occasionally elevated
Positive rheumatoid factor	Almost always	Never

Patients may also develop subcutaneous nodules that feel firm and fixed and are often found on the proximal side of the elbow (LeBlond et al, 2015).

Systemic symptoms may include fatigue, malaise, anorexia, weight loss, and anemia. RA in older adults may appear atypically; that is, large joints are affected more often, and the onset may be more sudden than in younger adults. Fatigue, weakness, and fever may be present (Table 21.1). Patients with long-term RA may develop comorbidities such as Sjögren syndrome, Felty syndrome, and pericarditis (Ishchenko and Lories, 2016).

Nursing Care Guidelines for the Older Adult with Rheumatoid Arthritis

Recognize cues (assessment). A careful nursing history is taken. Questions are asked about family history and constitutional symptoms, including fever, anorexia, weight loss, fatigue, and the duration of joint stiffness. On physical examination, the affected joints are inspected for symmetric involvement, pain, tenderness, swelling, heat, erythema, and deformity. For patients with long-term complicated RA, assessment should also include examination of the eye for scleritis and corneal ulcers, the lungs for pneumonitis, and a cardiac examination for the presence of pericarditis (Ishchenko and Lories, 2016).

Analyze cues and prioritize hypotheses (patient problems). Patient problems for a patient with RA include the following:
- Pain resulting from swollen, inflamed joint tissue.
- Reduced mobility as a result of joint deformities and inflammation.
- Fatigue is a result of the systemic disease process.
- Inadequate nutrition as a result of loss of appetite.
- Inadequate bathing/dressing/feeding/toileting self-care in ADLs is a result of the loss of motion and strength in painful, swollen joints.
- Distorted body image as a result of the gradual onset of joint deformities.

Generate solutions (planning). Prevention of joint deformities, control of symptoms, and maintenance of the patient's abilities to have an active lifestyle are the focus of intervention for a patient with RA. Outcomes for the older patient include the following:
1. The patient will maintain maximal joint motion in the affected joints with minimum deformities.
2. The patient's pain related to inflammation will be controlled.
3. The patient will be able to maintain optimal functional status.

Take actions (nursing interventions). Older patients with RA and their families require extensive education to cope effectively with the chronic nature of this disease. The nurse needs to discuss with them pain management, drug therapies, maintenance of self-care activities, promotion of safe mobility, methods of joint protection and precautions, and management of overall health.

Education on pain management includes information on appropriate drugs that have been prescribed and OTC remedies that a patient may be using. The patient is informed that stress and anxiety may cause muscle tension that may worsen joint pain. Progressive relaxation and guided imagery are taught to decrease anxiety and stress. Application of heat and cold to the affected joints decreases cutaneous nerve stimulation. Ice packs are applied to joints during periods of acute inflammation.

Moist heat is useful for relaxing muscles and increasing joint mobility.

The role of the nurse in drug management is to teach the older patient about the action, side effects, and special precautions related to the specific drugs. Table 21.2 presents multiple drugs classically used in the treatment of arthritis. In addition to those drugs listed in Table 21.2, newer pharmacologic and biologic agents are being researched and developed for use in patients with RA.

The drug management of RA is directed at disease management and symptom control. Drugs selected for relief of pain and inflammation include corticosteroids, analgesics, and NSAIDs. Corticosteroids, along with drugs known as *disease-modifying antirheumatic drugs* (DMARDs), are prescribed to aid with disease control. Concern exists about extended corticosteroid use because of the multiple side effects of long-term use, such as infection, peptic ulcer disease, and osteoporosis. Aspirin, an NSAID, is no longer a first line of treatment for RA because of its toxic effects at effective doses (Yaseen, 2024).

The conventional DMARDs, which suppress the immune response, include drugs such as methotrexate, leflunomide, hydroxychloroquine, and sulfasalazine (Dunkin, 2022). The newer DMARDs, which are biologic agents, are used if the conventional DMARDs were ineffective in controlling RA; they are administered subcutaneously, intravenously, and orally. Drugs known as *tumor necrosis factor* (TNF) inhibitors (i.e., infliximab, adalimumab, and etanercept) are effective for the treatment of RA in combination with methotrexate, DMARDs, or corticosteroids (Chan, 2023). Numerous side effects are reported to be caused by TNF inhibitors and include infections, potential worsening of heart failure, and demyelinating disease. Janus kinase (JAK) inhibitors are the newest class of antirheumatics in that they prevent cell signaling; thereby reducing inflammation. Currently, there are three JAK inhibitors: tofacitinib, baricitinib, and upadacitinib. Nurses need to educate patients about the numerous side effects of these drugs and stress the importance of not taking any OTC drugs without the permission of their health care provider.

Fatigue and decreased mobility of the joints of the upper extremities contribute to self-care deficits. Occupational therapists work with older patients to improve joint function and prevent disability. The modalities used include exercises, splints, methods to protect joints, and assistive devices. Splints may be used to protect joints, maintain joint function, and decrease pain. The nurse reinforces the use of these devices and monitors their correct use.

Limitations in mobility because of pain and joint stiffness may lead to disuse and greater disability. To prevent excessive disability, the patient is taught body mechanics and proper body alignment and is given recommendations for an exercise program. Using good body mechanics and keeping the body in a position of optimal alignment decreases joint stress and fatigue. Physical therapists prescribe individualized therapeutic exercise programs, which include strengthening and stretching exercises, range-of-motion exercises, and endurance training.

Fatigue is a common constitutional symptom of RA. Fatigue may interfere with the older adult's achievement of optimal functional independence. Methods used to decrease fatigue include balancing rest with activity, scheduling short rest periods, practicing relaxation techniques, and adapting the environment to simplify work. Coping with chronic illness, pain, deformity, and alterations in body image may predispose a patient to depression. If clinical depression occurs, medical evaluation and treatment are indicated.

The joint deformities and alteration in body image may negatively affect sexual function. The nurse should be aware of this and openly discuss issues of sexuality and methods of maintaining physical intimacy. Suggestions may include using analgesics before sexual activity, planning rest periods before sexual activity, assuming alternative positions, and encouraging alternative methods of maintaining physical intimacy.

Adults with RA require many types of support to cope with this chronic, disabling disease. The nurse's role is to provide the older adult with information about available resources so that optimal levels of functioning can be reached.

A good resource is the Arthritis Foundation (https://www.arthritis.org/), which publishes educational materials that address exercise programs, work simplification, and the disease process. Support groups and self-help classes taught in 6-week sessions are conducted by local chapters. The content of the classes includes self-efficacy, exercise, pain management, depression, stress management, and nontraditional therapies.

Evaluate outcomes (evaluation). The older adult with RA should experience minimum discomfort and be able to maintain an acceptable level of function and mobility. With advances in drug therapy and active participation by the patient in activities to prevent joint deformities, the patient should experience less deformity, increased comfort levels, and a better understanding of the disease process.

Gouty Arthritis

Gout is a disease in which acute attacks of arthritis pain occur because of elevated levels of serum uric acid. During acute gout attacks, joint inflammation is caused by sodium urate crystals in the joint. Gout is classified as either *primary* or *acquired*. Primary gout is an inborn disease of purine metabolism. Acquired gout is caused by drugs that affect the excretion of uric acid. These drugs include diuretics, levodopa-carbidopa, and low-dose aspirin (Kuo et al, 2015). Gout usually occurs in the middle years but also affects older adults; it is more prevalent in males than in females.

In gout, excessive production or decreased urinary excretion of uric acid may occur. The excess monosodium urate salts are deposited in joints and surrounding connective tissue. The deposits of the uric acid crystals are called *tophi,* often found on the helix of the ear, on the olecranon bursa, and over the Heberden nodes in patients with coexisting OA (Fig. 21.11).

Gout may manifest as an acute or chronic condition. The onset of gout is sudden and manifested by an acute attack of pain in one or more joints. The most commonly affected area is the great toe, known as *podagra*. Other joints and periarticular structures affected by gout include the ankle, knee, wrist, and the olecranon bursa (Kuo et al, 2015). The affected joint becomes hot, reddened, and tender. The pain may be severe and interfere with mobility, self-care, and functional abilities. Chills

TABLE 21.2 Drugs Used in the Treatment for Rheumatoid Arthritis

Drug	Rationale for Use	Side Effects	Nursing Implications
Salicylates: aspirin	Used in the early disease phase; analgesic, antipyretic, and anti-inflammatory	Gastrointestinal irritation; slight elevation of liver enzyme levels; tinnitus (reversible)	Administer with milk or food. Teach the use of enteric-coated tablets. Evaluate for gastrointestinal pain or bleeding, as well as tinnitus.
NSAIDs Long term: diclofenac, fenoprofen, flurbiprofen, ibuprofen, indomethacin, ketoprofen, meclofenamate, mefenamic acid, nabumetone, naproxen, oxaprozin, piroxicam, salsalate, sulindac, tolmetin	Used when salicylates are ineffective; analgesic, antipyretic, and anti-inflammatory actions; generally inhibit prostaglandin synthesis	Gastrointestinal irritation; diarrhea; fluid retention, edema; interstitial nephritis; nephrotic syndrome; dizziness, tachycardia, blurred vision, headaches; cholestatic hepatitis; bone marrow depression	Must be administered for 1–2 weeks before a therapeutic response is seen. Administer with food or antacids. Assess for gastrointestinal pain and occult bleeding. Teach the patient to avoid alcohol. Evaluate renal and hepatic function regularly.
Short-term: phenylbutazone	Specific for adjunctive use	Same as above	Same as above; a 1-week trial is suggested. Evaluate CBC. Use with caution in older adults.
Oxyphenbutazone	Effective for articular symptoms in some patients	Same as above	Same as above; use under close medical supervision.
Antimalarials: hydroxychloroquine sulfate, hydroxychloroquine phosphate	Used for severe destructive disease; 3–6 months needed to reach therapeutic levels	Gastrointestinal irritation; skin rash and changes; retinal changes; bone marrow depression	Advise ophthalmologic examination every 4–6 weeks. Allow 6–8 weeks for therapeutic effects to begin. Evaluate CBC regularly. Assess for gastrointestinal effects, headaches, dizziness, hearing effects, and hepatotoxic effects. Evaluate for water and sodium retention.
Auranofin	Effects cumulative, slow onset of effects (8–14 weeks); dosage may be gradually decreased after remission	Proteinuria; interstitial fibrosis; metallic taste	Teach skin care. Evaluate gastrointestinal discomfort. Check urine for blood and protein.
Penicillamine	As effective as gold sodium thiomalate but more toxic; unknown mechanism of action; effects seen in 2 months	Gastrointestinal irritation; taste alterations; blood dyscrasias; skin rash; stomatitis; nephrotic syndrome, glomerulonephritis; autoimmune syndrome; proteinuria	Evaluate CBC, liver, and renal function weekly for 2 months and then monthly. Teach the patient to report a sore throat or fever. Take it between meals because food decreases absorption.
Antirheumatics: gold sodium thiomalate, aurothioglucose	Used when salicylates and NSAIDs fail; remission-inducing action suppresses inflammation	Skin rashes, pruritus; stomatitis; diarrhea; blood dyscrasias; hepatitis	Give with NSAIDs until efficacy is reached. Assess CBC and renal and liver function often.
Steroids: systemic prednisone, prednisolone, hydrocortisone	Symptom relief for months to years for certain prolonged conditions	Multiple toxic effects, including osteoporosis, gastric ulcers, risk of infection susceptibility, hirsutism, emotional lability, edema, moon facies, hypokalemia, cataracts, glaucoma	Teach the patient not to stop the drug abruptly. Administer for short periods and taper the dose slowly. Monitor for side effects, including hypertension and hyperglycemia.
Intraarticular	Used when only one or two joints are involved; used for pain relief or to increase function; benefits last 2 weeks to several months. The joints most amenable are the ankles, knees, hips, shoulders, and hands	Same as above	Teach the patient that the effects may be short lived. Advise that administration is limited to two to four infections per year per joint.
Immunosuppressives: azathioprine, methotrexate, cyclophosphamide	Used with advanced disease, affect immune system to decrease inflammation, teratogenic potential	Hepatitis, cirrhosis; gastrointestinal ulcers; susceptibility to infection; bone marrow suppression; alopecia; skin rash	Evaluate CBC, liver function, and renal function weekly. Assess older adults closely for signs of toxicity.
Capsaicin cream, gel, liquid, patch	Topical for pain	Irritation of the skin and other mucous membranes	Avoid contact with the eyes, nares, or other mucous membranes to avoid a burning sensation. Avoid using heat sources to prevent burns

CBC, complete blood cell count; NSAIDs, nonsteroidal anti-inflammatory drugs.
Modified from Roberts, D. (2013). Arthritis and connective tissue disorders. In L. Schoenly (Ed.), *Core curriculum for orthopaedic nursing* (7th ed.). Pitman, NJ: National Association of Orthopaedic Nurses, pp 340–346.

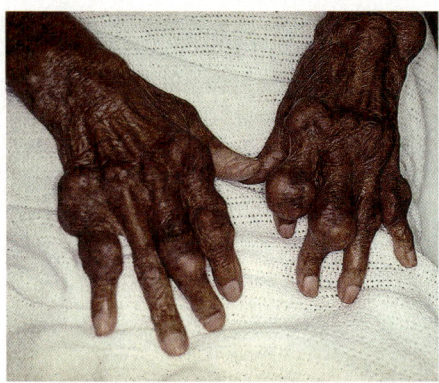

Fig. 21.11 Tophaceous gout. (Courtesy John Cook, MD. From Goldstein, B. G., & Goldstein, A. E. [1997]. *Practical dermatology* [2nd ed.]. St Louis, MO: Mosby.)

and fever may also be present. Acute attacks of gout usually subside in 7 days, regardless of treatment. In chronic gout, the uric acid crystals cause bone destruction and deformity. Uric acid crystals may also be deposited in the kidney and cause nephrolithiasis.

Nursing Care Guidelines for the Older Adult with Gout

Recognize cues (assessment). The onset of an acute gout attack is identified by the presence of warmth, swelling, cutaneous erythema, and severe pain in the affected joint. The initial attack is usually in one joint, and in nearly half of patients, it will involve the first metatarsophalangeal joint. In older females, however, the initial presentation often begins in multiple joints (West and O'Dell, 2015). The pain is intense, and the joint is sensitive to even the slightest touch. Other symptoms may include fever, chills, and malaise. The intervals between initial attacks and subsequent acute episodes will vary, but the attacks usually become more frequent and involve more joints.

Patients with chronic gouty arthritis usually report 10 or more years of previous acute gout attacks. The involved joints are chronically uncomfortable and swollen, although the intensity of the pain is less than in acute episodes. Tophi may or may not be detected on a physical examination (Igel et al, 2017). A nursing assessment should identify other risk factors or conditions that may predispose the patient to the development of gout. These factors include obesity, hypertension, alcohol ingestion, use of diuretics, recent trauma, hyperlipidemia, diabetes mellitus, chronic kidney disease, and organ transplants.

Analyze cues and prioritize hypotheses (patient problems). Patient problems for a patient with gouty arthritis include the following:
- Pain, acute or chronic, resulting from joint inflammation and swelling
- Reduced mobility resulting from joint deformity and discomfort secondary to the disease process
- Potential for reduced stamina resulting from pain

Generate solutions (planning). The overall management plan for an older adult with gouty arthritis, either acute or chronic, is to decrease the pain and other associated symptoms. Expected outcomes for a patient with gout include the following:
1. The patient will verbalize increased comfort and pain relief with the use of appropriate analgesics and NSAIDs.
2. The patient will be able to verbalize understanding of the disease process.
3. The patient will incorporate appropriate diet modifications and lifestyle changes, such as weight loss and the avoidance of alcohol and food products high in purine.
4. The patient will modify his or her activity and rest pattern based on the limitations imposed by the pain.
5. The patient will incorporate health practices to minimize recurrent attacks.

Take actions (nursing interventions). In the acute phase, the goal of nursing management is to relieve pain. During an acute attack of gout, the pain may be so severe that the patient is unable to bear weight or to tolerate clothing or blankets on the affected joint. Colchicine is an effective medicine for the treatment of pain and inflammation in acute gout; severe pain subsides within 48 hours. The use of NSAIDs, especially indomethacin, provides relief comparable with that provided by colchicine. Other pain relief measures include analgesics, elevation of the affected extremity, immobilization of the joint, and applying heat or ice packs to the area.

Nursing interventions for chronic gout also focus on pain relief measures and the prevention of recurrent attacks of gout. This is accomplished through patient education. Because obesity and diets high in protein have been linked to gout, information about the role of dietary habits should be provided. Foods high in purines, for example, shellfish and organ meats, should be avoided. Alcoholic beverages should also be avoided. Obese patients should have weight-reduction diets or programs recommended. A consultation with a dietitian for diet modifications may be helpful.

A xanthine oxidase inhibitor such as allopurinol or febuxostat is the drug of choice for patients with chronic gout symptoms (Feng et al, 2015). Probenecid, a uricosuric agent, is another drug that may be used. Patients must be closely monitored for renal function during drug therapy. To discourage the formation of renal stones, the patient should be encouraged to have a daily intake of 2–3 liters (L) of fluid unless contraindicated. The patient should also be instructed to avoid salicylates, which could inhibit drug effects.

Evaluate outcomes (evaluation). Patients with acute or chronic gout should be able to maintain a healthy lifestyle, incorporating the changes suggested during treatment. The patient must understand the drug therapy for acute attacks and chronic treatments. Pain management should allow a patient to participate fully in ADLs and allow for full mobility.

Osteoporosis

Osteoporosis is considered the most common metabolic bone disorder, affecting more than 10 million people in the United States (Bone Health and Osteoporosis Foundation [BHOF], n.d.). Common among postmenopausal females, bone fractures occur every year secondary to osteoporosis (Prah et al, 2017). The disease primarily affects females but also occurs in one in six males. Osteoporosis is commonly referred to as *porous bone disease* or *brittle bone disease* and is characterized by a reduction in bone mass and a loss of bone strength.

Bone is constantly remodeling itself throughout life, and the process of bone maintenance is constant. Old bone cells are removed (resorbed) by osteoclasts, and new bone cells are formed by osteoblasts. The complete process of bone remodeling takes 4–8 months. Bone mass is accumulated in the early part of life; bone mineral density (BMD) increases until approximately age 30, when peak bone mass is attained. Anything that interferes with the normal process of bone remodeling may lead to the development of osteoporosis. Conditions that contribute to this process include renal or hepatic failure and endocrine disorders such as hyperthyroidism, hyperparathyroidism, type 1 diabetes mellitus, RA, and chronic kidney disease. Other risk factors include heredity and genetic predisposition, lifestyle factors, and age. With osteoporosis, the bone remodeling process is altered, and the rate of bone resorption exceeds the rate of bone formation, which leads to decreased bone mass.

Osteoporosis is classified as primary osteoporosis and secondary osteoporosis. Although the cause of primary osteoporosis is not clearly understood, it is further classified into postmenopausal (type 1) osteoporosis and age-associated (type 2) osteoporosis. Type 1 osteoporosis is related to menopausal estrogen deficiency and is seen in females between the ages of 51 and 75. In type 1 osteoporosis, the trabecular bone in the vertebral column, hips, and wrists is weakened. Because type I osteoporosis is related to estrogen deficiency, it is seen six times more often in females than in males. Type 2 osteoporosis occurs in both males and females older than age 70 and causes a gradual loss of cortical bone. Because this cortical bone provides support in the body, weakening of the bone is a predisposing factor in hip fractures. Age-related changes in vitamin D synthesis that result in decreased calcium absorption are thought to be the cause of type 2 osteoporosis.

Secondary osteoporosis, seen in 15% of cases, is the result of diseases such as hyperthyroidism, hyperparathyroidism, gastrointestinal disorders, neoplasms, and alcoholism. In females, early oophorectomy is a cause of secondary osteoporosis. Long-term use of corticosteroids, methotrexate, aluminum-containing antacids, phenytoin, and heparin may result in secondary osteoporosis. Prolonged immobility, which causes calcium excretion, is also a cause of secondary osteoporosis (Prah et al, 2017).

Certain risk factors for the development of osteoporosis have been identified (Box 21.1). Risk factors that can be modified with lifestyle changes involve calcium intake, exercise, cigarette smoking, and consumption of alcoholic beverages and excessive caffeine products (Prah et al, 2017). Age, race, gender, and body frame are risk factors that cannot be changed. The nurse may educate the older patient about these risk factors, making suggestions to modify lifestyle and nutrition. Three key essentials in preventing osteoporosis throughout life are appropriate diet, exercise, and lifestyle changes (Prah et al, 2017).

Osteoporosis is called a "silent killer" because, frequently, no clinical symptoms appear until fractures occur. The initial complaint may be back pain or fatigue. The fatigue results from the increased demand on muscles to keep the body in an upright position with decreased bone mass. Osteoporotic fractures are most commonly seen in the vertebrae of the thoracic spine, the femoral neck, and the wrist. Fractures may occur with routine activities such as bending, lifting, coughing, and straining during defecation. Osteoporosis of the spinal vertebrae causes a loss of height of 1–2.5 inches. Also seen is the "dowager's hump," or kyphosis, which results from the vertebrae sliding on top of each other (Fig. 21.12). Conventional radiography may provide evidence of osteoporosis, although it is often performed retrospectively after a fracture. Unfortunately, at least 30% of bone mass must be lost before the disease is apparent on standard radiography. For the evaluation of bone mass in individuals suspected of having osteoporosis or in those considered at risk for the development of the disease, a determination of BMD appears irrefutable. Bone densitometry is commonly performed with dual-energy X-ray absorptiometry (DEXA). This procedure is simple, noninvasive, uses a low radiation dose, and is completed in less than 30 minutes. Many physician offices are now equipped with a

> **BOX 21.1 Risk Factors for the Development of Osteoporosis**
>
> - Female gender
> - Increasing age
> - White race
> - Thin body frame
> - History of bilateral oophorectomy
> - History of anorexia
> - Family history of osteoporosis
> - Long-term use of certain drugs such as corticosteroids, phenytoin, and phenobarbital
> - Chronic conditions such as hyperthyroidism, hyperparathyroidism, and rheumatoid arthritis
> - Alcoholism
> - Cigarette smoking
> - Calcium intake below daily requirements

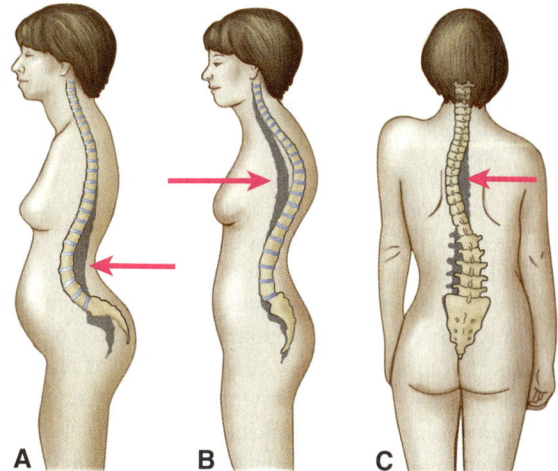

Fig. 21.12 Abnormal spinal curvatures. **A,** Lordosis. **B,** Kyphosis. **C,** Scoliosis. (From Patton, K. T., & Thibodeau, G. A. [2014]. *The human body in health & disease* [6th ed.]. St. Louis, MO: Elsevier.)

DEXA machine for quick and simple screening of patients. Measurement sites include the hip or lumbar spine and peripheral sites such as the wrist. Scores computed from the testing compare the older patient's score with those of normal young adults for peak bone mass and compare the older patient's score with those of gender-matched and age-matched control subjects. The T-score obtained from DEXA is a measure of how much an individual's bone mass differs (in standard deviation) from the bone mass of a healthy 20–29-year-old person. The score obtained defines bone loss as normal, osteopenia, or osteoporosis. If a patient's T-score is −2.5 or less, it is indicative of osteoporosis (Mackey and Whitaker, 2015).

To more clearly establish the candidacy of patients for pharmacologic treatment of osteoporosis, the BHOF recommends that clinicians use the Fracture Risk Assessment Tool (FRAX) developed by the World Health Organization (BHOF, n.d.). FRAX can be accessed as a web-based algorithm that combines risk factors for developing osteoporosis with BMD results. The tool has been designed to be used in males and postmenopausal females between the ages of 40 and 90 years. The limitations of using the FRAX tool are that the calculated score underestimates fracture risk in patients with recent fractures, multiple osteoporosis-related fractures, and those at increased risk for falling (Cosman et al, 2014). Laboratory blood studies are obtained to differentiate osteoporosis from other diseases that may cause bone loss. Complete blood cell count (CBC) and levels of serum calcium, serum phosphorus, alkaline phosphatase, and urinary calcium are all normal in osteoporosis.

Measures to address osteoporosis should be directed at minimizing bone loss in older adults and preserving the current level of bone mass. Patient education and the development of awareness of the disease are critical for prevention and risk reduction. Elimination of lifestyle risk factors, nutritional counseling, and pharmacologic management are strategies used to prevent osteoporosis (Mackey and Whitaker, 2015).

Adequate nutritional intake of calcium should be instituted in early childhood and continued throughout the life span. The current recommendation for daily calcium intake is 1000 mg for males and premenopausal females aged 25 to 49, 1,500 mg for postmenopausal females who are not taking estrogen, 1000 mg for postmenopausal females taking estrogen, and 1,500 mg for males and females older than 65 years (Mackey and Whitaker, 2015). Milk, either low-fat or nonfat, is a good source of calcium and vitamin D. Table 21.3 identifies dietary sources of calcium. Many of these food items are also good sources of vitamin D, which is essential for the synthesis of calcium.

For individuals unable to consume adequate calcium, supplements are recommended. Various forms of calcium supplements are available. Calcium carbonate is thought to be the best supplement because it contains 40% elemental calcium, is the least expensive, and requires taking the least number of tablets. Patients, however, may find calcium citrate, which contains only 20% elemental calcium, to cause fewer gastrointestinal side effects, thus making it more tolerable for long-term therapy. Calcium supplements should be taken with meals and followed by at least 10 ounces (oz.) of water to promote absorption. No more than 600 milligrams (mg) of calcium should be taken in a single dose because absorption is compromised with higher doses. The Bone Health Osteoporosis Foundation (BHOF) currently recommends that patients at risk take vitamin D replacement 800–1000 international units per day in addition to calcium (Mackey and Whitaker, 2015; LeBoff et al, 2022).

Exercise programs that include weight bearing and resistance have been shown to prevent bone loss. Exercises should be performed three times a week for 30–60 minutes for the best results. Postural exercises to prevent or minimize kyphotic deformity are also of benefit to older adults. Moderation in any exercise program is always recommended.

TABLE 21.3 Dietary Sources of Calcium

Food	Serving	Calcium Content (mg)
Milk		
Skim	8 oz	299
2% fat	8 oz	297
Whole	8 oz	291
Cheeses		
Swiss	1 oz	272
Processed American	1 oz	174
Mozzarella	1.5 oz	333
Cottage cheese	1 oz	135
Other Dairy Products		
Yogurt, plain, low-fat	8 oz	415
Ice cream, vanilla	1 cup	168
Ice milk, vanilla	1 cup	274
Frozen yogurt, vanilla	1 cup	206
Seafood		
Oysters	1 cup	226
Pink salmon, canned with bones	3 oz	167
Vegetables		
Collards, frozen or fresh	1 cup	357
Broccoli, fresh	1 cup	42
Turnip greens	1 cup	198
Mustard greens	1 cup	104
Kale, cooked	1 cup	94
Dried Beans (cooked and drained)		
Navy beans	1 cup	90
Pinto beans	1 cup	86
Red kidney beans, canned	1 cup	74
Other Foods		
Blackstrap molasses	2 tbsp	274
Tofu	4 oz	108
Orange juice, calcium fortified	6 oz	261

oz, ounce; *tbsp*, tablespoon.

Modified from National Institutes of Health, Office of Dietary Supplements. (2017). *Sources of calcium*. Retrieved February 12, 2024 from https://ods.od.nih.gov/factsheets/Calcium-HealthProfessional/#h3.

According to the BHOF *Clinician's Guide to Prevention and Treatment of Osteoporosis,* pharmacologic treatment for osteoporosis is recommended for patients who have had a vertebral or hip fracture, a T-score of −2.5 or less, and a 10-year high probability of hip fracture (>/= 3%) or a 10-year probability of a major osteoporosis-related fracture occurring (>/= 20%), as indicated by the score on the US-adapted FRAX score (LeBoff et al, 2022). Bisphosphonates (alendronate, risedronate, and zoledronic acid) are recommended by the American College of Physicians as the initial treatment for osteoporosis in males with primary osteoporosis and in post-menopausal females (Qaseem et al, 2023). The biphosphonates are also classified as antiresorptive drugs. They are known for their ability to slow bone breakdown by inhibiting osteoclasts, thereby preventing bone resorption. Patients should be instructed on the importance of following drug guidelines when taking oral bisphosphonates. Special instructions include taking the drug daily, 1 hour before any food or drug. It must be taken with 6–8 ounces of water, and the patient must remain upright for at least 30 minutes after taking the drug. Nurses should also instruct patients about the long-term side effects of bisphosphonates, including bone fractures, which patients may not recognize as a drug side effect but misinterpret as progression of the disease. Denosumab, also recommended for the prevention and treatment of osteoporosis, is an injectable agent that needs to be administered twice a year. It is contraindicated in patients with a known history of hypocalcemia, so calcium and vitamin D deficiencies need to be corrected before a patient is started on denosumab (LeBoff et al, 2022).

Denosumab, a RANK ligand inhibitor, is recommended if bisphosphonates are contraindicated or if patients experience adverse effects (Qaseem et al, 2023). Denosumab is a monoclonal antibody with a potent antiresorptive property (LeBoff et al, 2022). It is administered intravenously or intramuscularly (Hildebrand and Kasi, 2022). Periodic monitoring of vitamin D levels, serum calcium, phosphorous, magnesium, and serum creatinine is needed. The adverse effects of osteonecrosis of the jaw are lower than with bisphosphonates. Teriparatide, a synthetic parathyroid hormone that helps stimulate bone formation, is indicated for the treatment of patients at high risk of fracture from osteoporosis. This drug has been shown to be effective in increasing BMD in patients with osteoporosis related to long-term glucocorticoid therapy (Mackey and Whitaker, 2015). Upon discontinuation of teriparatide, rapid bone loss can occur (LeBoff et al, 2022). It is recommended that an antiresorptive agent be started.

Another antiresorptive drug used to treat osteoporosis is calcitonin in a parenteral or nasal spray preparation. Oral administration is not appropriate because the drug is a polypeptide hormone and is destroyed in the gastrointestinal tract. The nasal spray preparation is a formulation of synthetic salmon calcitonin, and it has been approved for use in the treatment of osteoporosis in females who are at least 5 years postmenopausal, have low bone density, and are not candidates for estrogen replacement therapy (ERT). Calcitonin is generally taken daily in one puff, alternatingly through the nares. Because the drug may elicit a systemic allergic reaction in certain individuals, intradermal skin testing should precede delivery of the initial dose. Systemic adverse effects of the nasal route are reported as being minimal but may include nasal discomfort, occasional rhinitis, and itching of the nasal mucosa.

Since it was first reported, it has been recommended that the use of estrogen or hormone replacement therapy in postmenopausal females with moderately severe menopausal symptoms be limited on the basis of the findings of the Women's Health Initiative, which found that there is an increased risk for breast cancer, myocardial infarction, stroke, invasive breast cancer, pulmonary embolism, and DVT. Nonestrogen therapies are recommended first for the treatment of osteoporosis (LeBoff et al, 2022).

Nursing Care Guidelines for the Older Adult with Osteoporosis

Recognize cues (assessment). Nursing assessment of older patients should include taking a thorough family health history and determining the presence of risk factors, the level of exercise, alcohol and caffeine intake, and smoking. Females should be assessed for age of onset of menopause, use of ERT, date of last mammography, and history of breast or uterine cancer. All patients should be asked about their lifelong intake of calcium, history of fractures, presence of pain, and history of falls. A physical examination includes the determination of the presence of kyphosis, gait impairments, muscle weakness, and cognitive impairments (Prah et al, 2017).

Analyze cues and prioritize hypotheses (patient problems)
Patient problems for an older patient with osteoporosis include the following:

- Inadequate nutrition resulting from a decreased intake of calcium and vitamin D
- Potential for injury resulting from weakening of the bones
- Pain resulting from inadequate pain relief secondary to bone fractures
- Distorted body image resulting from spinal deformities and loss of height
- Need for patient teaching resulting from a lack of previous exposure to disease processes, risk factors, and measures of prevention

Generate solutions (planning). Awareness of the risk factors and education about the lifetime prevention of osteoporosis and its complications, such as falls and fractures, are the most important aspects of planning the care of older adults with osteoporosis. Expected outcomes for a patient with osteoporosis include the following:

1. The patient will demonstrate taking precautions at home and in the community to prevent falls and activities that may result in fractures.
2. The patient will report an adequate level of pain control in the presence of bone fractures.
3. The patient will consume nutritional supplements, food products, and drugs recommended or prescribed for meeting dietary needs, as evidenced by a diet log.
4. The patient will verbalize acceptance of changes brought about by the disease and an understanding of the treatment and prevention of further deformities (see Health Promotion box).

HEALTH PROMOTION AND ILLNESS PREVENTION
Musculoskeletal Function: Osteoporosis

Health Promotion
- Routine weight-bearing exercises that do not stress the joints, such as walking
- Achievement of ideal body weight
- Initiation of a weight-training program
- Smoking cessation
- Decreased intake of alcohol and caffeine

Disease Prevention
- Participation in a regular program of weight-bearing exercises
- Avoidance of injury and falls
- Maintenance of adequate dietary intake of calcium and supplementation with oral calcium supplements, as indicated
- Consideration of hormone replacement therapy
- Little to no intake of alcohol and caffeine
- Avoidance of smoking

Take actions (nursing interventions). The nurse's role focuses on patient education about the disease process, strategies to prevent further injury or deformity, and measures to promote decreased bone loss. Education should emphasize the identification and minimization of controllable risk factors. These include cigarette smoking, excessive consumption of alcohol, and caffeine intake. Exercise programs that will place some stress on the bones and, thus, strengthen them; for example, walking and lifting light weights, are recommended. Additional information for osteoporosis education and programs can be found through the BHOF (https://www.bonehealthandosteoporosis.org/).

Compression fractures of the vertebrae may cause pain, loss of function, and disturbance in body image brought about by the gradual loss of height caused by multiple fractures. Control of pain is achieved through the use of analgesics, NSAIDs, positioning, and relaxation techniques. Other pain management modalities include transcutaneous electrical nerve stimulation (TENS), various back supports or braces, and formal pain management consultations. Positive body image may be promoted through discussions of acceptance of changes that have occurred, with a focus on prevention of further injury and deformity (Corrarino, 2015).

Nursing care or an older adult with a hip fracture or other fracture secondary to osteoporosis includes the interventions previously noted in this chapter.

Evaluate outcomes (evaluation). An older patient with osteoporosis should be able to describe measures that can be taken to decrease the potential for further bone loss as well as measures that can be taken to maintain a safe living environment so that the risk of injury resulting from falls is reduced. The patient will be able to describe the benefits of an appropriate diet, lifestyle modifications, and diet supplements or drugs, if needed. The older adult will also be able to participate in regular exercise programs and identify resources available for the prevention of disease (see Nursing Care Plan: Osteoporosis With Fractured Thoracic Vertebrae).

NURSING CARE PLAN
Osteoporosis With Fractured Thoracic Vertebrae

Clinical Situation

Mrs. R is a 79-year-old widow who has severe osteoporosis and who recently fractured her T4 and T5 vertebrae. After the fracture, she complained of severe pain, which has limited her daily activity and caused her to spend most of the day in bed. The period of bed rest has left her weak. Before the fracture, she was independent in terms of mobility and self-care. She drove and participated in activities with her friends on a regular basis. She is referred to the home care agency for pain management and physical therapy to upgrade her skills for performing ADLs and to promote endurance.

Mrs. R has no other health problems. She lives alone in a two-story house. The bathroom is on the second floor. Since the fracture, Mrs. R has stayed on the second floor all day except for one trip a day to the kitchen on the first floor to fix a meal. Mrs. R's major support is her daughter, who lives in another state. She has several close friends, but they are unable to help her because of their health problems.

On the admission visit, the nurse finds Mrs. R's house to be in an unsafe condition. The rooms and stairs are cluttered with papers, boxes, and other objects. Mrs. R tells the nurse that her pain has somewhat improved, but it still limits her ability to take care of herself and her home. She also tells the nurse, "I don't understand this osteoporosis; how did that cause my fractures?"

Analyze Cues and Prioritize Hypotheses (Patient Problems)
- Potential for injury resulting from an unsafe environment
- Need for patient teaching resulting from a lack of exposure to osteoporosis
- Reduced mobility resulting from pain and musculoskeletal impairment
- Pain resulting from inadequate knowledge of pain management
- Inadequate bathing and dressing self-care (bathing and dressing lower extremities) resulting from pain and prolonged immobility

Generate Solutions (Planning)
- The patient will remain free from fractures or other injuries and will verbalize unsafe features of her home and a plan to correct them.
- The patient will verbalize basic information about the disease process, outcomes, and treatment.
- The patient will safely walk 100 feet using a pickup walker and will participate in a daily exercise program.
- The patient will verbalize that pain is tolerable. Pain will not interfere with the ability to participate in daily activities.
- The patient will bathe and dress her lower extremities with the use of assistive devices.

Take Actions (Nursing Interventions)
- Discuss outcomes of an unsafe environment: risks of falling and fracture as a result of a cluttered environment.
- Use homemakers and friends to reduce clutter and encourage the use of safety aids.
- Teach safe transfer and ambulation techniques, the wearing of sturdy supportive footwear, the avoidance of lifting heavy objects, and how to bend from the knees when lifting.
- Provide information and instruction on osteoporosis, including the pathophysiology of the disease, treatment regimen, drug schedule, doses, and side effects.

> **NURSING CARE PLAN—cont'd**
>
> - Stress the importance of dietary calcium intake and provide information on foods that are high in calcium.
> - Consult with physical therapy for a program of muscle strengthening, endurance development, stair training, and regular exercise.
> - Reinforce physical therapy training.
> - Give positive feedback for gains made.
> - Instruct the patient to make limited trips up and down stairs until strength is improved.
> - Instruct the patient on taking pain drugs before the exercise program and the need for regular rest periods throughout the day.
>
> - Assess pain and the effectiveness of prescribed drugs.
> - Instruct the patient to take pain drugs before activities and on a regular basis until pain diminishes.
> - Instruct the patient on the use of diversional activities and relaxation techniques.
> - Assist the patient in setting short-term, realistic goals.
> - Consult with an occupational therapist for specific assistive devices.
> - Instruct the patient on the use of assistive devices.
> - Provide assistance, supervision, and teaching, as needed, to promote self-care.

Paget's Disease

Paget's disease (osteitis deformans) is an inflammatory disease of the bone in which both osteoclasts and osteoblasts proliferate. The processes of bone formation and bone resorption do not always proceed at the same rate. The cause of Paget's disease is not known. Recent evidence supports the theory that a viral infection of the osteoclasts causes the disease. A possible familial predisposition to Paget's disease also exists. This disease occurs most often in males older than 40 years; a higher incidence occurs in individuals older than 80 years. Paget's disease is predominant in people of European descent; it is a condition that is rarely found in Asians and Africans (Ralston, 2013).

Increased activity of osteoclasts leads to increased bone resorption. Bone formation is increased to compensate. This abnormal remodeling causes deformed and enlarged bones. Vascularity in the abnormal bones is increased, which results in excessive warmth over the bones involved. Bones affected by the disease are structurally weak and prone to pathologic fractures (Ralston, 2013).

The onset of Paget's disease is insidious. The bones most often involved are the pelvis, femur, skull, tibia, and spine. The first symptom is bone pain, which is not relieved with rest and movement. The intensity of the pain varies from mild to severe; the quality may be stabbing or dull. If the bones of the skull are involved, headaches and conductive hearing loss may occur. Barreling of the chest, kyphosis, skull enlargement, and bowing of the tibia and femur are commonly seen bone deformities. The bowing of the legs and kyphosis lead to a reduction in height.

The prognosis for patients with Paget's disease is not favorable because of the complications that may develop. These include pathologic fractures and loss of hearing related to changes in the temporal bone. The overgrowth of the spinal vertebrae may cause cord compression and paralysis.

Nursing Care Guidelines for the Older Adult with Paget's Disease

Recognize cues (assessment). Nursing assessment should include taking a thorough health history; information about a known family history of the disease should also be elicited. The nurse should assess for warmth, deformity, pain, and erythema over the long bones; assess the range of motion in joints; and evaluate the presence of any weakness, ataxia, or hearing loss.

Analyze cues and prioritize hypotheses (patient problems). Patient problems for an older patient with Paget's disease include the following:

- Pain resulting from bone deformity and possible joint involvement
- Reduced mobility resulting from bone deformity, fracture, or pain
- Potential for injury resulting from limitations in mobility and altered bone metabolism
- Distorted body image resulting from deformities and disturbances in function

Generate solutions (planning). Nursing care for the patient should focus primarily on pain management, if necessary, and the issues of chronic disease. Addressing the alterations in body image and impaired mobility is also critical. Expected outcomes include the following:

1. The patient will achieve a satisfactory comfort level with pain management techniques and drugs.
2. The patient will modify the home environment and take precautions in the community to prevent injuries.
3. The patient will verbalize an understanding of the chronic nature of the disease and appropriate therapies.
4. The patient will make positive coping statements related to a potential altered body image.

Take actions (nursing interventions). Nursing care for a patient with Paget's disease includes education regarding the disease and treatment. Pain management should be addressed; pain is usually the presenting symptom. The pain is usually a deep, aching type of bone pain that may worsen with activity, especially with weight-bearing activities in patients with spinal or lower extremity deformities. For symptomatic patients, first-line drugs are nitrogen-containing bisphosphonates, such as alendronate, pamidronate, risedronate, and zoledronic acid (Ralston, 2013). Patients may also be prescribed vitamin D if the 25-hydroxy vitamin D level is found to be subclinical (Ralston, 2013). Various methods of pain relief may be tried, including the use of NSAIDs and analgesics. Other nursing interventions include instructing an older patient on the use of heat or cold therapy, rest, and other pain relief measures.

The patient's safety and mobility issues should be assessed. Instruction on simple exercises, the use of assistive devices, or consultation with physical or occupational therapists may be of benefit. Occasionally, the patient's disease may involve the hip or knee joint, resulting in chronic, severe pain, and deformity. Arthroplasty may be recommended to correct the deformity and relieve pain.

Helping the patient maintain mobility and independence with daily activities may also positively affect the patient's body image and attitude toward the chronic disease. Discussions of long-term prognosis and treatment may offer encouragement.

Evaluate outcomes (evaluation). Abnormal bone remodeling results in brittle bones, deformities, and pain. Ensure the patient's pain is controlled and they are able to perform ADLs. Evaluate their tolerance to physical and/or occupational therapy treatments. When teaching patients with Paget's disease, ensure their understanding of the importance of therapy for the prevention of pain, deformity, and loss of function. Patients may benefit from adaptive equipment such as canes, walkers, or shoe lifts when limb shortening has occurred (Ralston, 2013).

Osteomyelitis

Osteomyelitis is an infection of the bone that may be either acute or chronic. Acute osteomyelitis resolves in 4 weeks when treated with antibiotics. Chronic osteomyelitis lasts longer than 4 weeks and does not respond to initial treatment with antibiotics.

Invasion of bone by microorganisms is the cause of osteomyelitis. Microorganisms enter the body directly through an open fracture or stage IV pressure ulcer. Bloodborne bacteria from distant sources, such as urinary tract infections, may indirectly inoculate bones. *Staphylococcus aureus* is the most common bacterium seen in osteomyelitis (Oliphant, 2015). Other causative agents are Gram-negative bacteria such as *Escherichia coli* and *Pseudomonas aeruginosa*. Osteomyelitis is seen most often in older adults as a complication of a stage IV pressure ulcer.

Bacteria infiltrate bone through the blood supply and lodge in an area of bone where circulation is sluggish. The bacteria multiply, resulting in an inflammatory response. Pus and vascular congestion develop, causing increased pressure in the bones, which leads to ischemia and vascular compromise. Necrotic bone separates from living bone. The devitalized areas are called *sequestra* (Oliphant, 2015).

In an older adult with osteomyelitis associated with a bone injury, the presenting signs are localized pain, tenderness on palpation, erythema, warmth to the touch, and edema. In osteomyelitis associated with infected pressure ulcers, the symptoms may be subtle changes in mental status, low-grade fever, chills, and increased purulent wound drainage. These signs and symptoms may go unnoticed until sepsis occurs (Oliphant, 2015).

If treated early, osteomyelitis has a good prognosis. The older adult may not have the classic signs of infection. Often, the first sign of osteomyelitis may be sepsis; in these cases, the prognosis is poor.

Nursing Care Guidelines for the Older Adult with Osteomyelitis

Recognize cues (assessment). The nurse caring for older adults with osteomyelitis or for those at risk of developing osteomyelitis involves being aware of the subtlety of the presenting signs and symptoms of infection. Presenting symptoms vary in older adults and range from severe, acute onset to a clinical picture of a chronic, subacute illness with minimal pain. Nursing assessment should focus on identifying risk factors predisposing a patient to osteomyelitis, examining any preexisting incisions, especially those related to the insertion of a prosthetic device, wounds, decubitus ulcers, or ulcers related to peripheral vascular disease (PVD) or infections, and monitoring vital signs and diagnostic test results (Oliphant, 2015). Another potential site for the development of osteomyelitis is the oral cavity, in association with poor dentition and periodontal disease (Mears and Edwards, 2016). Close inspection of the mouth to look for eroding teeth and ill-fitting dentures and partials, which may contribute to dental abscesses, is important for the prevention of mandibular osteomyelitis (Mears and Edwards, 2016).

Analyze cues and prioritize hypotheses (patient problems) Patient problems for a patient with osteomyelitis include the following:
- Pain resulting from swelling and tenderness
- Reduced skin integrity resulting from infected wounds
- Reduced mobility resulting from lower extremity pain

Generate solutions (planning). The planning of care for a patient with osteomyelitis should include a multidisciplinary approach. Treatment for this condition may be prolonged and, therefore, may require additional emotional and physical support. The long-term treatment for this problem requires family and significant others to be involved in the planning process. Expected outcomes include the following:
1. The patient will report minimum discomfort and adequate pain control.
2. The patient will verbalize an understanding of the need for long-term therapy to eliminate infection.
3. The patient will demonstrate safe and independent mobility.
4. The patient will exhibit intact skin surfaces and no evidence of further infection.

Take actions (nursing interventions). Prevention of osteomyelitis includes using sterile technique during dressing changes and following strict wound precautions. A patient with infected pressure ulcers will most likely be functionally impaired and return to a long-term care setting for the completion of intravenous antibiotic treatment (Oliphant, 2015). Older patients with osteomyelitis as a result of other causes will be discharged while receiving oral antibiotics. Discharge planning involves teaching about the importance of completing the course of oral antibiotics, methods of preventing infection, and specific techniques of wound management. An alternative treatment is a surgically implanted drug pump to deliver continuous antibiotics to the infection site.

The long-term treatment of chronic osteomyelitis creates psychological coping issues. Lengthy hospitalizations, immobility, and dependence may lead to feelings of anger and decreased self-worth. To help patients cope more effectively, the nurse should allow them to make informed decisions about care and should consult with therapeutic recreation specialists for diversional activities. Prolonged immobility may lead to complications of immobility and self-care deficits. To prevent these problems, physical and occupational therapists should be consulted to provide individualized exercise programs that promote optimal functioning and prevent disability.

Evaluate outcomes (evaluation). Patients with osteomyelitis should participate fully in all aspects of care. Any wounds or other potential sources of infection should show progressive healing. The patient should be able to verbalize understanding of the chronic nature of treatment, and documentation should include the patient's involvement in wound care or antibiotic therapy. For older patients who may have difficulty adjusting to the extended hospitalization required for therapy, the nurse should facilitate appropriate consultations.

Amputation

Amputation of the lower extremity is a common surgical procedure in older patients. The level of amputation depends on the extent of the disease process. PVD, infections, neoplasms, and traumatic injury may all lead to lower extremity amputation; however, PVD is the most common cause in older adults (Jaramillo, 2021). Atherosclerosis and diabetes are predisposing factors in the development of PVD (Amputee Coalition, n.d.).

In PVD, chronic obstruction of the arteries results in inadequate circulation, which causes tissue hypoxia. When the tissues are inadequately perfused for prolonged periods, atrophy of the underlying tissue occurs. This decreased circulation leads to delayed healing of injured feet or lower extremities. When ischemic ulcers do not heal, infection and necrosis, or gangrene develop.

Gangrene manifests as a blackened area. The temperature in the affected area is lower than that of the unaffected area, and pain may be present. With the chronically infected extremity ulcer, the ulcer persists despite treatment with antibiotics.

Nursing Care Guidelines for the Older Adult with Amputation

Recognize cues (assessment). Before the surgical procedure, a complete nursing assessment is performed to determine the presence of other diseases and their effect on function. The focus of this assessment is on mobility and self-care abilities. How does the patient walk? Are assistive devices required? What is the extent of your self-care abilities? Assessment of the affected limb includes determining peripheral pulses, temperature, sensation, and movement. The specific characteristics of the ulcer or gangrenous area are noted, including location, size, and color. The individual's perception of the surgery is ascertained. Older patients should be asked how they feel about the impending surgical procedure and how they see the amputation affecting their health and lifestyle.

Analyze cues and prioritize hypotheses (patient problems). Patient problems for an older patient undergoing amputation include the following:

- Pain secondary to the surgical procedure and phantom limb sensation
- Distorted body image resulting from amputation, impaired mobility, and prolonged immobilization
- Potential for reduced skin integrity resulting from the disease process, surgical procedure, and immobility
- Reduced mobility resulting from the loss of an extremity
- Reduced stamina resulting from immobility
- Inadequate coping resulting from loss

Generate solutions (planning). Nursing care for the patient undergoing amputation includes planning for the patient's preoperative, postoperative, and rehabilitative periods. Multidisciplinary planning is critical for the patient's recovery and long-term prognosis. Expected outcomes include the following:

1. The patient will report pain relief with the administration of analgesics.
2. The patient will demonstrate acceptance of body image changes, as evidenced by positive statements regarding the body and active involvement in treatment of the stump.
3. The patient's incisional area will remain clean and without evidence of infection.
4. The patient will safely perform self-care activities within his or her activity and energy expenditure limitations.

Take actions (nursing interventions). Patient education plays an important nursing role in preventing amputation. Because the majority of amputations are a result of PVD, patients need knowledge of how to control the factors that lead to amputation. Patients with diabetes and PVD are taught how to inspect and care for their feet and lower extremities. Instructions include information on promptly notifying a health care provider if changes occur in temperature, sensation, and color. If a sore develops, prompt treatment must be sought. Methods to protect the lower extremity from injury are included in the teaching plan.

Preoperative care. Amputation has a major negative effect on an individual's body image and has the potential to lead to ineffective coping. To assist with adjustment in the postoperative phase, the nurse provides extensive information about the surgical procedure, including the purpose of the amputation, the potential use of prosthesis, and the rehabilitation program. To assist in the rehabilitation phase, the nurse teaches exercises to strengthen the upper extremities. Postoperative care, including positioning, turning, compression bandaging, and pain control, is discussed. Patients also require information about phantom sensations and phantom limb pain. *Phantom limb sensation* is the feeling of tingling, itching, or aching in the limb that no longer exists; *phantom limb pain* is a painful sensation that occurs in the limb that no longer exists; both of these conditions may become chronic.

Postoperative care. Routine postoperative care is provided in the immediate postoperative period. Patients are monitored carefully for complications that may be a result of preoperative health problems. Complications include hemorrhages and infections. Postoperative dressing depends on the type of prosthesis that will be used. The patient has either an immediate prosthetic fitting or a delayed prosthetic fitting. Because older adults may be debilitated by multiple chronic illnesses and the chronic condition that caused the amputation, they will probably have a delayed prosthetic fitting. Dressings are either rigid or soft in delayed prosthetic fittings. The rigid dressing may be made from either plastic or plaster. The advantage of this type of dressing is that it decreases edema. Soft dressings consist of gauze covered with an elastic wrap that acts as a compression dressing. The compression dressing is used to support the tissues, to decrease pain and edema, and to promote the shrinking of the stump. The soft dressing is changed daily using a sterile technique. The wound is assessed for signs and symptoms of infection. A dry dressing is applied directly to the suture site.

In the immediate postoperative period (48–72 hours), pain medication is given on a regular schedule. Because of age-related changes in pharmacokinetics and pharmacodynamics, older patients receiving opiates should be monitored closely for response and side effects. The effect of opiates may last longer and may also result in excessive sedation, confusion, or respiratory depression. Initial doses should be lower than those used for younger adults. However, on the basis of the individual's pain relief and tolerance, doses may be increased. Morphine sulfate is the drug used most often in this phase of care.

Rehabilitative care. The rehabilitative phase starts immediately after surgery with the application of the dressing. The dressing is important for prosthesis fitting because it shapes the stump for the prosthesis. The compression dressing is worn continuously and removed at least two times a day. Care is taken to properly apply the dressing. It should be wrapped snugly and securely, but not so tightly that it impairs circulation. A *stump shrinker,* a continuous tube of elasticized fabric closed at one end, may be used instead of the wrap.

Physical therapy begins when the patient's condition is stable. Nursing goals for this phase include preventing complications and assisting the patient in reaching an optimal level of functioning. The physical therapy program includes active range of motion, upper extremity strengthening, and gait training. In older adults, walkers are used for ambulation rather than crutches because crutches require greater upper extremity strength and endurance. The nurse reinforces the importance of the exercise program and assists the patient in practicing safe transfer techniques.

Prosthetic fitting and adaptation. Not all older adults are candidates for prostheses. Multiple chronic illnesses may result in a state of debilitation in which the patient will not have the strength and reserve to complete a program of intense prosthetic training. These patients are taught transfer techniques and wheelchair mobility.

Prosthetic fitting is delayed until the stump is healed and well shaped. The fitting is performed by a prosthetist (who makes a mold of the stump). As the stump shrinks, adjustments are made in the prosthesis. The patient is instructed to assess the stump daily for signs of irritation from an ill-fitting prosthesis.

The physical therapist and prosthetist instruct the older patient on the use of the prosthesis. The physical therapist also works on gait training. The nurse reinforces the teaching and provides the older patient with reinforcement on performance.

The individual who has had an amputation experiences loss and a major threat to body image. The normal response to loss is grief. The grieving process and adjustment to the loss are an individualized response characterized by vacillations in the recognized stages of grief: denial, isolation, anger, bargaining, depression, and acceptance.

Body image is an individual's subjective perception of the body. Gradual changes in body image are easier to adapt to than those that have an abrupt onset, as in the case of change experienced by an individual who has had an amputation. The adaptation to the change in body image does not always reflect the extent of the injury, but it is related to that individual's feelings toward himself or herself as a total person. The role of the nurse is to help the amputee discover a new self. Traumatic changes in body image may be characterized by revulsion in viewing the amputation. Viewing the amputation and looking in the mirror at the total self-picture may be difficult. Accepting the body changes is a gradual process. The nurse must allow the patient time to work through this process. The nurse may ask broad, open-ended questions about the body changes, for example, "How do you see yourself?" and "How do you think others see you?" (Touhy and Jett, 2016). Talking with other amputees on a one-on-one basis and in support groups is helpful for patients in adapting to changes in body image. The nurse should give positive but realistic feedback about the older patient's progress in functional abilities (see Nursing Care Plan: Amputation).

Evaluate outcomes (evaluation). Evaluation is based on the achievement of expected outcomes, as evidenced by the patient exhibiting a positive outlook about body changes, performing self-care and other activities safely and adequately, and experiencing pain relief over time, until eventually an analgesic pain drug is not needed. Documentation of these activities is critical for the multidisciplinary evaluation of the older patient's progress and is used as the basis for further care planning.

NURSING CARE PLAN

Amputation

Clinical Situation

Mr. C is a 78-year-old retired male truck driver with a medical history of type 2 diabetes mellitus, PVD, and a chronic right foot ulcer. Because the foot ulcer did not respond to conservative treatment, he underwent a right below-the-knee amputation. Before this surgical procedure, Mr. C had been hospitalized for 3 weeks for the treatment of the foot ulcer. During the hospitalization, he became weak and deconditioned. He now requires assistance with eating and ADLs, and maximum assistance for transfers. Mr. C complains of phantom limb pain and requires a pain drug every 4–6 hours.

The prolonged illness, hospitalization, and amputation have caused Mr. C to feel hopeless. He has told the nurses he is tired of being in the hospital, sick, and in pain. Mr. C has also verbalized feelings about not being the male he once was. He does not initiate any self-care and needs encouragement to complete self-care. Mr. C has a supportive wife and family. His wife has RA and thinks it will be difficult for her to care for her husband unless he participates in his care and is rehabilitated with his prosthesis. Mr. C is stable 2 days postoperatively and is beginning physical therapy for preprosthetic training.

Analyze Cues and Prioritize Hypotheses (Patient Problems)
- Distorted body image resulting from amputation, impaired mobility, and prolonged hospitalization
- Pain resulting from the surgical procedure and phantom limb sensation
- Potential for reduced skin integrity resulting from disease processes, surgical procedures, age-related changes, and immobility

> **NURSING CARE PLAN—cont'd**
>
> - Reduced mobility resulting from below-the-knee amputation and prolonged immobility
> - Reduced stamina resulting from prolonged immobility, deconditioning, and disease processes
> - Inadequate coping resulting from amputation
> - Inadequate family coping resulting from the spouse's chronic illness and disability
>
> **Generate Solutions (Planning)**
> - The patient will verbalize feelings of acceptance of a change in body image.
> - The patient will verbalize that pain is tolerable.
> - Pain will not interfere with the ability to participate in ADLs.
> - The incision will heal without signs or symptoms of infection.
> - Skin will remain free from pressure ulcers.
> - The patient will transfer independently and walk 10 feet with a pickup walker.
> - Range of motion will remain within normal limits.
> - Flexion contracture will not develop.
> - The patient will attend and participate in a daily therapy program with a normal physiologic response.
> - The patient will use effective coping strategies and participate in a rehabilitation program.
> - The family will use effective coping strategies and support the patient's participation in the rehabilitation process.
>
> **Take Actions (Nursing Interventions)**
> - Allow verbalization of feelings; actively listen to feelings.
> - Give positive feedback for progress made in self-care and mobility and for aspects of general appearance.
> - Encourage normal activities such as dressing in street clothes.
> - Encourage participation in support groups.
> - Assess the pain and effectiveness of drugs.
> - Administer pain drugs as ordered.
> - Provide diversional activities and alternative treatments, such as relaxation techniques.
> - Assess incision and pressure areas (use a risk assessment scale) daily for the signs of infection or pressure ulcers.
> - Change surgical dressing using aseptic technique.
> - Reposition every 2 hours; position to keep pressure off bony prominences.
> - Teach the patient how to change positions.
> - Provide adequate caloric, protein, and fluid intake.
> - Wrap stump with compression dressing or stump shrinker.
> - Consult with physical therapy for a program of muscle strengthening, transfer training, and gait training.
> - Reinforce physical therapy training.
> - Give positive feedback for gains made.
> - Teach transfer techniques; assist with transfers.
> - Teach the safe use of a walker.
> - Give pain drugs 30–60 minutes before therapy.
> - Do not elevate the stump on pillows.
> - Keep the stump in good alignment; prevent flexion contractures.
> - Reinforce the use of active range-of-motion exercises.
> - Encourage lying on the abdomen for 30 minutes two times a day.
> - Encourage participation in the therapy program.
> - Gradually increase activity.
> - Allow at least 60 minutes of rest after therapy.
> - Monitor vital signs before, during, and after therapy.
> - Assist the patient in identifying previously successful coping skills.
> - Suggest and describe effective coping skills.
> - Encourage activities that enhance self-esteem.
> - Encourage the use of support systems.
> - Encourage participation in an amputation support group; include the family, especially the spouse, in the support group.
> - Encourage the spouse's verbalization of feelings when the patient is not present.
> - Suggest and describe effective coping skills to her.
> - Suggest taking time to care for herself.

Polymyalgia Rheumatica

Polymyalgia rheumatica (PMR) is a chronic inflammatory condition characterized by the sudden onset of muscle stiffness and aching (myalgia) in the neck, shoulders, and pelvic girdle. The disease occurs after the age of 50, most often in those 65 years of age or older. Females are affected more compared with males (Hancock et al, 2014). The cause of PMR is not known. Infection and an altered immune response have been suggested but not proven as the cause. Likewise, a genetic predisposition is suggested but not confirmed. The pathophysiology of PMR is not clearly understood.

The clinical presentation of PMR is similar to that of RA and OA. Symptoms include muscle stiffness and aching in the neck, shoulders, and pelvic girdle (Buttgereit et al, 2016). The muscle stiffness is present in the morning and lasts more than 1 hour. Constitutional symptoms such as fatigue, fever, often with night sweating, malaise, anorexia, depression, and weight loss may be present (Saad et al, 2023). Initially, the pain may be limited to one area, but it generally develops in a symmetric fashion. Objective signs of muscle weakness are not present on physical examination. Check for signs of carpal tunnel syndrome, such as paresthesia of the thumb and index finger. Look for swelling with pitting edema in the ankles and the top of the feet (González-Gay and Pina, 2015).

Diagnostics indicative of PMR are an elevated erythrocyte sedimentation rate (ESR) and C-reactive protein (CRP). Patients with PMR generally are found to be anemic. PMR is treated with corticosteroids that are tapered over time. Symptoms of aching, stiffness, and fatigue may begin to resolve in about 1–2 days, and patients will remain on long-term corticosteroids until the laboratory values return to normal. Treatment may last 1 to 3 years for PMR (Dejaco et al, 2015). This marked improvement so soon after the initiation of treatment is not seen in RA or OA.

Nursing Care Guidelines for the Older Adult with Polymyalgia Rheumatica

Recognize cues (assessment). A thorough history of the patient's symptoms, physical examination, and functional assessment is important in determining the effects of the disease on functional abilities.

Analyze cues and prioritize hypotheses (patient problems). Patient problems for a patient with PMR include the following:
- Pain resulting from muscle stiffness and aching
- Reduced mobility resulting from pain and muscle stiffness

- Fatigue resulting from systemic symptoms
- Inadequate self-care resulting from muscle stiffness
- Inadequate coping resulting from the chronic nature of the disease

Generate solutions (planning). Expected outcomes for an older patient with PMR include the following:

1. The patient will report pain relief with the initiation of treatment.
2. The patient will correctly describe pharmacologic therapy, including the purpose, action, and side effects of prescribed drugs.
3. The patient will establish an activity and rest pattern based on the limitations imposed by the disease.
4. The patient will incorporate effective coping strategies into disease management.
5. The patient will correctly state the treatment rationale and prognosis.

Take actions (nursing interventions). The medical diagnosis of PMR is difficult to make because its symptoms are similar to those of RA and OA. It is often misdiagnosed. The older patient who has been to many physicians in an attempt to receive the correct diagnosis and proper treatment may be frustrated, angry, and worn out. The nurse should listen to the patient's concerns and give information to the patient about the disease and the treatment plan. This includes information about the treatment with corticosteroids and their side effects. The nurse monitors the patient for the development of side effects from long-term corticosteroid use, such as infection, osteoporosis, fractures, and diabetes mellitus. The older patient should be reassured that the dose of drug will be tapered and that eventually the symptoms will subside; however, it should be emphasized that the drug needs to be continued despite the patient becoming symptom-free. Patients should also be informed that it is common to have a relapse of PMR and that, now that they are familiar with the disease presentation, they should report any new onset of symptoms right away to their care providers (Patil and Dasgupta, 2013).

Evaluate outcomes (evaluation). Patients with PMR need to understand the chronic nature of the disease and be able to maintain functional abilities. Pain management is necessary for the older patient to perform ADLs, so the patient will need to be familiar with the drugs and their side effects. Providing appropriate education about the disease and symptom management will assist in acceptance. Documentation of education, pain assessment, and functional abilities is important for the ongoing planning and care of the patient.

Foot Problems

The foot is often overlooked in the assessment and care of older adults. Foot problems, especially pain, are common in older adults. The incidence and severity of foot problems increase with age. After the age of 65, 75% of the population complains of foot problems. More than 80% of those older than the age of 55 demonstrate arthritic changes on radiography. Foot problems may cause an unsteady gait and may result in falls (Violand, 2017).

The foot is a complex structure composed of 26 bones, 33 joints, and numerous ligaments, tendons, and muscles. The foot is necessary for ambulation. During standing and ambulation, the foot provides body support and absorbs shock. Painful feet may be the result of congenital deformities, weak structures, injuries, and diseases such as diabetes, RA, and OA. Ill-fitting shoes cause foot pain by crowding the toes and impeding normal movement. With aging, feet show signs of wear and tear. The cushioning layer of fat on the soles of feet becomes thin. Years of walking cause the metatarsal bones to spread and the ligaments to stretch, which results in a widening of the feet.

Corns

Corns are thickened and hardened dead or hyperkeratotic tissue that develops over bony protuberances. Corns often cause localized pain. Ill-fitting or loose shoes that constantly place pressure on bony prominences cause corns. Soft corns are produced by the bony prominence of one toe rubbing against the adjacent toe in the web space between the toes. Soft corns are macerated because of moisture in the web space. Hard corns, also known as *heloma durum,* have a dry mass of keratosis with a central hard core (Fig. 21.13). Heloma durum is found on the plantar side of the foot often over the fifth metatarsal and the surrounding metatarsal head (Feldman, 2017). Warm water soaks are used to soften corns before gently rubbing with a pumice stone or callus file. Another treatment is gentle debridement by a podiatrist. To relieve pain and prevent the development of corns, moleskin or cotton pads are placed over areas subjected to rubbing and pressure (Feldman, 2017). Wider and softer shoes are recommended; older females should avoid wearing high-heeled shoes. Use of topical applications of salicylic acid should be avoided in older adults because these may cause irritation, burns, or infection, especially in those with diabetes and impaired circulation, especially in diabetics, as skin damage could occur without the patient's knowledge (Romano, 2016).

Calluses

Calluses, or plantar keratoses, are dead tissue found on the plantar surfaces of the feet. They form under the metatarsal heads, most commonly the second and third heads. Calluses are also common in people who have bunions (Hashmi, 2013). About 50% of people older than 65 years have some degree of plantar calluses. The aging changes of decreased toe function and decreased fat padding contribute to their development. Soft-soled shoes with additional cushioned insoles are recommended. Treatment is the same as for corns.

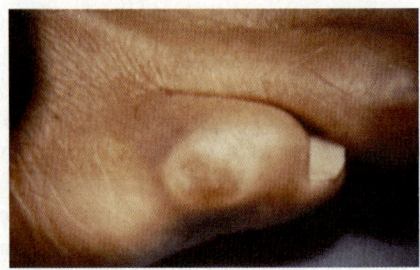

Fig. 21.13 Hard corn with keratotic buildup. (From Coughlin, M. J., Mann, R. A., & Saltzman, C. L. [2007]. *Surgery of the foot and ankle* [Vol. 2, 8th ed.]. Philadelphia, PA: Elsevier.)

Bunions

Bunions, or *hallux valgus,* have the greatest prevalence among those older than 50 years, and females experience them four times more often compared with males because females tend to wear narrow, pointed, high-heeled shoes. Arthritis and other age-related changes, such as ligament and tendon atrophy, predispose older adults to bunions.

Bunions appear as bony protuberances on the side of the great toe (Fig. 21.14). With bunions, the large toe angles laterally toward the second toe. As the great toe rubs against the shoe, the bursa becomes inflamed, which results in bursitis and pain. Initial treatment of bunions involves wearing soft leather shoes that are flat, wide, and laced up. Walking or running shoes with a wide toe box prevent rubbing on the bunion. Moleskin bunion pads may be used to protect the bony protrusion. NSAIDs may be prescribed to reduce inflammation and pain. Surgical interventions are used after conservative treatment has failed. The surgical procedure includes the removal of the bursa sac and the correction of the bony deformity.

Hammertoe

Hammertoe is a deformity of the second toe. The metatarsophalangeal joint is dorsiflexed, the proximal interphalangeal joint is plantar flexed, and callus formation occurs on the dorsum of the proximal interphalangeal joint and the end of the affected toe. The result is a toe that has a clawlike appearance (Fig. 21.15). Improperly fitted shoes, muscle weakness, and arthritis place older adults at risk for hammertoe. Symptoms include pain and burning on the bottom of the foot and problems walking in shoes. Initially, pain may be relieved with the use of a moleskin toe pad. Other treatments for hammertoe include metatarsal arch support, orthotics, splints, and passive manual stretching of the proximal interphalangeal joint. A surgical correction is performed if conservative treatment is ineffective.

Nail Disorders

Toenail problems are common in older adults. Older adults with problems with their nails should be referred to a podiatrist.

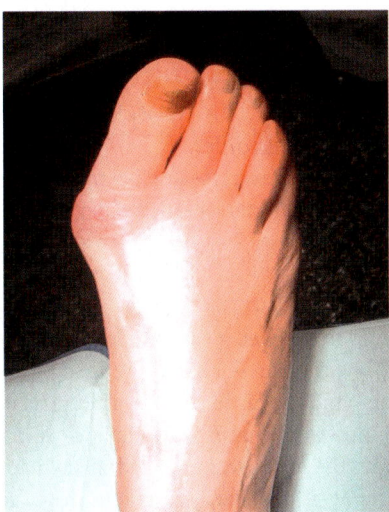

Fig. 21.14 Hallux valgus angulation of the first three toes and wide, flat metatarsus. (© Cyberprout/CC-BY-SA-1.0, via Wikimedia Commons.)

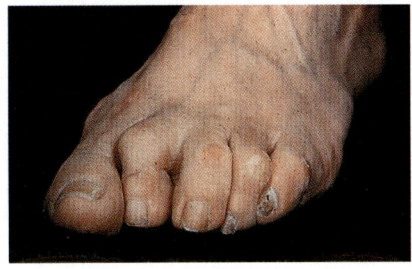

Fig. 21.15 Hammertoe associated with hallux valgus. (Courtesy Charles W. Bradley, DPM, MPA, and Caroline Harvey, DPM, California College of Podiatric Medicine.)

Onychauxis is described as hypertrophic nails whose borders curve into the soft tissue of the toes. This disorder may cause nail bed ulcers, infection, and pain.

Onychomycosis is a localized fungal infection of the toenail that is seen most frequently in older adults. Degeneration of the nail plate causes changes in the growth and appearance of the nail. Onychomycotic nails may have simple scaling or may be totally destroyed by the fungus. Initially, the nail becomes brittle and hypertrophic. The nails may be white, yellow, or brown in color. Ridges and pitting of the nail are common. Generally, the infection spreads between the nails. Predisposing factors for onychomycosis are moisture, ill-fitting footwear, recurrent trauma, and diabetes.

Treatment of onychomycosis is difficult because of the composition of the nail and the involvement of the nail matrix. Topical antifungals such as clotrimazole are generally used for several months. Oral antifungal agents such as terbinafine and itraconazole are generally not used in older adults because many older adults have a decreased pedal blood supply. The older patient with onychomycosis who does not respond to topical antifungal agents should be referred to a podiatrist. The podiatrist will debride the nail at periodic intervals.

Patient Education

The nurse should educate the older adult about the predisposing factors, prevention, and treatment of onychomycosis and the need for ongoing foot care, including inspection of feet for signs of infection and the application of the drug.

The nurse has an important role in educating patients about proper foot care and footwear. Well-fitting shoes are essential for the prevention of foot problems. The shoes should not crowd the toes and should be of the correct length and width. Shoes that are too short or narrow may force the great toe into a position of hallux valgus. Shoes should be wide enough to allow bending of the toes and movement of the foot muscles. Adequate arch support should be provided. Older females should avoid wearing high heels (Farndon et al, 2015).

Patients should be taught foot care that includes daily hygiene and changing of socks. Socks or stockings should be loose enough to avoid the development of pressure ulcers. Toenails should be trimmed with nail clippers; patients with impaired vision, impaired mobility, or self-care deficits may require assistance to perform this task safely. The nails should be trimmed straight across so that the development of ingrown toenails and infections can be prevented. If the foot problems persist, a podiatrist should be consulted (Violand, 2017).

Muscle Cramps

Idiopathic muscle cramps without muscle weakness are common in older adults. The cramps may start during rest or after minor exercise. Muscle cramps generally affect the calf or foot muscles, producing plantar flexion of the foot or toes. They occur most frequently at night, during sleep.

Stretching the affected muscles for several minutes at bedtime may prevent muscle cramps. If cramping occurs, stretching will generally relieve the discomfort. Calf muscles should be stretched, with two or three 1-minute intervals and 1-minute rest periods between stretches. Stretching exercises improve muscle flexibility and reduce motor activity in the affected muscles.

Quinine sulfate is sometimes prescribed for muscle cramps; however, its effectiveness has been questioned. The side effects of quinine therapy for muscle cramps may increase the concentration of digoxin, and an overdose may cause confusion.

SUMMARY

Problems with the musculoskeletal system may have a great effect on the day-to-day lives of older adults. Conditions such as OA, RA, PMR, osteoporosis, and fractures may result in functional disability, chronic pain, and a decreased quality of life. The role of the nurse working with older patients with musculoskeletal disorders is to promote safe, optimal functioning with regard to mobility and self-care. Interventions to promote comfort and relieve pain are critical to the maintenance of function. To prevent serious disability, it is essential that patients resume activity as soon as possible after episodes of acute illness. A key nursing role is to educate patients about the importance of musculoskeletal activity in maintaining function.

HOME CARE

1. Assessment of the musculoskeletal system includes examination of bones, muscles, and joints in homebound older adults.
2. Instruct caregivers and homebound older adults about reportable signs and symptoms related to the musculoskeletal system disease or disorder being treated and when to report these changes to the home care nurse or physician.
3. Instruct caregivers and homebound older adults on the name, dose, frequency, side effects, and indications of both the prescribed and over-the-counter drugs being used to treat the identified musculoskeletal problem.
4. Musculoskeletal problems increase safety hazards (e.g., falls) in homebound older adults.
5. Assess for functional impairments, such as the inability to provide self-care and perform IADLs. If necessary, have a social worker identify community resources for additional assistance with identified impairments, such as transportation and food preparation.
6. Assess the activity tolerance level, which may be affected by musculoskeletal problems.
7. Instruct caregivers and homebound older adults about the diagnosed musculoskeletal disease or disorder, focusing on self-care measures that maintain or promote independence.
8. Have the physical therapist and the occupational therapist evaluate and teach caregivers and homebound older adults how to adapt to the environment based on the specific musculoskeletal problem (e.g., gait training, use of handheld devices to assist with eating, splints, and prostheses).
9. Encourage ambulation in a safe manner. Stretching exercises that improve posture should be part of the nursing interventions.
10. An exercise program may be suggested after consulting with the physician.
11. Instruct caregivers and homebound older adults on the necessity of calcium supplements and exercise to maintain proper skeletal function and prevent bone loss.

KEY POINTS

- A high incidence of musculoskeletal disorders exists among older adults.
- Musculoskeletal disorders are a major cause of functional impairment in older adults.
- Age-related changes in the musculoskeletal system may predispose older adults to falls.
- The most common sites of fractures in older adults are the hips, wrists (Colles fracture), and vertebrae.
- Demographic factors associated with osteoporosis include female gender, age, and White race.
- Lower extremity amputations in older adults are most often the result of PVD or diabetes.
- The symptoms of OA, RA, gouty arthritis, and PMR are similar, but treatments differ.
- Physical activity and exercise are key to preventing disability from musculoskeletal disorders in older adults.

CLINICAL JUDGMENT EXERCISES

1. An 83-year-old female has suffered a musculoskeletal injury that requires a period of bed rest and limited mobility. How will age affect her ability to tolerate a period of decreased mobility? Explain.
2. You are caring for two patients: a 74-year-old male with gouty arthritis and a 68-year-old female with RA. What aspects of their care will be similar? What aspects will be different?
3. A 72-year-old male lived a fairly sedentary lifestyle as an accountant. Now that he is retired, he recognizes the need to be active to maintain his health for as long as possible. He is concerned, however, that it is too late for him to start exercising because he has never engaged in such activities. What encouragement, if any, can you give to him, and what suggestions can you make for an exercise program?

REFERENCES

Ackermann, L., Schwenk, E. S., Lev, Y., & Weitz, H. (2021). Update on medical management of acute hip fracture. *Cleveland Clinic Journal of Medicine, 88*(4), 237–347. doi:10.3949/ccjm.88a.20149.

Agency for Healthcare Research and Quality (AHRQ). (2017). Chapter 1. Introduction and program overview. In *The falls management program: A quality improvement initiative for nursing facilities*. Retrieved from https://www.ahrq.gov/patient-safety/settings/long-term-care/resource/injuries/fallspx/man1.html. Accessed February 16, 2024.

Allen, K. D., Choong, P. F., Davis, A. M., Dowsey, M. M., Dziedzic, K. S., Emery, C., et al. (2016). Osteoarthritis: models for appropriate care across the disease continuum. *Best Practice & Research: Clinical Rheumatology, 30*(3), 503–535. doi:10.1016/j.berh.2016.09.003.

American Academy of Orthopaedic Surgeons (AAOS). (2020). *Care of casts and splints*. OrthoInfo [website]. Retrieved from https://orthoinfo.aaos.org/en/recovery/care-of-casts-and-splints/. Accessed February 12, 2024.

American Academy of Orthopaedic Surgeons (AAOS). (2021). Management of hip fractures in older adults. Evidence-based clinical practice guideline. Retrieved from https://www.aaos.org/hipfxcpg. Accessed February 12, 2024.

American Geriatrics Society Health in Aging Foundation (AGS). (2022). *Fractures*. HealthinAging.org [website]. Retrieved from https://www.healthinaging.org/a-z-topic/fractures/basic-facts. Accessed February 12, 2024.

Amputee Coalition. (n.d.). *Limb loss statistics*. Retrieved from https://www.amputee-coalition.org/resources/limb-loss-statistics/. Accessed February 12, 2024.

Ashford, S., & Williard, J. (2014). Osteoarthritis: A review. *The Nurse Practitioner, 39*(5), 1–8. doi:10.1097/01.NPR.0000445886.71205.c4.

Ayhan, E., Kesmezacar, H., & Akgun, I. (2014). Intraarticular injections (corticosteroid, hyaluronic acid, platelet rich plasma) for the knee osteoarthritis. *World Journal of Orthopedics, 5*(3), 351. doi:10.5312/wjo.v5.i3.351.

Bhatia, D., Bejarano, T., & Novo, M. (2013). Current interventions in the management of knee osteoarthritis. *Journal of Pharmacy and Bioallied Sciences, 5*(1), 30–38. doi:10.4103/0975-7406.106561.

Bone Health & Osteoporosis Foundation (BHOF). (n.d.). *Module A: Osteoporosis basics*. Retrieved from https://cme.nof.org/system/files/Module%20A.pdf. Accessed February 12, 2024.

Browne, K. L., & Merrill, E. (2015). Musculoskeletal management matters: Principles of assessment and triage for the nurse practitioner. *The Journal for Nurse Practitioners, 11*(10), 929–939. doi:10.1016/j.nurpra.2015.08.036.

Bullock, M. W. (2021). *Infection and your joint replacement*. American Association of Hip and Knee Surgeons (AAHKS). Retrieved from https://hipknee.aahks.org/wp-content/uploads/2021/07/FINAL-Infection-and-Your-Joint-Replacement-7-8-21.pdf. Accessed February 12, 2024.

Buttgereit, F., Dejaco, C., Matteson, E. L., & Dasgupta, B. (2016). Polymyalgia rheumatica and giant cell arteritis: A systematic review. *JAMA, 315*(22), 2442–2458. doi:10.1001/jama.2016.5444.

Centers for Disease Control and Prevention (CDC). (2016). *Hip fractures among older adults*. Retrieved from https://www.cdc.gov/falls/hip-fractures.html. Accessed February 12, 2024.

Centers for Disease Control and Prevention (CDC). (2023). *Facts about falls*. Retrieved from https://www.cdc.gov/falls/facts.html. Accessed February 12, 2024.

Chan, K. K. (2023). *Tumor necrosis factor (TNF) inhibitors*. American College of Rheumatology. Retrieved from https://rheumatology.org/patients/tumor-necrosis-factor-tnf-inhibitors. Accessed February 12, 2024.

Corrarino, J. E. (2015). Fracture repair: Mechanisms and management. *The Journal for Nurse Practitioners, 11*(10), 960–967. doi:10.1016/j.nurpra.2015.07.009.

Cosman, F., de Beur, S. J., LeBoff, M. S., Lewiecki, E. M., Tanner, B., Randall, S., et al. (2014). Clinician's guide to prevention and treatment of osteoporosis. *Osteoporosis International, 25*(10), 2359–2381. doi:10.1007/s00198-014-2794-2.

Dejaco, C., Singh, Y. P., Perel, P., Hutchings, A., Camellino, D., Mackie, S., et al. (2015). 2015 Recommendations for the management of polymyalgia rheumatica: A European League Against Rheumatism/American College of Rheumatology collaborative initiative. *Arthritis & Rheumatology, 67*(10), 2569–2580. doi:10.1002/art.39333.

Della Rocca, G. J., Moylan, K. C., Crist, B. D., Volgas, D. A., Stannard, J. P., & Mehr, D. A. (2013). Comanagement of geriatric patients with hip fractures: A retrospective, controlled cohort study. *Geriatric Orthopaedic Surgery & Rehabilitation, 4*(1), 10–15. doi:10.1177/2151458513495238.

Derry, S., Wiffen, P. J., Kalso, E. A., Bell, R. F., Aldington, D., Phillips, T. (2017). Topical analgesics for acute and chronic pain in adults – an overview of Cochrane Reviews. *Cochrane Database Systematic Reviews, 5*(5), CD008609. doi:10.1002/14651858.CD008609.pub2.

Dunkin, M. A. (2022). *Treatments for rheumatoid arthritis*. Arthritis Foundation. Retrieved from https://www.arthritis.org/health-wellness/treatment/treatment-plan/disease-management/treatments-for-rheumatoid-arthritis. Accessed February 12, 2024.

Emmerson, B. R., Varacallo, M., & Inman, D. (2023). Hip fracture overview. In *StatPearls* [Internet]. Treasure Island, FL: StatPearls Publishing. Retrieved from https://www.ncbi.nlm.nih.gov/books/NBK557514/. Accessed February 12, 2024.

Ensrud, K. E. (2013). Epidemiology of fracture risk with advancing age. *The Journals of Gerontology: Series A, Biological Sciences and Medical Sciences, 68*(10), 1236–1242. doi:10.1093/Gerona/glt092.

Farndon, L., Concannon, M., & Stephenson, J. (2015). A survey to investigate the association of pain, foot disability and quality of life with corns. *Journal of Foot and Ankle Research, 8*, 70. doi:10.1186/s13047-015-0131-4.

Feldman, N. J. (2017). Corns and calluses. In F. J. Domingo, J. Golding, M. B. Stephens, & R. A. Baldor (Eds.), *5-minute clinical consult, the 2017* (25th ed.). Philadelphia, PA: Lippincott Williams & Wilkins Health.

Feng, X., Li, Y., & Gao, W. (2015). Significance of the initiation time of urate-lowering therapy in gout patients: A retrospective research. *Joint Bone Spine, 82*(6), 428–431. doi:10.1016/j.jbspin.2015.02.021.

Fischer, S. J., & Gray, J. L. (2020). *Hip fractures*. OrthoInfo [website]. American Academy of Orthopaedic Surgeons. Retrieved from https://orthoinfo.aaos.org/en/diseases--conditions/hip-fractures/. Accessed February 12, 2024.

Forster, R., & Stewart, M. (2016). Anticoagulants (extended duration) for prevention of venous thromboembolism following total hip or knee replacement or hip fracture repair. *Cochrane Database of Systematic Reviews, 3*(3), CD004179. doi:10.1002/14651858.CD004179.pub2.

Githens, M. F., & Lowe, J. A. (2022). *Clavicle fracture (broken collarbone)*. OrthoInfo [website]. American Academy of Orthopaedic Surgeons. Retrieved from https://orthoinfo.aaos.org/en/diseases—conditions/clavicle-fracture-broken-collarbone/. Accessed February 12, 2024.

González-Gay, M. A., & Pina, T. (2015). Giant cell arteritis and polymyalgia rheumatica: An update. *Current Rheumatology Reports, 17*(2), 6. doi:10.1007/s11926-014-0480-1.

Gray-Miceli, D. (2017). Impaired mobility and functional decline in older adults: Evidence to facilitate a practice change. *Nursing Clinics of North America, 52*(3), 469–487. doi:10.1016/j.cnur.2017.05.002.

Hancock, A. T., Mallen, C. D., Muller, S., Belcher, J., Roddy, E., Helliwell, T., et al. (2014). Risk of vascular events in patients with polymyalgia rheumatica. *CMAJ, 186*(13), E495–E501. doi:10.1503/cmaj.140266.

Hashmi, F. (2013). Calluses, corns and heel fissures. *Dermatological Nursing, 12*(1), 36–40.

Hildebrand, G. K., & Kasi, A. (2022). Denosumab. In *StatPearls* [Internet]. Treasure Island, FL: StatPearls Publishing. Retrieved from https://www.ncbi.nlm.nih.gov/books/NBK535388/. Accessed February 12, 2024.

Hootman, J. M., Helmick, C. G., Barbour, K. E., Theis, K. A., & Boring, M. A. (2016). Updated projected prevalence of self-reported doctor-diagnosed arthritis and arthritis-attributable activity limitation among US adults, 2015–2040. *Arthritis & Rheumatology, 68*(7), 1582–1587. doi:10.1002/art.39692.

Igel, T. F., Krasnokutsky, S., & Pillinger, M. H. (2017). Recent advances in understanding and managing gout. *F1000Research, 6*, 247. doi:10.12688/f1000research.9402.1.

Ikpeze, T. C., Mohney, S., & Elfar, J. C. (2017). Initial preoperative management of geriatric hip fractures. *Geriatric Orthopaedic Surgery & Rehabilitation, 8*(1), 64–66. doi:10.1177/2151458516681145.

Ishchenko, A., & Lories, R. J. (2016). Safety and efficacy of biological disease-modifying antirheumatic drugs in older rheumatoid arthritis patients: Staying the distance. *Drugs & Aging, 33*(6), 387–398. doi:10.1007/s40266-016-0374-1.

Jaramillo, C. A. (2021). Geriatrics. In D. X. Cifu, B. C. Eapen, J. S. Johns, K. Kowalske, H. L. Lew, M. A. Miller, & G. Worsowic (Eds.), *Braddom's physical medicine and rehabilitation* (6th ed.). Philadelphia, PA: Elsevier.

Kalff, R., Ewald, C., Waschke, A., Gobisch, L., & Hopf, C. (2013). Degenerative lumbar spinal stenosis in older people: Current treatment options. *Deutsches Arzteblatt International, 110*(37), 613–624. doi:10.3238/arztebl.2013.0613.

Kuo, C. F., Grainge, M. J., Mallen, C., Zhang, W., & Doherty, M. (2015). Rising burden of gout in the UK but continuing suboptimal management: A nationwide population study. *Annals of the Rheumatic Diseases, 74*(4), 661–667. doi:10.1136/annrheumdis-2013-204463.

LeBlond, R. F., Brown, D. D., Suneja, M., & Szot, J. F. (2015). *DeGowin's diagnostic examination* (10th ed.). New York: McGraw-Hill Medical.

LeBoff, M. S., Greenspan, S. L., Insogna, K. L., Lewiecki, E. M., Saag, K. G., Singer, A. J., et al. (2022). The clinician's guide to prevention and treatment of osteoporosis. *Osteoporosis International, 33*(10), 2049–2102. doi:10.1007/s00198-021-05900-y.

Lee, S. Y., Kim, T. H., Oh, J. K., Lee, S. J., & Park, M. S. (2015). Lumbar stenosis: A recent update by review of literature. *Asian Spine Journal, 9*(5), 818–828. doi:10.4184/asj.2015.9.5.818.

Mackey, P. A., & Whitaker, M. D. (2015). Osteoporosis: A therapeutic update. *The Journal for Nurse Practitioners, 11*(10), 1011–1017. doi:10.1016/j.nurpra.2015.08.010.

Manini, T. M., Gundermann, D. M., & Clark, B. C. (2016). Aging of the muscles and joints. In J. B. Halter, J. G. Ouslander, S. Studenski, K. P. High, S. Asthana, M. A. Supiano, & C. Ritchie. (Eds.), *Hazzard's geriatric medicine and gerontology* (7th ed.). New York: McGraw-Hill Medical.

Mears, S. C., & Edwards, P. K. (2016). Bone and joint infections in older adults. *Clinics in Geriatric Medicine, 32*(3), 555–570. doi:10.1016/j.cger.2016.02.003.

National Institute on Aging (NIA). (2022). *Falls and fractures in older adults: Causes and prevention*. National Institutes of Health. Retrieved from https://www.nia.nih.gov/health/falls-and-falls-prevention/falls-and-fractures-older-adults-causes-and-prevention. Accessed February 12, 2024.

O'Connell, S., Bashar, K., Broderick, B. J., Sheehan, J., Quondamatteo, F., Walsh, S. R., et al. (2016). The use of intermittent pneumatic compression in orthopedic and neurosurgical postoperative patients: A systematic review and meta-analysis. *Annals of Surgery, 263*(5), 888–889. doi:10.1097/SLA.0000000000001530.

Oliphant, C. M. (2015). Management of orthopedic infections. *The Journal for Nurse Practitioners, 11*(10), 1036–1042. doi:10.1016/j.nurpra.2015.07.015.

Onat, Ş. Ş., Ekiz, T., Biçer, S., & Özgirgin, N. (2015). The differential diagnosis of atypical localized osteoarthritis in elderly patients: A case report. *Journal of Physical Medicine & Rehabilitation Sciences, 18*, 58–62.

Park, D. K. (2021). *Lumbar spinal stenosis*. OrthoInfo [website]. American Academy of Orthopaedic Surgeons (AAOS). Retrieved from https://orthoinfo.aaos.org/en/diseases--conditions/lumbar-spinal-stenosis/. Accessed February 12, 2024.

Patil, P., & Dasgupta, B. (2013). Polymyalgia rheumatica in older adults. *Aging Health, 9*(5), 483–495. doi:10.2217/ahe.13.50.

Prah, A., Richards, E., Griggs, R., & Simpson, V. (2017). Enhancing osteoporosis efforts through lifestyle modifications and goal-setting techniques. *The Journal for Nurse Practitioners, 13*(8), 552–561. doi:10.1016/j.nurpra.2017.07.015.

Qaseem, A., Hicks, L. A., Etxeandia-Ikobaltzeta, I., Shamliyan, T., Cooney, T. G., Cross, J. T., Jr, et al. (2023). Pharmacologic treatment of primary osteoporosis or low bone mass to prevent fractures in adults: A living clinical guideline from the American College of Physicians. *Annals of Internal Medicine, 176*(2), 224–238. doi:10.7326/M22-1034.

Ralston, S. H. (2013). Clinical practice. Paget's disease of bone. *New England Journal of Medicine, 368*(7), 644–650. doi:10.1056/NEJMcp1204713.

Romano, M. I. (2016). Corns and calluses. In T. M. Buttaro & J. Trybulski (Eds.), *Primary care: A collaborative practice* (pp. 268–269.e1). St. Louis, MO: Elsevier.

Saad, E. R., Papadopoulos, P. J., Floravanti, G., & Samuels, A. J. (2023). *Polymyalgia rheumatica (PMR)*. Medscape [website]. Retrieved from http://emedicine.medscape.com/article/330815-overview. Accessed February 12, 2024.

Schweich, P. (2023). Patient education: Cast and splint care (beyond the basics). In K. Boutis & M. Ganetsky (Eds.), *UpToDate*. Wolters Kluwer. Retrieved from https://www.uptodate.com/contents/cast-and-splint-care-beyond-the-basics/print. Accessed February 12, 2024.

Shelton, L. R. (2013). A closer look at osteoarthritis. *The Nurse Practitioner, 38*(7), 30–37. doi:10.1097/01.NPR.0000431178.49311.42.

Taylor-Piliae, R. E., Peterson, R., & Mohler, M. J. (2017). Clinical and community strategies to prevent falls and fall-related injuries among community-dwelling older adults. *Nursing Clinics of North America, 52*(3), 489–497. doi:10.1016/j.cnur.2017.04.004.

Touhy, T., & Jett, K. (2016). *Towards healthy aging: Human needs and nursing response* (9th ed.). St. Louis, MO: Elsevier.

Violand, M. (2017). Putting a healthy foot forward. *The Journal for Nurse Practitioners, 13*(7), 499–500. doi:10.1016/j.nurpra.2017.04.003.

Wedro, B. (2022). *Broken bone (types of bone fractures)*. MedicineNet [website]. Retrieved from https://www.medicinenet.com/broken_bone_types_of_bone_fractures/article.htm. Accessed February 12, 2024.

West, S. G., & O'Dell, J. R. (2015). *Rheumatology secrets* (3rd ed.). Philadelphia, PA: Elsevier.

Yang, H. (2023). *Spinal stenosis*. American College of Rheumatology. Retrieved from https://rheumatology.org/patients/spinal-stenosis. Accessed February 12, 2024.

Yaseen, Kinanah (2024). Rheumatoid Arthritis (RA). https://www.merckmanuals.com/professional/musculoskeletal-and-connective-tissue-disorders/joint-disorders/rheumatoid-arthritis-ra. (Accessed 01 June 2024).

Yung, R. (2017). Chapter 121: Rheumatoid arthritis and other autoimmune diseases. In J. B. Halter, J. G. Ouslander, S. Studenski, K. P. High, S. Asthana, M. A. Supiano, & C. Ritchie. (Eds.), *Hazzard's geriatric medicine and gerontology* (7th ed.). New York: McGraw-Hill.

22

Cognitive and Neurologic Function

Jennifer J. Yeager, PhD, MSN, RN

http://evolve.elsevier.com/Yeager/gerontologic/

LEARNING OBJECTIVES

On completion of this chapter, the reader will be able to:

1. Compare structural changes in the brain and nerve function associated with aging.
2. Describe functional changes in the neurologic system during the aging process.
3. Compare normal, age-related changes of the neurologic system with those associated with cognitive and neurologic disorders.
4. Differentiate the symptoms of depression, delirium, dementia, and other cognitive and neurologic disorders.
5. Describe the symptoms and associated diagnostic tests and interventions related to common cognitive and neurologic disorders in older adults.
6. Apply the nursing process to the development of a plan of care for patients with common cognitive and neurologic disorders.
7. Analyze evidence-based practices that enhance the management of patients with cognitive and neurologic disorders.

WHAT WOULD YOU DO?

What would you do if you were faced with the following situations?

- Your 72-year-old patient, admitted yesterday for intravenous (IV) antibiotics to treat a urinary tract infection (UTI), is lethargic and has slurred speech when responding to questions. Their responses are not always appropriate to the question. What is going on?

- A 68-year-old is brought to the emergency department (ED) via ambulance with an ischemic stroke. The family states that symptoms began when the evening news began, about 45 minutes ago. How would you determine whether the patient was appropriate for a tissue plasminogen activator (TPA)?

The number of Americans at the age of 65 and older continues to grow rapidly. There has been a 38% increase in older adults since 2010. The old adult population is expected to grow by 22% by 2040 (Administration for Community Living [ACL], 2022). Considering this projection, it is essential that nurses stay abreast of the most recent findings regarding the development, manifestations, and treatment of cognitive and neurologic problems among older adults. The brain is a complex organ composed of more than a billion nerves and many specialized areas (Maldonado and Alsayouri, 2023). For nurses caring for older persons, an understanding of basic neurologic function, normal age-related changes, and common disorders is necessary to assist nurses in providing safe, effective, and evidence-based nursing interventions.

The nervous system undergoes many neurophysiologic changes as a person ages. The changes do not affect all older individuals equally or occur at the same age. Additionally, these changes do not always result in a loss of neurologic function. An individual's environment, genetics (Maisese, 2022a), lifestyle, and nutritional intake are some of the many factors that affect the neurologic system. To understand the most common chronic neurologic diseases that occur with aging, and their management, a brief review of the brain and spinal cord and associated age-related changes is necessary. For a more in-depth review of the neurologic system, please refer to a pathophysiology text.

THE CENTRAL NERVOUS SYSTEM

The central nervous system (CNS) is composed of the brain and spinal cord. The brain is responsible for responses, sensation, movement, emotions, communication, thought processing, and memory. The spinal cord is responsible for signal transmission between the body and the brain and controls simple reflexes that do not require input from the brain (Banasik, 2022).

Previous authors: Lois VonCannon, MSN, RN, and Ramesh C. Upadhyaya, RN, CRRN, MSN, MBA, PhD-C.

The Brain

The brain is divided into specialized structures, including the parietal lobe, occipital lobe, cerebellum, brain stem, temporal lobe, and frontal lobe (Fig. 22.1). While each lobe is primarily responsible for specific functions, most activities require coordination of multiple areas. For example, although the occipital lobe is essential to visual processing, parts of the parietal, temporal, and frontal lobes also process complex visual stimuli. Visual, tactile, and motor activities of the left side of the body are predominantly directed by the right hemisphere and vice versa. Certain complex functions involve both hemispheres but are directed predominantly by one (referred to as cerebral dominance). For example, the left hemisphere is typically dominant for language, and the right is dominant for spatial attention. The primary sensory areas receive somesthetic, auditory, visual, and gustatory stimuli from the thalamus, which receives stimuli from peripheral receptors in sensory organs. Sensory stimuli are further processed in association areas that relate to one or more senses. The primary motor cortex generates voluntary body movements, while motor association areas help plan and execute complex motor activity (National Institute of Neurological Disorders and Stroke, 2024).

Neurons and Neurotransmitters

The neuron is the basic unit of the CNS and functions to transmit impulses. Some neurons are motor neurons, and some are sensory neurons. Each neuron has a cell body (soma), dendrites, and a single axon (Fig. 22.2). Synapses are structural and functional junctions between two neurons. These are the points at which the nerve impulse is transmitted from one neuron to another or from neuron to efferent organ. Neurotransmitters are chemical messengers that enhance or inhibit nerve impulses. These substances are necessary in the synaptic transmission of information from one neuron to another (Table 22.1; Fig. 22.3).

Changes with Aging

With age, the brain begins to atrophy, and there is a decrease in overall brain weight. The amount of gray and white matter decreases by about 1%–0.5% per year; the age at which this begins to occur varies between individuals. Nerve fibers in the brain may decrease (there is individual variation); nerve axons develop swelling at their ends, and dendrites shrink, resulting in a decrease in signal transmission. Additionally, there is a decrease in norepinephrine and dopamine secretion and an increase in monoamine oxidase activity. This manifests as short-term memory loss, reduced speed of learning, increased processing time to learn new material, increased reaction time, diminished abstract reasoning, and impaired perception (Banasik, 2022; Maiese, 2024a).

Spinal Cord

The spinal cord is a bundle of nerve pathways that carries information between the brain and the rest of the body. The spinal cord controls coordinated movements, such as walking and urination, and is the center for deep tendon reflexes. The spinal cord is protected by the spine, which consists of 33 vertebrae. Between each vertebra are cartilaginous disks

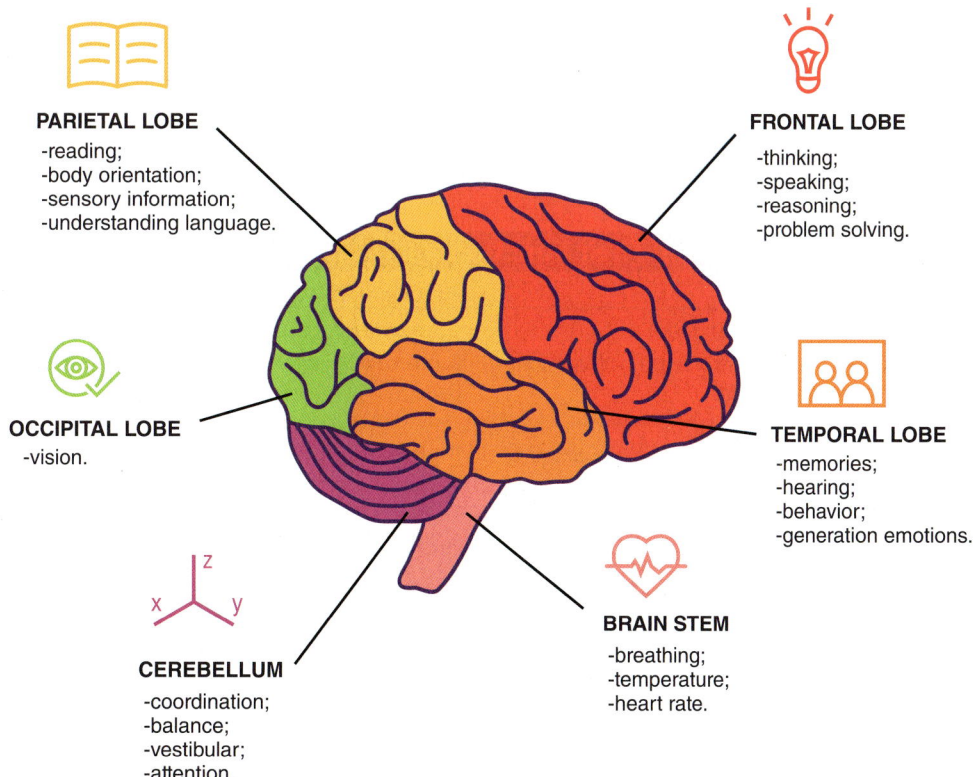

Fig. 22.1 Functional areas of the brain, lateral view. (From iStock #1056971922; marina_ua.)

PART V Nursing Care of Physiologic and Psychological Disorders

that cushion the spine and provide flexibility. Extending from the spinal cord between each vertebra are 31 pairs of spinal nerves. The anterior root carries motor commands to skeletal muscle, and the posterior root caries sensory information (i.e., pain, temperature, vibration, and limb position) (Maiese, 2024b).

Changes with Aging

With age, the intervertebral disks become hard and brittle, and lose the ability to cushion the spine and provide flexibility. Subsequently, pressure is applied to the spinal nerve roots and may cause injury. Injury can result in decreased sensation, strength, and balance (Maiese, 2024a).

Evaluation of Cognitive Function

Evaluation of cognition is a required part of Medicare's annual wellness visit. If cognitive impairment is observed during the visit or reported by the patient, family, or others, further evaluation is necessary. Evaluation includes a detailed history and physical examination, as well as the administration of screening tools (Centers for Medicare and Medicaid Services [CMS], 2023a). Most often, the Mini-Mental Status Exam (MMSE) or Montreal Cognitive Assessment (MoCA) are used to determine the presence of cognitive impairment. It is important to note that the U.S. Preventive Services Task Force (2020) does not recommend screening for cognitive impairment unless symptoms are observed or reported.

Montreal Cognitive Assessment

The Montreal Cognitive Assessment (MoCA) was developed as a quick screening tool for mild cognitive impairment (MCI). The 30-item tool assesses the domains of orientation to time and place, short-term memory, visuospatial abilities, executive functions, attention, concentration, and language. Research indicates the MoCA can discriminate reliably between normal subjects, participants with MCI, and those with dementia. The score for MCI ranges between 19 and 25, and for mild AD, it

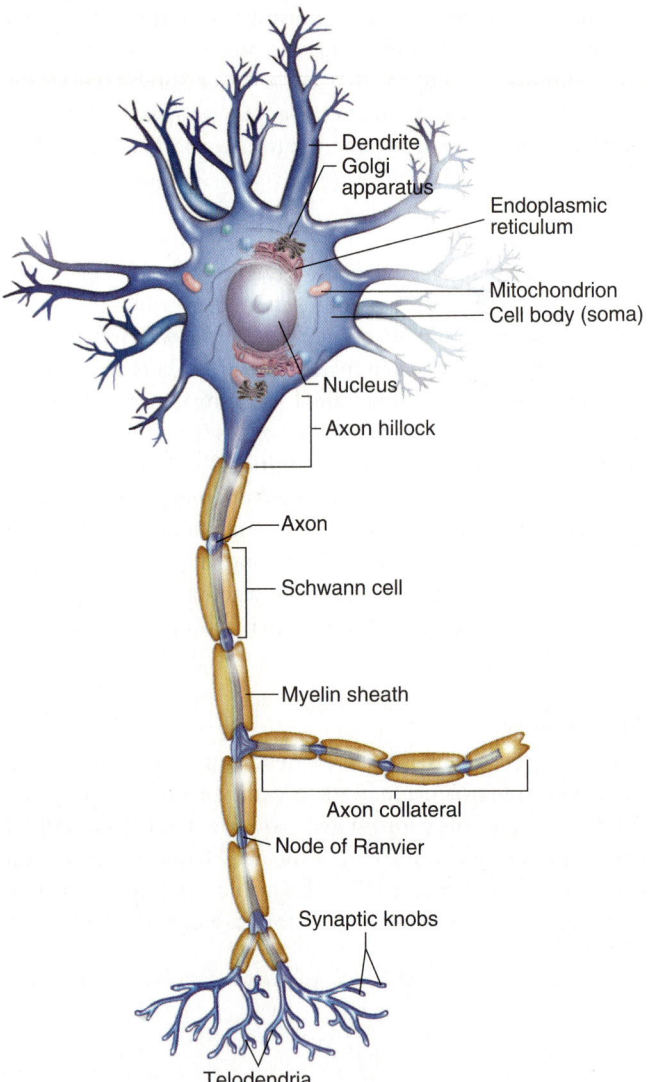

Fig. 22.2 Neuron with composite parts. (Modified from Patton, K. T., Thibodeau, G. A., & Douglas, M. M. [2012]. *Essentials of anatomy & physiology.* St. Louis, MO: Elsevier.)

TABLE 22.1 Neurotransmitters and Their Function

Neurotransmitter	Functions	Associated Disorders
Glutamate (Glu)	Involved in learning and memory	Increased (results in death of neurons): epilepsy, stroke, Lou Gehrig disease
Acetylcholine (ACh) In the central and peripheral nervous systems	Cognition, learning, attention, and memory. Voluntary muscle movement.	Decreased ACh secreting neurons: Alzheimer disease Decreased ACh receptors: myasthenia gravis (MG)
Dopamine (DA)	Important in memory, learning, behavior (reward, motivation), control of movement	Dopamine depletion in the Substantia Nigra: Parkinson disease Abnormalities in transmission: depression Excessive amounts in the frontal lobes: schizophrenia
Norepinephrine (NE)	Regulates mood, vigilance, stress, and memory	Post-traumatic stress disorder; Parkinson disease (PTSD)
Epinephrine (Epi)	Involved in "fight or flight"	
Gamma-aminobutyric acid (GABA)	Primary inhibitory messenger Contributes to motor control and vision	Reduced activity: anxiety disorder If it inhibits cells too much: epilepsy
Serotonin (5-HT)	Helps regulate mood, behavior, sleep, and memory	Elevated in schizophrenia

Data from Vaskovic, J. (2022). *Neurotransmitters.* Kenhub [website]. Retrieved from https://www.kenhub.com/en/library/anatomy/neurotransmitters; Berry, J. (2023). *What are neurotransmitters?* MedicalNewsToday [website]. Retrieved from https://www.medicalnewstoday.com/articles/326649; Kerr, L. M., Huether, S. E., & Sugerman, R. A. (2017). Structure and function of the neurologic system. In S. Huether & K. McCance (Eds.), *Understanding pathophysiology* (6th ed., pp. 307–336). St. Louis: Elsevier.

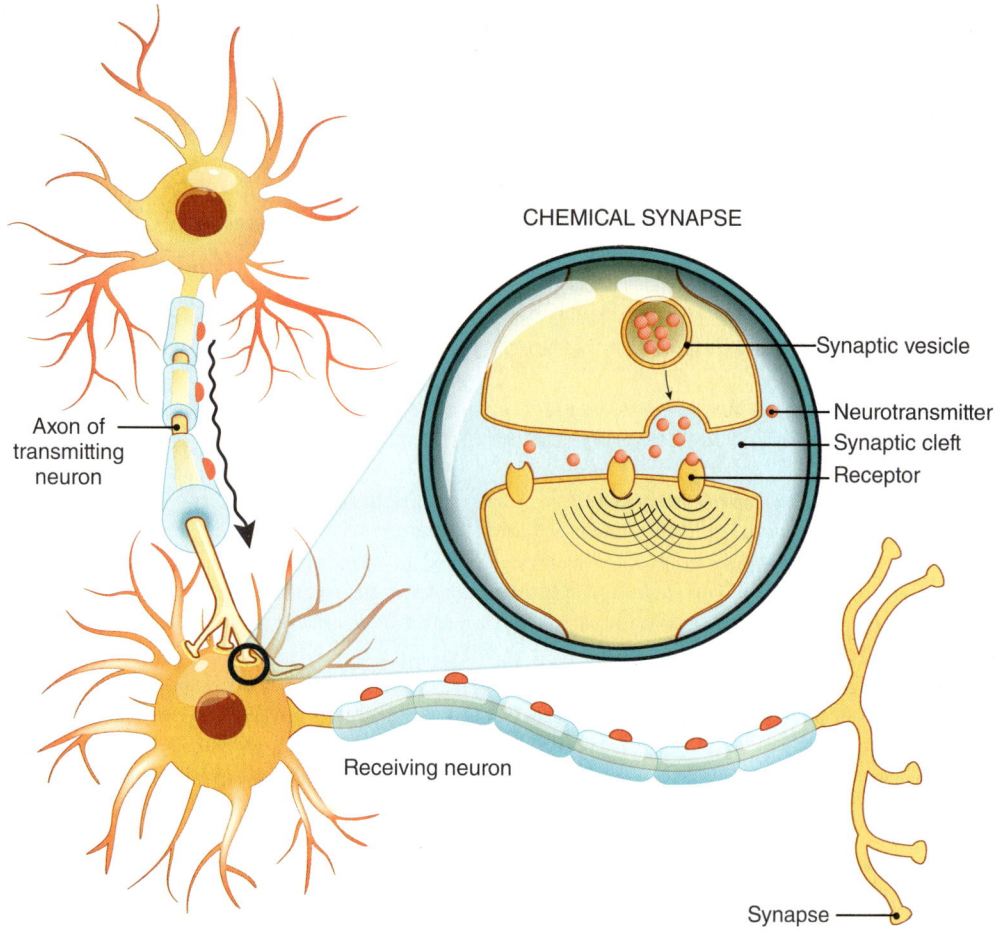

Fig. 22.3 Neuron communication. (From iStock #1163216973; ttsz.)

ranges from 11 to 21. The tool is free to use, however, training is required. Further information on the tool can be found at https://mocacognition.com/.

Mini-Mental State Examination

The most commonly used screening tool is the MMSE; also referred to as the Folstein MMSE. This 30-item tool provides a quantitative evaluation of cognitive impairment and can be used to record changes over time. Questions on the tools relate to orientation to time and place, attention and calculation, language, and visual construction. A score of 18–24 indicates MCI. A score less than 17 indicates severe impairment (Dementia Care Central, 2022).

Depression Assessment

It is advised that screening for depression should be done along with an evaluation of cognitive function. Studies have shown that depression is common in people with MCI and AD. Since depression can cause memory impairment, it is essential to screen for depression and develop an appropriate plan of care based on the results (Wood et al, 2018). The Geriatric Depression Scale (GDS) short form is a 15-question scale that can be used to evaluate for depression in healthy, ill, and mild to moderately cognitively impaired older adults. Scores of 0–4 are considered normal, 5–8 indicate mild depression, 9–11 show moderate depression, and 12–15 suggest severe depression (Greenberg, n.d.).

Cognitive Function in Typical Aging

Mild forgetfulness may affect both young and old people and should not be confused with cognitive impairment. Normal aging results in slower information processing and increased trouble multitasking, but memory, skills, and knowledge are stable (Table 22.2). While 40% of older adults experience some memory loss after the age of 65, it is still unlikely they have dementia, and most can live their lives without interruption. A decline in cognitive function is an effect of disease, not an effect of the normal aging process. Older adults can do things to help keep their brains healthy (Centers for Disease Control and Prevention [CDC], 2023a):

- Smoking cessation
- Maintain adequate blood pressure control
- Be physically active
- Maintain a healthy weight
- Eat a healthy and balanced diet (e.g., Mediterranean diet)
- Get enough sleep (7–9 hours)
- Stay engaged socially
- Manage blood sugar and control diabetes

TABLE 22.2 Signs of Dementia Compared to Normal Aging*

Signs of Alzheimer Dementia	Typical Age-Related Changes
Memory loss that disrupts daily life: One of the most common signs of AD, especially in the early stages, is forgetting recently learned information. Others include asking the same questions over and over and increasingly needing to rely on memory aids (e.g., reminder notes or electronic devices) or family members for things that used to be handled on one's own.	Sometimes forgetting names or appointments, but remembering them later
Challenges in planning or solving problems: Some people experience changes in their ability to develop and follow a plan or work with numbers. They may have trouble following a familiar recipe or keeping track of monthly bills. They may have difficulty concentrating and take much longer to do things than they did before.	Making occasional errors when managing finances or household bills
Difficulty completing familiar tasks: People with AD often find it hard to complete daily tasks. Sometimes, people have trouble driving to a familiar location, organizing a grocery list, or remembering the rules of a favorite game.	Occasionally needing help using microwave settings or recording a television show
Confusion with time or place: People living with Alzheimers can lose track of dates, seasons, and the passage of time. They may have trouble understanding something if it is not happening immediately. Sometimes they forget where they are or how they got there.	Getting confused about the day of the week but figuring it out later
Trouble understanding visual images and spatial relationships: For some people, having vision problems is a sign of AD. They may also have problems judging distance and determining color and contrast, causing issues with driving.	Vision changes related to cataracts
New problems with words in speaking or writing: People living with AD may have trouble following or joining a conversation. They may stop in the middle of a conversation and have no idea how to continue, or they may repeat themselves. They may struggle with vocabulary, have trouble naming a familiar object, or use the wrong name (e.g., calling a watch a "hand clock").	Sometimes having trouble finding the right word
Misplacing things and losing the ability to retrace steps: People living with AD may put things in unusual places. They may lose things and be unable to go back over their steps to find them. They may accuse others of stealing, especially as the disease progresses.	Misplacing things from time to time and retracing steps to find them
Decreased or poor judgment: Individuals may experience changes in judgment or decision-making. For example, they may use poor judgment when dealing with money or pay less attention to grooming or keeping themselves clean.	Making a bad decision or mistake once in a while, such as neglecting to schedule an oil change for a car
Withdrawal from work or social activities: People living with AD may experience changes in their ability to hold or follow a conversation. As a result, they may withdraw from hobbies, social activities, or other engagements. They may have trouble keeping up with a favorite sports team or activity.	Sometimes feeling uninterested in family and social obligations
Changes in mood, personality, and behavior: The mood and personalities of people living with AD can change. They can become confused, suspicious, depressed, fearful, or anxious. They may be easily upset at home, at work, with friends, or when out of their comfort zones.	Developing very specific ways of doing things and becoming irritable when a routine is disrupted

*For more information about the symptoms of Alzheimers, visit alz.org/alzheimers-dementia/10_signs.
From Alzheimer's Association. (2023). 2023 Alzheimer's disease facts and figures. *Alzheimers Dement, 19*(4), 1598–1695. Retrieved from https://www.alz.org/media/Documents/alzheimers-facts-and-figures.pdf.

COGNITIVE DISORDERS ASSOCIATED WITH ALTERED THOUGHT PROCESSES

Several cognitive disorders are associated with altered thought processes in older adults. These include the three *D*s—depression, delirium, and dementia (Table 22.3)—as well as cranial tumors, subdural hematomas, and normal pressure hydrocephalus. It is often difficult to accurately diagnose the underlying cause of altered thought processes in older adults because of the similarity in their presentations. Nevertheless, accurate assessment and diagnosis are essential for ensuring appropriate treatment to improve or potentially reverse the underlying pathophysiologic condition contributing to the individual's impaired cognition.

Depression

In general, 1%–5% of community-dwelling older adults experience major depression; the number rises to 13.5% for those needing home care and 11.5% for hospitalized older adults. Drugs to treat depression and/or psychotherapy improve symptoms in most older adults. (CDC, 2022). Older adults have a high risk for depression due to multiple factors unique to older adults, including multiple chronic conditions (80% of older adults have at least one chronic condition), decreased functional ability, reduced mobility, chronic pain, financial issues following retirement, abuse, caregiver stress, sedentary lifestyle, and social isolation (National Council on Aging [NCOA], 2022).

However, depression in older adults is often undertreated or inappropriately treated, as depression is often seen as a normal part of aging. Additionally, the diagnosis of depression is stigmatized. Because of this, older adults may not accept the diagnosis or its treatment. Untreated depression in older adults can lead to suffering, impaired function, and an overall decreased quality of life (QoL) (Devita et al, 2022).

Clinical Manifestations

Depression is a mood disorder and a chronic medical condition that often has an atypical presentation in older adults. Depression may be found as part of an evaluation of cognitive function. Signs and symptoms of depression in older adults

TABLE 22.3 Clinical Features of Depression, Delirium, and Dementia

Clinical Feature	Depression	Delirium	Dementia
Onset	Can be abrupt or associated with life events	Sudden onset	Months to years
Duration	Weeks to months	Hours to days	Long-term or lifetime
Mood	Consistent; sadness, anxiety, irritability	Labile; suspicious, mood swings	Fluctuating; depressed, apathetic, uninterested
Behavior	Variable; may have psychomotor retardation or agitation	Variable; hypokinetic or hyperkinetic	Variable with psychomotor retardation or agitation
Cognition			
Orientation	Selected disorientation	Impaired with variable severity	Slow decline over time
Alertness	Normal	Lethargic or hypervigilant	Generally normal
Memory	Selective impairment	Impairment of recent memory and attentiveness	Early, recent, and later remote memory impairment
Thought processes	Intact with themes of hopelessness, helplessness, and self-depreciation	Difficulty maintaining concentration; disorganized; fragmented	Impoverished; impaired abstract thinking; word-finding difficulties; impaired judgment
Perception	Normal	Possible visual, auditory, and tactile hallucinations or delusions	Misperceptions not generally present
Speech and language	Normal to slowed	Slurred, forced, or rambling	Disordered; word-finding difficulties
Mini-Mental State Examination	Performance fluctuates over time	Acute fluctuations	Moderately stable with decreasing scores over time

include apathy, persistent sadness, irritability, fatigue, low energy, feelings of guilt and worthlessness, hopelessness, loss of interest in activities once enjoyed, trouble concentrating and other cognitive changes, insomnia, oversleeping, overeating, or anorexia, slower speech or movement, persistent digestive problems, physical pains that do not respond to treatment, and recurring thoughts of death. (NCOA, 2022). Additional symptoms include "cognitive deficits involving executive functions, such as problem-solving, planning, decision-making, and inhibition, along with selective and sustained attention and working memory impairment. Other deficits, involving some aspects of episodic memory and visuospatial functions, may be secondary to executive dysfunction" (Devita et al, 2022, p. 2871).

Diagnosis of Depression in the Older Adult

Assessment of the older adult presenting with somatic complaints, cognitive difficulties, and functional changes should include a thorough history. Additionally, the use of a standardized screening tool, such as the Geriatric Depression Scale (GDS), can not only help with the diagnosis of depression but also assess the response to treatment. Other components of the depression workup include a thorough physical examination, laboratory evaluation (complete blood count, complete metabolic panel with liver function studies, thyroid function tests, vitamin B12 and folate, syphilis screening, and urine drug screen), and neuroimaging to determine the presence of cerebral abnormalities (Tampi and Tampi, 2022).

Treatment of Depression

There are multiple treatment approaches for depression, and no one therapy is right for everyone. Treatment includes antidepressant drugs, psychotherapy, and electroconvulsive therapy.

Psychotherapeutic options. Cognitive behavioral therapy (CBT), reminiscence therapy (RT), and interpersonal psychotherapy (IPT) plus antidepressants appear to have a positive effect on depression in older adults.

Cognitive behavioral therapy. CBT targets thoughts and feelings and their relationship to behavior and promotes modification of unhelpful thinking and behavioral patterns that impair function (American Psychological Association, 2023).

Reminiscence therapy. RT helps older adults cope by helping them reflect on their life stories from childhood to the present. Through reflection, the older adult can appreciate the past and present and develop a balanced and satisfied perspective of their life. It can help the older adult cope with changes and feel at peace with their life choices and experiences (American Psychological Association, 2023).

Interpersonal psychotherapy. IPT helps to improve dysfunctional relationships and distressing events that are directly related to depressive symptoms. It helps the older adult learn strategies to communicate their needs and emotions, as well as helping them develop problem-solving skills. IPT should be combined with a second-generation antidepressant (American Psychological Association, 2023).

Drug therapy. Pharmacotherapy of depression needs to consider the older adult's response to previous treatments, current medications (prescribed, over-the-counter [OTC], and supplements), and concurrent medical conditions (Devita et al, 2022). Due to their side-effect profile and safety, second-generation antidepressants (selective serotonin reuptake inhibitors [SSRIs], serotonin-norepinephrine reuptake inhibitors [SNRIs], or norepinephrine/dopamine reuptake inhibitors [NDRIs]) are considered first-line drugs to treat depression in older adults. Second-generation antidepressants regulate the neurotransmitters serotonin, norepinephrine, and dopamine, which are involved in brain functions related to mood and behavior (American Psychological Association, 2023).

Second-generation antidepressants. SSRIs help regulate the amount of serotonin that is active in the synapses between neurons. SNRIs regulate levels of both serotonin and norepinephrine. NDRIs help regulate both norepinephrine and dopamine levels (American Psychological Association, 2023). These drugs have fewer anticholinergic side effects than first-generation antidepressants (with the exclusion of paroxetine; Devita et al, 2022). Side effects of these drugs include headaches, nausea, diarrhea, sleep disturbances, drowsiness, and hyponatremia. Due to their interactions with other drugs, dosing should begin low and slowly increase until the desired benefits are reached (American Psychological Association, 2023).

Second-generation antidepressants can be safely used in older adults with cognitive impairment and cardiovascular disease (CVD) (Devita et al, 2022). Duloxetine is the only antidepressant that the Food and Drug Administration (FDA) has approved for the treatment of neuropathic pain (Bugos, 2023). Mirtazapine is particularly useful for treating anorexia and insomnia in older adults with depression. "Vortioxetine, a multimodal serotonin modulator, seems to be promising for elderly people since it also has a positive effect on cognition, independently of the improvement in depression" (Devita et al, 2022, p. 2872).

New treatments. New drug therapies that have demonstrated a significant reduction in depression in older adults include ketamine (an N-methyl-D-aspartate receptor [NMDAR] antagonist) and esketamine (ESK) (a mirror image of ketamine that is known to have a higher affinity for NMDAR). Adverse effects of these drugs include perceptual disturbance, derealization, altered body perception, altered time perception, palpitations, flushing, dizziness, paresthesia, fatigue, and sleepiness. These effects are dose-dependent and transient (Tampi and Tampi, 2022).

Repetitive transcranial magnetic stimulation (rTMS) has been approved as a treatment for depression in older adults who have failed a trial of medications. rTMS uses magnets to activate specific regions of the brain, does not require anesthesia, and does not induce seizures like electroconvulsive therapy (ECT). It has few adverse effects on cognition. Older adults receiving rTMS may experience discomfort from scalp or facial muscle twitching and headaches (National Institute on Aging [NIA], 2021; Tampi and Tampi, 2022).

Electroconvulsive therapy. ECT is reserved for refractory depression. During ECT, mild electrical impulses are used to stimulate the brain. ECT has been in use since the 1940s. It is a safe and effective treatment for major depression (NCOA, 2022). Rhee et al (2021) conducted an observational study examining the effects of ECT on suicide and mortality risk in older adults; they concluded that ECT resulted in remission in 50%–70% of those treated and was associated with lower mortality and an initial reduction in suicide attempts that waned over time. ECT is associated with transiently increased blood pressure and arrhythmias. Other side effects include confusion and some anterograde memory impairment (Dominiak et al, 2021).

Delirium

Delirium presents as a disturbance in attention, cognition, affective expression, and motor behavior. The onset of the disturbance is rapid (hours to days) and typically fluctuates over the course of the day. Delirium is associated with poor outcomes, an increased risk of morbidity and mortality, loss of autonomy, an increased length of hospital stays and expenses. Older adults are at increased risk of delirium due to multiple medical conditions and increased sensitivity to drugs (Fuchs et al, 2020).

Risk Factors

The risk factors for delirium include advanced age, underlying neurocognitive disorders (i.e., dementia, stroke, and Parkinson disease), polypharmacy and multiple medical conditions, withdrawal syndrome, frailty, malnutrition, immobility, advanced cancer, untreated pain, immobilization, indwelling Foley catheter, fractures, visual and auditory impairments, sleep deprivation, and organ failure (Francis and Young, 2023).

Clinical Manifestations

Symptoms of delirium fluctuate and may include difficulty maintaining concentration or attention to external stimuli and a language disturbance, including slurred, forced, or rambling speech. Disorganized thinking demonstrated by tangential reasoning and conversation is often the presenting symptom. Other common symptoms of delirium include the following (Grover and Avasthi, 2018):

- Clouding of consciousness or fluctuation of awareness
- Misperceptions, illusions, or hallucinations
- Disorientation to persons, place, and time
- Impaired memory (may be both short- and long-term)
- Increased or decreased physical activity
- Impaired judgment and executive function
- Disturbances in the sleep-wake cycle

Management

Many interventions are used to prevent delirium in hospitalized patients. Assessment with the use of a validated instrument such as the Confusion Assessment Method (CAM) is the first-line treatment for preventing and treating delirium. The CAM is a standardized evidence-based tool that enables health-care personnel to identify and recognize delirium quickly and accurately in multiple settings. The CAM includes four features (onset, attention, thinking, and consciousness) found to have the greatest ability to distinguish delirium from other types of cognitive impairment (Tran et al, 2021). Additionally, delirium management includes rapid diagnosis and treatment of the underlying cause.

Nonpharmacologic interventions. A therapeutic environment includes frequent reassurance and memory cues (calendar, clock, and family photos); clear communication; caregiver consistency; decreased stimuli (noise reduction, adequate lighting, not rushing the patient); decreased stress and anxiety through frequent reassurance and providing daily routine; maintaining comfort (eyeglasses, hearing aids, and personal belongings); re-establishing the sleep-wake cycle by controlling night-time noise and unnecessary disruptions; ensuring adequate food and fluid intake; ensuring elimination needs are met; providing for physical activity, ambulation, and range of motion; and avoiding chemical or physical restraint. Drugs should be used as a last resort (Oh et al, 2017).

Pharmacotherapy. Most studies do not show any benefit from using pharmacologic interventions for delirium. Studies of the use of antipsychotics demonstrated no significant difference in incidence, duration, severity, or reduction in mortality when antipsychotics were used. In fact, the use of antipsychotics may contribute to an increase in adverse effects and poor outcomes (Oh et al, 2017). However, if there is a risk of patient harm due to agitation, haloperidol may be considered (Francis and Young, 2023).

Dementia

Dementia is a syndrome of gradual and progressive cognitive decline. It has been defined as an alteration in memory in addition to an acquired persistent alteration in intellectual function (e.g., orientation, calculation, attention, and motor skills) compromising multiple cognitive domains. In dementia, individuals are unable to do the things they used to do because of the mental changes associated with this disease process. Dementia may involve language deficits, apraxia (difficulty with the manipulation of objects), agnosia (inability to recognize familiar objects), agraphia (difficulty drawing objects), and impaired executive function (Alzheimer's Association, 2023).

Although dementia is more common in older people than in younger persons, it is not part of the normal aging process. Dementia is usually a condition occurring in later life because of changes in neurologic function caused by a disease process. AD is the most common, followed by vascular dementia (VaD), dementia with Lewy bodies (DLB), frontotemporal dementia (FTD), mixed dementia, and dementia caused by reversible causes.

Reversible Dementia

Reversible dementia occurs when other pathologic conditions masquerade as dementia (i.e., drug side effects, depression, untreated sleep apnea, delirium, vitamin deficiency [B-1 is Korsakoff syndrome from chronic alcohol misuse], and thyroid disease; Alzheimer's Association, 2023). It is important to identify and treat the underlying causes of dementia symptoms (CDC, 2019). The mnemonic DEMENTIA is a useful tool to remember reversible causes of dementia (Home Care Assistance Roseville, 2022; Assisting Hands Home Care, 2022):

Drugs: drugs for Parkinson disease, asthma, overactive bladder, and chronic obstructive pulmonary disease (COPD) have side effects that may affect cognitive abilities.
Emotional disorders: signs of depression, such as confusion and difficulty thinking, are often mistaken for signs of dementia.
Metabolic disorders: persons with hyper- or hypothyroidism, hypercalcemia, and adrenal insufficiency may have confusion and fatigue that is misinterpreted as dementia.
Ear and eye problems: vision and hearing loss associated with aging may lead to difficulty processing information and confusion.
Nutritional deficiencies: deficiencies in vitamin C, B, and D vitamins, as well as magnesium, may result in confusion, altered memory, and anxiety.
Toxins/tumors: persons with COPD who inhale toxins (such as those in cleaning products) may have shortness of breath and confusion. Persons who drink alcohol in excess may develop cognitive deficits and confusion that resemble dementia. Brain tumors can lead to difficulty recalling memories and problem-solving.
Infections: altered mental status secondary to infection can mimic dementia. The most common infections experienced by older adults include pneumonia, influenza, cellulitis, infections of the gastrointestinal (GI) tract, and UTIs.
Anemia: older adults with anemia may think slowly and forget things easily.

Alzheimer Disease

AD is the most common form of dementia. AD is a slowly progressive neurodegenerative disease whose main characteristic is the accumulation of the protein beta-amyloid (plaques) outside neurons and twisted strands of the protein tau (tangles) inside neurons in the brain. These changes are accompanied by the death of neurons and damage to brain tissue, resulting in atrophy. The presence of beta-amyloid and tau proteins is thought to activate the immune system, causing inflammation in the brain. Finally, AD decreases the brain's ability to metabolize glucose. The deposits of beta-amyloid and tau proteins are visible on a positron emission tomography (PET) scan. Persons with AD survive on average, 4–8 years after diagnosis (Alzheimer's Association, 2023).

The personal and public costs of AD are high. Medicare costs for beneficiaries with AD are expected to exceed their ability to absorb the cost. Costs are estimated to soar from $259 billion in 2017 to $1.1 trillion by 2050 for caring for patients with AD and other types of dementia. Approximately 4% of people in the United States live in extended-care facilities; 75% of the people with AD will be admitted to a nursing home by age 80. The changing demographics of our society and the anticipated growth of the older adult population during the next few decades have created a need for health-care providers to develop age-related interventions that address the mental-health needs of an aging population (Alzheimer's Association, 2023).

Risk factors. Research has focused on genetic, nutritional, viral, environmental, and other causes of AD. Age is the single most-important risk factor for the development of AD, as the number of people with the disease doubles every 5 years beyond the age of 65. After the age of 85, the risk is nearly one-third. Additionally, there is a link between head injuries and the future development of AD. Overall healthy aging (eating healthy, remaining active, avoiding excessive alcohol, and avoiding tobacco) is important as damage to the heart and blood vessels has been linked to the development of AD, as well as vascular dementia following a stroke (Alzheimer's Association, 2023).

> **EVIDENCE-BASED PRACTICE**
>
> *Function and Behavior-Focused Care for Nursing Home Residents*
>
> **Background**
> Neuropsychiatric symptoms are present in nearly two-thirds of nursing home residents with dementia. Additionally, residents with dementia are frequently disabled; within 6 months of nursing home admission, most residents with dementia experience functional decline in activities of daily living (ADLs). Assistance with care is often perceived as a threat that results in resistance to care and other behavioral symptoms. "Promoting maximum level of resident participation in their own care activities decreases the risk of behavioral symptoms while optimizing function" (p. 1422).
>
> **Sample/Setting**
> Twelve (12) nursing homes (6 treatment and 6 control) and 336 residents (173 treatment and 163 control) with moderate to severe cognitive impairment.
>
> **Methods**
> A clustered, randomized controlled trial with a repeated-measures design was implemented in 12 nursing homes randomized to either the Function and Behavior Focused Care for the Cognitively Impaired (FBFC-CI) intervention or the Function and Behavior Focused Care Education (FBFC-ED) educational control.
>
> **Findings**
> The mean age of participants was 82.6, primarily female, and based on the MMSE, they experienced moderate to severe cognitive impairment. "There was a significantly greater increase in time spent in total activity ($P = .004$), moderate activity ($P = .012$), light activity ($P = .002$), and a decrease in resistiveness to care ($P = .004$) in the treatment versus control group at 4 months," (p. 1426), but not at 12 months. There was no change in mood, agitation, and the use of psychotropic medications.
>
> **Implications**
> "This study provides some support for the use of the FBFC-CI Intervention to increase time spent in physical activity and decrease resistive behaviors during care commonly noted among nursing home residents with moderate to severe cognitive impairment. ... Small increases in physical activity (sitting up in a chair rather than remaining bedbound) may affect QoL of the resident as well as his or her caregiving needs. Any decrease in resistiveness to care may positively influence staff response to residents" (p. 1427).

Data from Galik, E. M., Resnick, B., Holmes, S. D., Vigne, E., Lynch, K., Ellis, J., Zhu, S., & Barr, E. (2021). A cluster randomized controlled trial testing the impact of function and behavior focused care for nursing home residents with dementia. *Journal of the American Medical Directors Association, 22*(7), 1421–1428.e4.

Genetic factors. While researchers have not identified a specific gene directly linked to the development of AD, a genetic variant of the apolipoprotein e4 (APOE) gene on chromosome 19 increases a person's risk of developing AD. However, it should be noted that inheriting the gene does not mean a person will develop AD (NIA, 2023a). So, while having a first-degree relative with Alzheimer increases the risk, environmental and other factors play a role as well. Considering this, genetic testing for AD is not recommended, even though it is available (Alzheimer's Association, 2023).

Clinical manifestations. Early symptoms of AD include difficulty remembering recent conversations, names, or events. This may be accompanied by apathy and depression. Later symptoms include impaired communication, disorientation, confusion, poor judgment, and behavioral changes. End-stage symptoms include difficulty speaking, swallowing, and walking (Alzheimer's Association, 2023).

AD is divided into several phases: preclinical AD, MCI due to AD, and AD dementia. AD dementia is further divided into phases, namely, mild, moderate, and severe (Fig. 22.4) (Alzheimer's Association, 2023).

Preclinical Alzheimer disease. In preclinical AD, the person has not developed any symptoms. However, brain changes are visible on PET scans. Tau proteins may also be found in cerebrospinal fluid (CSF). In this phase, the brain is compensating for changes, and the person functions normally. It should be noted that some persons never advance beyond this stage, as beta-amyloid plaques were found on autopsy, but the individual never had memory problems while alive. Because of this, the use of PET scans and CSF analysis is not recommended as screening tools (Alzheimer's Association, 2023).

MCI due to Alzheimer disease. In this phase, in addition to changes noted on PET scans, proteins are found in the CSF. Subtle changes in memory, language, and thinking are also present. The brain is no longer able to compensate for neuronal death. For the person with MCI, their friends and family notice these changes, but others may not. The person is still able to carry out their daily activities. About 15% of persons with MCI advance to AD in 2 years; by 5 years, one-third progress to AD; others have no additional decline (Alzheimer's Association, 2023).

Alzheimer dementia. Persons with AD have noticeable changes in memory, language, and thinking; they may also experience behavioral symptoms that impair their ability to

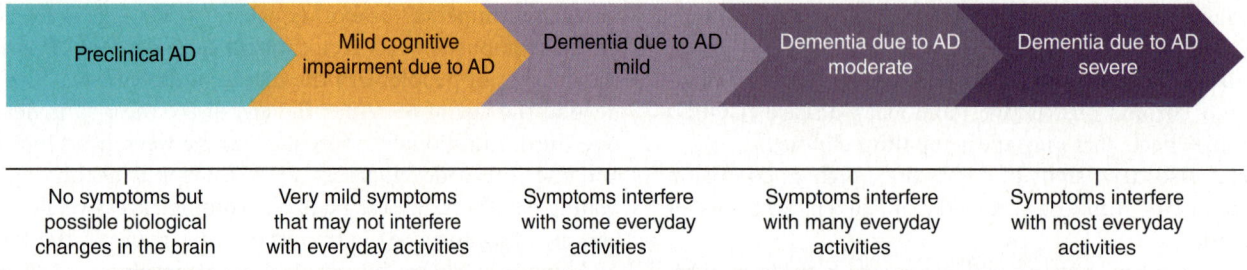

Fig. 22.4 Alzheimer disease continuum. Note: Although these arrows are of equal size, the components of the AD continuum are not equal in duration. (Redrawn from Alzheimer's Association. [2023]. 2023 Alzheimer's disease facts and figures. *Alzheimer's & Dement, 19*[4], 1598–1695.)

complete instrumental ADLs (IADLs). The rate of progression of AD varies from person to person. As AD progresses, the symptoms experienced by persons with AD change (Alzheimer's Association, 2023).

Mild Alzheimer dementia. In this state, persons with AD can complete ADLs independently but need assistance with IADLs. With assistance (such as handling finances), they can remain independent and safe. Many can still do some work, drive, and participate in social activities (Alzheimer's Association, 2023).

Moderate Alzheimer dementia. This stage is often the longest. Memory and language problems worsen and the person is more confused and finds it hard to complete multistep tasks (i.e., ADLs). The person with AD in this stage may become incontinent and may have personal changes and behavioral issues, such as paranoia and agitation, and they may begin to have problems recognizing family and friends (Alzheimer's Association, 2023).

Severe Alzheimer dementia. In this final stage, communication is greatly reduced. Persons with severe AD require around-the-clock care. Some people become bed-bound, making them at risk for developing blood clots, pressure injuries, and skin infections. Significant neuronal damage in multiple parts of the brain also makes swallowing difficult, increasing the risk for aspiration and aspiration pneumonia. Aspiration pneumonia is a contributing cause of death for many persons with severe AD (Alzheimer's Association, 2023).

Diagnostic evaluation. If cognitive impairment is observed during the visit or reported, as stated previously, evaluation includes a detailed history and physical examination, as well as the administration of screening tools. Additionally, blood (i.e., complete blood count [CBC], thyroid studies, B-12, human immunodeficiency virus [HIV] serology, and chemistry panel), urine, CSF (typically only performed in atypical and rapidly progressive dementia), and scans (computed tomography [CT], magnetic resonance imaging [MRI], or PET) are ordered to rule out reversible causes.

Pharmacological management. Several drugs are approved by the FDA to treat AD. Donepezil, rivastigmine, galantamine, and memantine temporarily treat the symptoms of AD and may control some cognitive and behavioral symptoms of dementia, but they do not alter the underlying neurodegeneration causing the disease. Donepezil, rivastigmine, and galantamine are cholinesterase inhibitors that improve symptoms by increasing the neurotransmitter acetylcholine in the brain. The most common side effects of these drugs are headache, nausea, vomiting, diarrhea, weight loss, indigestion, and muscle weakness. Memantine is an NMDAR antagonist that targets glutamate, which damages neurons. Side effects of this drug include dizziness, headache, diarrhea, constipation, and confusion (Alzheimer's Association, 2023; NIA, 2023b). As AD progresses, the brain produces less acetylcholine; it is thought that these drugs become less effective (NIA, 2023b).

In 2021, the FDA approved aducanumab, the first drug developed to treat AD by reducing the beta-amyloid plaques in the brain. Aducanumab is appropriate for some people with MCI and mild AD. This drug is associated with brain swelling or bleeding. Other side effects include headaches, dizziness, falls, diarrhea, and confusion (NIA, 2023b). Patients on aducanumab need to be closely monitored for these serious side effects. It should be noted that aducanumab received accelerated approval. If clinical benefits cannot be verified in postapproval trials, drug approval will be withdrawn (Alzheimer's Association, 2023).

Another drug, lecanemab, received approval on July 6 2023 (Stewart, 2023). The drug appears to slow the progression of cognitive decline. It works by preventing amyloid plaques in the brain from clumping (Mayo Clinic Staff, 2024a). However, like aducanumab, it can cause brain swelling (Howard, 2023).

Nonpharmacological management. The goal of nonpharmacological management of AD is to maintain or improve cognitive function, QoL social engagement, and the ability to perform ADLs. As AD progresses, family caregivers must be trained to manage the day-to-day care needs of the person with dementia (Alzheimer's Association, 2023). Caregivers also need support, which can be found in support groups, counseling, and spiritual communities. Family caregivers need to spend time with friends and family (Mayo Clinic Staff, 2024a).

Vascular Dementia

In general, 5%–10% of people with dementia have vascular dementia (VaD). VaD is a result of blockage of blood vessels in the brain, resulting in ischemia. The most common cause is a stroke. The determining factor in the development of dementia in persons who have experienced a stroke is the location and number of infarcts (Alzheimer's Association, 2023).

Risk factors. Atherosclerotic changes in the vasculature and increasing age are the primary risk factors for developing VaD. Additional factors include smoking, uncontrolled hypertension (HTN), obesity, a sedentary lifestyle, and excessive alcohol consumption (Alzheimer's Association, n.d.).

Clinical manifestations. Symptoms of VaD vary widely depending on the severity of damage and the part of the brain affected. Symptoms may include slowed thoughts or decision-making capability and poor judgment, as well as difficulty planning and organizing, confusion, disorientation, and trouble speaking or understanding speech. Persons with VaD also experience impaired motor function, which manifests as a slowed gait and poor balance. A person with VaD may also have numbness or paralysis on one side of the face or body. Persons with global small vessel disease (SVD) may have uncontrolled laughing or crying, impaired social functioning, inattention, and word-finding difficulty (Alzheimer's Association, 2023; Alzheimer's Association, n.d.).

Diagnostic studies. Neuroimaging usually reveals one or more areas of cerebral infarction in persons with VaD (Alzheimer's Association, 2023).

Treatment. Research has indicated that the same drugs used to treat AD also offer some benefit to people with VaD. Of major importance is adherence to treatment plans designed to control the underlying disease processes (i.e., HTN, hyperlipidemia, and DM); studies have shown this helps improve outcomes and slow the progression of the disease (Alzheimer's Association, n.d.).

Dementia with Lewy Bodies

DLB is a progressive, degenerative brain disorder. People with DLB experience a decline in thinking, reasoning, and independent functioning. In DLB, abnormal clumps of the protein alpha-synuclein aggregate in neurons of the cortex. DLB develops in about 5% of persons with dementia. Most people with DLB also have the pathology of AD (Alzheimer's Association, n.d.).

Risk factors. No risk factors or causes are currently known for DLB (Alzheimer's Association, n.d.).

Clinical manifestations. The clinical manifestations of DLB are like those of AD; however, early symptoms of rapid eye movement (REM) sleep disturbances occur in DLB, as well as visual hallucinations and visuospatial impairment. In people with DLB, cognition and other symptoms fluctuate during the day and from day to day. Disturbances in motor function occur, like those seen in Parkinson disease (i.e., slow movement, tremor at rest, and rigidity). While persons with DLB may not experience early problems with memory, memory loss ultimately occurs at some point in the disease progression (Alzheimer's Association, 2023; Alzheimer's Association, n.d.).

Diagnostic studies. There is no single test to diagnose DLB. Essentially, it is a diagnosis of exclusion based on the healthcare provider's clinical judgment and assessment. The only way to definitively diagnose DLB is through autopsy (Alzheimer's Association, n.d.).

Management. The management of patients with DLB focuses on symptomatic relief when psychiatric and behavioral symptoms become distressing. Treatment for DLB is essential in the event of gait and balance alterations. The use of cholinesterase inhibitors has been supported in DLB, as has the use of antidepressants, especially SSRIs. Antipsychotic drugs should be used with extreme caution, as they may cause serious side effects in around 50% of patients. These side effects include sudden onset of altered mental status, impaired swallowing, delusions, or hallucinations, and worsening of Parkinson-like symptoms (Alzheimer's Association, n.d.).

Frontotemporal Degeneration

Frontotemporal lobar degeneration (FTD) is an overarching term for a group of disorders encompassing several subtypes, including behavioral-variant FTD (bvFTD), primary progressive aphasia (PPA), Pick's disease, corticobasal degeneration (CBD), and progressive supranuclear palsy (PSP). In this disease, nerve cells become markedly atrophied in the frontal and temporal lobes of the brain. Additionally, the outer layers of the brain become "spongy," and there are abnormal deposits of tau protein or the transactive response (TAR) deoxyribonucleic acid DNA-binding protein, TDP-43. People with FTD typically develop it younger (45–60 years of age), and then people typically develop AD. In adults over the age of 65, FTD accounts for about 3% of those with dementia; in adults under the age of 65, FTD accounts for about 10% of dementia cases (Alzheimer's Association, 2023).

Risk factors. There are no known risk factors for the development of FTD. In roughly a third of the cases, it is inherited. Genetic testing and counseling are available for persons with a family history (Alzheimer's Association, n.d.).

Clinical manifestations. Early manifestations of FTD include "marked changes in personality and behavior and/or difficulty with producing or comprehending language" (Alzheimer's Association, 2023, p. 7; Alzheimer's Association, n.d.):

- *bvFTD:* In this subtype, symptoms can develop when the person is as young as 20 years old, or as old as 80 years old. Nerve cells are primarily lost in the areas controlling conduct, judgment, empathy, and foresight.
- *PPA:* In this subtype, symptoms typically appear before the age of 65, however, it can occur after. PPA affects language skills, speaking, writing, and comprehension. There are two variants of PPA, namely, 1) the semantic variant, where persons lose the ability to understand or formulate words, and 2) the nonfluent/agrammatical variant, where a person's speaking is hesitant, labored, or ungrammatical.
- *Corticobasal syndrome:* This subtype causes a person's arms and legs to become stiff and uncoordinated.
- *PSP:* This subtype causes muscle stiffness, difficulty walking, and changes in posture. The eyes are also affected.

The progress of FTD varies from person to person. Ultimately, the person with FTD becomes wheelchair-bound and then bedbound. The person develops dysphagia and incontinence of the bowel and bladder. They develop pressure injuries, UTIs, and pneumonia, eventually resulting in death (Alzheimer's Association, n.d.).

Diagnostic studies. Diagnoses of FTD and PPA are based on a specialist's clinical judgment and neurological assessment and evaluation of the person's behavior combined with an MRI or PET scan (Alzheimer's Association, n.d.).

Management. There is no specific treatment for FTD or any subtype. Interventions, both nonpharmacological and pharmacological, should be implemented to reduce agitation, irritability, and depression.

Normal Pressure Hydrocephalus

Normal pressure hydrocephalus (NPH) occurs most often in persons in their 60s to 70s. In NPH, CSF circulates to the cerebral subarachnoid space, enlarging the ventricles but causing no rise in the CSF pressure.

Risk factors. The cause of NPH is unknown in most cases; however, tumors, head injury, hemorrhage, infection, and inflammation of the brain may contribute to the development of NPH (Alzheimer's Association, n.d.).

Clinical manifestations. The hallmark symptoms of NPH include (Alzheimer's Association, n.d.):

- Gait disturbance with the body bent forward, legs wide apart, and shuffling gait
- Mild dementia, involving loss of interest in ADLs, inability to complete routine tasks, forgetfulness, and short-term memory loss
- Decline in the ability to complete IADLs, apathy, reduced concentration, and changes in personality and behavior
- Urinary incontinence; incontinence appears later than difficulty walking and cognitive decline

Diagnostic studies. NPH is often misdiagnosed as AD, Creutzfeldt-Jakob disease (CJD), or Parkinson disease (PD), as persons with NPH do not always present with all "hallmark symptoms." Confirmation of NPH can be done via MRI or CT scan combined with a neurologic exam by a specialist (Alzheimer's Association, n.d.).

Management. Treatment involves placing a shunt to drain CSF from the brain to the abdomen. Placing the shunt can improve walking, but cognitive changes and incontinence are less likely to improve. Additionally, placing a shunt does not help all people with NPH, and its benefit declines over time (Alzheimer's Association, n.d.).

Hippocampal Sclerosis

Hippocampal sclerosis (HS), also referred to as hippocampal sclerosis of aging (HS-A), affects the oldest old, those 85 and older. HS involves the shrinkage and hardening of the hippocampal region of the brain. The hippocampus plays a "key role in forming memories. HS brain changes are often accompanied by the accumulation of the misfolded protein TDP-43" (Alzheimer's Association, 2023, p. 7). Memory loss is the primary symptom.

Mixed Dementia

Mixed dementia occurs when a person has more than one cause of dementia. It is thought that 50% or more of people diagnosed with AD also have VaD, or DLB. Symptoms of mixed dementia depend on the areas of the brain affected and the underlying pathological condition (Alzheimer's Association, 2023). Management is dependent on the type of dementia involved. Health-care providers who believe AD is part of the cause of dementia prescribe drugs approved to treat AD (Alzheimer's Association, n.d.).

Person-Centered Care

Person-centered care (PCC) is designed to help the person with dementia maintain a sense of purpose and a sense of self. "PCC is a philosophy of care built around the needs of the individual and contingent upon knowing the person through an interpersonal relationship" (Fazio et al, 2018, p.S10). It incorporates the person's goals, preferences, and values and involves coordination of care across health-care systems and between providers. Providers are accountable for providing care that supports the person's health and wellbeing (CMS, n.d.). Although there are various models of PCC for the person with dementia, Fazio et al (2018) identified the following practice recommendations:
- Know the person living with dementia.
- Recognize and accept the person's reality.
- Identify and support ongoing opportunities for meaningful engagement.
- Build and nurture authentic, caring relationships.
- Create and maintain a supportive community for individuals, families, and staff.
- Evaluate care practices regularly and make appropriate changes (p. S18).

P.I.E.C.E.S. P.I.E.C.E.S. stands for the physical, intellectual, emotional, capabilities, environment, and social evaluation needed to determine the cause of behavioral and psychological symptoms of dementia (BPSD) (Baycrest, n.d.).

Physical. There are many physical triggers for BPSD. Eliminate as many as can be determined, including pain, sensory impairment (visual or auditory impairment), difficulty walking, being either too hot or too cold, and medication side effects (Baycrest, n.d.).

Intellectual. The underlying disease process leading to dementia results in cognitive impairment that can cause agitation and other BPSDs. When evaluating the effect of cognitive impairment on BPSD, remember the 7As (Baycrest, n.d.):
- **A**nosognosia is the lack of insight or awareness.
- **A**mnesia is the loss of memories such as facts, experiences, or information.
- **A**ltered perception is the inability to recognize themselves.
- **A**phasia is a problem with language:
  - Expressive: know what you want to say but cannot say what you mean
  - Receptive: hear the voice or see the print but cannot make sense of the words
  - Anomic: trouble using the correct word for places, objects, or events
  - Global: cannot speak, understand speech, read, or write
- **A**pathy is the absence or suppression of interest or motivation.
- **A**gnosia is the loss of the ability to recognize objects, faces, voices, or places but still have the ability to think, speak, and interact with the world normally.
- **A**praxia is a motor speech disorder where messages from the brain to the mouth are disrupted. The person is unable to move their mouth, lips, or tongue to the right place to make sounds correctly, even though their muscles are not weak (Baycrest, n.d.).

Emotional. The emotional causes of BPSD include anxiety and depression. Persons with dementia have altered anxiety thresholds. To a person with dementia, the world is frightening and a place where they no longer have control. Persons with emotional causes of BPSD may be upset or follow their caregivers constantly (referred to as shadowing) (Baycrest, n.d.).

Capabilities. Caregivers need to assess the person with dementia and determine what they can do themselves. Tasks may take longer, but it provides a sense of control and a sense of self if the person with dementia is allowed to complete as many tasks as possible by themselves (Baycrest, n.d.).

Environment. Environmental factors may trigger BPSD. Ensure the environment is not cluttered; create clear, open, and safe spaces for the person with dementia to navigate. Ensure there are no shadows in the room that could be frightening, but also make sure it is not so bright as to be overly stimulating. Too many people or too much noise can be confusing. Persons with environmental triggers of BPSD may shout or be agitated (Baycrest, n.d.).

Social. Persons with dementia are not able to express themselves as they once were. Ensure the person is provided with activities that are meaningful for the person with dementia. It is important to understand the person's previous occupation, routines, interests, skills, social and family roles, cultural background, and spirituality. This information should be used to plan individualized activities that meet the person's needs

(Baycrest, n.d.; Best Practice Advocacy Centre New Zealand [bpac^nz], 2020).

Behavioral and Psychological Symptoms of Dementia

BPSD are attempts by the person to communicate. At some point during the trajectory of dementia, most persons with dementia develop BPSD. Therefore, it is paramount that the nurse understand what the person with dementia is trying to convey. BPSD can be organized into five categories (PsychDB, 2024).

- Apathy: lack of initiative
- Psychosis: delusions and hallucinations
- Aggression/agitation: verbal and physical
- Hyperactivity: pacing, restlessness, and disinhibition
- Affective: dysphoria, elation, irritability, and anxiety

Nonpharmacological Measures

Nonpharmacological measures are first-line therapy in the treatment of BPSD (Table 22.4). Effective interventions focus on addressing the needs a person with dementia can no longer express. This approach can be guided by the need-driven dementia-compromised behavior model, developed by a group of nurses with the purpose of elevating the standard of care for persons with dementia. The model reframes the prevailing viewpoint on BPSD. Caregivers are directed to identify triggers (such as pain or the need for toileting) leading to BPSD, instead of extinguishing these behaviors with physical or chemical restraints, thus rendering person-centered, holistic care (Algase et al, 1996).

Dementia results in the loss of the ability to communicate needs. According to Algase et al (1996), the expressed behavior is a result of background factors and proximal factors that, when combined, result in dementia-compromised behaviors. The need-driven dementia-compromised behavior model conceptualizes behavioral issues in nursing home residents as expressions of unmet needs. Understanding the interplay between BPSD and unmet needs is paramount, as individuals with significant dementia are dependent on others to meet their needs (Fig. 22.5).

Antipsychotics

In 2012, CMS launched an initiative to reduce the off-label prescribing of antipsychotics in long-term care. At the time, CMS reported 23.9% of residents received antipsychotic drugs, and 83% of them were prescribed off label, many for reasons identified on boxed warnings NOT to administer them:

> "Elderly patients with dementia-related psychosis treated with antipsychotic drugs are at an increased risk of death. Antipsychotics are not approved for the treatment of patients with dementia-related psychosis."

Guidelines suggest that some atypical antipsychotics can be considered, but only if the resident behaviors result in "significant distress for the patient or pose a safety risk for the persons with dementia or those around them" (Kirkham et al, 2017, p. 170). Antipsychotic use in persons with dementia is associated with "increased risks of mortality, stroke, and more common side effects such as falls, sedation, and cognitive decline" (Kirkham et al, 2017, p. 170). Additionally, current evidence shows there is little benefit when prescribing antipsychotics for BPSD, and significant adverse effects. The APA has drawn up guidelines for the appropriate use of antipsychotics in long-term care (Reus et al, 2016) (Box 22.1). Since the implementation of this program, there has been a 39% decrease (down to 14.5% of residents) in the prescribing of antipsychotic drugs in long-term care (CMS, 2023b).

Nursing Care Guidelines for the Person with Dementia

The goal of nursing care is to promote patient function, independence, and maximal QoL for as long as possible. The nurse teaches and assists family members with home care, provides supportive care, and serves as a patient advocate.

Recognize cues (assessment). The nurse caring for the patient with dementia should perform a complete nursing assessment, including psychological and neurological status, using evidence-based tools. Baseline data should be collected and used to monitor disease progression and help determine nursing interventions. Gather data to help identify the underlying causes of BPSD (i.e., hunger, thirst, pain, or needing to use the restroom), or altered mental status (i.e., dehydration, malnutrition, or infection). Monitor for nonverbal cues to anticipate the person's needs (i.e., assess for grimacing, crying, and pointing).

Analyze cues and prioritize hypotheses (patient problems). Assessment data should be analyzed, and patient problems should be identified and prioritized. Patient problems relating to the person with dementia include:

- Aggression
- Anxiety
- Caregiver burden
- Communication is impaired
- Confusion
- Dysphagia
- Harm to others or potential for harm
- IADLs
- Potential for injury
- Insomnia
- Isolation

Generate solutions (planning). Expected outcomes for the older adult with dementia are to a maintain maximal level of independence in self-care, remain free from injury, have underlying needs expressed as BPSD addressed, be involved in activities and socialization, and be free from infection secondary to dysphagia. The person's family will utilize appropriate resources and support services to care for the person with dementia.

Take actions (nursing interventions)

- Know the likes, dislikes, values, beliefs, and abilities of a person with dementia.
- Recognize behavior as communication; accept the person's perspective and feelings.
- Identify and support opportunities for meaningful experiences and interactions that incorporate the person's preferences.
- Build caring relationships in which you demonstrate respect by "doing with" rather than "doing for" the person.
- Create and maintain a supportive community that incorporates the person, family members, and staff in care.

TABLE 22.4 Possible Nonpharmacological Approaches for Behavioral and Psychological Symptoms of Dementia

Behavior	Presentation	Nonpharmacological Management Strategy
Agitation and aggression	Occurs in approximately 60% of people with dementia. Can be verbal, e.g., complaining, moaning, angry statements, threats, or physical, e.g., resistiveness to caregivers, restlessness, spitting, or hitting out.	May be due to underlying depression, unmet needs, boredom, discomfort, perceived threat, or violation of personal space. Make environmental or management modifications to resolve these issues. Nonspecific calming and positive experience interventions may be beneficial, such as music or touch therapy, e.g., hand massage, a mechanical pet, or a twiddle muff (sleeve or glove with attached materials, buttons, etc., for sensory stimulation).
Apathy	Estimated to occur in 55%–90% of people with dementia; most frequently vascular, Lewy body dementia (LBD), and frontotemporal lobar dementia (FTLD). Presents as a lack of initiative, motivation, drive, aimlessness, and reduced emotional response. Reduced motivation can be a feature of depression, but a pure apathy syndrome can be distinguished from depression by the absence of sadness and other signs of psychological distress.	Reading to the person and encouraging them to ask questions, small group, and individual activities, e.g., puzzles, games, sensory stories, may all be helpful. Music, exercise, multisensory stimulation with touch, smell, and sound, and spending time with pets can also be effective. The key is to provide enriched prompts and cues to overcome the apathy and generate positive behavior.
Depression	Occurs in approximately 20% of people with dementia but is more prevalent in the early stages. May present as sadness, tearfulness, pessimistic thoughts, withdrawal, inactivity, or fatigue.	Recommend exercise, social connection, and engaging activities. Cognitive behavioral therapy (CBT) may be helpful in the early stages. Severe depression requires input from a clinician with experience managing patients with dementia.
Anxiety	Estimated to occur in 16%–35% of people with dementia. One of the most disabling BPSDs. In later-stage dementia, this may be an exaggerated response to separation from family, a different setting, or a reduced capacity to make sense of the environment.	Focus on identifying and eliminating the trigger rather than symptom control. Maintain structure and routine and reduce the need for stressful decision-making. Assess if sensory overstimulation may be contributing. Music and CBT have the greatest amount of evidence showing benefits.
Psychotic symptoms	Approximately 25% of people with dementia will experience psychosis, causing delusions, or hallucinations. In dementia, delusions are usually reflective of the underlying memory loss or changes in perception, e.g., accusations of theft of personal items, infidelity of a spouse, or that family members are imposters, rather than delusions normally associated with mania or schizophrenia. Vivid visual hallucinations are common, particularly in LBD, but auditory hallucinations are less common.	Often causes more distress for the caregivers/family than the patient. Potentially reversible causes of psychosis include sensory or vision loss, overstimulation, delirium, the initiation of a new medicine, or substance misuse. Confirm that the patient's claims are not occurring, e.g., items are not being stolen. Use memory aids, e.g., photographs, to cue the person to reality. Distraction can sometimes be effective.
Wandering	Sometimes related to agitation. Wandering may be circular, pacing between two points, random, or direct to a location without diversion. Often one of the most challenging and problematic BPSD due to safety concerns.	Wandering can have positive effects via exercise, e.g., improving sleep, mood, and general health, and may prevent the person from feeling confined. Consider how to make wandering safe: supervised walks, secured space to roam, exercise equipment, and GPS watch. Try to determine if there is a purpose to the wandering, e.g., trying to return home, looking for a person, or escaping a perceived threat.
Nocturnal disruption	Sleep disturbances can occur secondary to depression, anxiety, agitation, or pain and may cause other BPSD to be exacerbated at night, e.g., wandering. Occurs more frequently in people with LBD. Sundowning, i.e., increased agitation in the late afternoon, is also common. A sleep/wake reversal can sometimes be the cause; a form of sleep phase-shift.	Assess for underlying causes, including thirst or hunger. Restrict caffeine in the evening, limit fluid intake in the hours before bed, establish a night-time routine, minimize light and noise intrusion, and ensure adequate stimulating activities during the daytime.
Disinhibited behavior	Typically occurs due to reduced impulse control. May be exacerbated by impaired judgment, reduced awareness of the environment, or a lack of understanding of the effect on others. Inappropriate sexual behavior or verbal or physical behavior ordinarily considered "rude" can occur. Reduced privacy, lack of personal affection, absence of a sexual partner, misinterpretation of assistance provided by caregivers, and dopaminergic medicines, e.g., to treat Parkinson's disease, delusions, or hallucinations, may contribute to the behavior.	Avoid reflexive responses that may humiliate the patient. People with dementia can often learn what is appropriate and what is not with clear messages, but it may take longer to do so. Identify triggers, e.g., a caregiver performing a particular task, and, where possible, modify environmental factors, e.g., temperature control, to avoid overheating. Use distraction and redirection techniques to divert the patient's focus, e.g., provide a craft activity or puzzle. Ensure the patient has privacy if sexual behaviors are prominent.

Sources: 1. NSW Ministry of Health and Royal Australian and New Zealand College of Psychiatrists. *Assessment and management of people with behavioural and psychological symptoms of dementia (BPSD).* 2022. Retrieved from https://www.health.nsw.gov.au/mentalhealth/resources/Publications/ass-mgmt-bpsd-handbook-dec-22.pdf. Accessed August, 2024. 2. Guideline Adaption Committee. *Clinical practice guidelines and principles of care for people with dementia.* 2016. Retrieved from https://cdpc.sydney.edu.au/wp-content/uploads/2019/06/CDPC-Dementia-Guidelines_WEB.pdf. 3. Burns, K., Jayasinha, R., & Brodaty, H. (2014). *A clinician's field guide to good practice.* Retrieved from https://dementiaresearch.org.au/wp-content/uploads/2020/07/A_Clinicians_Field_Guide_to_Good_Practice_Managing_Behavioural_and_Psychological_Symptoms_of_Dementia.pdf. In: Best Practice Advocacy Centre New Zealand (bpac[nz]). (2020). *Managing the behavioural and psychological symptoms of dementia.* Retrieved from https://bpac.org.nz/2020/docs/bpsd.pdf.

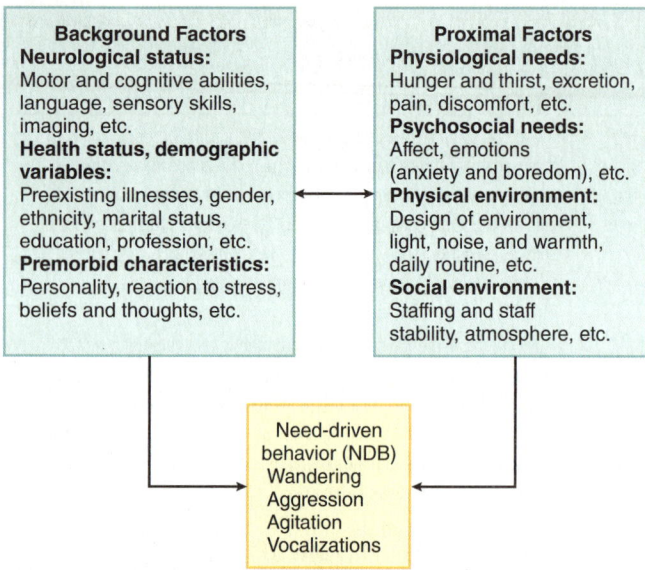

Fig. 22.5 Need-driven dementia-compromised behavior model. (Modified from Holle, D., Roes, M., Buscher, I., et al. [2014]. Process evaluation of the implementation of dementia-specific case conferences in nursing homes [FallDem]: Study protocol for a randomized controlled trial. *Trials, 15*, 485.)

- Regularly evaluate care practices and programs, sharing findings with other health-care team members and making changes as needed.
- Clarify the personal values and preferences related to advance directives.
- Engage in effective communication practices:
  - Avoid elderspeak (i.e., terms such as sweetie, honey, or dear).
  - Speak in a calm voice and allow for pauses between ideas.
  - Give the person time to respond so they do not feel hurried or rushed.
  - Avoid corrective speech (i.e., if patients are not oriented to date or place, gently incorporate the information into conversation rather than overtly correcting them).
  - Call patients by their preferred names.
  - Introduce yourself with each encounter.
  - Narrate actions, saying what you are doing and why.
  - Provide choices.
  - Approach the person with dementia from the front at eye level.
  - Use gentle touch to get the person's attention and to provide a transition from one activity to the next.
  - Avoid triggers that are known to update or agitate the person with dementia.

BOX 22.1 The American Psychiatric Association Practice Guideline on the Use of Antipsychotics to Treat Agitation or Psychosis in Patients With Dementia

When using practice guidelines, it is important to remember that they are not updated annually and are not patient-specific. Guidelines do not substitute for clinical judgment or supersede the patient's personal and sociocultural preferences.

APA Practice Guideline Statements
Assessment of Behavioral/Psychological Symptoms of Dementia
Statement 1. The APA recommends that patients with dementia* be assessed for the type, frequency, severity, pattern, and timing of symptoms. (1C)
Statement 2. The APA recommends that patients with dementia be assessed for pain and other potentially modifiable contributors to symptoms, as well as for factors such as the subtype of dementia, that may influence choices of treatment. (1C)
Statement 3. The APA recommends that in patients with dementia with agitation or psychosis, the response to treatment be assessed with a quantitative measure. (1C)

Development of a Comprehensive Treatment Plan
Statement 4. The APA recommends that patients with dementia have a documented comprehensive treatment plan that includes appropriate person-centered nonpharmacological and pharmacological interventions, as indicated. (1C)

Assessment of the Benefits and Risks of Antipsychotic Treatment for the Patient
Statement 5. The APA recommends that nonemergency antipsychotic medication should only be used for the treatment of agitation or psychosis in patients with dementia when symptoms are severe, are dangerous, and/or cause significant distress to the patient. (1B)
Statement 6. The APA recommends reviewing the clinical response to nonpharmacological interventions prior to the nonemergency use of an antipsychotic medication to treat agitation or psychosis in patients with dementia. (1C)
Statement 7. The APA recommends that before nonemergency treatment with an antipsychotic medication is initiated in patients with dementia, the potential risks and benefits from antipsychotic medication be assessed by the clinician and discussed with the patient (if clinically feasible) as well as with the patient's surrogate decision-maker (if relevant) with input from family or others involved with the patient. (1C)

Dosing, Duration, and Monitoring of Antipsychotic Treatment
Statement 8. The APA recommends that if a risk/benefit assessment favors the use of an antipsychotic medication for behavioral/psychological symptoms in patients with dementia, treatment should be initiated at a low dose to be titrated up to the minimum effective dose as tolerated. (1B)
Statement 9. The APA recommends that if a patient with dementia experiences a clinically significant side effect of antipsychotic treatment, the potential risks and benefits of antipsychotic medication should be reviewed by the clinician to determine if tapering and discontinuation of the medication are indicated. (1C)
Statement 10. The APA recommends that in patients with dementia with agitation or psychosis, if there is no clinically significant response after a 4-week trial of an adequate dose of an antipsychotic drug, the medication should be tapered and withdrawn. (1B)
Statement 11. The APA recommends that in a patient who has shown a positive response to treatment, decision-making about possible tapering of antipsychotic medication should be accompanied by a discussion with the patient (if clinically feasible) as well as with the patient's surrogate decision-maker (if relevant), with input from family or others involved with the patient. The aim of such a discussion is to elicit their preferences and concerns and to review the initial goals, observed benefits and side effects of antipsychotic treatment, and potential risks of continued exposure to antipsychotics, as well as past experience with antipsychotic medication trials and tapering attempts. (1C)
Statement 12. APA recommends that in patients with dementia who show an adequate response of behavioral/psychological symptoms to treatment with an antipsychotic drug, an attempt to taper and withdraw the drug should be made within 4 months of initiation, unless the patient experienced a recurrence of symptoms with prior attempts at tapering antipsychotic medication. (1C)

BOX 22.1 The American Psychiatric Association Practice Guideline on the Use of Antipsychotics to Treat Agitation or Psychosis in Patients With Dementia—cont'd

Statement 13. APA recommends that in patients with dementia whose antipsychotic medication is being tapered, assessment of symptoms should occur at least monthly during the taper and for at least 4 months after medication discontinuation to identify signs of recurrence and trigger a reassessment of the benefits and risks of antipsychotic treatment. (1C)

Use of Specific Antipsychotic Medications, Depending on Clinical Context

Statement 14. The APA recommends that in the absence of delirium, if nonemergency antipsychotic medication treatment is indicated, haloperidol should not be used as a first-line agent. (1B)

Statement 15. The APA recommends that in patients with dementia with agitation or psychosis, a long-acting injectable antipsychotic medication should not be utilized unless it is otherwise indicated for a co-occurring chronic psychotic disorder. (1B)

The strength of recommendations reflecting the level of confidence in the evidence supporting each statement is as follows:

A = high
B = moderate
C = low

*Throughout this guideline, we use the term *dementia*, which was used in the evidence that was considered in developing these recommendations. These recommendations are also meant to apply to individuals with major neurocognitive disorder (MND), as defined in the American Psychiatric Association's *Diagnostic and Statistical Manual of Mental Disorders*, 5th ed. (DSM–5).
Reprinted with permission from the American Journal of Psychiatry, 173:5, Text Excerpt: "Guideline Statements," pages 543-546 (Copyright © 2016). American Psychiatric Association. All Rights Reserved.

- Repeat, reassure, and redirect.
- Maintain a consistent routine.
- Promote sensory stimulation with appropriate activities, such as activity kits, sewing cards, word search puzzles, adult coloring books, and towel folding.
- Encourage the person with dementia to participate as much as they can in performing ADLs.
- Simplify the presentation of the food, offer small, frequent meals, limit mealtime distractions, demonstrate the use of utensils as needed, and provide cues.
- Assist with ambulation and minimize the amount of time the person spends in bed or in a chair.
- Schedule range of motion and other exercises.
- Offer regular toileting.
- Create an environment free of hazards and safe for mobility.
- Provide the family with appropriate resources to either provide effective care for the person with dementia or cope with the progression of dementia.

Evaluate outcomes (evaluation). Evaluation is a continual process when caring for persons with dementia. Interventions should be evaluated and compared to baselines, on an ongoing basis for efficacy. Successful and unsuccessful interventions should be communicated to other caregivers and family members to aid in the continuity of care.

Resources

The physical and mental strain placed on family caregivers can be significantly reduced if available resources are identified and used. Community resources become increasingly important as the primary caregiver grows more isolated and overextended. The nurse should identify appropriate community resources available to the patient and family and encourage family members to participate as the need becomes critical. These resources may include community mental-health centers, adult day-care centers, respite services, local Alzheimer's Associations and support groups, medical information and referral programs, and other family support groups specific to the disease type. Additionally, through the *eldercare* locator, a public service of the U.S. Administration on Aging (AoA), individuals can find resources in their area by entering their zip code into the search bar (https://eldercare.acl.gov/Public/About/Aging_Network/AAA.aspx).

Family Support Groups

A significant increase in family support groups has created a network to help families faced with caring for a loved one with dementia. These support groups offer a variety of services, ranging from assisting family members to cope with the inevitable losses faced by patients with dementia to emotional support and respite.

Respite Services

Respite service is provided to family members requiring temporary relief from the pressures of continuous caregiving. These services may prevent the premature institutionalization of individuals with dementia because of caregiver stress. Respite can be provided in the home by friends, other family members, volunteers, or paid caregivers.

Adult Day Care

Adult day-care centers help keep people with dementia in the community by providing family respite, promoting activity, and encouraging the retention of previously learned skills. Some centers provide planned activities, such as music and art programs, specialized social work, nursing, and physical and occupational therapy services. Meals are often provided. Adult day-care centers allow family members to work during the day, do errands, rest, and yet be involved in important areas of their loved ones' lives.

Home Health Care

Home health care may provide nursing, physical and occupational therapies, the services of social workers, and personal-care services to patients in their homes in the later stages of dementia. Home-health personnel may help with direct-care needs, including meals and shopping, drugs, cleaning, laundry, transportation, an appraisal of a person's condition, and companionship.

However, unless the individual has an established need for skilled nursing or therapy, Medicare does not cover these services.

Long-Term Care Services

Some long-term care facilities may offer the ability for persons with dementia to stay overnight, for a few days, or for a few weeks. This affords the caregivers the opportunity to take a vacation while their loved one stays in a supervised, safe environment. The cost varies and is not usually covered by insurance or Medicare.

Legal Services

Legal services are necessary when family members must consider questions related to the person's ability to handle finances and make decisions. It is important to set up a durable power of attorney (PoA) for financial matters and a health-care proxy for medical matters early in the disease process while the individual can still participate in decision-making. Legal guardianship is granted when the individual is no longer capable of making decisions for themselves. This requires that a physician or mental-health professional document that the patient does not understand the ramifications of decisions or behaviors.

Community Mental-Health Centers

Community mental-health centers may have specialized geriatric programs that provide a wide range of services. These services may include comprehensive assessment, psychiatric evaluations, and individual, group, and family counseling. In addition, case-management services available in community mental-health centers may assist in the identification of other community resources necessary to maintain individuals in the home.

Psychiatric Hospitals

Psychiatric hospitals offer assessment and behavior stabilization. In addition, an increasing number of geriatric psychiatric units can meet the multidimensional physiologic and mental-health needs of older adults with cognitive disorders. Psychiatric hospital placement usually occurs when an individual cannot be managed in a community setting, and more advanced assessment and behavior management techniques are required. Outcomes of geriatric psychiatric hospital placement may include drug management and behavior modification therapies in the hope of returning the older adult to their home or may result in placement in long-term care facilities.

OTHER COMMON PROBLEMS AND CONDITIONS

Suicide

There has been a progressive increase in suicide as people age, especially among males. Risk factors for suicide include (De Leo, 2022):
- Chronic pain
- Dependence on others
- Loneliness
- Feelings of abandonment
- Loss of meaning for life

Baby boomers (born between 1946 and 1964) have a higher suicide rate than other age cohorts. The Substance Abuse and Mental Health Services Administration (SAMHSA) has published the following list as warning signs of potential suicide (CDC, 2022):
- Talking about being a burden
- Being isolated
- Increased anxiety
- Talking about feeling trapped or in unbearable pain
- Increased substance use
- Looking for a way to access lethal means
- Increased anger or rage
- Extreme mood swings
- Expressing hopelessness
- Sleeping too little or too much
- Talking or posting about wanting to die
- Making plans for suicide

A single warning sign may not be an indicator of potential suicide; however, noting multiple signs, combined with risk-taking behavior, major life-changing events, chronic illness, and mental-health issues, could be an indicator of suicide risk (Tisdale, 2022). Box 22.2 provides a more in-depth look at suicide risk factors as well as protective factors against suicide.

Nursing Care Guidelines for the Person with Suicidal Ideation

Recognize cues (assessment). Conducting the assessment in an environment free of distractions and disruptions will help allay the anxiety and fear patients face when discussing such a sensitive topic. During the assessment, the nurse should use active listening skills, maintain eye contact, and appear genuine and nonjudgmental. Open-ended questions should be used to begin questioning and gain trust. It is important to determine the extent of suicidal ideation, the presence of a specific plan, weather preparations have been made, and the method the person plans to use. The Columbia Suicide Severity Rating Scale (C-SSRS) is one of many reliable tools that can be used to determine suicide risk (Fig. 22.6). The C-SSRS is available in different versions to use in a variety of settings, as well as a version for persons with cognitive impairment (Tan et al, 2021).

Analyze cues and prioritize hypotheses (patient problems). Patient problems for older adults at risk for suicide include the following:
- Decreased ability to cope
- Grieving
- Social isolation
- Injury
- Risk for self-harm

Generate solutions (planning). Planning care for an older adult patient with suicidal ideation requires a strong interpersonal connection with the patient. Expected outcomes include the following (Martin, 2024):
1. The patient will establish a safety plan with the nurse, including the identification of triggers, coping strategies, and emergency contacts.
2. The patient will identify at least one meaningful goal for the future, fostering a sense of purpose and hope.

BOX 22.2 Risk and Protective Factors of Suicide

Circumstances That Increase Suicide Risk

Individual Risk Factors

These personal factors contribute to the risk:
- Previous suicide attempt
- History of depression and other mental illnesses
- Serious illness, such as chronic pain
- Criminal/legal problems
- Job/financial problems or loss
- Impulsive or aggressive tendencies
- Substance use
- Current or prior history of adverse childhood experiences
- Sense of hopelessness
- Violence victimization and/or perpetration

Relationship Risk Factors

These harmful or hurtful experiences within relationships contribute to risk:
- Bullying
- Family/loved one's history of suicide
- Loss of relationships
- High conflict or violent relationships
- Social isolation

Community Risk Factors

These challenging issues within a person's community contribute to risk:
- Lack of access to healthcare
- Suicide clusters in the community
- Stress of acculturation
- Community violence
- Historical trauma
- Discrimination

Societal Risk Factors

These cultural and environmental factors within the larger society contribute to risk:
- Stigma associated with help-seeking and mental illness
- Easy access to lethal means of suicide among people at risk
- Unsafe media portrayals of suicide

Circumstances That Protect Against Suicide Risk

Individual Protective Factors

These personal factors protect against suicide risk:
- Effective coping and problem-solving skills
- Reasons for living (e.g., family, friends, pets, etc.)
- Strong sense of cultural identity

Relationship Protective Factors

These healthy relationship experiences protect against suicide risk:
- Support from partners, friends, and family
- Feeling connected to others

Community Protective Factors

These supportive community experiences protect against suicide risk:
- Feeling connected to school, community, and other social institutions
- Availability of consistent and high-quality physical and behavioral healthcare

Societal Protective Factors

These cultural and environmental factors within the larger society protect against suicide risk:
- Reduced access to lethal means of suicide among people at risk
- Cultural, religious, or moral objections to suicide

From Centers for Disease Control and Prevention (CDC), & National Center for Injury Prevention and Control. (2022). *Suicide prevention: Risk and protective factors.* Retrieved from https://www.cdc.gov/suicide/risk-factors/index.html.

Question	Past month	
1. Have you wished you were dead or wished you could go to sleep and not wake up?		
2. Have you actually had any thoughts about killing yourself?		
If YES to 2, answer questions 3, 4, 5, and 6 If NO to 2, go directly to question 6		
3. Have you thought about how you might do this?		
4. Have you had any intention of acting on these thoughts of killing yourself, as opposed to you have the thought but definitely would not act on them?	High risk	
5. Have you started to work out or worked out the details of how to kill yourself? Do you intend to carry out this plan?	High risk	
(Always ask question 6)	Lifetime	Past 3 months
6. Have you done anything, started to do anything, or prepared to do anything to end your life? *Example: Collected pills, obtained a gun, gave away valuables, wrote a will or suicide note, held a gun but changed your mind, cut yourself, tried to hang yourself, etc.*		High risk

Fig. 22.6 Questions for assessing the risk for suicide: Columbia Suicide Severity Rating Scale. (Redrawn from The Columbia Lighthouse Project, 2016. http://cssrs.columbia.edu/.)

3. The patient will adhere to a no-suicide contract and verbalize a desire to live.
4. The patient will demonstrate improved emotional regulation and employ at least two healthy strategies for managing emotional pain.
5. The patient will exhibit a reduction in self-destructive behaviors through the implementation of healthier coping mechanisms.

Take actions (nursing interventions). Appropriate actions may include the following (Gulanick and Myers, 2022):

- Provide a safe environment: Suicide precautions are used to prevent the patient from acting on sudden self-destructive impulses. These measures include removing potentially harmful objects (e.g., electrical appliances, sharp instruments, belts and ties, glass items, and medications) and always maintaining visual contact with the patient.
- Provide supervision and always maintain observation and awareness of the patient: The degree of supervision is defined by the degree of risk. Suicide may be an impulsive act with little or no warning. The patient may need direct observation by health-care staff at frequent intervals, as often as 30 minutes or less.
- Develop a written contract stating that the patient will not act on impulse to do self-harm (review and update as needed): A written or verbal agreement establishes permission to discuss the subject, makes a commitment not to act on impulse, and defines a plan of action in case an impulse occurs.
- Provide opportunities for the patient to express concerns, fears, feelings, and expectations in a nonjudgmental environment: The patient benefits from talking about suicidal thoughts with trusted staff. Patients need the opportunity to discuss suicidal thoughts and intentions to harm themselves. Verbalization of these feelings may lessen their intensity. Patients also need to see that staff members are open to discussing suicidal thoughts.
- Assist the patient with problem-solving in a constructive manner: Patients learn to recognize situational, interpersonal, or emotional triggers; learn to assess a problem; and implement problem-solving measures before reacting.
- Discourage the patient from making decisions when under severe stress: Patients can learn to identify mood changes that signal problems with impulsivity or signal a deepening depressive state. At these times, deciding not to make a decision may be best.
- Refer the patient and family for additional and ongoing support: Recovery from a suicide attempt will likely require involvement from many sources, including community-based mental-health resources, crisis lines, spiritual support, financial aid, housing, and welfare resources. Recovery may require psychological insight that builds slowly.
- Instruct the patient on the appropriate use of medications: Drug therapy may help the patient manage underlying health problems such as depression.
- Teach the patient cognitive behavioral self-management responses to suicidal thoughts: Patients are better able to recognize and respond to early thoughts of suicide. The patient can be taught to identify negative self-talk or automatic thoughts that lead to suicidal ideas. Then the patient learns how to develop positive approaches and positive self-talk to counter those negative ideas.
- Teach patients to use self-expression methods to manage suicidal feelings: Patients are better able to recognize and safely manage suicidal feelings by using methods such as keeping journals and calling hotlines.

Evaluate outcomes (evaluation). Unfortunately, despite excellent nursing assessment and intervention, older adults do continue to commit suicide at a distressingly high rate. Older adults ages 85 and older have the highest suicide rate: 22.4 per 100,000; older adults aged 75–84 follow closely at 19.6 per 100,000 (CDC, 2023b). When an older adult has committed suicide, the nurse's focus shifts to assisting family and friends in coping with the resulting grief and trauma. A psychological autopsy, or the processing of events and behaviors surrounding the patient's suicide, may be useful to both the health-care professionals and the patient's family and friends. Family and friends may also be encouraged to obtain assistance from support groups.

Parkinson Disease

Parkinson disease (PD) is a progressive disorder resulting from the degeneration of dopaminergic neurons in the substantia nigra, the part of the brain that controls movement. With degeneration, the nerve cells are no longer able to produce dopamine. The depletion of dopamine produces the hallmark symptoms associated with the disease, including tremor, rigidity, bradykinesia, and impaired balance and coordination (American Association of Neurological Surgeons [AANS], 2024). Degeneration of nerve cells results from deposits of a protein called alpha-synuclein (α-syn), which "become organized into insoluble amyloid fibrils" (Vidović and Rikalovic, 2022, Introduction). These deposits are called Lewy bodies.

Motor activity occurs because of the integrated actions originating from the cerebral cortex, basal ganglia, and cerebellum. The main area in the brain affected by PD is the basal ganglia. The basal ganglia controls both muscle tone and the process of voluntary movement. This is accomplished through the secretion of the excitatory neurotransmitter acetylcholine (ACh) and the inhibitory neurotransmitter dopamine. ACh is produced in the basal ganglia and transmits excitatory messages throughout this area. Dopamine inhibits the function of ACh in the basal ganglia to control fine and voluntary movements. Therefore, it is the dopamine–ACh balance that produces normal motor function (Fig. 22.7). In PD, there is dopamine depletion in the basal ganglia, while the ACh-secreting neurons remain active. This creates an imbalance between excitatory and inhibitory neural activity and is the cause of symptoms such as hypertonia (tremors and rigidity) and akinesia in PD.

Risk Factors

Approximately 60,000 people per year are diagnosed with PD. The risk of PD increases with age, and the peak onset is after the age of 55 (AANS, 2024). Genetics are the cause of 10%–15% of PD cases. The most common genetic mutation linked to PD is a mutation in leucine-rich repeat kinase 2 (LRRK2; also known

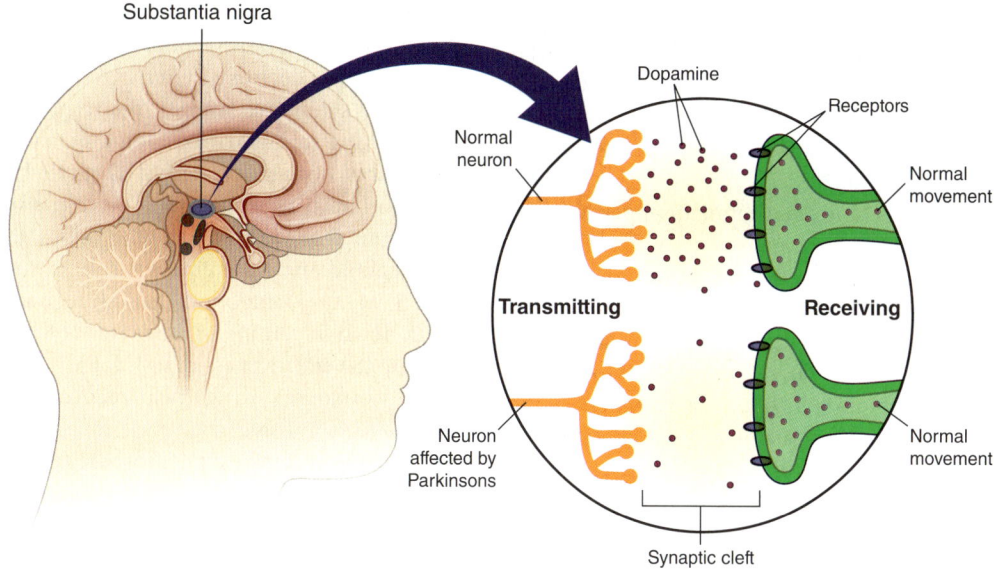

Fig. 22.7 Dopaminergic pathways of the brain.

as PARK8). This mutation is responsible for about 2% of autosomal-dominant inherited PD (Gonzalez-Usigli, 2022). The environment and lifestyle also play a role in the development of PD. Environmental factors include head injury, place of residence, exposure to pesticides and herbicides, exposure to Agent Orange, and industrial pollution (i.e., heavy metals, detergents, and solvents). Other factors include increasing age, ethnicity (White), and sex; PD is more common in males (Gonzalez-Usigli, 2022; Johns Hopkins Medicine, n.d.).

Clinical Manifestations

Signs and symptoms begin subtly, including a resting tremor of one hand. This may be the only initial symptom. The tremor is reduced with movement and absent during sleep. As the degeneration of dopaminergic neurons progresses, so do the symptoms (Box 22.3). PD is categorized into five stages.

Stage one. During stage one, the person has mild symptoms that generally do not interfere with daily activities. Tremor and other movement symptoms (rigidity and bradykinesia) occur on one side of the body only. Changes in posture and balance, walking, and facial expressions occur (Allarakha, 2022; Parkinson's Foundation, n.d.).

Stage two. Symptoms begin to increase in stage two. Tremor, rigidity, and bradykinesia affect both sides of the body or the midline (such as the neck and the trunk). Difficulty with walking and balance, as well as poor posture, may be apparent. Facial expressivity worsens. This is referred to as "masked facies." The person can live alone, but daily tasks are more difficult and take longer (Allarakha, 2022; Parkinson's Foundation, n.d.).

Stage three. Stage three is considered mid-stage. Loss of balance (such as unsteadiness as the person turns or when they are pushed from standing) is the hallmark. Falls are more common. Motor symptoms continue to worsen. Although the person is still physically capable of leading an independent life, ADLs

BOX 22.3 Postural and Gait Terms for Parkinson's Disease

Akinesia: Absence or difficulty producing movement
Ataxia: Loss of balance
Athetosis: Abnormal involuntary movements that are slow, repetitive, and sinuous
Bradykinesia: Slowing down of movement
Festination: Walking in rapid, short, shuffling steps
Hypokinesia: Decreased motor activity
Myoclonus: Jerking, involuntary movement of arms and legs, usually occurring during sleep
Postural instability: Difficulty with balance
Propulsive gait: During walking, steps become faster and faster with progressively shorter steps that pass from walking to a running pace and may precipitate falling forward
Retropulsion: Walking that is propelled backwards

Data from WebMD Editorial Contributors. (2022). *Glossary of Parkinson's disease terms*. WebMD [website]. Retrieved from https://www.webmd.com/parkinsons-disease/parkinsons-glossary.

(eating, bathing, and dressing) are impaired. Disability is mild to moderate at this stage (Allarakha, 2022; Parkinson's Foundation, n.d.).

Stage four. At this point, symptoms are fully developed and severely disabling. The person is still able to walk and stand without assistance but may need to ambulate with a cane/walker for safety. The person needs significant help with ADLs and is unable to live alone (Allarakha, 2022; Parkinson's Foundation, n.d.).

Stage five. This is the most advanced and debilitating stage. Stiffness in the legs may make it impossible to stand or walk. The person is bedridden or confined to a wheelchair unless aided. Around-the-clock care is required for all activities (Allarakha, 2022; Parkinson's Foundation, n.d.).

Diagnostic Studies

No specific studies can be used to diagnose PD. The diagnosis is based primarily on the clinical features of the disorder, history, and physical examination, including a neurological exam. Patients with PD typically exhibit the following during a neurological exam (Gonzalez-Usigli, 2022):

- Finger-to-nose coordination: the tremor disappears in the extremity being tested
- Rapidly alternating movements: the patient cannot perform the task
- Reflexes: normal, but tremor and rigidity interfere with testing

Diagnostic and laboratory studies may be ordered to rule out other causes of the symptoms, including a complete blood ccount (CBC), which may reveal anemia; a blood chemistry profile may show low albumin and protein levels. Drug screens may be done to rule out toxic causes of the symptoms. An MRI and PET scan of the brain may also help to rule out other causes (Mayo Clinic Staff, 2024b).

A new test, the alpha-synuclein seed amplification assay (αSyn-SAA), is being evaluated to determine its ability to detect the disease before symptoms begin. Spinal fluid is examined for clumps of the protein alpha-synuclein, which is found in Lewy bodies. Initial tests indicate it is sensitive for detecting those at risk for PD (Mayo Clinic Staff, 2024b).

Management

Treatment is aimed at relieving clinical manifestations, increasing the individual's ability to perform ADLs, and decreasing the risk for injury. This is accomplished using drugs, surgery, and rehabilitation aimed at optimizing the patient's functional level. A team approach is essential for a high-quality care of PD patients.

Drugs. Many drugs are used to treat the symptoms of PD (Table 22.5). First-line treatment with carbidopa/levodopa. Levodopa converts to dopamine in the brain, helping to control movement; carbidopa prevents levodopa from breaking down in the bloodstream before it reaches the brain. Carbidopa can also help reduce the nausea and vomiting associated with levodopa. It may take several months before feeling the full benefit of the drug. It is recommended that patients take 4-5 doses a day to prevent fluctuating blood levels that can lead to fluctuating symptoms. Carbidopa levodopa should not be taken with iron-containing supplements, such as multivitamins, as iron can reduce the absorption of the drug.

Side effects of carbidopa levodopa include nausea and vomiting, dizziness, and trouble concentrating. Patients taking the drug should be told to notify their health-care provider if they have unusual changes in behavior (i.e., gambling, hypersexuality, or other addictive types of behaviors), visual hallucinations, or suicidal thoughts.

Persons taking levodopa, dopamine agonists, and amantadine should not stop the drugs suddenly, or they may experience life-threatening withdrawal symptoms, referred to as dopamine agonist withdrawal syndrome (DAWS). Withdrawal symptoms include convulsions, dyspnea, panic attacks, diaphoresis, agitation, pain, tachycardia, high fever, orthostatic hypotension, loss of bladder control, and severe muscle stiffness.

Amantadine (an NMDAR antagonist) is given to improve dyskinesias that occur secondary to cumulative exposure to levodopa and to decrease tremors.

As PD symptoms worsen, the response to levodopa wears off, resulting in fluctuating motor symptoms and dyskinesias. When this occurs, a catechol O-methyltransferase (COMT) inhibitor, such as entacapone or tolcapone, is added. These drugs inhibit the breakdown of levodopa and dopamine.

Selegiline and rasagiline are selective monoamine oxidase type B (MAO-B) inhibitors that inhibit one of the enzymes that break down dopamine in the brain. The drugs are used to help prolong the effectiveness of levodopa.

Anticholinergic drugs help reduce tremors. However, adverse effects include cognitive impairment and dry mouth. Benztropine and trihexyphenidyl are the most commonly used anticholinergics.

Surgical therapy. If drug therapy is not effective or side effects become intolerable, deep-brain stimulation or lesional surgery may be considered.

Deep-brain stimulation involves placing electrodes in certain areas of the brain that interrupt the disorganized electrical signals causing the symptoms of PD. It can significantly improve stiffness, tremors, dyskinesia, and slowness. However, it does not cure PD or stop the progression of the disease, and it does not improve memory problems, depression, anxiety, dysphagia, and ataxia. Although the dose of drugs used to treat PD can be reduced after surgery, they cannot be stopped.

Lesional surgeries, such as thalamotomy and pallidotomy, which destroy targeted areas in the brain associated with specific PD symptoms, are rarely performed anymore due to their long recovery times and irreversible nature.

Nursing Care Guidelines for the Person with Parkinson Disease

Recognize cues (assessment).

- Assess functional status and activity tolerance; determine the need for assistive devices and rehabilitative services.
- Assess for the hallmark signs of PD: tremor, rigidity, bradykinesia, decreased facial expression, impaired balance, and coordination.
- Assess for dysphagia.
- Assess for signs of aspiration.
- Monitor food and fluid intake.
- Perform nutritional screening.
- Assess for signs and symptoms of constipation.
- Assess for alterations in verbal and written communication.
- Assess the emotional response to the diagnosis.

Analyze cues and prioritize hypotheses (patient problems).

Priority patient problems for an individual with PD include the following:

- Decreased functional mobility
- Inadequate communication
- Inadequate nutrition
- Potential for injury
- Constipation
- Decreased ability to cope

TABLE 22.5 Drugs Used to Treat Parkinson Disease

Drug Classification and Example	Mechanism of Action	Indications	Common Side Effects	Nursing Implications
Anticholinergics Trihexyphenidyl benztropine	Inhibit the action of endogenous acetylcholine and muscarine agonists to block the excitatory effect of the cholinergic system	Ease tremors and dystonia; may be used to treat drooling in advanced disease	Blurred vision, dry mouth, constipation, cognitive problems, and hallucinations	Usually contraindicated in patients with acute-angle glaucoma and tachycardia; monitor pulse and blood pressure during periods of dosage adjustment; administer with meals; do not withdraw the drug suddenly
Dopaminergics Levodopa is taken with carbidopa, a decarboxylase inhibitor	Cause the release of dopamine in the central nervous system (CNS)	Controls slow movements and stiff, rigid body parts With long-term use may develop restlessness, confusion, or unusual movements—changing the amount and timing of the drug may prevent this	Dizziness, ataxia, insomnia, and leg edema Orthostatic hypotension, nausea, hallucinations, dystonia, and dyskinesia	Monitor the patient for postural hypotension; do not administer at bedtime Monitor blood pressure: use elastic stockings to increase venous return; monitor patient for urinary retention
Dopamine Agonists Apomorphine, pramipexole, rotigotine, and ropinirole	Active dopamine receptors in the CNS	Fluctuation of manifestations, dyskinesia, and dystonia	Hallucinations, mental fogginess, orthostatic hypotension, and confusion Orthostatic hypotension, nausea, and insomnia	Monitor blood pressure and mental status Monitor blood pressure; do not administer at bedtime
Amantadine		Used to treat slowness, stiffness, and tremor May ease involuntary dyskinesia	Confusion and memory loss	
Catechol-O-Methyltransferase (COMT) Inhibitor Tolcapone, entacapone, and opicapone	Inhibit the enzyme that breaks down levodopa	Adjunct treatment to extend the benefit of levodopa	Diarrhea and harmless urine discoloration. Tolcapone can cause liver disease Nausea and headache	Monitor liver enzymes Monitor for levodopa side effects
MAO-B Inhibitors Selegiline, rasagiline Safinamide is an adjunctive medication prescribed when levodopa and carbidopa have breakthrough symptoms	Inhibit monoamine oxidase B, an enzyme that converts chemical by-products in the brain into neurotoxins that prevent substantia nigra cell death	May slow the progression of Parkinson's disease (PD) early on	Nausea, dizziness, fainting, and stomach pain Headache, joint pain, indigestion, and depression	Monitor for levodopa side effects, as selegiline may increase the effect of levodopa
Adenosine Receptor Antagonist Istradefylline	Blocks the brain chemical adenosine to boost the signaling of dopamine	Adjunct to treat time when symptoms return between doses of carbidopa-levodopa	Dyskinesia, dizziness, constipation, nausea, hallucinations, and insomnia	

Data from WebMD Editorial Contributors. (2022). *Medications for Parkinson's disease*. WebMD [website]. Available at: https://www.webmd.com/parkinsons-disease/guide/drug-treatments; Sivanandy, P., Leey, T. C., Xiang, T. C., et al. (2021). Systematic review on Parkinson's disease medications, emphasizing on three recently approved drugs to control Parkinson's symptoms. *Int J Environ Res Public Health*, 19(1), 364.

Generate solutions (planning). Expected outcomes for a patient with PD include the following:

1. The patient will maintain an effective communication pattern.
2. The patient will maintain physical functioning and mobility and will not sustain injury.
3. The patient will maintain effective coping by demonstrating the use of coping strategies that enhance individual and family functioning.
4. The patient will maintain socialization by participating in activities.
5. The patient will verbalize satisfactory effects from drugs and safely manage the drug schedule.

Care planning and expected outcomes for a patient with PD frequently need revision because of changes in the patient's status.

Take actions (nursing interventions). Nursing care includes teaching patients the importance of performing active range-of-motion exercises twice a day, walking at least 4 times a day, and using an assistive device when recommended to prevent injuries associated with falls. Because PD leads to rigidity of the facial muscles, mouth, and general functioning of individuals, assessment of communication skills, speech, and writing is needed.

Consultation with a speech pathologist may be necessary if the patient develops dysphagia. Assessment of nutritional status and self-feeding abilities is crucial for preventing aspiration, respiratory complications, and nutritional imbalance. Nurses are also responsible for monitoring the intake of foods high in bulk and fluids.

Patient education includes the following:
- Teaching preventive measures for malnutrition, falls and other environmental hazards, constipation, skin breakdown from incontinence, and joint contractures
- Teaching gait training and exercises for improving ambulation, swallowing, speech, and self-care

Referral to community agencies and resources is also helpful. Some of the resources specifically available to individuals and families affected by PD include those from the American Parkinson Association (APA). Recommendations of appropriate internet sites for further information are also helpful. The nurse should encourage families and patients to communicate with their primary care provider when they have questions about PD and encourage them to keep a diary to track the symptoms as well as the effects and side effects of drugs.

Evaluate outcomes (evaluation). PD is a progressive terminal disease that has no cure. Therefore, the evaluation of nursing interventions should focus on the maintenance of function and engagement in activities for as long as possible. Evaluation is based on documentation of the achievement of expected outcomes, as evidenced by an older adult patient exhibiting intact skin, appropriate body weight, effective communication, effective coping, and knowledge of appropriate self-care practices. The participation of family members in continued care and rehabilitation is also noted. Specific problems are documented, as is any teaching.

Next-Generation NCLEX® Examination-Style Case Study

Phase 1, Question 1

Scenario: A patient presents to the Senior Health Center with their oldest child.

Nurses' Notes

0845:
A 75-year-old patient presents for an annual physical and a follow-up on laboratory work that was done recently. Patient reports feeling generally well, yet experiences frequent minor aches in the shoulders, hips, and knees due to arthritis. Patient has also noted a tremor in the left hand, which developed a couple of months ago.

History: The patient grew up in the Midwest on a dairy farm. Their childhood health history was unremarkable other than sustaining a fracture of the arm and 2 concussions when playing football as a high school and college athlete. The patient left college when they were drafted to serve in Vietnam in 1962. Following honorable discharge from the Army, they worked as an exterminator until retirement. The spouse died 10 years ago. They have 3 adult children living; one lives close to the patient. The patient has lived in the same single-story ranch-style home for 25 years. There is no current history of smoking, but patient states they smoked about one-half pack per day while in the Army. The patient drinks a glass of wine on celebratory occasions. The patient has a history of hypertension (HTN); osteoarthritis (OA) of shoulders, hips, and knees; and atrial fibrillation (AFib). Medications include atenolol 100 mg each day, rivaroxaban 20 mg each evening with dinner, and acetaminophen arthritis 650 mg twice daily as needed for joint pain, which "usually helps."

Nurses' Notes

Physical exam: Alert and oriented to person, place, time, and situation. No apparent distress. Heart with regular rate and rhythm. Normal S_1 S_2. Capillary refill <2 seconds. Peripheral pulses 3+. Lungs are clear to auscultation throughout. Respirations are even and unlabored. Bowel sounds normoactive throughout. Strength of 5 in all extremities. Stiffness is noted in the upper extremities with passive range of motion. Cogwheel rigidity of the left-upper extremity. Rhythmic pill-rolling tremor present in the left hand—improves with movement. Reflexes are intact bilaterally in the upper and lower extremities. Gait is slow with a shortened step and reduced arm swing.

Vital signs: Blood pressure: 180/90 mm Hg; pulse: 88; respiration: 16; temperature: 97.1° (36.17°C); oxygen saturation: 98% on room air; weight: 196 pounds; height: 5'11" (BMI: 27.3).

Next-Generation NCLEX® Examination-Style Case Study—cont'd

| Health History | **Laboratory Profile** | Health-Care Provider's Orders | Nurses' Notes |

Laboratory Test	Result (Day of Appointment)	Reference Range
Glucose	95 mg/dL	74–106 mg/dL
Calcium (Ca^{+2})	9.2 mg/dL	9.0–10.5 mg/dL
Sodium (Na^+)	1138 mEq/L	136–145 mEq/L
Potassium (K^+)	4.2 mEq/L	3.5–5.0 mEq/L
Blood urea nitrogen (BUN)	28 mg/dL **H**	10–20 mg/dL
Creatinine (Cr)	1.9 mg/dL **H**	0.6–1.2 mg/dL
Albumin (Alb)	3.6 g/dL	3.5–5.0 g/dL
Total protein (TP)	6.7 g/dL	6.4–8.3 g/dL
Alanine transaminase (ALT)	30 U/L	4–36 U/L
Aspartate transaminase (AST)	32 U/L	0–35 U/L
Total bilirubin	0.8 mg/dL	0.3–1.0 mg/dL

Highlight the assessment findings that require follow-up by the nurse.

Phase 1, Question 2

For each assessment finding listed, indicate with an "X" whether it is associated with PD or OA. Some findings may be associated with both conditions.

Assessment Finding	Parkinson Disease	Osteoarthritis
Served in Vietnam		
Played football		
Stiffness with range of motion		
Cogwheel rigidity		
Pill-rolling tremor		
Frequent minor aches in shoulders		
Gait abnormality		
Acetaminophen relieves discomfort		

Phase 2, Question 1

Scenario: Following an MRI that shows no abnormalities, the provider starts the patient on carbidopa 25 mg/levodopa 100 mg 3 times per day. The patient returns to the primary-care provider 3 months later, accompanied by their oldest adult child.

| Health History | **Nurses' Notes** | Health-Care Provider's Orders | Laboratory Profile |

1345:
Patient presents for follow-up. Previous MRI reported no abnormalities. Previous CBC with differential was unremarkable. The patient reports having somewhat adhered to a medication regimen for 3 months. Reports increased issues with balance and has fallen twice since their last visit, sustaining bruising but no broken bones or head injuries. Is no longer driving as they do not trust reflexes and tremor/rigidity interfere. The patient relies on the oldest child for transportation, shopping, and housekeeping, who reports that the patient becomes easily frustrated when others must assist. States tremor and rigidity are worse, and nutrition intake has decreased. The patient requires assistance with activities of daily living and has begun to use a 4-pronged cane. The patient denies incontinence.

| Health History | **Nurses' Notes** | Health-Care Provider's Orders | Laboratory Profile |

History remains unchanged from previous visits.

Physical exam: Alert and oriented to person, place, time, and situation. Masked facies. Heart rhythm is irregular. Normal S_1 S_2. Capillary refill <2 seconds. Peripheral pulses 3+. Lungs with diminished sounds in the right base; otherwise clear to auscultation. Respirations are unlabored, occasional dry cough. Bowel sounds normoactive throughout. Strength of 4 for all extremities. Stiffness is noted with passive range of motion. Cogwheel rigidity bilateral upper extremities. Reflexes 3+. Rhythmic pill-rolling tremor present bilateral upper extremities; has developed tremors of the jaw/chin. Gait is shuffling with a shortened step and reduced arm swing. Stooped posture. Unsteady with turns.

Vital signs: Blood pressure: 130/82 mm Hg; pulse: 98 and irregular; respiration: 20; temperature: 98.9° (37.17°C); oxygen saturation: 94% on room air; weight: 184 pounds; height: 5'11" (BMI: 25.7).

Home medications include atenolol 100 mg each day, rivaroxaban 20 mg each evening with dinner, entacapone 200 mg 4 times daily with carbidopa/levodopa ER 25/100 mg 4 times daily, and acetaminophen arthritis 650 mg two times daily as needed for joint pain. Reports rash with last treatment with amoxicillin clavulanate several years ago.

Tinetti gait and balance—<18 high risk for falls
MoCA—22/30 but unable to complete Trail Making or copying the cube
GDS—6
Lawton—4
Katz—3
Chest X-ray on site—atelectasis right lower lobe.
Repeat CBC ordered.
Health-care provider has ordered admission to the hospital.

| Health History | **Laboratory Profile** | Health-Care Provider's Orders | Nurses' Notes |

Laboratory Test	Result (Day of Appointment)	Reference Range
WBC	13.6 x 10^9/L **H**	4.5–12 x 10^9/L
RBC	4.51 cells/mL	4.5–5.9 cells/mL
Hgb	14.3 g/dL	13.5–17.5 g/dL
Hct	43.2%	40–55%
Platelet count	256 x 10^9/L	150–450 x 10^9/L
RDW	13.0%	11.8–14.5%
MCV	88.8 fL **H**	74–87 fL
MCH	30.3 pg **H**	24–29 pg
Neutrophils	65% **H**	40–60%
Lymphocytes	20%	20–40%
Monocytes	3%	2–8%
Eosinophils	1%	1–4%
Basophils	1%	0.5–1%
Bands	10% **H**	0–3%

Based on the information provided, select the 2 priority patient problems.
- ❑ Decreased functional mobility
- ❑ Stiffness with range of motion
- ❑ Inadequate nutrition
- ❑ Potential for injury
- ❑ Potential for social isolation
- ❑ Decreased ability to cope
- ❑ Potential for pneumonia

Continued

Next-Generation NCLEX® Examination-Style Case Study—cont'd

Phase 2, Question 2
For each potential nursing intervention, indicate with an "X" whether the intervention is indicated or contraindicated for the care of the patient.

Nursing Intervention	Indicated	Contraindicated
Administer ceftriaxone plus azithromycin as ordered		
Administer paroxetine as ordered		
Administer atenolol as ordered		
Teach about the intake of protein		
Encourage the patient to drive		
Require family members to don a mask when visiting		
Request a referral to home health		
Request a referral to occupational therapy		

Phase 3, Question 1
Scenario: The patient is seen by the health care provider one year later.

Health History | **Nurses' Notes** | **Health-Care Provider's Orders** | **Laboratory Profile**

1010:
The patient presents for an annual evaluation. Has kept all appointments unless hospitalized.
The patient is in a wheelchair, although is able to use a walker with standby assistance at home. Requires full-time assistance with care.
The patient has sold their house and moved in with their oldest child and their family of 4 in a large, 2-story home. The patient's bedroom is on the ground floor and has a private bathroom that has been fitted with safety rails and a walk-in tub. The patient has been hospitalized 3 times in the past year. The patient fell 10 months ago and sustained a right-shoulder fracture. The patient has also been hospitalized twice for pneumonia, most recently 2 weeks ago. The patient has become incontinent of urine.
The patient was continent of stool until several days ago, when diarrhea developed. A family member states the diarrhea is watery and foul-smelling. They noticed a few flecks of blood on the last adult protective brief.

Advance directives: The oldest child has both general PoA and PoA for health care. Out-of-hospital do-not-resuscitate (DNR) was completed during the last hospitalization. The patient has a living will in place stating that no artificial ventilation or feeding tubes are desired.

Physical exam: Alert and oriented to person and place. Uncertain of the date and situation. Masked facies. Red, scaly, oily patches of skin in the beard area, sides of the nares, and eyebrows. Heart with regular rhythm. Normal S_1 S_2. Capillary refill <3 seconds. Peripheral pulses 3+. Lungs with diminished sounds bilateral bases, otherwise clear to auscultation. Respirations are unlabored, with frequent cough. Bowel sounds hyperactive throughout. Strength of 3 in all extremities. Stiffness in all joints—unable to fully extend any extremity. Cogwheel rigidity bilateral upper extremities. Reflexes 3+. Tremor present bilateral upper extremities; tremor of the jaw/chin present. Stooped posture with a shuffling gait and feet not clearing the floor when using a walker. Requires assistance to get up from the chair. A gait belt is used.

Health History | **Nurses' Notes** | **Health-Care Provider's Orders** | **Laboratory Profile**

Vital signs: Blood pressure: 110/70 mm Hg; pulse: 88 and regular; respiration: 22; temperature: 98.5° (36.94°C); oxygen saturation: 93% on room air; weight: 145 pounds; height: 5'11" (BMI: 20.22).
The patient has had medication changes during their recent hospitalization.
Home medications include atenolol 50 mg each day, acetaminophen arthritis 650 mg twice daily as needed for joint pain, levodopa/carbidopa/entacapone 150/37.5/200 mg 5 times daily, and mirtazapine 15 mg each bedtime. Allergy: penicillin.
Modified Caregiver Strain Index—13 discussed options to reduce strain, including regular breaks as able, ensuring they maintain their own physical health, joining a support group, and accessing community services for help.
The health-care provider diagnoses pneumonia and a *Clostridium difficile* infection.

For each body system below, select the nursing intervention that will be implemented in the care of the patient at this time. Each body system may support more than one nursing intervention.

System	Possible Interventions
Musculoskeletal	☐ Use a gait belt when transferring from bed to chair ☐ Maintain strict bedrest ☐ Use a cane for ambulation
Respiratory	☐ Apply oxygen via nasal cannula at 2 L as ordered ☐ Listen to lung sounds every 2 hours ☐ Monitor pulse oximetry
Gastrointestinal	☐ Monitor perineal skin condition ☐ Prepare patient for colonoscopy ☐ Implement contact precautions

Phase 3, Question 2
Which statement indicates the caregiver has developed a definitive plan to reduce strain? (Select all that apply; one, some, or all may be correct).
☐ "I have to keep providing care; I promised I would not put my parents in a nursing home."
☐ "I have a monthly spa day scheduled to get a massage."
☐ "I can't expect my partner to help out; this isn't their parent."
☐ "My sibling is coming to stay with my parent soon so our family can go on a cruise."
☐ "Dad will be going to adult day care once a week so I can have free time."
☐ "I don't know what I am going to do when caring for him gets too hard."
☐ "A support group meets in the library each week; I'm thinking about going."
☐ "I will talk to my siblings to see if we can work out something to give me a break."

Cerebrovascular Accident

A disruption in the normal blood supply to the brain tissue causes a cerebrovascular accident (CVA). CVAs occur suddenly and produce focal neurologic deficits. In strokes, 80% are ischemic, resulting from thrombosis or embolism. The remaining 20% are hemorrhagic in nature, resulting from vascular rupture. They are medical emergencies that should be treated immediately to prevent permanent neurologic deficits and disability (Fig. 22.8). A transient ischemic attack (TIA) consists of similar symptoms but lasts less than an hour and shows no evidence of acute cerebral infarction on MRI (Alexandrov and Krishnaiah, 2023).

Risk Factors

Strokes are the fifth leading cause of death and the most common cause of neurological disability in the United States (Alexandrov and Krishnaiah, 2023). Health conditions that increase the risk for CVA include previous stroke or TIA, HTN, hypercholesterolemia, coronary artery disease (CAD), diabetes, obesity, and sickle cell disease (SCD). Modifiable behaviors that increase the risk of stroke include a diet high in saturated fats, transfat, and cholesterol, a sedentary lifestyle, drinking alcohol in excess, and tobacco use. Table 22.6 summarizes stroke prevention.

Nonmodifiable factors increasing the risk for stroke include genetics, family health history, age (risk increases with age; the chance of having a stroke doubles every 10 years after age 55), sex (stroke is more common in males; however, females are more likely to die from stroke than males), race, or ethnicity (non-Hispanic Black or Pacific Islanders are more likely to die from stroke; the risk of having a stroke is almost twice as high for Blacks than Whites [CDC, 2023c]).

Clinical Manifestations

Initial stroke symptoms have a sudden onset. Clinical manifestations vary according to the cerebral vessel involved (Alexandrov and Krishnaiah, 2023):

- **Internal carotid:** contralateral motor and sensory deficits of the arm, leg, and face. In dominant hemispheric CVA, aphasia occurs. In nondominant hemispheric CVA, apraxia, agnosia, and unilateral neglect occur, as well as homonymous hemianopia (loss of one-half of the visual field in each eye).
- **Middle cerebral artery:** drowsiness, stupor, coma, contralateral hemiplegia, sensory deficits of arm and face, aphasia, and homonymous hemianopia may be seen.
- **Anterior cerebral artery:** contralateral weakness or paralysis and sensory loss of the foot and leg, loss of ability in decision-making and voluntary actions, and urinary incontinence.
- **Vertebral artery:** pain in the face, nose, or eye; numbness or weakness of the face on the ipsilateral side; problems with gait; dysphagia; and dysarthria (difficulty speaking).

Other symptoms may also reflect the type of stroke: A sudden, severe headache suggests a subarachnoid hemorrhage. Impaired consciousness accompanied by headaches, nausea, and vomiting suggests increased intracranial pressure. An increase in intracranial pressure can occur 48–72 hours following a large ischemic stroke or early on in a hemorrhagic stroke. Fatal brain herniation may occur if pressure is not reduced (Alexandrov and Krishnaiah, 2023).

Complications

Complications following a stroke include insomnia, confusion, depression, incontinence, atelectasis, pneumonia, and dysphagia. Dysphagia can lead to aspiration, dehydration, and malnutrition.

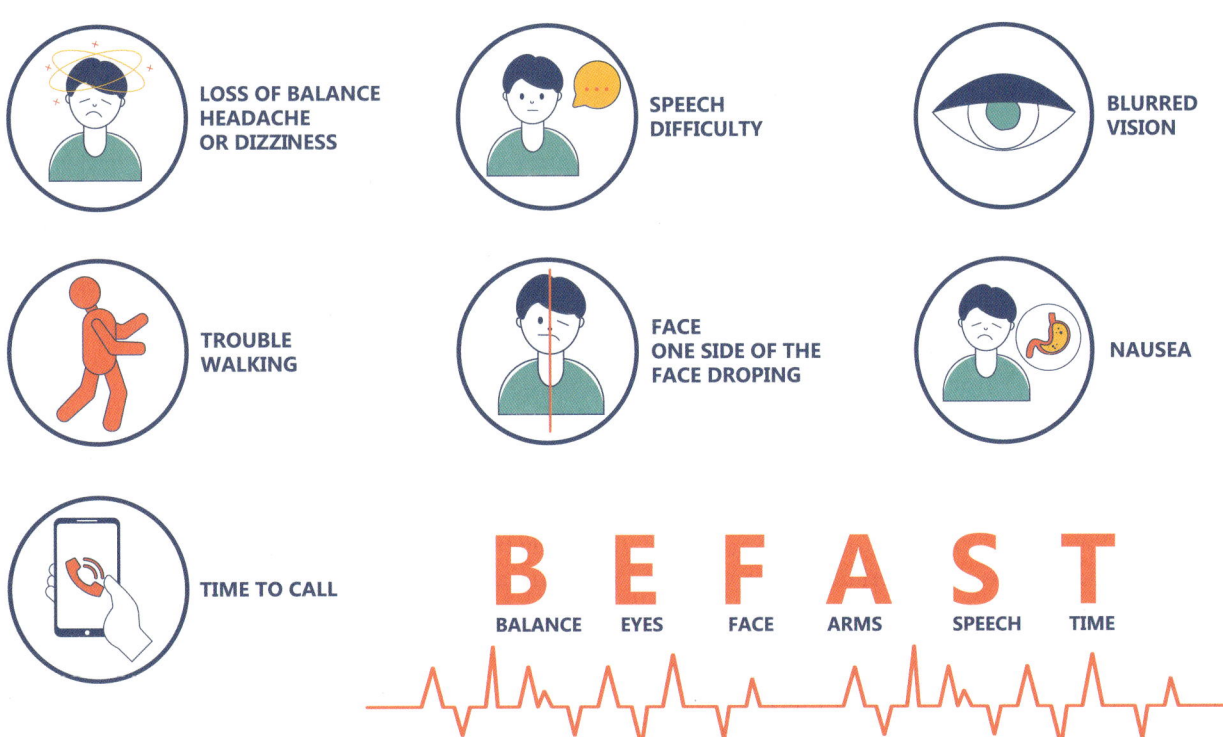

Fig. 22.8 Symptoms and action on stroke. (From iStock #1480614643; Elena Yakovlieva.)

TABLE 22.6 Preventing Stroke

Modifiable Risk Factor	Recommendations
Use multidisciplinary care teams to personalize care for patients and employ shared decision-making with the patient to develop care plans that incorporate a patient's wishes, goals, and concerns.	
Hypertension (HTN)	Every 10-mm Hg reduction in systolic blood pressure and 5-mm Hg reduction in diastolic blood pressure reduces the risk of stroke by 41%.
Diabetes mellitus (DM)	A hemoglobin A1c of ≤7% is recommended. Metformin—the first-line medication for type 2 DM (T2DM) patients—also has potential benefits for clinical atherosclerotic disease.
Obesity	The risk of ischemic stroke is increased by 22% for overweight individuals and by 64% in obese individuals as compared to normal-weight individuals. Losing as little as 5–10 pounds can make a significant difference in risk.
Impaired lipid profile	LDL target of < 55 mg/dL for extreme risk, < 70 mg/dL for very high risk, < 100 mg/dL for high and moderate risk, and < 130 mg/dL for low-risk individuals. Fibrates are recommended for triglycerides >200 mg/dL and HDL < 40 mg/dL.
Atrial fibrillation (AFib)	AFib leads to about a 1.9% risk of stroke per year and is responsible for as many as 1 in 6 strokes. Screening for and diagnosing AFib and starting appropriate blood-thinning medications to reduce recurrent events is recommended.
Mitral stenosis	Maintain adequate anticoagulation.
Asymptomatic carotid artery stenosis (ACAS)	Adhere to treatment with daily aspirin and *statin* drugs.
Lifestyle choices—diet, exercise, smoking, alcohol, and illegal drugs	The American Heart Association (AHA) recommends a diet that has an increased intake of fruits, vegetables, and whole grains and a limited intake of sugar, saturated fat, transfat, and red meat. Regular exercise (aiming for being active for at least 150 minutes a week) has been shown to reduce stroke risk by half. Smoking has been associated with an increased risk of ischemic stroke and intracranial bleeds. It is one of the leading preventable risk factors for stroke. It takes 2–4 years after smoking cessation for the excess risk to go down. Chronic alcohol use and heavy drinking are risk factors for stroke. There is a protective effect from light to moderate consumption (likely due to an increase in high-density lipoprotein (HDL) and a decrease in platelet aggregation) and an increased risk of stroke with heavy alcohol consumption (due to a hypercoagulable state, alcohol-induced HTN, cardiomyopathy, and AFib). Avoid street drugs such as cocaine and methamphetamines, as they increase the risk of stroke.
Obstructive sleep apnea (OSA)	Adhere to recommended treatment for OSA.

Data from Centers for Disease Control and Prevention (CDC). (2022). *Prevent stroke: What you can do*. Retrieved from https://www.cdc.gov/stroke/prevention.htm; American Stroke Association. (2023). *Risk factors under your control*. Retrieved from https://www.stroke.org/en/about-stroke/stroke-risk-factors/risk-factors-under-your-control; Sabih, A., Tadi, P., & Kumar, A. (2023). Stroke prevention. In *StatPearls* [website]. Treasure Island, FL: StatPearls Publishing. Retrieved from https://www.statpearls.com/ArticleLibrary/viewarticle/29556.

Complications of immobility include deep vein thrombosis (DVT) and pulmonary embolism (PE), deconditioning, sarcopenia, UIT, pressure injury, and contractures. The ability to complete ADLs may be decreased (Alexandrov and Krishnaiah, 2023).

Diagnostic Evaluation

Evaluation for stroke should occur in patients with sudden neurologic deficits associated with a specific cerebral artery, sudden severe headache, unexplained coma, or sudden altered consciousness. When a stroke is suspected, the National Institutes of Health Stroke Scale (NIHSS) (https://www.aclsmedicaltraining.com/nih-stroke-scale/), a 15-item scale, may be used to grade severity and follow changes over time. The scale evaluates "the patient's level of consciousness and language function and to identify motor and sensory deficits by asking the patient to answer questions and to perform physical and mental tasks" (Alexandrov and Krishnaiah, 2023, Evaluation of Stroke section). The scale can also be used to determine the appropriate therapeutic regimen.

When a patient presents with symptoms of stroke, fingerstick blood glucose should be determined to rule out hypoglycemia. If the patient is taking anticoagulants, platelet count, international normalized ratio (INR), and partial thromboplastin should be measured.

Neuroimaging, particularly MRI, can differentiate between ischemic and hemorrhagic strokes, as well as determine the presence of increased intracranial pressure. However, a CT can often be completed quicker than an MRI.

If the determination of stroke is unclear, further testing is required to rule out other causes, such as metabolic encephalopathy, infection, dehydration, or a postictal state. These diagnostic tests include (Alexandrov and Krishnaiah, 2023):

- Comprehensive metabolic panel and CBC with differential, liver function tests (LFTs), and ammonia level
- Arterial blood gasses
- Blood and urine culture
- Toxicology
- Electrocardiography
- Chest X-ray
- Imaging tests to evaluate for tumors, hemorrhage, edema, bone trauma, and hydrocephalus
- Echocardiography to evaluate for the presence of clots, pumping and structural abnormalities, and valve disorders
- (EEG)

Management

Medical and pharmacologic therapy during acute stroke.
The immediate goal for acute management of stroke during

evaluation is to stabilize the patient and complete an assessment, including all imaging and laboratory studies, within 60 minutes of arrival at the emergency department. The initial focus is on the need for airway support and supplemental oxygen for saturation <94%. Hypoglycemia (blood glucose <60 mg/dL) and hyperglycemia (blood glucose should be lowered to 140–180 mg/dL) must also be managed quickly (Alexandrov and Krishnaiah, 2023; Jauch et al, 2022).

Reduction of blood pressure should only occur if there are signs of end organ damage (i.e., acute MI and acute kidney failure) or if the patient is to receive tissue plasminogen activator or thrombectomy. Otherwise, areas of cerebral ischemia may require high blood pressure to maintain perfusion (Alexandrov and Krishnaiah, 2023).

Guidelines for tissue plasminogen activator (Box 22.4) are to decrease blood pressure to <180/105 mm Hg before drug administration. Labetalol 10–20 mg IV push over 1–2 minutes may be administered, or an infusion of nicardipine (maximum 15 mg/hr) or clevidipine (maximum 21 mg/hr), titrated until the desired blood pressure goal is reached. In cases where tissue plasminogen activator is not administered, it is recommended that decreasing the blood pressure by 15% in the first 24 hours is ideal, if two readings 15 minutes apart are ≥220 mm Hg systolic or ≥120 mm Hg diastolic (Alexandrov and Krishnaiah, 2023).

The American Stroke Association (ASA) Guidelines for the Early Management of Patients with Acute Ischemic Stroke (stroke.org/AISToolkit; Powers et al, 2019) recommend the administration of alteplase within 4.5 hours of stroke onset, as this allows for the most favorable outcomes. Alteplase (a tissue plasminogen activator, or tPA) should be administered even if thrombectomy is being considered.

Alteplase works to dissolve the clots blocking arterial blood flow in the brain. The risks of thrombolytic therapy include intracerebral hemorrhage, which can be fatal (Caplan, 2023).

Mechanical thrombectomy removes the clot in the artery. A thrombectomy can reduce long-term disability from a stroke. The procedure is most beneficial if it can be performed within 6 hours of the onset of stroke symptoms, but it can be beneficial up to 24 hours after symptom onset in specific situations (Caplan, 2023).

When thrombolytic therapy is not an option, other early treatments include antiplatelets and anticoagulants. Antiplatelets include aspirin (81 or 325 mg daily), clopidogrel (75 mg daily), and ticagrelor (90 mg twice daily). Antiplatelets do not dissolve existing clots, they prevent new clots from forming. Most people who experience a TIA are given aspirin. Persons who have had a minor ischemic stroke or those who have had a TIA and are considered high risk for a stroke may be prescribed short-term (i.e., 21–90 days) dual antiplatelet therapy with aspirin (25 mg) plus dipyridamole extended release (200 mg) twice daily (Alexandrov and Krishnaiah, 2023; Caplan, 2023).

It should be noted that genetic testing for CYP450 polymorphisms is recommended to determine if a patient has impaired metabolism of clopidogrel due to a reduction in CYP2C19 prior to initiation of therapy with the drug (Alexandrov and Krishnaiah, 2023).

Anticoagulants make the blood less likely to clot. Heparin and low-molecular-weight heparin are injectable anticoagulants.

> **BOX 22.4 Fibrinolytic Therapy**
>
> The American Heart Association/American Stroke Association (AHA/ASA) inclusion guidelines for the administration of alteplase (rt-PA) in under 3 hours are as follows:
>
> - Diagnosis of ischemic stroke causing measurable neurologic deficit
> - Neurologic signs not clearing spontaneously to baseline
> - Neurologic signs not minor and isolated
> - Symptoms not suggestive of subarachnoid hemorrhage
> - No head trauma or prior stroke in the past 3 months
> - No myocardial infarction (MI) in past 3 months
> - No gastrointestinal/genitourinary hemorrhage in the previous 21 days
> - No arterial puncture at a noncompressible site during the past 7 days
> - No major surgery in the past 14 days
> - No history of prior intracranial bleeding
> - Systolic blood pressure under 185 mm Hg, and diastolic blood pressure under 110 mm Hg
> - No evidence of acute trauma or bleeding
> - Not taking an oral anticoagulant, or if so, INR under 1.7
> - If taking heparin within 48 hours, a normal activated prothrombin time (aPT)
> - Platelet count of more than 100,000/μL
> - Blood glucose greater than 50 mg/dL (2.7 mmol)
> - CT scan does not show evidence of multilobar infarction (hypodensity over one-third hemisphere) or intracerebral hemorrhage
> - The patient and family understand the potential risks and benefits of therapy
>
> Fibrinolytic therapy administered 3–4.5 hours after the onset of symptoms was found to improve neurologic outcomes in carefully selected patients. Eligibility criteria for treatment during this later period are like those for earlier treatment but are more stringent, with any one of the following serving as an additional exclusion criterion:
>
> - Age older than 80 years
> - Use of oral anticoagulants, regardless of the INR
> - Baseline score on the National Institutes of Health Stroke Scale (NIHSS) greater than 25
> - History of stroke and diabetes

Modified from Adams H. P., Jr., del Zoppo, G., Alberts, M. J., Bhatt, D. L., Brass, L., Furlan, A., et al. (2007). Guidelines for the early management of adults with ischemic stroke: a guideline from the American Heart Association/American Stroke Association Stroke Council, Clinical Cardiology Council, Cardiovascular Radiology and Intervention Council, and the Atherosclerotic Peripheral Vascular Disease and Quality of Care Outcomes in Research Interdisciplinary Working Groups: The American Academy of Neurology affirms the value of this guideline as an educational tool for neurologists. *Stroke, 38*(5), 1655–1711, Table 11; and Jauch, E. C., Kasab, S. A., & Stettle, B. (2022). *Ischemic stroke treatment & management.* Medscape [website]. Retrieved from https://emedicine.medscape.com/article/1916852-treatment#d11.

Warfarin (a vitamin K antagonist), dabigatran (a direct thrombin inhibitor), apixaban (a direct factor Xa inhibitor), and rivaroxaban (a direct Factor Xa inhibitor) are oral anticoagulants. However, due to the risk of bleeding, anticoagulants are only used for certain types of strokes (i.e., cardioembolism or arterial dissection) in high-risk individuals (i.e., those with valvular disease or severe heart failure).

Long-term stroke management. Long-term management, or supportive care, includes (Alexandrov and Krishnaiah, 2023):
- Controlling hyperglycemia and fever, if present
- Screening for dysphagia before patients begin to eat, drink, or receive medications

- If needed, enteral nutrition should be started within 7 days of an acute stroke
- Intermittent compression devices are recommended for immobile patients to prevent deep vein thrombosis
- Implement measures to prevent pressure injuries early
- Initiate physical, occupational, and speech therapy to maximize function and prevent joint contractures
- If tolerated, maintain systolic blood pressure <120 mm Hg to prevent recurrent stroke
- Often, following a stroke, patients experience depression that can interfere with recovery; treatment should be initiated to aid in rehabilitation
- Treatment with atorvastatin or rosuvastatin is recommended for patients with evidence of atherosclerosis and an LDL ≥100 mg/dL; the LDL target level is <70 mg/dL

Nursing Care Guidelines for the Person with Stroke

Recognize cues (assessment). Complete a thorough history and physical examination to determine the presence of common signs and symptoms of a stroke.
- Facial numbness/weakness
- Change in mental status
- Trouble speaking or understanding speech (dysarthria [difficulty forming words], expressive aphasia [unable to form understandable words], and receptive aphasia [unable to comprehend the spoken words])
- Visual disturbances (homonymous hemianopsia [loss of half of the visual field] and loss of peripheral vision)
- Hemiparesis or hemiplegia
- Ataxia (unsteady gait)
- Dysphagia
- Paresthesia

Perform a neurological exam to determine the location of the stroke and establish baseline function. Include cranial nerve testing, range of motion and muscle strength, the presence of sensation and vibratory sense, cerebellar function, gait, language, mental status, and level of consciousness. Complete the NIHSS.

Perform a peripheral vascular exam, including palpation of carotid, radial, femoral, and posterior tibial pulses.

Analyze cues and prioritize hypotheses (patient problems). Priority patient problems for an individual with a CVA include:
- Clotting - deep vein thrombosis or pulmonary embolus
- Dysphagia
- Elimination - UTI
- Intestinal bleeding
- Myocardial tissue injury
- Pressure injuries
- Falls
- Depression
- Malnutrition
- Reduced perfusion - heart failure

Generate solutions (planning). Outcomes for an older adult with a CVA include the following (SimpleNursing, n.d.):
- Maintain optimal oxygenation and prevent respiratory complications, such as pneumonia or atelectasis.
- Improve the patient's ability to perform ADLs such as bathing, grooming, dressing, and feeding.
- Prevent complications such as DVT, pressure ulcers, contractures, aspiration, or falls.
- Alleviate pain and discomfort associated with stroke, such as headaches, muscle spasms, or neuropathic pain.
- Provide emotional and psychological support to the patient and family, and address depression, anxiety, or other psychological effects of stroke.
- Prevent future strokes by managing modifiable risk factors such as HTN, DM, or hyperlipidemia.
- Improve the patient's ability to express themselves and understand language.

Take actions (nursing interventions). Management of the respiratory system is a priority following a stroke. Provide oxygen for saturations <90% and maintain at 95% (Maxwell, 2018). Other airway support includes suction as needed, encouraging deep breathing, and positioning to prevent aspiration. Early mobility will help prevent atelectasis and pneumonia. Patients on the ventilator need oral care every 2 hours to prevent ventilator associated pneumonia, as well as suctioning and proper positioning.

Additional nursing interventions include the following:
- Encourage active range of motion on the unaffected side and passive range of motion on the affected side.
- Turn the patient every 2 hours.
- Monitor the lower extremities for thrombophlebitis resulting from immobilization.
- Encourage the use of the unaffected arm for ADLs.
- Teach the patient to put clothing on the affected side first.
- Have the patient resume an oral diet only after they have successfully completed a swallowing evaluation. The patient may need thickened liquids or foods with the consistency of oatmeal and may need to chew on the unaffected side of the mouth. This is sometimes referred to as a *dysphagia diet*.
- Collaborate with occupational and physical therapists for rehabilitation.
- Try alternative methods of communication with the patient who has aphasia.
- Teach the patient with homonymous hemianopia to adapt to the deficit by turning the head side to side to fully scan the visual field.
- The nurse also needs to educate the patient and family about:
  - CVA and CVA prevention
  - Community resources
  - Physical care and the need for psychosocial support
  - Drugs

HOME CARE

1. Assess sensorimotor function. A decline in this function is the most notable change in older adults and may be the cause of other changes, such as slowed reaction time.
2. Memory impairment may compromise the teaching of homebound patients, so the nurse may have to use alternative approaches and rely on family and significant others involved in caregiving.
3. Assess for signs of impaired emotional control, diminished initiative, withdrawal, or other changes, which may be initial signs of brain dysfunction.

> **HOME CARE—cont'd**
>
> 4. Altered thought processes occur with cognitive decline or disturbances in cognitive function, both of which occur in homebound patients with dementia, depression, delirium, or amnesic disorders.
> 5. The effects of aging must be considered when interpreting laboratory tests and alerting physicians about abnormal results.
> 6. Instruct caregivers about the dosages and side effects of drugs, especially tranquilizers and antidepressants that are used in managing symptoms caused by dementia.
> 7. Instruct caregivers on methods to manage behavioral problems and caregiver stress.
> 8. Use social workers to assess community resources for caregivers and patients with dementia.
> 9. Assess the home environment of the older person with cognitive impairment for safety hazards and provide caregivers with tips and strategies for reducing and eliminating the identified hazards.

Evaluate outcomes (evaluation). Patient progress occurs in small increments, and interventions are modified to assist patients in meeting their goals. Evaluation criteria include the following:

- Maintenance and improvement of cerebral tissue perfusion
- Avoidance of respiratory complications
- Prevention of aspiration from food, fluids, and secretions
- Prevention of contractures
- Prevention of edema in the affected extremity
- Maintenance of skin integrity
- Achievement of independence
- Pain management
- Increased ability to communicate, express feelings, and understand others
- Prevention of fecal and urinary incontinence
- Establishment of a normal voiding pattern
- Compensation for sensory deficits and physical and intellectual losses
- Participation by family members in the rehabilitation process

Anxiety

Anxiety is common among older adults. In general, 14%–17% of older adults are diagnosed with anxiety. However, only about one-third of older adults diagnosed with anxiety receive mental health care for the condition. Genetics may predispose a person to developing anxiety; females have twice the risk of being diagnosed with anxiety than males (Pelham, 2023).

Older adults face multiple factors that can cause anxiety, including multiple medical conditions, financial insecurity, retirement, loss of a loved one, loss of independence, limited physical mobility, sleep disturbances, and other issues impacting QoL that may also lead to isolation. Additionally, medications to treat asthma and COPD, hypothyroidism, seizure disorder, and PD can cause anxiety (WebMD Editorial Contributors, 2023; Pelham, 2023). Persons with dementia have a high prevalence of anxiety, which negatively impacts cognition and overall QoL (Subramanyam et al, 2018).

Signs and Symptoms of Anxiety

Extreme, lasting, and uncontrollable worries that do not match reality are the hallmark of generalized anxiety disorder. Other symptoms of anxiety include avoiding previously enjoyed activities, insomnia, anorexia, restlessness, trouble focusing, intrusive thoughts, trembling, sweating, palpitations, muscle tension, irritability, stomach aches, and headaches (NCOA, 2022; Pelham, 2023).

In addition to anxiety, older adults may develop phobias; debilitating, life-limiting fears about falling, becoming terminally ill, and dying; and social anxiety. The COVID-19 pandemic increased mental health conditions among older adults (Pelham, 2023).

Diagnostic Evaluation

Evaluation of the older adult with anxiety includes laboratory studies (CBC, chemistry panel, thyroid panel, urinalysis, and drug screening), imaging as needed (chest X-ray and echo), and ECG. A scale should be used to assist in the diagnosis, such as the Beck Anxiety Inventory (BAI) or the Hamilton Anxiety Rating Scale (HAM-A). The Geriatric Anxiety Inventory (GAI) is the gold standard for assessing anxiety in older adults (Subramanyam et al, 2018).

Nonpharmacological Treatment

Nonpharmacological measures are the first-line treatment for anxiety in older adults. These include lifestyle modifications and the elimination of known triggers. A structured daily routine is key (Subramanyam et al, 2018).

Regular physical exercise, such as walking, swimming, and playing games, helps to improve cerebral blood flow and metabolism. Exercise does not need to be strenuous. Persons with limited functional ability and those who are wheelchair-bound benefit from stretching (Subramanyam et al, 2018).

With age, there is a shorter nighttime sleep phase, and sleep becomes fragmented. Older adults should be taught about sleep hygiene as well as the changes in sleep patterns that accompany aging (Subramanyam et al, 2018).

Older adults often have compromised nutrition related to social isolation, medical conditions, and medications. Ensuring adequate nutrition and intake of vitamins and minerals can help manage anxiety (Subramanyam et al, 2018).

Psychotherapeutic options. CBT utilizes cognitive restructuring to help identify maladaptive behaviors that are addressed using the principle of antecedents-behavior-consequences to try and change old patterns (Subramanyam et al, 2018).

Mindfulness helps the individual focus on the now, moving from taste, smell, vision, and hearing to emotions, reactions, and physical responses to stimuli. Mindfulness seeks to find harmony between mind and body (Subramanyam et al, 2018).

Other therapies to target anxiety include behavioral therapies such as relaxation therapy and systemic desensitization, as well as yoga, art therapy, dance therapy, music therapy, cognitive rehabilitation, and social networking (Subramanyam et al, 2018).

Pharmacological Treatment

The first-line pharmacological treatment for anxiety is SSRIs, while the second-line treatment is SNRIs. Response to pharmacotherapy may take as long as 12 weeks. Hyponatremia (sodium <135 mmol/L), commonly associated with SSRIs, and SNRIs can result in nausea, malaise, lethargy, and confusion. Sodium levels <115 mmol/L can result in disorientation, seizures, coma, respiratory depression, and death. Hyponatremia should be corrected as soon as possible (Subramanyam et al, 2018).

Benzodiazepines should only be used for a short time (2–4 weeks), then tapered off. Benzodiazepines result in an increased risk of falls, dissociative phenomena, and confusion in older adults. Additionally, benzodiazepines can cause paradoxical agitation in older adults (Subramanyam et al, 2018).

Nursing Care Guidelines for the Person with Anxiety Disorder

Recognize cues (assessment). Older adult patients with anxiety disorders are usually able to describe their anxiety without the nurse needing to probe extensively. They may also exhibit behavioral clues such as pacing, irritability, and fidgeting. When patients lack insight into their anxiety, the nurse may find it helpful to describe the symptoms observed as indicating anxiety. The nurse should also assess associated changes such as sleeping habits and appetite, the presence or absence of depression, and any reports of physical pain that may accompany the anxiety.

Somatic complaints are often seen in older adult patients experiencing anxiety. This may be attributed to the physical toll that anxiety takes on the physical systems or to a patient being more comfortable reporting a physical health concern than a mental health concern. If the nurse believes the somatic concerns may be related to anxiety, a thorough anxiety assessment should be conducted.

Analyze cues and prioritize hypotheses (patient problems). Patient problems for older adults with an anxiety disorder usually include the following:
- Anxiety resulting from a situational crisis
- Inadequate coping resulting from perceived vulnerability

Generate solutions (planning). Expected outcomes include the following:
1. The patient identifies their own anxiety and coping patterns.
2. The patient reports an increase in psychological and physiologic comfort.
3. The patient demonstrates effective coping skills, as evidenced by his or her ability to solve problems and meet self-care needs.
4. The patient demonstrates the use of appropriate relaxation techniques.

Take actions (nursing interventions). The nurse may intervene with older adults experiencing anxiety in a number of ways. It may be helpful to assist patients in examining their own "worst-case scenario." By developing strategies that could be used to cope with the worst possible situation, patients may feel an increased ability to cope with their current situation. Relaxation strategies such as progressive muscle relaxation, breathing techniques, therapeutic use of music, and exercise are useful in helping patients alleviate the acute anxiety states that are most distressing to them. The nurse should help patients learn to identify increasing anxiety early in the anxiety cycle so that they can take steps to reduce it to a lower level. Family education may also be beneficial to obtain support systems for patients. Patients experiencing moderate to panic-level anxiety may need a referral for pharmacologic therapy. Patients who continue to experience distress because of anxiety may benefit from psychotherapy. Behavior modification techniques are especially effective with phobic disorders.

Evaluate outcomes (evaluation). The nurse may evaluate the care that has been provided to patients experiencing anxiety by monitoring their progress toward achieving the expected outcomes and documenting the results. The effectiveness of any health teaching is evident in a patient's ability to use relaxation techniques and constructive problem solving.

Schizophrenia

Older adults living with chronic schizophrenia are a public health concern worldwide. Older adults with schizophrenia have a shorter life expectancy; the risk of mortality is two to three times greater than that of the general population. Additionally, due to lifestyle factors, older adults with schizophrenia also experience an increased incidence of heart failure, COPD, and hypothyroidism. Older adults with schizophrenia have a twofold increased risk of developing dementia before the age of 80 compared to the general population. This increased risk is due to age, low educational level, cognitive dysfunction, cardiovascular disease, polypharmacy, and a history of substance use disorder (Khan and Rajji, 2019).

The symptoms of schizophrenia are typically divided into three categories: psychotic, negative, and cognitive.

Psychotic (Positive) Symptoms

Psychotic symptoms include changes in the way a person thinks, acts, and experiences the world. People with psychotic symptoms may lose a shared sense of reality with others and experience the world in a distorted way (National Institute of Mental Health [NIMH], 2024; Treatment Advocacy Center, 2022). The symptoms include:
- Hallucinations: a person sees, hears, smells, tastes, or feels things that are not actually there
- Delusions: a person has strong beliefs that are not true and may seem irrational to others
- Thought disorders: a person has ways of thinking that are unusual or illogical; people with thought disorders may have trouble organizing their thoughts and speech
- Movement disorders: a person exhibits abnormal, agitated body movements

Negative Symptoms

Negative symptoms are associated with disruptions to normal emotions and behaviors, loss of interest or enjoyment in ADLs, and withdrawal from social life. The symptoms include (NIMH, 2024; Treatment Advocacy Center, 2022):
- Flat affect (reduced expression of emotions via facial expression or voice tone)
- Reduced feelings of pleasure in everyday life
- Difficulty beginning and sustaining activities
- Talking in a dull voice and showing limited facial expression
- In extreme cases, a person might stop moving or talking for a while, which is a rare condition called catatonia

Cognitive Symptoms

For some patients, the cognitive symptoms of schizophrenia are subtle, but for others, they are more severe, and patients may notice changes in their memory or other aspects of thinking. Symptoms include (NIMH, 2024; Treatment Advocacy Center, 2022):
- Poor "executive functioning" (the ability to understand information and use it to make decisions)
- Trouble focusing or paying attention
- Problems with "working memory" (the ability to use information immediately after learning it)

Treatment of Schizophrenia

Treatment focuses on managing symptoms so people can function in the day-to-day world. Treatment includes antipsychotic medications and nonpharmacological psychosocial treatments.

Antipsychotic medications. Antipsychotic medications reduce the intensity and frequency of symptoms. Side effects of antipsychotic medications include tardive dyskinesia, orthostatic hypotension, weight gain, dry mouth, constipation, urinary retention, blurred vision, restlessness, and drowsiness. Older adults experience more adverse effects from antipsychotic medications than younger adults due to reduced renal and hepatic blood flow, reduced glomerular filtration rate, and an increased ratio of fat to muscle mass (Khan and Rajji, 2019; Rolin, 2021).

Risperidone is the first-line treatment for older adults. Olanzapine is effective but has increased anticholinergic side effects. Due to their side effects, antipsychotic drugs should be used at the lowest possible dose in older adults (Khan and Rajji, 2019).

Nonpharmacological psychosocial treatments. Nonpharmacologic interventions reduce psychotic symptoms and augment pharmacotherapy. Cognitive-behavioral therapy is used to resolve social problems, psychotic and negative symptoms, and mood in older adults. Bilateral electroconvulsive therapy has shown efficacy in the maintenance treatment of schizophrenia in older adults (Khan and Rajji, 2019).

Nursing Care Guidelines for the Person with Schizophrenia

Recognize cues (assessment). The reader is referred to a general psychiatric nursing textbook for a complete review of the assessment process for individuals with a diagnosis of schizophrenia.

Analyze cues and prioritize hypotheses (patient problems). Patient problems appropriate to the older adult with schizophrenia include the following:
- Social isolation resulting from altered mental status
- Anxiety resulting from unconscious conflict with reality
- Inadequate coping resulting from unrealistic perceptions
- Altered sleep pattern resulting from psychological status

Generate solutions (planning). Schizophrenia is an illness that shows periods of exacerbation and remission. The goal of nursing intervention in individuals with schizophrenia is safe, effective treatment rather than a cure. The goals for the patient that the nurse should work toward are a reduction in symptoms and an improved QoL. Other goals include reducing patient anxiety (anxiety usually exacerbates the schizophrenic symptoms), building a therapeutic relationship with the patient, providing continuity of care, and eliciting the support of family and friends to enhance the patient's function and experience. Expected outcomes include the following:
1. The patient develops a trusting relationship, as evidenced by the presence of supportive significant others.
2. The patient maintains contact with mental-health caregivers, as evidenced by weekly meetings with a counselor.
3. The patient experiences a decrease in hallucinations and distress, as evidenced by verbalized reports of fewer hallucinations and feelings of distress, as well as demonstrations of methods to handle hallucinations.
4. The patient gets adequate sleep, as evidenced by reports of sleeping through the night or verbalizations of feeling rested after a night's sleep.

Take actions (nursing interventions). Nursing interventions for older adults with schizophrenia should provide a comprehensive approach to the maintenance of ADLs, nutrition, hygiene, health promotion, and reality orientation. Interventions that may be most essential in dealing with older adults with schizophrenia include providing adequate family or social support, responding to patient symptoms, using touch appropriately, and dealing with aggressive behavior.

If patients give evidence (verbal or nonverbal) of hallucinations or delusions, the nurse should focus on responding to the feelings without arguing about the reality of their perceptual experiences. For example, if a patient states that the television is broadcasting his or her thoughts, the nurse could respond by saying, "That must be frightening," rather than saying, "Now, Mr. D, you know that the television can't do that!" Attempting to argue perception with patients only escalates their anxiety. It may, however, be helpful to reorient patients without being confrontational.

Patients with schizophrenia may easily misinterpret touch by the nurse as being harmful or threatening to them. Therefore, the nurse should only touch the patient for a specific purpose and only with permission from the patient.

Older adults with schizophrenia may, at times, present a danger to themselves or others. The nurse should assess the level of danger that each patient presents. If the assessment shows that a patient has a potential for aggression, the nurse should take steps to deescalate the patient's anger and to provide safety for the patient and others.

Evaluate outcomes (evaluation). Evaluation is based on the achievement of the identified expected outcomes. The nature of the disorder may make it difficult for the nurse to establish a relationship with a patient; the nurse may therefore feel hopeless, frustrated, and inadequate while attempting to provide care. It is often helpful to establish short-term goals for patients with schizophrenia that are easily achievable and specific. The nurse is responsible for documenting progress toward achievement of the objectives as well as the level of safety achieved.

MENTAL HEALTH RESOURCES

With age, people experience multiple changes and losses that impact their mental health. Some older adults experience grief, social isolation, and loneliness. Without intervention, this can lead to mental illnesses such as depression and anxiety.

SAMHSA has many resources for older adults. These resources are beneficial for not just older adults but also their providers and caregivers. One of these resources is the E4 Center.

E4 Center

The mission of the E4 Center of Excellence for Behavioral Health Disparities in Aging's mission is to "engage, empower, and educate health-care providers and community-based organizations for equity in behavioral health for older adults and their families" (Substance Abuse and Mental Health Services Administration [SAMHSA], 2024, New Items section) (Fig. 22.9). The E4 Center has set goals and strategies for reducing behavioral health disparities for older adults:

- Develop knowledge, skills, and attitudes in the health-care workforce regarding aging.
- Catalyze partnerships for integrated health-care for older adults.
- Expedite the implementation of evidence-based programs.
- Provide resources for engaging, educating, and empowering older adults and families.
  For further information, visit https://e4center.org/.

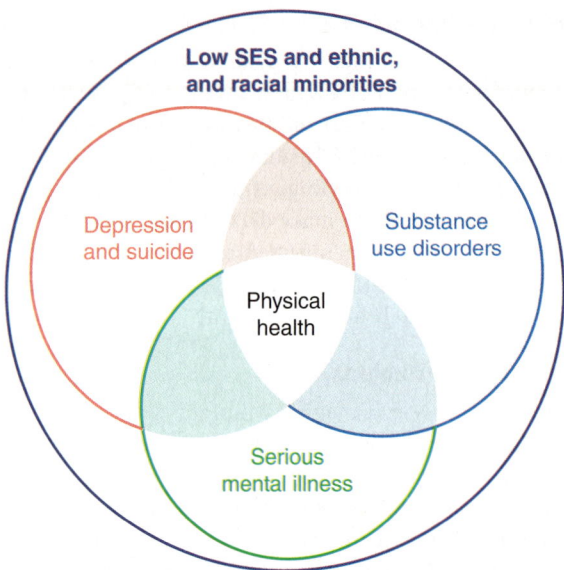

Fig. 22.9 E4 Center strategic priorities to reduce behavioral health disparities. (Redrawn from Substance Abuse and Mental Health Services Administration [SAMHSA], 2022.)

SUMMARY

Nurses caring for older adults face many challenges as the population of older adults continues to increase in the United States and around the world. A significant percentage of older adults have cognitive impairment, all of whom could benefit from nursing care focusing on their special needs. Those with cognitive impairments continue to be at high risk for limited access to appropriate and cost-effective care.

The practice of gerontologic nursing is collaborative and interdisciplinary in scope. This is necessitated by the vast complexity, diversity, and heterogeneity of older adults in terms of their physical and mental health conditions, health-care needs, past-life experiences, current lifestyles, culture, ethnicity, and resources. The family is an extremely important aspect of gerontologic practice, not only because many older adults live within a family setting but also because the family is becoming a primary provider of care.

The most serious health problems occur in those older than 80 years old, and this group is likely to be cared for by relatives who are older than 65 years of age. The blend of medical–surgical, psychiatric, and community health nursing skills and the expertise required to care for older adults with cognitive impairments provides unique and unlimited opportunities and challenges in nursing practice.

KEY POINTS

- The nervous system undergoes many neurophysiologic changes as a person ages. An individual's environment, genetics, lifestyle, and nutritional intake are some of the many factors that affect the neurologic system.
- Evaluation of cognition is a required part of Medicare's annal wellness visit. If cognitive impairment is observed during the visit or reported by the patient, family, or others, further evaluation is necessary.
- The Montreal Cognitive Assessment (MoCA) was developed as a quick screening tool for MCI. The tool assesses the domains of orientation to time and place, short-term memory, visuospatial abilities, executive functions, attention, concentration, and language.
- It is advised that screening for depression should be done along with an evaluation of cognitive function. Studies have shown that depression is common in people with MCI and AD.
- The Geriatric Depression Scale (GDS) short form is a 15-question scale that can be used to evaluate for depression in healthy, ill, and mild to moderately cognitively impaired older adults.
- Normal aging results in slower information processing and increased trouble multitasking, but memory, skills, and knowledge are stable.
- Several cognitive disorders are associated with altered thought processes in older adults. These include the three *D*s—depression, delirium, and dementia—as well as cranial tumors, subdural hematomas, and normal pressure hydrocephalus.
- Depression is a mood disorder and a chronic medical condition that often has an atypical presentation in older adults.
- There are multiple treatment approaches for depression, and no one therapy is right for everyone. Treatment includes antidepressant drugs, psychotherapy, and electroconvulsive therapy.

- Delirium presents as a disturbance in attention, cognition, affective expression, and motor behavior. Assessment with the use of a validated instrument such as the CAM is the first step in preventing and treating delirium.
- Delirium management includes rapid diagnosis and treatment of the underlying cause.
- Dementia is a syndrome of gradual and progressive cognitive decline. It has been defined as an alteration in memory in addition to an acquired persistent alteration in intellectual function (e.g., orientation, calculation, attention, and motor skills) compromising multiple cognitive domains.
- AD is the most common form of dementia. AD is a slowly progressive, neurodegenerative disease whose main characteristic is the accumulation of the protein beta-amyloid (plaques) outside neurons and twisted strands of the protein tau (tangles) inside neurons in the brain.
- Several drugs are approved by the FDA to treat AD. Donepezil, rivastigmine, galantamine, and memantine temporarily treat the symptoms of AD and may control some cognitive and behavioral symptoms of dementia, but do not alter the underlying neurodegeneration causing the disease.
- The goal of nonpharmacological management of AD is to maintain or improve cognitive function, QoL, social engagement, and the ability to perform activities of daily living ADLs.
- Iν γενεραλ, 5%–10% of people with dementia have VaD. VaD is a result of blockage of blood vessels in the brain, resulting in ischemia. Symptoms of VaD vary widely depending on the severity of damage and the part of the brain affected.
- Research has indicated that the same drugs used to treat AD also offer some benefit to people with VaD.
- Dementia with Lewy bodies (DLB) is a progressive, degenerative brain disorder. People with DLB experience a decline in thinking, reasoning, and independent functioning. In DLB, abnormal clumps of the protein alpha-synuclein aggregate in neurons of the cortex.
- Management of patients with DLB focuses on symptomatic relief when psychiatric and behavioral symptoms become distressing. The use of cholinesterase inhibitors has been supported in DLB, as has the use of antidepressants, especially the use of SSRIs. Antipsychotic drugs should be used with extreme caution, as they may cause serious side effects in around 50% of patients.
- FTD is an overarching term for a group of disorders encompassing several subtypes, including bvFTD, PPA, Pick's disease, CBD, and PSP.
- There is no specific treatment for FTD or any subtype. Interventions, both nonpharmacological and pharmacological, should be implemented to reduce agitation, irritability, and depression.
- Normal pressure hydrocephalus (NPH) occurs most often in persons in their 60s to 70s. In NPH, CSF circulates to the cerebral subarachnoid space, enlarging the ventricles but causing no rise in the CSF pressure. Treatment involves placing a shunt to drain CSF from the brain to the abdomen. Placing the shunt can improve walking, but cognitive changes and incontinence are less likely to improve.
- Mixed dementia occurs when a person has more than one cause of dementia. It is thought that 50% or more of people diagnosed with AD also have VaD, or DLB.
- Person-centered care is designed to help the person with dementia maintain a sense of purpose and a sense of self.
- BPSD are attempts by the person to communicate. At some point during the trajectory of dementia, most persons with dementia develop BPSD. Therefore, it is paramount that the nurse understand what the person with dementia is trying to convey.
- Nonpharmacological measures are first-line therapy in the treatment of BPSD.
- Guidelines suggest that some atypical antipsychotics can be considered as treatment for BPSD, but only if the resident behaviors result in "significant distress for the patient or pose a safety risk for the persons with dementia or those around them."
- The goal of nursing care is to promote patient function, independence, and maximal QoL for as long as possible.
- There has been a progressive increase in suicide as people age, especially among males.
- PD is a progressive disorder resulting from the degeneration of dopaminergic neurons in the substantia nigra, the part of the brain that controls movement. Treatment is aimed at relieving clinical manifestations, increasing the individual's ability to perform ADLs, and decreasing the risk for injury.
- A disruption in the normal blood supply to the brain tissue causes a CVA (stroke). CVAs occur suddenly and produce focal neurologic deficits. In strokes, 80% are ischemic, resulting from thrombosis or embolism. The remaining 20% are hemorrhagic in nature, resulting from vascular rupture.
- The immediate goal for acute management of stroke during evaluation is to stabilize the patient and complete an assessment, including all imaging and laboratory studies, within 60 minutes of arrival at the emergency department.
- The American Stroke Association (ASA) Guidelines for the Early Management of Patients with Acute Ischemic recommend the administration of alteplase within 4.5 hours of stroke onset, as this allows for the most favorable outcomes.
- Anxiety is common among older adults. Older adults face multiple factors that can cause anxiety, including multiple medical conditions, financial insecurity, retirement, loss of a loved one, loss of independence, limited physical mobility, sleep disturbances, and other issues impacting QoL that may also lead to isolation.
- Older adults living with chronic schizophrenia are a public-health concern worldwide. Older adults with schizophrenia have a shorter life expectancy; the risk of mortality is 2-3 times greater than that of the general population. Treatment focuses on managing symptoms so people can function in the day-to-day world.
- The mission of the E4 Center of Excellence for Behavioral Health Disparities in Aging's mission is to "engage, empower, and educate health-care providers and community-based organizations for equity in behavioral health for older adults and their families."

CASE STUDY

The patient is a 78-year-old African American who arrived in the ED lethargic, vomiting, unable to speak clearly, and with right-sided weakness. The patient has a medical history of HTN and T2DM. Their family reports that for the past 3 months they have been having right-sided weakness and slurred speech that resolved within an hour of onset. The patient also has glaucoma, gout, and a history of AFib (managed with drugs). The patient's family reported that they were taking the following drugs at home: digoxin, allopurinol, furosemide, neutral protamine Hagedorn (NPH), insulin twice a day, lisinopril, baby acetylsalicylic acid, potassium chloride, and eye drops.

The patient's partner reported that approximately 3 days ago, the patient stopped taking their blood pressure drugs (lisinopril and furosemide) because they had spent the money on a horse race. Two (2) nights ago, the patient started to experience more frequent numbness of the right arm and slurred speech but did not think it was important because it disappeared after several hours. Today, their partner had difficulty waking them up, and their adult child called the ambulance.

On admission, the patient's blood pressure was 220/120 mm Hg, heart rate was 126 beats/min, respiratory rate was 28 breaths/min, and temperature was 98.9° (37°C). They have right-sided hemiparesis and hemiplegia. Speech is slurred and, at times, incomprehensible. The patient can maintain their airway. Oxygen via nasal cannula is started at 2 L/min, and a peripheral intravenous (IV) line is started with normal saline at 80 mL/hr. A 12-lead ECG is obtained, and the patient is sent for CT of the head.

CLINICAL JUDGMENT EXERCISES

1. In the case study, which one of the patient's symptoms supports a diagnosis of stroke?
2. What risk factors does the patient have for the development of stroke?
3. Indicate the type of stroke most likely experienced by the patient and support your answer.
4. What evidence is presented to support the claim that the patient has experienced previous TIAs?
5. Why is AFib a risk factor for embolic stroke?
6. Identify a patient problem based on the patient's assessment and develop an appropriate plan of care.

REFERENCES

Administration for Community Living (ACL). (2022). *2021 profile of older Americans*. U.S. Department of Health and Human Services. Retrieved from https://acl.gov/aging-and-disability-in-america/data-and-research/profile-older-americans. Accessed August 12, 2024.

Alexandrov, A. V., & Krishnaiah, B. (2023). Overview of stroke. In *Merck manual professional version*. Merck & Co., Inc. Retrieved from https://www.merckmanuals.com/professional/neurologic-disorders/stroke/overview-of-stroke. Accessed August 12, 2024.

Algase, D. L., Beck, C., Kolanowski, A., Whall, A., Berent, S., Richards, K., et al. (1996). Need-driven dementia-compromised behavior: An alternative view of disruptive behavior. *American Journal of Alzheimer's Disease*, 11(6), 10–19. doi:10.1177/153331759601100603.

Allarakha, S. (2022). *What are the 5 stages of parkinson's disease?* MedicineNet [website]. Retrieved from https://www.medicinenet.com/what_are_the_5_stages_of_parkinsons_disease/article.htm. Accessed August 12, 2024.

Alzheimer's Association. (2023). 2023 Alzheimer's disease facts and figures. *Alzheimers Dement*, 19(4), 1598–1695. doi: 10.1002/alz.13016.

Alzheimer's Association. (n.d.). *Types of dementia*. Retrieved from https://www.alz.org/alzheimers-dementia/what-is-dementia/types-of-dementia. Accessed November 2, 2023.

American Association of Neurological Surgeons (AANS). (2024). *Parkinson's disease*. Retrieved from https://www.aans.org/en/Patients/Neurosurgical-Conditions-and-Treatments/Parkinsons-Disease. Accessed August 12, 2024.

American Psychological Association (APA). (2023). *Depression treatments for older adults*. Clinical Practice Guideline for the Treatment of Depression. Retrieved from https://www.apa.org/depression-guideline/older-adults. Accessed August 12, 2024.

Assisting Hands Home Care. (2022). *A mnemonic about reversible causes of dementia* [Blog]. Assisting Hands Home Care. Retrieved from https://assistinghands.com/66/ohio/columbus/blog/mnemonic-tool-to-remember-dementia-causes-that-are-reversible/. Accessed August 12, 2024.

Banasik, J. (2022). Structure and function of the nervous system. In J. Banasik (Ed.), *Pathophysiology* (7th ed., pp. 866–906). St. Louis: Elsevier.

Baycrest. (n.d.). *Managing behavioural and psychological symptoms of dementia (BPSD): Non-pharmacological intervention strategies*. Behavioural Supports Ontario. Retrieved from https://www.baycrest.org/Baycrest_Centre/media/content/Non-Pharmacological-Intervention.pdf. Accessed August 12, 2024.

Best Practice Advocacy Centre New Zealand (bpac[nz]). (2020). *Managing the behavioural and psychological symptoms of dementia*. Retrieved from https://bpac.org.nz/2020/bpsd.aspx. Accessed August 12, 2024.

Bugos, C. (2023). *New research shows most antidepressants don't work for chronic pain conditions*. Verywell Health [website]. Retrieved from https://www.verywellhealth.com/antidepressant-chronic-pain-7152653. Accessed August 12, 2024.

Caplan, L. R. (2023). Patient education: Ischemic stroke treatment (Beyond the Basics). In S. E. Kasner & J. F. Dashe (Eds.), *Up ToDate*. Waltham, MA: UpToDate, Inc. Retrieved from https://www.uptodate.com/contents/ischemic-stroke-treatment-beyond-the-basics. Accessed August 12, 2024.

Centers for Disease Control and Prevention (CDC). (2023a). *Recognizing symptoms of dementia and seeking help*. Retrieved from https://www.cdc.gov/aging/publications/features/dementia-not-normal-aging.html. Accessed August 12, 2024.

Centers for Disease Control and Prevention (CDC). (2023b). *Suicide data and statistics*. Retrieved from https://www.cdc.gov/suicide/facts/data.html?CDC_AAref_Val=https://www.cdc.gov/suicide/suicide-data-statistics.html. Accessed August 12, 2024.

Centers for Disease Control and Prevention (CDC). (2023c). *Know your risk for stroke*. Retrieved from https://www.cdc.gov/stroke/risk-factors/index.html. Accessed November 2, 2023.

Centers for Disease Control and Prevention (CDC). (2022). *Depression is not a normal part of growing older*. Retrieved from https://www.cdc.gov/aging/olderadultsandhealthyaging/depression-and-aging.html. Accessed November 2, 2023.

Centers for Disease Control and Prevention (CDC). (2019). *About dementia*. Retrieved from https://www.cdc.gov/aging/dementia/index.html. Accessed August 12, 2024.

Centers for Medicare & Medicaid Services (CMS). (2023a). *Cognitive assessment & care plan services*. Retrieved from https://www.cms.gov/cognitive. Accessed August 12, 2024.

Centers for Medicare & Medicaid Services (CMS). (2023b). *National partnership to improve dementia care in nursing homes*. Retrieved from https://www.cms.gov/medicare/provider-enrollment-and-certification/surveycertificationgeninfo/national-partnership-to-improve-dementia-care-in-nursing-homes. Accessed August 12, 2024.

Centers for Medicare & Medicaid Services (CMS). (n.d.). *Person-centered care*. Retrieved from https://www.cms.gov/priorities/innovation/key-concept/person-centered-care. Accessed August 12, 2024.

De Leo, D. (2022). Late-life suicide in an aging world. *Nature Aging*, 2(1), 7–12. doi:10.1038/s43587-021-00160-1.

Dementia Care Central. (2022). *Mini-mental state exam (MMSE) alzheimer's/dementia test: Administration, accuracy and scoring*. Retrieved from https://www.dementiacarecentral.com/mini-mental-state-exam/. Accessed August 12, 2024.

Devita, M., De Salvo, R., Ravelli, A., De Rui, M., Coin, A., Sergi, G., et al. (2022). Recognizing depression in the elderly: Practical guidance and challenges for clinical management. *Neuropsychiatric Disease and Treatment*, 18, 2867–2880. doi:10.2147/NDT.S347356.

Dominiak, M., Antosik-Wójcińska, A., Wojnar, M., & Mierzejewski, P. (2021). Electroconvulsive therapy and age: Effectiveness, safety and tolerability in the treatment of major depression among patients under and over 65 years of age. *Pharmaceuticals (Basel)*, 14(6), 582. doi:10.3390/ph14060582.

Fazio, S., Pace, D., Flinner, J., & Kallmyer, B. (2018). The fundamentals of person-centered care for individuals with dementia. *Gerontologist*, 58(Suppl. 1), S10–S19. doi:10.1093/geront/gnx122.

Francis, J. Jr., & Young, G. B. (2023). Patient education: Delirium (beyond the basics). In M. J. Aminoff, K. E. Schmader, & J. L. Wilterdink (Eds.), *UpToDate*. Waltham, MA: UpToDate Inc. Retrieved from https://www.uptodate.com/contents/delirium-beyond-the-basics. Accessed August 12, 2024.

Fuchs, S., Bode, L., Ernst, J., Marquetand, J., von Känel, R., & Böttger, S. (2020). Delirium in elderly patients: Prospective prevalence across hospital services. *General Hospital Psychiatry*, 67, 19–25. doi:10.1016/j.genhosppsych.2020.08.010.

Gonzalez-Usigli, H. A. (2022). Parkinson disease. In *Merck manual professional version*. Merck & Co., Inc. Retrieved from https://www.merckmanuals.com/professional/neurologic-disorders/movement-and-cerebellar-disorders/parkinson-disease. Accessed November 2, 2023.

Greenberg, S. A. (n.d.). *The geriatric depression scale (GDS)*. Hartford Institute for Geriatric Nursing. Retrieved from https://hign.org/consultgeri/try-this-series/geriatric-depression-scale-gds. Accessed August 12, 2024.

Grover, S., & Avasthi, A. (2018). Clinical practice guidelines for management of delirium in elderly. *Indian Journal of Psychiatry*, 60(Suppl. 3), S329–S340. doi:10.4103/0019-5545.224473.

Gulanick, M., & Myers, J. L. (2022). *Nursing care plans: Diagnoses, interventions, and outcomes* (10th ed., pp. 251–254). St. Louis: Elsevier.

Home Care Assistance Roseville. (2022). *What are some reversible causes of dementia? A mnemonic*. Home Care Assistance [website]. Retrieved from https://www.homecareassistanceroseville.com/easy-way-to-remember-reversible-causes-of-dementia/. Accessed August 12, 2024.

Howard, J. (2023). *FDA decision on experimental Alzheimer's drug expected this week*. CNN [website]. Retrieved from https://www.cnn.com/2023/01/02/health/lecanemab-fda-decision-expected/index.html. Accessed August 12, 2024.

Jauch, E. C., Almallouhi, E., & Holmstedt, C. A. (2022). *Acute management of stroke*. Medscape [website]. Retrieved from https://emedicine.medscape.com/article/1159752-overview. Accessed November 2, 2023.

Johns Hopkins Medicine. (n.d.). *Parkinson's disease risk factors and causes*. Retrieved from https://www.hopkinsmedicine.org/health/conditions-and-diseases/parkinsons-disease/parkinsons-disease-risk-factors-and-causes. Accessed August 12, 2024.

Khan, W. U., & Rajji, T. K. (2019). Schizophrenia in later life: Patient characteristics and treatment strategies. *Psychiatric times*, 36(3), 14–16. Retrieved from https://www.psychiatrictimes.com/view/schizophrenia-later-life-patient-characteristics-and-treatment-strategies. Accessed August 12, 2024.

Kirkham, J., Sherman, C., Velkers, C., Maxwell, C., Gill, S., Rochon, P., et al. (2017). Antipsychotic use in dementia. *Canadian Journal of Psychiatry*, 62(3), 170–181. doi:10.1177/0706743716673321.

Maiese, K. (2024a). Effects of aging on the nervous system. In: *Merck manual consumer version*. Merck & Co., Inc. Retrieved from https://www.merckmanuals.com/home/brain,-spinal-cord,-and-nerve-disorders/biology-of-the-nervous-system/effects-of-aging-on-the-nervous-system. Accessed August 12, 2024.

Maiese, K. (2024b). Spinal cord. In *Merck manual consumer version*. Merck & Co., Inc. Retrieved from https://www.merckmanuals.com/home/brain,-spinal-cord,-and-nerve-disorders/biology-of-the-nervous-system/spinal-cord. Accessed August 12, 2024.

Maldonado, K. A., & Alsayouri, K. (2023). Physiology, brain. In *StatPearls* [Internet]. Treasure Island, FL: StatPearls Publishing. Retrieved from https://www.ncbi.nlm.nih.gov/books/NBK551718/. Accessed August 12, 2024.

Martin, P. (2024). *6 suicidal ideation (hopelessness & impaired coping) nursing care plans*. Nurseslabs [website]. Retrieved from https://nurseslabs.com/suicide-behaviors-nursing-care-plans/#h-nursing-goals. Accessed August 12, 2024.

Maxwell, Y. L. (2018). *New BMJ guidance urges prudence with supplemental oxygen, especially in acute MI, stroke*. tctMD [website]. Retrieved from https://www.tctmd.com/news/new-bmj-guidance-urges-prudence-supplemental-oxygen-especially-acute-mi-stroke. Accessed August 12, 2024.

Mayo Clinic Staff. (2024a). *Dementia: Diagnosis & treatment*. Mayo Clinic [website]. Retrieved from https://www.mayoclinic.org/diseases-conditions/dementia/diagnosis-treatment/drc-20352019. Accessed August 12, 2024.

Mayo Clinic Staff. (2024b). *Parkinson's disease: Diagnosis & treatment*. Mayo Clinic [website]. Retrieved from https://www.mayoclinic.org/diseases-conditions/parkinsons-disease/diagnosis-treatment/drc-20376062. Accessed August 12, 2024.

National Council on Aging (NCOA). (2022). *How common is depression in older adults?* Retrieved from https://www.ncoa.org/article/how-common-is-depression-in-older-adults. Accessed August 12, 2024.

National Institute on Aging (NIA). (2023a). *Alzheimer's disease genetics fact sheet*. National Institutes of Health. Retrieved from https://www.nia.nih.gov/health/alzheimers-disease-genetics-fact-sheet. Accessed August 12, 2024.

National Institute on Aging (NIA). (2023b). *How is Alzheimer's disease treated?* National Institutes of Health. Retrieved from https://www.nia.nih.gov/health/how-alzheimers-disease-treated. Accessed August 12, 2024.

National Institute on Aging (NIA). (2021). *Depression and older adults*. National Institutes of Health. Retrieved from https://www.nia.nih.gov/health/depression-and-older-adults. Accessed August 12, 2024.

National Institute of Mental Health (NIMH). (2024). *Schizophrenia*. National Institutes of Health, U.S. Department of Health and Human Services. Retrieved from https://www.nimh.nih.gov/health/topics/schizophrenia. Accessed August 12, 2024.

National Institute of Neurological Disorders and Stroke. (2024). *Brain basics: Know your brain*. National Institutes of Health, U.S. Department of Health and Human Services. Retrieved from https://www.ninds.nih.gov/health-information/public-education/brain-basics/brain-basics-know-your-brain. Accessed August 12, 2024.

Oh, E. S., Fong, T. G., Hshieh, T. T., & Inouye, S. K. (2017). Delirium in older persons: Advances in diagnosis and treatment. *JAMA*, 318(12), 1161–1174. doi:10.1001/jama.2017.12067.

Parkinson's Foundation. (n.d.). *Stages of parkinson's*. Retrieved from https://www.parkinson.org/understanding-parkinsons/what-is-parkinsons/stages. Accessed August 12, 2024.

Pelham, V. (2023). *Anxiety in the golden years: What you should know*. Cedars-Sinai. Retrieved from https://www.cedars-sinai.org/blog/anxiety-in-the-golden-years.html. Accessed August 12, 2024.

Powers, W. J., Rabinstein, A. A., Ackerson, T., Adeoye, O. M., Bambakidis, N. C., Becker, K., et al. (2019). Guidelines for the early management of patients with acute ischemic stroke: 2019 update to the 2018 guidelines for the early management of acute ischemic stroke: A guideline for healthcare professionals from the American Heart Association/American Stroke Association. *Stroke*, 50(12), e344–e418. doi:10.1161/STR.0000000000000211.

PsychDB. (2024). *Behavioural and psychological symptoms of dementia (BPSD)*. Retrieved from https://www.psychdb.com/geri/dementia/1-bpsd. Accessed August 12, 2024.

Reus, V. I., Fochtmann, L. J., Eyler, A. E., Hilty, D. M., Horvitz-Lennon, M., Jibson, M. D., et al. (2016). The American Psychiatric Association Practice Guideline on the use of antipsychotics to treat agitation or psychosis in patients with dementia. *American Journal of Psychiatry*, 173(5), 543–546. doi:10.1176/appi.ajp.2015.173501.

Rhee, T. G., Sint, K., Olfson, M., Gerhard, T., Busch, S. H., & Wilkinson, S. T. (2021). Association of ECT with risks of all-cause mortality and suicide in older Medicare patients. *American Journal of Psychiatry*, 178(12), 1089–1097. doi:10.1176/appi.ajp.2021.21040351.

Rolin, D. (2021). *What guidance is there for clinicians who treat older adults with schizophrenia?* SMI Adviser [website]. Retrieved from https://smiadviser.org/knowledge_post/what-guidance-is-there-for-clinicians-who-treat-older-adults-with-schizophrenia. Accessed November 2, 2023.

SimpleNursing. (n.d.). *Nursing care plan for stroke*. SimpleNursing.com [website]. Retrieved from https://simplenursing.com/nursing-care-plan-stroke/. Accessed August 12, 2024.

Stewart, J. (2023 July 13). Leqembi FDA aproval history. Drugs.com. https://www.drugs.com/history/leqembi.html. Accessed October 24, 2024.

Subramanyam, A. A., Kedare, J., Singh, O. P., & Pinto, C. (2018). Clinical practice guidelines for geriatric anxiety disorders. *Indian Journal of Psychiatry*, 60(Suppl. 3), S371–S382. doi:10.4103/0019-5545.224476.

Substance Abuse and Mental Health Services Administration (SAMHSA). (2024). *Resources for older adults*. SAMHSA, U.S. Department of Health and Human Services. Retrieved from https://www.samhsa.gov/resources-serving-older-adults. Accessed August 12, 2024.

Tampi, R. R., & Tampi, D. J. (2022). The management of depression among older adults. *Psychiatric Times*, 39(4). Retrieved from https://www.psychiatrictimes.com/view/the-management-of-depression-among-older-adults. Accessed August 12, 2024.

Tan, R. Q., Lim, C. S., & Ong, H. S. (2021). Suicide risk assessment in elderly individuals. *Singapore Medical Journal*, 62(5), 244–247. doi:10.11622/smedj.2021065.

Tisdale, W., 3rd. (2022). *Suicide warning signs and prevention strategies for older adults*. Substance Abuse and Mental Health Services Administration (SAMHSA). Retrieved from https://www.samhsa.gov/blog/suicide-warning-signs-prevention-strategies-older-adults. Accessed August 12, 2024.

Tran, N. N., Hoang, T. P. N., & Ho, T. K. T. (2021). Diagnosis and risk factors for delirium in elderly patients in the emergency rooms and intensive care unit of the national geriatric hospital emergency department: A cross-sectional observational study. *International Journal of General Medicine*, 14, 6505–6515. doi:10.2147/IJGM.S325365.

Treatment Advocacy Center. (2022). *Schizophrenia – fact sheet*. Retrieved from https://www.treatmentadvocacycenter.org/evidence-and-research/learn-more-about/25-schizophrenia-fact-sheet. Accessed August 12, 2024.

U.S. Preventive Services Task Force. (2020). *Cognitive impairment in older adults: Screening. Final recommendation statement*. Retrieved from https://www.uspreventiveservicestaskforce.org/uspstf/recommendation/cognitive-impairment-in-older-adults-screening. Accessed August 12, 2024.

Vidović, M., & Rikalovic, M. G. (2022). Alpha-synuclein aggregation pathway in Parkinson's disease: Current status and novel therapeutic approaches. *Cells*, 11(11), 1732. doi:10.3390/cells11111732.

WebMD Editorial Contributors. (2023). *Understanding generalized anxiety disorder—diagnosis and treatment*. WebMD [website]. Retrieved from https://www.webmd.com/anxiety-panic/understanding-anxiety-treatment. Accessed November 15, 2023.

Wood, F. J., Nabi, A., & Adebekun, I. (2018). Screening for depression in patients with cognitive impairment: A local audit. *Progress in Neurology and Psychiatry*, 22(4), 23–26. Retrieved from https://wchh.onlinelibrary.wiley.com/doi/pdf/10.1002/pnp.519. Accessed August 12, 2024.

WEBSITES

Alzheimer's Association: https://www.alz.org/.
American Parkinson Disease Association: https://www.apdaparkinson.org/.
Association of Rehabilitation Nurses (ARN): http://www.rehabnurse.org/.
American Stroke Association: https://www.stroke.org/en/.
Family Caregiver Alliance: https://www.caregiver.org/.
Substance Abuse and Mental Health Services Administration (SAMHSA): https://www.samhsa.gov.

23
Endocrine Function

Mary B. Winton, PhD, MSN, RN

http://evolve.elsevier.com/Yeager/gerontologic/

LEARNING OBJECTIVES

On completion of this chapter, the reader will be able to:
1. Discuss the normal age-related physiologic changes in the endocrine system.
2. Describe the major characteristics of common endocrine disorders: metabolic syndrome, type 2 diabetes mellitus, hyperthyroidism, hypothyroidism, osteoporosis, and sexual dysfunction.
3. Apply the Clinical Judgment Measurement Model (nursing process) for older adults with endocrine disorders.

WHAT WOULD YOU DO?

What would you do if you were faced with the following situations?
- A 71-year-old patient presents to the clinic complaining of excessive urination, thirst, and hunger. The patient is actively involved in the community and eats foods that are easily obtained. The patient lives alone but has a family member who lives nearby. What would you do?
- Your 69-year-old patient tells you that lately they have been getting tired easily, has gained some weight despite eating less, and cannot get warm. What would you do?
- One of your patients, a 73-year-old male, is interested in a more romantic relationship with a friend and would like to see more often but is concerned about not being able to "get it up." How would you proceed?

Previously dominated by diabetes and thyroid disease, gerontologic endocrinology has recently been redefining itself through innovative insights developed from the mapping of the human genome (Bergman et al, 2013). Knowledge of aging endocrine physiology and genetic influences has begun to grow at a very fast pace. New animal models (Toivonen and Partridge, 2009) and genomic endocrine-related trait studies (Walter et al, 2011) have led to a robust subspecialty often referred to as the *endocrinology of aging* (Michael, 2010). Andropause, circadian dysrhythmias, dehydroepiandrosterone (DHEA) replacement, erectile dysfunction (ED), glucagon-like peptide 1 (GLP-1) replacement, male osteoporosis, menopause, metabolic syndrome, and metabolic presbycusis have joined the traditional topics of diabetes and thyroid disease.

The endocrine system is closely connected with the nervous system. When combined, they are referred to as the *neuroendocrine system*. Neuroendocrine aging is discussed in terms of decreased estrogen production in females (menopause), decreased testosterone production in males (andropause), decreased DHEA (adrenopause), and decreased growth hormone (GH)–insulin-like growth factor (IGF) (somatopause) (Jones and Boelaert, 2015) (Fig. 23.1). Endocrinologic aging involves increased molecular disorderliness of the endocrine regulatory mechanisms that result in reduced vitality of the overall person. This molecular dysregulation of neurohormones from or with the central nervous system (CNS) is one of the earliest measurable characteristics of endocrine aging.

ENDOCRINE PHYSIOLOGY IN OLDER ADULTS

The endocrine system comprises endocrine glands (without ducts) (Fig. 23.2), which secrete hormones that control numerous processes throughout the body. Table 23.1 outlines the major endocrine glands, their functions, and possible endocrine disorders due to aging. The endocrine system uses a delicate balance of chemical messengers in the bloodstream to maintain homeostasis and regulate mood, growth, organ function, metabolism, nutrition, and sexual activity (Jones and Boelaert, 2015). Dependent on a complex interplay of factors, many hormones are secreted in a cyclic pattern of minutes, hours, days, or months. Feedback control processes (Fig. 23.3) of these intricate gland–hormone–organ–tissue systems depend on the secretion and degradation of hormones classified by chemical structure and cell receptor type (Steil et al, 2011). Subtle changes to the endocrine system occur with aging (Veldhuis, 2013) because of reduced production and secretion of hormones and decreased tissue

---
Previous authors: Sue E. Meiner, EdD, APRN, BC, GNP, and Jean Benzel-Lindley, PhD, RN

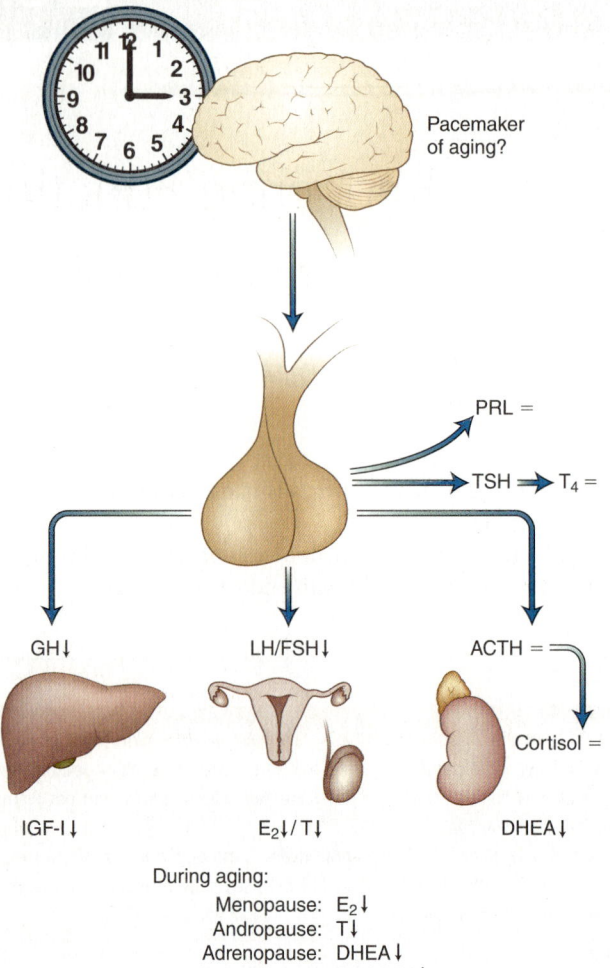

Fig. 23.1 During aging, declines in the activities of a number of hormonal systems occur. *Left,* A decrease in growth hormone (GH) release by the pituitary gland causes a decrease in the production of insulin-like growth factor 1 (IGF-1) by the liver and other organs (somatopause). *Middle,* A decrease in the release of gonadotropin luteinizing hormone (LH) and follicle-stimulating hormone (FSH) and decreased secretion at the gonadal level (from the ovaries, decreased estradiol [E_2]; from the testicle, decreased testosterone [T]) cause menopause and andropause, respectively. (Immediately after the initiation of menopause, serum LH and FSH levels increase sharply.) *Right,* The adrenocortical cells responsible for the production of dehydroepiandrosterone (DHEA) decrease in activity (adrenopause) without clinically evident changes in corticotropin (adrenocorticotropic hormone, ACTH) and cortisol secretion. A central pacemaker in the hypothalamus or higher brain areas (or both) is hypothesized, which, together with changes in the peripheral organs (the ovaries, testicles, and adrenal cortex), regulates the aging process of these endocrine axes. *PRL,* prolactin; T_4, thyroxine; *TSH,* thyroid-stimulating hormone. (From Melmed, S., Auchus, R. J., Goldfine, A. B., Koenig, R. J., & Rosen, C. J., [Eds.]. [2020]. *Williams textbook of endocrinology* [14th ed.]. Philadelphia, PA: Elsevier.)

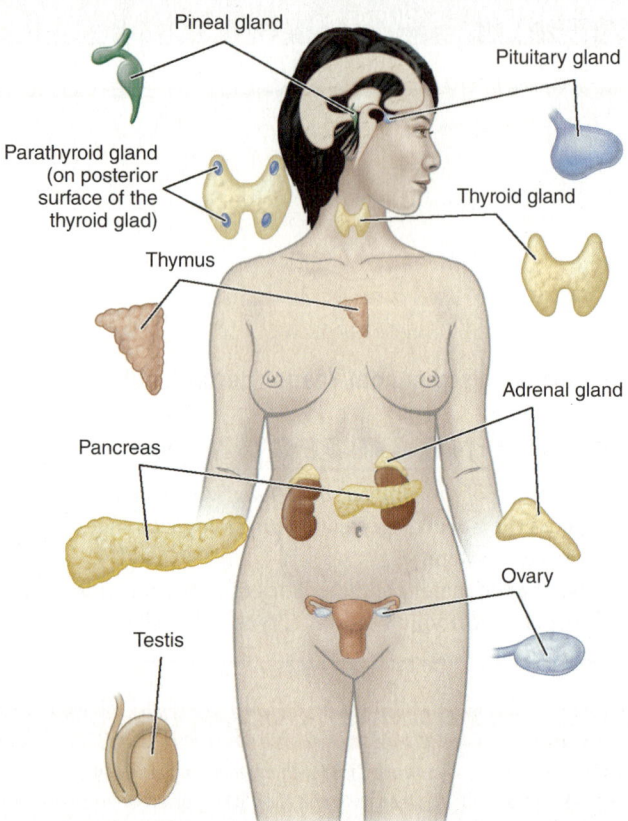

Fig. 23.2 Major endocrine glands. (From Applegate, E. [2011]. *The anatomy and physiology learning system* [4th ed.]. St. Louis, MO: Saunders.)

muscle mass, increased adipose tissue, compromised skin integrity, impaired insulin signaling, and impaired immune response (Jones and Boelarert, 2015). Also, disease processes may alter the older person in other body systems, such as the syndrome of inappropriate antidiuretic hormone secretion, which occurs with many types of tumors or infections. Therefore, this chapter discusses the typical aging changes of menopause, andropause, adrenopause, and somatopause physiology without discussing other potential superimposed pathophysiologic states.

Andropause and Menopause

Older adults experience a decline in the biosynthesis and balance of their sex hormones (andropause) as they age (Jones and Boelaert, 2015). Females experience menopause, a complete cessation of menstruation, due to a dramatic decline in estrogen (van den Beld et al, 2018). A decrease in testosterone in males can cause decreased libido and erectile dysfunction. In both genders, the activity of the hypothalamus–anterior pituitary–gonadal (testes and ovaries) axis declines. Both genders may experience hot flashes, night sweats, depression, and sexual dysfunction in response to age-related declines in androgen or estrogen (Felman, 2018). In contrast to the previous gender similarities in symptoms, laboratory values to determine the endocrine decline are unique to each sex: luteinizing hormone (LH) and testosterone are of primary importance in males, whereas follicle-stimulating hormone (FSH) and estrogen are of primary importance in females (van den Beld et al, 2018).

Hormone replacement therapy (HRT) in both genders is a hotly debated topic among health-care providers because risks

sensitivity to the hormone's action (Fig. 23.3) (Jones and Boelaert, 2015). Morbidity of the older adult may be attributed more to hormonal imbalance (Jones and Boelaert, 2015). Four categories classify endocrine pathology: hyporesponsiveness, hyposecretion, degradation changes, and hypersecretion. The endocrine system is elaborate and increases in complexity with the aging process (Table 23.2). The clinical manifestations of the imbalance include decreased bone remodeling, decreased lean

TABLE 23.1 Principal Endocrine Glands

Name	Location	Function	Aging Endocrine Disorder
Thyroid	Anterior aspect of neck	Basal metabolic rate, growth, nutrition	Obesity, hyperthyroidism, hypothyroidism, autoimmune thyroiditis, Graves' disease, euthyroid sick syndrome, thyrotoxicosis, thyroid storm, multinodular toxic goiter
Parathyroid	Back of each thyroid	Calcium and phosphorus metabolism, muscular irritability	Osteoporosis, osteomalacia, Paget disease, mineral imbalances (calcium, phosphate, magnesium)
Adrenal cortex	Above each kidney	Carbohydrate metabolism, salt–water balance, some sexual characteristics	Addison disease, Cushing syndrome, dehydration, electrolyte imbalance, acid-base imbalance, infection
Adrenal medulla	Embedded in kidney, surrounded by adrenal cortex	Sympathetic nervous system, carbohydrate metabolism	Metabolism
Anterior pituitary	Base of brain	Growth, sexual development, skin pigmentation, thyroid function, adrenocortical function (indirectly)	Hypopituitarism causing secondary dysfunction of other endocrine glands
Posterior pituitary	Attached to hypothalamus and anterior pituitary	Uterine contraction, water balance	Dehydration, diabetes insipidus, syndrome of inappropriate antidiuretic hormone
Testes	Scrotum	Secondary sexual characteristics and function, metabolism	Andropause
Ovaries	Pelvic cavity	Secondary sexual characteristics and function, metabolism	Andropause, menopause
Pancreas	Abdomen	Sugar metabolism	Hyperglycemia, hypoglycemia, diabetes mellitus
Pineal gland	Center of brain	Daily biologic clocks	Sleep disturbance
Thymus	Chest cavity	Influences immune system response	Immune senescence: reduced response to immunization, cancer, monoclonal gammopathy, increased autoantibodies
Hypothalamus	Brain	Regulates autonomic nervous system; influences hormone production, sleep, and appetite	Kwashiorkor, obesity, hypothermia, hyperthermia, sleep disturbance

Data from Stefanacci, R. G. (2022). *Physical changes with aging*. Merck Manual: Professional Version. Retrieved from https://www.merckmanuals.com/professional/geriatrics/approach-to-the-geriatric-patient/physical-changes-with-aging#v1130874l; Copstead, L. E. & Banasik, J. K. (2019). *Pathophysiology* (5th ed.). St, Louis, MO: Elsevier; Melmed, S., Auchus, A.B., Goldfine, A. B. Koenig, R. J., & Rosen, C. J., (2020). *Williams textbook of endocrinology* (14th ed.). Philadelphia, PA: Elsevier.

and benefits are unique to each patient. The ongoing debate over whether aging is a disease contributes to the controversy. Those who advocate estrogen and testosterone replacement cite the benefits of improvements in relation to bone density, libido, muscle mass, strength, visuospatial skills, depression, fatigue, hot flashes, irritability, mood, and sleep (Veldhuis, 2013). HRT is not without risks. Estrogen replacement increases the risk for venous thromboembolism and breast cancer (Marko, 2020). Testosterone replacement in andropause is complicated by adverse lipid effects, the risk for promoting prostate- and cardiovascular-related adverse events (AEs) (van den Beld et al, 2018), and the risk for erythrocytosis (Madsen et al, 2021). Although many clinicians continue to prescribe HRT, the benefit must outweigh the risks for developing AEs (Maggio et al, 2015).

Adrenopause

Weighing approximately 4 grams (g), the adrenal glands sit on top of the kidneys and are composed of the adrenal medulla and cortex. The hypothalamic-pituitary-adrenal axis regulates the body in response to stress and maintains homeostasis (Jones and Boelaert, 2015). A total loss of adrenocortical function causes death within days; however, age-related decreases in mineralocorticoids, glucocorticoids, and androgenic hormones manifest changes in body composition, skeletal mass, muscle strength, body weight, and metabolism (Jones and Boelaert, 2015). Age-related decreases in DHEA and aldosterone (Yiallouris et al, 2019) can produce fluid and electrolyte imbalances; impair glucose, protein, and fat metabolisms; impair immune and inflammatory responses; lower bone mass; and lower self-esteem. Other adrenal hormones either increase (epinephrine and norepinephrine) or have minimal change (cortisol) (Young, 2022). All in all, changes to the adrenal glands due to aging have a profound effect on the ability for older adults to adapt to stress, which can cause acute and chronic diseases (Yiallouris et al, 2019).

Somatopause

Somatotropin (a GH), an anabolic protein, is secreted from the hypothalamus–pituitary axis to stimulate the IGF-1 (van den Beld et al, 2018). A decrease in these GHs disrupts the somatotropic axis along the hypothalamic-pituitary axis, which results in somatopause. Somatopause is often spoken of from a neuroendocrine point of view because certain neurons in the hypothalamus secrete hormones (neurosecretion). Somatopause focuses on the neuron–hypothalamus–pituitary axis and the failure of CNS integration of the endocrine and

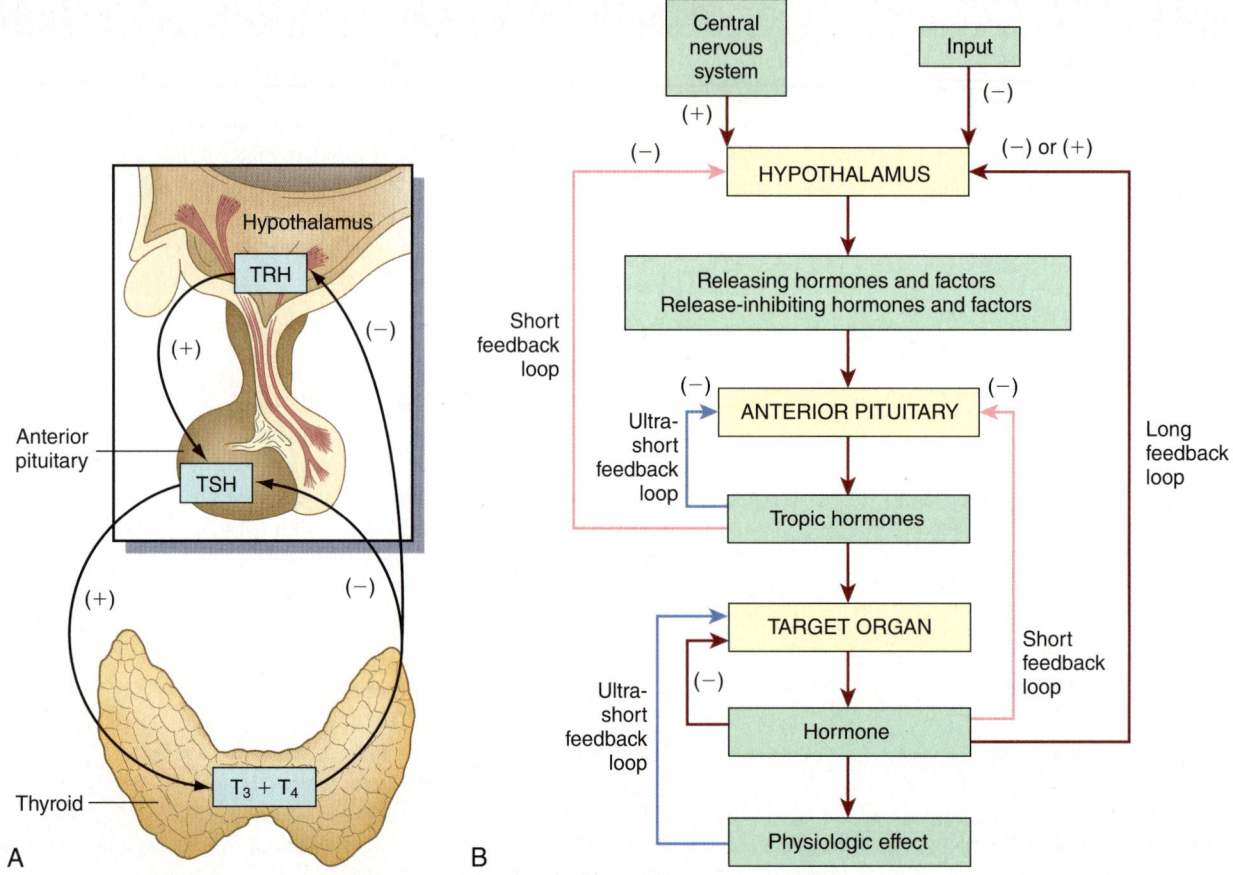

Fig. 23.3 Feedback loops. **A,** Endocrine feedback loops involving the hypothalamus–pituitary gland and end organs; in this example, the thyroid gland is illustrated (endocrine regulation). **B,** General model for control and negative feedback to hypothalamus–pituitary target organ systems. Negative feedback regulation is possible at three levels: target organ (ultrashort feedback), anterior pituitary (short feedback), and hypothalamus (long feedback). T_3, Triiodothyronine; T_4, tetraiodothyronine (thyroxine); *TRH*, thyroid-releasing hormone; *TSH*, thyroid-stimulating hormone. (From Huether, S. E., McCance, K. L., & Brashers, V. L. [Eds.]. [2020]. *Understanding pathophysiology* [7th ed.]. St. Louis, MO: Elsevier.)

TABLE 23.2	Aging Changes in the Endocrine System		
Hyporesponsiveness	**Hyposecretion**	**Degradation Changes**	**Hypersecretion**
Increased connective tissue, pigment, and structural changes in target tissue	Plasma insulin-like growth factor T_3	Thyroid hormones Cortisol Aldosterone	Norepinephrine Parathyroid hormone Atrial natriuretic peptide
Decreased receptor—ligand binding	Aldosterone Active renin Calcitonin Arginine vasopressin Growth hormone	Inactive to active renin conversion Norepinephrine clearance	Insulin Glucagon

Data from Carpenito, L. J. (2023). *Nursing diagnosis: Application to clinical practice* (16th ed.). Philadelphia: Lippincott Williams & Wilkins.

nervous systems, which causes peripheral endocrine gland insufficiency contributing to a disrupted feedback axis in aging (Di Somma et al, 2011). Like adrenopause, somatopause has been linked with several conditions, such as decreased muscle mass and bone density; thinning of the skin; dysfunction of the cardiovascular system and cognition; increased adipose tissue; and frailty and falls (Pamphlett et al, 2019). Current antiaging researchers who believe "you are as young as your oldest part" (Liantonio et al, 2013) have focused on various secretagogue compounds that stimulate pulsatile GH secretion and increase IGF-1 in older adults to levels approximating those found in young adults. Additionally, with the continued evolving epigenomic research, cellular rejuvenation could restore some function to aging cells (Gill et al, 2022). However, no single therapy exists to decrease or reverse somatopause (van den Beld et al, 2018).

COMMON ENDOCRINE PATHOPHYSIOLOGY IN OLDER ADULTS

Metabolic Syndrome–Diabetes Continuum

Pathophysiology

Metabolic syndrome (MetS) is a common multifactorial syndrome of aging due to chronic low inflammation that affects the body and is characterized by central obesity, elevated triglycerides, reduced high-density lipoprotein (HDL) cholesterol, hypertension, and/or hyperglycemia (Bonomini et al, 2015). Suspected endocrine influences on MetS include corticosteroid axis derangement, polycystic ovary syndrome, and dysglycemia. MetS, also known as insulin resistance syndrome, increases the risk for diabetes, stroke, and heart disease (National Heart, Lung, and Blood Institute, 2022). Insulin resistance (IR) causes increased production of inflammatory cytokines correlating with the development of type 2 diabetes mellitus (T2DM) and atherosclerotic vascular disease (ASCVD). The primary risk factors for the syndrome are abdominal obesity, hypertension, hyperglycemia, elevated triglycerides (TGs), and decreased HDL (National Heart, Lung, and Blood Institute, 2022). Additionally, some evidence exists for genetic influences through various gene polymorphisms.

Signs and Symptoms

MetS, according to the National Cholesterol Education Program/ (NCEP) Adult Treatment Panel-III (ATP III), is diagnosed when three of the following five criteria are met: obesity (waist circumference >40 inches in males or >34 inches in females), blood pressure of 130/85 mm Hg or higher, fasting plasma glucose of 110 mg dL or higher, TG 150 mg dL or higher, and HDL cholesterol of 40 mg dL or lower in males and 50 mg dL or lower in females (Olatunbosun, 2020).

Medical Management

Reducing risk factors for diabetes, coronary heart disease (CAD), and obesity are the primary therapeutic objectives in MetS (CDC and National Center for Chronic Disease Prevention and Health Promotion, 2010). Nutritional management for MetS should include meticulous attention to the amounts of low-saturated fats, *trans* fats, cholesterol, and simple sugars. The American Heart Association (AHA) recommends avoiding *trans* fats, reducing saturated fatty acids to less than 7% of daily caloric intake, reducing total daily sodium intake to less than 2300 mg, and increasing physical activity to 30 minutes of moderate to vigorous activity on most days of the week. These lifestyle changes, also termed *lifestyle medicine*, are beneficial to not only physical health but also mental health and stress reduction (Rippe, 2018). Box 23.1 provides additional details of habits and practices to promote a healthy lifestyle. When the risk is high, drug therapy for hypertension, elevated low-density lipoprotein (LDL) cholesterol, and diabetes should be incorporated into the regimen.

Clinical Judgment (Nursing Process) Applied to Metabolic Syndrome

The clinical judgment is applied to the MetS by focusing on the root causes of improper nutrition and inadequate physical activity, as detailed in Table 23.3.

> **BOX 23.1 Habits and Practices for a Healthy Lifestyle**
>
> **Physical Activity:** Moderate to vigorous physical activity improves quality of life, sleep, and general well-being. It decreases unhealthy weight gain and adiposity. It promotes cognitive functioning; thereby decreasing the risk for dementia. Fall-related injuries among older adults are decreased and regular activity lowers the risk for osteoarthritis and hypertension.
>
> **Nutrition:** Diets high in fruits, vegetables, whole grains, nonfat dairy, seafood, legumes, and nuts lessens the risk for cardiovascular disease, diabetes, obesity, and cancer.
>
> **Weight Management:** Balancing energy intake to prevent weight gain or increasing energy deficit for weight loss are the mainstay for treating obesity. Excess body weight is associated with cardiovascular disease, diabetes, arthritis, and cancer.
>
> **Tobacco Products:** Use of tobacco products significantly increases the risk for diabetes, heart disease, cerebrovascular accidents, and cancer. Secondhand smoke also increases the risk for these chronic diseases.
>
> **Stress, Anxiety, and Depression:** Lifestyle changes, such as increasing physical activity, have been demonstrated to decrease anxiety, depression, and promote sleep.

Data from Rippe, J. M. (2018). Lifestyle medicine: The health promoting power of daily habits and practices. *American Journal of Lifestyle Medicine, 12*(6), 499–512.

> **EVIDENCE-BASED PRACTICE**
>
> ***Chronic Low-Calorie Sweetener Use and Risk for Abdominal Obesity Among Older Adults: A Cohort Study***
>
> **Sample/Setting**
> Study sample includes 1454 adults 20 years of age and older at the start of the study in 1958, had at least one Baltimore Longitudinal Study of Aging (BLSA) visit, lived in the community, healthy, and had complete dietary record since 1984.
>
> **Methods**
> An observational continuous-enrollment cohort study was established in 1958, conducted by the National Institute on Aging (NIA). Anthropometric measures, use of low-calorie sweetener, and covariates (age, sex, race, behavioral factors that affect weight, smoking status, dietary intake of specific nutrients; e.g., fat, protein, fiber), quality of diet using Dietary Approaches to Stop Hypertension (DASH) score, and diabetes status from an oral glucose tolerance test were collected and analyzed. Statistical analysis used included marginal structural models to determine the associations of low-calorie sweetener use with body mass index (BMI), waist circumference, obesity, and abdominal obesity.
>
> **Findings**
> Participants who used low-calorie sweetener had higher BMI, larger waist circumference, and higher prevalence and incidence of abdominal obesity than low-calorie sweetener nonusers.
>
> **Implications**
> Use of low-calorie sweeteners may not be an effective means to control weight. The brain does not sense satiety with low-calorie sweeteners. Nonsatiety encourages one to compensate by overeating, which can lead to abdominal obesity. Low-calorie sweeteners implicated in weight gain include saccharin and sucralose. Furthermore, these sweeteners worsen glucose tolerance.

Data from Chia, C. W., Shardell, M., Tanaka, T., Liu, D. D., Gravenstein, K. S., Simonsick, E. M., et al. (2016). Chronic low-calorie sweetener use and risk of abdominal obesity among older adults: A cohort study. *PLoS One, 11*(11), e0167241.

TABLE 23.3 Metabolic Syndrome

Recognize Cues (Assessment)	Analyze Cues and Prioritize Hypotheses (Patient Problems)	Generate Solutions (Planning)	Take Actions (Nursing Interventions)	Evaluate Outcomes (Evaluation)
Nutrition 1. Mini nutritional assessment 2. Body mass index 3. Overweight: >10% over ideal 4. Obese: >20% over ideal 5. Triceps skin fold: >15 mm in males or >25 mm in females 6. Lifetime weight trends 7. Thyroid function 8. Drugs 9. Nutrition knowledge 10. Cultural issues 11. Comorbidities 12. Drugs 13. Social support network	1. Excessive nutrition	1. Use calorie count and dietary log. 2. Use satiety and emotional scale. 3. Adjust seasonings, as needed. 4. Introduce behavior modification techniques. 5. Provide teaching on drug and dietary recommendations of National Research Council Report for older adults.	1. Review log and weight weekly. 2. Eat only at kitchen table. 3. Drink 8 ounces of water before meal. 4. Limit fat, sweets, and alcohol. Eat low-calorie snacks. 5. Control portions, eat slowly, wait 15 seconds between bites.	1. Patient is able to list dietary rules and reasons. 2. Patient demonstrates slow, steady weight loss toward goal. 3. Patient lists drug effects and dietary implications.
Activity 1. Respiratory system 2. Cardiovascular system 3. Musculoskeletal system 4. Developmental status 5. Comorbidities 6. Drugs 7. Cultural issues 8. Social support network	1. Reduced stamina 2. Need for health teaching 3. Inadequate coping	1. Accommodate comorbidities, sensory deficits, safety concerns, financial aspects. 2. Address motivation, lifestyle, and environmental barriers. 3. Provide role models and social support. 4. Include aerobic and strength training.	1. Assess resting vital signs and 3 minutes after activity. 2. Reduce intensity or duration of activity if pulse takes longer than 3 to 4 minutes to return within six beats of baseline. 3. Begin with active range-of-motion exercises twice a day; add isometrics. Gradually increase tolerance from 15 minutes. 4. Provide support, safety, and fall protection. 5. Use personal incentives such as playing with grandchildren, returning to work, or going fishing. 6. Teach primary and secondary prevention related to aging and sensory deficits. 7. Teach stress-related signs and symptoms.	1. Patient will progress to specified activity level. 2. Patient is able to verbalize and engage in health maintenance behaviors. 3. Patient will make decisions and follow through with appropriate actions.

Data from McCuistion, L. E., Vuljoin-DiMaggio, K., Winton, M. B., & Yeager, J. J. (2023). *Pharmacology: A patient-centered nursing process approach* (11th ed.). St. Louis, MO: Elsevier; and Farinde, A. (2021). *Oral hypoglycemic agents.* Medscape [website]. Retrieved from https://emedicine.medscape.com/article/2172160-overview.

Type 2 Diabetes Mellitus

Pathophysiology

Patients with MetS are five times more likely to develop T2DM (Regufe et al, 2020). Metabolically distinct genetic influences play a pivotal role in diabetes among older adults and require a different approach (Cigolle et al, 2011). Often starting with MetS, the disease ultimately produces dysfunction and failure of various organs such as the heart, kidneys, nerves, eyes, and blood vessels (Regufe et al, 2020). Age-related changes combined with genetics and lifestyle factors can promote a hyperglycemic state. Hyperglycemia of T2DM is caused by impaired carbohydrate metabolism, decreased insulin release, dysregulation of hormonal secretions, and IR. As with MetS, the most important variables associated with T2DM are obesity and IR. Starting with a compensatory hyperinsulinemia that affects insulin receptors on target tissues, which leads to insulin resistance (IR) that produces hyperglycemia, T2DM is a disorder of relative insulin insufficiency. The pathophysiology of T2DM in contrast to type 1 diabetes mellitus involves defects in the cell membrane, receptors, or intracellular pathways (Figs. 23.4 and 23.5).

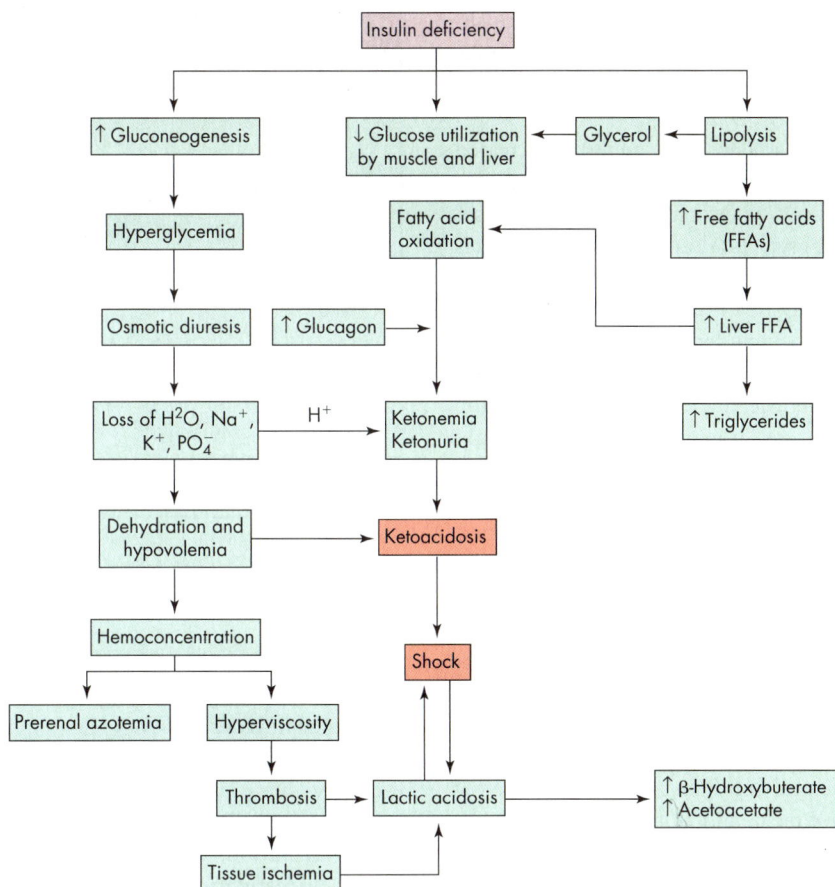

Fig. 23.4 Pathophysiology of insulin deficiency. (From Monahan, F. D., Sands J. K., Neighbors M., Marek, J. F., Green-Nigro, C. J. [2007]. *Phipps' medical-surgical nursing: Health and illness perspectives* [8th ed.]. St. Louis, MO: Mosby.)

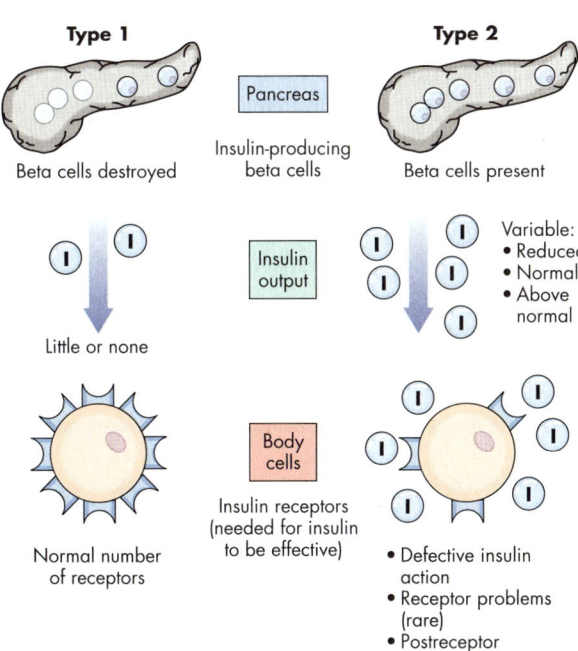

Fig. 23.5 Insulin defects in type 1 and type 2 diabetes mellitus. (From Monahan, F. D., Sands, J. K., Neighbors, M., Marek, J. F., Green-Nigro, C. J. [2007]. *Phipps' medical-surgical nursing: Health and illness perspectives* [8th ed.]. St. Louis, MO: Mosby.)

Signs and Symptoms

Nearly 50% of older adults are prediabetic, and 33% have diabetes (LeRoith et al, 2019). Of those with diabetes, more than 90% have T2DM. At the time of diagnosis, T2DM may be associated with symptoms of excessive thirst, hunger, and urination (i.e., polydipsia, polyphagia, and polyuria, respectively). However, older adults with T2DM often do not have classic symptomatology and will not complain of weight loss or fatigue along with these classic symptoms (Rejeski et al, 2012). Instead, they often describe symptoms of fatigue, blurred vision, weight change (gain or loss), and infections (Munshi, 2024). When questioned, older adults often attribute these changes to "aging." Individuals are often diagnosed with diabetes during a concurrent infection such as a major foot or leg wound, vaginitis, or urinary tract infection (UTI), or they may present with sexual dysfunction, numbness of the extremities, or vision changes.

Medical Management

Diabetes management for older adults is similar to that for younger adults. Hypoglycemia should be avoided. The appropriate goal for A glycated hemoglobin (A1C) is individualized with the following considerations: (1) older adult is fit and healthy; (2) older adult has a life expectancy greater than 10 years; (3) older adult has risks for hypoglycemia; and (4) older adult has the ability to follow the treatment regimen (Munshi, 2024). Generally, the goal for A1C in the healthy older population should be <7.5%; in frail, older adults with comorbidities, the A1C should be ≤8% ([ADA], 2020).

The risk for hypoglycemia among older adults is increased. Manifestations of hypoglycemia are often mistaken for other neurologic disorders, such as transient ischemic attacks (TIAs) (Munshi, 2024). A mild hypoglycemic event can lead to falls and fractures. Additionally, episodes of hypoglycemia increase the older adult's risk for cardiovascular events, dysrhythmias, and dementia.

Medical management also includes risk reduction by emphasizing cessation of smoking, controlling HTN, managing dyslipidemia, promoting exercise, and aspirin therapy (Munshi, 2024). Initial drug therapy among healthy older adults includes metformin along with lifestyle modification. If metformin is contraindicated or the patient is intolerant, then short-acting sulfonylurea (e.g., glipizide) is recommended; however, older adults are at an increased risk for hypoglycemia and weight gain (LeRoith et al, 2019). Other drugs that can be used as initial therapy include nonsulfonylurea secretagogues (e.g., repaglinide). Combination antidiabetic drugs may be more beneficial in controlling hyperglycemia than a single drug. Thiazolidinediones is not recommended for older adults due to the risk for fluid retention, weight gain, and increased risks of heart failure. Some oral antidiabetic drugs are listed in Table 23.4; dosages, drug effects, and nursing considerations are provided in Table 23.5. Insulin could be beneficial, especially if the A1C is >9%, fasting plasma glucose is >250 mg/dL, random glucose is consistently >300 mg/dL, or ketonuria is present. Insulin is further discussed later.

Nursing Care Guidelines for Type 2 Diabetes Mellitus

The clinical judgment (nursing process) in T2DM addresses the core defects of impaired insulin secretion and insulin action, as well as the prevention of vascular and microvascular complications of the eyes, heart, kidneys, and feet (Fig. 23.5). Lifestyle modifications based on the older adult's cognitive capacity and functional limitations are incorporated into the plan of care.

Recognize cues (assessment). Comprehensive nursing assessment of the older adult includes a thorough review of past medical, surgical, and family histories. The nurse should ask the patient about current drugs, particularly diuretics, β-blockers, anticonvulsants, antihypertensives, and steroids. Asking patients to bring in their prescription and over-the-counter drugs would help the nurse assess for potential problems related to drug interactions or for drugs that alter blood glucose levels. The nurse should determine the drug's name, type, dose, and schedule; if possible, the nurse should try to observe drug administration. Self-care abilities or restrictions, self-monitoring of blood glucose levels, and any history of hypoglycemia or hyperglycemia should be assessed.

Nutritional assessment includes a current weight measurement and recent patterns of loss or gain, typical dietary patterns, changes in the sense of taste or smell, dentition, and ability to shop for and prepare foods. Because uncontrolled diabetes affects the fluid and food balance, the nurse should assess patients for signs and symptoms of nausea, vomiting, hunger, and thirst, considering that hyperglycemia may produce subtle symptoms in older adults.

Assessment of elimination in an older adult with diabetes includes obtaining a history of urinary incontinence, urinary frequency, nocturia, polyuria, sexual dysfunction, and pain during urination. The nurse should evaluate for fecal incontinence, constipation, and diarrhea. Stress incontinence, which is more common in older adults, may be intensified by hyperglycemia.

Assessment of current living conditions is essential. The nurse should ask if the individual lives alone or with others, if living arrangements afford the ability to prepare food, and if adequate financial resources are available for food and shelter. Additionally, the nurse should determine whether transportation to healthcare services is available to the older adult patient.

It is important to assess a patient's learning ability before assessing knowledge of diabetes and its management. Cognitive function and learning styles vary, so knowing the patient's preferred learning style facilitates education. Some individuals prefer to learn by visual methods, others by listening, and still others by experiencing contact in a hands-on approach.

T2DM is associated with increased depression and memory problems in older adults (Munshi, 2024). These problems are often aggravated by uncontrolled diabetes or hyperglycemia. It is important for the nurse to evaluate current and past blood glucose results. The nurse should assess the older adult's ability to remember simple facts and his or her mood and level of anxiety. For example, the nurse may ask a patient to explain content that was just presented. If the patient cannot recall, the nurse needs to determine whether a learning or memory problem exists. Memory testing may be accomplished simply by asking patients to repeat number sequences or by making a short- or long-term memory assessment. The nurse should ask the older patient about neurologic symptoms such as numbness, tingling, blurred vision, headaches, and the inability to sense temperature, especially in the feet.

TABLE 23.4 Oral Antidiabetic Agents

Classification	Drugs
Thiazolinediones	Rosiglitazone Pioglitazone
Biguanides	Metformin Metformin extended-release
α-glucosidase inhibitors	Acarbose, miglitol
Sulfonylureas	Chlorpropamide (avoid in older adults) Glipizide Glimepiride Glyburide Tolazamide Tolbutamide
Nonsulfonylurea secretagogues	Nateglinide, repaglinide
Fixed-dose combinations	Multiple combination drugs with metformin are available.

Data from McCuistion, L. E., Vuljoin-DiMaggio, K., Winton, M. B., & Yeager, J. J. (2023). *Pharmacology: A patient-centered nursing process approach* (11th ed.). St. Louis, MO: Elsevier.

TABLE 23.5 Common Oral Drugs for Type 2 Diabetes Mellitus

Parameter	Biguanides	TZDs	Sulfonylureas	α-Glucosidase Inhibitors
Mechanism of actions	Decreased hepatic glucose Increased skeletal muscle sensitivity, increased intestinal glucose absorption	Increased insulin sensitivity	Increased insulin secretion Decreased hepatic glucose production	Decreased carbohydrate digestion and absorption from gastrointestinal tract
Glucose effects	Fasting and postprandial	Fasting and postprandial	Fasting and postprandial	Postprandial
Hypoglycemia as monotherapy	Usually not	No	Yes	No
Weight gain	No	Yes	Yes	No
Insulin levels	Decreased	Decreased	Increased	Decreased
Side effects	Gastrointestinal (self-limiting symptoms of nausea, diarrhea, anorexia). Serious effects include lactic acidosis and hepatotoxicity	Swelling and edema; weight gain Serious side effects include HF	Potential allergic reaction if patient has sulfa allergy Potential drug interactions (first-generation drugs) Nervousness, tremors, weight gain, and confusion Serious side effects include aplastic anemia, thrombocytopenia, seizures, and coma	Gastrointestinal (flatulence, abdominal distention, diarrhea)
Lipid effects	Decreased	Decreased	Increased or decreased	Decreased
Starting dose for a 70-kg person	Metformin 500 mg/d with evening meal	Varies with each drug: pioglitazone 15 to 30 mg/d in monotherapy rosiglitazone 4 mg/d in monotherapy	Varies with each drug: glyburide 1.25 to 2.5 mg/d with first meal of the day; glyburide, micronized 1.5 to 3 mg/d administered with first meal of the day; glipizide 5 mg/d 30 minutes before meal; glipizide ER 5 mg/d 30 minutes before first meal of the day; glimepiride 1 mg/d	Acarbose 25 mg/tid, with first bite of each meal
Maximum dose	2550 mg/d in divided doses with meals; can be divided	Pioglitazone 45 mg/d; rosiglitazone 8 mg/d, without regard to food	Varies with each agent: glyburide 20 mg/d in single or divided doses; glyburide, micronized 12 mg/d; glipizide 40 mg/d in divided doses; glipizide extended release 20 mg/d with first meal of the day; glimepiride 8 mg/d	150–300 mg/d in divided doses based on weight Must be taken with the first bite of food at each meal
Contraindications	Type 1 diabetes Renal dysfunction Hepatic dysfunction History of alcohol abuse Chronic conditions associated with hypoxia (asthma, chronic obstructive pulmonary disease, HF) Acute conditions associated with potential for hypoxia (surgery, acute myocardial infarction, HF) Situations associated with potential renal dysfunction (e.g., intravenous contrast media) DKA	Type 1 diabetes Class III or IV HF	Type 1 diabetes Hepatic dysfunction Avoid long-acting sulfonylureas to older adults DKA	Type 1 diabetes Inflammatory bowel disease DKA Bowel obstruction Cirrhosis Chronic conditions associated with maldigestion or malabsorption

d, Day; *DKA*, diabetic ketoacidosis; *HF*, heart failure; *kg*, kilogram; *mg*, milligram; *tid*, three times daily; *TZD*, thiazolidinediones.
Data from Carpenito, L. J. (2023). *Nursing diagnosis: Application to clinical practice* (16th ed.). Philadelphia: Lippincott Williams & Wilkins; and McAuley, D. F. (2017). *Diabetes*. GlobalRPh [website]. Retrieved July 20, 2023 from http://www.globalrph.com/diabetes.htm#Biguanides.

The nurse should assess the patient's skin condition, paying particular attention to the skin on the feet, legs, and elbows because these areas are at greatest risk for skin breakdown from pressure. The nurse should assess the skin for intactness, color, presence of swelling, discharge, odor, turgor, dryness, peeling, and lesions. Assessment of the skin in the perianal area may provide information on current skin status and general hygiene practices. Patients with hyperglycemia are prone to yeast and fungal infections in this area. Poor hygiene may predispose an individual to urinary or vaginal infections.

To assess circulation, the nurse should take an apical pulse, noting rate and rhythm; check pedal pulses bilaterally; and note the presence of hair on the lower extremities. The nurse should take blood pressure measurements with the patient in both the recumbent position and the sitting position; note any dizziness associated with a change of position; and assess the respiratory rate, depth, and chest sounds.

Analyze cues and prioritize hypotheses (patient problems). Problems for an older patient with T2DM include the following:
- Need for health teaching resulting from diabetes self-management and skills
- Decreased tissue perfusion - peripheral, resulting from decreased or interrupted arterial flow
- Potential for reduced skin integrity resulting from impaired circulation
- Inadequate or excessive nutrition resulting from decreased functional capacity, altered taste, and deficient knowledge
- Reduced sexual expression resulting from metabolic alterations
- Inadequate coping resulting from metabolic alteration or feelings of distress

Generate solutions (planning). The goal of nursing management for older adults with DM is the achievement and maintenance of desired blood glucose control, prevention of hypoglycemia and complications, and self-care management when feasible. Expected outcomes for the plan of care include the following:
1. The patient follows the plan of care by taking action based on professional advice, as evidenced by:
   a. Report of following prescribed regimen
   b. Correct modification of regimen as directed by a health professional
   c. Performance of self-screening currently and routinely
2. The patient shows evidence of successful individual coping, as evidenced by:
   a. Verbalization of a sense of control
   b. Verbalization of acceptance of the situation
   c. Use of available social support
3. The patient demonstrates increased knowledge of the American Diabetes Association (ADA) diet, as evidenced by:
   a. Verbalization of the rationale for a prescribed diet
   b. Setting goals for the diet
   c. Selection of foods recommended in the diet
4. The patient demonstrates an understanding of drug administration, as evidenced by:
   a. Statement of correct drug name, dose, and schedule
   b. Correct demonstration of drawing up and self-injection of insulin
   c. Description of side effects of the drug
5. The patient maintains peripheral circulation, as evidenced by:
   a. Pink, warm extremities without lesions or ulcers
   b. Verbalization of the need for daily skin and extremity inspections
6. The patient correctly demonstrates a foot-care regimen of foot cleansing and inspection techniques.
7. The patient verbalizes satisfaction with the degree of sexual functioning and ability.

The family or significant others should be involved in the care planning because they often provide the support and reinforcement needed for the long-term management of a chronic condition.

Take actions (nursing interventions). The nursing care of an older adult patient with T2DM is often complex. Usually, many issues must be dealt with; therefore, it is important to prioritize problems. In general, emergent issues or life-threatening crises such as severe hyperglycemia, hypoglycemia, and sepsis are top priorities. Once crises are resolved, the nurse may provide education to support diabetes management.

Education. The nurse provides or coordinates education on a variety of recommended diabetic topics such as drugs, pathophysiology of diabetes, monitoring of blood glucose levels, hypoglycemia and hyperglycemia, sick day management, foot care, eye care, complications, the diabetic diet, product supplies, and instructions on when to contact the health-care team. Teaching is facilitated if older patients and significant others are actively involved in learning (e.g., having patients demonstrate glucose monitoring or insulin injection techniques to the nurse). Teaching aids such as booklets and handouts may enhance learning. Resources for patient educational handouts may be obtained from the ADA, the National Diabetes Information Clearinghouse (NDIC), and commercial sources.

Diet. Although diet is the cornerstone of therapy for diabetes, it may be difficult to persuade older adults to change their dietary patterns. Other factors affecting dietary adherence include limited finances, social isolation, and lack of motivation (Wood, 2017). Dietary planning with a registered dietitian may be helpful in achieving dietary goals. Dietary goals include achieving good nutrition and reaching or maintaining the ideal body weight while decreasing the risk for hyperlipidemia, atherosclerosis, and hypertension. When a diet plan is established, nursing interventions are directed at supporting the dietitian's recommendations by assessing the patient's understanding of and adherence to the plan (see Nutritional Considerations box).

Insulin and oral hypoglycemic drugs. Simple is better when treating older adults to reduce the risk for hypoglycemic events. The ability of the older adult to self-manage (e.g., cognitive function) should be considered before initiating insulin. Many older patients have difficulty managing frequent glucose tests and insulin injections (ADA, 2018). Insulin therapy requires the older patient or their caregiver to give the insulin; therefore, the patient or the caregiver should have adequate visual, motor, and cognitive skills to properly administer the drug (ADA, 2018). Insulin doses should be individualized, and hypoglycemia should be avoided. Once-daily basal insulin is usually best and with minimal side effects (ADA, 2018). Written instructions about the drug regimen should be provided for a patient and his or her significant other.

NUTRITIONAL CONSIDERATIONS

Nutritional Goals for Patients With Diabetes Mellitus

Calories
Caloric intake should be individualized
Eat enough calories while maintaining their ideal weight
Do not focus on losing weight
Control blood sugar and avoid hypoglycemia

Protein
Approximately 12% to 20% of total calories
Recommended daily allowance: 0.8 grams per kilogram (g/kg) of body weight for adults (most adults consume twice the amount of protein needed)

Carbohydrates
Approximately 45% to 60% of total calories
Emphasis placed on total carbohydrate intake rather than eliminating simple sugars
Modest sucrose intake perhaps acceptable based on metabolic control
Consistent mealtime carbohydrate intake

Fats
No more than 30% of total calories
May need further reduction depending on lipid profile
Polyunsaturated fats: 6% to 8%
Saturated fats: 10%
Monounsaturated fats: remaining percentage

Fiber
25 g per 1000 kilocalories (kcal) for low-calorie intake
Up to 40 g/day

Sodium
3000 milligrams per day (mg/day) or less
May be reduced for medical conditions such as hypertension, congestive heart failure, and edema

Vitamins and Minerals
No specific recommendations

Data from Muñoz-Pareja, M., León-Muñoz, L. M., Guallar-Castillón, P., Graciani, A., López-García, E., Banegas, J. R., et al. (2012). The diet of diabetic patients in Spain in 2008 to 2010: Accordance with the main dietary recommendations—a cross-sectional study. *PLoS One, 7*(6), e39454.

The nurse should observe the patient and his or her significant other preparing the prescribed insulin dosages, observe the patient actually injecting insulin, and note if the patient draws up an accurate amount of insulin, injects it into an appropriate site, and discards the sharp needle in a puncture-proof container. Vision or manual dexterity problems common among older adults, which may interfere with proper insulin delivery, may be identified through observation. The patient's physician should be notified of visual concerns to obtain appropriate medical equipment for visually impaired persons.

Older patients may require two insulin injections daily to control blood glucose levels. Splitting the intermediate insulin dose or adding short-acting insulin may help prevent hypoglycemia and offer flexibility for older adults with eating pattern variations or decreased renal function. Home care or visiting nurse services may be useful to older adults in the initial phases of insulin therapy (Farmer et al, 2012).

Because hypoglycemia is the major complication of insulin and oral hypoglycemic therapy, patients should be instructed about this complication. Oral drugs are associated with other adverse effects such as rashes, itching, nausea, vomiting, liver damage, and increased urinary frequency and urgency. Routine medical visits that include laboratory testing for complications are important. Patients taking drugs that lower glucose levels should recognize the symptoms of mild hypoglycemia and test their blood glucose accordingly; if the result is abnormal, they should ingest a source of rapid-acting carbohydrates such as 4 ounces of orange juice. The early recognition and treatment of mild hypoglycemia prevents the more serious neuroglycopenic symptoms associated with moderate and severe hypoglycemia. Unrecognized and untreated hypoglycemia puts an individual with diabetes at risk for seizures and even death.

Emergency identification. Patients should be advised to carry medical emergency identification. If an individual who takes oral hypoglycemic experiences a major complication such as severe hypoglycemia, medical emergency identification facilitates treatment of the condition by healthcare workers or others (Table 23.6).

Monitoring. Monitoring the blood glucose level is recommended for older patients with T2DM because they tend to have higher renal thresholds. Blood glucose monitoring is used to achieve and maintain desired glucose goals, detect complications such as hyperglycemia and hypoglycemia, and educate patients about the effects of diet, drugs, activity, and stress (Mbaezue et al, 2010). Blood glucose monitoring is particularly important for individuals taking drugs that lower blood glucose levels (e.g., oral hypoglycemics and insulin). Among healthy older adults without comorbidities, the blood glucose should be between 140 and 150 mg/dL (Munshi, 2024). The glycemic goal should be higher at 160 to 170 mg/dL for those with significant comorbidities. Glucose monitoring devices are generally easy to use and reliable; however, practicing the glucose monitoring technique is important for ensuring the accuracy of test results.

Exercise. Exercise is a strategy for decreasing IR and hyperglycemia. It is beneficial for older adults from both physiologic

TABLE 23.6 Hypoglycemia Levels, Symptoms, and Treatment

Hypoglycemia Level	Symptoms	Treatment
Mild	Hunger, diaphoresis, nervousness, shakiness, tachycardia, and pale skin	15 g of carbohydrate 4 oz of juice (no sugar added)
Moderate	Headache, irritability, fatigue, blurred vision, and mood changes	15 g of carbohydrate; may repeat
Severe	Unresponsiveness, confusion, coma, and convulsions	Glucagon; intravenous glucose

Data from Carpenito L. J. (2023). *Nursing diagnosis: Application to clinical practice* (16th ed.). Philadelphia: Lippincott Williams & Wilkins.

and psychological perspectives. The assumption that older persons are not physically capable of or willing to exercise may result in neglect of this important aspect of care. Once the patient's capabilities and limitations are considered, an exercise program is personalized to the patient. Teaching topics should include the safety rules of exercising, which include wearing a medical alert bracelet, checking blood glucose before exercise, identifying hypoglycemia signs and symptoms, carrying a carbohydrate source, and avoiding dehydration. Exercise-related complications or injuries are more likely to occur in this population as a result of preexisting conditions such as cardiac, musculoskeletal, and ophthalmic diseases. Therefore, precautions and exercise modifications for older adults are indicated to help prevent problems.

Lifestyle changes. Lifestyle changes are often required for individuals with diabetes. It is difficult to manage a chronic illness that affects diet, exercise, weight, drugs, sexuality, and finances. Proper diabetes management requires knowledge, skills, and the organization of a team of experts that includes the patient as the core of the team. Avoidance of smoking and alcohol is believed to improve diabetes management. An older patient's ability to adapt to lifestyle changes must be evaluated *frequently* so that additional support can be provided when needed.

Sick day management. Older adults have a high incidence of chronic illness, and those with diabetes need to take special measures for "sick days." *Sick days* are generally defined as illness days that necessitate an alteration of typical treatment strategies (e.g., increasing drugs [insulin doses], meals, and fluids) or the initiation of medical interventions (e.g., antibiotics for infections). For example, when an individual with diabetes becomes ill with "stomach flu," the stress of even this common illness may precipitate severe hyperglycemia. The individual may detect significant hyperglycemia during routine blood glucose testing and should contact the health-care provider for specific instructions on increasing the insulin dosage. Individuals with nausea and vomiting are generally instructed to take 8 ounces of fluids (nondiet beverages) hourly and increase monitoring of blood glucose levels. Instructions from the provider usually indicate the levels of blood glucose that require an immediate call to the provider or a visit to the emergency department (see the Emergency Treatment box).

Skin alterations. Lower extremity amputations are a common yet preventable problem for individuals with diabetes. Individuals with diabetes who develop foot ulcers may be as high as 30% (Boulton, 2019). Foot ulcers increase the risk for amputation; up to 85% are preceded by foot ulcers. Foot ulcers occur usually due to trauma and can affect small and large vessels (Fig. 23.6). Prevention of foot ulcers is the key to proper foot management in older patients with diabetes. This is achieved through daily cleansing of the feet with nondrying agents, inspection of the feet, and prompt treatment of problems (see the Patient/Family Teaching box). When older adult patients are unable to inspect their own feet because of mobility or vision problems, significant others should be taught how to perform thorough inspections.

EMERGENCY TREATMENT

Sick Day Management for the Individual With Diabetes Mellitus

The term *sick days* refers to episodes of acute illness in individuals with diabetes, involving complications such as nausea, vomiting, and diarrhea. Illnesses trigger stress hormone production and result in hyperglycemia. With the onset of gastrointestinal symptoms, individuals with diabetes become easily dehydrated. If the patient's meal plan cannot be tolerated, easily digested foods such as plain soda, soups, popsicles, and crackers are taken instead. This diet may be supplemented with noncaloric liquids such as water or diet sodas to replace fluids lost from vomiting or diarrhea.

Individuals with diabetes must continue taking prescribed drugs such as insulin or oral hypoglycemic agents, ensure adequate hydration, and test blood sugar more often. Urine should be tested for ketones whenever the blood glucose level is >240 milligrams per deciliter (mg/dL). Other recommendations include obtaining and recording all temperatures, weights, and any interventions provided to the patient. Patients with diabetes should contact their health-care provider whenever they have questions or concerns or the treatment regimen is not working. Patients should seek emergent care of they have trouble breathing, have moderate to high ketones in the urine, blood sugar is <60, temperature >101° F for an extended period, decreasing alertness or ability to think, vomiting and/or diarrhea that persists for ≥6 hours (CDC, 2022).

Sick day management is important in individuals with T2DM because an untreated illness may lead to a complication called *hyperglycemic hyperosmolar nonketotic coma* (HHNC). This hyperglycemic condition is more common in older patients with T2DM, whereas patients with T1DM are more likely to experience diabetic ketoacidosis. HHNC is characterized by severe dehydration and hyperglycemia (blood glucose values ≥600 mg/dL; and hyperosmolarity of blood: ≥340 milliosmoles per liter [mOsm/L] of water]). Treatment for HHNC consists of insulin, intravenous fluids, and identification and treatment of the precipitating event (e.g., infection or cardiovascular problems) in the intensive care setting of a hospital.

PATIENT/FAMILY TEACHING

Prevention of Foot Ulcers in Individuals With Diabetes Mellitus

- Perform daily foot inspection.
- Perform daily foot hygiene using warm (not hot) soapy water to wash feet; pat feet dry.
- Gently apply mild skin cream to feet if dry or rough; do not apply between toes.
- Keep toenails trimmed straight across.
- Wear socks and proper-fitting shoes; do not go barefoot.
- Measure feet when purchasing new shoes; break them in gradually.
- Do not wear tight shoes or stockings that bind.
- Exercise regularly and maintain ideal body weight.
- Avoid smoking because it impairs circulation to the feet.
- Seek early interventions to problems (e.g., tenderness, redness, swelling, leakage of fluid).

Foot care is the same for older adults as for other persons with diabetes. Daily inspection and cleansing of feet with nondrying agents is important to eliminate potential infectious organisms. Lubrication of the feet (but not between the toes, where heat and lotions may be trapped and lead to infections)

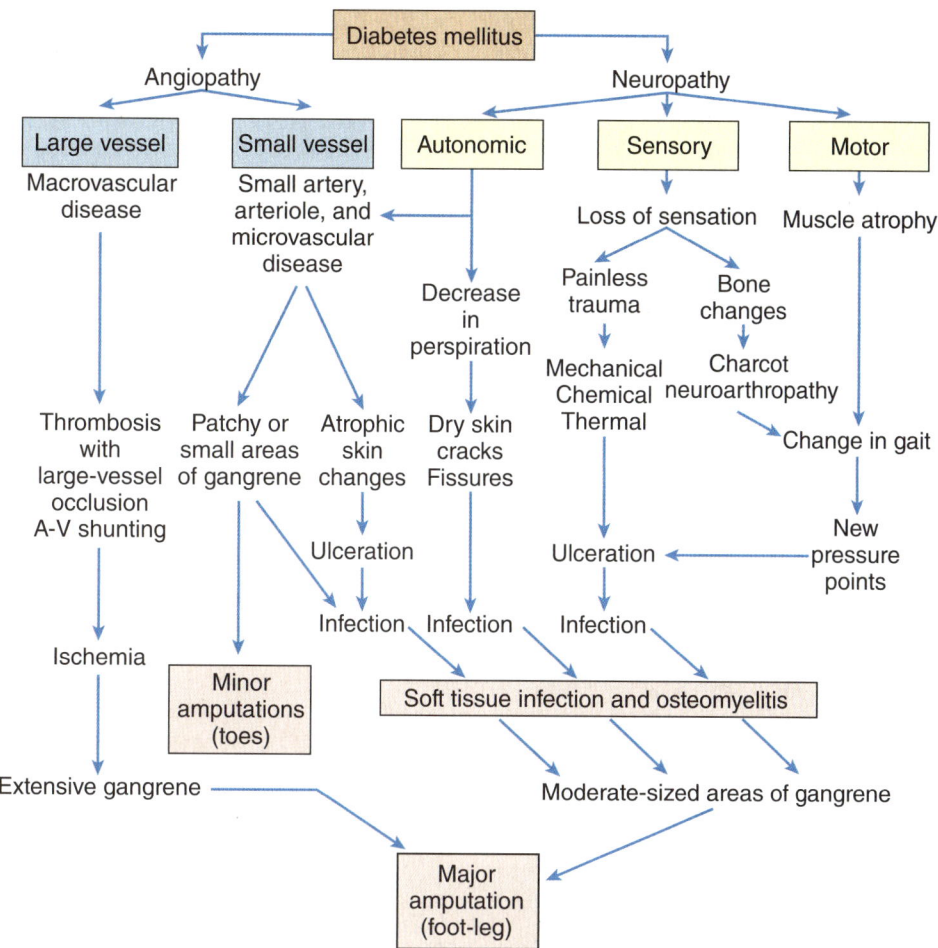

Fig. 23.6 How foot lesions of diabetes can lead to amputation. (From Levin, M. E., O'Neal, L. W., & Bowker, J. H. [1993]. *The diabetic foot* [5th ed.]. St. Louis, MO: Mosby.)

with unscented lotions is often needed to help decrease skin dryness and cracking. Appliances such as corn pads and drying agents such as alcohol should be avoided because they impair the integrity of the skin. Shoes need to be tested for a good fit. Patients or caretakers should cut nails straight across to prevent complications. Individuals with diabetes with foot neuropathy, significant hyperglycemia (blood glucose values of ≥250 mg/dL), or a history of foot infections should seek care at the first sign of a wound or infection to the feet.

Wound infections. Older adults with diabetes are at a higher risk for foot complications than those without diabetes because of changes in nerves and blood vessels. Because these foot problems are common, the phrase *diabetic foot syndrome* has come into use to describe the vascular and neurologic pathology associated with diabetes. Inadequate blood flow to the feet and nerve damage contribute to developing ulcers and infections. Hyperglycemia also plays a role in foot problems because blood glucose levels of ≥200 mg/dL are associated with an altered immune system leukocytic response.

The clinical symptoms of foot infections vary from no symptoms to fever, erythema, warmth, discharge with ulceration, and leukocytosis (Peters et al, 2012). The skin over and around the infection may appear white, pink, red, or shades of blue. Blood vessels may be distended and pronounced over the infection site. Nail beds may be pale, and show slowed capillary refilling when pressed. The shape of the foot may be altered by infection due to significant soft tissue swelling. Superficial inspection of a lesion may be deceptive because the outside appearance often does not reflect the extent of the problem beneath the skin's surface. Wound infections in older adults with diabetes are common and are serious events that require immediate attention. Infections may manifest symptoms such as pain, swelling, and redness or may be symptom-free and remain undetected until they are at an advanced stage. Significant delays may occur before the health-care provider is contacted and treatment is initiated, and infection may spread from the skin to fat, muscle, fascia, and bone (osteomyelitis).

Evaluate outcomes (evaluation). The nurse evaluates the effectiveness of the care plan for an older patient with diabetes by frequently measuring the achievement of established specific outcomes. For example, nutritional outcomes include food selection consistent with the prescribed meal plan. Achievement of weight change goals is measured over time with weight graphs. The patient may be asked to log his or her exercise and drug compliance to enable monitoring of progress with each activity.

Insulin injection site rotations may be tracked on a chart. The patient logs blood glucose values, which are then compared with corresponding laboratory results. Patients are examined to see whether they wear or carry medical alert bracelets or other emergency information. Patients may be asked to review their recent experiences with sick days and their management of fluids, nausea, vomiting, drugs, and testing.

An important principle of diabetes management is having the patient "take control" of the diabetes. Self-care activities such as daily inspection of the feet and basic diabetic foot care support this self-care approach. The nurse may help a patient evaluate the effectiveness of self-care activities by direct examination and interview techniques.

The nurse should positively reinforce effective diabetes management strategies used by an older patient. For example, when an older patient improves in foot care or the technique

NURSING CARE PLAN
Diabetes Mellitus With Foot Infection

Clinical Situation

Mr. J notices that his right foot aches slightly. Taking off his shoe, he can see that his foot is red and swollen with a small amount of purulent fluid draining from a lesion on his small toe. He can even see the indentations from his shoes on the skin of his feet. He is surprised that his foot looks this bad when he had no problems earlier. He makes an appointment with his primary care provider. The appointment is 2 days after he first noticed the problem. During those 2 days, Mr. J becomes increasingly tired. Despite drinking fluids continuously, he is thirsty all the time. At the visit with his physician, Mr. J is found to have 3+ edema in the affected foot, temperature of 101° F, and blood glucose level of 250 milligrams per deciliter (mg/dL). He is diagnosed with a diabetic foot infection. Mr. J first learns of his diagnosis of diabetes mellitus at this time.

The physician sends Mr. J to the local community hospital for inpatient admission. Hospitalization is necessary to treat the foot infection and his newly diagnosed diabetes.

Recognize Cues (Assessment)

- Right foot achy
- Right foot red and swollen with indentations from shoes
- Lesion to the small toe on right foot with small amount of purulent fluid
- Increasingly tired
- Thirsty all the time
- 3+ edema to right foot
- Temperature 101° F
- Blood glucose 250 mg/dL

Analyze Cues and Prioritize Hypotheses (Patient Problems)

- Infection resulting from microorganisms entering through the impaired skin
- Reduced skin integrity resulting from compromised innate defense (skin)
- Pain resulting from treatments for foot ulcer (e.g., biopsy, curettage, and debridement)
- Need for health teaching resulting from new experience with recently diagnosed diabetes mellitus
- Need for patient teaching resulting from new experience with foot care management

Generate Solutions and Evaluate Outcomes (Planning and Evaluation)

- Wound healing will occur, as demonstrated by decreasing size of wound and less purulent drainage, as well as laboratory values of complete blood cell count with differential and electrolytes within normal limits.
- Circulation to affected area will be maintained, as evidenced by normal skin color and temperature, presence of pedal pulses, and no evidence of edema.
- The patient will verbalize comfort after debridement procedures.
- The patient will maintain stable vital signs before, during, and after the procedure.
- The patient will verbalize and demonstrate understanding of diabetes and diabetes management, as evidenced by making appropriate diet selections, correctly and safely administering drugs, and accurately testing his blood glucose level.
- The patient will verbalize appropriate sick day management regimen.
- The patient will demonstrate daily foot care regimen of inspecting, cleansing, and using emollients.
- The patient will verbalize when to contact a physician if complications occur.
- The patient will achieve an optimal level of physical mobility, as evidenced by the ability to safely meet self-care needs.
- The patient will protect the affected extremity, as evidenced by the ability to adhere to weight-bearing restriction.
- The patient will verbalize reduced levels of anxiety with increasing knowledge and skill acquisition.

Take Actions (Nursing Interventions)

- Assess the wound at each dressing change for wound stage, epithelialization, color, edema, and discharge.
- Assess vital signs.
- Administer antibiotics, as prescribed.
- Administer physician-ordered intravenous fluids, insulin, and drugs.
- Notify the health-care provider of signs and symptoms of increased pain, swelling, drainage, or fever.
- Change linens, as needed, to maintain a clean wound environment.
- Provide pain control during debridement by medicating before procedures.
- Assess patient's vital signs and level of consciousness before administering drugs.
- Assess pain level, vital signs, and level of comfort and sedation after drug.
- Document the patient's tolerance of the procedure.
- Assess patient understanding of the condition.
- Monitor readiness and determine best methods for teaching and learning.
- Provide patient information on diabetes over span of his hospitalization, including topics such as T2DM; ADA diet; exercise; drugs; sick day management; monitoring; lifestyle factors (e.g., smoking and alcohol); complications, especially of hypoglycemia and hyperglycemia; and eye, kidney, nerve, foot, and vessel problems.
- Provide proper foot care teaching with demonstration, including topics such as daily inspection and cleansing, wearing shoes, avoidance of tape and drying chemicals, use of proper foot gear, applying emollients, keeping feet dry, and safe nail cutting.
- Have the patient perform a return demonstration.
- Instruct the patient on reportable signs and symptoms such as fever, pain, swelling, redness, and breaks in skin integrity.
- Instruct the patient not to bear weight on the infected foot.
- Set up the room to maximize patient independence in activities of daily living.
- Assess the patient's mood and coping mechanisms.
- Allow the patient to verbalize feelings about the diagnosis of the chronic disease of diabetes.
- Support the patient in self-care and management of diabetes by (1) encouraging involvement in self-care activities, (2) providing an environment conducive to relaxation, and (3) reassuring the patient when he safely or accurately performs self-care skills and techniques.

for insulin injections, the nurse needs to acknowledge the patient's skill. If a patient does not comply with management strategies, the situation needs to be reassessed so that adaptations can be made. An older patient may have cognitive, financial, or social support problems that hinder compliance.

Documentation of assessments — including patient responses to treatment measures, patient comprehension of teaching, and patient ability to self-manage treatment measures and diet, as well as other nursing interventions — is an essential component of care for older adult patients with diabetes.

Next-Generation NCLEX® Examination-Style Case Study

Phase 1, Question 1
Scenario: The nurse is caring for a 71-year-old patient in the emergency room. The nurse documents vital signs and assessment findings in the nurses' notes.

| Health History | **Nurses' Notes** | Physician's Orders | Laboratory Profile |

0730:
71-year-old patient brought in by a family member due to increased confusion and frequent urination. The daughter also reports the patient has been "sleeping all the time." The patient has a history of hypertension and was recently diagnosed with a urinary tract infection and started on amoxicillin. Vital signs: Temperature: 99.6° F; blood pressure: 134/86 mm Hg supine/left arm; pulse: 94 beats per minute; respiratory rate: 18 breaths per minute; oxygen saturation: 94% on room air. Patient is oriented to name only, speech clear and articulate. Skin warm and dry, decreased turgor, few ecchymoses to arms, wound 1 cm × 0.5 cm beside callus of right great toe with mild erythema, no exudate. Heart with S_1, S_2, no arrhythmia. Lungs with crackles to bases bilaterally. Abdomen rounded, active bowel sounds in all quadrants, nontender to palpation.

Select the four (4) findings that require *immediate* follow-up by the nurse.
- ☐ Increased confusion
- ☐ Frequent urination
- ☐ "Sleeping all the time"
- ☐ Temperature 99.6° F
- ☐ Blood pressure 134/86 mm Hg
- ☐ Wound to right foot 1 cm × 0.5 cm and erythematous
- ☐ Ecchymoses to right arm
- ☐ Decreased skin turgor
- ☐ Diminished lung sounds to bases

Phase 1, Question 2
For each clinical finding below, place an "X" in the appropriate column to specify if the finding is consistent with the disease process of diabetes in the older adult, hypothyroidism, or metabolic syndrome. Each column must have at least one response. Each finding may support more than one disease process.

Assessment Findings	Diabetes	Hypothyroidism	Metabolic Syndrome
Confusion			
Polyuria			
Wound			
Fatigue/Lethargy			

Phase 2, Question 1
Scenario: The nurse on the medical-surgical unit received a Situation, Background, Assessment, and Recommendation (SBAR) on the 71-year-old patient from the emergency department (ED) nurse. The nurse documents the following:

| Health History | **Nurses' Notes** | Physician's Orders | Laboratory Profile |

1030:
Received SBAR from the ED nurse: vital signs - blood pressure 128/74 mm Hg, pulse 99 beats per minute, respiratory rate 20 breaths/minute and unlabored, temperature 100.4° F, oxygen saturation 94% on room air. Oriented to person only, calm; family member at bedside. Lungs with crackles to bases bilaterally, heart tones with S_1, S_2, extremities without edema. Wound to right foot 1 cm × 0.5 cm with erythematous border and pustulant drainage. Voided 800 mL of clear yellow urine. Medications received in the ED: Regular insulin 15 units intravenously, intravenous fluids of 0.9% sodium chloride 500 mL bolus then 125 mL/hr, potassium chloride 50 mEq in 50 mL of 0.9% sodium chloride at 17 mL/hr still infusing.

| Health History | Nurses' Notes | Physician's Orders | **Laboratory Profile** |

Laboratory Test	Result	Reference Range
White blood cell (WBC)	13.2	3.8 to 10.4 10^3/microL
Hemoglobin (Hgb)	11.3 L	11.9 to 16.9 g/dL
Hematocrit (Hct)	33%	35 to 50%
Sodium	136	135 to 145 mEq/L
Potassium	3.6	3.5 to 5 mEq/L
Glucose	425 H	Adult: 74–106 mg/dL or 4.1–5.9 mmol/L Older adult: 60–90 years: 82–115 mg/dL or 4.6–6.4 mmol/L >90 years: 75–121 mg/dL or 4.2–6.7 mmol/L
Creatinine	1.2	0.6 to 1.3 mg/dL
Blood urea nitrogen (BUN)	29 H	6 to 20 mg/dL

Complete the following sentence by choosing from the lists of options.
Upon receiving the patient from the emergency department nurse, the medical-surgical nurse would first monitor the patient for ____1____ due to receiving ___2____.

Continued

Next-Generation NCLEX® Examination-Style Case Study—cont'd

Terms for Option 1	Terms for Option 2
Hypertension	Regular insulin
Hypoglycemia	Potassium chloride
Hyperkalemia	Intravenous fluids

Phase 2, Question 2

Scenario: The nurse on the medical-surgical unit is planning care for the 71-year-old patient. At 1100, the nurse documents new assessment findings.

Health History	**Nurses' Notes**	Physician's Orders	Laboratory Profile

1100:
Family member reported the patient is "acting weird and breathing funny." Upon assessment, patient's respirations are shallow at 10 breaths per minute. Difficult to arouse. Skin pale. Lungs with crackles to bases. Other vital signs: Temperature 99.8° F, blood pressure 109/68, pulse 136 per minute, oxygen saturation 88% on room air. Reported findings to the health-care provider.

For each intervention, indicate with an "X" whether the intervention is emergently indicated or contraindicated.

Nursing Intervention	Indicated	Contraindicated
Request order to administer 0.9% sodium chloride 1000 mL bolus		
Obtain glucose reading		
Prepare the patient for intubation		
Request order to administer 10% dextrose intravenous push		
Place patient in Trendelenburg position		
Request order for oxygen		

Phase 3, Question 1

Scenario: The health-care provider places the following orders:

Health History	Nurses' Notes	**Physician's Orders**	Laboratory Profile

1120:
- Oxygen 2 L per nasal cannula; titrate to maintain oxygen saturation > 90%
- Give 10% dextrose intravenous push, once
- Obtain bedside glucose 10 minutes after 10% dextrose IV push
- Laboratory tests: Complete blood count (CBC), complete metabolic panel (CMP)
- Diagnostic test: Chest x-ray
- Consult wound therapy

Select the three (3) actions the nurse will carry out immediately.
- ☐ Increase oxygen flow
- ☐ Obtain blood for laboratory studies
- ☐ Obtain bedside glucose 10 minutes after 10% dextrose IV push
- ☐ Consult wound therapy
- ☐ Give 10% dextrose IV push, once
- ☐ Obtain chest x-ray

Phase 3, Question 2

Scenario: The nurse completes the actions as ordered by the health-care provider, documents the results in the nurses' notes, and evaluates the outcome.

Health History	**Nurses' Notes**	Physician's Orders	Laboratory Profile

1110:
New orders received. Bedside glucose 24 mg/dL. Administered 10% dextrose IVP. Initiated oxygen at 2 L per nasal canula. CBC, CMP, chest x-ray, and wound consult ordered and pending.

1120:
Reassessed. Labs, x-ray, and wound consult still pending.

Health History	Nurses' Notes	Physician's Orders	**Laboratory Profile**

Laboratory Test	Result for 0730	Result for 1110	Result for 1120	Reference Range
Bedside glucose		24 **L**	146 **H**	80 to 130 mg/dL

For each new assessment finding, use an "X" to specify if the finding indicates that the patient's condition is improved, no change, or declined.

Assessment Finding	Improved	No Change	Declined
Blood pressure 116/72 mm Hg			
Pulmonary crackles to bilateral bases			
Respiratory rate 20 breaths per minute			
Pulse 90 beats per minute			
Oxygen saturation 95% on 2 L per nasal canula			
Bedside glucose 146			
Skin pale, cool, and diaphoretic			

Hyperthyroidism

Pathophysiology

The size of the thyroid gland is usually reduced among older adults. Additionally, there are increased fibrotic changes (Salvatore et al, 2020). Older adults without comorbidities usually have normal free thyroxine (T_4) and decreased free triiodothyronine (T_3), but the thyroid-stimulating hormone (TSH) may increase or decrease based on dietary iodine intake. Thyroid dysfunction (hyperthyroidism or hypothyroidism) can affect muscle strength, cardiovascular health, bone health, and cognition.

Primary hyperthyroidism involves hypersecretion (hyperfunctioning) of thyroid hormones, usually associated with an enlarged thyroid gland. Hyperthyroidism in older adults is often caused by multinodular and uninodular toxic goiter rather than Graves' disease, which is the most common cause in younger adults (Medeiros-Neto, 2016). Thyroid nodules are identified in 5% of people older than age 60, and 90% of nodules are benign (Fig. 23.7). Iodine-induced hyperthyroidism is another common type of hyperthyroidism among older patients using amiodarone, a cardiac drug containing iodine, which deposits in tissue and delivers iodine to the circulation over long periods. Another common cause of hyperthyroidism among older adults is excessive amounts of exogenous thyroid hormone in the treatment of hypothyroidism (Samuels, 2021).

Subclinical hyperthyroidism, a condition in which an otherwise healthy, asymptomatic patient has a suppressed serum Triiodothyronine level with normal T_4 and T_3 levels, has been associated with an increased incidence of atrial fibrillation and decreased bone mineral density. *Thyroid storm,* or thyrotoxic crisis, is a life-threatening syndrome consisting of fever, severe tachycardia, altered mental status, dehydration, and irritability. It is most commonly seen in persons with Graves' disease, but it may result from other causes of hyperthyroidism. It may be precipitated by a concurrent illness, withdrawal from antithyroid drugs, toxic nodular hyperthyroidism, or treatment with radioactive iodine (Jones and Boelaert, 2015).

Signs and Symptoms

The predominant symptoms of hyperthyroidism among older adults are related to their cardiovascular health. Symptoms such as tachycardia, atrial fibrillation, and hypertension are common findings (Samuels, 2021). Other symptoms include fatigue, weight loss, agitation, anorexia, or cognitive decline. An enlarged, palpable goiter is often present in older adults with hyperthyroidism.

Medical Management

Untreated hyperthyroidism increases the risks for heart failure, bone fractures, and cardiovascular events among older adults (Veldhuis, 2013). Treatment for hyperthyroidism includes antithyroid drugs and radioactive iodine (American Thyroid Association [ATA], n.d.). Rarely is surgical intervention required due to the risk for surgery to older adults. Adjunctive treatment, such as with β-adrenergic blockers, can slow the heart rate of tachycardia.

Nursing Care Guidelines for Hyperthyroidism

Table 23.7 details how to recognize and analyze cues, prioritize hypotheses, generate solutions, take action, and evaluate outcomes for hyperthyroidism.

Hypothyroidism

Pathophysiology

A common *hypofunctioning* endocrine state that results from inadequate thyroid hormone function is hypothyroidism. Diagnosis is based on sensitive, reliable serum TSH and T4 level assays. The most sensitive indication of hypothyroidism caused by *primary* thyroid gland failure is an elevation of the serum TSH level. The most specific test finding is a subnormal serum-free T_4 level because it corrects for abnormalities in the T_4-binding proteins. As the thyroid gland ages, it develops moderate atrophy, fibrosis, colloid nodules, and lymphocyte infiltration (Garg and Vanderpump, 2013). The production of T_4 decreases by about 30% between young adulthood and advanced age. However, serum levels are usually maintained because of the body's decreased use of T_4 as a correlate to the age-related decline in lean body mass. Hypofunctioning thyroid states may result from defects in hormone production, target tissues, or receptors. When the defect involves a hypofunctioning peripheral gland like the thyroid, it is called *primary hypothyroidism.* If the hypothyroid state is a result of a nonfunctional anterior pituitary gland, the condition is called *secondary* hypothyroidism. *Tertiary* hypothyroidism results from a defect in the hypothalamus.

Approximately 12% of the US population have hypothyroidism and older adults are at an increased risk, with *autoimmune thyroiditis* and overtreatment of hyperthyroidism being the main cause of hypothyroidism (Seabright, 2024). Overtreatment

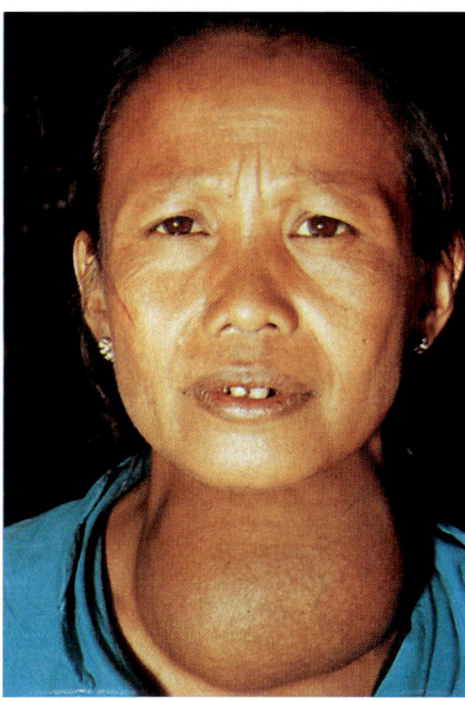

Fig. 23.7 Simple goiter. (Courtesy of Bergman, L.V. and Associates, Cold Spring, NY.)

TABLE 23.7　Hyperthyroidism

Recognize Cues (Assessment)	Analyze Cues and Prioritize Hypotheses (Patient Problems)	Generate Solutions (Planning)	Take Actions (Nursing Interventions)	Evaluate Outcomes (Evaluation)
1. Weight loss trends over 3 and 6 months 2. BMI 3. Serum albumin and thyroid-stimulating hormone 4. Mini nutritional assessment 5. Mini-Mental State Examination 6. Dysphagia 7. Manual dexterity 8. Financial resources 9. Dentition 10. Comorbidities 11. Drugs 12. Social support 13. Cultural influences 14. Tachycardia, defined as >90 beats/min 15. Fatigue	1. Inadequate nutrition 2. Potential for reduced cardiac tissue perfusion 3. Fatigue	1. Teach disease, treatment and monitoring. 2. Teach dietary recommendations of the National Research Council Report for those > 65 years. 3. Add 250- to 300-calorie snacks to increase body weight slowly. 4. Refer to Meals on Wheels, consultations, or other community resources as needed. 5. Monitor cardiovascular status.	1. Explain hyperthyroidism, complications, testing techniques, activity restrictions, dietary measures, drugs, radioactive iodine therapy (if needed), surgery (if needed), eye care for exophthalmos (if needed). 2. Facilitate specific meal plans, procurement, preparation, and social support. 3. Monitor for pulse rate <90 beats/min, respiratory rate < 22 breaths/min, normal blood pressure, bibasilar crackles, decreased urine output, pigmentation changes, cool or mottled skin, distended neck veins, decreased saturation of arterial oxygen (SaO_2).	1. Patient will increase intake as evidenced by gradual weight gain to normal range of body mass index. 2. Patient will maintain adequate cardiac output.

Data from Carpenito, L. J. (2023). *Nursing diagnosis: Application to clinical practice* (16th ed.). Philadelphia: Lippincott Williams & Wilkins.

and *drug-induced hypothyroidism* may occur with the use of lithium carbonate, amiodarone, and iodine (Orlander et al, 2022). Other causes of hypothyroidism include ablation of the thyroid gland with radioiodine or surgery for the treatment of hyperthyroidism and postsurgical or radiation treatment of head and neck cancer. Hypothalamic or pituitary problems are rarely originating causes (Schlumberger et al, 2012).

Signs and Symptoms

The clinical symptoms of hypothyroidism in older people are atypical compared with those of younger adults. Almost all cases of hypothyroidism in older adults are subclinical, inconspicuous, and progress slowly toward thyroid failure (Seabright, 2024). Because the condition is insidious, the symptoms are often attributed to aging. Older patients complain of fatigue, cold intolerance, weight gain, muscle cramps, paresthesia, and confusion (ATA, n.d.).

Medical Management

Treatment for hypothyroidism includes pure synthetic thyroxine (e.g., levothyroxine), which is instituted slowly so as not to place undue stress on the heart and the nervous system (ATA, n.d.). The usual starting dose is 25 micrograms (μg) per day. The drug is increased every 4 to 6 weeks until the serum levels of T_4 and TSH are within the normal range. For older adults without underlying cardiovascular or CNS disease, the initial dose may be higher.

Nursing Care Guidelines for Hypothyroidism

Recognizing and analyzing cues, prioritizing hypotheses, generating solutions, taking actions, and evaluating outcomes for hypothyroidism are detailed in Table 23.8.

Primary Osteoporosis

Pathophysiology

Osteoporosis is a legitimate concern in postmenopausal females and andropausal males because of the influence of systemic sex hormones on bone (Eastell, 2013). Found more frequently in postmenopausal females and older adults, osteoporosis is a disease characterized by low bone mass, leading to fragile bones that break easily. The aging skeleton is a metabolically active organ that experiences continuous remodeling, providing structural integrity, body support, protection of vital organs, and a reservoir of calcium and other minerals (Griffith, 2013). Low bone mass may result from a failure to reach peak bone mass as a young adult, increased bone resorption, or decreased bone formation; these three mechanisms are believed to play a role in osteoporosis.

Genetic influences on osteoblast function have recently improved our understanding of osteoporosis pathogenesis. Researchers have suggested that up to 80% of osteoporosis is genetically determined (Mäkitie et al, 2019), which supports the importance of family history in determining an individual's risk.

Hypersecretion of parathyroid hormone has also been shown to increase skeletal resorption in estrogen-deficient menopausal females; this same mechanism is believed to influence male osteoporosis (ATA, n.d.). Additionally, low vitamin D status in older persons contributes to bone loss mediated by the aging parathyroid gland, low daily exposure to natural sunlight, and reduced dietary intake. The primary role of calcium alone in maintaining bone mass in older persons continues to spur controversy. Osteopenia precedes osteoporosis, defined as bone mass <2.5 standard deviations below that of a young control population. Osteoporosis generally occurs in those in

TABLE 23.8 Hypothyroidism

Recognize Cues (Assessment)	Analyze Cues and Generate Hypotheses (Patient Problems)	Generate Solutions (Planning)	Take Actions (Nursing Interventions)	Evaluate Outcomes (Evaluation)
1. Fatigue on a scale of 1–10 2. Onset, pattern, and aggravating and relieving factors of fatigue 3. Effects of fatigue on activities of daily living (ADLs), instrumental ADLs (IADLs), mood, accident proneness, concentration, motivation, leisure activities, and libido 4. Depression Scale 5. Mini-Mental State Examination 6. Laboratory values of thyroid-stimulating hormone, hemoglobin, and hematocrit 7. Comorbidities 8. Drugs 9. Social support network 10. Weight as detailed in Table 23.3	1. Fatigue	1. Identify patient's energy patterns and teach energy conservation. 2. Facilitate prioritization and delegation of tasks. 3. Teach disease pathophysiology, drug management, and monitoring. 4. Facilitate appropriate community and financial resource use.	1. Explain patient's type of hypothyroidism, symptoms, complications, diagnostic tests, activity restrictions, dietary guidelines, lifelong therapy, and symptoms of accidental thyroid hormone overdose. 2. Work with patient to target ADLs and IADLs for patient performance, health care surrogate, and community services assistance.	1. Patient will achieve a balance of activity and rest. 2. Patient can verbalize pathophysiology, drug use, and monitoring required.

Data from Carpenito, L. J. (2023). *Nursing diagnosis: Application to clinical practice* (16th ed.). Philadelphia: Lippincott Williams & Wilkins.

the sixth decade or older. Divided into primary and secondary types based on etiology, osteoporosis involves both the appendicular and axial skeleton. Other endocrine disorders such as parathyroid disease, Cushing syndrome, hypogonadism, alcohol abuse, liver disease, and amenorrhea may cause secondary osteoporosis. Osteoporosis is diagnosed by dual-energy x-ray absorptiometry (DXA) of the proximal femur and lumbar spine because these scans are sensitive to subtle changes in mineral density.

Signs and Symptoms

Spontaneous fractures or those caused by minimum trauma, in addition to loss of height, necessitate DXA scanning in older patients because of the high incidence of occult osteoporosis. Because of its low cost and portability, ultrasonographic densitometry is frequently used on the heel; however, it is not considered as reliable as DXA scanning. A history of fractures after age 40, family history of osteoporosis, cigarette smoking, and low BMI have all been shown to correlate strongly with osteoporosis. Dorsal kyphosis, chronic back pain, and loss of height are common signs of primary osteoporosis in older persons (Van Meirhaeghe et al, 2013).

Medical Management

Calcium and vitamin D supplementation, exercise, and antiresorptive therapy are the cornerstones of medical therapy in primary osteoporosis (Elam et al, 2024). In the United States, the recommended intake for older adults is 1000 to 1200 mg/day of elemental calcium and 600 to 800 IU/day, and no more than 4000 IU/day, of vitamin D. Weight-bearing and muscle-strengthening exercises add minimally to bone density; however, they are important to maintain bone strength (Campbell, 2020). Additionally, a significant benefit is seen in improved posture, balance, and reduced falls. Estrogens, bisphosphonates, parathyroid hormone analogs (e.g., teriparatide), monoclonal antibodies (e.g., romosozumab), selective estrogen receptor modulators (e.g., raloxifene), and calcitonin are used in antiresorptive therapy based on the older patient's risk profile (Elam et al, 2024). However, patients at high risk for breast cancer should not take estrogen or selective estrogen receptor modulators to treat osteoporosis. Additionally, some clinicians choose a thiazide diuretic for those with hypertension as a comorbid condition because it decreases urinary calcium excretion, which slows bone loss; however, long-term use of thiazide diuretics can cause hyponatremia, which can exacerbate osteoporosis.

Nursing Care Guidelines for Osteoporosis

Recognizing and analyzing cues, prioritizing hypotheses, generating solutions, and evaluating outcomes for osteoporosis are detailed in Table 23.9.

Sexual Dysfunction

Erectile dysfunction (ED) and female sexual dysfunction (FSD) have garnered increased interest and research dollars in recent years as many older people strive to retain the vitality of their sexual function. Previously, sexual dysfunction was discreetly minimized or overlooked in the professional literature. A recent

TABLE 23.9	Osteoporosis			
Recognize Cues (Assessment)	**Analyze Cues and Prioritize Hypotheses (Patient Problems)**	**Generate Solutions (Planning)**	**Take Actions (Nursing Interventions)**	**Evaluate Outcomes (Evaluation)**
1. Use of hormone replacement therapy 2. Calcium and vitamin D intake 3. Exercise habits 4. Alcohol, caffeine, and protein intake 5. Current or past use of corticosteroids 6. History of thyroid, bowel, kidney, or liver disease 7. Use of excessive thyroid replacement 8. Weight as listed in Table 23.3 9. Comorbidities 10. Drugs 11. Social support 12. Cultural influences	1. Inadequate health maintenance	1. Teach disease and medical management and dietary recommendations of the National Research Council Report for those > 65 years. 2. Teach therapeutic lifestyle changes. 3. Ensure safety and fall awareness.	1. Teach pathophysiology, testing, drugs, monitoring, complications, sources of support and information, and fall precautions. 2. Provide for supervised meal planning, encourage food label reading, and calcium and vitamin D supplementation. 3. Have patient undergo postural retraining and weight-bearing exercises.	1. Patient will have an absence of fractures, no falls, and improved bone mineral density.

Data from Carpenito, L. J. (2023). *Nursing diagnosis: Application to clinical practice* (16th ed.). Philadelphia: Lippincott Williams & Wilkins.

cross-sectional study of males 40 to 88 years demonstrated the overall prevalence of ED to be 77% in males over 70 (Mola, 2015). FSD remains ill-defined, even though a relatively high rate of sexual dysfunction exists among postmenopausal females because of low desire, vaginal dryness, or inability to reach orgasm (Hughes et al, 2015) The effects of menopause appear to be incremental and additional to those characteristic of aging.

Pathophysiology

The causes of ED among males could be organic, psychological, or both, organic being vascular, hormonal, neurogenic, or anatomic (Mola, 2015). Hormonal changes associated with ED begin at 40 years old in the aging male and include decreased testosterone, decreased bioavailability of testosterone, increased sex hormone–binding globulin, decreased DHEA, mildly increased estradiol-17-β, decreased melatonin, and decreased GH and IGF-1 (Gratzke et al, 2010).

The female sexual response cycle comprises a neuroendocrine-mediated vascular and nonvascular smooth muscle relaxation, which results in increased pelvic blood flow, vaginal lubrication, and clitoral engorgement. As in males, these mechanisms in females are mediated by a combination of neuromuscular and vasocongestive events. More cases of females with FSD are seen by urologists. Some researchers think that androgen deficiency or relative inactivity of the adrenal enzyme 17, 20-lyase in females is the pathophysiologic entity responsible for FSD, which is often characterized by diminished libido, diminished arousal and orgasmic capabilities, and deficient androgen levels.

Signs and Symptoms

ED is the persistent inability to achieve or sustain an erection firm enough for sexual intercourse and penetration (Wincze and Weisberg, 2015). ED ranges from mild to severe and occurs in 50% of 65-year-old men and 75% of men older than 80 years.

FSD is a sexual arousal disorder that may develop as females age. Menopause and declining estrogen produce a thin and dry vaginal vault. As a result, the ability to become aroused may decline because of pain during sexual intercourse, which decreases the desire for sexual intercourse. Additionally, in FSD, neuroendocrine physiologic impairments interfere with the normal female sexual response and frequently bring about complaints of diminished sexual arousal, libido, genital sensation, and ability to achieve orgasm. Other physical contributors to FSD include vaginitis, cystitis, endometriosis, hypothyroidism, and diabetes mellitus. Drugs such as oral contraceptives, HRT, antihypertensives, antidepressants, or sedatives can cause a sexual arousal disorder as a side effect.

Medical Management

Medical management includes pharmacologic (e.g., phosphodiesterase type 5 inhibitors and alprostadil), nonpharmacologic (e.g., counseling, lifestyle modifications, vacuum constriction devices, and performing regular erection exercises), and surgery (Mola, 2015). Often, these drugs must continue to be taken, and additional medicine is added to address ED. Sildenafil, phentolamine, yohimbine, testosterone, and alprostadil are a few of the drugs prescribed to increase blood flow to the penis and thus correct ED.

Most males with ED may achieve erections by using a constriction device, with or without a vacuum device (Mola, 2015). These devices are among the least expensive treatments for ED, and they enable males to avoid the side effects of drug treatment. Constriction bands or rings made of metal, rubber, or leather are placed at the base of the penis to

TABLE 23.10 Sexual Dysfunction

Recognize Cues (Assessment)	Analyze Cues and Prioritize Hypotheses (Patient Problems)	Generate Solutions (Planning)	Take Actions (Nursing Interventions)	Evaluate Outcomes (Evaluation)
1. Genital anatomy 2. Sexual identity and sexual behaviors 3. Sex drive 4. Fatigue 5. Emotional lability 6. Painful intercourse 7. Cultural influences 8. Partner availability 9. Available private time 10. Baseline function 11. Couple's connectedness 12. Erectile dysfunction, ejaculatory dysfunction, or anorgasmia 13. Depression 14. Comorbidities 15. Fears related to sexually transmitted disease 16. Medications 17. Job or financial worries 18. Values or relationship conflicts 19. Alcohol or drug use 20. Energy level 21. Laboratory abnormalities	1. Inadequate sexuality pattern	1. Explore patient's patterns of functioning. 2. Discuss relationship between sexual functioning and life stressors. 3. Reaffirm need for candid discussion between partners. 4. Intensive therapy: refer patient to appropriate therapist, counselor, or physician.	1. Permission: convey a willingness to discuss sexual matters. 2. Limited information: provide some information on likely situations and treatments. 3. Specific suggestions: offer some specific instructions based on patient's acknowledged situation. 4. Identify and problem solve acute or chronic illness and other contributing factors.	1. Patient will achieve satisfactory sexual function.

Data from Carpenito, L. J. (2023). *Nursing diagnosis: Application to clinical practice* (16th ed.). Philadelphia: Lippincott Williams & Wilkins.

slow the outflow of blood. A constriction band used alone may produce an erection in a male with mild ED, especially if the problem is the maintenance of an erection. If that does not work, a constriction device may also be combined with a vacuum device. A vacuum device consists of a hollow chamber attached to a source of suction that fits over the penis, creating an air seal. Then suction applied to the chamber draws blood into the penis, producing an erection; a binding device is then applied to maintain the erection. Surgical implantation of firm rods or pump-operated devices is an option for males with a low risk for postoperative. Recently, sensate focus psychotherapy has gained some popularity because of its ability to mitigate compounding psychological factors that may overlie physiologic ED.

A multidisciplinary approach with pharmacologic and nonpharmacologic is needed to manage FSD. Nonpharmacologic means include lifestyle modifications (e.g., weight loss and healthy diet), physiotherapy (e.g., pelvic floor exercise), and psychotherapy (e.g., counseling) (Kershaw and Jha, 2022). Pharmacologically, females can use lubricants and vaginal moisturizers; hormones (e.g., estrogen and testosterone); and antidepressants (e.g., bupropion). Some drugs that can cause FSD (e.g., antihypertensives and sedatives) may need to be reduced.

Nursing Care Guidelines for Sexual Dysfunction

Recognizing and analyzing cues, prioritizing hypotheses, generating solutions, taking actions, and evaluating outcomes for sexual dysfunction are detailed in Table 23.10.

SUMMARY

This chapter discussed endocrine aging as an increased molecular disorderliness of the regulatory mechanisms, which results in reduced vitality of the overall person. It described a new ensemble view in terms of decreased estrogen production in females (menopause), decreased testosterone production in males (andropause), decreased adrenal function (adrenopause), and decreased GH–IGF-1 (somatopause). This chapter included current literature on aging endocrine physiology showing current knowledge. Finally, clinical judgment was applied to some of the most common endocrine diseases affecting older adults.

HOME CARE

1. Regularly assess homebound older adults diagnosed with endocrine disorders for signs and symptoms indicating exacerbation or instability.
2. Instruct caregivers and homebound older adults about reportable signs and symptoms related to the endocrine problems being monitored and about when to report these changes to the home care nurse or health-care provider.
3. Instruct caregivers and homebound older adults on types, dosage, and technique of administering insulin. Have caregivers and homebound older adults do a return demonstration of this skill. Ensure that they receive written instructions to assist them in the learning process.
4. Instruct caregivers and homebound older adults about laboratory indications used to evaluate endocrine disorders. Inform them of the results of the tests after the health-care provider has been notified.
5. Instruct caregivers and homebound older adults on safety tips related to insulin injection. Injecting insulin isophane and then switching to beef or pork insulin without a physician order results in altering the times of insulin action, initiation, peak insulin action, and duration of insulin action.
6. Instruct caregivers and homebound older adults on diabetes management.
7. Instruct caregivers and homebound older adults on the proper dosage of drugs used to treat hormone imbalances associated with endocrine disorders.

KEY POINTS

- The endocrine system is regulated by feedback systems that involve a chemical connection between structures of the brain, peripheral glands, and hormones. The feedback loops regulate hormone production. The majority of the endocrine system functions by a negative feedback loop.
- A hypofunctioning state is one that results when the endocrine gland does not secrete enough of its hormones.
- A hyperfunctioning state is one that results from excessive secretion of hormones.
- Endocrine pathology may also manifest in hormone resistance, a condition in which the tissue response to hormones is inadequate. Resistance may be caused by a genetic defect or may be acquired, as in the case of T2DM.
- Older adults experience andropause and menopause when a decline in biosyntheses of their dominant sex hormones occurs.
- Adrenopause and somatopause are changes that occur as the result of aging.
- MetS is rapidly increasing in the older population. It is caused by improper nutrition, inadequate physical activity, and obesity.
- T2DM is very common in the older population.
- The most important variables associated with T2DM are obesity and IR.
- Older individuals with T2DM should strive for proper control of their blood glucose levels to reduce the risk of potential complications.
- A comprehensive nursing assessment of older patients with T2DM includes assessment of the patient's feet, the patient's knowledge of diabetes management (e.g., diet, desirable weight, exercise, drugs, and treatment of hypoglycemia and hyperglycemia), the patient's learning style, and emergency identification.
- Management of serious wounds in older patients with diabetes optimally needs to involve a multidisciplinary health team.
- Thyroid disorders are more common among older adults and more difficult to diagnose than in the younger population.
- Primary hypothyroidism in older persons may often remain unnoticed or indiscernible. Symptoms of depression, apathy, decreased appetite, weight loss, and weakness should be investigated.
- Thyroid HRT is usually started at a low dose and increases slowly (4 to 6 weeks) with careful monitoring; follow-up appointments are essential for incremental dosing over several weeks.
- Hyperthyroidism may have an atypical presentation in older adults. Symptoms often include apathy, tiredness, weakness, anorexia, weight loss, angina, heart failure, atrial fibrillation, and absence of thyroid changes.
- Older adults need to be taught the actions and side effects of prescribed drugs and the need for lifelong monitoring of thyroid status.
- Both genders can have sexual dysfunction.
- A multidisciplinary approach is needed to manage those with sexual dysfunction.

CLINICAL JUDGMENT EXERCISES

1. Compare the endocrine gland function of a 72-year-old male with that of a 30-year-old male.
2. A 65-year-old female was recently diagnosed with MetS. She is sedentary, has a BMI >30, and has abdominal obesity. What three issues would you prepare to teach the patient about her condition?
3. A 74-year-old male was recently diagnosed with insulin-dependent diabetes mellitus. While teaching him to administer 70/30 Humulin insulin, you note that he cannot draw up the correct number of units into a syringe. What further information about your patient do you need before proceeding with your teaching plan?

REFERENCES

American Diabetes Association (ADA). (2018). 11. Older adults: Standards of medical care in diabetes – 2018. *Diabetes Care, 41*(Suppl. 1), S119–S125. doi:10.2337/dc18-SPPC01.

American Diabetes Association (ADA). (2020). 12. Older Adults: Standards of medical care in diabetes – 2020. *Diabetes Care, 43*(Suppl. 1), S152–S162. doi:10.2337/dc20-S012.

American Thyroid Association (ATA). (n.d.). *Older patients and thyroid disease*. Retrieved from https://www.thyroid.org/thyroid-disease-older-patient/. Accessed August 12, 2024.

Bergman, A., Heindel, J. J., Kasten, T., Kidd, K. A., Jobling, S., Neira, M., et al. (2013). The impact of endocrine disruption: A consensus statement on the state of the science. *Environmental Health Perspectives, 121*(4), A104–A106. doi:10.1289/ehp.1205448.

Bonomini, F., Rodella, L. F., & Rezzani, R. (2015). Metabolic syndrome, aging, and involvement of oxidative stress. *Aging and Disease, 6*(2), 109–120. doi:10.14336/AD.2014.0305.

Boulton, A. J. M. (2019). The diabetic foot. *Medicine, 47*(2), 100–105. doi:10.1016/j.mpmed.2018.11.001.

Campbell, B. J. (2020). *Exercise and bone health*. OrthoInfo [website]. American Academy of Orthopaedic Surgeons. Retrieved from https://orthoinfo.aaos.org/en/staying-healthy/exercise-and-bone-health/. Accessed August 12, 2024.

Centers for Disease Control and Prevention (CDC), & National Center for Chronic Disease Prevention and Health Promotion. (2010). *Can lifestyle modifications using therapeutic lifestyle changes (TLC) reduce weight and the risk for chronic disease? Research to Practice Series, No. 7*. Retrieved from https://stacks.cdc.gov/view/cdc/42271.

Centers for Disease Control and Prevention (CDC). (2022). *Managing sick days*. Retrieved from https://www.cdc.gov/diabetes/living-with/managing-sick-days.html. Accessed July 25, 2023.

Cigolle, C. T., Lee, P. G., Langa, K. M., Lee, Y. Y., Tian, Z., & Blaum, C. S. (2011). Geriatric conditions develop in middle-aged adults with diabetes. *Journal of General Internal Medicine, 26*(3), 272–279. doi:10.1007/s11606-010-1510-y.

Di Somma, C., Brunelli, V., Savanelli, M. C., Scarano, E., Savastano, S., Lombardi, G., et al. (2011). Somatopause: State of the art. *Minerva Endocrinologica, 36*(3), 243–255.

Eastell, R. (2013). Identification and management of osteoporosis in older adults. *Medicine, 41*(1), 47–52. doi:10.1016/j.mpmed.2012.10.007.

Elam, R. E. W., Jackson, N. N., Machua, W., & Carbone, L. D. (2024). *Osteoporosis treatment & management*. Medscape [website]. Retrieved from https://emedicine.medscape.com/article/330598-treatment#d8. Accessed August 12, 2024.

Farmer, A., Hardeman, W., Hughes, D., Prevost, A. T., Kim, Y., Craven, A., et al. (2012). An explanatory randomised controlled trial of a nurse-led, consultation-based intervention to support patients with adherence to taking glucose lowering drug for type 2 diabetes. *BMC Family Practice, 13*, 30. doi:10.1186/1471-2296-13-30.

Felman, A. (2018). *Is the male menopause real?* MedicalNewsToday [website]. Retrieved from https://www.medicalnewstoday.com/articles/266749. Accessed August 12, 2024.

Garg, A., & Vanderpump, M. P. J. (2013). Subclinical thyroid disease. *British Medical Bulletin, 107*(1), 101–116. doi:10.1093/bmb/ldt024.

Gill, D., Parry, A., Santos, F., Okkenhaug, H., Todd, C. D., Hernando-Herraez, I., et al. (2022). Multi-omic rejuvenation of human cells by maturation phase transient reprogramming. *eLife, 11*, e71624. doi:10.7554/eLife.71624.

Gratzke, C., Angulo, J., Chitaley, K., Dai, Y. T., Kim, N. N., Paick, J. S., et al. (2010). Anatomy, physiology, and pathophysiology of erectile dysfunction. *The Journal of Sexual Medicine, 7*(1 Pt 2), 445–475. doi:10.1111/j.1743-6109.2009.01624.x.

Griffith, J. F. (2013). Age-related physiological changes of the bone marrow and immune system. In G. Guglielmi, W. C. G. Peh, & A. Guermazi (Eds.), *Geriatric imaging* (pp. 891–904). New York: Springer.

Hughes, A. K., Rostant, O. S., & Pelon, S. (2015). Sexual problems among older women by age and race. *Journal of Women's Health, 24*(8), 663–669. doi:10.1089/jwh.2014.5010.

Jones, C. M., & Boelaert, K. (2015). The endocrinology of ageing: A mini-review. *Gerontology, 61*(4), 291–300. doi:10.1159/000367692.

Kershaw, V., & Jha, S. (2022). Female sexual dysfunction. *TOG: The Obstetrician & Gynaecologist, 24*(1), 12–23. doi:10.1111/tog.12778.

LeRoith, D., Biessels, G. J., Braithwaite, S. S., Casanueva, F. F., Draznin, B., Halter, J. B., et al. (2019). Treatment of diabetes in older adults: An Endocrine Society clinical practice guideline. *The Journal of Clinical Endocrinology and Metabolism, 104*(5), 1520–1574. doi:10.1210/jc.2019-00198.

Liantonio, A., Gramegna, G., Carbonara, G., Sblendorio, V. T., Pierno, S., Fraysse, B., et al. (2013). Growth hormone secretagogues exert differential effects on skeletal muscle calcium homeostasis in male rats depending on the peptidyl/nonpeptidyl structure. *Endocrinology, 154*(10), 3764–3775. doi:10.1210/en.2013-1334.

Madsen, M. C., van Dijk, D., Wiepjes, C. M., Conemans, E. B., Thijs, A., & den Heijer, M. (2021). Erythrocytosis in a large cohort of trans men using testosterone: A long-term follow-up study on prevalence, determinants, and exposure years. *The Journal of Clinical Endocrinology and Metaoblism, 106*(6), 1710–1717. doi:10.1210/clinem/dgab089.

Maggio, M., De Vita, F., Fisichella, A., Lauretani, F., Ticinesi, A., Cresini, G., et al. (2015). The role of the multiple hormonal dysregulation in the onset of "anemia of aging": Focus on testosterone, IGF-1, and thyroid hormones. *International Journal of Endocrinology, 2015*, 292574. doi:10.1155/2015/292574.

Mäkitie, R. E., Costantini, A., Kämpe, A, Alm, J. J., & Mäkitie, O. (2019). New insights into monogenic causes of osteoporosis. *Frontiers Endocrinology, 10*, 70. doi:10.3389/fendo.2019.00070.

Marko, K. I. (2020). *Medical management of menopausal symptoms*. SASGOG Pearls of Exxcellence [website]. The Society for Academic Specialists in General Obstetrics and Gynecology. Retrieved from https://www.exxcellence.org/list-of-pearls/. Accessed August 12, 2024.

Mbaezue, N., Mayberry, R., Gazmararian, J., Quarshie, A., Ivonye, C., & Heisler, M. (2010). The impact of health literacy on self-monitoring of blood glucose in patients with diabetes receiving care in an inner-city hospital. *Journal of the National Medical Association, 102*(1), 5–9. doi:10.1016/s0027-9684(15)30469-7.

Medeiros-Neto, G. (2016). Multinodular goiter. In K. R. Feingold, B. Anawalt, M. R. Blackman, A. Boyce, G. Chrousos, E. Corpas, et al. (Eds.), *Endotext* [Internet]. South Dartmouth, MA: MDText.com, Inc. Retrieved from https://www.ncbi.nlm.nih.gov/books/NBK285569/. Accessed August 12, 2024.

Michael, O. T. (2010). Endocrinology of aging: The convergence of reductionist science with systems biology and integrative medicine. *Frontiers in Endocrinology, 1*, 2. doi:10.3389/fendo.2010.00002.

Mola, J. R. (2015). Erectile dysfunction in the older adult male. *Urologic Nursing, 35*(2), 87–93. doi:10.7257/1053- 816X.2015.35.2.87.

Munshi, M. (2024). Treatment of type 2 diabetes mellitus in the older patient. In D. M. Nathan, K. E. Schmader, K. Rubinow, & J. Givens (Eds.). *UpToDate*. Waltham, MA: UpToDate, Inc. Retrieved from https://www.uptodate.com/contents/treatment-of-type-2-diabetes-mellitus-in-the-older-patient. Accessed August 12, 2024.

National Heart, Lung, and Blood Institute. (2022). *What is metabolic syndrome?* Retrieved from https://www.nhlbi.nih.gov/health/metabolic-syndrome. Accessed August 12, 2024.

Olatunbosun, S. T. (2020). *Insulin resistance differential diagnoses*. Medscape [website]. Retrieved from https://emedicine.medscape.com/article/122501-differential#. Accessed August 12, 2024.

Orlander, P. R., Varghese, J. M., & Nalk, S. (2022). *Hypothyroidism*. Medscape [website]. Retrieved from https://emedicine.medscape.com/article/122393-overview#a4. Accessed August 12, 2024.

Pamphlett, R., Jew, S. K., Doble, P. A., & Bishop, D. P. (2019). Elemental analysis of aging human pituitary glands implicates mercury as a contributor to the somatopause. *Frontiers in Endocrinology, 10*, 419. doi:10.3389/fendo.2019.00419.

Peters, E. J. G., Lipsky, B. A., Berendt, A. R., Embil, J. M., Lavery, L. A., Senneville, E., et al. (2012). A systematic review of the effectiveness of interventions in the management of infection in the diabetic foot. *Diabetes/Metabolism Research and Reviews, 28*(Suppl. 1), 142–162. doi:10.1002/dmrr.2247.

Regufe, V. M. G., Pinto, C. M. C. B., & Perez, P. M. V. H. C. (2020). Metabolic syndrome in type 2 diabetic patients: A review of current evidence. *Porto Biomedical Journal, 5*(6), e101. doi:10.1097/j.pbj.0000000000000101.

Rejeski, W. J., Ip, E. H., Bertoni, A. G., Bray, G. A., Evans, G., Gregg, E. W., et al. (2012). Lifestyle change and mobility in obese adults with type 2 diabetes. *New England Journal of Medicine, 366*(13), 1209–1217. doi:10.1056/NEJMoa1110294.

Rippe, J. M. (2018). Lifestyle medicine: The health promoting power of daily habits and practices. *American Journal of Lifestyle Medicine, 12*(6), 499–512. doi:10.1177/1559827618785554.

Salvatore, D., Cohen, R., Kopp, P. A., & Larsen, P. R. (2020). Thyroid physiology and diagnostic evaluation of patients with thyroid disorders. In S. Melmed, R. Koenig, C. C. Rosen, R. J. Aughus, & A.B. Goldfine, et al. (Eds.), *Williams textbook of endocrinology* (14th ed., pp 332–363.e6). Philadelphia: Elsevier.

Samuels, M. H. (2021). Hyperthyroidism in aging. In K. R. Feingold, B. Anawalt, M. R. Blackman, A. Boyce, G. Chrousos, E. Corpas, et al. (Eds.), *Endotext* [Internet]. South Dartmouth, MA: MDText.com, Inc. Retrieved from https://www.ncbi.nlm.nih.gov/books/NBK278986/. Accessed August 12, 2024.

Schlumberger, M., Catargi, B., Borget, I., Deandreis, D., Zerdoud, S., Bridji, B., et al. (2012). Strategies of radioiodine ablation in patients with low-risk thyroid cancer. *New England Journal of Medicine, 366*(18), 1663–1673. doi:10.1056/NEJMoa1108586.

Seabright, J. (2024). Thyroid function age-related changes. *Endocrinology advisor*. Retrieved from https://www.endocrinologyadvisor.com/ddi/do-thyroid-levels-change-with-age/. Accessed September 29, 2024.

Steil, G. M., Palerm, C. C., Kurtz, N., Voskanyan, G., Roy, A., Paz, S., et al. (2011). The effect of insulin feedback on closed loop glucose control. *The Journal of Clinical Endocrinology and Metabolism, 96*(5), 1402–1408. doi:10.1210/jc.2010-2578.

Toivonen, J. M., & Partridge, L. (2009). Endocrine regulation of aging and reproduction in Drosophilia. *Molecular and Cellular Endocrinology, 299*(1), 39–50. doi:10.1016/j.mce.2008.07.005.

van den Beld, A. W., Kaufman, J. M., Zillikens, M. C., Lamberts, S. W. J., Egan, J. M., & van der Lely, A. J. (2018). The physiology of endocrine systems with ageing. *The Lancet Diabetes Endocrinology, 6*(8), 647–658. doi:10.1016/S2213-8587(18)30026-3.

Van Meirhaeghe, J., Bastian, L., Boonen, S., Ranstam, J., Tillman, J. B., & Wardlaw, D. (2013). A randomized trial of balloon kyphoplasty and nonsurgical management for treating acute vertebral compression fractures: Vertebral body kyphosis correction and surgical parameters. *Spine (Phila, Pa 1976), 38*(12), 971–983. doi:10.1097/BRS.0b013e31828e8e22.

Veldhuis, J. D. (2013). Changes in pituitary function with ageing and implications for patient care. *Nature Reviews Endocrinology, 9*(4), 205–215. doi:10.1038/nrendo.2013.38.

Walter, S., Atzmon, G., Demerath, E. W., Garcia, M. E., Kaplan, R. C., Kumari, M., et al. (2011). A genome-wide association study of aging. *Neurobiology of Aging, 32*(11), 2109.e15–2109.e28. doi:10.1016/j.neurobiolaging.2011.05.026.

Wincze, J. P., & Weisberg, R. B. (2015). *Sexual dysfunction: A guide for assessment and treatment* (3rd ed.). New York: Guilford Publications, Inc.

Wood, C. (2017). Ensuring good nutrition for older patients in the community. *Journal of Community Nursing, 31*(3), 49–51.

Yiallouris, A., Tsioutis, C., Agapidaki, E., Zafeiri, M., Agouridis, A. P., Ntourakis, D., et al. (2019). Adrenal aging and its implications on stress responsiveness in humans. *Frontiers in Endocrinology, 10*, 54. doi:10.3389/fendo.2019.00054.

Young, W. F., Jr. (2022). Overview of endocrine disorders. In *Merck manual professional version*. Merck & Co., Inc. Retrieved from http://www.merckmanuals.com/professional/endocrine-and-metabolic-disorders/principles-of-endocrinology/overview-of-endocrine-disorders. Accessed August 12, 2024.

WEBSITES

American Association of Clinical Endocrinologists. http://www.aace.com.

American College of Obstetricians and Gynecologists. http://www.acog.com.

Food and Nutrition: Dietary Guidelines for Americans—USDA. http://www.health.gov/dietaryguidelines/.

North American Menopause Society. http://www.menopause.org.

National Institute of Diabetes and Digestive and Kidney Diseases of the National Institutes of Health. http://www.niddk.nih.gov.

Office of Disease Prevention and Health Promotion. http://health.gov.

Physical Activity Readiness Questionnaire (PAR-Q). https://www.nasm.org/docs/pdf/parqplus-2020.pdf?sfvrsn-401bf1af_24.

Systematic Evidence Review: Managing Overweight and Obesity in Adults. https://www.nhlbi.nih.gov/health-topics/managing-overweight-obesity-in-adults.

PART VI

Health Care Transitions

24

Health Care Delivery Settings and Older Adults

Martha Smith, DNP, APRN, FNP-BC

http://evolve.elsevier.com/Yeager/gerontologic/

LEARNING OBJECTIVES

On completion of this chapter, the reader will be able to:
1. Describe acute care hospital-use patterns in the older adult population.
2. Describe a functional model of nursing care.
3. Identify risks associated with the hospitalization of older adults.
4. Identify ways to modify the physical and social environment to improve care for hospitalized older adults.
5. Identify special considerations in caring for critically ill older adults and those suffering from trauma.
6. List adaptations that can be made to facilitate learning in older adults.
7. Describe the profile of a "typical" noninstitutionalized older adult, including common diagnoses and functional limitations.
8. Distinguish the categories and types of home care organizations in existence.
9. Explain the benefits of home care.
10. Analyze the effect of recent changes instituted by Medicare on home health agencies and home health patients.
11. Discuss the philosophy of hospice care and how it differs from traditional home health care.
12. List five common factors associated with institutionalization.
13. Identify the differences between the medical and psychosocial models of care for institutional long-term care.
14. Summarize key aspects of resident rights as they relate to the nursing facility.
15. List assessment components included in the minimum data set of the Resident Assessment Instrument.
16. Describe common clinical management programs in the nursing facility for skin problems, incontinence, nutritional problems, infection control, and mental health.
17. Differentiate types of nursing care delivery systems found in nursing facilities.
18. Describe assisted living, special care units, and subacute care units as specialty care settings of the nursing facility.

WHAT WOULD YOU DO?

What would you do if you were faced with the following situations?
- Your neighbor states her father-in-law has become forgetful and fails to take his drugs at least weekly. Last week he fell; aside from bruising, there were no serious injuries. But she is concerned and does not know where to turn for help. What advice can you offer her?
- Your new admission to the general medical floor is 92 years old. He is ambulatory with the assistance of a four-point cane; he is on standby to assist with activities of daily living (ADLs). You are concerned for his safety. What do you do?

By 2030, the World Health Organization (WHO) predicts one in six people worldwide will be 60 or older. In fact, the population of people who are 80 years of age or older is expected to triple by 2050 to reach 426 million. Therefore, it is now estimated that most of a nurse's career will be spent working with older adults, and almost all nurses will care for older adults in the acute care setting at some time. Older adults are a diverse, heterogeneous group in terms of age, life experiences, aging process, health habits, attitudes, and responses to illnesses. Nurses need to have specialized knowledge, skills, and abilities to care for older adults across all health-care delivery settings.

Previous author: Marie H. Thomas, RN, PhD, FNP-C, CNE

CHARACTERISTICS OF OLDER ADULTS IN ACUTE CARE

According to the Agency for Healthcare Research and Quality (AHRQ), the most common diagnoses for inpatient stays in the United States among those of the age of 75 or older are septicemia, heart failure, pneumonia, cardiac dysrhythmias, osteoarthritis, urinary tract infections, acute or nonspecific renal failure, cerebral infarction, fracture of the neck of the femur (hip) initial encounter, and acute myocardial infarction (McDermott and Roemer, 2021). The top five major causes of death in those older than 65 years are heart disease, malignant neoplasms, COVID-19, cerebrovascular disease, and Alzheimer disease (Centers for Disease Control and Prevention [CDC], 2021a).

Chronic conditions refer to chronic illness and impairments, and an individual's level of disability is typically categorized by the amount of assistance required in both basic ADLs and instrumental activities of daily living (IADLs). Arthritis, diabetes mellitus, hypertension, and heart disease are the most prevalent chronic diseases in older adults and are the leading causes of disability. The exacerbation of a chronic illness may precipitate hospitalization, and complications may profoundly affect the progress of a hospitalized patient. Because the acute event for which an older patient is hospitalized is frequently superimposed on a chronic condition or disease, this older age group is increasingly influencing the acute care environment and the professional caregiver skills required in this setting.

CHARACTERISTICS OF THE ACUTE CARE ENVIRONMENT

It is a challenge for caregivers to attend to the diverse needs of everyone admitted to the acute care setting. The older adult is not likely to be admitted to the hospital until a high level of acuity or complications exist. Reimbursement patterns can create additional complications that put stress on the care team, which, in turn, affect care. The intensity of care required for the typically emergent condition for which an older adult is admitted, compounded by the normal aging process, chronic illness, and impaired functional status, requires astute care planning and case management on the part of the health-care team. The health-care team's success in providing care is influenced by the philosophy of care, awareness of the risks of hospitalization, and safety features of the acute care environment.

Philosophy of Care

Rapidly rising costs and concerns over quality in acute care have fostered a climate in which the value and efficacy of hospitalization have come under increasing scrutiny. With an increasing number of hospitalized older adults, the focus on technology is being recognized as obscuring activities aimed at improving the function of those with chronic illness, physical disability, and cognitive impairment. Effective caregiving practices enable older adults to maintain or improve their independence and to return to their preferred living environment at discharge. However, in the hospital setting, health-care professionals may become so involved in addressing the acute condition that they fail to appreciate the underlying problems and how these, too, influence the patient's health and recovery.

The hospital is a highly technologic system that is in a good position to address both acute and chronic problems. The focus needs to be on not only the restoration of health but also the promotion and preservation of health. The value placed on technology fosters a task orientation that may detract from the holistic focus required for the care of older adults. Acute care centers have traditionally provided care within a medical model whose focus is on diagnosis and treatment rather than providing care within a functional model, which more broadly integrates all aspects of care. With older adults, particularly those hospitalized because of an exacerbation of a chronic illness, focusing on a functional model helps address concerns related to both their medical and functional stability. The medical model practiced in the hospital needs to be expanded to include this functional model, in which the main goal may not be curing the disease but rather managing the disease, with a focus on self-care and symptom management strategies.

The 4Ms (Fig. 24.1) is an initiative of The John A. Hartford Foundation and the Institute for Healthcare Improvement (IHI) in partnership with the American Hospital Association and the Catholic Health Association of the United States. The Age-Friendly Health System is a framework to guide hospitals, medical practices, nursing homes, home-care providers, retail pharmacy clinics, and others to deliver age-friendly care. It is meant to incorporate the 4Ms into current care. The aim is to cause no harm, follow essential evidence-based practices, and align with "What Matters" for older adults and their families. The 4Ms — What Matters, Medication, Mentation, and Mobility should determine care and facilitate decision-making with older adults. Therefore, older adults' wellness and strengths drive care rather than just the disease process (IHI, n.d.).

Risks of Hospitalization
Adverse Drug Reaction

An adverse drug reaction is "an unwanted, undesirable effect of a drug that occurs during usual clinical use" (Schatz and Weber, 2015, p. 5). Approximately one in six hospitalized older adults will experience an adverse drug reaction (Jennings et al, 2020). The most common drugs for reported adverse drug reactions are diuretics, systemic antimicrobials, antithrombotic agents, analgesics, and drugs for obstructive airway diseases. Polypharmacy, although poorly defined in the literature, is a common cause of iatrogenic illness among patients over 65 years of age and is associated with multimorbidity in older adult patients (Sirois et al, 2019). Hospitalized patients are often admitted with a large number of prescribed, over-the-counter, and homeopathic drugs that they have or have not been taking correctly or as prescribed before entering the acute care setting. Adjusting, removing, or adding to the number of drugs can put the older adult at risk for adverse drug reactions.

Hospital staff need to obtain an accurate drug history from patients, be aware of pharmacokinetic and pharmacodynamic changes related to aging, and have a working understanding of drug–disease, drug–drug, and drug–food interactions in older adults. Nurses should be particularly aware of drugs that may be high-risk when used in older adults and carefully monitor patients taking them for signs and symptoms of toxicity. Partnering with the pharmacy team to put into place pathways to identify high-risk drugs, interactions, and prescribing practices is necessary to ensure safe-drug prescribing for older adults in the hospital and during transitions in care (2019 American Geriatrics Society Beers Criteria® Update Expert Panel, 2019).

Falls

Somewhere between 700,000 and 1,000,000 people in the United States each year sustain a fall in the hospital (AHRQ, 2021).

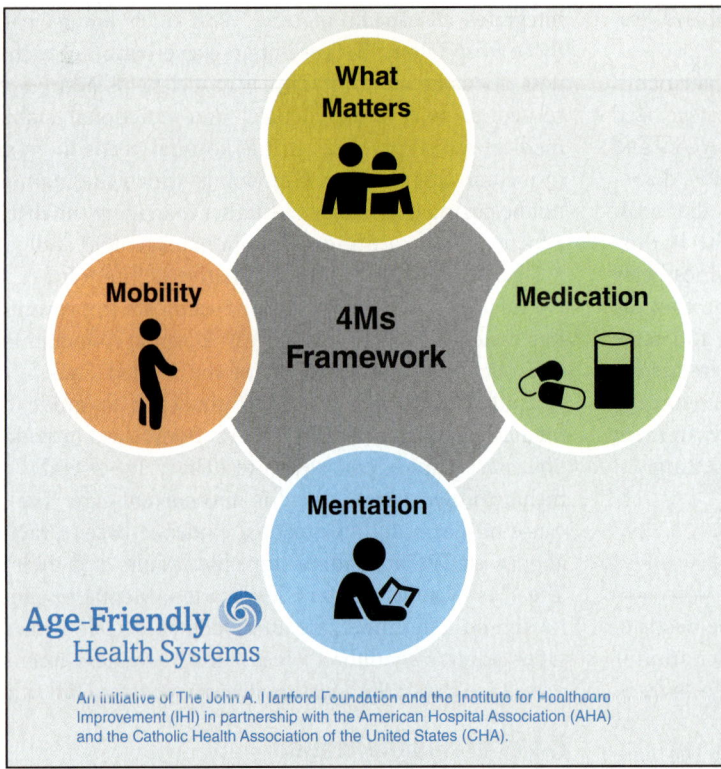

Fig. 24.1 The age-friendly 4Ms framework. (From Institute for Healthcare Improvement [IHI]. *Age-Friendly Health Systems.* An initiative of The John A. Hartford Foundation and the IHI in partnership with the American Hospital Association [AHA] and the Catholic Health Association of the United States [CHA]. Retrieved from https://www.ihi.org/Engage/Initiatives/Age-Friendly-Health-Systems/Pages/default.aspx.)

Each fall puts an individual at risk for lacerations, fractures, or internal bleeding, which leads to increased health-care utilization (see the Emergency Treatment box). According to research, one-third of falls can be prevented. To prevent falls, a patient's underlying fall-risk factors must be managed. Also, optimizing the hospital's physical design and environment is a priority. Risk factors for hospital falls include both intrinsic and extrinsic factors. Intrinsic factors include age-related physiologic changes and diseases, as well as drugs that affect cognition and balance. Extrinsic factors include environmental hazards such as the layout of older hospital rooms or cluttered hospital rooms, wheels on beds and chairs, and beds higher than what an older adult usually has at home. The hospital can be a dangerous and foreign place for older adults because of its unfamiliarity and because of changes in the patient's medical condition. The Joint Commission (2015) has emphasized the need to decrease the risk of falls, recommending the following:

- Raise awareness among staff of the need to prevent falls.
- Establish an interdisciplinary fall prevention team.
- Use standardized, validated tools to identify risk factors for falls.
- Develop individualized plans of care based on identified risk factors for falls.
- Use evidence-based practices and interventions.
- Conduct postfall huddles.
- Analyze contributing factors for falls on an ongoing basis to inform quality improvement efforts.

✚ EMERGENCY TREATMENT
Fall Assessment

- Before moving the patient, ask them what they think caused the fall and assess any associated symptoms.
- Conduct a comprehensive assessment, including vital signs (apical and radial pulses) and cranial nerves.
- Examine the skin for pallor, trauma, circulation, abrasion, bruising, and sensation.
- Check for sensation and movement in the lower extremities.
- Determine current level of consciousness and whether the patient experienced any loss of consciousness.
- Look for subtle cognitive changes.
- Observe for leg rotation, hip pain, shortening of the extremity, and pelvic or spinal pain.
- Identify points of pain or tenderness.
- Observe for warning signs of spinal cord injury, leg or pelvic fracture or head injury, numbness or tingling in the extremities, back pain, rib pain, or an external rotated or shortened leg.

Data from Hendrich, A. (2007). When a fall occurs: Four steps to take in response to a fall. *American Journal of Nursing, 107*(11). doi: 10.1097/01.NAJ.0000298064.12102.08

Infection

Older adults are generally more vulnerable to infections because of physiologic changes in the immune system and underlying chronic diseases. The CDC (2021b) estimates that 1 in 31 hospital patients and 1 in 43 nursing-home residents has a hospital-acquired infection (HAI) on any given day.

Slightly more than 33% of HAIs occur in the older patient population (Katz and Roghmann, 2016). This may be a low estimate because older adults with infections may have an atypical presentation, making infections more difficult to diagnose. Hospital-acquired pneumonia is the most common HAI (Monegro et al, 2023); symptoms in older adults are often mental status changes or confusion, making the diagnosis more challenging (Cristina et al, 2021).

UTIs are the second most frequent HAI (Cristina et al, 2021) although bacteriuria in an older adult is often asymptomatic. Subclinical infection and inflammation may occur with presenting symptoms such as acute confusion, functional capacity deterioration and falls, anorexia, or nausea rather than the classic symptoms of fever and dysuria. Increased instrumentation and manipulation, as well as decreased host-immune mechanisms, contribute to the increased risk of older adult patients developing sepsis originating from the urinary tract.

Since 2020, COVID-19 has been diagnosed in hospitals and nursing homes in the United States, which in elderly patients can lead to major complications such as mechanical ventilation and subsequently ventilator-associated pneumonia (Cristina et al, 2021). Higher mortality rates have been associated with advanced age and comorbidities. Other common sites of infection in hospitalized older adults include the gastrointestinal tract (*Clostridium difficile*), skin and soft tissues, and the bloodstream (CDC, 2021b). Older adults are at increased risk for colonization and infection with antibiotic-resistant strains of organisms such as methicillin-resistant *Staphylococcus aureus* (MRSA), vancomycin-resistant enterococcus (VRE), and multi-drug-resistant Gram-negative rods. Control of the spread of resistant strains of organisms continues to be a problem in institutional settings. Adhering to the basic principles of infection control is critical for nurses. It is essential to comply with proper hand washing, disinfection of the environment, and appropriate precautions, including personal protective equipment (PPE), when caring for patients infected or colonized with resistant strains.

Hazards of Immobility

Once hospitalized, 95% of an adult patient's time is spent in bed or a chair (Floegel et al, 2018). The resultant prolonged immobility is associated with loss of muscle mass, muscle strength, physical function, muscle protein synthesis, and cognitive function in older adults (Falvey et al, 2015). Skin breakdown, venous stasis, hospital-associated pneumonia, urinary incontinence, and retention, as well as fecal impaction, can all be hazards of this immobility. Therefore, this deconditioning results in prolonged hospitalization and can lead to early readmission. Gerontological nurses must be leaders in advocating more appropriate care and treatment for hospitalized older adults to prevent or at least reduce the occurrence of iatrogenic illness.

Safety Features

Older adults have a decreased ability to negotiate within and adapt to an unfamiliar environment. Multiple stimuli, such as contact with many departments and personnel or multiple room changes, may prompt confusion and exhaustion, resulting in the loss of crucial personal items necessary for maximum functioning, such as hearing aids, prostheses, dentures, and eyeglasses. The environment may be modified in many ways for older adult patients (Box 24.1). Some modifications require additional resources, but some changes require minimum creativity on the part of the nursing staff.

NURSING IN THE ACUTE CARE SETTING

The nursing staff provides the majority of health care delivered in the hospital. Nurses are considered an integral part of the health-care team and frequently provide leadership for this team. Nurses need to be at the forefront of identifying high-quality, cost-effective interventions and transitions in care to

BOX 24.1 Environmental Modifications

- Stabilized furnishings (e.g., removing or locking wheels)
- "Blue" fluorescent lighting
- Night lights
- Extra lighting in bathrooms
- Consistent lighting intensity
- Light switches that glow
- Solid-color designs for floors (i.e., avoidance of patterns)
- Nonskid, nonglare floor wax
- Carpeting with an uncut, low pile and padding underneath
- Contrasting color to identify boundaries between floor and wall
- Nonglossy wall surfaces
- Polarized window glass to decrease glare
- Nonglare glass over pictures; avoidance of abstract designs
- Rounded handrails for easy grasp in all areas where walking occurs; use of high-contrast colors in these areas
- Levers for doors and dressers instead of knobs
- Large-numbered, white-on-black (or black-on-white) clocks with nonglare glass
- Large-print calendars within patient's line of vision
- Telephones with large numbers
- Cases for glasses and prostheses attached to the bedside and within reach
- Amplified and hearing aid-compatible phones
- Pocket talker
- Beds that lower to a height that enables patients to sit on the edge with both feet on the floor
- Use of no side rails or half-rails to deter climbing over rails
- Bed or chair exit alarms
- Chairs with armrests
- Portable elevated toilet seats
- Grab bars in showers and around toilets

Data from American Association of Retired Persons (AARP). (2022). *AARP HomeFit guide*. Retrieved from https://www.aarp.org/livable-communities/housing/info-2020/homefit-guide-download.html; Hallstrom, L. (2022). *Keeping seniors safe: Home care services and tips for aging in place*. AgingCare [website]. Retrieved from https://www.agingcare.com/articles/making-home-safer-for-seniors-a-room-by-room-assessment-121363.htm.

prepare patients and families for discharge. The quality of the nursing care provided is influenced by the philosophy of nursing, the nursing-specific competency and expertise of the nursing staff, and the various aspects of the nursing role implemented in acute care.

Nursing-Specific Competency and Expertise

Developing nursing competency helps nursing staff customize the care provided to patients age 65 or older. It enhances the nurse's job performance and the quality of care delivered. The Centers for Medicare and Medicaid Services and The Joint Commission (2019) require documentation that all staff members (e.g., nurses, unlicensed assistive personnel, phlebotomists, and physical therapists) have a documented competency assessment that includes the special needs and behaviors of the specific patient age groups (e.g., geriatric, pediatric, and adolescent) that are provided care for in the assigned area. CMS and TJC further require that this be done on initial employment and then periodically reviewed.

A priority at the beginning of every hospitalization is the assessment of the older adult's baseline functional status so that an individual care plan can be developed (CMS and TJC, 2019). Systematic functional assessment in the acute care setting also provides a benchmark of a patient's progress as they move along the continuum of care, and it promotes systematic communication of the patient's health status between health-care settings (CMS and TJC, 2019). Assessment in the acute care setting includes recognition that older adults are in an unfamiliar environment, which is not conducive to optimal functioning at a time when reserves and homeostatic needs are compromised by acute illness. Many common assessment tools for ADLs and mental status assess areas of function that may not be easily evaluated at the time of admission or may not be significant at that time (i.e., assessing orientation when a calendar is not present in the room and the older adult's daily routines are disrupted). The primary goal of the acute care nurse is to maximize the older patient's independence by enhancing function. Functional strengths and weaknesses need to be identified. The care plan must provide for interventions that build on identified strengths and help the patient overcome identified weaknesses. Function integrates all aspects of the patient's condition; any change in functional status in an older adult should be interpreted as a classic sign of illness or as a complication of their illness. By knowing an older patient's baseline function, the nurse can assess new-onset signs or symptoms before they trigger a downward spiral of dependency and permanent impairment.

Advanced practice nurses certified as Adult Gerontology Nurse Practitioners (AGNP) are educationally prepared to be the leaders to guide staff in understanding the unique needs of older patients while enhancing skills to manage common geriatric syndromes. In order to attain this certification, one must have a master's degree in nursing or a Doctor of Nursing Practice degree from an accredited nursing program. In addition, the curriculum must include specialization in adult and gerontological nursing with clinical hours of supervision and practice within the adult gerontology role (APRN Consensus Workgroup and National Council of State Boards of Nursing APRN Advisory Committee, 2008).

The advanced practice nurse functions in the role of clinician, educator, consultant, and researcher. A growing number of acute care settings are recruiting and hiring advanced practice nurses to assist with the day-to-day assessment and management of patients in the acute care setting. Studies have demonstrated a significant decrease in the length of hospital stay when an advanced practice nurse is part of the care team (Kleinpell et al, 2019; Kapu et al, 2014; Kapu and Steaban, 2016; Moote et al, 2011). The advanced practice nurse can be instrumental in developing and implementing protocols for managing common geriatric syndromes.

Critical Care and Trauma Care

Older adults admitted to the hospital are often critically ill, and effective nursing care requires an understanding of their impaired homeostatic mechanisms, the diminished reserve capacity of their body systems, and their impaired immune response. Homeostatic mechanisms are altered with age so that the ability to generate a fever, to respond to alterations in tissue integrity, and to sense pain may be very different from those manifested by young or middle-aged adults in critical care (Merck Manual, 2024). The atypical and subtle nature of disease presentation becomes even more important in the intensive care unit (ICU), where the patient is often less able to articulate discomfort and new problems may arise quickly. The nurse must be aware that the most common presenting symptom of sepsis in older patients is acute mental status change (Tucker et al, 2013; Clifford et al, 2016). Astute observation for delirium is essential to aggressively managing its underlying cause. Delirium in this setting was referred to in the past as "ICU psychosis" and was thought to be caused by sensory overload or sensory deprivation. The causes are now recognized as multifactorial and, in this environment, are often secondary to acute illness, drugs, and the environment. Critically ill individuals are at particular risk for delirium because of impaired physical and mental defenses (Li et al, 2020) (Table 24.1).

Two additional issues for the critical care of older adults are the prevention of nutritional compromise and the recognition of adverse drug reactions. Up to 65% of hospitalized older adults are malnourished on admission or acquire nutritional deficits while hospitalized. In the critical care setting, patients are sicker and have ever-changing metabolic requirements that necessitate daily nutritional monitoring. Patients over 75 years of age admitted to the ICU after emergency surgery or for medical reasons have a mortality rate of up to 67% (Siobal et al, 2021). In 2020, researchers made the novel discovery that delirium-associated mortality had not changed over the past 30 years, in contrast to a decline in cardiovascular mortality observed in the past 40 years (Aung Thein et al, 2020). Clinical recognition of the pharmacokinetic and pharmacodynamic changes associated with aging is most important in the critical care setting, where more drugs are used to combat more problems. Drugs given in a critical care context may be lifesaving and life-threatening at the same time.

The most common traumatic injuries experienced by those older than the age of 65 result from falls, automobile accidents,

TABLE 24.1 Changes in Cognitive Status

	Delirium	Dementia	Depression
Onset	Sudden and acute	Insidious, subtle, and gradual; difficult to pinpoint	May be sudden or gradual, depending on course; may pinpoint date
Duration	Brief: often clears within 1 month or when the underlying disorder is resolved	2–20 years	Weeks to years; variable
Awareness	Clouded state of consciousness; disoriented	Alert and aware	Directed inward; self-absorbed
Mood/behavior	Easily distracted; incoherent speech; difficulty with attention and concentration; hallucinations and illusions; disturbed sleep-wake cycle; increased or decreased psychomotor activity; fluctuation of symptoms: lucid at times but often worse at night	Personality changes; emotionally labile; may become easily agitated, with catastrophic reactions	Often aware of cognitive problems; apathetic, with feelings of hopelessness or worthlessness; vague somatic complaints
Task performance	Often unable to carry out tasks; difficulty following directions	Tries hard to carry out activities; gradual loss of abilities	Able, but makes little effort
Mental function	Disorganized thinking; fluctuating impairments in memory, coherence, orientation, and perception	Impairments in memory, abstract thinking, judgment, and language; loss of common knowledge	Selective memory loss: "I don't know" answers on cognitive tests

and burns. Older adults suffer injuries of equivalent severity to those of younger persons; however, the consequences are more severe. It is essential to obtain a thorough history of an injury from the patient and their family, including the circumstances surrounding the event and the events leading up to the injury. Health-care professionals in the field need to realize that older adults do not tolerate hypoperfusion for long and may quickly go into cardiogenic shock and multisystem organ failure. Early hemodynamic monitoring is required. The vital signs of an older adult might be restored to normal, yet the person may still be in cardiogenic shock. As much as volume depletion is a concern, so is volume overload in patients with limited cardiac and renal reserves. Although insertion of a Foley catheter increases the risk of infection in older adults, it is justified for its value in monitoring volume status in critically ill older adults (CDC, 2024; Legome and Shockley, 2011; Fuchs et al, 2012). Additionally, studies have linked Foley catheter use and frailty to delirium in older ICU surgical patients (Saravana-Bawan et al, 2019; Fukushima et al, 2021).

Thermoregulatory mechanisms become impaired as a person ages, and older adults with trauma are particularly vulnerable. Care should be taken to reduce heat loss with the use of warm IV solutions, warm blankets, and proper environmental control. The degree of long-term recovery of older adults who survive injury is variable, and aggressive rehabilitation and social support are important factors in recovery. Research supports the fact that older adults are at greater risk for complications and higher mortality even when injuries are not severe (Legome and Shockley, 2011). Frailty is defined as the presence of at least three of the following criteria: decreased strength, exhaustion, slow walking speed, low physical activity, and unintentional weight loss associated with increased functional impairment, falls, prolonged hospitalizations, and death (Monkhouse, 2013). Frailty is associated with female gender, chronic disease, increased chronologic age, and decreased functional status. Frailty is a measure of vulnerability and indicates those at risk for increased mortality and institutionalization. Frail individuals have a limited capacity to respond to internal and external stressors (Hubbard and Woodhouse, 2010).

CONTINUITY OF CARE

Enhancement of the continuum of care from hospital to home is a goal shared by both hospital and home care personnel. Continuity of care involves assisting older adults to remain in the home and avoid institutionalization by having available resources that are responsive to their needs. The AHRQ (2022) defines a Patient-Centered Medical Home (PCMH) as a model of primary care that delivers the core functions of primary health care. The primary care medical home delivers comprehensive care that is patient-centered and coordinates care across all elements of the health-care system with accessible services while delivering safe and quality care based on evidence-based principles. The PCMH is a model of care led by a primary care provider (PCP) who provides continuous and coordinated care throughout a patient's lifetime to maximize health outcomes. A PCMH service includes preventive services, treatment of acute and chronic illnesses, and assistance with end-of-life issues. This care model promotes improved access and communication, care coordination and integration, and care quality and safety. The Patient Protection and Affordable Care Act (2010) endorsed a move toward the PCMH model with reimbursement incentives for PCMH care. The result of this change is to ensure that a continuum of care exists from hospital to home. Health-care providers should follow the "Plan, Do, Check, Act Cycle" (Box 24.2).

Benefits of Home Care

In survey after survey, older Americans choose "home" as their treatment place of choice. As a result of advances in technology, individuals who at one time could be treated only in the hospital can now be managed at home. Family, friends, and even patients themselves can be taught to manage enteral and parenteral feedings, central lines, pain control, antibiotic therapy, wound care, and urinary catheters with a minimum of assistance.

Among those older adults who can benefit from home care services are individuals who:
- Have chronic medical conditions with exacerbations such as congestive heart failure, chronic obstructive pulmonary

BOX 24.2 Plan, Do, Check, Act Cycle

Plan
- Gather data on admission.
- Identify goals for discharge.
- Identify specific functional problems.
- Validate that a problem exists.
- Structure problems by delineating components.

Do
- Gather information about resources.
- Select all possible options.
- Identify measurable objectives in terms of the patient's functional problems.
- Analyze each option for capacity to fulfill objectives.
- Identify advantages and disadvantages.

Check
- Compare alternatives for the probability of fulfilling discharge objectives.
- Project results of alternatives.
- Explore alternatives with the patient and family.
- Choose among alternatives.

Act
- Develop the discharge plan.
- Implement the plan.
- Evaluate and follow up on the plan.
- Revise the plan, as indicated.
- Update the resource file.

BOX 24.3 High-Risk Patient Indicators for Home Care Services

- Unexpected readmission to the hospital within 15–30 days
- Frequent readmissions
- Alteration of health-care problems or management
- Changes in mental status
- Nonadherent behavior before or during hospitalization
- Terminal or preterminal condition
- Seen in the hospital by a physical, occupational, or speech therapist
- After amputation
- After hip or knee replacement
- New assistive devices
- Foley catheter, ileal conduit, suprapubic catheter, and/or incontinence
- Complex health management regimen
- Enteral or parenteral feedings
- Ostomies or tubes of any kind
- Draining wounds
- After wound debridement or irrigation and debridement for pressure injury
- Pain management
- IV antibiotics
- Peripherally inserted central catheter
- IV chemotherapy
- Multiple drugs or a major drug change
- Ventilator dependence
- Low-air-loss bed or other complex medical equipment

---

disease (COPD), unstable diabetes, kidney, or liver disease with subsequent transplantation, or recent strokes
- Have chronic mental illnesses such as depression, schizophrenia, or other psychoses
- Need assistance with medical regimens to prevent readmission to an acute care facility
- Need continued treatment after discharge from a hospital or nursing facility (e.g., wound care, IV therapy, or physical therapy)
- Require short-term assistance at home after same-day or outpatient surgery, or are terminally ill and want hospice care to die with their families and to die with dignity in the comfort of their own homes

Home care is less expensive than hospitalization in most cases. For example, considerable savings may be achieved using home care services for infusion therapy services. Although home care services are being used because of financial considerations, sound medical and humane reasons also exist for treatment to take place in a person's home. Evidence suggests that people recover faster at home than in institutions, and hospital-acquired infections from exposure to multiple infectious processes are minimized in a person's home.

Box 24.3 lists patient characteristics that should suggest further evaluation for a home care referral. These characteristics alone do not warrant the need for home health care, but in combination with one another or with a new diagnosis that requires monitoring, they provide an excellent guideline to determine the need for services. The assessment may be done as a prehospitalization screening, at the time of admission to the hospital, after a patient's condition has changed, or as a patient is being discharged. What really matters is that the patient be assessed for home care needs before they leave the hospital.

Ideally, a patient is screened for home care needs at the time of admission to a hospital to ensure adequate time to plan for continuity of care. In most instances, unless a patient is already known to a home care agency, discharge planning occurs late in the hospital stay. As hospital lengths of stay become increasingly shorter, the time available to plan adequately for a patient's postdischarge care is limited. Home care agencies and hospital discharge planners or case managers need to develop a good working relationship to ensure that patients going home have continuity of care. To ensure a smooth transition, members of all disciplines who were caring for a patient in the hospital—nurses, physicians, physical therapists, social workers, and others—should provide qualitative and quantitative information about the patient's disposition at discharge. The same principles apply to the discharge process from Skilled Nursing Facilities (SNFs) or rehabilitation facilities.

In most cases, a social worker or case manager is responsible for notifying the home health agency of a patient's discharge. The home health agency requests information needed to ensure a smooth transition from the facility to home. In addition to demographics, necessary information includes the following:
- Identification of the PCP or the PCMH who will sign the home care orders
- Orders for home health-care treatments (e.g., wound care, IV therapy, physical therapy, occupational therapy, or speech therapy)
- Description of the patient's knowledge about the disease and treatment
- Summary of patient's independence with skills

- Quantitative measures of range of motion and patient response to treatment modalities
- Known social situations that could complicate or hinder home treatment plan
- List of supplies and drugs going home with patient
- Expectations for rehospitalization or follow-up clinic visits
- Anything that would enhance a timely and efficient response from a home care agency

Role of Home Care Agency

Admission to the home care agency begins with the referral intake. Referrals are called in to the home-care agency, and the agency confirms home care benefits; schedules the admission visit consistent with the expectations of the discharge planner, physician, or patient; and communicates the referral information to the nurse who will be admitting the patient into service. The patient must be admitted within 48 hours of discharge, according to Medicare regulations.

Nurses are assigned to patients in various ways. Some assignments are made according to geographic areas, the patient's special needs, or the nurse's specialty.

IMPLEMENTING THE PLAN OF TREATMENT

The Nurse's Role

The nurse conducts the initial evaluation visit after a patient is referred for home care. During the initial visit and throughout subsequent visits, the nurse assesses the patient's physical, functional, emotional, socioeconomic, and environmental well-being. Nurses initiate the care plan and make revisions as appropriate throughout the length of their stay in home care.

Other activities requiring the specialized skills of registered nurses (RNs) include the following:
- Health and self-care teaching
- Coordination and case management of complex care needs
- Drug administration (e.g., intramuscular and subcutaneous) and teaching about all drugs
- Wound and pressure injury care
- Urinary catheter care and teaching
- Ostomy care and teaching
- Postsurgical care
- Care of the terminally ill patient

Additional activities provided by some home care nurses are as follows:
- Case management
- IV therapy, enteral and parenteral nutrition, and chemotherapy
- Psychiatric nursing care

Characteristics of a Home-Care Nurse

Home health nursing is a subspecialty of community health nursing. It is community-based in that the focus is the patient and family, not an aggregate population. The American Nurses Association (ANA) has endorsed practice standards for home health nurses. As with other specialties, the standards address theory, research, ethics, and professional development. The ANA's statement on *The Scope of Home Health Nursing Practice* (ANA, 2014) presents the conceptual model for home health nursing. The model depicts the holistic practice of the home health nurse. Nurses who work in home care require a diverse set of skills and abilities. Most home care agencies require a nurse to have a minimum of 2 years of hospital experience before working as a home health nurse. Working in home care requires knowledge of acute and chronic disease processes and how they affect older adults. Knowledge of gerontology, pharmacokinetics in older adults, rehabilitation nursing, and principles and presentation of disease processes in older adults are areas in which home care nurses need to be competent. The home care nurse also needs to know adult learning principles and interpersonal communication techniques, and they must be aware of cultural differences and how they affect health and health care.

The home care nurse coordinates care with all disciplines involved with the case and reports findings, changes, and recommendations to the primary physician. The home care nurse also works cooperatively with community resources and governmental agencies if a situation warrants. The nurse, often the sole health-care provider who visits a patient's home, knows that observations made must be acted on immediately and that the instructions provided must last until the next visit. If emergency hospitalization is required, the nurse coordinates it with the family, the physician, the hospital, and emergency services.

Home care nurses need to be conscious of their own safety. Some neighborhoods are dangerous, and visits sometimes need to be made in the evening or at night. The home health nurse should never go into a situation that might be physically threatening or dangerous. The nurse must be self-reliant, self-assured, and comfortable providing care in the patient's locale. Always taking precautions, not just in potentially dangerous neighborhoods, will ensure the nurse's safety. In a recent position paper, TJC endorsed the role of the home health care nurse in managing patients in noninstitutional settings and preventing admissions and readmissions to the institutional setting (The Joint Commission, 2012).

Role of the Home-Health Aide

In 2022, approximately 3,715,500 home health aides (HHAs) were working in home health, with a projected increase of 22% between 2022 and 2032. Home Health Agencies (HHAs) are the second largest group of employees in home care (U.S. Bureau of Labor Statistics, 2022). Under the direction of an RN, HHAs assist patients with intermittent personal care services (e.g., ADLs and hygiene), take vital signs, perform simple duties (e.g., nonsterile dressing changes and Foley catheter care), assist with drugs that are normally self-administered, and report changes in patients' conditions or needs. The HHA is a nonprofessional caregiver who has completed a course of study and has been certified by an appropriate agency. In addition, an HHA is required to complete at least 12 hours of in-service training per year of employment. The HHA must demonstrate competency in certain required skills and subjects taught at in-service training at least once a year.

Because the HHA sees the patient more often than caregivers from other disciplines, they are one of the most important members of the home care team. The patient feels comfortable with the aide and often shares concerns that the nurse or therapist cannot elicit. The RN supervises the HHA on a bimonthly basis (Centers for Medicare and Medicaid Services [CMS], 2018).

Home health agencies also employ patient-care assistants (PCAs). PCAs are generally hired for private duty cases in which only a sitter is required (as opposed to someone who provides personal or skilled care). No formal or informal training is required, but individual agencies may provide orientation and some training. Duties performed by PCAs may include, but are not limited to, the following:
- Preparing light meals
- Helping the patient to the bathroom
- Assisting with dressing and ambulation
- Light housekeeping

OASIS

Outcome and Assessment Information Set (OASIS) is an assessment tool integrated into an agency's assessment form. It is used to monitor the outcomes of home care. OASIS is mandated by the CMS for all adult patients except maternity patients. Its purpose is to improve performance through an approach called outcome-based quality improvement (CMS, 2022a). OASIS was developed to help shape the future direction of Medicare reimbursement and the future of home health.

OASIS data are reported to regulatory bodies at least every 30 days. The completion and reporting of OASIS data are part of the conditions of participation for the Medicare program (CMS, 2022a). OASIS is intended to focus on outcomes of care, such as satisfaction and improved patient outcomes. OASIS data are completed on admission, discharge, interruption of services, and resumption of services. Surveyors who monitor agencies use the data for onsite reviews. They compare the data on OASIS with data from the assessment of a patient when visiting the patient at home.

COMMUNITY-BASED PROVIDERS

Community-based service providers are challenged to develop affordable and appropriate programs to assist older adults to remain in the home while maintaining their quality of life. Community-based services for older adults include home-health care, community-based alternative programs, respite care, adult day care programs, senior citizen centers, homemaker programs, home-delivered meals, and transportation, among many others (Box 24.4). In some areas, churches and neighborhoods have organized volunteer programs to help meet the needs of older adults who rarely leave home. Some of these programs rely on paid nurses and volunteers from the community.

To identify the needs of the older population, nurses in the community must have sharp assessment skills and knowledge of normal aging changes, chronic illnesses, and the effects of illnesses and treatments on older adults. They must also be aware of available community resources. Home health remains one way to help an older adult who has a physical or cognitive impairment stay at home. Because of changes in reimbursement for federal programs that provide services for older adults and limited funds for state programs, home health nurses are challenged to use interventions that are both effective and cost-efficient.

> **BOX 24.4 Services for Older Individuals**
>
> **Access Services**
> - Case management
> - Information and referral
> - Transportation
>
> **Community-Based Services**
> - Adult day care
> - Congregate nutrition programs
> - Elder abuse/protective services
> - Health screening/wellness promotion services
> - Housing services
> - Institutional respite care
> - Legal assistance
> - Multipurpose senior centers
> - Psychologic counseling
> - Retirement planning
>
> **In-Home Services**
> - Home-delivered meals
> - Home health services
> - Home hospice care
> - Homemaker services
> - Home maintenance, repair, or chore services
> - In-home respite care
> - Personal emergency response systems
> - Telephone monitoring and friendly visitors

FACTORS AFFECTING THE HEALTH CARE NEEDS OF OLDER ADULTS

Functional Status

The WHO's International Classification of Functioning, Disability and Health (ICF) defines the term "function" as an umbrella term, including all body structures and functions, activities, and participation in daily life. To standardize postacute care data, thereby improving Medicare beneficiary outcomes through care coordination, shared decision-making, and enhanced discharge planning, the Improving Medicare Post-Acute Care Transformation Act of 2014 (the IMPACT Act) was signed into law. The Act requires the submission of standardized data assessment data elements (SPADEs) by SNFs, Long-Term Care Hospitals (LTCHs), HHAs, and Inpatient Rehabilitation Facilities (IRFs). Commonly used assessment instruments will standardize data: the Minimum Data Set (MDS) for SNFs, the Long-Term Care Hospital CARE Data Set (LCDS) for LTCHs, the OASIS for HHAs, and the Inpatient Rehabilitation Facility Patient Assessment Instrument (IRF PAI) for IRFs. The gathering of this information permits communication among providers on specific domains that include functional status, cognitive function, and mental status. This shared decision-making and coordination of care will improve discharge planning and enhance rehabilitation outcomes.

Functional status is a term used to describe an individual's ability to perform the normal, expected, or required activities for self-care. It is a determinant of well-being and a measure of independence for older adults. Functional measures are much more useful in describing the service needs of older adults living in the community than are measures of acute and chronic illness. Because of their ability to predict service needs, functional measures are used to determine eligibility for many state-funded and federally funded, community-based, long-term care programs. Health-care providers frequently order physical or occupational therapy when a functional deficit exists.

Functional status determines whether an older adult needs home health care or whether a home health patient is recertified for home care services. The use of adaptive equipment as well as barriers to the patient's function should be noted. While assessing the patient's functional status, the nurse considers cognitive status, respiratory and cardiovascular status, and skin integrity. Deficits in these areas may impair the patient's ability to perform ADLs and IADLs safely. The patient's perception of self-care is also important because they may believe that no assistance is required when, in fact, a deficit exists.

For older adults, adapting to functional limitations is crucial for maintaining independence. The outcomes of severe functional impairments are costly (e.g., institutionalization). The nurse must assess for functional impairments. Early detection of limitations leads to interventions that help preserve function and avoid more severe disability. *Frailty*, as previously defined, has become a predictor for older adults. Frail older adults are more likely to require assistance in the home care setting or require a supervised care setting (Kojima et al, 2019).

Cognitive Function

A cognitive assessment can determine the need for a referral to a speech-language pathologist. Speech and language skills are readily assessed during an initial interview. Speech patterns should be noted. Assessing whether the patient can understand the spoken and written word is paramount to treatment. Determining if the patient can follow directions, such as a simple command, can determine comprehension. The nurse can also administer screening cognition tests to determine delirium or dementia.

Cognitive status is assessed on admission, with every nursing visit, and at discharge. Other disciplines are also responsible for reporting a change in cognition to the nurse or case manager. A change in cognitive status frequently signals a change in another body system. The nurse must establish a baseline assessment and be alert to deviations. Cognitive impairments may be reversible or irreversible, and health personnel are in a key position to detect any changes.

Cognitive impairments are associated with functional limitations. For example, individuals with deficits in memory, language, abstract thinking, and judgment have great difficulty executing ADLs or IADLs (e.g., shopping, paying bills, preparing meals, and personal care tasks), even though they may have no *physical* impairments or disabilities. Cognitively impaired individuals often need supervision and cueing, rather than physical assistance, to perform ADLs and IADLs.

Although cognitive impairment alone does not meet the criteria for home health-care services covered by Medicare, many states provide services for individuals with Alzheimer disease and related dementias through Medicaid and Medicare waiver programs. Medicare covers skilled nursing visits when (1) the skill is necessary to maintain the patient's health, (2) the cognitive impairment interferes with the patient's ability to perform the skill, and (3) no caregiver is present or able to perform the skill. An older adult who requires daily insulin injections but is unable to draw up or administer the insulin because of a cognitive impairment is an example of someone who qualifies for home health care.

Housing Options for Older Adults

Although older adults prefer to live independently, it is not always possible or appropriate; financial status, functional status, frailty, and physical health may dictate consideration of alternative housing options that provide a more protective and supportive environment. Table 24.2 describes the most common housing options for older adults. Each option has its advantages and disadvantages. The decision about which option is most appropriate depends on such factors as the amount and type of assistance an older person requires, financial resources, geographic mobility, preferences for privacy and social contact, and the types of housing available. The American Association of Retired Persons (AARP) has several publications that describe each of these options in greater detail, including issues to consider when evaluating each option.

Profile of Community- and Home-Based Services
Area Agencies on Aging

The major goal of the Older Americans Act (OAA) of 1965 was to remove barriers to independent living for older individuals and to ensure the availability of appropriate services for those in need. Through Title III, the Administration on Aging (AOA) and state and community programs were designed to meet the needs of older adults, especially those at risk for loss of independence. The OAA established a national network of federal, state, and Area Agencies on Aging (AAAs), which is responsible for providing a range of community services for older adults. States are divided into areas for planning and service administration. The OAA requires that each AAA designate community "focal points" as places where anyone in the community can receive information, services, and access to all community resources for older adults. Multipurpose senior citizen centers often serve as these focal points, but community centers, churches, hospitals, and town halls may also be designated as focal points. The types of services provided through the OAA and the AAAs include information and referral for medical and legal advice; psychologic counseling; preretirement and postretirement planning; programs to prevent abuse, neglect, and exploitation; programs to enrich life through educational and social activities; health screening and wellness promotion services; and nutrition services (Administration for Community Living, 2017).

TABLE 24.2 Housing Options for Older Adults

Type of Housing	Description of Housing
Accessory apartment	This is a self-contained apartment unit within a house that allows an individual to live independently without living alone. It generates additional income for older homeowners and allows older renters to live near relatives or friends and remain in a familiar community.
Assisted living facility (also called *board and care home; personal care home;* or *sheltered care, residential care,* or *domiciliary care facility*)	This is a rental housing arrangement that provides room, meals, utilities, laundry, and housekeeping services for a group of residents. Such facilities offer a homelike atmosphere in which residents share meals and have opportunities to interact. What distinguishes these facilities from simple boarding homes is that they provide protective oversight and regular contact with staff members. Some facilities offer additional services such as nonmedical personal care (e.g., bathing and grooming) and social and recreational activities. In many states, these facilities operate without specific regulation or licensure; therefore, the quality of service may vary greatly.
Congregate housing	Congregate housing was authorized in 1970 by the Housing and Urban Development Act. It is a group-living arrangement, usually an apartment complex that provides tenants with private living units (including kitchen facilities), housekeeping services, and meals served in a central dining room. It is different from board and care facilities in that it provides professional staff such as social workers, nutritionists, and activity therapists who organize social services and activities.
Elder Cottage Housing Opportunity (ECHO)	This is a small, self-contained portable unit that can be placed in the backyard or at the side of a single-family dwelling. The idea was developed in Australia (where it is called a "granny flat") to allow older adults to live near family and friends but still retain privacy and independence. ECHO units are distinct from mobile homes in that they are barrier-free and energy-efficient units specifically designed for older or disabled persons.
Foster home care	Foster care for adults is similar in concept to foster care for children. It is a social service administered by the state that places an older person who needs some protective oversight or assistance with personal care in a family environment. Foster families receive a stipend to provide board and care, and older patients have a chance to participate in family and community activities. Adult foster care is appropriate for older adults who cannot live independently but do not want or need institutional care.
Home sharing	Home sharing involves two or more unrelated people living together in a house or apartment. It may involve an older person and a younger person or two or more older people living together. The participants may share all living expenses, share rent only, or exchange services for rent. For the older homeowner, renting out a bedroom generates revenue that may make it possible to afford taxes and home expenses. Many older adults view home sharing as a practical alternative to moving in with adult children. Some communities provide house-matching programs, usually sponsored by local senior centers or the Area Agency on Aging.
Life care or continuing care retirement community (CCRC)	This is a facility designed to support the concept of "aging in place." It provides a continuum of living arrangements and care—from assistance with household chores to nursing facility care—all within a single retirement community. Residents live independently in apartments or houses and contract with the community for health and social services, as needed. If a resident's need for health and nursing care prohibits independent living, the individual can move from a residential unit to the community's health-care unit or nursing facility. In addition to providing shelter, meals, and health care, a CCRC provides a variety of services and activities (e.g., religious services, adult education classes, libraries, trips, and recreational and social programs). The key attribute of a CCRC is that it guarantees a lifetime commitment to the care of an individual if the person remains in the retirement community. The major disadvantage of a CCRC is that it can be expensive; most CCRCs require a nonrefundable entrance fee and charge a monthly assessment, which may increase.

Data from Hoyt, J. (2023). *Senior housing options and retirement guide.* SeniorLiving.org. [website]. Retrieved from https://www.seniorliving.org/housing/.

Multipurpose Senior Centers

Senior centers are community facilities that provide a broad range of services to older adults in the community. These services include (1) health screening; (2) health promotion and wellness programs; (3) social, educational, and recreational activities; (4) congregate meals; and (5) information and referral services for older individuals and their families. Relatively active and independent older adults primarily use senior centers because such centers do not provide nursing and custodial-care services. Older adults who require these types of services would benefit from attending an adult day care program. Funding for senior centers is provided primarily through the Older Americans Act (OAA) and agencies such as the United Way.

Adult Day Care Services

Adult day care services provide a variety of health and social services to older adults who live alone or with their families in the community. Most people who use adult day care services are physically frail, cognitively impaired, or both, and require supervision or assistance with ADLs. Adult day care programs help delay institutionalization for older adults who require some supervision but who do not need continuous care. This allows family members to maintain their lifestyles and employment and allows the older adult to remain in the home.

Most adult day care services operate 5 days a week during typical business hours. Charges vary with each facility, from per-week to per-day to per-half-day. Adult day care services vary considerably in terms of eligibility criteria and the types of services provided. Key services may include transportation to and from the facility, assistance with personal care, nursing and therapeutic services, meals, and recreational activities.

Adult day care services are not federally regulated but may be licensed or certified by the state. Certification is required to receive federal funding, such as Medicaid and OAA funding. Other funding sources include private pay, foundations, and long-term care insurance. Medicaid is a major funding source for most of these programs; however, participants usually pay part of the fee. Some facilities may accept only private pay or long-term care insurance. Other private sources of funding include religious organizations, businesses, and the United Way.

Some programs accept only patients with dementia. It is difficult to combine patients with dementia and patients who have no cognitive impairment. This situation requires extra staff and usually a larger facility with separate areas for the two different groups. The staff in these programs is trained to work with persons with dementia.

Respite Care

Respite care provides short-term relief or time off for persons providing home care to ill, disabled, or frail older adults. Adult day care services are a form of respite provided outside the home. Respite care is often provided at home or in institutional settings such as specially designated hospital or nursing facility units. Respite staff includes health professionals, trained volunteers, and PCAs. In-home and institutional respite may be provided on a regular schedule (e.g., 4 hours a week) or for longer time intervals (e.g., 1 week, a weekend, or on an intermittent basis). Private pay and state programs that target lower-income families are the two main funding sources for respite care.

Homemaker Services

Homemaker services include such things as housecleaning, laundry, food shopping, meal preparation, and running errands. Fees vary according to the type and frequency of services provided and are usually not covered by Medicare or Medicaid. These services are offered through home health agencies, Area Agencies on Aging (AAAs), the Department of Health and Human Services, and private companies and organizations that provide other services to older adults. Prices vary with the type of agency offering the homemaker services. In most states, no licensing or certification is required for the individual providing the care. Background checks and letters of recommendation are often the only qualifications for the positions.

Nutrition Services

Nutrition services provide older adults with inexpensive, nutritious meals at home or in group settings. Home delivery programs such as Meals-on-Wheels deliver hot meals to the home once or twice a day, 5 days a week, and can accommodate special diets. Some Meals-on-Wheels programs sell nutritional supplements at reduced rates to older adults who cannot leave the home. Congregate meal sites provide meals in group settings such as senior centers, churches, synagogues, schools, and senior housing. The advantage of congregate meal sites is that they provide social opportunities for older adults who are otherwise socially isolated. Most nutrition programs charge a minimum fee or ask for donations. Another advantage of home-delivered meals is that the volunteer delivering the meal can check on the older adult daily and report any problems to the supervisor. In some instances, a Meals-on-Wheels volunteer has been the first person to discover an older adult who fell in the home and was unable to seek assistance.

Transportation Services

Many communities provide transportation services for disabled older adults through public or private agencies. Transportation may be handled by volunteer drivers in cars or by a bus, taxi, train, or a public van equipped to accommodate wheelchairs. The fee for such transportation services is usually minimal and is often based on a sliding scale. In addition, many facilities that serve older adults (e.g., adult day care services, senior centers, and health facilities) have their own transportation services.

Telephone Monitoring and Friendly Visitors

Telephone monitoring programs provide regular phone contact (usually daily) to older persons who live alone or are alone during the day. The phone calls provide social contact as well as a check for those who are concerned about their health and safety. Friendly visitors make home visits for the purpose of companionship, assistance with correspondence, and needs assessment. Telephone monitoring staff and friendly visitors are volunteers who work through local community organizations such as churches, synagogues, senior centers, and social service agencies. Even if older adults live in areas where these formal services are not available, nurses can encourage informal telephone monitoring and visits by family members, friends, and neighbors. Telephone services that will call individuals to remind them to take their drugs are also available, usually for a monthly fee.

Personal Emergency Response Systems

Personal emergency response systems (PERSs) are home monitoring systems that allow older persons to obtain immediate assistance in emergent situations, for example, after a fall or when suffering life-threatening symptoms. A PERS consists of a small device worn on the body (encouraged to be a necklace) that, when triggered, will send an alarm to a central monitoring station. The central monitoring station then contacts predesignated persons or the police, who respond to the emergency. A PERS may be purchased or leased for a monthly fee. Because these devices are relatively expensive, they are not a practical alternative for older adults in middle-income groups. Those in lower-income groups or with dual eligibility will have it as part of a comprehensive home management plan. They are recommended with caution for persons with dementia because resetting the device is very difficult and the device may be triggered too often for nonemergencies. Newer devices include GPS that look like a wristwatch, so older adults with dementia or wandering tendencies can be found.

HOME HEALTH CARE

Home care consists of multiple health and social services delivered to recovering, chronically ill, or disabled individuals of all ages in their place of residence. There are three main categories of home care providers, known as *home care organizations* (National Association for Home Care and Hospice [NAHC], n.d.). Medicare-certified agencies include hospice, freestanding, and facility-based home health agencies.

Medicare, Medicaid, private insurance, managed care plans, and private pay cover home health services. Persons of all ages are eligible for home health services. Criteria for services vary based on the type of insurance. Most home health-care recipients are 65 or older. Medicare, the primary payer source for home health services, requires the home health patient to (1) have a skilled care need, (2) be homebound, (3) be unable to perform the skilled care alone and have no one in the home to provide care, and (4) require only intermittent care. If a caregiver is present, they must be unwilling or unable to provide the care needed. Being homebound means that the home health patient has a physical reason (e.g., being bedridden) or medical condition that limits their ability to leave home. The use of assistive devices or a wheelchair alone does not qualify an individual for homebound status. The home health patient is allowed to leave home for medical reasons, but it must be an *effort* to do so. In other words, if the patient could get to a physician's office to receive care on a regular basis, Medicare would deny the home health services. The patient must also have a physician's written plan of treatment for the service, specifying the frequency and duration of care provided.

Medicare establishes specific criteria for coverage by the physician, home health agency, disciplines providing care, and other entities (e.g., medical supply companies) that provide goods or services to the patient. The purpose of eligibility criteria is to ensure that Medicare dollars are being spent in the most cost-effective manner (CMS, 2018). Other payer sources (e.g., health maintenance organizations [HMOs] and private insurance) use Medicare criteria as a guideline for eligibility but have the flexibility to vary the criteria with individual circumstances.

Medicaid is delivered by each state and has its own criteria for reimbursement. Other funding sources for home health include social service block grants, OAA funds, and general state revenues. The dollar amount spent on home health by sources other than Medicare and Medicaid varies with each state. The U.S. Department of Veterans Affairs; the Veterans health-care program, TRICARE; and the VA Civilian Health and Medical Program (CHAMPVA) have their own coverage guidelines and payment methods for home health, and each covers different home health services (USA.gov, 2022).

Managed care companies have various methods for approving services related to home health care. The admissions assessment is usually approved first. Then, based on the diagnosis, the functional status of the home health patient, and the ability of the caregiver to provide help, the company assigns further home health visits. Other companies approve a specified number of visits based on the diagnosis and information from the referring physician. The home health agency stays in close communication with the managed care company to report progress and request any changes in the original care plan.

Home Health Agency

The predominant and most familiar provider of home care is the home health agency. Home health agencies have as their primary function the treatment or rehabilitation of patients through the intervention of skilled nurses or therapists. Patients admitted to a home health agency must be under a physician's supervision, and services must be provided in accordance with a physician's signed order. Home health agencies can provide a different combination of services. Skilled nursing and physical therapy may stand alone, that is, either the RN or physical therapist may serve as the case manager. Speech therapists, occupational therapists, and medical social workers are not allowed to admit patients to home health care but must work with a nurse or physical therapist. In addition, many agencies offer nutritional services on a limited basis. Agencies may also provide disposable medical supplies as appropriate for the diagnosis and treatment plan of a patient.

Proprietary Agencies

A proprietary or for-profit home care agency is designed to make money for its owners. Until 1982, proprietary home care agencies were not allowed to participate in Medicare. This was changed in response to a concern that not enough home care services were available to meet the demand. As a result, the Omnibus Budget Reconciliation Act (OBRA) of 1982 allowed proprietary home care agencies to become Medicare certified, but they were not allowed to make a profit on the Medicare portion of their business. Owners of a for-profit entity are stockholders in the corporation.

Facility-Based Agencies

A facility-based home care agency is a department or component of an organization. It may be a part of a skilled nursing facility (SNF) or rehabilitation center, or it may be hospital-based. Many agencies are hospital based, that is, they function as a department of the hospital. These agencies may or may not share clinical, financial, or management services with the hospital.

The first hospital-based home care agency was established in 1947. Its programs offered nursing care, housekeeping, and chore duties. In 1958, radiology services, nutritional services, and physical therapy were offered. With the enactment of Medicare and Medicaid in 1965, nurses were able to offer more home care to the sick and the disabled. Hospital-based home care agencies were few until the enactment of Medicare reform (OBRA, in 1987), when hospitals began to be paid for patients receiving Medicare benefits based on a diagnosis-related group (DRG). With shorter lengths of stay, hospitals established home care agencies or affiliated with existing home care agencies to provide options for patients who were going home with existing health-care needs. The Patient Protection and Affordable Care Act of 2010 made changes to Medicare reimbursement, resulting in a 5% reduction in reimbursement for home care visits.

What determines a facility-based home care agency from CMS's point of view is whether it receives an allocation of the institution's corporate overhead. A facility-based home care agency, according to The Joint Commission (2012), shows evidence of an organizational and functional relationship between the home care agency and the facility or public representation of the home care agency as a service of the facility.

Visiting Nurse Associations

A visiting nurse association (VNA), or community nursing service, is a community-based home care agency with a governing board consisting of community representatives. Because of their commitment to provide home care services to a defined community and their not-for-profit status, VNAs are often recipients of United Way or Community Givers funds.

OVERVIEW OF LONG-TERM CARE

Definition

Long-term care has several meanings in the gerontological nursing literature. The phrase is most accurately used to describe a collection of health, personal, and social services provided over a prolonged period. Of people over the age of 65, 70% will use some form of long-term care in their lifetime (Johnson, 2019). Recipients of long-term care services typically include older adults but may also include developmentally disabled persons, persons permanently impaired from traumatic injuries, and chronically ill younger persons. Services range from supportive care to very complex care. Long-term care settings may be categorized on a continuum according to the complexity of care provided and the amount of skilled care and services required by the residents served. Settings go from more structure to less structure as one moves from the institutional setting to community-based programs to the home setting. Table 24.3 illustrates this continuum of long-term care settings.

Persons living in nursing facilities are called *residents*. The facility is their permanent or temporary home. Some residents require nursing care until death. Other residents are admitted to an acute care hospital. They stay for a short time to recover from an acute illness, injury, or surgery, then return home. Medical, nursing, dietary, recreational, rehabilitative, social, and spiritual care is usually provided. All nursing facilities must function under the federal regulations set forth by the OBRA. Some facilities are also accredited by TJC.

Factors Associated with Institutionalization

As life expectancy and the size of the older adult population increase, the possibility of a person entering a nursing facility at some point also increases. Advanced age, living alone, female gender, utilizing home care, experiencing at least two falls during the previous 12 months, utilizing a walking aid, cognitive decline (<24 in mini-mental state examination [MMSE]), dementia, kidney disease, thyroid disease, and multimorbidity (at least two diseases) were all significantly associated with a higher institutionalization rate (Salminen et al, 2020).

Factors contributing to the need for institutionalization may be categorized according to the characteristics of the person, the characteristics of the person's support system, and the community resources available to the person.

Many older persons receive long-term care services in the home from relatives and friends, and in small group settings with intermediate levels of care. Despite an older person's preference to stay at home, admission to a nursing facility becomes necessary when the person's physical and mental capabilities deteriorate to a point where adequate family and community resources are no longer available (National Institute on Aging [NIA], 2017).

Medical and Psychosocial Models of Care

Nursing facilities evolved from the acute-care hospital system and the medical model. Like hospitals, nursing facilities were designed around the departments and professionals rather than the consumers they served. Although the organization of nursing facilities tends to be hierarchic and bureaucratic, alternative methods of staffing are being developed and implemented. In contrast, resident-centered care is a philosophy of care focused on the needs of the resident and is contingent upon knowing the person through an interpersonal relationship. This shift in focus challenges the traditional medical model of care, which tends to focus on schedules, processes, and staff and organizational needs. Everyone, including leadership, within the organization must commit to this shift in focus (Fazio et al, 2018).

This model is incongruent with changes mandated by the OBRA, with an emphasis on the social and psychologic health of nursing facility residents in addition to the traditional medical concerns. Residents' subjective evaluations of their quality of life need to be solicited and valued. Psychosocial models of care emphasize resident decision-making and the exercise of personal choice. The ideal long-term care facility is a combination of both medical and social models, not exclusively one or the other (Box 24.5). Creative strategies are necessary to enhance a resident's perception of autonomy (see the Evidence-Based Practice box). The baccalaureate-prepared nurse is in a wonderful position to combine their knowledge of medicine, nursing, psychology, and sociology into a model that truly provides individualized care to each resident in the nursing facility.

TABLE 24.3 Continuum of Settings in Which Long-Term Care is Provided

Institutional	Community	Home
Nursing facility	Adult day care center	Home health nursing
Group home	Senior center	Home health rehabilitation services
Board and care facility	Congregate meal programs	Homemaker
Assisted living	Hospice	Home-delivered meals
Continuing care retirement communities		Adaptive devices for the home environment
Hospice		Hospice

BOX 24.5 Major Regulatory "Level A" Requirements Defined by the Omnibus Budget Reconciliation Act of 1987

- Resident rights
- Admission, transfer, and discharge rights
- Resident behavior and facility practices
- Quality of life
- Resident assessment
- Quality of care
- Nursing services
- Dietary services
- Physician services
- Specialized rehabilitative services
- Dental services
- Pharmacy services
- Infection control
- Physical environment
- Administration

> **EVIDENCE-BASED PRACTICE**
>
> *Person-Centered Care*
>
> **Background and Objectives**
> Person-centered care is a philosophy of care built around the needs of the individual and contingent upon knowing the unique individual through an interpersonal relationship. This review article outlines the history, components, and impact of person-centered care practices.
>
> **Research Design and Methods**
> Through a literature review, published articles on person-centered measures and outcomes were examined.
>
> **Results**
> The history of person-centered care was described, the core principles of care for individuals with dementia were outlined, current tools to measure person-centered care approaches were reviewed, and the outcomes of intervention were discussed.
>
> **Discussion and Implications**
> Evidence-based practice recommendations for person-centered care for individuals with dementia are outlined. More research is needed to further assess the outcomes of person-centered care approaches and models.
>
> **Practice Recommendations for Person-Centered Care**
> *Know the person living with dementia*
> The individual living with dementia is more than a diagnosis. It is important to know the unique and complete person, including his/her values, beliefs, interests, abilities, likes, and dislikes—both past and present. This information should inform every interaction and experience.
>
> *Recognize and accept the person's reality*
> It is important to see the world from the perspective of the individual living with dementia. Doing so recognizes behavior as a form of communication, thereby promoting effective and empathetic communication that validates feelings and connects with the individual in his/her reality.
>
> *Identify and support ongoing opportunities for meaningful engagement*
> Every experience and interaction can be seen as an opportunity for engagement. Engagement should be meaningful to and purposeful for the individual living with dementia. It should support interests and preferences, allow for choice and success, and recognize that even when the dementia is most severe, the person can experience joy, comfort, and meaning in life.
>
> *Build and nurture authentic, caring relationships*
> Persons living with dementia should be part of relationships that treat them with dignity and respect and their individuality should always be supported. This type of caring relationship is about being present and concentrating on the interaction, rather than the task. It is about "doing with" rather than "doing for," as part of a supportive and mutually beneficial relationship.
>
> Create and maintain a supportive community for individuals, families, and staff.
>
> A supportive community allows for comfort and creates opportunities for success. It is a community that values each person and respects individual differences, celebrates accomplishments and occasions, and provides access to and opportunities for autonomy, engagement, and shared experiences.
>
> *Evaluate care practices regularly and make appropriate changes*
> Several tools are available to assess person-centered care practices for people living with dementia. It is important to regularly evaluate practices and models, share findings, and make changes to interactions, programs, and practices as needed.

Data from Fazio, S., Pace, D., Flinner, J., & Kallmyer, B. (2018). The fundamentals of person-centered care for individuals with dementia. *The Gerontologist, 58*(Suppl. 1), S10–S19.

CLINICAL ASPECTS OF THE NURSING FACILITY

Resident Rights

One of the accomplishments of the report of the Committee on Nursing Home Regulation of the Institute of Medicine (IOM) was to lay the foundation for greater regulatory support of resident rights in the nursing facility (IOM, 1986). The emphasis on resident rights was directly related to a revised view that residents really did have the right to autonomy and to be active participants and decision-makers in their care and life in the institutional setting.

Resident rights unique to the nursing facility are to be promoted in several ways. These include, but are not limited to, the following (CMS, 2022b):

- Establishment and maintenance of a resident council
- Public display of posters listing resident rights
- Public display of local ombudsman program information
- Public display of annual state inspection results
- Aggressive attempts to provide opportunities for residents to exercise their right to vote during public elections
- Manage your own money as well as get information on fees and services
- Provision of opportunities for competent residents to self-administer drugs
- Informed consent process for the use of side rails and chemical and physical restraints
- Informed consent process for withdrawal or withholding of life-sustaining treatments
- Grievance process whereby residents and families can challenge the care that is given

All departments within the nursing facility, including social services, activities, nursing, dietary, and maintenance, must share responsibility for ensuring the enforcement of these resident rights. Ideally, this effort will be the operational philosophy for all nursing facilities.

Regulatory enforcement focuses strongly on resident safety without always considering a resident's individual right to be autonomous and make a conscious decision to place themselves at risk (e.g., for falling) to retain some degree of independence. Each situation must be evaluated individually, and the legalities may be complicated.

Resident Assessment

Interdisciplinary functional assessment of residents is the cornerstone of clinical practice in this setting. The OBRA prescribed the method of resident assessment and care-plan development in an instrument known as the Resident Assessment Instrument (RAI). The RAI consists of three parts: (1) the minimum data set (MDS), (2) the resident assessment protocols (RAPs), and (3) the utilization guidelines specified by the CMS *MDS 3.0 RAI Manual* (CMS, 2023).

The MDS is a tool that includes a comprehensive assessment of residents. Categories include resident background information; cognitive, communication, hearing, and vision patterns; physical functioning and structural problems; mood, behavior, and activity pursuit patterns; psychosocial well-being; fecal and urinary continence; health conditions; disease diagnoses; oral, nutritional, and dental status; skin condition; drug use; and special treatments and procedures. This resident profile is used to develop an individualized, comprehensive care plan for each resident (Fig. 24.2).

Deadlines for completion of each section and care-planning decisions emanating from the assessment process are prescribed by regulation.

The specific method used to complete the RAI varies from facility to facility. Some facilities assign one nurse to complete all documentation related to the RAI; others distribute this responsibility among all the nurses. The RAI is completed for each resident on admission, annually, when a significant change of condition occurs (as defined by the CMS *MDS 3.0 RAI Manual*), and quarterly. For persons admitted for skilled care under Medicare Part A, the MDS and the RAI are completed at 5 or 14 days, 30 days, 60 days, and 90 days, and with any significant change.

Both licensed vocational or practical nurses and RNs may contribute to the RAI. However, only an RN can sign the document and function as the RN assessment coordinator (RAC). The RAC signs and certifies the completion of the assessment, not the accuracy of the assessment data (CMS, 2023). Contributions to the RAI are also made by the dietary supervisor, social worker, recreational therapist, medical records clerk, and physical and occupational therapists.

The overall goal of the RAI is to provide an ongoing, comprehensive assessment of a resident, emphasizing functional ability and both a physical and a psychosocial profile. It is also a key component in the development of a national database for long-term care.

Skin Care

Skin and nail care programs are important to a resident's overall health and quality of life. Skin care programs in the nursing facility are focused on the prevention and treatment of skin problems. Preventive strategies include prevention of pressure injury, skin tears, and dry skin or xerosis.

Other skin-related problems commonly occurring and treated in this setting include MRSA infections, ischemic ulcers,

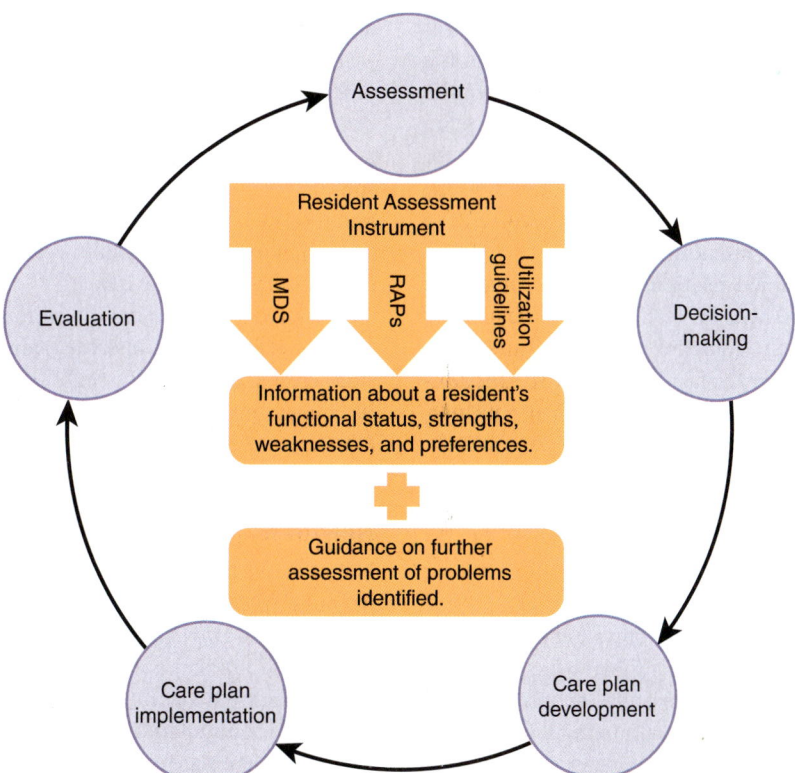

Fig. 24.2 The Resident Assessment Instrument (RAI) is comprised of the Minimum Data Set (MDS), Care Area Assessments (CAAs), and RAI Utilization Guidelines. These instruments provide data on the resident's functional status, strengths, weaknesses, and preferences. (Modified from Centers for Medicare and Medicaid Services [CMS]. 2019.)

dermatitis, eczema, herpes zoster, scabies, pediculosis, bullous pemphigoid, and skin tumors. The prevention of skin tears, pressure injuries, and ischemic ulcers is an ongoing challenge for the staff in nursing facilities. The development of pressure injuries during a person's stay in a nursing facility is considered an indicator of poor quality of care, although research and current knowledge of pressure injury etiology do not support this view as totally accurate. Aggressive and appropriate preventive measures are initiated to address each resident's specific and unique risk factors.

Most nursing facilities have a structured skin care program coordinated by an RN that involves all nursing department staff plus a physical therapist, occupational therapist, and dietitian. On admission, a resident's skin is thoroughly assessed. Individual risk for developing pressure injuries is established, and preventive interventions are initiated as appropriate. These may include a special mattress, positioning devices, vitamin and nutritional supplements, skin lubricants, and a schedule for repositioning the resident in beds and chairs. The certified nursing assistant (CNA) plays a key role in providing effective preventive skin care by assisting the resident in routine bathing, toileting, and maintenance of schedules for turning and repositioning. The individualized care plan, developed by the interdisciplinary team, provides specific instructions concerning the preventive treatment measures for each resident.

Based on the physical examination as well as RAI data, a care plan is initiated. Individual states have varying regulations concerning the required frequency of the nurse's clinical staging and routine assessment of pressure injuries. Most facilities require at least weekly monitoring by an RN. The nurse measures and stages the pressure injury and evaluates the efficacy of the treatment plan. The director of nursing may also work with the medical director or individual health-care providers practicing in the facility to coordinate and standardize treatments for various stages of pressure injuries. Another alternative is to intervene in skin problems on a case-by-case basis according to the preference of the resident's attending physician.

Facilities may have sustained relationships with companies that manufacture specialized beds for residents with stage III or IV pressure injuries. Often, the company provides a nurse consultant as a clinical resource for the facility. The nurse functioning as the skin-care program coordinator might meet routinely with the consultant. The two nurses often work collaboratively, along with the dietitian and physical therapist, to treat skin problems. Consistently following a treatment plan is essential for positive outcomes.

Incontinence

As functional dependence increases, the prevalence of incontinence increases. This common health problem has financial, physical, and psychosocial consequences, and incontinence is a common reason for placing a person in a nursing facility.

Caring for an incontinent resident is expensive; it requires more nursing time and frequent linen and clothing changes. Physical consequences of incontinence include skin breakdown, UTIs, an increased risk of falling, and consequent hip fractures. Urinary incontinence is one of the most psychologically distressing health problems faced by older adults. It may lead to decreased self-esteem and social isolation (Gümüşsoy et al, 2019). One of the features of the OBRA was the inclusion of specific standards and recommendations for the assessment and treatment of urinary incontinence. Clinical programs in nursing facilities are directed at the prevention, treatment, and management of incontinence. Prevention is aimed at reducing the risk of developing urinary incontinence among at-risk residents of nursing facilities. Preventive measures include assessment of individual patterns of elimination so that anticipatory assistance with toileting may be provided, aggressive staff response to residents' requests for assistance in toileting, and arrangement of the physical environment to minimize the physical effort involved in getting to the bathroom.

Treatment programs are resident-oriented and focus on creating changes in the function of the lower urinary tract. Treatments include surgery, pharmacologic interventions, bladder training, pelvic muscle exercises, and biofeedback procedures (McDaniel et al, 2020). It is important to identify those residents who can benefit from these therapies.

Management programs for urinary incontinence are the dominant forms of intervention in nursing facilities. Some residents benefit from programs that involve behavioral approaches such as scheduled toileting, habit training, and prompted voiding. These approaches focus on changing the behavior of the caregiver and the resident to minimize incontinence. However, residents with dementia and other MCIs may not benefit from these interventions; the use of incontinence pads and protective undergarments is necessary for these individuals. External condom catheters may be helpful for males.

Intermittent self-catheterization may be appropriate for residents who are cognitively intact and have adequate manual dexterity. Long-term, indwelling catheterization is indicated for residents who cannot empty their bladders and have not responded to other treatments. Residents who are terminally ill and those with pressure injuries may also benefit from indwelling catheterization. Indwelling catheterization is used only after other interventions have failed.

Effective management of urinary incontinence involves a well-coordinated and sustained effort between licensed nursing staff, CNAs, and activity staff. The nurse must play a key role in managing incontinence and preventing complications; management and treatment must be directed at the cause of incontinence.

Nutrition

Nutritional deficiencies contribute to adverse clinical outcomes in nursing facility residents. Protein-calorie undernutrition results from two broad categories of factors: those causing inadequate intake and those causing increased nutritional requirements (Corcoran et al, 2019).

The older population is the single largest demographic group at disproportionate risk of inadequate diet and malnutrition. Aging is associated with a decline in multiple physiologic functions that may affect nutritional status, including reduced lean body mass and a resultant decrease in basal metabolic rate, decreased gastric secretion of digestive juices and changes in the oral cavity, sensory function deficits, changes in fluid and electrolyte regulation, and chronic illness. Medication, hospitalization, and other social determinants may also contribute to nutritional inadequacy. The nutritional status of older people is an important determinant of quality of life, morbidity, and mortality (Acar Tek and Karaçil-Ermumcu, 2018). Contributing factors include loss of manual dexterity, pain, dementia-related illnesses, certain drugs, and chronic medical disorders. Culture, religion, and personal choice also affect how and what a person eats. A resident's appetite is affected by personal comfort and unpleasant odors, sights, and sounds. Meeting a resident's nutritional needs requires the involvement of the entire health-care team. The health-care provider, dietitian, nurse, speech and language pathologist, occupational therapist, social worker, and nursing assistant all play roles in the assessment of individual needs, care planning, care-plan implementation, and care-plan evaluation. The resident is always included, and the resident's family may also provide important information.

Increased nutritional requirements may be a consequence of hyperactivity in some persons with dementia-related illnesses. Infectious illnesses, periods of recovery after surgical interventions that require tissue healing, and recovery from pressure injuries also increase the nutritional requirements of nursing facility residents.

Various clinical interventions are directed at the nutritional support of residents, including programs focused on maintaining adequate caloric intake and effective identification of residents requiring supplemental nutritional support.

Enhancement of the dining experience through improved esthetics, improved dining room service, attractive food preparation, and increased sensitivity to the social nature of mealtimes is directed toward the maintenance of adequate caloric intake. Other strategies related to this goal include increasing staff assistance for residents who need help with eating and improving staff techniques for aiding with eating. Sensitivity to dental needs and the provision of the textures of foods most easily and safely consumed by each resident are additional strategies.

In nursing facilities, the most common program for prompt identification of residents requiring supplemental nutritional support consists of routine weighing. Weights are taken daily, weekly, biweekly, or monthly, depending on the severity of weight loss or gain experienced by a resident. Interdisciplinary team members, including the nurse, restorative nursing assistant (a CNA with 30 hours of formal training beyond CNA with a focus on direct restorative care and delegated formalized therapy tasks as assigned to continue an ongoing formalized therapy program), dietitian, and speech and language pathologist, may meet routinely to review weight changes and develop interventions directed at supplemental nutritional support. In addition to the strategies already described, changes in therapeutic diets and the use of nutritional products (e.g., Ensure), vitamin supplements, and enteral nutrition products may be considered. Laboratory tests are often ordered to help monitor a resident's nutritional status.

Compliance with the OBRA requires aggressive monitoring of the variables of nutritional status, with attention focused on unintended weight loss. The functional implications of reduced caloric intake are to be considered. Any unintended weight loss of 5% or greater in 30 days, 7.5% in 90 days, or 10% in 180 days (CMS, 2008) is an indicator of poor quality of care. Any weight loss or gain must be carefully monitored. The reasons for the loss or gain and the interventions taken must be documented.

Drug Administration

One of the basic services provided in nursing facilities is drug administration through oral, IV, intramuscular, subcutaneous, and enteral routes. In the nursing facility, the licensed nurse is often responsible for the administration, documentation, storage, ordering, cart stocking, and destruction of many drugs. In some states, medication aids are used to administer drugs. The RN is responsible for monitoring the drug's therapeutic effects, side effects, and any allergic reactions. The RN also monitors and evaluates the skills of medication aides on an ongoing basis. Because most nursing facilities do not have an onsite pharmacy, the nursing staff is responsible for drug-related functions that would be handled by the pharmacy staff in an acute care hospital.

Monitoring for the clinical manifestations of polypharmacy, the occurrence of adverse drug reactions, and the overuse of "as required" (PRN) drug orders have increasingly been emphasized since the enactment of the OBRA. The pharmacist contributes to this monitoring effort through a monthly drug review of each resident's medical record, and the nurse has numerous structured opportunities to monitor for these drug-related problems. These opportunities include routine interactions with residents while administering drugs and assessment at quarterly care-planning conferences, monthly reviews of psychotropic drug regimens, and completion of the long form of the MDS. Facilities must have policies and procedures to monitor for drug interactions and side effects.

The routine use of certain drugs, including long-acting benzodiazepines, hypnotics, sedatives, anxiolytics, and antipsychotics, has been curtailed since the enactment of the OBRA. Recommended drug dosages and indications for the use of such drugs are given to federal and state survey teams to assist them in the survey and inspection process of each nursing facility (CMS, 2018).

Residents have the right to participate in decisions about care and treatment. They must be informed of any changes in their drug regimens. Nurses must document their ongoing instructions to each resident (or the resident's legal representative) regarding the initiation of new drug therapy and changes in drug dosages. If a resident is cognitively intact, the opportunity to self-administer drugs is to be provided (CMS, 2018). Facilities must have and follow policies and procedures for identifying and following up on errors in drug administration.

Rehabilitation

The provision of rehabilitation programs in nursing facilities has increased over the past 20 years. Factors contributing to this growth in rehabilitation include the OBRA regulatory mandate that facilities provide services directed at achieving the highest practicable level of physical, mental, and psychosocial well-being for residents; the growth of the subacute level of care, including nursing facility participation in managed-care programs; and sustained political will to control the growth of health-care expenditures.

Rehabilitation teams in nursing facilities consist of the physician, physical therapists, occupational therapists, speech and language pathologists, and facility interdisciplinary team members, including the nurse, social services representative, activity coordinator, and clinical dietitian. Ideally, a medical director with rehabilitation training and experience coordinates the rehabilitation team.

For facilities receiving funds from Medicare, managed-care organizations, or private insurance groups, weekly rehabilitation meetings are held to review clinical cases. Residents and family members participate in these meetings to mutually set goals and review progress. Weekly meetings promote communication, effective discharge planning, and resident and family education.

Rehabilitation programs may be categorized into two groups:
(1) The more intensive rehabilitation programs are reimbursed through the Medicare Part A program, managed-care organizations, or private insurance groups. Some of these intensive rehabilitation programs seek credentialing from TJC and the Commission for Accreditation of Rehabilitation Facilities (CARF) to be recognized as benchmark quality programs. Intensive rehabilitation includes daily or twice-daily therapy sessions involving two or more therapy specialties. These sessions are directed toward returning a resident to a prior level of function and residence in the community. Endurance building, strengthening, ADL training, treatment of aphasia and dysphasia, cognitive testing and retraining, new disability adaptation training (e.g., after a stroke or an amputation), and training with new adaptive equipment are therapeutic components of these programs.
(2) The less-intensive rehabilitation programs that exist in nursing facilities are reimbursed through the Medicare Part B program or private payments, or they are part of the basic services offered by the nursing facility. These services include restorative nursing programs involving ambulation, ADLs, self-feeding, and range of motion. Such programs are provided by specially trained CNAs or facility nursing staff. These programs are established, revised, and supervised by the physical and occupational therapists and the speech and language pathologists. Program goals are focused on the maintenance of functional gains achieved during the more intensive rehabilitation program, regaining a level of function lost because of a short-term illness, and preventing unnecessary loss of function.

Facilities must provide the required rehabilitation services or obtain them from an outside source. The needs of the individual resident are based on a comprehensive assessment. The goal is to help the resident maintain or regain the highest possible level of physical, mental, and psychosocial well-being.

Infection Control

The development and spread of infections are major health and safety hazards in nursing facilities. A written program to protect residents, staff, and visitors from infection is required. Facility policies and procedures must include the use of standard precautions and transmission-based precautions, as outlined by the CDC. They must also follow the Occupational Safety and Health Administration's (OSHA) Bloodborne Pathogen Standard.

The OBRA requires nursing facilities to have an infection control program designed to provide a safe, sanitary, and comfortable environment; its purpose is to help prevent the development and transmission of disease. Facilities must have policies and procedures for investigating, controlling, and preventing infections. Records of incidents and corrective action taken related to infections must be maintained. The infection control program should quickly identify new infections. Special attention is given to residents at high risk of infection (e.g., those who are immobilized, have invasive devices or procedures, have pressure injuries, have been recently discharged from the hospital, have decreased mental status, or are nutritionally compromised). The program must also include measures to prevent outbreaks of communicable diseases, including COVID-19, tuberculosis (TB), influenza, hepatitis, scabies, *C. diff*, and MRSA. Preventive measures involve TB testing and screening programs for residents and staff. The facility must have procedures for following up on any positive results. Programs to make annual influenza vaccinations and pneumococcal pneumonia vaccinations available as appropriate are also in place. The CDC is continuously updating recommendations for COVID-19. Nursing facilities must adhere to updated recommendations based on outbreaks, including testing recommendations (CDC, 2023).

According to OSHA, employees at risk for exposure to bloodborne pathogens must receive free information and training on employment and annually thereafter. Employers must make the hepatitis B vaccine available to employees within 10 working days of being hired. Personal protective equipment such as gloves, goggles, face shields, gowns, shoe covers, and surgical caps must be made available free of charge to employees; they must also receive instructions on when and how to use these equipment.

An infection control committee consisting of staff members representing each department meets either monthly or quarterly to review data describing the prevalence and incidence rates of infection. This committee discusses any new or proposed revisions in policies and procedures. Typically, one nurse is designated as the infection control nurse and is responsible for coordinating surveillance, data-collection activities, and ongoing educational sessions for the facility. The infection control nurse is the facility's resource for information related to the infection control program. It is this person's responsibility to obtain and use current information from the CDC, OSHA, CMS, and the state's department of health to ensure that the facility's infection control program is effective and meets standards. The facility's medical director and consulting pharmacist are also valuable resources.

Every department and employee has the responsibility to know and follow the policies and procedures outlined in the infection control program. Policies and procedures include hand washing, standard precautions, respiratory protection, the Bloodborne Pathogen Standard, linen handling, housekeeping, hazardous waste disposal, and proper use of disinfectants, antiseptics, and germicides.

Mental Health

Among the aged and institutionalized population, mental health issues of particular concern include a variety of behavioral problems that may jeopardize the safety of the resident or other residents (e.g., wandering, kicking, or hitting). Because the residents live in a community setting, disruptive behaviors are not just an issue for the affected resident. The disruptive behaviors of one resident adversely affect other residents.

Residents manifesting disruptive behavior commonly have dementia-related illnesses. More than 60% of nursing facility residents have some degree of cognitive deficit. These deficits frequently precipitate behaviors that are difficult to understand and ameliorate. The use of physical and chemical restraints is restricted, and emphasis is placed on using behavioral interventions and environmental modifications (see section on Special Care Units). Doors may have alarms to deter wandering, and exercise, music, massage, low-stimulation environments, lighting, and aromatherapy may be used to decrease agitation.

Most importantly, nurses are learning ways to determine causes of the disruptive behaviors by assessing for pain, hunger, infection, and inappropriate environmental stimulation. Psychotropic drugs are used only as a last resort, and the side effects must be carefully monitored. It is important to know the type of dementia a resident with disruptive behaviors has been diagnosed with. All dementia is not Alzheimer disease, and residents with other types of dementia may experience adverse responses to psychotropic drugs.

End-of-Life Care

The nurse working in a nursing facility is responsible for helping the entire health-care team meet the physical, spiritual, and psychosocial needs of dying residents. Ministering to the residents' families is an important part of this care. Knowledge about a resident's culture and religious beliefs helps the team provide more effective and compassionate care. Some facilities provide hospice training for staff. Hospice programs may also provide care to residents in the nursing facility.

MANAGEMENT ASPECTS OF THE NURSING FACILITY

The Nursing Department

The nursing department is the largest department in the nursing facility. The director of nursing is responsible for managing the entire nursing staff. This consists of RNs, licensed vocational or practical nurses, CNAs, and, if employed by the facility, gerontological nurse practitioners. In some facilities, nurse managers (usually RNs) assist the director of nursing in managing and carrying out the functions of the nursing department. Nurse managers may be responsible for a specified shift, a nursing unit, or specific nursing department functions such as infection control, restorative nursing, total quality management (TQM), and nursing education. Some facilities use unit-charged nurses. These are usually RNs, but in some areas, they are licensed vocational or practical nurses. Some facilities employ nurse practitioners to provide clinical expertise and serve as a valuable resource for the nursing staff. Nurse practitioners often work closely with the medical director and the resident's PCP to manage the resident's day-to-day care. They may write orders for drugs and treatment following collaborative practice protocols.

In 2021, there were 131,320 RNs and 235,720 licensed vocational/licensed practical nurses were working in nursing facilities. CNAs are the largest employee group in the nursing departments and facilities as a whole; nursing assistants provide as much as 80% to 90% of direct care for long-term care residents (Xiao et al, 2021).

Working in a nursing facility presents rewards, opportunities, and challenges for nurses. Rewards include the chance to establish long-term relationships with residents and family members and an opportunity to work in a setting that has a holistic orientation toward resident care. Nurses employed in nursing facilities have many opportunities to use their professional skills as clinicians, teachers, and managers. They are part of an interdisciplinary team that provides a broad spectrum of health-care services. The nurse frequently takes a leadership role in developing policies and procedures, assessing resident care needs, developing and implementing care plans, and evaluating outcomes. Excellent assessment and critical thinking skills are very important. A qualified, creative nurse can advance from staff nurse to charge nurse to nurse manager. Opportunities to chair committees on topics such as TQM, infection control, restorative nursing, and pharmacy are also available. Opportunities for professional growth continue to increase in this evolving, challenging area of health care. However, nurses who choose long-term care as a career must be willing to function in a highly regulated industry. Funding for innovative programs and services is often limited, and in some geographic areas, employees' salaries are lower than in acute care settings.

Nursing Care Delivery Systems

Several nursing-care delivery systems are found in nursing facilities. There are pros and cons for each delivery system. Unfortunately, the system most likely to be in place is the one that is least expensive. Federal regulations regarding staffing requirements for nursing facilities are broad and vague. They are not based on resident acuity and allow the individual facility to determine whether it can provide the care required for any given resident. A few, if any, states have required staffing ratios that are more stringent than the federal requirements.

One nursing-care delivery system is functional nursing. The jobs of licensed nurses and CNAs are determined according to work tasks. For example, these may include an MDS nurse, an admission nurse, a medication nurse, a treatment nurse, a restorative nursing assistant, and possibly a dining assistant. CNAs may take groupings of rooms as an assignment for a variable period. A charge nurse functions as the first-line manager. This care delivery system is widely used because it can carry out basic care somewhat efficiently while maintaining only the minimum staffing levels required by regulations. However, if verbal communication between staff members is poor and written documentation is inadequate, many resident issues and care needs go unaddressed.

Team nursing is a more integrated care delivery system than functional nursing. The licensed nurse, working with a group of residents (usually 30–50), provides drugs and treatments to residents, functions as charge nurse or first-line supervisor to the CNAs, and maintains the required documentation for the residents. The licensed nurse may change the resident group assignments on a scheduled basis, usually weekly or monthly. CNAs may change every week or every month. The team nursing system has several advantages. Long-term continuity cannot be provided when CNAs and licensed nurses frequently change group assignments. Staff do not form attachments to residents, and residents, particularly those with memory loss, often have difficulty coping with these changes (i.e., remembering new names and faces and adjusting to the expectations of new personnel). The other major disadvantage of this system is the burden placed on one licensed nurse to administer drugs and treatments safely and efficiently to 50 residents, thoroughly assess episodic health problems, and meet documentation requirements.

A third delivery system is primary team nursing, which is also called *total patient care*. This involves the combination of a licensed nurse and a CNA working together to care for approximately 10 to 15 residents. This team provides all nursing care, including admissions, assistance with ADLs, and the administration of drugs and treatments. The main disadvantage is that too few staff members are available to meet all the residents' needs, and a risk of inadequate coverage exists when some staff are on break.

Regardless of the care delivery system used, the RN practicing in the nursing facility is challenged to work effectively with licensed vocational or practical nurses and CNAs, incorporating them into a professional practice model. It is essential that the RN practicing in this setting has excellent supervisory and management skills. The leadership positions in the department of nursing are held by RNs; these positions include director of nursing services and, increasingly, director of staff development. The baccalaureate-level nurse is the best prepared to fill these positions and significantly affect the quality of care and the quality of life of many residents.

SPECIALTY CARE SETTINGS
Assisted-Living Programs

Assisted-living facilities are an increasingly attractive long-term care setting, placed between home care and the nursing facility in the continuum of long-term care (NIA, 2017). Regulations are minimal, so great diversity exists in the types of service delivery models used, the types of services offered, and the setting within which assisted living is provided.

Assisted-living settings are homelike and offer an array of services, including meals, assistance with bathing and dressing, social and recreational programs, personal laundry and housekeeping services, transportation, 24-hour security, an emergency call system, health checks, drug administration, and minor medical treatments (NIA, 2017). Many services are purchased individually, as needed by the resident.

A professional nurse can provide a broad and holistic array of services to residents in assisted living facilities. Many opportunities exist to incorporate both health promotion and illness care into the model. Resident education may delay admission to long-term care. The professional nurse may help coordinate the services provided by various departments, for example, activities, social services, physical and occupational therapy, and housekeeping. As the need for assisted living facilities continues to grow, so will the opportunity for professional nurses to define their contributions and enhance the services offered to frail older adults.

Special Care Units

Since the 1980s, the popularity of specialized units for persons with dementia has expanded. A *Special care unit* (SCU) is the designation given to freestanding facilities or units within nursing facilities that specialize in the care of people with Alzheimer disease and other types of dementia-related illnesses. Behavioral manifestations of dementia are managed in the environment without the use of chemical or physical restraints, whenever possible.

It is advisable for SCUs to have objective, measurable criteria for admission. An objective discharge policy should also be in place. These admission and discharge criteria are helpful to both nursing staff and families who are reluctant to transfer residents to another care setting when a particular resident can no longer benefit from the specialized milieu of the SCU and no longer requires a secured unit. Admission criteria also deter SCU placement for residents without dementia who have other behavioral problems.

SCUs have physical environmental features that control stimuli and maximize safety while minimizing environmental barriers to freedom of movement (e.g., door alarms and outside fencing to facilitate safe wandering). Program features emphasize nutrition (e.g., finger foods and portable foods), structured daily activities, family involvement, and special staff training in behavioral manifestations of dementia and communication with residents who have dementia. An interdisciplinary team coordinates services and care.

Employment opportunities for the nurse in the SCU are like those in a traditional nursing facility. The SCU is a desirable work setting if the nurse has an interest in the health-care needs of persons with Alzheimer disease and other dementia-related illnesses that have behavioral manifestations. It is not a work setting that everyone can enjoy. Nurses who work with these special resident populations are able to provide valuable consultation regarding persons with Alzheimer disease to nurses practicing in other settings, including hospitals, home care, and nursing facilities.

Subacute Care

The growth of subacute care has been spurred by the belief that patients in acute medical or rehabilitation hospital units could be treated effectively in less-costly settings. With increased political awareness of the rising costs of the Medicare and Medicaid programs, the prospect of significant savings provided by subacute care is an attractive one. Insurance companies are looking for less-costly settings to provide patient care. It is estimated that subacute care could eventually replace almost 50% of current acute-care hospital lengths of stay.

Subacute care is an industry category rather than a reimbursement or regulatory category. Professional organizations have developed guidelines for the clinical and business development of this level of care. Facilities with subacute care programs can obtain accreditation through TJC and CARF. These accreditations are granted to facilities with well-defined subacute care programs. Care may be reimbursed through Medicare, HMO benefits, private payments, or Medicaid.

Persons in a subacute care unit are stable and no longer acutely ill or require daily physician visits MW (Dietrich, A. 2024). They may require services such as rehabilitation, IV drug therapy, parenteral nutrition, complex respiratory care, and wound management.

The nursing facility has not traditionally been considered a setting in which aggressive rehabilitative services or acute care treatments such as intense rehabilitation, ventilator care, and IV infusion therapy are provided. Subacute care is a growing industry in which services such as these are offered to older persons, patients of managed care organizations, and patients whose private insurance company has contracted with a nursing facility to provide care. To care for such patients, the nursing staff requires a level of clinical skill beyond what is typically needed in the nursing facility. Staffing levels, particularly those related to licensed nurses, are higher in response to the increased patient acuity. The involvement of the health-care provider has also significantly increased.

INNOVATIONS IN THE NURSING FACILITY

Creativity in "Everyday" Nursing Facilities

All that is required to put a little life and love into any nursing facility is some creative thinking, a desire to make life better for residents, and adequate funding. As in similar endeavors, obtaining the financial resources can be the most difficult aspect of this process. However, the innovative nurse accepts this challenge and looks beyond the usual sources to obtain the necessary resources to develop and support new interventions.

Nursing facilities all over the country have acquired dogs, cats, and other animals that can live in the facility and serve as loving companions to the residents. More functionally capable residents can sometimes take primary responsibility for walking and feeding these pets. Aviaries containing tiny birds provide hours of enjoyment for many residents. Music therapy, touch therapy, and aromatherapy are among the innovative activities currently being used in nursing facilities. Indoor and outdoor gardening projects are therapeutic for many residents.

CASE STUDY

The following situation depicts how a team of home care providers, coupled with a determined patient, can accomplish more than any one discipline working independently.

Situation

Mr. G is a 75-year-old husband, father, and grandfather who suffered a hip fracture after falling at home. He was admitted to the hospital with multiple complications after open reduction internal fixation (ORIF) repair, including delirium, pressure injury, and subsequent subacute rehabilitation. He is being discharged after 3 months of care. He has been discharged home with home health care for wound management and physical therapy. His vital signs on admission to home health were stable and within normal limits. He has had increased confusion with the transition home. He is not able to manage his drugs or wound care independently. His wife is frail and has difficulty with her own drug and mobility concerns. He has been discharged with the following drugs:

- Docusate (Colace) 240 mg po, daily
- Bisacodyl (Dulcolax) suppository, ½ to 1 rectally, every morning as needed (PRN)
- Famotidine (Pepcid) 40 mg po, every hour of sleep (qhs) PRN
- Enteric-coated aspirin, 325 mg po, daily
- Warfarin 5 mg daily, alternating with 2.5 mg

The home health nurse is charged with creating a plan of care to meet the needs of Mr. G and his family. His children and grandchildren are not available to provide hands-on care or manage his drugs.

To meet the needs of Mr. G, the following services were ordered:

- Nursing—three times weekly skilled nursing visits to manage wound care, assess drug management, and coordinate labs for warfarin
- Physical therapy—three times weekly visits to improve stamina, stability, and improve gait
- Medical social work—three times a month to assist with community resources and possible placement in a nursing facility
- HHA service—three or four times a week to assist with personal care

Because of Mrs. G's comorbidities and minimal ability to care for her husband, he will need assistance longer.

The HHA worked with physical and occupational therapists to reinforce the exercises and safe transfer techniques. Because the aide was assisting with personal care, they were able to reinforce physical and occupational therapy exercises while assisting with transfers, walking, and bathing. The aide reported that Mr. G wanted to use the bathtub and recommended that placement of the commode in the tub could allow Mr. G to transfer safely to the commode and then into the tub. This observation and recommendation from the HHA greatly enhanced Mrs. G's progression with self-care activities.

The team members worked together to identify how Mr. G and his wife could manage at home independently but are struggling. The social worker has a meeting with Mr. and Mrs. G to discuss long-term options. The family comes to a planning meeting and can identify ways to assist with the care of their patients. Referrals are made to the Area on Aging to plan for assistive services in the home supplemented by family care.

Nurse Practitioners in the Nursing Facility

Over the past two decades, many studies have been conducted to evaluate the effect of the nurse practitioner on older adult residents of nursing facilities. Long-term care facilities that use nurse practitioners can provide more timely care to acutely ill residents. The use of nurse practitioners in collaboration with physicians has been shown to reduce emergency department transfers, hospital days, and subacute days. Several HMOs are using physician–nurse practitioner teams to provide primary care to nursing facility residents.

A nurse practitioner hired by a facility must have the full support of administration to have a real effect on care. They must be free to be an educational resource for staff without being required to participate in staff evaluations. The nurse practitioner must also have the full support of the facility medical director, who serves as a resource for the practitioner and sanctions their services and expertise.

Despite studies demonstrating the cost-effectiveness of nurse practitioners in nursing facilities, a few facilities currently employ them on a full-time basis. The major employment opportunities are with groups of physicians who have a large nursing facility practice. These nurse practitioners may go on rounds with the physician or see nursing facility residents independently on alternate months, whereas the physician sees residents in the intervening months. Medicare reimburses both the physician and the nurse practitioner for this method of overseeing residents. In addition to seeing residents in the nursing facility, the practitioner may handle telephone calls from nursing facilities, triage problems, diagnose problems, and prescribe treatments and drugs as needed.

THE FUTURE OF THE NURSING FACILITY

The future of the nursing facility is complicated and uncertain. Its destiny is intimately linked to public policy regarding healthcare reform, long-term care, and mechanisms of reimbursement. Certain aspects of this service setting are flourishing, including subacute care and SCUs for the cognitively impaired. As the number of adults reaching retirement age increases and their need for assistance grows, it is essential for the professional nurse to play a dominant role in improving and transforming this practice setting. Nurses can prepare themselves to play a role in nursing facility transformation through increased education in gerontological nursing, nursing administration, health-care regulation, and public policy related to long-term care.

Nurses need to be leaders in helping shape the future of how and where long-term health care is provided. Being creative in a highly regulated industry is a significant challenge. Professional nurses who conceptualize their practice as including care for the whole person, principles of health promotion and disease prevention, and creative use of the organizational and social environment to achieve health outcomes will make valuable contributions to society. Through such efforts by nurses and other like-minded professionals committed to achieving excellence, the nursing facility will be a place where people truly can live out their days with dignity, integrity, and a sense of personal autonomy.

HOSPICE

Dying is the final phase in the trajectory of a chronic illness. Terminal illnesses, such as certain cancers and acquired immunodeficiency syndrome (AIDS), remain incurable. However, because of pharmacologic and technologic advances in treatments, many cancers and AIDS are now considered chronic illnesses. Many chronically ill persons choose to remain in their homes during the last phase of their illness to prepare for their deaths in familiar surroundings, together with family and friends. Hospice provides care and services to terminally ill persons and their families, which can provide a choice for the terminally ill person to die in a facility or at home.

Hospice Philosophy

Hospice is a special kind of medically directed compassionate care for dying individuals and their families. It is a concept of care, not a particular place or building. The care is designed to address the physical, emotional, psychologic, and spiritual needs of dying persons and to provide support services for their families during both the dying and bereavement processes. The goal of hospice is to provide comfort care, not a cure. Individuals with incurable or irreversible diseases who do not respond to treatment may choose hospice care. In addition, when a person and their family have decided to stop pursuing aggressive medical treatment, hospice is an appropriate choice.

Hospice and Palliative Care

A clarification of the terms commonly used in the end-of-life literature and clinical practice is necessary. In the United States, the terms *hospice* and *palliative care* are frequently used. *Palliative care* refers to a broader concept—it is therapy aimed at relieving or reducing the intensity of uncomfortable symptoms; it is not aimed at producing a cure. *Hospice* refers to a specific type of palliative care. Because of reimbursement policies such as the Medicare hospice benefit (discussed later in this chapter), American hospices are mandated to include specific services and are subject to the eligibility requirements that patients have a terminal diagnosis and a 6-month prognosis. Palliative and hospice care both have the goal of comfort, not cure. However, palliative care is provided in settings outside a hospice program and is currently not subject to the same regulations as hospice programs.

In Canada, the term *palliative care* is pervasive, and *hospice* usually refers to a particular agency or program. Many of the international journals on palliative care originate from Canada, the United Kingdom, and the United States. Therefore, it is critical to understand the meaning of the terms used in the literature about end-of-life care in the respective country of origin. In addition, the health-care delivery systems and the private versus governmental insurance programs also differ among the countries. Terminally ill persons, families, and health-care providers in Canada and the United Kingdom do not have the constraints of the 6-month prognosis that is required by the US system.

A widely accepted definition of palliative care, developed by the WHO, reads in part: Palliative care is the active total care of patients whose disease is not responsive to curative treatment. Control of pain, of other symptoms, and of psychologic, social, and spiritual problems is paramount. The goal of palliative care is achievement of the best possible quality of life for patients and families. It affirms life and regards dying as a normal process. Palliative care neither hastens nor postpones death. It emphasizes relief of pain and other distressing symptoms, integrates the physical, psychologic, and spiritual aspects of patient care, and offers a support system to help the family cope during the patient's illness and in their own bereavement with a team approach to care that focuses on quality of life versus quantity (WHO, n.d.).

Since the 1990s, tremendous interest in palliative care and end-of-life issues has grown throughout the world. Palliative medicine is a recognized medical specialty in the United Kingdom and Canada. In the United States, numerous initiatives, federal funding, and financial support from private foundations are available for research and innovative programs regarding end-of-life issues. As research-based knowledge continues to grow, interventions to achieve the outcomes of high-quality end-of-life care for all may become a reality.

Hospice Services

In 2018, approximately 4639 Medicare-certified hospices in the United States served 1.55 million Medicare enrollees (National Hospice and Palliative Care Organization [NHPCO], n.d.). In 2018, 50.7% of Medicare decedents were in hospice care at the time of their deaths.

Top diagnoses of enrollees were cancer (29.6%), followed by circulatory/heart disease (17.4%), and dementia (15.6%). Services provided by a comprehensive hospice program include physician services; nursing care; medical social work; counseling services and spiritual care; CNA services; additional therapies, as needed (e.g., physical, occupational, and speech therapy); inpatient care related to difficulty in managing symptoms; drugs; supplies; equipment; volunteers; respite services; continuous care in times of crisis; and bereavement services. These services constitute a basic level of hospice care established through the development of the NHPCO's *Standards of practice for hospice programs: professional development and resource series* and the federally mandated operating standards for Medicare certification for hospice programs (NHPCO, 2018).

Hospice services are provided by an interdisciplinary team consisting of the patient's own physician, hospice physicians, nurses, HHAs, medical social workers, chaplains, bereavement coordinators, and volunteers. Team members use their skills and expertise to meet the needs of dying persons and their families. These needs may include teaching family and friends how to administer drugs, helping dying persons maintain as much mobility and activity as possible, and listening to and responding to a dying person's needs. Help from the hospice team is available 24 hours a day. One member of the team is always on call and will make home visits as needed. However, the dying person and their family direct the care and are directly involved in the decision-making processes.

Hospice professionals anticipate problems and concerns, including preparing a family for the loss of a dying person. After the patient's death, various types of bereavement services are available: individual and family counseling, bereavement volunteer visits, support groups, and grief classes. The bereaved family members determine their level of participation in any of the activities and services offered.

Historically, most hospice programs in the United States have followed the home care model. This means that the interdisciplinary team provides routine hospice care in a terminally ill person's own home. In contrast to traditional home health care, it is not necessary for a terminally ill person to be homebound or to have a skilled nursing need. A family member or friend is usually designated as the primary family caregiver. Family members provide the 24-hour care of the dying person, and the hospice team consults and supports the family in their commitment to care for the hospice patient. However, the creativity and innovation of the hospice team enable many dying individuals to remain in their homes without family caregivers.

Based on the needs of a dying person and their family, other levels of care are also available. Inpatient care is available when the patient experiences acute or severe pain or symptom management problems. Inpatient respite care provides family caregivers with release time from the daily care of the patient. This type of respite care is usually limited to 5 consecutive days. Continuous care is reserved for times of crisis. This service is provided in the patient's home by nurses and HHAs. It allows for up to 24-hour care.

Medicare Benefit

Hospice services are a fully covered Medicare benefit. Anyone covered by Medicare Part A is eligible for hospice care. The following three conditions must be met to qualify for the Medicare hospice benefit. First, a terminally ill person's physician and the hospice medical director must certify that the patient is terminally ill and has a life expectancy of 6 months or less. Second, a patient must choose to receive care from a hospice instead of receiving standard Medicare benefits. Third, care must be provided by a Medicare-certified hospice program. The Medicare benefit pays for two 90-day periods of hospice care and an unlimited number of 60-day periods if the patient is reassessed and recertified as terminally ill at the beginning of each period. Hospice patients may change their minds at any time, discontinue hospice care, and return to the cure-oriented care covered by standard Medicare benefits (NHPCO, n.d.).

The Medicare hospice benefit covers pain and symptom control drugs for a terminal illness. Durable medical equipment needed to care for a patient in the home is also covered. The Medicare hospice benefit does not pay for treatment or services unrelated to the terminal illness. Attending physician charges continue to be reimbursed in part through Medicare Part B coverage. The standard Medicare benefit program continues to cover costs necessary to treat unrelated conditions that the hospice patient may have concurrently with the terminal diagnosis (NHPCO, n.d.).

HMOs are not required by law to provide hospice services. However, most HMOs do provide these end-of-life services. In addition, HMOs that receive Medicare funding are required to inform their members who are Medicare beneficiaries of Medicare-certified hospice programs located in their geographic area. If such a person chooses hospice care, they do not need to leave the HMO and will continue to receive HMO benefits not covered by Medicare (NHPCO, n.d.). Most private insurance companies and Medicaid also provide hospice benefits.

Location of Care

In the United States, hospice care is primarily provided in the home. However, other sites include hospital-based units, free-standing independent facilities, and long-term care facilities (nursing facilities). The use of these facilities is based on the needs of a dying patient and their family and on the type of services offered in the patient's geographic area.

The hospice team recognizes that circumstances change. For example, a dying person and their family may initially choose to care for the dying person at home with the support of the hospice. Later, the primary caregiver may become exhausted or sick and be unable to provide that care any longer. The hospice team will assist the family in choosing an alternative to home-based hospice care. The transition between locations of care should be seamless with the assistance of the hospice team.

SUMMARY

Although nurses work in a variety of practice settings, they are working primarily with older adults. Nurses need to provide competent, evidence-based care. The growing number of gerontological-certified basic and advanced practice nurses will help in the endeavor, as will the inclusion of more gerontological content in nursing school curricula. New acute care models will improve the care of hospitalized older adults, as will the development and dissemination of protocols that guide the assessment and treatment of commonly encountered geriatric syndromes.

Attitudes affect care delivery, and a nurse's respect and care for the special needs of older adults are essential. The diverse roles of acute care nurses working with older patients include those of practitioner, advocate, collaborator, educator, and case manager. In addition to ensuring safe and restorative health care in the hospital, the nurse must also address the learning needs, decision-making, and ethical and legal issues involved in caring for older persons.

The health-care needs of a growing, noninstitutionalized older adult population, coupled with rapid changes in today's health-care delivery system, demand continued exploration of alternative services and delivery mechanisms that support the care of older persons in home and community settings.

The need for programs and services aimed at supporting older persons and their caregivers in a community setting will continue to grow. Options for care must expand, and nontraditional alternatives must be developed for use by various health-care personnel. The reimbursement structure is currently challenged and will clearly continue to be challenged to accommodate these developments.

The entire long-term care industry is one of the greatest challenges not only to society at large but also to all health-care professionals. Attempts at regulating nursing facilities for the benefit of residents' overall health and well-being are an important yet modest step toward reform. Professional nurses must combine caring with innovative leadership to continue to make positive changes in this setting.

KEY POINTS

- Adults older than the age of 65 account for 47% of the country's inpatient days; the average length of hospital stay is 2 days longer than that of younger patients.
- The physical and social environment in which care occurs must be modified to facilitate maintenance of function and reduce the incidence of iatrogenic complications.
- Three conditions that require special attention during the hospitalization of older adults are falls, changes in cognitive status, and incontinence.
- New models of acute nursing care have emerged that are demonstrating improvements in the quality of the nursing care provided to hospitalized patients.
- Increasing numbers of older adults are discharged from hospitals with significant needs related to medical care and functional impairments; therefore, home health care for older adults is becoming more common and more complex.
- Older adults, family members, and health-care providers, including nurses, must learn about hospice care to make timely and appropriate referrals.
- Terminally ill older adults and their families are not maximizing the benefits of hospice care because of late referrals and misunderstandings of the Medicare hospice benefit.
- The Medicare hospice benefit covers (1) services and visits by all hospice staff, (2) durable medical equipment, (3) supplies needed for the plan of care, (4) drugs related to the terminal diagnosis (may involve a small copayment at the discretion of the individual hospice), and (5) dietary supplements.
- Home care is often chosen as a preferred treatment site because people want to remain in their homes, home care is usually less expensive than hospitalization, and home care minimizes exposure to multiple infectious processes. In addition, technology has evolved to support complex treatments in the home.
- Assessment for home care should be done early in a patient's hospital stay. Hospital discharge planners and home care managers must work together to ensure the continuity of care necessary for a timely and effective discharge.
- The home care nurse assesses the physical, functional, emotional, socioeconomic, and environmental well-being of patients. The nurse works in collaboration with all other members of the home care team whose services are needed to address the home care plan of treatment.
- Hospice nurses perform comprehensive, holistic assessments that are similar to those of home health nurses. In

- addition, the spiritual dimension is an important component of hospice care. In hospice, the terminally ill person and their family are the unit of care. Therefore, all assessments by members of the interdisciplinary hospice team address both as a unit.
- Residents in nursing facilities may be categorized according to their length of stay as short- or long-term residents.
- Risk factors associated with institutionalization include advanced age, physical disability, mental impairment, White race, living without a spouse, frailty, depression, and the presence of chronic medical conditions.
- The MDS includes a comprehensive and interdisciplinary assessment of residents.
- The RN plays a key role in all clinical programs, including programs for skin care, management of incontinence, nutrition, infection control, and the promotion of mental health.
- Nursing care delivery systems in nursing facilities include functional nursing, team nursing, and primary team nursing.
- Assisted-living programs, SCUs for dementia, and subacute care units provide unique opportunities for RNs who wish to specialize in one aspect of the care provided in institutional settings.
- Recent innovations in the nursing facility involve self-governance programs for residents, nursing education programs, and the use of nurse practitioners.

CLINICAL JUDGMENT EXERCISES

1. An 85-year-old is admitted to the acute care unit. How will you modify or adapt the environment to meet the needs of this patient? Why will you need to make these modifications?
2. A 92-year-old patient is ready for discharge, but they are having difficulty understanding discharge instructions. What interventions for the transition in care can you implement for this patient and family?
3. A 79-year-old with mild dementia is living with their 92-year-old spouse in their 55-year-old home. The spouse lives with multiple chronic conditions, including diabetes and heart failure. Their children and other family members live out of state. How will you determine what interventions are appropriate for this couple?
4. Symptom management is a critical part of hospice nursing care. What strategies can you implement to ensure adequate pain control along with managing the complications of opioid use?
5. What is OASIS, and how is it used in home health care?
6. A 96-year-old is living in the community and is no longer able to manage their personal care, nutritional needs, and drugs. What care environment is best suited to improve safety while letting them age in place?

REFERENCES

Acar Tek, N., & Karaçil-Ermumcu, M. Ş. (2018). Determinants of health-related quality of life in home dwelling elderly population: Appetite and nutritional status. *The Journal of Nutrition, Health & Aging, 22*(8), 996–1002. doi:10.1007/s12603-018-1066-9.

Administration for Community Living. (2017). *Administration on aging*. Retrieved from https://acl.gov/about-acl/administration-aging. Accessed July 25, 2023.

Agency for Healthcare Research and Quality (AHRQ). (2022). *Defining the PCMH*. Retrieved from https://www.ahrq.gov/ncepcr/research/care-coordination/pcmh/define.html. Accessed July 25, 2023.

Agency for Healthcare Research and Quality (ARHQ). (2021). *Preventing falls in hospitals: A toolkit for improving quality of care*. Rockville, MD: AHRQ. Retrieved from https://www.ahrq.gov/patient-safety/settings/hospital/fall-prevention/toolkit/index.html. Accessed July 25, 2023.

2019 American Geriatrics Society Beers Criteria® Update Expert Panel. (2019). American Geriatrics Society 2019 Updated AGS Beers Criteria® for potentially inappropriate medication use in older adults. *Journal of the American Geriatrics Society, 67*(4), 674–694. doi:10.1111/jgs.15767.

American Nurses Association (ANA). (2014). *Home health nursing: Scope and standards of practice* (2nd ed.). Silver Spring, MD: American Nurses Association.

APRN Consensus Workgroup and National Council of State Boards of Nursing APRN Advisory Committee. (2008). *Consensus model for APRN regulation: Licensure, accreditation, certification & education*. Retrieved from https://www.ncsbn.org/public-files/Consensus_Model_for_APRN_Regulation_July_2008.pdf. Accessed July 25, 2023.

Aung Thein, M. Z., Pereira, J. V., Nitchingham, A., & Caplan, G. A. (2020). A call to action for delirium research: Meta-analysis and regression of delirium associated mortality. *BMC Geriatrics, 20*(1), 325. doi:10.1186/s12877-020-01723-4.

Centers for Disease Control and Prevention (CDC). (2023). *Interim infection prevention and control recommendations for healthcare personnel during the coronavirus disease 2019 (COVID-19) pandemic*. Retrieved from https://www.cdc.gov/coronavirus/2019-ncov/hcp/infection-control-recommendations.html. Accessed July 25, 2023.

Centers for Disease Control and Prevention (CDC). (2021a). *Underlying cause of death, 1999-2020*. CDC WONDER Online Database. Retrieved from https://www.cdc.gov/healthcare-associated-infections/.

Centers for Disease Control and Prevention (CDC). (2021b). *2020 National and state healthcare-associated infections progress report. Executive summary*. Retrieved from https://www.cdc.gov/hai/pdfs/progress-report/2020-Progress-Report-Executive-Summary-H.pdf. Accessed July 25, 2023.

Centers for Disease Control and Prevention (CDC). (2024). *Catheter-associated urinary tract infections (CAUTI) prevention guideline*. https://www.cdc.gov/infection-control/hcp/cauti/index.html. Accessed July 29, 2024.

Centers for Medicare and Medicaid Services (CMS). (2023). *Minimum data set (MDS) 3.0 resident assessment instrument (RAI) manual*. Retrieved from https://www.cms.gov/Medicare/Quality-Initiatives-

Patient-Assessment-Instruments/NursingHomeQualityInits/ MDS30RAIManual. Accessed July 25, 2023.

Centers for Medicare and Medicaid Services (CMS). (2022a). *OASIS data sets*. Retrieved from https://www.cms.gov/Medicare/Quality-Initiatives-Patient-Assessment-Instruments/HomeHealthQualityInits/OASIS-Data-Sets. Accessed July 25, 2023.

Centers for Medicare and Medicaid Services (CMS). (2022b). *Medicare coverage of skilled nursing facility care*. Baltimore, MD: CMS. Retrieved from https://www.medicare.gov/Pubs/pdf/10153-Medicare-Skilled-Nursing-Facility-Care.pdf. Accessed July 25, 2023.

Centers for Medicare and Medicaid Services (CMS), & The Joint Commission (TJC). (2019). *Specifications manual for national hospital inpatient quality measures*. Retrieved from https://www.jointcommission.org/-/media/tjc/documents/measurement/specification-manuals/hiqr_specsman_july2019_v5_6.pdf. Accessed July 25, 2023.

Centers for Medicare and Medicaid Services (CMS). (2018). *CMS-3819-F medicare and medicaid program: Conditions of participation for home health agencies (HHA) interpretive guidelines*. Retrieved from https://www.cms.gov/Medicare/Provider-Enrollment-and-Certification/SurveyCertificationGenInfo/Downloads/QSO18-25-HHA.pdf. Accessed July 25, 2023.

Centers for Medicare and Medicaid Services (CMS). (2008). *CMS manual system*. Washington, DC: Department of Health & Human Services, Centers for Medicare & Medicaid Services. Retrieved from https://www.cms.gov/regulations-and-guidance/guidance/transmittals/downloads/r36soma.pdf. Accessed July 25, 2023.

Clifford, K. M., Dy-Boarman, E. A., Haase, K. K., Maxvill, K., Pass, S. E., & Alvarez, C.A. (2016). Challenges with diagnosing and managing sepsis in older adults. *Expert Review of Anti-infective Therapy*, 14(2), 231–241. doi:10.1586/14787210.2016.1135052.

Corcoran, C., Murphy, C., Culligan, E. P., Walton, J., & Sleator, R. D. (2019). Malnutrition in the elderly. *Science Progress*, 102(2), 171–180. doi:10.1177/0036850419854290.

Cristina, M. L., Spagnolo, A. M., Giribone, L., Demartini, A., & Sartini, M. (2021). Epidemiology and prevention of healthcare-associated infections in geriatric patients: A narrative review. *International Journal of Environmental Research and Public Health*, 18(10), 5333. doi:10.3390/ijerph18105333.

Dietrich, A. (2024). *What is sub-acute care?* https://www.nurse.com/nursing-resources/definitions/what-is-sub-acute-care/. Accessed August 25, 2024.

Falvey, J. R., Mangione, K. K., & Stevens-Lapsley, J. E. (2015). Rethinking hospital-associated deconditioning: Proposed paradigm shift. *Physical Therapy*, 95(9), 1307–1315. doi:10.2522/ptj.20140511.

Fazio, S., Pace, D., Flinner, J., & Kallmyer, B. (2018). The fundamentals of person-centered care for individuals with dementia. *The Gerontologist*, 58(Suppl. 1), S10–S19. doi:10.1093/geront/gnx122.

Floegel, T. A., Dickinson, J. M., DerAnanian, C., McCarthy, M., Hooker, S. P., & Buman, M. P. (2018). Association of posture and ambulation with function 30 days after hospital discharge in older adults with heart failure. *Journal of Cardiac Failure*, 24(2), 126–130. doi:10.1016/j.cardfail.2018.01.001.

Fuchs, L., Chronaki, C. E., Park, S., Novack, V., Baumfeld, Y., Scott, D., et al. (2012). ICU admission characteristics and mortality rates among elderly and very elderly patients. *Intensive Care Medicine*, 38(10), 1654–1661. doi:10.1007/s00134-012-2629-6.

Fukushima, T., Shoji, K., Tanaka, A., Aoyagi, Y., Okui, S., Sekiguchi, M., et al. (2021). Indwelling catheters increase altered mental status and urinary tract infection risk: A retrospective Cohort Study. *Annals of Medicine and Surgery*, 64, 102186. doi:10.1016/j.amsu.2021.102186.

Gümüşsoy, S., Kavlak, O., & Dönmez, S. (2019). Investigation of body image, self-esteem, and quality of life in women with urinary incontinence. *International Journal of Nursing Practice*, 25(5), e12762. doi:10.1111/ijn.12762.

Hubbard, R. E., & Woodhouse, K. W. (2010). Frailty, inflammation and the elderly. *Biogerontology*, 11(5), 635–641. doi:10.1007/s10522-010-9292-5.

Institute for Healthcare Improvement (IHI). (n.d.). *Age-friendly health systems*. Retrieved from https://www.ihi.org/Engage/Initiatives/Age-Friendly-Health-Systems/Pages/default.aspx. Accessed July 25, 2023.

Institute of Medicine. (1986). *Improving the quality of care in nursing homes*. Washington, DC: National Academies Press.

Jennings, E. L. M., Murphy, K. D., Gallagher, P., & O'Mahony, D. (2020). In-hospital adverse drug reactions in older adults; prevalence, presentation and associated drugs—a systematic review and meta-analysis. *Age and Ageing*, 49(6), 948–958. doi:10.1093/ageing/afaa188.

Johnson, R. W. (2019). *What is the lifetime risk of needing and receiving long-term services and supports?* U.S. Department of Health and Human Services, Office of the Assistant Secretary for Planning and Evaluation, Office of Disability, Aging and Long-Term Care Policy (DALTCP) and the Urban Institute. Retrieved from https://aspe.hhs.gov/reports/what-lifetime-risk-needing-receiving-long-term-services-supports-0. Accessed July 25, 2023.

Kapu, A. N., Kleinpell, R., & Pilon, B. (2014). Quality and financial impact of adding nurse practitioners to inpatient care teams. *The Journal of Nursing Administration*, 44(2), 87–96. doi:10.1097/NNA.0000000000000031.

Kapu, A. N., & Steaban, R. (2016). Adding nurse practitioners to inpatient teams: Making the financial case for success. *Nurse Leader*, 14(3), 198–202. doi:10.1016/j.mnl.2015.10.001.

Katz, M. J., & Roghmann, M. C. (2016). Healthcare-associated infections in the elderly: What's new. *Current Opinion in Infectious Diseases*, 29(4), 388–393. doi:10.1097/QCO.0000000000000283.

Kleinpell, R. M., Grabenkort, W. R., Kapu, A. N., Constantine, R., & Sicoutris, C. (2019). Nurse practitioners and physician assistants in acute and critical care: A concise review of the literature and data 2008-2018. *Critical Care Medicine*, 47(10), 1442–1449. doi:10.1097/CCM.0000000000003925.

Kojima, G., Liljas, A. E. M., & Iliffe, S. (2019). Frailty syndrome: implications and challenges for health care policy. *Risk Management and Healthcare Policy*, 12, 23–30. doi:10.2147/RMHP.S168750.

Legome, E., & Shockley, L. W. (Eds.). (2011). *Trauma: A comprehensive medicine approach*. New York, NY: Cambridge University Press.

Li, X., Zhang, L., Gong, F., & Ai, Y. (2020). Incidence and risk factors for delirium in older patients following intensive care unit admission: A prospective observational study. *The Journal of Nursing Research*, 28(4), e101. doi:10.1097/jnr.0000000000000384.

McDaniel, C., Ratnani, I., Fatima, S., Abid, M. H., & Surani, S. (2020). Urinary incontinence in older adults takes collaborative nursing efforts to improve. *Cureus*, 12(7): e9161. doi:10.7759/cureus.9161.

McDermott, K. W., & Roemer, M. (2021). *Most frequent principal diagnoses for inpatient stays in U.S. hospitals, 2018* [Statistical Brief #277]. Retrieved from https://www.hcup-us.ahrq.gov/reports/statbriefs/sb277-Top-Reasons-Hospital-Stays-2018.pdf. Accessed July 25, 2023.

Merck Manual. (2024). *Geriatrics*. Merck Manual Professional Version [website]. Retrieved from http://www.merckmanuals.com/professional/geriatrics. Accessed July 29, 2024.

Monegro, A. F., Muppidi, V., Regunath, H., & National Library of Medicine (NIH). (2023). Hospital-acquired infections. In *StatPearls* [Internet]. Retrieved from https://www.ncbi.nlm.nih.gov/books/NBK441857/. Accessed July 29, 2024.

Monkhouse, D. (2013). Advances in critical care for the older patient. *Reviews in Clinical Gerontology*, 23(2), 118–130. doi:10.1017/S0959259812000226.

Moote, M., Krsek, C., Kleinpell, R., & Todd, B. (2011). Physician assistant and nurse practitioner utilization in academic medical centers. *American Journal of Medical Quality*, 26(6), 452–460. doi:10.1177/1062860611402984.

National Association for Home Care & Hospice (NAHC). (n.d.). *About NAHC.* Retrieved from https://www.nahc.org/about/. Accessed July 25, 2023.

National Hospice and Palliative Care Organization (NHPCO). (2018). *Standards of practice for hospice programs: Professional development and resource series.* Alexandria, VA: NHPCO. Retrieved from https://www.nhpco.org/wp-content/uploads/2019/04/Standards_Hospice_2018.pdf. Accessed July 25, 2023.

National Hospice and Palliative Care Organization (NHPCO). (n.d.). *Medicare hospice benefit.* Retrieved from https://www.nhpco.org/hospice-care-overview/medicare-hospice-benefit-info/. Accessed July 25, 2023.

National Institute on Aging (NIA). (2017). *What is long-term care?* Retrieved from https://www.nia.nih.gov/health/what-long-term-care. Accessed July 25, 2023.

Patient Protection and Affordable Care Act of 2010, Pub. L. No. 111-148, 124 Stat. 119. (2010). Retrieved from https://www.congress.gov/111/plaws/publ148/PLAW-111publ148.pdf. Accessed July 25, 2023.

Salminen, M., Laine, J., Vahlberg, T., Viikari, P., Wuorela, M., Viitanen, M., et al. (2020). Factors associated with institutionalization among home-dwelling patients of Urgent Geriatric Outpatient Clinic: A 3-year follow-up study. *European Geriatric Medicine*, 11(5), 745–751. doi:10.1007/s41999-020-00338-7.

Saravana-Bawan, B., Warkentin, L. M., Rucker, D., Carr, F., Churchill, T. A., & Khadaroo, R. G. (2019). Incidence and predictors of postoperative delirium in the older acute care surgery population: A prospective study. *Canadian Journal of Surgery*, 62(1), 33–38. doi:10.1503/cjs.016817.

Schatz, S. N., & Weber, R. J. (2015). Adverse drug reactions. In *Pharmacotherapy self-assessment program (PSAP): CNS/pharmacy practice* (pp. 1–26). Lenexa, KS: ACCP. Retrieved from https://www.accp.com/docs/bookstore/psap/2015b2.samplechapter.pdf. Accessed July 25, 2023.

Siobal, M. S., Baltz, J. E., & Wright, J. (2021). *A guide to the nutritional assessment and treatment of the critically ill patient* (2nd ed.). Irving, TX: American Association for Respiratory Care. Retrieved from https://www.aarc.org/wp-content/uploads/2014/11/nutrition_guide.pdf. Accessed July 25, 2023.

Sirois, C., Domingues, N. S., Laroche, M. L., Zongo, A., Lunghi, C., Guénette, L., et al. (2019). Polypharmacy definitions for multimorbid older adults need stronger foundations to guide research, clinical practice and public health. *Pharmacy*, 7(3), 126. doi:10.3390/pharmacy7030126.

The Joint Commission (TJC). (2015, September 28). Preventing falls and fall-related injuries in health care facilities. *Sentinel Event Alert*, Issue 55. Retrieved from https://www.jointcommission.org/-/media/tjc/documents/resources/patient-safety-topics/sentinel-event/sea_55_falls_4_26_16.pdf. Accessed July 25, 2023.

The Joint Commission (TJC). (2012). *Improving patient and worker safety: Opportunities for synergy, collaboration and innovation.* Oakbrook Terrace, IL: TJC. Retrieved from https://www.jointcommission.org/-/media/tjc/documents/resources/patient-safety-topics/work-place-violence-prevention/updated-wsps-monograph-final-42020.pdf. Accessed July 25, 2023.

Tucker, G., Clark, N. K., & Abraham, I. (2013). Enhancing ED triage to accommodate the special needs of geriatric patients. *Journal of Emergency Nursing*, 39(3), 309–314. doi:10.1016/j.jen.2010.07.007.

USA.gov. (2022). *Veterans health.* Retrieved from https://www.usa.gov/veterans-health. Accessed July 25, 2023.

U.S. Bureau of Labor Statistics. (2022). *Occupational outlook handbook: Home health and personal care aides.* Retrieved from https://www.bls.gov/ooh/healthcare/home-health-aides-and-personal-care-aides.htm#tab-4. Accessed July 24, 2024.

World Health Organization. (n.d.). *Palliative care.* Retrieved from https://www.who.int/health-topics/palliative-care. Accessed July 25, 2023.

Xiao, C., Winstead, V., Townsend, C., & Jablonski, R. A. (2021). Certified nursing assistants' perceived workplace violence in long-term care facilities: A qualitative analysis. *Workplace Health & Safety*, 69(8), 366–374. doi:10.1177/2165079920986159.

25

Chronic Illness and Rehabilitation

Martha Smith, DNP, APRN, FNP-BC

http://evolve.elsevier.com/Yeager/gerontologic/

LEARNING OBJECTIVES

On completion of this chapter, the reader will be able to:
1. Define chronic illness and its relationship to rehabilitation.
2. Identify potential goals for an older adult with chronic illness.
3. Plan interventions that support an older adult's adaptation to a chronic illness or disability.
4. Describe the nurse's role in assisting older adults in managing chronic conditions.
5. Identify opportunities for change in the health care system to improve care for older adults with chronic illness and disability.

WHAT WOULD YOU DO?

What would you do if you were faced with the following situations?
- You are admitting a 75-year-old who was diagnosed with chronic obstructive pulmonary disease (COPD) 10 years ago. The patient presents with an exacerbation of COPD and pneumonia. They state that their energy has not returned since their last time in the hospital. The patient requires 2 L of oxygen at all times. What are important interventions for him?
- An 80-year-old with a history of coronary artery disease and new diagnosis of heart failure reports difficulty getting around. They also have osteoporosis with a history of spinal fractures and arthritis. The patient's family wants them to move into a long-term care facility upon hospital discharge. The patient wants to know your opinion. What do you say?

CHRONICITY

Chronic disease is defined by the Centers for Disease Control and Prevention (CDC) as a condition lasting at least 1 year or more that limits activities of daily living (ADLs), requires ongoing medical attention, or both (CDC, n.d.). Heart disease, cancer, and diabetes lead the nation in causes of death and disability. Chronic diseases are also responsible for 90% of the nation's $4.1 trillion annual health care costs.

Chronic disease affects the physical, psychological, and social aspects of the lives of individuals and families. A person's lifestyle, interactions, and relationships with others may change. Many older adults with chronic illness have limitations in mobility and are unable to be out in the community, and this decreased outside contact leads to social isolation. This may lead to being homebound or moving into long-term care. Individuals with chronic illness may perceive themselves as a burden, and families often experience caregiver stress. The individual is often stigmatized or acquires a label such as "that cancer patient" or "that person with chronic pain." The disease becomes the patient's identity.

It is important to differentiate between the terms *chronic disease* and *chronic illness*. Often, both health care providers and the general public use these terms interchangeably. *Disease* refers to a condition viewed from a pathophysiologic model such as an alteration in structure and function; it is a physical dysfunction of the body. *Illness* is what the individuals (and their families) experience, that is, how the disease is perceived, lived with, and responded to by individuals and families (Larsen, 2013). As health care providers, we can often modify the disease process or assist the patient in achieving optimal health; however, it is often the illness experience that we can most influence.

Just as the terms *chronic disease* and *illness* are complex, so is defining them. An early national group, the Commission on Chronic Illness (1957), defined *chronic illness* as:

All impairments or deviations from normal that have one or more of the following characteristics: (a) are permanent, (b) leave residual disability, (c) are caused by nonreversible pathological alteration, (d) require special training of the client for rehabilitation, and (e) may be expected to require a long period of supervision, observation, or care.

Previous authors: Beth Culross, PhD, RN, GCNS-BC, CRRN, FNGNA, and Ramesh C. Upadhyaya, RN, CRRN, MSN, MBA, PhD-C.

The CDC (Bernell and Howard, 2016) defined chronic disease as follows:

Noncommunicable illnesses that are prolonged in duration, do not resolve spontaneously, and are rarely cured completely.

The World Health Organization (WHO) also recognizes that noncommunicable disease refers to chronic disease (WHO, 2023). According to the WHO, these are diseases that cannot be passed from person to person and are slow in progression with a long duration. *Chronic condition* is another term used interchangeably but may mean slightly different things (Bernell and Howard, 2016). The suggestion by Bernell and Howard (2016) is to refer to the definition of "chronic" to help us understand. Simply stated, this is a disease or condition that will reoccur time and again over a long period of time.

Both the early definition from the Commission on Chronic Illness and the CDC definition emphasize the physicality of chronic disease, in other words, the pathology. Neither definition addresses the total experience of the individual or the family. It is important for the nurse to consider the illness-related issues that the patient and family experience. Understanding the perception of and response to the disease will allow for a more individualized plan of care. With over $4.1 trillion annually, chronic disease leads the nation in health care costs (CDC, 2020). Six out of 10 adults have at least one chronic illness, and 4 out of 10 have two or more.

As shown in Table 25.1, for 2020, heart disease was the leading cause of death, followed by cancer. COVID-19, newly added, was the third leading cause of death (CDC, 2020).

TABLE 25.1 Percentage of Deaths From Leading Causes Among Persons Aged 65 and Over: The United States, 2020*

15 Leading Causes of Death	Deaths	Crude Rate Per 100,000
Diseases of the heart	556,665	1,000.1
Malignant neoplasms	440,753	791.9
COVID-19	282,836	508.2
Cerebrovascular diseases	137,392	246.8
Alzheimer disease	132,741	238.5
Chronic lower respiratory diseases	128,712	231.2
Diabetes mellitus	72,194	129.7
Accidents (unintentional injuries)	62,796	112.8
Nephritis, nephrotic syndrome, and nephrosis	42,675	76.7
Influenza and pneumonia	42,511	76.4
Parkinson disease	39,316	70.6
Essential hypertension and hypertensive renal disease	34,344	61.7
Septicemia	29,630	53.2
Chronic liver disease and cirrhosis	19,367	34.8
Pneumonitis due to solids and liquids	15,659	28.1

*Based on a population of 55,659,365 persons.
Data from Centers for Disease Control and Prevention (CDC). (2022). *Underlying cause of death, 1999-2020.* CDC WONDER Database [Internet]. Retrieved from https://wonder.cdc.gov/Deaths-by-Underlying-Cause.html.

The continuing increase in the prevalence of chronic conditions is caused by many factors. Primary among them are lifesaving and life-extending technologies not previously available, an expanding population of older adults, and, as a result, increasing life expectancy. Individuals who would have succumbed to an acute illness in the past now recover, age, and live with a chronic condition. The young adult with a spinal cord injury, who years ago would not have survived, may now have a normal life span because of lifesaving technology and preventive health care. Think about the very-low-birth-weight infants of today who would not have survived in earlier years; they are now flourishing and growing into adulthood, or they survive with chronic health problems. The individual diagnosed with cancer, heart disease, or other condition can now expect to live into "old age," as formerly acute conditions have now become chronic in nature.

Even though the prevalence of chronic conditions has increased, most health care services remain oriented toward acute illnesses. The current US health care system was largely developed in the two decades after World War II. It was designed to provide acute, episodic, and curative care and was never intended to address the needs of those with chronic conditions. Overall, the health care system does a reputable job of caring for those with acute illnesses or injuries. However, it is a health care system that does not know how to care for older adults with chronic obstructive pulmonary disease (COPD), Parkinson disease, longstanding heart disease, or cancer. The health-care system applies the "acute care model" to those individuals with chronic conditions, and, as a result, a mismatch exists between the needs of older adults and what the system can provide. This conflict results in fragmented care, inadequate or inappropriate care from the system, and dissatisfaction on the part of the patient.

Prevalence of Chronic Illness

In the United States in 2018, 70.4% of all Medicare enrollees had two or more chronic illnesses (CDC, n.d.). Nearly 95% of older adults (60 and older) had at least one chronic illness (National Council on Aging, 2024). Hypertension was the most prevalent chronic illness among older adults, with 58% reporting it. High cholesterol was a close second, with 47% of older adults. Next, 37% of older adults were treated for arthritis. Ischemic heart disease was found in 29% of older adults. Diabetes was reported in 27% of older adults. Then, chronic kidney disease, heart failure, depression, Alzheimer with dementia, and COPD rounded out the top ten.

With the increasing number of individuals with chronic conditions, the health care system must do a better job of caring for them. Nursing care, in particular, needs to focus on increasing functional ability, preventing complications, promoting the highest quality of life (QoL), and, when the end stage of life occurs, providing comfort and dignity in dying. A key role for the nurse caring for an older adult with a chronic condition is to help the patient achieve optimal physical and psychosocial health.

Individuals with chronic conditions typically have repeated hospitalizations to treat exacerbations of their illness. According to the Agency for Healthcare Research and Quality (AHRQ, 2021), the most common diagnoses for inpatient stays in the

TABLE 25.2 Top Five Principal Diagnoses Among Nonmaternal and Nonneonatal Inpatient Stays by Sex-Age Group, 2018

	MALES				FEMALES		
Rank	Principal Diagnosis	Number of Stays	Rate per 100,000 Population	Rank	Principal Diagnosis	Number of Stays	Rate per 100,000 Population
Ages 65–74 years		**2,873,400**	**20,074.1**		**Ages 65–74 years**	**2,857,100**	**17,546.0**
1	Septicemia	258,100	1,803.1	1	Osteoarthritis	259,800	1,595.3
2	Osteoarthritis	172,500	1,205.0	2	Septicemia	234,000	1,436.8
3	Heart failure	140,400	980.9	3	Heart failure	113,600	697.7
4	Acute myocardial infarction	111,000	775.6	4	COPD and bronchiectasis	94,300	579.1
5	Cardiac dysrhythmias	94,300	659.1	5	Cardiac dysrhythmias	76,900	472.3
Age 75+ years		**3,233,700**	**37,421.6**		**Age 75+ years**	**4,273,700**	**34,090.0**
1	Septicemia	348,500	4,033.3	1	Septicemia	397,500	3,171.1
2	Heart failure	248,700	2,877.7	2	Heart failure	307,000	2,448.5
3	Pneumonia	128,000	1,481.7	3	Urinary tract infections	173,000	1,379.8
4	Acute and unspecified renal failure	106,000	1,226.7	4	Osteoarthritis	159,200	1,270.0
5	Cardiac dysrhythmias	104,600	1,210.5	5	Pneumonia	159,000	1,268.3

COPD, Chronic obstructive pulmonary disease
Modified from McDermott, K. W., & Roemer, M. (2021). *Most frequent principal diagnoses for inpatient stays in U.S. hospitals, 2018*. HCUP Statistical Brief #277. Rockville, MD: Agency for Healthcare Research and Quality. https://www.hcup-us.ahrq.gov/reports/statbriefs/sb277-Top-Reasons-Hospital-Stays-2018.pdf. Source: Agency for Healthcare Research and Quality (AHRQ), Healthcare Cost and Utilization Project (HCUP), National Inpatient Sample (NIS), 2018.

United States in those 75 or older are septicemia, heart failure, pneumonia, cardiac dysrhythmias, osteoarthritis, urinary tract infections, acute or nonspecific renal failure, cerebral infarction, fracture of the neck of the femur (hip) initial encounter, and acute myocardial infarction. Table 25.2 further describes the diagnosis with age- and gender-specific numbers.

The Illness Experience

Understanding each individual's priorities for health and well-being with the diagnosis of a chronic disease and subsequent management provides the foundation for identifying meaningful outcomes in care and opportunities to align care with personal values (Tuzzio et al, 2021).

Just as each individual and his or her disease process are unique, so, too, are the meanings and experiences of that disease for the individual and his or her family. However, the educational background of most health care professionals is one that fits with the medical model and does not consider the different illness perceptions and behaviors of individuals. We have been taught that patients have diseases, and the degree of their pathology dictates their treatment. Health care has even developed algorithms that tell us how and what care to provide. Nonetheless, having a chronic illness is not a black-and-white, quantifiable concept. The course of a chronic illness varies from one individual to another. The nurse must understand the outlying variables that affect the disease, including socioeconomic factors, psychosocial factors, culture, and other contributing comorbid diseases or illnesses.

Health Within Illness

Health care providers typically view an older person who is ill within a disease framework. This framework is an acute-care framework that "fixes and cures." However, we know that chronic conditions are not cured and probably cannot be "fixed."

In caring for older adults with chronic illnesses, health care professionals need a paradigm shift in attitude. After learning and mastering the requirements imposed by the condition, older adults often view themselves as "well." The disease is only one component of their life and is not their identity. The physical traits of chronic illness should not determine an older adult's state of wellness. Many older adults are now more involved in their health care than ever before and accept responsibility for their wellness. They seek education about health promotion and the management of their illness. The nurse is in a position to support older adults by working with them to identify areas that may hinder progress along the wellness continuum and by teaching self-care management in these areas (Review Appendix A for resources).

Cultural Competency

According to the 2020 U.S. Census, approximately 40% of the population is racially and ethnically diverse. Concepts of health and illness are deeply rooted in culture, race, and ethnicity and influence an individual's (and family's) illness perceptions and health and illness behavior (AHRQ, 2020). Ethnic minorities do not necessarily subscribe to the values or tenets associated with this country's medical system. Additionally, each culture is not homogeneous, and variations and subcultures exist within each.

With the increase in the numbers of ethnically and culturally diverse older adults, health care providers need to be better attuned to their needs.

A number of nursing frameworks can assist health care providers in providing culturally competent care. The website of the Transcultural Nursing Society (http://www.tcns.org) provides information about six different theories and models. Madeline Leininger's Culture Care Theory (Leininger, 1996) is based on developing nursing care with the intention of reaching positive health outcomes based on a plan that includes and considers the needs of populations and individuals with diverse cultural backgrounds.

Quality of Life and Health-Related Quality of Life

Advancements in health care have increased interest in the QoL of persons with chronic illnesses. Multiple definitions of QoL exist, but most include physical, psychological, and social components; disease and treatment-related symptoms; and spirituality. However, no consensus on the definition exists. The following definition, although somewhat older, fits well with regard to older adults. QoL is challenging to measure due to the complex nature of the concept and the generally subjective evaluation. According to the CDC (2021), QoL has meaning to a multitude of groups from every academic discipline and walk of life and may be viewed differently by each. It is made up of multiple domains that include health, jobs, housing, education, community, culture, and spirituality. The complexity of health and function in chronic illness, particularly if one believes that health can be present within illness, suggests that neither "good" health nor functional abilities are necessary for QoL. QoL is determined by the individual, not the health care provider.

Adding to the complexity of the issue, most researchers draw a distinction between QoL and health-related QoL (HRQoL). HRQoL is a multidimensional concept that has been used along with well-being to measure the effect of chronic illness, the treatments, and the corresponding related disabilities. The domains of HRQoL include physical, emotional, mental, and social functions (CDC, 2021).

How QoL and HRQoL intersect is salient to the patient with chronic illness and those providing care. For example, a person who has adjusted to a wheelchair for mobility might perceive his HRQoL and his QoL as excellent, whereas the health care provider may not rate the person's HRQoL high because a wheelchair may not be that person's optimal state of function and wellness. The subjective and objective components of both of these concepts are important.

Adherence in Chronic Illness

Adherence is described by (Fernandez-Lazaro et al, 2019) as the degree to which a person's behavior, including taking medication, implementing lifestyle changes, and adhering to dietary recommendations, matches with the health-care provider's recommendations. Common themes are noted in the literature regarding successful current and emerging practice models to successfully treat and support patients with multiple chronic conditions (MCCs) (Savitz and Bayliss, 2021). Patient-centered care involving a team-based approach, including care coordination, community partnerships, shared decision-making, home-based supports, and understanding patient treatment burden such as assessment of social risk factors, all ranked high in approaches to improve care.

Patient-Centered Approach

The patient-centered approach focuses on the relationship between the patient and the multidisciplinary team. Patient-centered care includes creating individualized interventions with patient input with regular meetings and feedback, sharing care plans with the multidisciplinary teams, and providing referrals (Poitras et al, 2018). The multidisciplinary team supports self-management with educational resources, taking into consideration the patient's situation, utilizing techniques to enhance motivation, and sharing decision-making. Access to home-based care further enhances patient-centered care because it meets the patient with MCCs, where most patients are more comfortable, in their home. COVID has afforded an increased uptake of home care, such as hospital at home, home visits, virtual visits, home-based palliative care, and remote monitoring (Savitz and Bayliss, 2021). A patient-centered approach provides holistic care by utilizing a complexity lens to address the needs of patients with MCCs, including social risk factors and the need for support for patients and caregivers outside of clinical encounters, while engaging community resources.

> ### EVIDENCE-BASED PRACTICE
>
> ### *Scoping Review of Interventions for Older Adults Transitioning from Hospital to Home*
>
> **Background/Objectives**
> Older adults are at high risk for adverse outcomes as they transition from hospital to home. Transitional care interventions primarily focus on care coordination and medication management and may miss key components. The objective of this study is to examine the current scope of hospital-to-home transitional care interventions that impact health-related outcomes and to examine other key components, including engagement by older adults and their caregivers.
>
> **Design**
> Scoping review
>
> **Methods**
> Eligible articles focused on hospital transition to home intervention, measured primary outcomes posthospitalization, used randomized controlled trial designs, and included primarily adults aged 60 years and older. Articles included in this review were reviewed in full, and all data were extracted that related to the study objective, setting, population, sample, intervention, primary and secondary outcomes, and main results.
>
> **Results**
> Five hundred sixty-seven records were identified by title. Forty-four articles were deemed eligible and included. The most common transitional care intervention components were care continuity and coordination, medication management, symptom recognition, and self-management. A few studies reported a focus on caregiver needs or goals. Common modes of intervention delivery included by phone, in person while the patient was hospitalized, and in person in the community following hospital discharge. The most common outcomes were readmission and mortality.
>
> **Conclusion**
> To improve outcomes beyond healthcare utilization, a paradigm shift is required in the design and study of care transition interventions. Future interventions should explore methods or novel interventions for caregiver engagement; leverage an interdisciplinary team or care coordination hub with engagement from underrepresented specialties such as social work and occupational therapy; and examine opportunities for interventions designed specifically to address older adult and caregiver-reported needs and their well-being.

Data from Liebzeit, D., Rutkowski, R., Arbaje, A. I., Fields, B., & Werner, N. E. (2021). A scoping review of interventions for older adults transitioning from hospital to home. *Journal of the American Geriatrics Society, 69*(10), 2950–2962.

Psychosocial Needs of Older Adults With Chronic Illness

Management of the physiologic changes caused by the disease process is the primary indicator of control of the disease. Controlling the symptoms, maintaining comfort, and preventing crises are major tasks for the patient and the provider to work on together. For this to be met, the nurse needs to understand how the patient perceives the disease, is experiencing it as an illness, and what the current standard of practice is.

Understanding the relationship among the older adult's social, psychological, and physiologic needs is important for health care providers. Each older adult and their family are unique, and the presence of one or more chronic illnesses further illuminates their uniqueness. The end result of understanding the patient's unique situation assists the health care provider in establishing interventions that support psychosocial adaptation.

Adaptation

Adaptation implies that an event or something unusual or different that has occurred is perceived as a threat or stressor to the individual and merits a reaction, a change, or a behavior by an individual (Stanton and Revenson, 2011). Other authors have seen adaptation as good QoL, well-being, vitality, positive effect, life satisfaction, and global self-esteem (Sharpe and Curran, 2006). Adaptation is a complex, multidimensional, and holistic concept. Consensus exists regarding the centrality of an individual's appraisal of their adjustment; it is *their* adjustment and their perception, not the health care professional's (Hoyt and Stanton, 2012).

Just as frameworks or models are helpful in caring for those with acute, episodic disease, they may be helpful in caring for those with chronic illness as well. Three frameworks for practice are discussed here, although more are described in the literature. These frameworks demonstrate the importance of controlling symptoms, managing the trajectory of the disease process, and engaging the patient in self-care.

Chronic Illness and QoL

Around 1975, nursing pioneers were working with dying patients and determining through research what kind of "care" those patients wanted. Their work provided a rudimentary framework that addressed the issues and concerns of patients with chronic illness. The framework was simple but was an early attempt to examine the psychosocial needs of patients versus their physical needs. Basic to patient care was an understanding of the key physical and psychosocial problems:

- The prevention of medical crises and their management if they occur
- Controlling symptoms
- Carrying out the medical regimen
- Prevention of, or living with, social isolation
- Adjustment to change in the disease
- Attempts to normalize interactions and lifestyle
- Funding
- Confronting attendant psychological, marital, and familial problems (Strauss, 1984)

Trajectory Framework

Corbin and Strauss (1991) developed the trajectory framework to assist nurses in (1) gaining insight into the chronic illness experience of the patient, (2) integrating existing literature about chronicity into their practice, and (3) providing direction for building nursing models that guide practice, teaching, research, and policy making. A *trajectory* is defined as the course of an illness over time plus the actions that patients, families, and health care providers use to manage that course. The illness trajectory is set in motion by the pathology of the patient, but the actions taken by the health care providers, patient, and family may modify the course. Even if two older adults have the same chronic condition, the illness trajectory of each individual is different and takes into account the uniqueness of the individual.

Nine phases—pre-trajectory, trajectory, stable, unstable, acute, crisis, comeback, downward, and dying—are described in the trajectory model, and although the trajectory could be conceived as a continuum, it is not linear. Patients may move through a phase, regress to a former phase, or plateau for an extended period.

Chronic Care Model

The Chronic Care Model was developed by Wagner (1998) to assist with the management of multiple chronic diseases and improve outcomes by providing a method of care coordination to improve patient self-care. There are six essential elements to the model:

1. Health System: The health system must support a culture focused on mechanisms to promote safety and quality care. The system must also be prepared to seek improvement in chronic illness management and look for improvements to reduce errors and improve communication.
2. Delivery System Design: The design of the system defines roles and tasks, is based on evidence-based care, and provides clinical case management. Care is based on the complexity of the patient and is proactive and more preventative in nature than reactive to crisis events.
3. Decision Support: Decisions are made using evidence-based guidelines. Patients are taught the guidelines to understand the underlying principles of treatment decisions. Patients are also encouraged to learn and participate in care.
4. Clinical Information Systems: A comprehensive system of communication is important for maintaining records of information. This is also important to be able to share information among providers and patients to enhance care, provide reminders of services, summarize care, and track changes. A comprehensive system can also be used to gather information about groups or populations to add to the evidence of care and create quality improvement plans.
5. Self-Management Support: The patient is central to the management of chronic illness. This element of the model empowers the patient to take responsibility for his or her own care. This is a collaboration with the providers to set priorities, educate, establish goals, and create a plan of care that can be monitored, evaluated, and changed together.
6. Community: Developing partnerships within the community leads to more effective programs. The intent of this essential

is to fill gaps that exist in services and advocate for policies to improve care. Health systems may partner with local organizations. Agencies at the state level may be able to provide material or help for managing diseases based on guidelines. National organizations can also contribute by helping to promote self-care strategies.

The Chronic Care Model brings in multiple elements of care to help the patient be educated, informed, and an active participant in the treatment plan. It also encompasses the community, the health system, and a proactive health care team (Wagner, 1998).

As we look at chronic illness and the older adult, a number of phenomena that may be experienced by individuals and families need to be considered. When considering the trajectory of disease and the multiple entities that may be involved in the care of the older adult with chronic illness, more than one framework may be needed to coordinate care and improve outcomes.

Powerlessness

An older adult's self-concept may be affected if he or she feels unable to control an illness or disability or feels that self-care patterns have contributed to the present disorder. Feelings of powerlessness may be a result of normal aging changes, an altered body image, or numerous losses. Older people grieve the loss of function or the loss of their former selves. How they grieve depends on the individuals, and the significance of the loss also influences the grieving process. The result of powerlessness is a loss of hope. In addition, older adults who feel powerless may lose their independence to family members or health care professionals who take over and make decisions for them. This cycle of powerlessness, loss of control, and dependence may be perpetuated by well-meaning caregivers.

Stigma

Stigma is defined as "a mark of shame or discredit or an identifying mark or characteristic" (*Merriam-Webster Dictionary*, 2024), and it may be a significant factor in many chronic illnesses and disabilities. Individuals with chronic illness present deviations from what many people expect in social exchanges (Stuenkel and Wong, 2013). American values of youth, attractiveness, and personal accomplishment provide daily examples of how those with chronic illness are different. A disease characteristic or having a disease with an unknown etiology may contribute to the stigma. Thus, the individual may be stigmatized by society.

However, older adults with the chronic illnesses may inflict the stigma on themselves. They may feel ashamed of their disability, disease, physical condition, and other factors. As a result, they become reclusive and socially isolated from others.

Social Isolation

Under normal circumstances, older adults are at increased risk of social isolation compared to younger adults (Courtin and Knapp, 2017). The pandemic that began in 2019 of the severe acute respiratory syndrome coronavirus 2 (SARS-CoV-2), which causes COVID-19, has further magnified social isolation in the elderly. Social isolation increases a person's risk of premature death from all causes, rivaling that of physical inactivity, obesity, and smoking (National Academies of Sciences, Engineering, and Medicine, 2020).

Chronic disease and social isolation have a reciprocal relationship. Older adults experiencing social isolation are at 50% more likely to have dementia. Social isolation increases a person's risk of heart disease by 29% and stroke by 32%. Heart failure patients who face social isolation have a 68% increased risk of being hospitalized and 57% more likely to have an emergency department visit, and are at nearly four times increased risk of death.

Social isolation may occur as an illness or disability becomes more severe or debilitating. This isolation may be initiated by the individual or by society. From the individual's perspective, it may become too difficult to functionally participate in activities, too complex to keep up with a medical regimen when away from home, or too difficult to manage physical symptoms such as pain or fatigue. Thus, the individual initiates the isolation and withdraws or limits social contact. This may be a difficult decision for individuals and their families, or it may be a relief to stay within the "safe" confines of their homes, where they may have more control.

Conversely, others may withdraw from the individual and family experiencing chronic illness. Friends may tire of hearing about the physical limitations of their friend or acquaintance. The long-term time frame or the individual with recurring cancer over a number of years, for example, may cause others to withdraw. Stigma might also be involved, and others may pull away from individuals with "unpleasant" diagnoses such as HIV and AIDS. Regardless of how or why social isolation occurs, the result is that basic needs for intimacy may be unmet.

Nursing Interventions to Assist Psychosocial Adaptation

The ability of older adults to cope with the issues and problems encountered in the course of living with and managing a chronic illness determines the nurse's role and the type of interventions needed. It is the role of the nurse to collaborate with the patient to develop an individualized plan that meets the needs, expectations, and perceptions of the patient. The Chronic Care Model is a consideration here. The Chronic Care Model is based on educating and providing a treatment plan that allows the patient to be in charge of the management of the chronic illness and have open communication with health care providers (Wagner, 1998). Independence is a major concern, especially for older persons in the American culture, where it is highly valued. The older adult who can have increased independence in the management of their care will be more knowledgeable and be able to prevent complications.

Adaptation is an individual process and depends on the circumstances of the disability. Developmental changes, life transitions, and meaning placed on the disability or illness influence this ongoing process. Interventions may include supporting existing relationships or referring older adults who have lost significant relationships to a senior center where they can establish new relationships. The nurse may also explore interventions that meet spiritual needs. The nurse may refer and encourage older adults to participate in formal or informal learning opportunities available in the community.

The COVID pandemic has prompted online interventions requiring technological savvy, such as virtual social support, telehealth, and online exercises that have been shown to be beneficial in combating social isolation (Rodrigues et al, 2022).

The group process is one way to assist patients in their psychosocial adaptation. Self-help groups provide a support system in which older adults redefine themselves, focus on issues, adjust to new roles, or learn about their disease processes and how others manage (Touhy and Jett, 2020).

Changes in positions within the family affect family duties and responsibilities. Successful coping requires a positive attitude toward new roles and the ability to obtain a feeling of independence and security. Traditional roles are often masked in the hospital, and patients may think that everything will be fine on returning home. However, the transition from hospital to home is often difficult for patients and their families. They discover how much has changed and begin to face their losses. Roles may need to be renegotiated, and those that are no longer applicable must be acknowledged and mourned (Hibbard et al, 1996).

The nurse should guide, educate, and support older adults and their families in developing positive coping strategies. Understanding the illness and what to expect is directly related to the ability to cope. In providing support to older adults and their families, the nurse assists them in identifying their feelings. A reduction in the distress that accompanies chronic illness or disability may be achieved with nursing interventions that encourage an active problem-solving and coping orientation that interrupts avoidant, passive coping patterns. Direct questions such as "How are you dealing with this illness? What helps you deal with this change in your family? What interferes with your ability to deal with this illness?" will provide an indication of a patient's coping strategies and their effectiveness (Twibell, 1998). The nurse should also observe older adults and family members for signs of stress that may result from ineffective coping.

One of the most difficult tasks in adaptation is balancing hope and realism. A patient and his or her family may need to express frustration and anger with the course of the illness and rehabilitation. By setting mutually agreed upon goals, divided into small increments, the nurse and the older adult may succeed in achieving them. Sharing goals with family members may elicit their support or assist them in accepting the need to avoid active involvement (Twibell, 1998). Personal coping also involves problem-solving. The nurse serves as a resource for older adults and their families in solving care management problems.

A supportive social network has also been found to have a significant effect on stress (Tremethick, 1997). The roles of the home, neighborhood, friends, and family need to be considered in assessing the adequacy of social support. Referrals for day care, home health nursing, temporary long-term care, or respite care may be needed.

Another obstacle is understanding and coping with role reversals. The nurse should guide older adults in finding tasks and responsibilities within their new roles and assist in conflict resolution as old roles are redefined. Chronic illness requires long-term adaptation on the part of older adults and their families. Ongoing support by health care professionals is crucial for the older adults and their families to find enough strength to continue coping.

Physiologic Needs of Chronically Ill Older Adults

A thorough nursing health history includes a comprehensive review of body systems as well as a medication and treatment review. The medication review should include both prescription drugs and over-the-counter medications. An older adult may have more than one physician prescribing drugs and additionally may be using nonprescription remedies.

Pain

A major issue with chronic disorders is the management of pain. In evaluating pain, the nurse should note its characteristics, location, and intensity (on a scale of 1–10). The nurse should make an assessment of causes of possible discomfort other than the chronic illness. In addition to pharmacologic therapy, the nurse may teach the patient relaxation techniques, deep breathing exercises, guided imagery, and visualization. These techniques may relieve muscular and emotional tension, enhance the sense of control, and possibly improve coping abilities.

Fatigue

Older adults living with a chronic disorder often experience fatigue. Fatigue may be unpredictable, making it difficult to manage or alleviate. The nurse should help older adults identify causes and patterns of fatigue. Older persons may need to be taught how to conserve energy to enjoy meaningful activities. Emphasizing the benefits of periodic rest, a slower pace of activity, and more time to complete tasks may help older patients cope and feel in control. The nurse should encourage older adults to choose where to expend energy and should respect the priorities established.

Immobility and Activity Intolerance

Activity may be the most important factor in maintaining or recovering health and wellness in the older adult. Physical activity and psychosocial interaction are important in maintaining chronically ill older adults on the continuum of wellness. Inactivity may result from functional loss, and as activity levels decline, even more function may be lost. Problems as a result of inactivity are compounded when patients, families, and health care professionals display reduced expectations of activity. One possible nursing goal may be to prevent complications of prolonged inactivity during an acute exacerbation of illness.

Sexual Activity

Aging, in and of itself, causes changes to the reproductive system in both males and females. Chronic disease may further affect the sexual activity and functioning of the older adult. These changes in a patient's sexual life may cause psychological distress. Effects of the condition, medications, treatments, fatigue, changes in body image, and the feeling that one is no longer attractive may present difficult emotional barriers. Open communication between partners, including frank discussions of needs and feelings, may result in helpful adjustments in sexual practices and a deeper commitment to the relationship. Counseling partners or individual patients may smooth over these transitions. In addition to a medication review, a sexual history provides the nurse with insight into a patient's needs. The nurse should create an open, accepting atmosphere to facilitate a discussion of sexuality and provide information in a nonjudgmental manner. Only when concerns are identified and discussed can problem solving occur.

Effect of Chronic Illness on Family and Caregivers

More and more families are faced with providing care for older family members with chronic illness because of the rapidly aging population and the present ability to manage chronic illness. Family caregivers constitute the overwhelming majority of unpaid caregivers and provide the equivalent of billions of dollars of care annually (Family Caregiver Alliance, n.d.). Studies have enhanced our awareness of family caregiver stress and the difficulty of balancing caregiving with activities such as personal time or social activities. The primary family caregiver often receives little help from siblings or children and considers institutionalization only when he or she is physically or emotionally exhausted.

Situational factors related to caring for adults with chronic illnesses contribute to caregiver stress. As noted previously, chronic illnesses are present for a long period and have an uncertain course. Periods of improvement, stability, and exacerbations in the trajectory of the illness cause uncertainty. Anticipation of these phases may also produce stress. Some chronic conditions develop slowly, and planning for crisis periods is possible. Advance notice of impending stress may allow the caregiver to activate coping strategies and reduce the stress experienced. However, anticipation may also be related to fear of the worst possible outcome.

The characteristics of a chronic illness may contribute to caregivers' stress. Caregivers report stress when, for example, the patient does not recognize family members or does not remember previous relationships because of cognitive changes. Behavioral problems resulting from illness also contribute to stress. The patient's functional ability and the type and amount of care needed affect caregiver stress. Ongoing care or the perception that ongoing care is needed may be physically and psychologically draining. When a caregiver is faced with a spouse's illness, the marital relationship may be affected. The quality of the past and present relationship contributes to how a spousal caregiver copes. In questioning a spousal caregiver, the nurse should determine whether unresolved marital problems exist because these problems may affect the caregiver's reactions to the caregiving experience. Interventions that focus on resolution of issues in relationships and identification of negative coping skills may improve relationships and decrease the possibility of depression in spousal caregivers.

Role strain is a problematic feature inherent in balancing the role as primary caregiver with other roles within the family network. Most caregivers feel a strong sense of responsibility to caregiving, and although most have a family system in place, it is rarely used as a source of support. Maintaining a healthy sense of self and successfully coping with role strain requires a balance of caregiving and caring for one's self. Personal activities may include work outside the home. Many caregivers experience work conflicts that result in changes in work schedules or performance.

Caregivers may feel powerless when they seem to have no control over events and perceive the stressors in their life as irreversible. Fewer than 15% of all "helper days of care" for people needing help with ADLs are provided by paid caregivers or sources outside the family. Factors that influence coping with caregiver stress and powerlessness are personal characteristics (e.g., age, gender, marital status, health, and social roles) and include knowledge of the illness, knowledge of available resources, personal perceptions, and coping strategies. Female caregivers experience a greater sense of burden and stress than male caregivers. The caregiving burden and feelings of being overwhelmed are related to a subsequent decline in mental and physical health (Family Caregiver Alliance, n.d.). Assumption of a role previously assigned to an older adult with chronic illness may significantly affect stress levels.

Nursing Implications of Caregiver Stress

Effective nursing care of a patient with a chronic illness requires providing care not only to the identified patient but also to the caregiver. The caregiver's personal characteristics, social and emotional support, financial resources, and perception of the caregiving situation should be assessed in relation to feelings of powerlessness. Personal coping strategies, including the ability to solve problems in managing care, need to be explored by the nurse. Questions such as "Many family member caregivers have trouble with [such and such]. Have you found that to be true for you?" may help the nurse determine stressors and problem-solving abilities in a nonthreatening manner.

Support may be obtained from other resources, such as community social service agencies, local church members, visiting nurse organizations, and other family members. Support groups for caregivers are also becoming more prevalent. Group participation decreases the sense of isolation and may help a caregiver cope with new situations. The nurse should provide information about the illness and reassurance that feelings of frustration or helplessness are not unusual reactions. Referral to a social worker may be necessary to provide detailed information regarding Medicare coverage and Medicaid eligibility, as well as other means of obtaining assistance in the health care system. Stress may be reduced by the use of adult day care or home health nursing. Temporary placement in a nursing facility provides the caregiver much-needed respite.

Caring for older adults with chronic conditions requires long-term adaptation on the part of family members. To continue in a caregiving role, a family member caregiver needs ongoing support by all involved health care professionals.

REHABILITATION

Effective rehabilitation is a person-centered process, with interventions specific to the individual's needs and personalized monitoring of progress associated with the intervention, updating the goals and actions as needed (Wade, 2020). Rehabilitation is a philosophy of care that promotes an optimal QoL in those with chronic illness.

Gerontologic rehabilitation nursing is a specialty practice that focuses on restoring and maintaining optimal function while considering holistically the unique effects of aging on the person. The gerontological rehabilitation nurse acts as an advocate, educator, consultant, practitioner, and researcher (Association of Rehabilitation Nurses [ARN], 2015). Interestingly, the specialty did not arise from gerontologic nursing but from rehabilitation nursing as a subspecialty. It was seen as a need because of the large number of older adults with more disease-related conditions rather than injury or trauma conditions. Clearly, these older patients needed a different approach to their care. The main goal of the gerontologic rehabilitation nurse is to assist the older adult in achieving their personal optimal level of health and well-being by providing holistic care in a therapeutic environment (ARN, 2015). What is unique about the role is that these nurses consider the special needs, roles, social relationships, and potential comorbidities that occur in the aging process.

Centenarians, the so-called elite-old, are the fastest growing segment of our population, followed by the age group that is 85 years or older, the oldest-old (U.S. Census Bureau, 2022). Strokes occur more commonly after the age of 65 years, and the incidence of stroke doubles and every decade after the age of 55 years (Yousufuddin and Young, 2019). Hip fractures peak in the eighth decade of life and are expected to double by the year 2040 (Ethans and MacKnight, 1998). Older drivers are involved in more crashes per mile driven compared with middle-aged drivers (Foley and Mitchell, 1997). These data suggest an increasing need for rehabilitation with a gerontologic focus. Rehabilitation planning should begin at the time an older adult is first seen or hospitalized.

The growth of the older population has specific implications for disability, and it affects the nurses who provide preventive, restorative, and rehabilitation services to this population. Age-related physiologic changes may slow recovery and increase residual debilitation from an acute illness or injury. Age-related changes also increase the likelihood of physical limitations from a chronic illness. Studies agree that older adults are more likely to be functionally impaired in ADLs and mobility.

Care Environments

Rehabilitation services are offered in a variety of settings. Therapy in acute medical–surgical units may assist a patient in maintaining strength when confined to bed. However, the acute medical environment offers little opportunity to apply skills learned in therapy and often emphasizes inactivity. Rehabilitation services lasting 1–3 hours a day are available in intermediate rehabilitation facilities and skilled care facilities (Fig. 25.1). This environment is suitable for an older adult who has the goal of returning home, who is unable to tolerate more therapy, or who requires only one therapy discipline. Intensive rehabilitation (3 hours of therapy or more) is available in the rehabilitation units of acute care hospitals, freestanding rehabilitation hospitals, and some geriatric assessment or rehabilitation units.

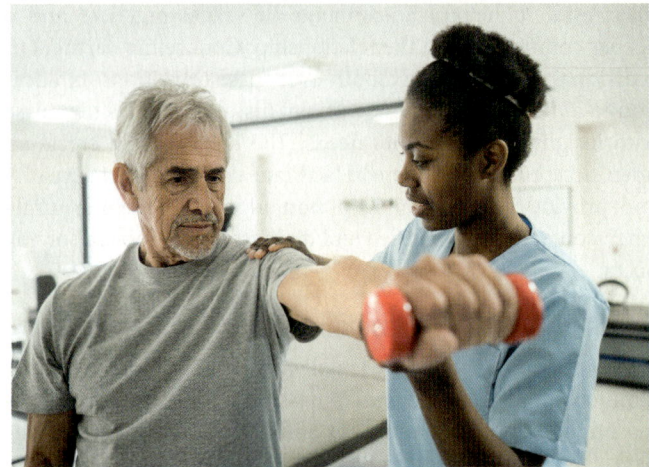

Fig. 25.1 Older adult receiving therapy in a rehabilitation setting. (From iStock.com/andresr.)

Outpatient rehabilitation therapy services may be available to older adults in their homes.

Reimbursement Issues

Medicare becomes available to older adults at the age of 65, regardless of whether they continue to work. Part A, or basic coverage (inpatient hospital coverage), is without cost to those who qualify. Part B (more comprehensive coverage) is available for a monthly premium with deductibles. A variety of private insurance plans are available to cover the "Medigap," or the 20% of service costs not reimbursed under Medicare guidelines. Medicare is a fee-for-service delivery system. Medicare also contracts with health maintenance organizations (HMOs). HMOs provide the full range of Medicare benefits and may offer additional benefits at little or no additional charge.

Medicaid is a state-specific medical care source of funding for people with low incomes. It varies from state to state, but generally the costs of inpatient, outpatient, home health, and nursing facility rehabilitation services are partially reimbursed. Increasing fiscal constraints in local, state, and federal agencies will affect rehabilitation reimbursement and may further decrease resources available to older adults.

Public Policy and Legislation

Nurses have the power to influence public policy and legislation by advocating for the needs of older adults with disabilities and supporting and conducting relevant nursing research. The process of national public policymaking started in 1951, when the first White House Conference on Aging was held. This conference made the problems of older adults visible and, since then, has been held each decade. The Older Americans Act of 1965 (last amended in 2006) introduced the concept of a focal point for services for older adults. Also in 1965, Medicare and Medicaid were established and have been revised in subsequent years. In 1982, the Tax Equity and Fiscal Responsibility Act introduced prospective reimbursement for hospitals under Medicare diagnosis-related groups.

The Americans with Disabilities Act (ADA) of 1990 outlawed discrimination on the basis of disability in employment, in programs and services provided by state and local governments, and in the provision of goods and services provided by private companies and commercial facilities (ADA, 2009). However, the ADA did not eliminate the discrimination inherent in the current system of risk-based health insurance. The Patient Protection and Affordable Care Act of 2010 has changed the issues of quality, access, and cost significantly since passage. This legislation and its accompanied parts provide a set of health benefits available and affordable to most citizens of the United States (Patient Protection and Affordable Care Act, 2010).

The National Council on Disability (NCD), founded in 1978, champions the disability movement. The NCD strives to ensure full participation, equal opportunity, independent living, and economic self-sufficiency for all Americans with disabilities. Currently, 54 million Americans (of all ages) are listed as disabled (http://www.ncd.gov).

Enhancement of Fitness and Function

The goal of caring for older adults with disabilities is to maintain or improve function. Maintaining mobility, even when hospitalized, may prevent or decrease the effects of deconditioning. Referral of the older adult to physical therapy assists the nurse in developing and implementing an exercise plan. Many activities that older adults enjoy—for example, walking, swimming, cycling, rowing, and dancing—may be incorporated into exercise and endurance training. In teaching older adults that deconditioning can be reversed, the nurse should stress that activity and exercise not only increase muscle strength and endurance but also help reduce diastolic blood pressure, body fat, and the risk of coronary artery disease. Other benefits include increased bone mineral density, improved joint flexibility, and improved mental health.

Many of the nation's chronic health problems could be reduced by an increase in physical activity. Finding ways to increase fitness levels at all ages is a national public health priority.

Older adults often think that they are too old to begin and sustain a program of exercise. However, even a small amount of time (at least 30 minutes several times a week) may improve health. In 1998, the National Institute on Aging produced their first guidelines for older adults and exercise, titled *Exercise: A Guide from the National Institute on Aging* (National Institute on Aging [NIA], 1998). The updated guide, *Exercise and Physical Activity: Your Everyday Guide from the National Institute on Aging*, was published in 2009 (NIA, 2009). The guide was reprinted in 2013. The guide lists four types of exercises important for older adults. These include endurance training, which is an exercise to increase breathing and heart rate; strength training, which builds muscles and increases muscle strength; balance exercises, which improve standing and gait; and flexibility exercises, which keep the body limber. Further information regarding exercising with chronic conditions can be found at: https://www.nia.nih.gov/health/exercising-chronic-conditions.

Functional Assessment

Regular, comprehensive assessment of older adults is a central principle of gerontologic care. Function is a useful measure in the diagnosis of illness and self-care deficits. Functional assessment may help older adults, their families, and health care providers identify problem areas and plan appropriate interventions that assist in treatment or the provision of support measures.

Similarly, in rehabilitation, progress is noted through assessments. In rehabilitation, assessment tools measure the functional status of patients. This functional assessment is incorporated into the initial nursing assessment and provides information about a patient's level of functioning before any planned rehabilitation program begins. Establishing a patient's baseline level of functioning helps the nurse identify the patient's strengths and rehabilitation potential.

The Impact Act of 2014

To standardize post-acute care data, thereby improving Medicare beneficiary outcomes through care coordination, shared decision-making, and enhanced discharge planning, the Improving Medicare Post-Acute Care Transformation Act of 2014 (the IMPACT Act) was signed into law (Centers for Medicare and Medicaid Services, 2021). The Act requires the submission of standardized data assessment data elements (SPADEs) by Skilled Nursing Facilities (SNFs), Long-Term Care Hospitals (LTCHs), Home Health Agencies (HHAs), as well as Inpatient Rehabilitation Facilities (IRFs). Commonly used assessment instruments will standardize data: The Minimum Data Set (MDS) for SNFs, the Long-Term Care Hospital CARE Data Set (LCDS) for LTCHs, the Outcome and Assessment Information Set (OASIS) for HHAs, and the Inpatient Rehabilitation Facility Patient Assessment Instrument (IRF PAI) for IRFs (Table 25.3).

Keys for Completing a Functional Assessment

To successfully complete a functional assessment:

- The nurse should be aware of a patient's mental status before assessment. For example, some people with cognitive impairment deny any and all problems, whereas people with depression may just respond, "I don't know."
- The assessment approach should be adapted to the degree of potential or actual disability. Healthy older adults may not need to be assessed in all areas. Older adults with complex problems need specific assessments of their abilities and disabilities.
- Self-reported data and observation may be used along with data from a functional assessment tool. Some older adults may deny any functional difficulty or may minimize the amount of assistance needed. The nurse should ask the older adult what they can do rather than what they cannot do.
- The nurse should screen for safety factors that limit older adults in their self-care or in their ability to remain in their home independently: (1) confusion, (2) safety awareness, (3) toileting, (4) continence, (5) depression or poor motivation, (6) falls, and (7) transfer ability. The most important physical task for an older adult is the ability to transfer in and out of a bed or chair. A person who cannot transfer from bed to

TABLE 25.3 IMPACT Act Measures

IMPACT Act Domain	IMPACT Act Measure	PAC Setting Adopted
Skin Integrity and Changes in Skin Integrity	Percent of Residents or Patients with Pressure Ulcers that are New or Worsened (Short Stay) Replaced with Changes in Skin Integrity Post-Acute Care: Pressure Ulcer/Injury	IRF, LTCH, SNF, HH
Functional Status, Cognitive Function, and Changes in Function and Cognitive Function	• Application of Percent of LTCH Hospital Patients with an Admission and Discharge Functional Assessment and a Care Plan that Addresses Function • Percent of LTCH Hospital Patients with an Admission and Discharge Functional Assessment and a Care Plan that Addresses Function • Change in Self-Care Score for Medical Rehabilitation Patients • Change in Mobility Score for Medical Rehabilitation Patients • Change in Discharge Self-Care Score for Medical Rehabilitation Patients • Change in Discharge Mobility Score for Medical Rehabilitation Patients	• IRF, LTCH, SNF, HH • LTCH • IRF, SNF • IRF, SNF • IRF, SNF • IRF, SNF
Medication Reconciliation	Drug Regimen Review	IRF, LTCH, SNF, HH
Incidence of Major Falls	Application of the Percent of Residents Experiencing One or More Falls with Major Injury (Long Stay)	IRF, LTCH, SNF, HH
Transfer of Health Information and Care Preferences when an Individual Transitions	Under Development	IRF, LTCH, SNF, HH
Resource Use Measures, including Total Estimated Medicare Spending Per Beneficiary	Medicare Spending Per Beneficiary	IRF, LTCH, SNF, HH
Discharge to the Community	Discharge to the Community	IRF, LTCH, SNF, HH
All-Condition Risk-Adjusted Potentially Preventable Hospital Readmissions Rates	Potentially Preventable 30-Day Post-Discharge Readmission	IRF, LTCH, SNF, HH

PAC, postacute care; *LTCH*, long-term care hospital; *SNF*, skilled nursing facility; *HHA*, home health agency; *IRF*, inpatient rehabilitation facility.
From Centers for Medicare and Medicaid Services (CMS). (2021). IMPACT Act of 2014 data standardization & cross setting measures. Retrieved from https://www.cms.gov/Medicare/Quality-Initiatives-Patient-Assessment-Instruments/Post-Acute-Care-Quality-Initiatives/IMPACT-Act-of-2014/IMPACT-Act-of-2014-Data-Standardization-and-Cross-Setting-Measures.

chair or chair to toilet cannot be left alone for long periods of time.
- A geriatric assessment must consider older adults' values and beliefs. An older patient's cultural and spiritual beliefs, feelings regarding health practices, and beliefs about QoL issues should be incorporated into the care plan.

Health Promotion

The WHO defines health promotion as the practice of empowering people to exert control over and improve, their health (WHO, n.d.[b]). It not only focuses on individual behavior but also includes social and environmental interventions.

Research over the years has demonstrated that pursuing a healthy lifestyle and making lifestyle changes prevents disease; however, health care providers and patients continue to have difficulty implementing needed changes in lifestyle. Although existing chronic disease and disability cannot be eliminated, health promotion within rehabilitation allows older adults to achieve a maximum level of functioning and increase longevity. Health promotion in chronic illness involves behavioral change for positive lifestyle activities, accepting one's condition and making the necessary adjustments, decreasing the risk of secondary disabilities, and preventing further disease, all while striving for optimal health.

Determining the reasons why an older adult participates in rehabilitation may provide the nurse with insight to further promote health in the patient. Some authors have promoted

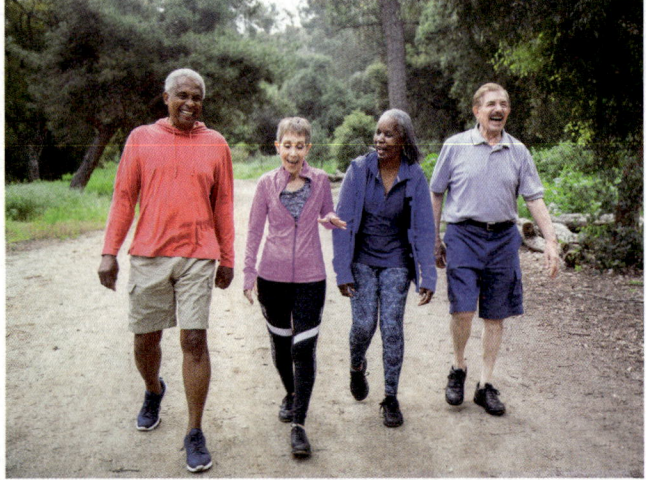

Fig. 25.2 Group of older adults walking and practicing health promotion. (From iStock.com/adamkaz.)

self-efficacy as a major determinant of behavior (Resnick, 2002). Other studies have found that fitness, health, independence, and socialization are important incentives for older adults (Lavie and Milani, 1997; McWilliam et al, 1996) (Fig. 25.2). Motivational assessment tools may be used in rehabilitation programs to facilitate the planning of interventions that enhance participation and compliance.

As Calloway stated, "nurses have been leaders in health promotion since the time of Florence Nightingale, whose pioneering work with the use of statistics demonstrated the positive effect of improved sanitation on the health of injured soldiers" (Calloway, 2007).

Management of Disabling Disorders

It is important for the nurse to understand the normal physiologic effects of aging and their effect on rehabilitation. For example, a cardiac rehabilitation program should focus on exercise training, education, secondary prevention, and vocational counseling. Modifications in exercise training may be needed for older adults with other physical impairments.

Peripheral vascular disease frequently limits activities of endurance. A graded reconditioning program to increase endurance is the most successful. If amputation is required, rehabilitation goals and candidacy for prosthetics should be determined by premorbid function, the condition of the residual limb, and the goals of the amputee.

An older adult incapacitated by COPD can improve QoL and ease functional tasks through pulmonary rehabilitation. Success depends on the patient's motivation because improvement may occur in symptom management but not in pulmonary function testing.

The acute presentation of neurologic disorders in older patients is confounded by comorbid conditions. The risk of stroke increases with age. With an increased incidence of hypertension, atrial fibrillation, and heart disease, an older adult with a stroke is at greater risk for compromised cerebral perfusion. Functionally, an older adult who survives a brain injury needs more personal assistance. Discharge to a long-term care facility, rather than home, is more likely as a person ages (Saposnik and Black, 2009).

Life Issues

For those with lifelong conditions, complications and continued deterioration of function may go unrecognized as a result of an inadequate transition from pediatric to adult health services. People with disabilities treated by rehabilitation are usually not "sick" but have a narrower margin of health. Many persons with disabilities state that they must constantly educate health professionals about the idiosyncrasies of their condition and their unique needs when treatment is prescribed.

A wide range of responses to disability exist. An individual who has had arthritis for many years may attach little significance to the condition. An individual faced with a long rehabilitation after a stroke may respond with shock, fear, and disbelief. The human spirit is remarkably resilient, adjusting to seemingly unbearable circumstances. In time, most people (in their own ways) come to accept the reality of their condition.

A person with a chronic illness or disability finds that taking health or ability for granted is no longer possible. Symptoms may spoil plans for the day, week, or month. Side effects from medication may present a variety of problems, from dry mouth to ataxia. A short trip to the store may be impossible if the day is windy or the sidewalks are wet or icy. As discussed previously, fatigue is a constant companion for many older adults with chronic disabilities.

Older adults must also reorganize their lives to enhance their functional abilities and rehabilitation. The nurse may assist older adults with organization. For example, calendars, schedules, and lists may assist with organizing self-care activities. Home blood glucose and blood pressure monitoring, weight measurement, self-assessments of physical condition based on the specific illness, and records of findings are examples. Organizing medications and treatments might include establishing a schedule for medications or treatments such as catheterization, toileting, or home dialysis. Organizing for working with health care professionals might include establishing a means to make and keep appointments, preparing for a visit, and obtaining the information needed to improve self-care.

The nurse should help older adult patients maximize financial resources by interpreting insurance coverage and making referrals to community agencies. Most assistive devices, handrails, canes, walkers, and hearing aids are paid for out of pocket. The nurse should encourage patients to shop around, ask questions, try the equipment, and inquire about service and the cost of repairs. Used equipment may be purchased at medical supply stores or privately from individuals. Nurses need to influence legislators regarding the insurance industry's coverage of monitoring equipment, adaptive equipment, and supplies needed to maintain health. The NCD periodically reviews Medicare and Medicaid benefit packages to ensure the inclusion of assistive technologies that accurately reflect contemporary health and medical practices. The NCD also recommends that the insurance term *medical necessity* be clarified to include the concept of maintaining and improving the functional capacity of individuals.

Nursing Strategies

In addition to helping older adults with rehabilitation, the nurse may assist the patient in setting and achieving goals that facilitate reintegration into their former environments. As with all patients, old or young, the patient should be in agreement regarding all goals. The goals cannot be imposed by health-care providers. Potential goals for older adults in rehabilitation include the following:

- Improving range of motion
- Improving endurance and tolerance for activity
- Restoring functional ability to an acceptable level
- Improving ambulation (if appropriate)
- Maintaining safety

An important tenet of rehabilitation is setting goals; however, the goals must be the patient's goals, not the health care provider's goals of care. Often, health care providers make assumptions as to what is most important for patients (often what is most important for themselves) as opposed to listening to the patient and identifying his or her priorities. Drawing up a contract with a patient may clarify expectations. The strategy of providing homelike routines is consistent with teaching patients how to live with their illnesses and disabilities. Incorporating a patient's normal routine into teaching content can provide a sense of security that facilitates learning. Showing interest by listening to older adult patients and involving them in all decision-making increases their confidence in their ability to achieve care outcomes.

CASE STUDY

Mrs. W is a 75-year-old female admitted to a skilled nursing facility for rehabilitation after a cerebrovascular accident (CVA) resulting in right hemiparesis. She has had a history of hypertension. In addition to the hemiparesis, she displays fatigue and emotional lability. She receives physical and occupational therapy twice a day. Her goal is to return home and be with her husband. The priorities in her care are to (1) prevent complications and permanent disabilities, (2) help her achieve independence in ADLs, (3) support the coping process and integration of changes into her self-concept, and (4) provide information about the CVA, prognosis, and treatment.

The nursing staff assists Mrs. W in turning and repositioning until she masters bed mobility in physical therapy. Mrs. W becomes tearful and frustrated with her attempts at self-care. She is upset with the length of time and effort needed to complete tasks. The nurse supports Mrs. W by anticipating the time required for self-care and getting her started. The nurse provides assistance only as necessary, maintaining a supportive but firm attitude. The nurse praises Mrs. W's efforts, and slowly Mrs. W gains a sense of self-worth that encourages her continued endeavors. She loudly expresses her feelings about her body. She refers to the affected side as "it." The nurse acknowledges Mrs. W's feelings about the betrayal of her body but retains a matter-of-fact attitude that Mrs. W can still use the unaffected side and learn to control the affected side. The staff uses words such as *weak, affected, right,* and *left* to treat that side as a part of her body. Small gains in function are celebrated. Mrs. W is also referred to social services for additional support.

After 60 days, Mrs. W is independent in ambulation with a quad cane and independent in self-care. She is able to assist in meal preparation in the sitting position. She is discharged home with her husband. Follow-up home care includes an assessment of the home environment by the occupational therapist and additional physical therapy in the home. Homemaker assistance is not necessary because of family support.

SUMMARY

Our health care system is based on acute and episodic care and does not fit with long-term chronic disease and disability. The aging of the population and the increasing prevalence of chronic diseases will continue to challenge the health care system. In an ever-changing health care environment (from technology and medications to changes in payer sources), it is important to consider the chronic illness, the functional status of the older adult, and the perception of the older adult. Considering the potential trajectory of the disease and the components of the Chronic Care Model to help increase knowledge and independence, nurses can improve the QoL for patients with chronic illness.

KEY POINTS

- Health care providers need to understand the unique illness experience of each older adult and his or her chronic condition.
- It is important to recognize that health may exist within illness.
- Regular, comprehensive assessment, both physical and psychosocial, is a central principle of the care of older adults.
- Assessing what is meaningful to older adults helps the nurse plan interventions to support psychosocial adjustment to a chronic condition or illness.
- Rehabilitation of older adults focuses on improving functional ability.
- Health promotion incentives that are important to older adults are fitness, health, independence, and socialization.

CLINICAL JUDGMENT EXERCISE

1. An 83-year-old female, independent and in relatively good health, has had a nagging cough for the past several months. She is concerned that the cough may indicate a serious illness. She is reluctant to seek help because she does not want to prolong her life if it means a loss of quality. Make a judgment about where she fits within the illness trajectory, and explain how a nurse can be of assistance.

REFERENCES

Agency for Healthcare Research and Quality (AHRQ). (2020). Consider culture, customs, and beliefs: Tool #10. In *AHRQ health literacy universal precautions toolkit* (3rd ed.). Retrieved from https://www.ahrq.gov/health-literacy/improve/precautions/tool10.html. Accessed August 14, 2024.

Agency for Healthcare Research and Quality (AHRQ). (2021). *HCUP fast stats - Most common diagnoses for inpatient stays*. Healthcare Cost and Utilization Project. Retrieved from https://datatools.ahrq.gov/hcup-fast-stats/. Accessed August 14, 2024.

Americans with Disabilities Act (ADA). (2009) Americans with Disabilities Act of 1990, as amended. Retrieved from https://www.ada.gov/law-and-regs/ada/. Accessed August 14, 2024.

Association of Rehabilitation Nurses (ARN). (2015). *What does a gerontological rehabilitation nurse do?* Retrieved from https://rehabnurse.org/about/roles/gerontological-rehab-nurse. Accessed August 14, 2024.

Bernell, S., & Howard, S. W. (2016). Use your words carefully: What is a chronic disease? *Frontiers in Public Health, 4,* 159. doi:10.3389/fpubh.2016.00159.

Calloway, S. (2007). Mental health promotion: Is nursing dropping the ball? *Journal of Professional Nursing, 23*(2), 105–109. doi:10.1016/j.profnurs.2006.07.005.

Centers for Disease Control and Prevention (CDC). (2020). *Underlying cause of death, 1999-2020.* CDC WONDER database. Retrieved from https://wonder.cdc.gov/Deaths-by-Underlying-Cause.html. Accessed August 14, 2024.

Centers for Disease Control and Prevention (CDC). (2021). *Health-related quality of life (HRQOL)*. Retrieved from https://archive.cdc.gov/#/details?url=https://www.cdc.gov/hrqol/index.htm. Accessed August 14, 2024.

Centers for Disease Control and Prevention (CDC). (n.d.). *Chronic disease indicators* [database]. Retrieved from https://nccd.cdc.gov/cdi/rdPage.aspx?rdReport=DPH_CDI.ExploreByLocation&rdRequestForwarding=Form. Accessed August 14, 2024.

Centers for Medicare and Medicaid Services (CMS). (2021). *IMPACT act of 2014 data standardization & cross setting measures*. Retrieved from https://www.cms.gov/Medicare/Quality-Initiatives-Patient-Assessment-Instruments/Post-Acute-Care-Quality-Initiatives/IMPACT-Act-of-2014/IMPACT-Act-of-2014-Data-Standardization-and-Cross-Setting-Measures. Accessed July 28, 2023.

Commission on Chronic Illness. (1957). *Chronic illness in the United States, volume I: Prevention of chronic illness*. Cambridge, MA: Harvard University Press.

Corbin, J. M., & Strauss, A. (1991). A nursing model for chronic illness management based upon the Trajectory Framework. *Scholarly Inquiry for Nursing Practice, 5*(3), 155–174.

Courtin, E., & Knapp, M. (2017). Social isolation, loneliness and health in old age: A scoping review. *Health & Social Care in the Community, 25*(3), 799–812. doi:10.1111/hsc.12311.

Ethans, K. D., & MacKnight, C. (1998). Hip fracture in the elderly. An interdisciplinary team approach to rehabilitation. *Postgraduate Medicine, 103*(1), 157–158, 163–164, 167–170. doi:10.3810/pgm.1998.01.277.

Family Caregiver Alliance. (n.d.). *Caring for yourself: Strategies and support for your well-being as a caregiver*. Retrieved from https://www.caregiver.org/caregiving-issues-and-strategies. Accessed August 14, 2024.

Fernandez-Lazaro, C. I., Garcia-Gonzalez, J. M., Adams, D. P., Fernandez-Lazaro, D., Mielgo-Ayuso, J., Caballero-Garcia, A., et al. (2019). Adherence to treatment and related factors among patients with chronic conditions in primary care: A cross-sectional study. *BMP Primary Care, 20*(132), 1–12. doi: 10.1186/s12875-019-1019-3.

Foley, K. T., & Mitchell, S. J. (1997). The elderly driver: What physicians need to know. *Cleveland Clinic Journal of Medicine, 64*(8), 423–428. doi:10.3949/ccjm.64.8.423.

Hibbard, J., Neufeld, A., & Harrison, M. J. (1996). Gender differences in the support networks of caregivers. *Journal of Gerontological Nursing, 22*(9), 15–23. doi:10.3928/0098-9134-19960901-08.

Hoyt, M., & Stanton, A. L. (2012). Adjustment to chronic illness: Theory and research. In A. Baum, T. A. Revenson, & J. E. Singer (Eds.), *Handbook of health psychology* (2nd ed.). New York: Taylor & Francis.

Larsen, P. (2013). Chronicity. In I. Lubkin & P. Larsen (Eds.), *Chronic illness: Impact and intervention* (8th ed.). Sudbury, MA: Jones & Bartlett.

Lavie, C. J., & Milani, R. V. (1997). Benefits of cardiac rehabilitation and exercise training in elderly women. *The American Journal of Cardiology, 79*(5), 664–666. doi:10.1016/s0002-9149(96)00835-1.

Leininger, M. (1996). Culture care theory, research, and practice. *Nursing Science Quarterly, 9*(2), 71–78. doi:10.1177/089431849600900208.

McWilliam, C. L., Stewart, M., Brown, J. B., Desai, K., & Coderre, P. (1996). Creating health with chronic illness. *Advances in Nursing Science, 18*(3), 1–15. doi:10.1097/00012272-199603000-00002.

Merriam-Webster Dictionary. (2024). Definition of stigma. Merriam-Webster.com [website]. Retrieved from https://www.merriam-webster.com/dictionary/stigma. Accessed August 14, 2024.

National Academies of Sciences, Engineering and Medicine. (2020). *Social isolation and loneliness in older adults: Opportunities for the health care system*. Washington, DC: The National Academies Press.

National Council on Aging. (2024). *The top 10 most common chronic conditions in older adults*. Retrieved from https://www.ncoa.org/article/the-top-10-most-common-chronic-conditions-in-older-adults. Accessed August 14, 2024.

National Institute on Aging (NIA). (1998). *Exercise: A guide from the national institute on aging*. NIH Publication No. 01-4258. Washington, DC: National Institute on Aging.

National Institute on Aging (NIA). (2009). *Exercise & physical activity: Your everyday guide from the national institute on aging at NIH*. NIH Publication No. 09-4258. Washington, DC: National Institute on Aging.

Patient Protection and Affordable Care Act. (2010). Pub. L. No. 111-148, 124 Stat. 119. Retrieved from https://www.congress.gov/111/plaws/publ148/PLAW-111publ148.pdf. Accessed August 14, 2024.

Poitras, M. E., Maltais, M. E., Bestard-Denommé, L., Stewart, M., & Fortin, M. (2018). What are the effective elements in patient-centered and multimorbidity care? A scoping review. *BMC Health Services Research, 18*(1), 446. doi:10.1186/s12913-018-3213-8.

Resnick, B. (2002). Geriatric rehabilitation: The influence of efficacy beliefs and motivation. *Rehabilitation Nursing, 27*(4), 152–159. doi:10.1002/j.2048-7940.2002.tb02224.x.

Rodrigues, N. G., Han, C. Q. Y., Su, Y., Klainin-Yobas, P., & Wu, X. V. (2022). Psychological impacts and online interventions of social isolation amongst older adults during COVID-19 pandemic: A scoping review. *Journal of Advanced Nursing, 78*(3), 609–644. doi:10.1111/jan.15063.

Saposnik, G., & Black, S. (2009). Stroke in the very elderly: Hospital care, case fatality and disposition. *Cerebrovascular Diseases (Basel, Switzerland), 27*(6), 537–543. doi:10.1159/000214216.

Savitz, L. A., & Bayliss, E. A. (2021). Emerging models of care for individuals with multiple chronic conditions. *Health Services Research, 56 Suppl 1*(Suppl. 1), 980–989. doi:10.1111/1475-6773.13774.

Sharpe, L., & Curran, L. (2006). Understanding the process of adjustment to illness. *Social Science & Medicine, 62*(5), 1153–1166. doi:10.1016/j.socscimed.2005.07.010.

Stanton, A. L., & Revenson, T. A. (2011). Adjustment to chronic disease: Progress and promise in research. In H. S. Friedman (Ed.), *The oxford handbook of health psychology* (pp. 241–268). New York: Oxford University Press.

Strauss, A. L. (1984). *Chronic illness and the quality of life* (2nd ed.). St. Louis: C.V. Mosby.

Stuenkel, D., & Wong, V. (2013). Stigma. In I. Lubkin & P. D. Larsen (Eds.), *Chronic illness: Impact and intervention* (8th ed.). Sudbury, MA: Jones & Bartlett.

Touhy, T. A., & Jett, K. (2020). *Ebersole & Hess' toward healthy aging: Human needs & nursing response* (10th ed.). St. Louis: Elsevier.

Tremethick, M. J. (1997). Thriving, not just surviving. The importance of social support among the elderly. *Journal of Psychosocial Nursing and Mental Health Services, 35*(9), 27–31. doi:10.3928/0279-3695-19970901-16.

Tuzzio, L., Berry, A. L., Gleason, K., Barrow, J., Bayliss, E. A., Gray, M. F., et al. (2021). Aligning care with the personal values of patients with complex care needs. *Health Services Research, 56*(5), 1037–1044. doi:10.1111/1475-6773.13862.

Twibell, R. S. (1998). Family coping during critical illness. *Dimensions of Critical Care Nursing, 17*(2), 100–112. doi:10.1097/00003465-199803000-00008.

U.S. Census Bureau. (2022). *Population projections*. Retrieved from www.census.gov/programs-surveys/popproj.html. Accessed August 14, 2024.

Wade, D. T. (2020). What is rehabilitation? An empirical investigation leading to an evidence-based description. *Clinical Rehabilitation, 34*(5), 571–583. doi:10.1177/0269215520905112.

Wagner, E. H. (1998). Chronic disease management: What will it take to improve care for chronic illness? *Effective Clinical Practice*, *1*(1), 2–4.

World Health Organization (WHO). (2023). *Noncommunicable diseases*. Retrieved from https://www.who.int/news-room/fact-sheets/detail/noncommunicable-diseases. Accessed August 14, 2024.

World Health Organization (WHO). (n.d.[b]). *Health promotion*. Retrieved from https://www.who.int/westernpacific/about/how-we-work/programmes/health-promotion. Accessed August 14, 2024.

Yousufuddin, M., & Young, N. (2019). Aging and ischemic stroke. *Aging*, *11*(9), 2542–2544. doi:10.18632/aging.101931.

26

Cancer

Mary B. Winton, PhD, MSN, RN

http://evolve.elsevier.com/Yeager/gerontologic/

LEARNING OBJECTIVES

On completion of this chapter, the reader will be able to:
1. Describe the physiologic and environmental factors contributing to the increased risk for cancer in older adults.
2. Identify the malignancies most commonly associated with older adults.
3. Discuss cancer prevention and early detection among older adults.
4. Create therapeutic nursing plans of care on the principles of cancer treatment for older adults.
5. Develop strategies to manage symptoms of cancer treatment experienced by older adults.
6. Discuss unique dimensions of psychosocial problems encountered by older adults with cancer.
7. Analyze ethical concerns related to caring for older adults with cancer.
8. Identify appropriate resources for older adults with cancer.

WHAT WOULD YOU DO?

What would you do if you were faced with the following situations?
- Your parent is diagnosed with cancer. What are your concerns?
- Your older adult patient is diagnosed with breast cancer and voices the most concern over the side effects of treatment. How do you respond?

"Cancer is a group of diseases characterized by the uncontrolled growth and spread of abnormal cells" (American Cancer Society [ACS], 2022a, p. 1). The risk for developing cancer increases with age. One of the most important risk factors for cancer is advanced age; 1000 per 100,000 diagnoses are in age groups 60 years and older (National Cancer Institute [NCI], 2021). Although cancer is the second leading cause of death in older adults (Centers for Disease Control and Prevention [CDC], 2023a), overall cancer deaths declined in males and females (2.3% and 1.9%, respectively) per year during the years of 2015 to 2019 (Cronin et al, 2022). The most common cancers in older adults are lung cancer, prostate and breast cancers, and colon and rectal cancers (Van Herck et al, 2021).

In the United States, the population of those 65 years or older has grown to 47.8 million, accounting for 14.9% of the total population. By 2040, the number of persons older than 65 is expected to surpass 82 million. The oldest-old population (those aged 85 or older) has grown to 6.3 million and is expected to reach 14.6 million by 2040 (Administration for Community Living, 2022). As the number of older adults increases, so does the prevalence of cancer; the number of new cancer diagnoses is expected to increase by 49% by the year 2050 (Weir et al, 2021), with 66 years being the median age of a cancer diagnosis (NCI, 2021).

INCIDENCE

Cancer incidence refers to the number of new cases in the general population in a specified period, usually a year. The leading types of cancer in males are lung, prostate, and colorectal cancers. The leading types of cancer in females are lung, breast, and colorectal cancers (Table 26.1). Mortality is the rate of deaths per number of incidences. Many persons survive cancer; some cancers have relatively high incidence rates and relatively low death rates.

The ACS (2022a) estimates that approximately 16.9 million Americans alive today have a history of invasive cancer. This is an increase from 15.5 million Americans in 2018. Of the survivors, some may be completely cured, whereas others still have some evidence of disease. Deaths related to cancer have steadily declined; however, the numbers are expected to increase due to the aging population (Weir et al, 2021). The likelihood of developing any type of invasive cancer during one's lifetime is approximately 40% for males and 39% for females (ACS, 2022a). The 5-year survival rate for all cancers is 68% for Whites and 63% for Blacks. The improvement in survival reflects progress in diagnosing certain cancers at an earlier stage and improvements in treatment. However, many older adults have comorbidities affecting survival, including diabetes, end-stage kidney disease, obesity, and immunodeficiencies (Williams et al, 2016). It is estimated that 57% of those with a diagnosis of cancer are 65 or older (ACS, 2022a).

TABLE 26.1 Leading Sites of New Cancer Cases and Deaths (2024 Estimates)

Male			Female		
Estimated New Cases					
Prostate	299,010	29%	Breast	310,720	32%
Lung and bronchus	116,310	11%	Lung and bronchus	118,270	12%
Colon and rectum	81,540	8%	Colon and rectum	71,270	7%
Urinary bladder	63,070	6%	Uterine corpus	67,880	7%
Melanoma of the skin	59,170	6%	Melanoma of the skin	41,470	4%
Kidney and renal pelvis	52,380	5%	Non-Hodgkin lymphoma	36,030	4%
Non-Hodgkin lymphoma	44,590	4%	Pancreas	31,910	3%
Oral cavity and pharynx	41,510	4%	Thyroid	31,520	3%
Leukemia	36,450	4%	Kidney and renal pelvis	29,230	3%
Pancreas	34,530	3%	Leukemia	26,320	3%
All sites	**1,029,080**		**All sites**	**972,060**	
Estimated Deaths					
Lung and bronchus	65,790	20%	Lung and bronchus	59,280	21%
Prostate	35,250	11%	Breast	42,250	15%
Colon and rectum	28,700	9%	Pancreas	24,480	8%
Pancreas	27,270	8%	Colon and rectum	24,310	8%
Liver and intrahepatic bile duct	19,120	6%	Uterine corpus	13,250	5%
Leukemia	13,640	4%	Ovary	12,740	4%
Esophagus	12,880	4%	Liver and intrahepatic bile duct	10,720	4%
Urinary bladder	12,290	4%	Leukemia	10,030	3%
Non-Hodgkin lymphoma	11,780	4%	Non-Hodgkin lymphoma	8,360	3%
Brain and other nervous system	10,690	3%	Brain and other nervous system	8,070	3%
All sites	**322,800**		**All sites**	**288,920**	

Note: Estimates are rounded to the nearest 10, and cases exclude basal cell and squamous cell skin cancers and in situ carcinoma except urinary bladder. Estimates to not include Puerto Rico or other U.S. territories. Ranking is based on modeled projections and may differ from the most recent observed data.

Modified from American Cancer Society. (2024). *Cancer facts & figures 2024*. Atlanta: American Cancer Society. Retrieved from https://www.cancer.org/research/cancer-facts-statistics/all-cancer-facts-figures/2024-cancer-facts-figures.html. Accessed May 8, 2024.

Lung cancer remains the leading cause of cancer-related death for both males and females. Lung cancer–related deaths have declined across all races and genders; however, Black males and females are more likely to develop and die of lung cancer than persons of any other racial or ethnic group, despite the fact that they smoke fewer cigarettes.

RACIAL AND ETHNIC PATTERNS

Cancer affects people of all racial and ethnic groups; however, the incidence of cancer for all cancer sites was highest among Whites (466/100,000), Blacks (455/100,000), and American Indian/Alaska natives (452.6/100,000) (ACS, 2022a). The Hispanic population was second lowest in cancer incidence rates with 348.3 per 100,000 population, and Asian/Pacific Islanders had the lowest cancer incidence rates at 294.5 per 100,000.

Racial and ethnic group age cohorts demonstrate different patterns of cancer incidence. Age is an important factor, especially when environmental influences are evaluated in cases in which persons of the same race and ethnicity had different exposures as children; any examination of patterns of cancer among racial or ethnic groups should include age and environmental considerations.

Because the incidence of cancer has demonstrated patterns by race and ethnicity, both of these factors are important in determining which groups are at risk. Race and ethnicity are highly correlated with socioeconomic status. Persons living in poverty tend to lack education, employment, adequate housing, good nutrition, preventive health practices, and access to health care. Within any one race or cultural group, economic status is the major determinant of cancer risk and outcome. Economic status as a risk factor for cancer is demonstrated globally. For most cancers, notable geographic variations in incidence rates exist and reflect socioeconomic differences, particularly differences between developing and developed countries. Addressing issues of poverty among groups of people, regardless of their race or ethnic origin, will lead to decreased cancer incidence and increased survival rates (ACS, 2022a).

As mentioned earlier, the White population has a higher overall cancer incidence rate than any other racial or ethnic group in America (ACS, 2022a). The top four cancers among White males are prostate, lung, colorectal, and renal cancers. The three highest incidence rates for cancer among White females include breast, lung, and colorectal cancers. Breast cancer among non-Hispanic Whites is higher than any other racial or ethnic group. Death rates due to cancer are highest for lung, breast, and prostate cancers.

The second highest overall incidence rate of cancer occurs among non-Hispanic Blacks (ACS, 2022a). The incidence rate for lung and prostate cancers is higher among Black males than any other racial or ethnic group. The third leading cause of cancer among Black males is colorectal cancer. Black females have the second highest incidence rate for breast cancer than other racial or ethnic groups. The second and third leading incidence rates among Black females are lung and colorectal cancers. In the United States, Black males and females have higher cancer death rates compared with other races and ethnicities.

Cancer incidence rates vary considerably among the subgroups of Asian/Pacific Islanders. Although Asian/Pacific Islanders have lower rates overall than other groups, they do have higher death and incidence rates than non-Hispanic Whites for certain cancers, especially liver and stomach cancers in both genders (ACS, 2022a). In males, the top three cancers among Chinese, Filipinos, Hawaiians, and Japanese are prostate, lung, and colorectal cancers; among Koreans, lung, stomach, and colorectal cancers; and Vietnamese, lung, liver, and prostate cancers. Stomach cancer rates among Korean males and liver cancer rates among Vietnamese males are higher than those among males of any other racial or ethnic group. The top three cancers among Asian/Pacific Islander females are breast, lung, and colorectal cancers, with the following exceptions: stomach cancer is the leading cancer in Japanese and Korean females, and the cervix in Vietnamese females. The incidence rate of cervical cancer for Vietnamese females is more than 2.5 times higher than that for any other racial or ethnic group. Asian Americans have the highest overall incidence of liver, bile duct, and stomach cancers for both males and females (ACS, 2022a).

American Indian/Alaskan Natives have the highest cancer incidence rates among any racial group for kidney/pelvic, colorectal, liver, and lung cancers (ACS, 2022a). The mortality rate is higher in this subgroup than in any other racial or ethnic group for kidney/pelvic, liver, and stomach cancers.

The leading cancers among Hispanic males and females are the same as those among Whites—lung, prostate, breast, and colorectal cancers (ACS, 2022a). Other cancers commonly diagnosed among Hispanics include cancers of the urinary bladder and stomach in males and cervical cancer in females. Similar to White subgroups, the leading cause of death is attributed to lung, prostate, and breast cancers. (See the Cultural Awareness box.)

CULTURAL AWARENESS
Cultural Considerations in Breast Cancer Screening

Mammography screening for early detection of breast cancer has been shown to be an effective method for reducing mortality in older females.

Data for 2018 indicate the rates of screening mammography range from 66% to 74%. Screening is lowest for American Indian, Alaska Native (66%) and Asian American (71%) and Hispanics (71%) (Susan G. Komen, 2023). Additionally, those without insurance have less frequent mammography than those with insurance (39% versus 75%). Other perceived barriers to mammograms include low education level, lack of access to healthcare, language differences, and lack of child or elder care.

Since the COVID-19 pandemic emergency response in March 2020, the rate of screening mammography has sharply declined by 87%, and the recovery rate to prepandemic screening levels have been slow to recover (Patt et al, 2022). Additionally, recovery rate increased slightly more among the White population compared with any other racial and ethnic groups, closely followed by Blacks.

The following strategies have been identified to reduce barriers to early detection of breast cancer (Susan G. Komen, 2023; Guide to Community Preventive Services, 2020):

- Remove financial barriers
- Improve healthcare access
- Remove language barriers
- Engage community partners to increase screening services
- Ensure healthcare providers are culturally sensitive
- Conduct research to identify culturally appropriate messages and intervention strategies for each of the at-risk groups to influence their early detection behaviors
- Use the media to increase knowledge and promote positive early detection practices among older females from culturally diverse backgrounds
- Offer services in nonclinical settings, such as mobile mammography

AGING AND ITS RELATIONSHIP TO CANCER

One of the main risk factors for cancer is aging (Berben et al, 2021). There are two schools of thought related to the development of cancer. These are not mutually exclusive. First, it is thought that cancer develops from inherited or acquired genetic mutations due to environmental insults or errors in DNA replication. (Vassilev and DePamphilis, 2017, p. 33). This thought correlates well with cancer and aging. Second, "cancer results from cancer stem cells that retain their ability to proliferate repeatedly without losing their ability to initiate uncontrolled growth, leading to cancer" (Vassilev and DePamphilis, 2017, p. 33). This school of thought points to leukemia as a theoretical exemplar. Regardless of the underlying mechanism of cancer, cancer cells have the following distinct characteristics (Vassilev and DePamphilis, 2017):

- Self-sufficiency in growth signals
- Insensitivity to antigrowth signals
- Evasion of apoptosis
- Unlimited proliferation
- Sustained angiogenesis
- Invasion of local tissues and metastasis to distant sites
- Utilization of abnormal metabolic pathways to *generate* energy
- Evasion of the immune system
- Genome instability
- Chronic inflammation

The process of cancer growth is believed to occur in three stages: tumor initiation, tumor promotion, and tumor progression (Fig. 26.1). *Tumor initiation* results from the activation of a protooncogene or the inactivation of a tumor-suppressor gene from exposure to an external agent that causes mutation of genetic material. The mutations are nonlethal, but they are passed on to future cell generations during replication. An initiated cell will continue to produce the mutations with each replication; however, the mutations alone are not enough to lead to cancer. Precancerous cell growth begins when an initiated cell encounters a promoting agent. Thus, the second stage in cancer development is called *tumor promotion*. Tumor promotion involves selective clonal expansion of initiated cells. Promoting agents are external or environmental agents. Many substances may be considered promoters of cancer; they may come from a variety of sources, including air, water, or soil; and they may be naturally occurring or chemically produced (e.g., dichlorodiphenyltrichloroethane, cigarette smoke, or polychlorinated biphenyls). Promoting agents share the common property of

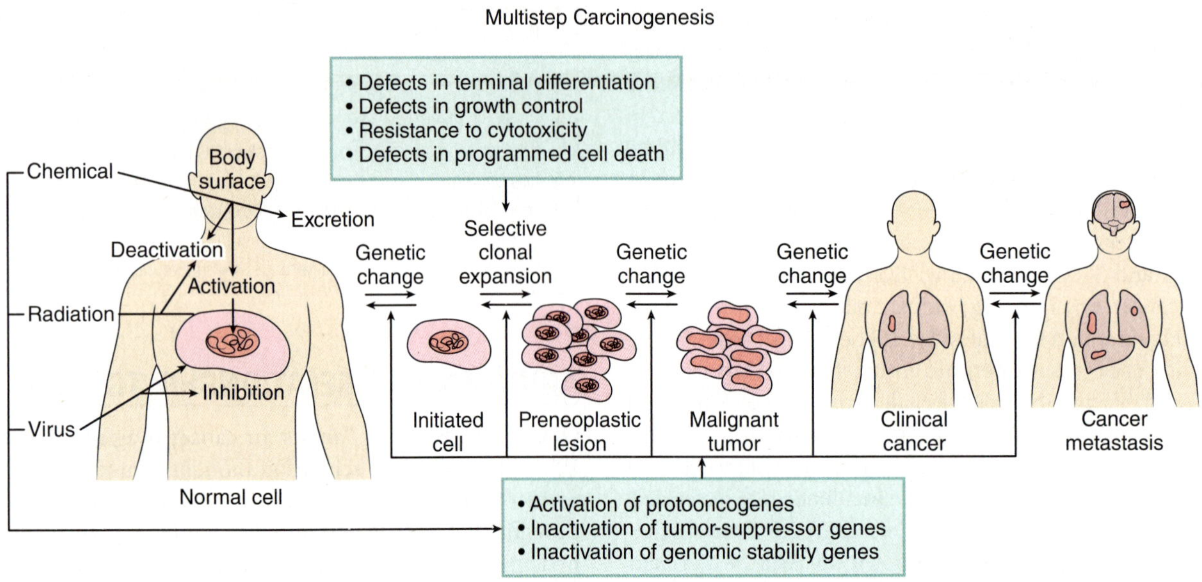

Fig. 26.1 Stages of carcinogenesis. (Redrawn from Hofseth, L. J., Weston, A., & Harris, C. C. [2017]. Chemical carcinogenesis. In R. C. Bast Jr., C. M. Croce, W. N. Hait, W. K. Hong, D. W. Kufe, M. Piccart-Gebhart, et al. [Eds.], *Holland-Frei cancer medicine* [9th ed.]. Hoboken, NJ: John Wiley & Sons, Inc.)

inducing replication of an initiated mutant cell, thus transforming the initiated cell into a precancerous cell. Promotion is dose-dependent in its effect, and although promotion may transform a cell immediately after initiation, promotion is thought to be most successful when it involves repeated exposure to an initiated cell (Saria, 2018; Weston and Harris, 2003).

Finally, *tumor progression* is the third stage in cancer growth. With tumor progression, the malignant phenotype is expressed, and malignant cells tend to acquire more aggressive characteristics over time. Malignant cells secrete proteases that facilitate tumor invasion of surrounding tissue. Genomic instability and uncontrolled growth are characteristics of malignant conversion (Saria, 2018; Weston and Harris, 2003).

Within normal human DNA material are genes that code cell growth–regulating substances. Oncogenes are genes that produce abnormal codes for growth-regulating substances. Oncogenes are believed to play a role in the development of cancers because, once activated, oncogenes interfere with normal physiologic regulation of cell growth. Oncogene activation is believed to result in excessive production of cell growth–regulating substances. Because oncogenes can cause improper regulation of cell growth, they can cause cancerous transformation in normal cells. The mechanism controlling oncogene activation is unclear; however, activation appears tightly controlled. The immune system is believed to play an important role in controlling oncogenes.

In 2003, researchers identified the sequence of the human genome as part of the Human Genome Project. Each cell in the human body contains about 20,500 genes. Genes are the blueprints that direct growth and development. They are arranged in pairs and made of genetic material called *DNA*. The totality of one's genes is known as a *genome*. Genomics is the study of what genes do and their interaction with each other.

A growing area of cancer research, cancer genome research, studies the differences in genes found in tumors to understand which ones are important in the development and proliferation of a tumor. Researchers collect thousands of samples from different types of tumors to find a tumor's genetic "fingerprint." Different genes are involved in different tumor types, and understanding what genes are important to cancer development has led to improvements in detecting, diagnosing, and treating cancer.

Studying or "mapping" the cancer genome helps researchers understand the mutated genes that lead to cancer. By identifying mutated genes that cause cancer to develop or spread, researchers hope to develop drugs that target those specific genes to stop the cancer's growth. Also, identifying the genes responsible for cancer helps researchers and doctors develop tests to detect cancer earlier. The identification of many mutated genes in breast cancer, colon cancer, melanoma, and other cancers has led to the development of tests that can determine which treatment will be the most effective, as well as the development of several new treatments that target mutated genes. For example, trastuzumab is a drug used to treat breast cancers with a specific genetic mutation that causes tumors to have too much of a protein called HER2; additionally, lung cancer patients with a specific gene mutation involving the *ROS1* gene often respond well to treatment with crizotinib, a targeted therapy (NCI, n.d.).

The Cancer Genome Atlas (TCGA) project is one of the biggest efforts to map the cancer genome. The National Cancer Institute and the National Human Genome Research Institute started this project. As part of TCGA, researchers collect tissue samples from patients treated at cancer centers across the United States. By studying these tissue samples and comparing them with tissue samples from people who do not have cancer, researchers have identified cancer types and subtypes based on their genetics, which may lead to better tests for diagnosing cancer, as well as more effective treatments (NCI, n.d.).

Several mechanisms have been proposed to explain the way in which the aging process directly influences the cancerous transformation of cells:

- Aging increases the duration of exposure to substances that may act as promoting agents. The effects of promoters are dose-dependent; a significant dose may accumulate in older adults over decades. Also, cellular transformations and the progression of cancer cells occur over time. Cancer cells grow at various rates, and in some cases, significant time is needed for the small cluster of cancer cells to grow large enough to cause signs and symptoms.
- Aging cells demonstrate a tendency toward abnormal growth. Aged cells are more vulnerable to damage; thus, aging likely increases the susceptibility of cells to substances that cause genetic mutations.
- Once a carcinogen damages an aged cell, it is more difficult to repair it.
- Oncogene activation might be increased in older persons, resulting in decreased regulation of cell growth and the development of cancer cells.
- Decreased immune surveillance, or immunosenescence, may contribute to increased development of cancers and their progression, are needed (Ribatti, 2017).

Aging and Cancer Prevention

The risk for cancer, either increased or decreased, frequently reflects changes in the habits of a specific birth cohort (Weir et al, 2021). Because most cancers are the result of lifelong exposure, the risk for developing malignant disease after age 65 is probably already determined by the time one reaches that age. Frequently, cancer risk is similar for a given birth cohort within specific environmental boundaries. Although it appears difficult to undo or reverse the cellular damage sustained in younger years, prolonged exposure to promoting agents is, nonetheless, needed for the initiated cells to be transformed. If exposure to promoters can be avoided or reduced and antipromoters can be used, cancerous transformation may not occur or may be delayed.

Interference with the promotion stage of cancer would seem to offer the best prospects for cancer prevention (Weir et al, 2021). Only recently has research included the search for interventions that halt the promotion phase. It is currently believed instituting lifestyle medicine (i.e., consuming fresh fruits and vegetables and maintaining ideal body weight) can be employed as preventive measures against cancer (Rippe, 2018). It is possible to decrease behaviors earlier in life that promote a predisposition to certain types of cancer; for example, limiting the number of severe sunburns in youth and reducing exposure by applying sunscreen may be ways to interfere with the promotion stage of cancer. Secondary to this, various vitamins and minerals contained in foods are being examined for their effects on the promotion phase. Older adults should be encouraged to consume the recommended daily requirements of fruits and vegetables because dietary habits may be beneficial in slowing or halting the cancer process. Additionally, evaluation of environmental risk factors may lead to specifically targeted education and screening programs among selected high-risk cohorts.

COMMON MALIGNANCIES IN OLDER ADULTS

Lung Cancer

Lung cancer is the most common type of cancer and the leading cause of cancer death in both males and females (ACS, 2022a). It occurs most often in older adults; more than 75% of all cancer diagnoses occur in persons over the age of 60 (White et al, 2019). It is estimated that there were nearly 237,000 new cases of lung cancer and about 130,000 deaths associated with lung cancer in 2022. Lung cancer–related deaths have declined across all races and genders; however, White, Black, and American Indian/Alaska Native subgroups are more likely to develop lung cancer and die of it than persons of Asian/Pacific Islander or Hispanic subgroups (ACS, 2022a).

Risk Factors

Smoking (e.g., cigarettes, pipes, or cigars) is, by far, the most important risk factor in the development of lung cancer, both for active smokers and nonsmokers exposed to secondhand smoke (ACS, 2022a). Tobacco smoke is considered a cancer promoter, demonstrating a *dose-response relationship*; that is, the risk for lung cancer increases with the number of cigarettes smoked. The greatest lifetime cumulative exposure to cigarette smoking occurs between ages 70 and 80. It has been known for some time that the risk for lung cancer decreases over time for ex-smokers; the risk for lung cancer is increased for both current and former smokers compared with nonsmokers (Tindle et al, 2018).

Other risk factors include exposure to certain industrial substances such as asbestos, chromium, nickel, arsenic, soot, tar, or radon. Radiation exposure from occupational, medical, and environmental sources is also a risk factor. Air pollution contains several substances that, with repeated exposure, may increase the risk for lung cancer (American Lung Association [ALA], n.d.). The risk for developing lung cancer is increased for those with a family history of the disease and persons infected with the human immunodeficiency virus (HIV) (ACS, 2022b). Most lung diseases are chronic and diminish the quality of life (QoL) for those persons living with HIV.

Signs and Symptoms

More than one-fourth of individuals diagnosed with lung cancer have no presenting symptoms. When symptoms do occur, they may be vague and attributed to other problems, especially in older adults with underlying lung or other chronic illnesses. Others present with symptoms that develop when the tumor becomes large and the cancer metastasizes to other organs. The classic clinical presentation of lung cancer is a persistent cough, sputum streaked with blood, chest pain, fatigue, weight loss, recurring respiratory infections, shortness of breath, and hoarseness. This constellation of symptoms is also associated with cigarette smoking, and its significance as an indicator of cancer may be overlooked (ALA, n.d.).

Early Detection

Low-dose spiral computed tomography (CT) screening of current or former (quit within 15 years) smokers between the ages 55 and 74 who have at least a 30-pack-year smoking history has been shown to reduce lung cancer mortality by about 20%. The ACS recommends shared decision-making between the healthcare provider, the patient, and their family concerning the benefits, uncertainties, and harms associated with lung cancer screening (ALA, n.d.).

Treatment

Options for treatment include surgery, radiation therapy, and chemotherapy, depending on the type and stage of disease. Lung cancer is classified into two basic types: small cell lung cancer (SCLC; 13% of cases) and non–small cell lung cancer (NSCLC; 84% of cases). In the case of early NSCLC, surgery is the treatment of choice, sometimes in combination with chemotherapy, other times with radiation. In advanced NSCLC, treatment is with chemotherapy and targeted drugs. In patients with SCLC, chemotherapy is used alone or combined with radiation. Cancer stage and molecular characteristics of NSCLC and SCLC determine treatment choices (ALA, n.d.).

Breast Cancer

Breast cancer is the most common neoplasm in females, increasing in incidence with advancing age. The incidence of breast cancer decreases after age 80, although this may be attributed to a decrease in cancer screening as opposed to an actual decrease in cancer development.

Breast cancer is the leading cause of cancer-related death in females ages 55 to 74. The primary presenting symptom is a lump in the breast (ACS, 2022c).

Although all females are at risk for developing breast cancer, the older a female is, the greater her chances are of developing breast cancer. Breast cancer is more common in White females than in other racial or ethnic groups. According to the most recent data, death rates are continuing to decline in White females; Black females of all ages have the highest mortality rates from breast cancer. Asians/Pacific Islanders have the lowest incidence of breast cancer in the United States (ACS, 2022c).

Risk Factors

The risk for breast cancer increases with age. Dominant risk factors appear to be related to duration and intensity of exposure to hormonal influences, especially estrogen and include early menarche (before age 12), late menopause (after age 55), lengthy exposure to postmenopausal estrogen, recent use of oral contraceptives, and never having given birth or having first given live birth at a late age (after age 30). Additional risk factors for the development of breast cancer include female gender, a personal or family history of breast cancer (5% to 10% of breast cancers have a genetic predisposition), a history of benign breast disease or dense breast tissue, excessive alcohol use, and smoking. Obesity, weight gain after menopause, type 2 diabetes, and a sedentary lifestyle have also been shown to increase the risk for developing breast cancer (ACS, 2022c).

A major advance in understanding breast cancer is that the disease has a genetic basis. Approximately 5% to 10% of breast cancers are hereditary (ACS, 2021). The genes involved in most inherited breast cancers are *BRCA1* and *BRCA2*. These are tumor-suppressor genes that also serve to protect and preserve DNA. Mutation of these genes has been linked to hereditary breast and ovarian cancer. A female's risk for developing breast cancer, ovarian cancer, or both is greatly increased if *BRCA1* or *BRCA2* mutation is inherited. By the age of 80, females with *BRCA1* or *BRCA2* mutations have up to 70% chance of developing breast cancer. Males have about a 1% chance of being diagnosed with breast cancer (CDC, 2023b).

Genetic tests are available to check for *BRCA1* and *BRCA2* mutations. Federal and state laws help ensure the privacy of a person's genetic information and provide protection against discrimination in health insurance and employment practices. Currently, many research studies are being conducted to discover newer and better ways of detecting, treating, and preventing cancer in carriers of *BRCA1* and *BRCA2* mutations (ACS, 2022c).

Signs and Symptoms

Malignant lumps are hard and fixed, with irregular borders, and are sometimes described as "frozen peas." Nipple retraction or elevation may be caused by tumor fixation involving underlying tissues. Skin dimpling may also be present, usually because of tumor invasion into the ligaments and fixation on the chest wall. Localized erythema and warmth may be present and are related to inflammation. Characteristically, edema appears as "orange peel" skin. Pain is not usually a presenting symptom unless the disease is locally advanced.

Early Detection

Among average-risk females, routine clinical breast exams or breast self-examination for detecting early breast cancer is no longer recommended. There is not enough supporting evidence "that these tests help find breast cancer early when women also get screening mammograms, … women should be familiar with how their breasts normally look and feel and report any changes to a health care provider right away" (ACS, 2022c).

Mammography can detect breast tumors before they manifest physical signs. Mammography screening is more accurate for older females because breast tissue tends to be less dense than that in younger females, making tumors easier to visualize. The ACS recommends annual mammography screening for females after age 40 until age 54; those over age 55 may change to biennial mammography if they choose. Mammography should continue "as long as overall health is good and life expectancy is 10 or more years" (ACS, 2022c).

Treatment

Breast cancer treatment should be multidisciplinary. Surgery — either breast-conserving surgery or mastectomy — is indicated for removal of the primary tumor. Radiation to the breast is recommended for most patients having breast-conserving surgery; radiation may also be recommended for females undergoing mastectomy, for large tumors, or for node-involved breast cancers. Because breast cancer metastasizes early in the course of the disease, axillary lymph nodes are removed and evaluated for the presence of cancer; another alternative is sentinel node biopsy. Treatment may also involve chemotherapy (before or after surgery), hormone (antiestrogen) therapy, and/or targeted therapy (ACS, 2022c).

As with everyone, older females should be given information and support to help make treatment decisions. Breast cancer should be treated promptly, but it is not an emergency. Nurses should provide a supportive atmosphere and encourage family members to participate in treatment decisions.

Survival

The 5-year survival rate for localized breast cancer, when caught early, is 99%; for regional breast cancer, the 5-year survival rate is 90%. It is important for females to realize everyone with breast cancer is different and that survival rates are not a predictor of treatment success. Risk factors, cancer stage, and treatment choice all play into the success of any given therapy.

Prostate Cancer

Prostate cancer is usually adenocarcinoma that develops slowly in the gland cells of the prostate (ACS, 2019a). Other types of cancer cells include small cell carcinomas and neuroendocrine tumors. Prostate cancer is rare before the age of 40; the average age at diagnosis is 66 (ACS, 2023a). About 12.5% or one in eight males will develop prostate cancer. Although prostate cancer is a serious disease, most males do not die of it. The 5-year survival rate for all stages of prostate cancer is 96.8% (NCI, 2023a).

Risk Factors

Prostate cancer is a disease of aging. Six of 10 cases of prostate cancer occur in persons over the age of 65. Black males develop prostate cancer more often than Asian American and Hispanic males. Other risk factors include a family history of prostate cancer and occupational exposure to carcinogens. Smoking increases the risk for fatal prostate cancer (ACS, 2023b).

Signs and Symptoms

Prostate cancer is asymptomatic in its early stages. Signs and symptoms of cancer are related to the increased growth of the prostate that surrounds the urethra; they include weak or interrupted urine flow, difficulty or inability to begin urine flow, difficulty stopping urine flow, and urinary frequency, especially at night. Many of these symptoms are like those of infection or benign prostatic hypertrophy. As the cancer progresses, additional signs and symptoms include pain in the hips, spine, and ribs (from bony metastases), impotence, weakness or numbness in the lower extremities, and bowel and bladder incontinence (ACS, 2019a).

Early Detection

"No organizations presently endorse routine prostate cancer screening for males at average risk, because of concerns about the high rate of overdiagnosis (detecting disease that would never have caused symptoms), along with the significant potential for serious side effects associated with prostate cancer treatment" (ACS, 2019a). The ACS recommends that males at average risk and who have a life expectancy of at least 10 years begin discussing the risks and benefits of screening for prostate cancer with their doctor at age 50 to make an informed decision. Those at high risk for developing prostate cancer (Black males, or those with a close relative diagnosed with prostate cancer before the age of 65) should have this discussion beginning at age 45 (ACS, 2019a).

Treatment

Multiple methods of treatment may be used, either alone or in combination, to manage prostate cancer: active surveillance, surgery, external beam radiation, or radioactive seed implants. In advanced cases, hormonal therapy may be used with surgery or radiation. The choice of treatment is determined by the patient's age, comorbidities, stage, and tumor grade, the likelihood of a cure, and the patient's inclination (ACS, 2019a).

Active surveillance involves digital rectal examination, periodic biopsy, and serial prostate-specific antigen testing. Should signs and symptoms change, treatment options may be readdressed. The primary surgery for prostate cancer is radical prostatectomy, which involves the removal of the prostate and surrounding tissue. After surgery, males may develop incontinence and impotence. When the cancer has not spread beyond the prostate, radiation therapy may be effective. It may also be used in conjunction with hormone therapy, after surgery, or with advanced cancer to relieve symptoms (ACS, 2022d).

Hormone therapy is an adjunct to radiation therapy or may be used alone in patients who are not candidates for surgery or radiation. It may also be used in cases where cancer has returned or to shrink tumors so that radiation therapy is more effective. The objective of hormone therapy is to reduce circulating androgens in the body or to prevent androgens from reaching the prostate. The objective can be accomplished by using several methods: orchiectomy, luteinizing hormone (LH)–releasing hormone analogs, LH-releasing hormone antagonists, antiandrogens, and androgen-suppressing drugs. All forms of hormone therapy have similar side effects: reduced libido, impotence, shrinking of the sex organs, hot flashes, breast tenderness, osteoporosis, anemia, decreased alertness, decreased muscle mass and weight gain, elevated cholesterol, fatigue, and depression (ACS, 2022d).

Chemotherapy is not the first-line therapy for prostate cancer, although it may be used in cases of metastasis. Chemotherapy targets the rapidly dividing cancer cells. However, other cells in the body (e.g., bone marrow, mucous membranes, hair follicles) divide rapidly as well, leading to side effects, such as hair loss, oral lesions, anorexia, nausea and vomiting, diarrhea, immunosuppression, easy bruising or bleeding, and fatigue (ACS, 2022d).

Vaccine therapy is an individualized treatment designed for advanced-stage prostate cancer. White blood cells (WBCs) from the patient are exposed to prostatic acid phosphatase from the cancer cells; the exposed cells are then put back into the patient intravenously to stimulate the patient's immune system to attack the cancer cells (ACS, 2022d). The vaccine hasn't been shown to stop prostate cancer from growing, but it seems to help males live an average of several months longer. The cost is prohibitive ($93,000 per course of treatment).

Colorectal Cancer

Colorectal cancer is the third most common cancer, accounting for 8.6% of all cancer diagnoses. An individual's lifetime risk for developing colorectal cancer is 4.3%. Death rates are declining because of a decrease in the number of cases. Early screening with polyp removal, early diagnosis and treatment leading to cure, and improvements in treatment are the reasons for the declining rates. Five-year survival is nearly 65%. The median age at diagnosis for colorectal cancer is 67; the median age at death is 73 (NCI, 2023b).

Risk Factors

A personal or family history of colorectal cancer, polyps, or inflammatory bowel disease has been associated with increased colorectal cancer risk, as have type 2 diabetes. Lifestyle choices linked to the development of colorectal cancer include eating a diet high in red meat and processed meats, low calcium intake, moderate to heavy alcohol consumption, and very low intake of fruits, vegetables, and whole-grain fiber. Obesity and a sedentary lifestyle have also been associated with colorectal cancer (ACS, 2022a).

Signs and Symptoms

In the early stages, colorectal cancer may not manifest any symptoms. As the disease advances, presenting signs and symptoms include a change in bowel habits or stool shape, the feeling that the bowel is not completely empty, abdominal cramping or pain, decreased appetite, and weight loss. In some cases, the cancer causes blood loss that leads to anemia, resulting in symptoms such as weakness and fatigue (ACS, 2022a).

Early Detection

According to the ACS guidelines for the early detection of colorectal cancer, starting at age 45, both males and females of average risk should have yearly guaiac-based fecal occult blood tests and flexible sigmoidoscopy every 5 years, *or* colonoscopy every 10 years, *or* double-contrast barium enema every 5 years, *or* CT colonography every 5 years. Although inexpensive and low-risk, fecal occult blood testing may miss polyps, and some cancers may produce false-positive test results; however, it has been proven effective in clinical trials (ACS, 2020a). Screening is appropriate for older adults at high risk, but care should be taken to ensure proper testing.

Treatment

Cancer stage guides treatment, although surgery is the treatment of choice for colorectal cancer. The extent of surgery is determined by the location of the cancer and the involvement of lymph nodes. Surgical procedures include the removal of the cancer and segments of the major arterial and venous blood suppliers to the affected area. Permanent colostomy is seldom needed for colon cancer. For localized cancers, surgery is frequently curative. Radiation therapy may take place before surgery to shrink the size of the tumor or after surgery to reduce the chance of recurrence. Radiation has also been used in situations where patients are not surgical candidates and for palliative pain relief. Chemotherapy before surgery may help shrink the tumor; chemotherapy after surgery is beneficial for patients with cancer that has spread to the lymph nodes or cancer that has penetrated the bowel wall (ACS, 2020b).

Targeted therapies attack cancer cells directly. Unlike standard chemotherapy, which targets all rapidly dividing cells, targeted therapy interferes with specific molecules (e.g., protein enzymes, and growth factor receptors) required for the cancer cells to replicate. Targeted therapies are used for treating advanced colorectal cancer, and immunotherapy is a newer option for some advanced colorectal cancers (ACS, 2020b).

SCREENING AND EARLY DETECTION: ISSUES FOR OLDER ADULTS

Primary prevention of cancer is desirable and is affected by changes in lifestyle (Rippe, 2018). Older adults are likely to have had a lifetime of exposure to risk factors;. However, changing lifestyles is advantageous for them, the changes may not reverse the effects of previous exposure. Furthermore, changing habits developed over a lifetime is difficult despite demonstrable benefits. Given the difficulty of cancer prevention, detection of cancer at an early stage may greatly improve survival rates. Screening asymptomatic persons at risk is feasible in many common malignancies, including breast, lung, cervical, prostate, and colorectal cancers.

When considering a cancer screening program, the healthcare provider should use a structured approach by assessing three factors relevant to the risks and benefits (Kotwal and Walter, 2020):

1. Assess the life expectancy and health of the older adult. Several tools (i.e., eprognosis.org) are available to estimate life expectancy
2. Individualize the risks and benefits of specific cancer screening tests in the context of the older adult's life expectancy
3. Assess the older adult's overall values and preferences regarding their health

Current efforts at advancing the science and technology of screening have resulted in greater accuracy of many screening tests. The accuracy of screening may be increased by the recognition of highly sensitive tumor-specific circulating markers (e.g., carcinoembryonic antigen for colorectal adenocarcinoma); the development of imaging techniques capable of finding smaller lesions (e.g., 3D mammography); and the identification of early molecular changes in cancer specimens (e.g., at the cellular level using Papanicolaou tests for cervical cancer). Given the limited effectiveness of primary prevention for older adults, screening asymptomatic persons at risk for cancer may be the most promising way to reduce the number of cancer deaths in older adults.

Yet another question to consider with a screening program is the prevalence of the disease in the population. The more prevalent the disease, the more beneficial a screening program will be. Because cancer is more common in older adults, screening is generally beneficial. Cancer incidence increases with age; thus, the positive predictive value of screening tests (i.e., the proportion of persons screened who actually have the disease) is likely to increase. Additionally, screening older adults with comorbid conditions at the time of cancer diagnosis may result in elective treatment at an early stage of the disease, thus reducing the possibility of serious treatment-related morbidity and deaths.

Recommendations on planning major screening programs for older adults should consider the risks and benefits of pursuing cancer screening among older adults (Kotwal and Walter, 2020). Screening guidelines vary greatly among different national organizations. Differences among recommendations are caused by the lack of cancer screening trials that include older adults. The lack of evidence-based criteria for screening older adults makes choosing screening protocols difficult. A decision-making process considering each older adult's personal preference and health should be used rather than relying only on age guidelines for cancer screening and detection methods. Screening should not be conducted without intent or the ability to follow up on the findings with a complete evaluation and treatment. Screening is costly and useless if no follow-up occurs. Other factors influencing the decision to screen an older adult include comorbidity, functional ability, and life expectancy.

Considerable uncertainty exists concerning cancer screening tests in older adults, as illustrated by the different age cutoffs recommended by various guideline panels. A framework to guide individualized cancer screening decisions in older patients may be more useful to the practicing nurse than age guidelines. Like many medical decisions, cancer screening decisions require weighing quantitative information, such as the risk for cancer death and the likelihood of beneficial and adverse screening outcomes and qualitative factors such as individual patients' values and preferences.

The potential benefits of screening are presented as the number needed to prevent one cancer-specific death based on the estimated life expectancy during which a patient will be screened. Estimates reveal substantial variability in the likelihood of benefit for patients of similar ages with varying life expectancies. In fact, patients with life expectancies of less than 10 years are unlikely to derive any survival benefit from cancer screening (Kotwal and Walter, 2020). The likelihood of potential harm from screening according to patient factors and test characteristics must also be considered. Some of the greatest harms of screening are detecting cancers that would never have become clinically significant. This becomes more likely as life expectancy decreases.

Finally, because many cancer screening decisions in older adults cannot be made solely based on quantitative estimates of benefits and harms, considering the estimated outcomes according to the patient's own values and preferences is the final step in making informed screening decisions. As more and more cancers occur in older people, oncologists are increasingly confronted with the necessity of integrating geriatric parameters into the treatment of their patients. In general, the United States Preventive Services Task Force recommends the following screenings for older adults (NCI, 2020):
- Colorectal cancer screening through age 75
- Breast cancer screening through age 74
- Cervical cancer screening through age 65

Nurses working with older adults should examine the role of cancer screening and the potential benefits for the population assigned to their care. The decision to screen or not to screen should be an active one made after thoughtful consideration within the context of a multidisciplinary healthcare team. Screening guidelines, individual circumstances, potential complications of aggressive evaluation workups, and associated costs are all factors to consider when screening older adults. The International Society of Geriatric Oncology Nursing and Allied Health Interest Group (SIOG NAH), with other oncology organizations, joined forces to update position statements for nursing care of older adults with hematology-oncology/cancer disorders (Puts et al, 2021). The four general roles of oncology nurses include for them to:
1. advocate for older adult's special needs for individualized care plans for cancer treatment
2. identify knowledge and skills required to provide daily care to older adults with oncology needs
3. recognize issues related to older adults
4. provide support to older adults during and after cancer treatment.

As a group, older persons generally require more individualized health teaching about cancer risk and detection. Older persons may lack an awareness of the risks for cancer associated with advanced age and may not know the warning signs of cancer. They may be reluctant to report physical complaints that could be indicative of cancer. Additionally, many older persons are concerned about, and even fear, the diagnosis of cancer and its effect on their overall well-being and functional status. Nursing considerations when caring for older adults include teaching them early warning signs of cancer:
- Change in bowel or bladder habits
- A sore that does not heal
- Unusual bleeding or discharge
- Thickening or lump in the breast or elsewhere
- Indigestion or difficulty swallowing
- Obvious change in a wart or mole
- Nagging cough or hoarseness

MAJOR TREATMENT MODALITIES

The five types of cancer treatment include (1) surgery, (2) radiation therapy, (3) chemotherapy, (4) targeted therapy, (5) immunotherapy, (6) hormone therapy, and (7) bone marrow/stem transplant (Cancer.Net, n.d.). Each form of treatment may be used alone or in combination. The type and stage of the cancer, the unique biophysiologic characteristics of the cancer cells, and an older patient's overall health status determine treatment selection at the time of diagnosis. Treatment goals also help determine the type of therapy. Cancer therapies may be directed at a *cure* or elimination of the disease, control or minimization of the disease, or *palliation* or relief of the symptoms. Adjuvant therapies following standard therapies have been developed that include many of the same modalities used for the initial cancer treatment. Therapies include hormones, immunotherapy, radiation, and targeted therapy (Pietrangelo, 2021).

Hormone therapy slows the growth of cancer cells that rely on the body's natural hormones for survival (ACS, 2020c). For hormone therapy to be effective, cancer cells must contain receptors for the specific hormone. Immunotherapy assists the person's own immune system to target cancer cells. Cancer cells survive by evading or disguising themselves from one's natural immune system. Medications used for immunotherapy have several functions (Welsh, 2023):

- Aids the immune system to recognize cancer cells
- Activate and amplify the natural immune system
- Prevent cancer cells from hiding from the natural immune system
- Alter cancer cell's signals

Radiation therapy is a common form of cancer treatment among older adults. It provides a curative option by targeting the specific location of cancer cells while decreasing toxicity to the surrounding healthy cells (Rosenblatt et al, 2017). Targeted therapy affects specific genes and proteins that allow cancer cells to grow (Cancer.Net, 2020a). Targeted therapy usually has fewer effects on healthy cells, reducing side effects.

Cancer treatment among older adults tends to be more complicated and challenging than among young adults (Cancer.Net, 2019). Older adults usually have chronic medical conditions, are on multiple medications, have poor healing processes, and longer recovery times. For decades, decisions to treat older adults with cancer were no different than other age groups. But, with continued research with a focus on older adults, age is no longer the only factor in deciding on cancer treatment. Cancer care has changed dramatically over the years; however, many older adults remember friends or relatives who were treated with now-outdated therapies that had devastating side effects. Because cancer is so prevalent in older adults, many have some information about cancer, but it is often misinformation. The nurse should ensure that patients and families have accurate information and a clear understanding of the treatment options offered.

Surgery

Surgery, the oldest method of treating cancer, is indicated for most solid tumors. Initially, with the use of sophisticated biopsy and exploratory techniques, surgery is used to diagnose and assess the extent of the disease, examine the tumor type, and stage the disease. The primary treatment goal of surgery is to remove the tumor when localized, thus preventing regional or distant metastasis. Surgery may also be indicated for palliative care in cases where the size or location of the tumor may create such problems as compression of surrounding tissues and organs, leading to pain, necrosis, or organ failure; large primary or metastatic tumors can be reduced with surgery. Surgery may be indicated for placing treatment-related devices such as implanted access devices, shunts, or drains. Additionally, surgery may be indicated for rehabilitation or restorative purposes, such as breast reconstruction after a mastectomy. Surgery is not a treatment of choice for disseminated diseases such as metastases of multiple small tumors in diffuse locations (e.g., when breast cancer metastasizes in the lungs) or for diseases that are disseminated from the onset, for example, leukemia.

In the past, surgical treatment of cancer involved extensive radical procedures. Such procedures were necessary to treat large, often neglected cancers. Poor understanding of patterns of metastatic spread and little knowledge of the benefits of adjuvant therapy contributed to the focus on radical operations. Greater insight into the pathophysiology of cancer and the development of additional therapies has led to more sophisticated surgical techniques. Early detection of smaller tumors has also contributed to the decline in high-intensity procedures. Lower-intensity surgeries result in fewer complications and improved QoL (Montroni et al, 2022).

The curability of cancer in older adults is largely predicted by an individual's ability to tolerate major surgery. Age alone should not be a determinant of surgical risk; instead, biological age examining the fitness or the frailty of older adults is a better predictor for complications (Berben et al, 2021). Careful preoperative assessment is critical because older adults are at risk for more complications. An in-depth evaluation of the status of the respiratory, cardiovascular, hepatic, immunologic, renal, nutritional, and central nervous systems is mandatory. The severity of underlying cancer and comorbid conditions is an important factor to consider in the decision regarding surgical therapy. Additionally, a patient's rehabilitation potential should be evaluated, particularly if the intended surgery will significantly alter normal physiologic function. Some surgical procedures may produce physiologic alterations beyond an older adult's adaptive capabilities. Arthritic changes and diminished visual acuity are two common problems in older adults that may make the management of surgical complications and postoperative care difficult (e.g., after colostomy creation). Older patients generally have a higher surgical risk than younger patients; however, through careful preoperative assessment to identify risks, older patients may be offered appropriate supportive therapies that minimize complications.

Postoperative priorities should include preventing respiratory complications and promoting cardiac and renal function. Because of the overall reduced compensatory reserves in these systems, older adults are susceptible to many serious complications, including congestive heart failure, electrolyte imbalances, hypoxia, dehydration, and venous thromboembolism. Using invasive lines and catheters may tax an aging immune system and predispose older patients to sepsis. The overall stress of surgery, including anesthesia and other centrally acting medications, may predispose older adults to the development of delirium. Bowel complications may include paralytic ileus and constipation. Decreased mobility and inadequate nutrition are risk factors for pressure ulcers. Careful, complete, and ongoing assessment of all body systems provides the foundation for the nurse to accurately diagnose, plan, implement, and evaluate nursing care during the postoperative period.

Radiation Therapy

Like all cancer therapies, radiation therapy is used for several different purposes. Radiation therapy may be curative for the treatment of several cancers, including skin, prostate, colorectal, lung, cervical, and Hodgkin's cancers. Radiation therapy may also be indicated as an adjuvant therapy to prevent recurrence of breast cancer after lumpectomy. In some cases, radiation therapy may be used to control cancers, adding months or years to an individual's life. Radiation therapy and chemotherapy may also be used before surgery to shrink the tumor. Often, recurrent breast and lung cancers can be controlled with radiation therapy in combination with chemotherapy, surgery, or both. Radiation therapy may also be used for palliative care. It relieves pain and prevents pathologic fractures associated with bone metastasis from breast, lung, and prostate tumors. Palliative radiation therapy is given for the relief of central nervous system symptoms caused by brain metastasis or spinal cord compression. In some cases, palliative radiation therapy may be given before a problem manifests itself, as in the treatment of vertebral lesions when spinal cord compression is imminent. According to the American Cancer Society (2019b), approximately half of all cancer patients receive radiation therapy during their treatments.

Therapeutic doses of radiation therapy are calculated to destroy or delay the growth of malignant cells without destroying normal tissue. Radiation effects at the cellular level may be either direct or indirect. Direct effects occur when key molecules within the cell — the DNA or RNA — are damaged. Indirect effects occur when charged particles (free radicals) are created by radiation therapy, which causes damage to cellular DNA.

The administration of radiation therapy may involve external or internal techniques. External beam therapy, which is radiation from a source at a distance from the body, is used to treat specific parts of the body, and mostly in an outpatient setting (NCI, 2019a). Rotation of the target site or the radiation beam makes delivering a high dose to the tumor possible. Yet, only part of the dose reaches the surrounding noncancerous tissue. Internal therapy involves radiation from a source placed within the body or a body cavity. Internal therapy can consist of a solid source inserted into target areas for a predetermined period; this is also called brachytherapy, a local treatment. Another internal therapy consists of liquid and is a systemic therapy that is administered orally, intramuscularly, or intravenously.

The associated side effects of radiation therapy are contingent on the health of older adults before radiation therapy. Increased frailty increases the risk for side effects, such as myelosuppression and fatigue. Geriatric screening tools can improve decision-making to minimize potential side effects (Rostoft et al, 2021). Unless severely debilitated, older adults tolerate radiotherapy with minimal side effects (Gosney, 2017). Age cannot be used as a predictor of how patients will respond to radiation therapy treatment.

Chemotherapy

For some cancers, chemotherapy may be the only treatment option available. Chemotherapy is often administered in addition to surgery or radiation (ACS, 2019c). It can also be used with targeted therapy, immunotherapy, or hormone therapy. Chemotherapy is a systemic treatment since the drugs travel throughout the body to kill cancer cells. Several chemotherapeutic drugs are often administered together to increase the killing power while minimizing drug resistance to any one drug.

Chemotherapy objectives include cure, control, and palliation (ACS, 2019c). In general, the survival of older persons who receive chemotherapy is significantly longer than that of untreated older persons, even though dose adjustments may be needed to control toxicity. Table 26.2 lists commonly prescribed chemotherapeutic agents by drug classification and mechanism of action.

Pharmacokinetics

Pharmacokinetics refers to the movement of drugs throughout the body, including absorption, distribution, metabolism, and excretion. For oral chemotherapeutic agents, age-related changes in the digestive tract appear to have little effect on the absorptive capacity of the intestine. Age-related changes in body composition — decreased total body water and increased body fat — may affect drug distribution; however, no consequences for chemotherapeutic agents have been demonstrated. The liver is the main site of metabolism for many chemotherapeutic agents. A reduction in cytochrome P-450 drug metabolizing enzymes occurs with aging, which may reduce hepatic drug clearance in older adults. The age-related decline in kidney function has been demonstrated to have clinical consequences for drug dosing. Toxic drug levels have been demonstrated for agents primarily excreted by the kidney (Merchan and Jhaveri, 2023). The dosage of chemotherapeutic agents may need to be adjusted to account for age-related kidney changes.

Pharmacodynamics

Pharmacodynamics refers to the interactions between the chemotherapeutic agents and their cellular targets, including the processes that modulate the activity of the agents. All agents act at the cellular level; however, their mechanisms of action vary, as do their respective administration guidelines and side effect profiles. Nurses caring for patients receiving chemotherapeutics should understand the specific actions and side effects of individual agents.

Targeted Therapy

Targeted cancer therapies are drugs that block the growth and spread of cancer by interfering with specific molecules (*molecular targets*) involved in the growth, progression, and spread of cancer. Targeted therapies differ from standard chemotherapy in several ways:

- They act on specific molecular targets associated with cancer, whereas most standard chemotherapies act on all rapidly dividing normal and cancerous cells.
- They are deliberately chosen or designed to interact with their target, whereas many standard chemotherapies were identified because they kill cells.
- Targeted therapies are often cytostatic (they block tumor cell proliferation), whereas standard chemotherapy agents are cytotoxic (they kill tumor cells).

Targeted therapies are the current focus of much anticancer drug development. They are a cornerstone of precision medicine, which uses information about a person's genes and proteins to prevent, diagnose, and treat disease (NCI, 2022a).

TABLE 26.2 Major Chemotherapeutic Agents

Drug Classification	Major Mechanism of Action	Drugs
Alkylating agents	Highly reactive compounds that act against already formed nucleic acids by cross-linking strands, thereby preventing RNA transcription and DNA replication. These agents are considered cell-cycle nonspecific.	Altretamine Bendamustine Busulfan Carboplatin Carmustine Chlorambucil Cisplatin Cyclophosphamide Dacarbazine Lomustine Melphalan Oxaliplatin Temozolomide Thiotepa
Antimetabolites	Analogs of normal metabolites and act by interfering with synthesis of chromosomal nucleic acid. Some agents block an enzyme necessary for synthesis of essential factors, whereas others are incorporated into RNA or DNA, thus preventing cellular replication. Pyrimidine analogs, purine analogs, and folic acid antagonists are three major subgroups of antimetabolites, which are considered cell-cycle specific.	Azacitidine 5-fluorouracil (5-FU) 6-mercaptopurine (6-MP) Capecitabine Cytarabine Decitabine Floxuridine Fludarabine Gemcitabine Hydroxyurea Methotrexate Nelarabine Pemetrexed Pralatrexate

Antitumor antibiotics	Natural products of various strains of soil fungi. These agents bind to DNA, preventing DNA synthesis, and are active in all phases of the cell cycle. They are divided into anthracyclines and non-anthracyclines.	*Anthracyclines:*
		  Daunorubicin
		  Doxorubicin
		  Epirubicin
		  Idarubicin
		  Valrubicin
		Non-anthracyclines:
		  Bleomycin
		  Dactinomycin
		  Mitomycin-C
		  Mitoxantrone (also acts as a topoisomerase II inhibitor)

Topoisomerase inhibitors	Plant alkaloids and interfere with enzymes called topoisomerases, which help separate the strands of DNA so they can be copied. Used to treat certain leukemias, as well as lung, ovarian, gastrointestinal, and other cancers. Grouped according to which type of enzyme they affect.	*Topoisomerase I inhibitors:*
		  Topotecan
		  Irinotecan
		Topoisomerase II inhibitors:
		  Etoposide (VP-16)
		  Teniposide
		  Mitoxantrone (also acts as an antitumor antibiotic)

Mitotic inhibitors	Compounds derived from natural products, such as plants (plant alkaloids). They work by stopping cells from dividing to form new cells but can damage cells in all phases by keeping enzymes from making proteins needed for cell reproduction. They are further divided into taxanes and vinca alkaloids.	*Taxanes:*
		  Cabazitaxel
		  Docetaxel
		  Estramustine
		  Paclitaxel
		Vinca alkaloids:
		  Vinblastine
		  Vincristine
		  Vinorelbine

Data from American Cancer Society. (2019). *How chemotherapy drugs work.* Retrieved from https://www.cancer.org/cancer/managing-cancer/treatment-types/chemotherapy/how-chemotherapy-drugs-work.html. Accessed December 15, 2023.

Immunotherapy

Immunotherapy is a cancer treatment designed to help the immune system fight cancer. Immunotherapy is a type of biological therapy, that is, a type of treatment that uses substances made from living organisms to treat cancer. Many different types of immunotherapy are used to treat cancer. They include (NCI, 2019b):

- Monoclonal antibodies are drugs designed to bind to specific targets in the body. They can cause an immune response that destroys cancer cells. Other types of monoclonal antibodies can "mark" cancer cells, making it easier for the immune system to find and destroy them.
- Adoptive cell transfer is a treatment that attempts to boost the natural ability of the body's T cells to fight cancer. T cells most active against the specific cancer are isolated from the patient's body and grown in large batches in the laboratory. After immunosuppression, the T cells grown in the laboratory are returned to the patient as an intravenous (IV) infusion.
- Cytokines are proteins that are made by the body's cells. They play important roles in the body's normal immune responses and in the immune system's ability to respond to cancer. The two main types of cytokines used to treat cancer are interferons and interleukins.
- Treatment vaccines work against cancer by boosting the body's immune system's response to cancer cells. Treatment vaccines are different from the ones that help prevent disease.
- Bacillus Calmette-Guérin (BCG) is an immunotherapy used to treat bladder cancer. It is a weakened form of the bacteria that causes tuberculosis. When inserted directly into the bladder with a catheter, BCG causes an immune response against cancer cells.

Hormone Therapy

Hormones are natural substances the body makes to regulate the activities of cells and organs (Cancer.Net, 2023). Some cancer cells use these hormones for their own survival. Common cancers treated with hormone therapy include cancers of the breast, thyroid, prostate, uterine, and adrenal. Hormone therapy is oftentimes used in conjunction with other cancer treatments such as chemotherapy, radiation, or surgery. Hormone therapies act on the body in various ways, such as:

- Production of hormones is prevented by the body
- Mechanism of actions are altered in the body
- The binding of cancer cells to hormones is blocked

Bone Marrow/Stem Transplant

A bone marrow transplant is also called a stem transplant. The bone marrow is replaced with healthy stem cells (Cancer.Net, 2020b). It is used for certain cancers, such as leukemia, myeloma, and lymphoma. Before stem transplant, chemotherapy is administered with or without radiation to eradicate as many cancer cells as possible.

COMMON PHYSIOLOGIC COMPLICATIONS

Cancer treatments are aimed at destroying cancer cells. Because most treatment pharmacodynamics include the prevention of cell division, actively dividing cell types are particularly vulnerable and may exhibit side effects. Actively dividing cell types most likely to exhibit side effects include those in hematopoietic tissue, the gastrointestinal (GI) tract, and hair follicles. Chemotherapy side effects are specific to the type of agent, dosage, and duration of use (see Nursing Care Plan box). Radiation-related side effects depend on the location of the radiation field, intensity of the dose, and duration of the therapy. In most cases, side effects are reversible.

NURSING CARE PLAN
Myelosuppressive Toxicities of Chemotherapy

Clinical Situation

Mr. K is a 69-year-old male recently diagnosed with SCLC. He lives with his wife in a modest home. Mr. K had no functional limitations before his diagnosis of cancer. He had 4 weeks of dry cough, fatigue, and weakness. CT of the chest revealed a 4-centimeter mass. His oncologist prescribes a chemotherapy regimen of cyclophosphamide, doxorubicin, and etoposide. As with many chemotherapy regimens, a primary side effect is myelosuppression, resulting in decreased red blood cells (RBCs), WBCs, and platelets. Because the therapy is given in the ambulatory care clinic, Mr. K and his wife will need to provide self-care for monitoring and managing the myelosuppressive effects of the agents.

Recognize Cues (Assessment)
- Advanced age
- 4-centimeter lung mass
- Fatigue and weakness
- Functional activities of daily (ADLs) living intact

Analyze Cues and Prioritize Hypotheses (Patient Problems)
- Potential for infection resulting from bone marrow depression (granulocytopenia) secondary to chemotherapy
- Potential for injury bleeding caused by bone marrow depression (thrombocytopenia) secondary to chemotherapy
- Inadequate peripheral tissue perfusion
- Potential for injury, fall from worsening fatigue and weakness

Generate Solutions and Evaluate Outcomes (Planning)
- The patient will remain free of infection.
- The patient will remain free of injury and bleeding incidents.
- The patient will not experience hypoxia, activity intolerance, or malaise.

Take Actions (Nursing Interventions)
- Monitor complete blood cell count and differential (absolute neutrophil count should remain > 500 cells/mm^3).
- Instruct the patient and family ways to avoid infection, such as:
  - Perform frequent oral hygiene using soft bristle toothbrush and low-alcohol mouthwash to minimize abrasions.
  - Lubricate dry areas using skin emollients and artificial tears to avoid skin tears.
  - Maintain adequate hydration.
  - Restrict visitors with infections.
  - Avoid large crowds.

Continued

> **NURSING CARE PLAN—cont'd**
> - Maintain proper hygiene.
> - Report temperature > 100° F.
> - Avoid trauma.
> - Instruct ways to avoid bruising or bleeding, such as:
>   - Use a soft bristle toothbrush and low-alcohol mouthwash and avoid flossing and use of toothpicks.
>   - Avoid tightly fitting or constrictive clothing.
>   - Use a nail file or emery board; avoid clipping or pulling hangnails.
>   - Use an electric razor for shaving.
> - Prevent constipation; use stool softeners and maintain adequate fluid intake.
> - Report minor bleeding such as petechiae, ecchymosis, epistaxis, and occult blood in stool, urine, or emesis.
> - Instruct the patient and family ways to preserve energy:
>   - Increase rest and sleep periods.
>   - Alternate rest and activity periods.
>   - Incorporate foods into the diet that are high in iron, such as eggs, lean meat, green leafy vegetables, carrots, and raisins.
>   - Modify roles and responsibilities, as needed.

Bone Marrow Suppression

Chemotherapy is designed to kill rapidly growing cells, such as cancer cells, but affects all rapidly growing cells, including hair follicles, the GI tract, and bone marrow. Bone marrow suppression is a decrease in the ability of the bone marrow to manufacture hematopoietic stem cells that differentiate into the RBCs, WBCs, and platelets that the body needs (Eldridge, 2023).

- *Red blood cells* contain hemoglobin that carries oxygen to every cell in the body and return carbon dioxide to the lungs. Hypoxia occurs if there are not enough RBCs to deliver oxygen to all body tissues.
- *White blood cells* are the body's defense system, providing protection from bacteria, viruses, and other foreign substances, such as cancer cells. Neutropenia refers to a deficiency of one particular type of WBC known as a neutrophil. Without adequate neutrophils, we are predisposed to infection.
- *Platelets* are responsible for creating blood clots. A deficiency of platelets can lead to bleeding and is referred to as thrombocytopenia.

The symptoms of bone marrow suppression depend on the type of blood cells affected. In general, a blood cell deficiency results in fatigue and weakness (Eldridge, 2023).

Chemotherapy-Induced Anemia

A decreased level of RBCs during chemotherapy is referred to *as chemotherapy-induced anemia*. The production of too few RBCs to carry oxygen results in fatigue, lightheadedness or dizziness, pallor, shortness of breath, tachycardia, or palpitations.

Anemia should improve once chemotherapy is completed; however, a medication to stimulate RBC production may be prescribed along with iron supplements. At times, a blood transfusion may be necessary. Anemia is a treatable cause of fatigue; unfortunately, there are many causes of cancer fatigue, and anemia is only one of these (Eldridge, 2023).

Chemotherapy-Induced Neutropenia

A low level of neutrophils during chemotherapy is referred to as *chemotherapy-induced neutropenia*. Suppression of the number of neutrophils is most important in raising the risk for infection. Most of the symptoms of neutropenia are related to infections and may include fever greater than 100.5° F, chills, cough, shortness of breath, and redness or drainage at the site of an injury. Persons receiving chemotherapy should be instructed to avoid situations that could result in infection, such as spending time with people who are ill or shopping in crowded malls. In the setting of neutropenia, chemotherapy treatment may be delayed, or medications prescribed to prevent infection or stimulate the production of WBCs (Eldridge, 2023).

Chemotherapy-Induced Thrombocytopenia

A low platelet count caused by chemotherapy is referred to *as chemotherapy-induced thrombocytopenia*. Thrombocytopenia can result in bleeding. Signs of thrombocytopenia include easy bruising, petechiae, joint and muscle pain, blood in urine or stools, or heavy menstrual periods (if menopause has not been reached). If bleeding is present, platelet transfusion or medications to stimulate the bone marrow to make more platelets may be prescribed (Eldridge, 2023).

Coping With Bone Marrow Suppression

Patients receiving chemotherapy should be taught to (Eldridge, 2023):
- Wash hands properly
- Call the healthcare provider with any signs of infection, such as a fever > 100.5° F, coughing, chills, shortness of breath, or pain with urination
- Rest when feeling tired
- Stand up slowly after resting
- Avoid medications such as aspirin and ibuprofen that can increase bleeding
- Take care to avoid situations where injuries may occur

Nausea and Vomiting

Nausea is a subjectively experienced stomach distress that may be described as a heaviness, pressure, or sinking feeling in the epigastric or sternal region. It is often associated with such physical signs as pallor, sweating, and chills. Most often, patients refer to nausea when describing "feeling sick." *Vomiting* is the ejection of stomach contents through the mouth. Nausea and vomiting are two separate and distinct events;. However, they frequently occur together, so it is important for the nurse to distinguish between the two when taking a patient history and planning care.

Chemotherapy-induced nausea and vomiting (CINV) are among its most distressing side effects. Not all chemotherapeutic agents cause nausea and vomiting, and those that have high emetic potential do not cause equal distress in all persons. Considerable variation exists among patients and types of agents. Some patients may expect to develop nausea and vomiting and may begin to experience symptoms before chemotherapy starts; this is referred to as *anticipatory nausea and vomiting*. Because many older adults likely have friends or family members who were treated with older therapies, nurses should reassure patients that management of this side effect has changed for the better.

Nausea may lead to decreased nutritional intake, whereas vomiting may lead to severe metabolic complications, including dehydration and metabolic alkalosis. Older adults are less tolerant of dehydration than younger persons and may manifest acute confusion in response. Dehydration may create a metabolic crisis necessitating resuscitation with IV fluid administration. Additionally, chemotherapeutic agents excreted by the kidney may build toxic levels, which could lead to increased side effects and renal failure, particularly when agents with known nephrotoxic side effects are used. Electrolyte imbalances may aggravate cardiac problems and precipitate drug toxicity if a patient is taking medication to manage a cardiac condition. Episodes of severe vomiting may require the dosage of chemotherapy to be reduced or treatment to be postponed.

Current pharmacologic management of CINV includes corticosteroids, serotonin antagonists, dopamine antagonists, neurokinin 1 receptor antagonists, cannabinoids, and antianxiety drugs (Fleishman, 2018).

Nursing care should begin with an in-depth emetic history and a preventive plan. Characteristics that have been linked with CINV include susceptibility to motion sickness, history of severe nausea during pregnancy, and poor emetic control during prior treatments. Nurses should evaluate the degree and duration of episodes of nausea and vomiting and monitor for signs of dehydration. Long-term nutritional compromise may result from poorly controlled nausea; consultation with a dietitian may be helpful (see Nutritional Considerations box).

Chemotherapy-Induced Oral Mucositis

Chemotherapy-induced oral mucositis is caused by the destruction of rapidly proliferating mucosal cells in the oral cavity, resulting in inflammation, ulceration, pain, and bleeding. Several chemotherapeutic agents are known to cause severe chemotherapy-induced oral mucositis. Evidence suggests that older adults are at increased risk for severe chemotherapy-induced oral mucositis. Radiation therapy that includes mucosal tissue in the radiation field may lead to dose-related oral mucositis, which generally clears when therapy is complete.

A dentist should evaluate dental and oral care needs before treatment begins, and treatment should be delayed until any dental problems are resolved. Patients should understand the

NUTRITIONAL CONSIDERATIONS

Nutritional Consequences of Cancer Treatment

The nutritional consequences of cancer treatment may be devastating, resulting in the older adult's inability to tolerate treatment and compromising their QoL. Specific consequences are related to the type of treatment. Nurses should be aware of possible nutritional consequences and complete a nutritional assessment early in the course of therapy. Early assessment provides a baseline for high-risk persons. Patients should be weighed at regular intervals. Individuals at the highest risk for nutritional compromise are those experiencing weight losses of 1% to 2% in 1 week, 5% in 1 month, 7.5% in 3 months, and > 10% in 6 months.

Treatment	Possible Nutritional Consequences	Treatment	Possible Nutritional Consequences

Chemotherapy	• Taste alterations
	• Decreased tolerance to protein-rich foods
	• Mucositis and esophagitis
	  • Difficulty chewing
	  • Difficulty swallowing
	• GI distress
	  • Dehydration
	  • Electrolyte imbalance
	  • GI bleed
	• Decreased caloric intake
	• Weight loss
		Radiation therapy of the lung	• Dyspnea
			• Anorexia
			• GI distress
			• Decreased appetite
			• Generalized malaise

		Radiation therapy of the abdomen	• GI distress • Abdominal cramps • Decreased appetite

		Surgical resection of oropharynx	• Postoperative changes
			  • Dysphagia
			  • Difficulty chewing
			  • Taste alterations
			• Possible need for tube feedings

		Esophagectomy, esophagogastrectomy, or esophageal reconstruction	• Gastric stasis • Steatorrhea • Diarrhea • Decreased appetite

Radiation therapy of the head and neck	• Taste alterations
	• Xerostomia
	• Mucositis and esophagitis
	• Dysphagia
	• Decreased appetite
		Gastrectomy (partial or complete)	• Dumping syndrome
			  • Abdominal cramps
			  • Early satiety
			  • Malabsorption of fats, iron, B_{12}, and calcium

		Intestinal resection	• Malnutrition • Malabsorption of nutrients, such as B_{12}, iron, fat, and electrolytes • Weight loss
Radiation therapy of the esophagus	• Dysphagia • Pharyngitis • Esophagitis • GI distress • Anorexia	Pancreatectomy	• Insufficient exocrine function and malabsorption • Insufficient endocrine function, which can lead to endocrine disorders, such as diabetes mellitus

importance of good oral hygiene with a soft bristle toothbrush and avoid products with alcohol, which dry the mucous membranes and increase the risk for cracking, bleeding, and infection. If toothpaste irritates the mouth, a half-teaspoon of salt in four cups of water can be used instead. Gargling with a solution made from one quart of water, with a half-teaspoon of salt and a half-teaspoon of baking soda, may soothe mucus membranes. Prescription products are also available, and patients should be instructed to speak to their healthcare provider if oral mucositis persists despite conservative treatment. The patient's mouth, lips, and tongue should be assessed for early signs of inflammation. Severe oral mucositis may result in decreased oral intake, which, in turn, may lead to dehydration and cause a metabolic crisis that may necessitate resuscitation with IV fluid administration. Also, severe oral mucositis may result in a decreased appetite, leading to nutritional compromise and, hence, decreased ability to tolerate treatment (Fleishman, 2018). Older persons generally become less tolerant of dehydration and nutritional depletion with age.

Anorexia and Cachexia

Many patients receiving cancer treatments complain of anorexia, a general loss of appetite. Contributing factors include chemotherapeutic agents, radiation therapy, especially to the head and neck area, pain medications, and chemotherapy-induced oral mucositis. Decreased appetite leads to decreased caloric intake and weight loss. Severe weight loss, with loss of muscle and general weakness, or cachexia, has been linked to poor outcomes; patients with significant weight loss have more complications and decreased survival rates. Anorexia and cachexia may also contribute to decreased immune function, increasing the risk for infectious complications. Patients may require medications to offset these side effects of chemotherapeutics (Weaver, 2021).

Dietary consultation and frequent weight monitoring are necessary to maintain optimal weight. The nutritional goal for patients with cancer or on cancer treatment is to provide the best possible QoL while controlling symptoms such as anorexia and cachexia (NCI, 2023c). A registered dietitian working with family members and the healthcare team can determine the best means of improving patient nutrition. The nurse should remember that food choices and eating patterns have strong cultural influences, and planning nutritional diets with patients and their families is critical to successful outcomes.

Diarrhea

Diarrhea results from the destruction of the actively dividing intestinal epithelial cells of the GI tract. When these cells are destroyed, atrophy of the intestinal mucosa occurs, resulting in the shortening or denuding of the intestinal villi. When the villi and microvilli become flattened, the absorptive surface area is reduced, and intestinal contents move rapidly through the gut, resulting in frequent liquid stools. Absorption of nutrients is decreased, and patients are at risk for dehydration and malnutrition. Circulatory collapse may occur, especially in older adults with cardiovascular disease. Diarrhea may aggravate perirectal problems such as hemorrhoids and may cause pain, bleeding, and infection.

Assessment of diarrhea includes the number of stools per day, their consistency, and their color. Older patients may be reluctant to discuss diarrhea, ignoring their symptoms until dehydration becomes a problem. To control diarrhea, patients should be instructed to eat small, frequent meals and avoid coffee, tea, alcohol, and sweets. They should be advised to eat low-fiber foods and avoid fried, greasy, or spicy foods, as well as milk and milk products. Patients should also be instructed to increase the potassium in their diet and drink plenty of room-temperature clear liquids (Fleishman, 2018). Chemotherapy is usually administered unless diarrhea is severe, resulting in dehydration.

Alopecia

Alopecia is a common complication of chemotherapy. Hair loss may range from thinning scalp hair to total body hair loss, including eyelashes, eyebrows, and pubic hair. The degree of alopecia depends on both the chemical agent and the dose. Chemotherapy-induced hair loss occurs rapidly and becomes apparent over a 2- to 3-week period after initiation of treatment. Chemotherapy-induced hair loss is temporary in most cases, and hair begins to grow slowly after treatment has been completed. Radiation-induced hair loss occurs when the scalp is in the radiation field. Hair loss is permanent if the radiation dose causes irreversible destruction of the hair follicles; otherwise, hair loss is temporary. To date, no type of hair care product or practice has been shown to satisfactorily prevent or reduce hair loss.

Although the physiologic consequences of alopecia are minimal, the emotional distress may be enormous. Hair greatly contributes to body image and sexuality. Wigs and hairpieces should be purchased *before* total hair loss occurs. Often, patients are too embarrassed to shop for hair replacements when they are bald. Once the hair is gone, it may be difficult to match color, texture, or style (Fleishman, 2018). The nurse should not assume that hair loss is an issue only for females; males may be equally devastated by hair loss. For instance, an older, completely bald male was mortified when he lost his big, bushy eyebrows, but the local university theater created a pair of high-quality eyebrows for him as a temporary relief.

OLDER ADULTS' EXPERIENCE OF CANCER

Older adults may already be experiencing significant cognitive and functional difficulties when diagnosed with cancer (Ornstein et al, 2020). They may also have financial strains and social isolation. These and other factors must be considered as they may determine how older adults tolerate cancer treatments and health outcomes.

Quality of Life

Historically, length of survival has been the most important consideration in measuring the outcome of cancer treatment. Recently, efforts have been made to address not only the length of life but also the circumstances of life — quality and quantity. For an older adult experiencing cancer in the context of a life mostly lived, quality is a very — if not the most — important consideration.

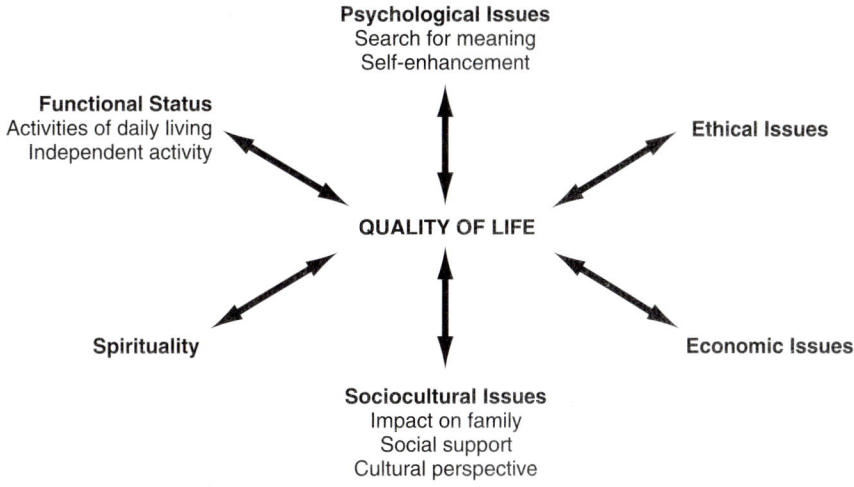

Fig. 26.2 Quality of life as a multidimensional concept.

Determining the QoL goes beyond evaluating the severity of symptoms (such as nausea, pain, or fatigue) to considering the degree of functional status reflected in the person's ability to perform ADLs. Quality of life is a multidimensional concept that includes not only functional status and the severity of symptoms but also the patient's ideas about psychological development, sociocultural issues, ethical issues, economic issues, and spirituality.

Fig. 26.2 depicts the multidimensional nature of QoL. Attitudes in three categories — physical well-being, psychological well-being, and interpersonal well-being — have been demonstrated to be the primary determinants of overall QoL for older adults (Padilla et al, 1990). The three categories mentioned by Padilla et al can be further divided into nine domains (health perception, autonomy, role/activity, relationships, attitude/adaptation, emotional comfort, spirituality, home/neighborhood, and financial security) (van Leeuwen et al, 2019). These nine domains are often intertwined and are often affected by the status of one or more domains at a given time. Also, in older adults, QoL factors are shown to be rated differently by males and females; for males, vitality and personal resources are most important, whereas for females, psychosocial well-being is most important (Dibble et al, 1998).

QoL evaluation is relevant to both curative and palliative care. In curative care, information obtained from a QoL assessment helps guide the selection of therapeutic strategies that result in a more normal life. Older adults may need special QoL consideration when choosing a treatment. A moderate treatment that provides relatively symptom-free disease control may be a better QoL choice for an older adult than a rigorous treatment that statistically offers a prolonged disease-free period. In palliative care, QoL assessment provides insight into areas that may require intervention, such as family counseling, financial planning, and management of depression.

Most studies evaluating treatment modalities or chemotherapeutic agents include some measures of a person's QoL. Historically, these studies focused on measures of functional status, primarily assessing the ability of patients to perform various ADLs and survival prediction (Baik et al, 2018) using the Palliative Performance Scale. The nurse plays a central role in supporting an older patient's QoL. Nurses manage disease-related symptoms and treatment-related side effects. Few studies have focused on the older adult's perception of health status while receiving cancer treatment. However, Steele et al (2005) found that even patients with terminal illnesses can have a good QoL when proper resources such as hospice care are initiated.

EVIDENCE-BASED PRACTICE

Symptom Management Guide for Home Health Nurses Caring for Cancer Patients

Background
Most patients with cancer manage their symptoms at home with support from home health nurses. Improved support and management from nurses can facilitate improved QoL and decreased use of healthcare services.

Sample/Setting
The sample encompassed six nursing agencies within a regional home care authority in Canada. The study involved 50 patient records, 14 interviews, and 150 survey responses.

Methods
This mixed methods study, guided by the Knowledge-to-Action Framework, "assessed factors influencing home care nurses' use of 15 evidence-informed symptom practice guides for providing telephone or in-home nursing services to [patients] with cancer" (p. 224). A chart audit was conducted to determine patient characteristics. Home health staff participated in semistructured interviews to determine "(1) current practice for providing symptoms support, (2) potential factors likely to influence use of 15 evidence-informed symptom practice guides, (3) need for local adaptation of the practice guises, and (4) strategies to implement the practice guides" (p. 225). Additionally, a barriers survey was administered to identify factors influencing use of the evidence-informed practice guides.

Findings
Average age of patients was 62.4 years. Of the 50 patients, 15 experienced one symptom, 11 two symptoms, and 22 three or more symptoms. Identified symptoms included nausea/vomiting, constipation, fatigue, loss of appetite, pain, diarrhea, mouth sores, anxiety, and/or depression. Nurses typically provided symptom management Monday through Friday, during normal business hours. However, patients could call 24 hours a day, 7 days a week.

Continued

> ### EVIDENCE-BASED PRACTICE—cont'd
>
> Barriers to using the symptom practice guides included length and complexity of the guides; inability for a single symptom practice guide to address multiple symptoms or symptom clusters; and inadequate space for additional comments. Facilitators to using the practice guides included comprehensive and evidence-based; systematic approach, relevance to current home care nursing practice; user-friendly format with plain language; and more efficient assessment.
>
> #### Implications
> The nurses felt barriers to adopting the guides could be overcome through education, clear organizational mandates for using them, and integration with documentation system. Overall, the symptom guides were well received by the nurses. Implementation of these guides has the "potential to narrow the know-do gap by providing nurses with user-friendly, evidence-based tools to guide their practice" (p. 233).

Data from Ludwig, C., Bennis, C., Carley, M., Gifford, W., Kuziemsky, C., Lafreniere-Davis, N., et al. (2017). Managing symptoms during cancer treatments: Barriers and facilitators to home care nurses using symptom practice guides. *Home Health Care Management & Practice, 29*(4), 224–234.

Depression

Depression is often associated with higher mortality, especially among older adults with cancer (Borza et al, 2022). The immune and neuroendocrine functions may be altered due to depression. Those with advanced disease may not be able to cope and have a decreased desire to live.

Depressive symptoms may result from side effects of medications used to control cancer. Depressive symptoms are especially associated with hormone therapy and cortisone medications, two medication groups frequently prescribed for cancer treatment (Massa et al, 2021). Additionally, older adults may have underlying diseases that are controlled by medications. Depressive symptoms are associated with many drugs used to manage chronic illness. Additionally, depressive symptoms are known to increase with an increased number of medications taken.

Nurses should assess the older adult's risk for depression. Tools, such as the 15-item Geriatric Depression Scale, can help healthcare providers identify and assess for depression among older adults (Borza et al, 2022). Older adults with cancer should be educated about the psychological implications of having cancer. An understanding of how the experience of cancer may affect such things as feelings of well-being, interpersonal relationships, and self-fulfillment is needed as much as an understanding of the schedule for taking medications. Older patients and their family members should be encouraged to discuss the effects of cancer on family functioning. Individual evaluation of depressive symptoms is needed if an older person is suspected of experiencing depression. Nurses should refer older patients for further evaluation for depression when symptoms last longer than a week, worsen rather than improve, or interfere with the ability to carry out daily routines or cooperate with treatment plans. Management of cancer-related depression should be individualized and may include supportive interventions, cognitive intervention, psychotherapy, and psychopharmacology.

Grief and Loss

Grief is a natural and expected human reaction to loss. An older adult who is being treated for cancer may experience multiple losses, including loss of energy, loss of a body part, loss of functional ability, loss of self-esteem, and loss of control. The losses associated with cancer may overlap other losses frequently experienced by older adults, including the loss of a spouse, friends, or family; changes in living arrangements; and physical losses of vision, hearing, or mobility.

Although grief is a universal human reaction, the subject and the intensity of grief are determined by the meaning an individual places on the loss. Grieving is a human imperative, but how people grieve varies. There is no one way to grieve, and no one timetable for grief exists. Understanding the practices of different cultures can help healthcare providers assess and develop appropriate methods to treat people who are grieving (NCI, 2022b).

The healthcare literature often reports that denial is among the initial responses to loss, including losses associated with a diagnosis of cancer. Denial is believed to protect people by providing them with the time needed to assimilate the effect of the diagnosis. Most people need some time to allow the diagnosis of cancer to reach conscious awareness. The information about the diagnosis is allowed into the awareness in increments that are tolerable to the person. However, a continued denial of the diagnosis can lead to an unhealthy grieving process (Hasdenteufel and Quintard, 2022).

Nurses should support older patients and families by patiently repeating information when asked, validating what the family has heard, and determining what the information means to them as individuals and as a family unit. The ongoing process of assessing a patient's and family's understanding of the information should spur nursing interventions. Patients and families should be allowed to come to their own level of understanding of the diagnosis. Nurses should validate the patient's feelings of grief and loss. Grief cannot be prevented, and nurses should give the individual permission to grieve in reaction to loss. Some older adults may have unresolved grief or complications associated with grieving or loss.

Healthcare providers, including nurses need to be alert to signs and symptoms of ongoing grief to minimize emotional and physical complications (Tofthagen et al, 2017). The following are examples of interventions that may help those who are grieving (CancerCare, 2018; Oates and Maani-Fogelman, 2022; Tofthagen et al, 2017):

- Be aware of available community resources for patients and family members to be referred for unresolved grief.
- Allow patients and family members time to express their feelings. Older adults may need more time to become aware of and express their feelings. Sometimes, they also need more time to complete activities. Providing extra time shows concern and respect for their needs.
- Pointing out signs of sadness or changes in behavior may help the person become aware of feelings and may help the person feel more comfortable talking about their feelings.
- Spending time with the person. When an older adult has lost something or someone special, especially a spouse, feelings of loneliness may last for a long time.

- Ask the person to talk about their loss. Older people, especially those who have experienced several losses over a short period, are often helped by sharing memories related to the losses.
- Watch for signs of prolonged grieving or depression and implement preventive therapies.
- Older adults often have more than one loss to deal with. Talking about each loss may help identify the person's feelings. Separating losses from one another may also help the person feel less overwhelmed and more able to cope with emotional distress.

Social Isolation and Loneliness

The health and well-being of older adults may be negatively impacted by social isolation and loneliness (WHO, 2021). Social isolation is an objective state noted by having few social contacts, and loneliness is subjective in that the person has negative feelings or pain because the need for social connection is unmet. Social isolation and loneliness negatively impact the health of older adults. Their physical and mental health declines, their QoL becomes subpar, and their lives are shortened. Conditions such as cardiovascular disease and stroke may be more likely in those who are isolated or lonely. Furthermore, mental health disorders, such as dementia, depression, anxiety, and suicide, are higher among those who are socially isolated, further exacerbating the feeling of loneliness. Not only do physical and mental health disorders are exacerbated by social isolation and loneliness, but social isolation may also cause these same medical problems (National Academies of Sciences, Engineering, and Medicine, 2020). Older adults with frailty, including those with dementia, are also at risk for social isolation and loneliness. Many older adults fear embarrassment or stigma due to cognitive deficits or certain health conditions.

Older adults with cancer may be further isolated because of the treatment's side effects, extended hospitalization, and limited network of people (Karam, 2021). Treatment-related side effects may interfere with the ability to drive or use public transportation, sit comfortably at a social gathering, or eat in restaurants. Patients fear alienating their social network if they discuss their distress and concerns. As mentioned earlier, patients with cancer have a higher cancer-related mortality rate when socially isolated than those who are not isolated. Isolation brings constant stress, and stress increases the inflammatory response, which can impede treatments. Older adults should be assessed for social isolation and loneliness as a standard part of their health care. A comprehensive geriatric assessment is a multidimensional and interdisciplinary tool that evaluates health domains, such as mental health, cognition, functionality, and social status (Berben et al, 2021).

The availability of social contacts may decline as family members and friends die or relocate (Tilden and Weinert, 1987). The recent loss of a spouse or partner may lead to social isolation, and the person may withdraw because of feelings of awkwardness or loneliness. Many older adults feel unsafe going places alone. Social isolation does not reflect being restricted to a single place, such as a home. Many older adults live a lifetime in a neighborhood only to find that the neighbors have moved, the area has changed and become less safe, and the social network in the neighborhood or town has slowly disappeared over time. Older adults may perceive themselves as disconnected from the unfamiliar people in the neighborhood.

Family members may not live in geographic proximity, decreasing the ability to visit or seek assistance. It may be necessary to relocate an older adult during cancer treatment. When an older adult is relocated to live with family or in a residential care facility, he or she needs assistance developing and maintaining social contacts.

Older adults may substitute interaction with healthcare personnel for meaningful social interaction. A clinic or home care visit may be an older adult's only social contact for an extended period of time. Nurses should evaluate the older adult's need for social interaction; assess the person's level of social activity before the cancer diagnosis and determine whether it was satisfactory; ask what has changed regarding social activities since the cancer diagnosis; determine what, if anything, has changed regarding social activities as the person has gotten older; and work with the patient and family to identify strategies for maintaining social activities and contacts. Nurses should explore the importance of various activities described by the older patient. Many older adults value religious activities such as church attendance or prayer groups. In addition to meeting social needs, religious activities help meet spiritual needs.

Resources and Support

An important component of nursing care for older adults is awareness of resources and referrals to appropriate agencies or support groups. Both cancer patients and their families have found support groups sponsored by local church groups, hospitals, home health agencies, and hospices helpful. Nurses should have up-to-date listings for the groups in their areas.

- The American Association of Retired Persons (AARP) and Grief and Loss, a national organization founded in 1973 to promote QoL for older people, provide resources. The website on grief and loss includes community resources offering support to people grieving the death of a loved one. The website also has information on coping with the loss of a loved one and making plans such as funeral arrangements and financial decisions after a person's death: http://www.aarp.org/families/grief_loss.
- The National Association for Home Care and Hospice (NAHC) seeks to heighten the public visibility of hospice services. NAHC offers a few helpful, practical publications for people considering hospice, including consumer guides, fact sheets, historical perspectives, and other background information. The website offers information from the legislative, regulatory, research, legal, and public relations departments, including "Home Care and Hospice Facts and Stats": https://www.nahc.org/.
- The U.S. National Hospice and Palliative Care Organization (NHPCO) offers information on local hospice and palliative care programs across America. NHPCO is committed to improving end-of-life care and expanding access to hospice care to improve the QoL for dying people and their loved ones: https://www.nhpco.org/.

- The American Society of Clinical Oncology (ASCO) offers resources for oncology professionals: http://www.asco.org.

Older persons are also using web resources. Those related to cancer include the following:
- National Cancer Institute: http://www.cancer.gov
- American Cancer Society: http://www.cancer.org
- National Breast Cancer Foundation: http://www.nationalbreastcancer.org
- Prostate Cancer Foundation: https://www.pcf.org
- American Lung Association: http://www.lung.org

SUMMARY

The incidence of most cancers increases with advancing age. The Oncology Nursing Society has outlined the knowledge nurses need to provide holistic care for older adults with cancer, including the physiology of aging, geriatric assessment, symptom management, and end-of-life care (Puts et al, 2021). Cancer prevention and screening programs for older adults require special attention to ethical issues. Decisions to screen older adults should be made on an individual basis.

Older adults are more vulnerable to the development of cancer. Because the aging cell has been exposed to a lifetime of potentially carcinogenic substances, it is more susceptible to damage and is less able to repair damage. In general, older adults can tolerate cancer treatment when careful attention is paid to dosage adjustments and comorbid factors. The experience of cancer for the older adult is unique. Cancer in the older adult is cancer in the context of a life mostly lived.

HOME CARE

1. Instruct homebound older adults and their caregivers to be aware of and report symptoms associated with the warning signs of cancer.
2. Educate older adults about cancer screening and self-examination.
3. Breast cancer is a disease of older women, thus breast screening is a lifelong process. Instruct homebound older women on the American Cancer Society's breast self-examination guidelines.
4. Assess nonspecific symptoms such as indigestion, loss of appetite, and weight loss in both older males and older females. These warning signs are seen in cancer of the stomach, colon, and rectum.
5. Instruct caregivers and homebound older adults with cancer about general comfort measures to promote rest and sleep, with the goal of increasing pain tolerance.
6. Assess for side effects of cancer treatment therapies (e.g., radiation therapy, chemotherapy) and report to a physician, as needed, for treatment recommendations.
7. Instruct caregivers and homebound older adults on measures to reduce the side effects of cancer treatment therapies.
8. Refer patients with advanced cancer to palliative care early in their cancer care.

KEY POINTS

- Three leading causes of cancer deaths in older adult females are lung, breast, and colorectal cancers; in males, the leading causes of cancer deaths are lung, colorectal, and prostate cancers.
- Aging cells show a tendency toward aberration as they replicate, probably because of the failure of growth control mechanisms. Altered growth control mechanisms make the aging cell more vulnerable to damage, leading to cancer development.
- Clinical manifestations of cancer in older adults may be mistakenly attributed to normal, age-related changes. Older adults should be made aware of the warning signs of cancer and report symptoms associated with them to a healthcare provider.
- Nurses caring for older adults have a major responsibility to recommend strategies aimed at the prevention and early detection of cancer in this age group.
- Major treatment modalities for cancer include surgery, radiation therapy, chemotherapy, targeted therapy, and immunotherapy. Therapy with these modalities may be used alone or in combination; therapy may be curative or palliative.
- Functional status of an older adult is the most important consideration in selecting a treatment goal and modality. Age alone is not a good predictor of treatment tolerance or response.
- Older adults generally have fewer reserves, and greater attention should be given to the status of major organs, including the kidneys, liver, heart, lungs, and GI system. Maintaining fluid, electrolyte balance, and caloric intake is critical to treatment outcomes for older adults.
- Older adults are especially vulnerable to the nephrologic and hematologic toxicity of chemotherapeutic agents.
- Psychosocial care of older adults with cancer includes addressing issues related to QoL, depression, loss and grief, and social isolation.
- The cancer experience for each older adult is unique. Cancer in an older adult is in the context of a life mostly lived.

CLINICAL JUDGMENT EXERCISES

1. You are asked to make a 30-minute presentation at a senior center on the benefits and risks of cancer screening in older adults. Prepare a topical outline for the presentation.
2. The director of oncology services asks you to develop a procedure for functional assessment of older adults with cancer. Develop the procedure and include any functional assessment parameters and instruments to be used.
3. The family cancer support group has asked you to facilitate a discussion on family considerations when an older family member has cancer. Prepare a list of the points that you would discuss with the group.

REFERENCES

Administration for Community Living. (2022). *2021 profile of older Americans*. Retrieved from https://www.acl.gov/aging-and-disability-in-america/data-and-research/profile-older-americans. Accessed December 15, 2023.

American Cancer Society (ACS). (2023a). *Key statistics for prostate cancer*. Retrieved from https://www.cancer.org/cancer/prostate-cancer/about/key-statistics.html. Accessed December 15, 2023.

American Cancer Society (ACS). (2023b). *Survival rates for prostate cancer*. Retrieved from https://www.cancer.org/cancer/types/prostate-cancer/detection-diagnosis-staging/survival-rates.html. Accessed December 15, 2023.

American Cancer Society (ACS). (2022a). *Cancer facts & figures 2022*. Retrieved from https://www.cancer.org/content/dam/cancer-org/research/cancer-facts-and-statistics/annual-cancer-facts-and-figures/2022/2022-cancer-facts-and-figures.pdf. Accessed December 15, 2023.

American Cancer Society (ACS). (2022b). *HIV and cancer*. Retrieved from https://www.cancer.org/cancer/cancer-causes/infectious-agents/hiv-infection-aids/hiv-aids-and-cancer.html. Accessed December 15, 2023.

American Cancer Society (ACS). (2022c). *American cancer society recommendations for the early detection of breast cancer*. Retrieved from https://www.cancer.org/cancer/breast-cancer/screening-tests-and-early-detection/american-cancer-society-recommendations-for-the-early-detection-of-breast-cancer.html. Accessed December 15, 2023.

American Cancer Society (ACS). (2022d). *Hormone therapy for prostate cancer*. Retrieved from https://www.cancer.org/cancer/prostate-cancer/treating/hormone-therapy.html. Accessed December 15, 2023.

American Cancer Society (ACS). (2021). *Breast cancer risk factors you cannot change*. Retrieved from https://www.cancer.org/cancer/breast-cancer/risk-and-prevention/breast-cancer-risk-factors-you-cannot-change.html. Accessed December 15, 2023.

American Cancer Society (ACS). (2020a). *American cancer society guideline for colorectal cancer screening*. Retrieved from https://www.cancer.org/cancer/types/colon-rectal-cancer/detection-diagnosis-staging/acs-recommendations.html. Accessed December 15, 2023.

American Cancer Society (ACS). (2020b). *Treating colorectal cancer*. Retrieved from https://www.cancer.org/content/dam/CRC/PDF/Public/8607.00.pdf. Accessed December 15, 2023.

American Cancer Society (ACS). (2020c). *Hormone therapy*. Retrieved from https://www.cancer.org/cancer/managing-cancer/treatment-types/hormone-therapy.html. Accessed December 15, 2023.

American Cancer Society (ACS). (2019a). *What is prostate cancer?* Retrieved from https://www.cancer.org/cancer/prostate-cancer/about/what-is-prostate-cancer.html. Accessed December 15, 2023.

American Cancer Society (ACS). (2019b). *How radiation therapy is used to treat cancer*. Retrieved from https://www.cancer.org/treatment/treatments-and-side-effects/treatment-types/radiation/basics.html#written_by. Accessed December 15, 2023.

American Cancer Society (ACS). (2019c). *How is chemotherapy used to treat cancer?* Retrieved from https://www.cancer.org/content/dam/CRC/PDF/Public/8417.00.pdf. Accessed December 15, 2023.

American Lung Association (ALA). (n.d.). *Lung cancer trends brief*. Retrieved from https://www.lung.org/research/trends-in-lung-disease/lung-cancer-trends-brief. Accessed December 15, 2023.

Baik, D., Russell, D., Jordan, L., Dooley, F., Bowles, K. H., & Creber, R. M. M. (2018). Using the palliative performance scale to estimate survival for patients at the end of life: A systematic review of the literature. *Journal of Palliative Medicine, 21*(11), 1651–1661. doi:10.1089/jpm.2018.0141.

Berben, L., Floris, G., Wildiers, H., & Hatse, S. (2021). Cancer and aging: Two tightly interconnected biological processes. *Cancers, 13*(6), 1400. doi:10.3390/cancers13061400.

Borza, T., Harneshaug, M., Kirkhus, L., Benth, J. S., Selbæk, G., Bergh, S., et al. (2022). The course of depressive symptoms and mortality in older patients with cancer. *Aging & Mental Health, 26*(6), 1153–1160. doi:10.1080/13607863.2021.1932739.

CancerCare. (2018). *How to help someone who is grieving*. Retrieved from https://www.cancercare.org/publications/67-how_to_help_someone_who_is_grieving. Accessed December 15, 2023.

Cancer.Net. (2023). *What is hormone therapy*. Retrieved from https://www.cancer.net/navigating-cancer-care/how-cancer-treated/hormone-therapy/what-hormone-therapy. Accessed December 15, 2023.

Cancer.Net. (2020a). *What is personalized cancer medicine?* Retrieved from https://www.cancer.net/navigating-cancer-care/how-cancer-treated/personalized-and-targeted-therapies/what-personalized-cancer-medicine. Accessed December 15, 2023.

Cancer.Net. (2020b). *What is a bone marrow transplant (stem cell transplant)?* Retrieved from https://www.cancer.net/navigating-cancer-care/how-cancer-treated/bone-marrowstem-cell-transplantation/what-bone-marrow-transplant-stem-cell-transplant. Accessed December 15, 2023.

Cancer.Net. (2019). *Cancer care decisions for older adults*. Retrieved from https://www.cancer.net/navigating-cancer-care/adults-65/cancer-care-decisions-older-adults. Accessed December 15, 2023.

Cancer.Net. (n.d.). *How cancer is treated*. Retrieved from https://www.cancer.net/navigating-cancer-care/how-cancer-treated. Accessed December 15, 2023.

Centers for Disease Control and Prevention (CDC). (2023a). *Older persons' health*. Retrieved from https://www.cdc.gov/nchs/fastats/older-american-health.htm. Accessed December 15, 2023.

Centers for Disease Control and Prevention (CDC). (2023b). *Breast cancer in men*. Retrieved from https://www.cdc.gov/breast-cancer/about/men.html. Accessed December 15, 2023.

Cronin, K. A., Scott, S., Firth, A. U., Sung, H., Henley, S. J., Sherman, R. L., et al. (2022). Annual report to the nation on the status of cancer, part 1: National cancer statistics. *Cancer, 128*(24), 4251–4284. doi:10.1002/cncr.34479.

Dibble, S. L., Padilla, G. V., Dodd, M. J., & Miaskowski, C. (1998). Gender differences in the dimensions of quality of life. *Oncology Nursing Forum, 25*(3), 577–583.

Eldridge, L. (2023). *An overview of myelosuppression: Consequences of chemotherapy induced myelosuppression*. VeryWellHealth.com [website]. Retrieved from https://www.verywellhealth.com/what-is-myelosuppression-2249131. Accessed December 15, 2023.

Fleishman, S. B. (2018). *Understanding and managing chemotherapy side effects*. CancerCare Connect Booklet Series. New York: Cancer*Care*.org. Retrieved from https://media.cancercare.org/publications/original/24-ccc_chemo_side_effects.pdf. Accessed December 15, 2023.

Gosney, M. A. (2017). Geriatric oncology. In H. M. Fillit, K. Rockwood, & J. Young (Eds.). *Brocklehurst's textbook of geriatric medicine and gerontology* (8th ed., pp. 772–780). Philadelphia: Elsevier.

Guide to Community Preventive Services. (2020). *Cancer screening: Interventions engaging community health workers – breast cancer*. Retrieved from https://www.thecommunityguide.org/findings/cancer-screening-interventions-engaging-community-health-workers-breast-cancer. Accessed December 15, 2023.

Hasdenteufel, M., & Quintard, B. (2022). Psychosocial factors affecting the bereavement experience of relatives of palliative-stage cancer patients: A systematic review. *BMC Palliative Care, 21*(1), 212. doi:10.1186/s12904-022-01096-y.

Karam, S. (2021). *Being apart doesn't mean fighting cancer alone: Social isolation in patients with cancer*. The Oncology Nursing Society. Retrieved from https://voice.ons.org/news-and-views/being-apart-doesnt-mean-fighting-cancer-alone. Accessed December 15, 2023.

Kotwal, A. A., & Walter, L. C. (2020). Cancer screening among older adults: A geriatrician's perspective on breast, cervical, colon, prostate, and lung cancer screening. *Current Oncology Reports, 22*(11), 108. doi:10.1007/s11912-020-00968-x.

Massa, E., Donisi, C., Liscia, N., Madeddu, C., Impera, V., Mariani, S., et al. (2021). The difficult task of diagnosing depression in elderly people with cancer: A systematic review. *Clinical Practice and Epidemiology in Mental Health, 17*(1), 295–306. doi:10.2174/17450 17902117010295.

Merchan, J. R., & Jhaveri, K. D. (2023). Chemotherapy nephrotoxicity and dose modification in patients with kidney impairment: Molecularly targeted agents and immunotherapies. In R. E. Drews, J. S. Berns, S. Shah, and A. Q. Lam (Eds.), *UpToDate*. Waltham, MA: UpToDate, Inc. Retrieved from https://www.uptodate.com/contents/chemotherapy-nephrotoxicity-and-dose-modification-in-patients-with-kidney-impairment-molecularly-targeted-agents-and-immunotherapies?topicRef=2834&source=see_link. Accessed December 15, 2023.

Montroni, I., Ugolini, G., Saur, N. M., Rostoft, S., Spinelli, A., Van Leeuwen, B. L., et al. (2022). Quality of life in older adults after major cancer surgery: The GOSAFE international study. *Journal of the National Cancer Institute, 114*(7), 969–978. doi:10.1093/jnci/djac071.

National Academies of Sciences, Engineering, and Medicine. (2020). *Social isolation and loneliness in older adults: Opportunities for the health care system*. Washington, DC: The National Academies Press. doi:10.17226/25663.

National Cancer Institute (NCI). (2023a). *Cancer stat facts: Prostate cancer*. Retrieved from https://seer.cancer.gov/statfacts/html/prost.html. Accessed December 15, 2023.

National Cancer Institute (NCI). (2023b). *Cancer stat facts: Colorectal cancer*. Retrieved from https://seer.cancer.gov/statfacts/html/colorect.html. Accessed December 15, 2023.

National Cancer Institute (NCI). (2023c). *Nutrition in cancer care (PDQ®) – Patient version*. National Cancer Institute. Retrieved from https://www.cancer.gov/about-cancer/treatment/side-effects/appetite-loss/nutrition-pdq. Accessed December 15, 2023.

National Cancer Institute (NCI). (2022a). *Targeted therapy to treat cancer*. Retrieved from https://www.cancer.gov/about-cancer/treatment/types/targeted-therapies/targeted-therapies-fact-sheet. Accessed December 15, 2023.

National Cancer Institute (NCI). (2022b). *Grief, bereavement, and coping with loss (PDQ®) – Health professional version*. Retrieved from https://www.cancer.gov/about-cancer/advanced-cancer/caregivers/planning/bereavement-hp-pdq. Accessed December 15, 2023.

National Cancer Institute (NCI). (2021). *Age and cancer risk*. Retrieved from https://www.cancer.gov/about-cancer/causes-prevention/risk/age. Accessed December 15, 2023.

National Cancer Institute (NCI). (2020). *Many older adults screened unnecessarily for common cancers*. Retrieved from https://www.cancer.gov/news-events/cancer-currents-blog/2020/screening-cancer-older-adults-unnecessary. Accessed December 15, 2023.

National Cancer Institute (NCI). (2019a). *Radiation therapy to treat cancer*. Retrieved from https://www.cancer.gov/about-cancer/treatment/types/radiation-therapy. Accessed December 15, 2023.

National Cancer Institute (NCI). (2019b). *Immunotherapy to treat cancer*. Retrieved from https://www.cancer.gov/about-cancer/treatment/types/immunotherapy. Accessed December 15, 2023.

National Cancer Institute (NCI). (n.d.). *Cancer genomics overview*. Retrieved from https://www.cancer.gov/about-nci/organization/ccg/cancer-genomics-overview. Accessed December 15, 2023.

Oates, J. R., & Maani-Fogelman, P. A. (2022). *Nursing grief and loss*. StatPearls [Internet]. Retrieved from https://www.ncbi.nlm.nih.gov/books/NBK518989/. Accessed December 15, 2023.

Ornstein, K. A., Liu, B., Schwartz, R. M., Smith, C. B., Alpert, N., & Taioli, E. (2020). Cancer in the context of aging: Health characteristics, function and caregiving needs prior to a new cancer diagnosis in a national sample of older adults. *Journal of Geriatric Oncology, 11*(1), 75–81. doi:10.1016/j.jgo.2019.03.019.

Padilla, G. V., Ferrell, B., Grant, M. M., & Rhiner, M. (1990). Defining the content domain of quality of life for cancer patients with pain. *Cancer Nursing, 13*(2), 108–115.

Patt, D., Gordan, L., Patel, K., Okon, T., Ferreyros, N., Markward, N., et al. (2022). Considerations to increase rates of breast cancer screening across populations. *The American Journal of Managed Care, 28*(3 Spec. No.), SP136–SP138. doi:10.37765/ajmc.2022.88855.

Pietrangelo, A. (2021). *What is adjuvant chemotherapy, and when is it needed?* Healthline [website]. Retrieved from https://www.healthline.com/health/cancer/adjuvant-chemotherapy. Accessed December 15, 2023.

Puts, M., Strohschein, F., Oldenmenger, W., Haase, K., Newton, L., Fitch, M., et al. (2021). Position statement on oncology and cancer nursing care for older adults with cancer and their caregivers of the International Society of Geriatric Oncology Nursing and Allied Health Interest group, the Canadian Association of Nurses in Oncology and Aging special Interest Group, and the European Oncology Nursing Society. *Journal of Geriatric Oncology, 12*(7), 1000–1004. doi:10.1016/j.jgo.2021.03.010.

Ribatti, D. (2017). The concept of immune surveillance against tumors. The first theories. *Oncotarget, 8*(4), 7175–7180. doi:10.18632/oncotarget.12739.

Rippe, J. M. (2018). Lifestyle medicine: The health promoting power of daily habits and practices. *American Journal of Lifestyle Medicine, 12*(6), 499–512. doi:10.1177/1559827618785554.

Rosenblatt, E., Zubizarreta, E., Camacho, R., & Vikram, B. (2017). Radiotherapy in cancer care. In E. Rosenblatt & E. Zubizarreta (Eds.), *Radiotherapy in cancer care: Facing the global challenge* (pp. 13–28). Vienna, Austria: International Atomic Energy Agency. Retrieved from https://www-pub.iaea.org/MTCD/Publications/PDF/P1638_web.pdf. Accessed December 15, 2023.

Rostoft, S., O'Donovan, A., Soubeyran, P., Alibhai, S. M. H., & Hamaker, M. E. (2021). Geriatric assessment and management in cancer. *Journal of Clinical Oncology, 39*(19), 2058–2067. doi:10.1200/JCO.21.00089.

Saria, M. G. (2018). Overview of cancer. In J. L. Watson (Ed.), *Your guide to cancer prevention* (pp. 1–12). Pittsburgh, PA: Oncology Nursing Society.

Steele, L. L., Mills, B., Hardin, S. R., & Hussey, L. C. (2005). The quality of life of hospice patients: Patient and provider perceptions. *The American Journal of Hospice & Palliative Care, 22*(2), 95–110. doi:10.1177/104990910502200205.

Susan G. Komen. (2023). *How do breast cancer screening rates compare among different groups in the U.S.?* Susan G. Komen [website]. Retrieved from https://www.komen.org/breast-cancer/screening/screening-disparities/. Accessed December 15, 2023.

Tilden, V. P., & Weinert, C. (1987). Social support and the chronically ill individual. *The Nursing Clinics of North America, 22*(3), 613–620.

Tindle, H. A., Duncan, M. S., Greevy, R. A., Vasan, R. S., Kundu, S., Massion, P. P., et al. (2018). Lifetime smoking history and risk of lung cancer: Results from the Framingham Heart Study. *Journal of the National Cancer Institute, 110*(11), 1201–1207. doi:10.1093/jnci/djy041.

Tofthagen, C. S., Kip, K., Witt, A., & McMillan, S. C. (2017). Complicated grief: Risk factors, interventions, and resources for oncology nurses. *Clinical Journal of Oncology Nursing, 21*(3), 331–337. doi:10.1188/17.CJON.331-337.

Van Herck, Y., Feyaerts, A., Alibhai, S., Papamichael, D., Decoster, L, Lambrechts, Y., et al. (2021). Is cancer biology different in older patients? *The Lancet Healthy Longevity, 2*(10), e663–e677. doi:10.1016/S2666-7568(21)00179-3.

van Leeuwen, K. M., van Loon, M. S., van Nes, F. A., Bosmans, J. E., de Vet, H. C. W., Ket, J. C. F., et al. (2019). What does quality of life mean to older adults? A thematic synthesis. *PLoS One, 14*(3), e0213263. doi:10.1371/journal.pone.0213263.

Vassilev, A., & DePamphilis, M. L. (2017). Links between DNA replication, stem cells, and cancer. *Genes, 8*(2), 45. doi:10.3390/genes8020045.

Weaver, C. H. (2021). *Anorexia and weight loss.* CancerConnect [website]. Retrieved from https://news.cancerconnect.com/treatment-care/anorexia-and-weight-loss. Accessed December 15, 2023.

Weir, H. K., Thompson, T. D., Stewart, S. L., & White, M. C. (2021). Cancer incidence projections in the United States between 2015 and 2050. *Preventing Chronic Disease, 18*, E59. doi:10.5888/pcd18.210006.

Welsh, J. (2023). *Immunotherapy for cancer: What are my options?* Verywellhealth.com [website]. Retrieved from https://www.verywellhealth.com/immunotherapy-for-cancer-7963397. Accessed December 15, 2023.

Weston, A., & Harris, C. C. (2003). Multistage carcinogenesis. In D. W. Kufe, R. E. Pollock, R. R. Weichselbaum, R. C. Bast, Jr., T. S. Gansler, J. F. Holland, et al. (Eds.), *Holland-Frei cancer medicine* (6th ed.). Hamilton, Ontario: BC Decker. Retrieved from https://www.ncbi.nlm.nih.gov/books/NBK13982/. Accessed December 15, 2023.

White, M. C., Holman, D. M., Goodman, R. A., & Richardson, L. C. (2019). Cancer risk among older adults: Time for cancer prevention to go silver. *The Gerontologist, 59*(Suppl. 1), S1–S6. doi:10.1093/geront/gnz038.

Williams, G. R., Mackenzie, A., Magnuson, A., Olin, R., Chapman, A., Mohile, S., et al. (2016). Comorbidity in older adults with cancer. *Journal of Geriatric Oncology, 7*(4), 249–257. doi:10.1016/j.jgo.2015.12.002.

World Health Organization (WHO). (2021). *Social isolation and loneliness among older people: Advocacy brief.* Retrieved from https://www.who.int/publications/i/item/9789240030749. Accessed December 15, 2023.

27

Loss and End-of-Life Issues

Jerilyn Bumpas, DNP, MSN, RN and Jennifer J Yeager, PhD, MSN, RN

http://evolve.elsevier.com/Yeager/gerontologic/

LEARNING OBJECTIVES

On completion of this chapter, the reader will be able to:
1. Distinguish between loss, bereavement, grief, and mourning.
2. Discuss factors that may affect the length of bereavement.
3. Identify physical, psychologic, social, and spiritual aspects of normal grief responses.
4. Discuss the tasks of mourning.
5. Describe nursing care activities for assisting bereaved older adults.
6. Explain age-related changes that affect older adults who are dying.
7. Describe nursing strategies for assisting dying older adults and their families.
8. Discuss the philosophy of palliative care.

WHAT WOULD YOU DO?

What would you do if you were faced with the following situations?
- An 85-year-old WWII veteran with prostate cancer with metastasis to the bones has been receiving chemotherapy and radiation for 2 years, but the disease has progressed. He was admitted to the acute care setting for management of postchemotherapy side effects. His oncologist is the admitting physician and has initiated his admitting orders. You are in report when you hear the code call for this patient. He is a full code and was well into being coded when his niece walked in and stated that he was a do not resuscitate (DNR), and the doctor didn't write the order! What do you do?
- A 90-year-old female is in the late stages of the dying process. Her partner of 40 years is at her bedside in the nursing home and has been her primary caregiver since she became ill. The patient's family has come and demands that their wishes be followed, not her partner's. The family will not talk to the partner. What do you do?

Loss is a natural part of life and aging. The longer people live, the more losses they experience. Losses commonly associated with aging include moving from employment into retirement, from a lifelong home to a smaller home or senior apartment, from being very active to being less so, from health to chronic illness, from marriage to widowhood, and from extensive social networks to smaller circles of family and friends. These transitions are considered losses in American society and are often viewed negatively. Successful aging requires learning to deal with these losses and adapting to the changes over time. Life transitions a, such as the death of a loved one, can act as catalysts for learning new skills and experiencing personal growth.

DEFINITIONS

The terms *loss, bereavement, grief,* and *mourning* are often used interchangeably, but these words convey different meanings (PDQ® Supportive and Palliative Care Editorial Board, 2021; Cancer.net Editorial Board, 2022; Doka, 2013):
- *Loss* is a broad term that connotes losing or being deprived of something, such as one's health, home, or relationship.
- *Bereavement* is the objective situation of having experienced a loss.
- *Grief* is the emotional/affective response to loss.
- *Mourning* is learning how to live with one's loss and grief. It is influenced by the individual's culture, religion, and environment. It is the public expression of grief.

Losses

Losses may involve a person, thing, relationship, or situation (Corless, 2010). Gradual and abrupt life-changing events such as retirement, change of residence, health problems, loss of pets, and the inability to drive are losses that evoke varying responses of grief. With age, people experience more losses. Over time, these losses take a personal toll and can lead to depression (Familydoctor.org editorial staff, 2022).

Bereavement

Bereavement is the objective reality of loss (PDQ® Supportive and Palliative Care Editorial Board, 2021). The death of one's spouse or life partner is usually the most significant loss that an older adult may experience. It involves the loss of a companion who often is one's best friend, sexual partner, and partner in decision-making

---

Previous authors: Linda Bub MSN, RN, GCNS-BC, Cindy R. Morgan, RN, MSN, CHC, CHPN, and Ramesh C. Upadhyaya, RN, CRRN, MSN, MBA, PhD-C.

and household management, as well as a contributing source to one's definition of self and identity (Balk, 2013).

Purrington (2021) conducted a systematic review of spousal bereavement in older adults and uncovered five characteristics that either facilitated or inhibited psychologic adjustment to loss: preloss spousal relationship, social support, finding meaning and spirituality in loss, the surviving spouse's personality traits and death characteristics.

Purrington determined that the findings supported the concepts of "making meaning" from the loss and that social support should be incorporated into therapeutic work with bereaved spouses to help facilitate psychologic adjustments.

Grief

Grief is a powerful and sometimes overwhelming natural emotion that people experience at a time of great loss. Grief emotions can manifest differently depending on the person (Cancer.net Editorial Board, 2022). It may affect a person physically, socially, behaviorally, or cognitively by changing behaviors and the older adult's ability to function. It may stem from the death of a loved one, a drastic change in a person's life circumstances, a severe or terminal medical diagnosis, or any other sudden or great loss. Grief is an important risk factor for depression in older adults. With increasing age and the burden of grief, depression severity increases (Schladitz et al, 2021).

PATIENT/FAMILY TEACHING
Grief Responses

Grief is natural. A person's response to grief is individual, fluctuates in intensity over time, and may vary between different losses. In cases of death, grief depends on our relationship with the person, how and why the person died, and how the loss affects our ability to perform activities of daily living.

There is no "normal grief." However, certain emotions and behaviors have been identified as common manifestations of grief:

Emotional	Behavioral	Physical
Shock, denial, numbness	Crying unexpectedly	Exhaustion/fatigue
Sadness, anxiety guilt, fear	Sleep changes (increase or decrease)	Decreased energy
Anger (at others or God)	Not eating/weight changes	Memory problems
Irritability, frustration	Withdrawing from others	Stomach and intestinal upset
	Restlessness, difficulty concentrating, trouble making decisions	Pain and headaches

Abnormal symptoms should be discussed with a health-care professional. These include the use of drugs, alcohol, violence, and suicidal thoughts.

There is no set duration for grief, although research has shown that 18 to 24 months is typical. Special days and anniversaries (i.e., anniversary of death, birthdays, and holidays) may result in a surge of emotion.

Table from Center for Integrated Healthcare. (2020). Bereavement, grief & mourning. Mental Illness Research Education and Clinical Center, U.S. Department of Veterans Affairs [website]. Retrieved from https://www.mirecc.va.gov/cih-visn2/Documents/Patient_Education_Handouts/Bereavement_Grief_and_Mourning_Version_4.pdf; data from Perng, A., & Renz, S. (2018). Identifying and treating complicated grief in older adults. *The Journal for Nurse Practitioners, 14*(4), 289-295.

There are no set categories for grief responses; they vary from author to author. For the purposes of further discussion, responses to grief are addressed following the holistic biopsychosocial and spiritual model. The interconnectedness between emotional instability and physical manifestation illustrates how a state of emotional health can profoundly affect our physical and spiritual health (Social Work Portal. n.d.) (Fig. 27.1).

Physical Symptoms

Physical symptoms are commonly associated with acute grief responses. Tearfulness, crying, loss of appetite, feelings of hollowness in the stomach, decreased energy, fatigue, lethargy, and sleep difficulties are common symptoms of grief. Other physical sensations may include tension, weight loss or gain, sighing, feeling of something being stuck in the throat, tightness in the chest or throat, heart palpitations, restlessness, shortness of breath, and dry mouth (Corr and Corr, 2013; Florida Crisis Consortium, n.d.; ReachOut Australia, n.d.).

Psychologic Responses

Studies of grief responses have consistently identified common psychologic responses. Feelings of sadness are the emotions most often mentioned (Florida Crisis Consortium, n.d.; ReachOut Australia, n.d.). Other common feelings include guilt, anxiety, anger, depression, apathy, helplessness, and loneliness. Guilt and regret regarding one's relationship with the person who has died may be especially troublesome (Florida Crisis Consortium, n.d.; ReachOut Australia, n.d.). Shock and disbelief may immediately follow the death. The bereaved person may also display diminished self-concern, a preoccupation with the deceased, and a yearning for their presence. Some older adults become confused and unable to concentrate after the death of someone significant to them. Waves of acute grief may come when least expected (Hairston and Pathak, 2019). How the grief response manifests itself is individually determined by sociocultural fandtion to the quality of the relationship between the deceased and the mourner. For some older adults, the grief experience may include feelings of relief and emancipation, especially after prolonged suffering or a difficult relationship.

Social Responses

The social changes that follow the loss of a loved one depend on the type of relationship and the definition of social roles within the relationship. Widowhood is the loss that generally has the greatest effect on social role change, but any loss of a person within one's household is especially difficult. In addition to deep psychologic pain, the bereaved person must often learn new skills and roles to manage tasks of daily living. All these social changes occur at a time when withdrawal, a lack of interest in activities, and a lack of energy make decision-making and action very difficult. Socialization and interaction patterns also change. If an older couple often socializes with other couples, widowhood may dramatically change the type and style of interaction. For others with strong social support and established patterns of independent interaction outside the lost relationship, the adjustment process toward creating new social roles and interactions may occur more quickly.

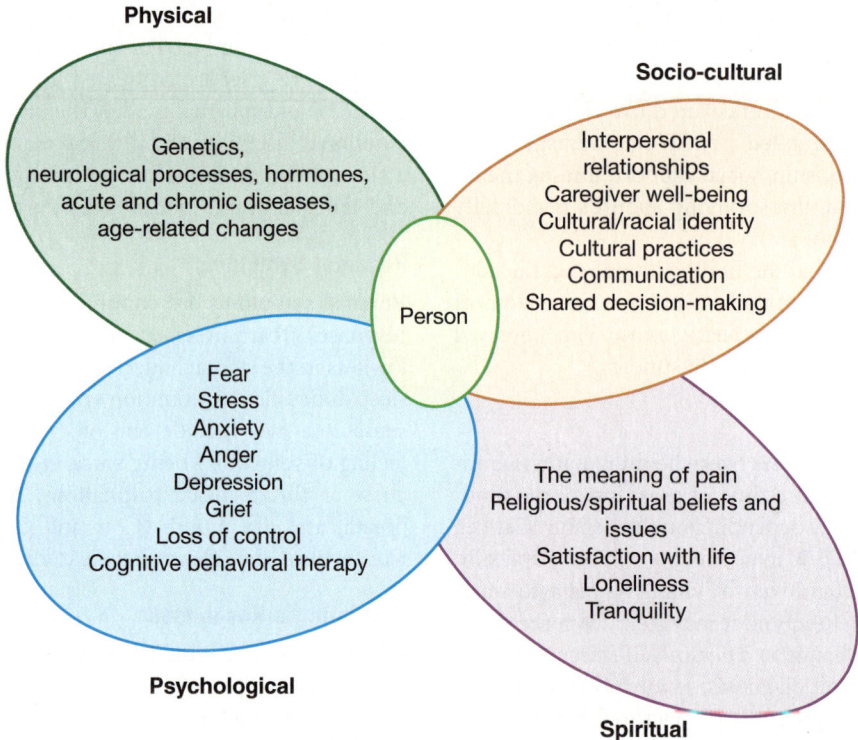

Fig. 27.1 Holistic biopsychosocial spiritual model. The interplay between model components and their intersection at the person (patient) receiving care.

Over the last 10 years, lesbian, gay, bisexual, transgender, queer, and others (LGBTQ+) individuals have been able to have more open relationships and are now encouraged to be part of the dying process with their partners. This has implications for the nurse and understanding personal biases and understanding disenfranchised populations and how they grieve; continued discrimination in health-care creates added burdens during the grieving process. It is vital that nurses understand that LGBTQ+ partners grieve differently because of previous experiences with discrimination. They often have little interaction with family due to homophobia; therefore, they rely on their community or friends for support (Patlamazoglou et al, 2018). It is also suggested that social support and community are vital components of coping among the LGBTQ+ during bereavement, particularly for older adults.

There are specific considerations to be aware of when caring for LGBTQ+ individuals at the end-of-life or when supporting them during bereavement. It may not be evident or known that a person is LGBTQ+, so it is important that care is given, and communication conducted in an inclusive, affirmative, and respectful way. Nurses must avoid making assumptions (Nolan et al, 2021).

Spiritual Aspects

Death causes people to ponder the existential issues of life and to examine the meaning of not only the lost loved one's life but also their own. Spiritual issues may surface as the person searches for meaning. Anger at God, sometimes followed by a crisis of faith and meaning, may accompany bereavement. It may be important for the bereaved to view the death of their loved one as a transition to a life with God in the spirit. Meaning in life is highly individualized, but the importance of finding meaning in life is more universal. What a person finds meaningful is not as important as the ability to look back on life, see that it has been meaningful, and understand that life can continue to be meaningful even in its last stages (Mendoza, 2020).

Religion and spirituality can provide a stabilizing influence during grief. One's religious institution may provide a sense of belonging in times of need. Some may experience a deep inner sense of peace that they are being cared for by a higher power. For others, however, the grief experience may precipitate a crisis in their beliefs and values. Comments that are intended to be comforting, offered by friends and family (i.e., "God will never give you more than you can handle" and "Everything happens for a reason") often contribute to spiritual distress (Mendoza, 2020). Gender, social class, ethnicity, and culture may influence one's spiritual response to grief (Gire, 2014).

Nurses should remember that grief is integrated into the whole person. Interventions directed at one category will affect the other areas; thus, an approach that separates the mind, body, and spirit is not advocated. Instead, an interconnected biopsychosocial spiritual approach is recommended.

See Box 27.1 for information on grief and loss during the recent COVID-19 pandemic.

Types of Grief

Various blogs and magazines propose multiple types of grief, ranging from five types (anticipatory, acute, normal, complicated, and disenfranchised) (Ernstmeyer & Christman, 2021)

> **BOX 27.1 Grief and Loss During the COVID-19 Pandemic**
>
> The world is united in grief as, by August 1, 2022, more than 6.4 million deaths (Kaiser Family Foundation, 2023) occurred secondary to COVID-19. The pandemic has changed not only how we live, but also how we die. The dying process has become complicated not only for patients with the disease, but also for individuals dying from other causes, and those who are left behind and grieving (Bauld et al, 2021).
>
> The high rates of death during the COVID-19 pandemic have thrown the question of a "good or bad death" into sharp focus as countries across the globe have struggled with multiple peaks of morbidity and mortality. COVID-19 fatalities exemplify "bad deaths" and are distinguished by physical discomfort, difficulty breathing, social isolation, psychologic distress, and care that may differ with the patient's preferences. Surviving loved ones experience symptoms of depression, anxiety, and anger. The grief experienced by surviving loved ones is worsened by the decreased access to supports for coping and simultaneous stressors including social isolation, financial uncertainty about the future, lack of routine, and the loss of face-to-face mourning rituals that provide a sense of community (Carr et al, 2020).
>
> Şahn and Büken (2020) examined what older adults believe are important aspects of a "good death." Older adults placed importance on psychosocial and spiritual aspects, personal control, and the clinical aspects of death. The authors concluded that decisions regarding the end of life, dignity, and the desire for a "good death" are equally essential rights for all people of all age groups.
>
> The World Health Organization (WHO) has called for palliative care to be "accessible to all" and an "essential component of primary health-care worldwide" providing quality end-of-life care including a full range of considerations involved in a holistic assessment of a patient's palliative care needs (Damarell et al, 2020).
>
> Palliative care improves the quality of life of patients and that of their families who are facing challenges associated with life-threatening illness, whether physical, psychologic, social, or spiritual. The quality of life of caregivers improves as well. Each year, an estimated 40 million people are in need of palliative care; 78% of the people live in low- and middle-income countries. Worldwide, only about 14% of people who need palliative care currently receive it (WHO, 2020).
>
> Grief is a normal response during and following disaster or another traumatic event. The COVID-19 pandemic made grief especially overwhelming as most individuals were not allowed to be with their loved ones as they died. Issues such as social distancing, orders to stay at home, limits to the size of gatherings changed family gatherings and funeral services. During the pandemic, family and friends of those who died of COVID-19 often felt social avoidance and isolation, as those who would normally have reached out to them, did not (Centers for Disease Control and Prevention [CDC], 2021).
>
> The CDC offers multiple resources for those experiencing grief and loss during the pandemic: https://www.cdc.gov/mentalhealth/index.htm. Nurses and health-care workers have a crucial role in the care of people with advanced diseases and should provide evidence-based palliative and end-of-life care (Quinn, 2022).

to upward of 16 types (normal, anticipatory, complicated, chronic, delayed, distorted, cumulative, exaggerated, secondary loss, masked grief, disenfranchised, traumatic, collective, inhibited abbreviated, and absent [Kelly, 2021]). However, for the purpose of discussion, bereavement research has clustered evidence into anticipatory grief, normal or common grief, complicated grief, and prolonged/persistent/complex grief (PDQ Supportive and Palliative Care Editorial Board, 2022).

Anticipatory grief. Anticipatory grief occurs "in anticipation of an impending loss" (PDQ Supportive and Palliative Care Editorial Board, 2022, p. 4). Both the family and the person who is dying can experience anticipatory grief. Symptoms of anticipatory grief include depression, heightened concern for the person who is dying, "rehearsal" of the death, attempts to adjust to the implications of their loved one's death, anxiety and worry, and irritability (Fanjul, 2022).

Normal or common grief. A person experiencing normal grief gradually works towards acceptance and continues with their daily routine despite difficulties. Symptoms of normal grief include numbness, shock, disbelief, and denial occurring in the immediate period following death. These symptoms are expressed by crying, sighing, having dreams of the person who has died, and going places that remind the person of their loved one (PDQ Supportive and Palliative Care Editorial Board, 2022).

Normal grief includes waves of grief. These occur with reminders of the person who has died, such as cultural or social holidays, the anniversary of the death, and when personal items of the deceased are given away. Symptoms often decrease after 6 months and resolve in 1 to 2 years (PDQ Supportive and Palliative Care Editorial Board, 2022).

Chronic or complicated grief. In complicated grief, the person experiences the same symptoms as someone experiencing normal grief, but the symptoms extend beyond 1 or 2 years. The symptoms are more persistent than in normal grief (PDQ Supportive and Palliative Care Editorial Board, 2022).

Prolonged/persistent/complex grief. The *Diagnostic and Statistical Manual of Mental Disorders,* 5th edition (DSM-5), identifies persistent complex bereavement disorder and prolonged grief disorder as diagnostic codes. The full diagnostic criteria are lengthy and include (but are not limited to) intense sorrow and emotional pain, difficulty accepting the death, a desire to die and be with the deceased, and difficulty planning for the future. The person experiencing prolonged/persistent/complex grief is unable to maintain social and occupational functioning (PDQ Supportive and Palliative Care Editorial Board, 2022).

As professionals and as a society, it is important to support healthy grieving, as well as help others understand that each person deals with grief differently and at their own pace (Sutton, 2022). Factors influencing how a person grieves include the griever's support system, sociocultural and religious background, education, economic status, and cultural practices. An individual's physical state also influences the grief response. Important physical factors are using drugs and sedatives, nutritional state, adequacy of rest and sleep, exercise, and general physical health. Nurses need to be aware of how all these factors affect the family of the person who is dying, as well as the dying person.

Mourning

Mourning was defined earlier as the "public expression of grief." It may include ritualistic activities such as wearing dark clothes during bereavement, lighting candles for the dead, and processes related to learning how to live with one's loss and grief.

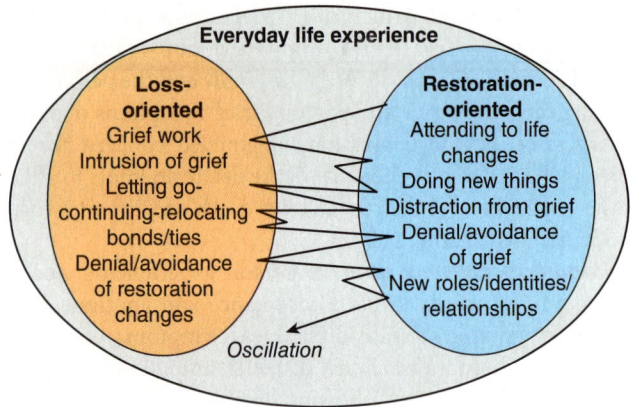

Fig. 27.2 Dual-process model. (Redrawn from Stroebe, M. S., & Schut, H. [1999]. The Dual Process Model of coping with bereavement: Rationale and description. *Death Studies, 23*[3], 197-224.)

Mourning is often prescribed by social and cultural norms that indicate acceptable coping behaviors in a person's society (Corless, 2010). The emphasis in this section will be on the process of learning to live with the loss of a loved one. The complexity of the mourning process does not lend itself to a single theory.

The dual process model of coping with bereavement (Fig. 27.2) provides a flexible approach to interpreting and managing grief. The model describes how a bereaved person copes with the experience of loss in everyday life, along with other lifestyle changes that develop because of that loss. The dual process model is based on the principle that when people are grieving, they waver (oscillate) between loss-oriented and restoration-oriented behaviors. Loss-oriented behavior occurs when the person encounters something that makes them think of their loved one, and they begin to focus on their grief and pain. Restoration-oriented behavior occurs with distraction, where the person focuses on their daily life and routines. Regardless of whether persons are in loss-oriented or restoration-oriented states, they oscillate between positive and negative thought processes until, over time, they become more focused on making meaning (Funeral Guide, 2021; Stroebe and Schut, 2010).

The tasks of mourning defined by Worden (2009) are useful descriptions of mourning among older adults. He described the following four tasks of mourning:
1. Accept the reality of the loss
2. Experience the pain of grief
3. Adjust to an environment without the deceased
4. Withdraw emotional energy and reinvest it in other relationships

The first task, accepting the reality of the loss, involves coming to the realization that the person is dead, that they will not return, and that reunion, at least in life as we know it, is impossible. The second task, experiencing the pain of grief, is necessary to prevent the grief from becoming distorted. Sociocultural customs that discourage open expression of grief often contribute to unresolved grief. The third task, adjusting to an environment where the deceased is missing, involves developing new skills and assuming the roles for which the deceased was responsible. The last task, withdrawal of emotional energy and reinvestment in another relationship, entails withdrawing emotional attachment to the deceased and loving another person in a similar way. For many, this last task is the most difficult.

It is critical that older adults who have experienced loss acknowledge the pain associated with grief and loss and adjust to an environment where their loved one is absent. Individual expression of pain depends partly on culture and the quality of the relationship with the lost loved one. Guilt may accompany the pain of grief.

Adjusting to one's environment after the loss of a loved one involves learning new roles, such as those previously assumed by the deceased, and new ways of interacting with others in one's social environment. This adjustment may be especially difficult if the loved one lost is the spouse and the social network consists primarily of other couples.

The final task, emotionally reinvesting in other relationships and moving on with life, gives the bereaved person permission to invest emotionally in others without being disloyal to the deceased. Although Worden (2009) pointed out that, in one sense, mourning is never over, he also stated that, in losses that involve a great deal of emotional attachment, the process takes at least a year before the wrenching pain subsides. Some older spouses have reported that they feel as though they will never "get over" their loss but that they have learned to live with it (Lund, 1989).

In contrast to detaching or "letting go" of the deceased, Klass et al (2006) viewed the bond between survivors and the deceased as dynamic rather than static. Their research suggested that a bereaved person finds a way to redefine their relationship with the deceased, thereby continuing the bond. The bond continues by talking to the deceased when visiting their grave, keeping keepsakes, maintaining favorite rituals that were shared, and carrying on the person's legacy through charity work (Frazer Consultants. 2018).

Meaning Making Out of Loss

Burbank (1992) found that the major source of meaning in life among older persons came from relationships with family members. When loved ones die, the meaning derived from these relationships changes. Personal beliefs and attitudes, including cultural and religious ones, influence the meaning of the loss, and have a significant effect on responses to that loss. For this reason, it is important that health-care providers explore the perceptions of the bereaved to understand and assist them as they mourn their loss.

Neimeyer (2000) proposed that reconstructing the meaning in a person's life after the death of a loved one is an important process of mourning. The bereaved are encouraged to find or create new meaning in their lives and in the death of the deceased. This is a cognitive process affected by one's social context as well as one's individual resources.

The multiple definitions of meaning, however, require further clarification. Holland et al (2006) found that the terms *sense-making* and *benefit-finding* were central to finding meaning. Their research indicated that better outcomes came from making sense of the death and the resulting life of the survivor, such as reordering life priorities and becoming more empathetic.

Building on the work by Holland et al (2006), researchers further operationalized "meaning" and "grief" to include *identity change* and *purpose in life* because they found that an important facet of meaning is the significance that some aspect of one's life experience "matters" (Hibberd, 2013).

The work of making sense of loss has changed little from the previous works of Burbank (1992), Neimeyer (2000), and Holland et al. (2006). Brandt (2021) reiterates that navigating and making meaning from loss can help people learn to value life. The goal of nursing care for older adults who are grieving and mourning is not to "make them feel better" quickly, although nurses are often tempted to do so. Nurses should assist and support bereaved persons through the grieving process, recognizing that pain is a normal and healthy response to loss and allowing bereaved persons to accomplish the tasks of mourning in their own way.

APPROACHING DEATH

Comfort Theory

Comfort theory is a midrange nursing theory developed by Katharine Kolcaba during the 1990s. In this theory, *comfort* is defined as "the immediate experience of being strengthened through having the needs for relief, ease, and transcendence met in four contexts of experience (physical, psychospiritual, social, and environmental)" (as quoted in Kolcaba and DiMarco, 2005, p. 188). Comfort is composed of three components:

1. *Relief* occurs when specific comfort needs are met
2. *Ease* is the absence of discomfort
3. *Transcendence* occurs when a patient can rise above their discomfort when it cannot be completely relieved

The theory recognizes the importance of patient involvement in identifying their needs. Comfort is the holistic outcome of nursing interventions (Fig. 27.3) (Kolcaba and DiMarco, 2005). Comfort theory has direct application for gerontological nurses who practice in medical/surgical environments and those in hospice and palliative care.

General Health-Care Needs

Regardless of needs that arise from specific diseases and functional problems, dying individuals have general health-care needs that must be addressed. General nursing interventions to meet these needs include

1. Stabilizing and supporting vital functions and facilitating integrated functioning
2. Determining functional deviation and adjusting treatment
3. Relieving distressing symptoms and suffering
4. Assisting patient and family interaction
5. Supporting a patient and their family in coping with the realities of death

Common physical problems and symptoms encountered by terminally ill patients include pain, dyspnea, constipation, delirium, altered urinary elimination patterns, altered skin integrity, loss of appetite, dry mouth, nausea and vomiting, restlessness and sleeplessness, difficulty swallowing, and nutritional problems (Derby et al, 2010). Family coping and stress, safety needs, and self-care deficits are other important problems (Weitzner et al, 1997). Age-related changes and comorbid conditions combined with these general health-care needs of dying older adults and their families make the provision of high-quality nursing care especially challenging. Skillful assessments and creative nursing strategies addressing multiple physical, psychosocial, and spiritual needs are necessary.

Effects of Age-Related Changes

Nursing care aimed at meeting the physical needs of older persons who are dying is no different from the meticulous care needed by any other patient with a debilitating condition. Age-related changes and the effects of long-term chronic illnesses predispose older persons to a greater risk for problems in hygiene and skin care, nutrition, elimination, mobility and transfers, rest and sleep, pain management, respiration, and cognitive and behavioral functioning. Only the areas that pose special problems for older persons are discussed in this section.

Age-related changes in the integumentary and vascular systems, coupled with alterations in nutrition, elimination, and

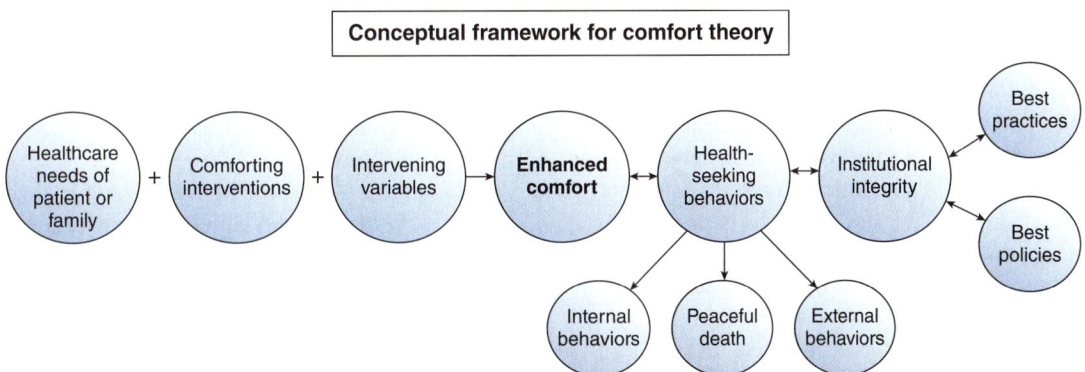

Fig. 27.3 Conceptual framework for Kolcaba's comfort theory. (Copyright © K. Kolcaba, 2007. TheComfortLine.com.)

mobility, quickly lead to skin breakdown. Loss of the subcutaneous fat layer and a decrease in sebaceous gland activity cause the skin to become thin and dry, which makes it more susceptible to the hazards of immobility. Pressure injuries are a problem for older, debilitated patients and are often quick to form and slow to heal. Sometimes, even the best skin care and positioning cannot prevent the formation of pressure injuries at the end of life (Carlsson and Gunningberg, 2017; Hughes et al, 2005).

Chest wall rigidity, decreased ciliary activity, and decreased coughing and gagging reflexes all predispose older persons to respiratory problems, especially pneumonia. Aspiration pneumonia is a common problem in older patients who cannot feed themselves and have difficulty maintaining an upright position. The decreased effectiveness of the immune system and the often nonspecific presentation of pneumonia symptoms may complicate the diagnosis and treatment of pneumonia in older adults. Shortness of breath and altered respiratory patterns in sleep, such as Cheyne-Stokes respirations or sleep apnea, are more prevalent among older persons and may become problematic if these patients are seriously ill or dying.

Digestive changes associated with age include decreased amounts of saliva, digestive fluids, and enzymes, decreased peristaltic activity, and decreased absorption through the intestinal wall. These changes predispose an older person who is dying to additional problems with maintaining adequate nutritional status and bowel function. They are exacerbated by immobility and often contribute to constipation, fecal impaction, and sometimes diarrhea. Although health-care professionals often downplay the seriousness of constipation, this problem may cause much discomfort to the dying person and contribute to other life-threatening complications.

Changes in vision and hearing commonly accompanying advancing age reduce the stimulation older persons receive from the environment. This is complicated by the usual practice of removing eyeglasses and hearing aids from patients who are ill and well-meaning attempts to provide a quiet, darkened, and peaceful environment. Sensory deprivation may lead to mental confusion among healthy individuals and is of even greater importance among older adults who are dying.

Environmental changes and unfamiliar people and settings also confuse older adults. Because hospitalization or a move to a nursing facility is often a part of the dying experience for older persons, the acute confusion that may result from such a move may be permanent.

Older adults seem to be more susceptible to the development of persistent pain, and medications acting on peripheral sensitization are less effective. Pathologic changes in the central nervous system are responsible for different pain processing and response to treatment (Tinnirello et al, 2021).

"Pain and discomfort at the end of life are frequently underrecognized and undertreated" (Sinha et al, 2023, para 1). All reports of pain and discomfort need to be addressed by the nurse. Management of pain includes pharmacologic and nonpharmacologic interventions. Pharmacologic interventions include nonsteroidal antiinflammatory drugs, acetaminophen, opioid analgesics, and adjuvant drugs. Nonpharmacologic interventions include avoiding pain triggers, positioning and supports, artificial tears, pressure-relieving devices, and oral care (Sinha et al, 2023).

Age-related changes in pharmacokinetics and pharmacodynamics lead to atypical drug responses. Because drugs are so widely used as an essential part of medical treatment, their effectiveness, side effects, and reactions need to be closely monitored. Physiologic changes associated with dying, for example, circulatory changes, increase the difficulty in managing drug regimens. Sleep patterns are also disturbed by physiologic changes, pain, and changes in the environment. Although sedative-hypnotics may be appropriate in some instances, they need to be prescribed with caution and monitored carefully, as they may cause new problems such as incontinence or delirium. Nonpharmacologic therapies should be used first before the use of medications. Psychologic causes of sleeplessness should also be explored. For example, if an older adult fears dying alone in their sleep or if they have unfinished business to resolve with their families, sedative-hypnotics are not the best answer. Instead, a careful assessment of the cause of sleeplessness must be followed by appropriate treatment aimed at the cause (Bettinger et al, 2017).

Nursing Care Guidelines for the Older Adult Who Is Dying

Excellent nursing care of the older adult who is dying begins with assessment. Delivering high-quality nursing care to older adults who are dying may be one of the most challenging and rewarding of all nursing experiences. It requires knowledge of the complexities of gerontological and end-of-life nursing combined with the knowledge, skill, and compassion necessary to deliver holistic care to both dying patients and their families (National Consensus Project for Quality Palliative Care, 2018).

Recognize Cues (Assessment)

As with other nursing care, nurses must make careful and ongoing holistic assessments of patient needs. Special attention must be given to potential problem areas such as skin integrity, respiratory status, nutrition, elimination, sensory abilities, cognitive functioning, comfort, and rest.

Measuring the effectiveness of palliative care interventions requires assessment tools that are reliable and valid. These tools should evaluate the impact of interventions (AHRQ, 2021).

Various frameworks may be used to assess a patient receiving palliative care. Nurses working in palliative care settings should be familiar with the assessment frameworks used by their organization.

One common assessment framework is identified by the mnemonic 'PEPSI COLA' (NursingAnswers.net, 2018) (Table 27.1). The PEPSI-COLA tool is intentionally holistic and comprehensive in its structure. It covers many palliative care activities and concerns and aligns well with the WHO's definition of quality palliative care. It was developed out of the Gold Standards Framework (https://www.goldstandardsframework.org.uk/). Components of this framework include physical needs, emotional needs, personal needs, social needs, information and communication needs, control and autonomy needs,

TABLE 27.1 PEPSI COLA Framework

	Topics to Consider	Questions to Ask
P	Physical needs: • Symptom assessment • Medication assessment (including side effects) • Identify and cease nonessential treatments	• What are your main physical problems? • How do these problems affect you? • What have you tried to manage these problems? • Are you taking your medication as prescribed? • What other treatments are you using? • Are you using any nonprescribed treatments?
E	Emotional needs: • Psychologic assessment (e.g., depression, anxiety, fears) • Understand patient's expectations of care/death • Coping mechanisms; including attempts to avoid uncomfortable thoughts/feelings • Altered body image • Relationships with others • Disturbed sleep	• Is there something that worries you most? • Have you recently lost interest in the things you once enjoyed? (Nurses should have the patient explain these interests if they are able) • Are you experiencing distress at present? How would you describe this distress? (Nurses may use a tool such as the Distress Thermometer) • How do you normally cope with stress? • Have you had difficulty coping in the past? • What forms of support do you think you have? • Would you like to speak to a professional who can provide emotional support (e.g., a counsellor, etc)?
P	Personal needs: • Sociocultural background and spiritual background, as described earlier in this chapter • Needs related to ethnicity, language, sexuality, etc	• How do you make sense of what is happening to you? • What can we do to help with your personal concerns? • Would you find it helpful to speak with somebody about these issues (e.g., a support group, patient information service, etc)? • How does your condition affect your ability to meet your personal needs?
S	Social needs: • Relationships with others • Welfare rights • Carer assessment	Ask the following questions as applicable to the individual patient: • How are you managing at home? • How are you managing at work? • How are you managing financially? • How are your close personal relationships? • Is there anyone who is dependent on you? • Do you have any legal concerns or issues?
I	Information and communication needs: • What information does the patient have, and need? • Is the patient's advance care documentation in order? • Does the patient understand their plan of care? • Determine patient's wishes for depth of information • Is the mode of communication and language used appropriate?	• Have you been asked if you would like to be included in correspondence between members of your multidisciplinary team? • Do you know who your key worker is, and how to contact them if needed? (If appropriate). • Do you feel you have been informed of all the relevant information? Is there anything else you would like to know? • Do you know how to access further information when you require it? • Have you been informed of the patient support groups relevant to you?
C	Control and autonomy needs: • Mental capacity to make decisions (as described in an earlier chapter) • Engagement in treatment options and plans • Identification of the patient's preferred place of care • Recap on advance care documentation	• Nurses may use a standard tool to assess the patient's decision-making capacity. • Have you discussed and documented your wishes for your future care? • If yes to the above question, where is this documentation located? Who has access to it? • Do you have a hand-held copy of your advance care plan/s or patient records (if you would like one)? • If your health deteriorated, where would you like to be cared for?
O	Out-of-hours needs: • Identification of appropriate out-of-hours services • Identification of preferred priorities for care • Transfer information, including ambulance services	• Are you (and your family/carer, as appropriate) aware of who you can call for out-of-hours advice and assistance? • Do you (and your family/carer, as appropriate) know how to contact services out-of-hours? • Do you (and your family/carer, as appropriate) know the transfer services available to you?
L	Living with your illness: • Rehabilitation support (to promote quality of life) • Referral to other agencies • End-of-life care planning	• How are you managing with your daily living tasks? • How is your appetite, mobility, swallowing, communication, diet, sleep, etc? • Have you been informed of the variety of support services available to you? • Have you been given the opportunity to discuss your future, expectations, goals, etc?
A	After-care needs: • Funeral arrangements • Family/carer bereavement risk assessment • Future support of the family	• Are there funeral arrangements in place? • Do you have information for bereavement services? • Are there any additional services your family requires?

From NursingAnswers.net. (2018). *Palliative care lecture: Holistic assessment and care.* Retrieved from https://nursinganswers.net/lectures/nursing/palliative-care/3-detailed.php?vref=1. Adapted from Thomas, K. (2009). *Holistic patient assessment: PEPSI COLA aide memoire.* Gold Standards Framework Centre.

out-of-hours needs, living with the illness, and aftercare needs (Damarell et al, 2020).

Another assessment tool for palliative care is the Palliative Performance Scale version 2 (PPSv2) (Anderson et al, 1996). This tool is useful for identifying and tracking the care needs of patients receiving palliative care. It is a quick means of describing the patient's functional level while receiving palliative care. Patients are scored from 0% to 100% on ambulation, activity and evidence of disease, self-care, intake, and level of consciousness. Table 27.2 provides a brief overview of selected additional assessment tools used in palliative care and hospice.

The psychosocial needs of the person who is dying, their family, and caregivers must also be carefully assessed. Spiritual and psychosocial needs are interrelated and affect each other. Questions to guide the assessment of spiritual needs include asking the person what is important to them, encouraging them to talk about their feelings, and reflecting on the meaning of their life (Curie, 2022; Doka, 1993).

The hierarchy of a dying person's needs, based on Maslow's hierarchy of needs framework, may assist nurses in identifying a dying older person's specific needs at each level (Touhy and Jett, 2020) (Fig. 27.4). Care can be structured around Maslow's

TABLE 27.2	Selected Palliative Care and Hospice Assessment Tools
Assessment Tool	**Use/Description**
Functional Assessment Staging Test (FAST)	A reliable and valid assessment tool to categorize the functional abilities of persons with dementia can be used to help monitor treatment and changes in condition[1]
Karnofsky Performance Status (KPS)	A reliable and valid assessment tool to identify functional abilities, impairments, and needs of persons with serious illness. It is useful to compare the effectiveness of therapies and prognosis.[2]
Brief Fatigue Inventory	A reliable and valid assessment tool to identify the severity and impact of fatigue on activity, mood, work, and relationships in patients with serious illness[3]
McGill Pain Inventory – Short Form	A reliable and valid assessment tool to discriminate among different pain diagnoses based on location and intensity, quality, pain pattern, and alleviating and aggravating factors[4]
Palliative Care Outcome Scale (POS)	A reliable and valid assessment tool to determine palliative care needs in physical, psychological, and spiritual domains[5]
Memorial Symptom Assessment Scale (MSAS)	A reliable and valid assessment tool for the evaluation of symptom prevalence, characteristics, and distress[6]

References:
1. Sclan, S. G., & Reisberg, B. (1992). Functional assessment staging (FAST) in Alzheimer's disease: Reliability, validity, and ordinality. *International Psychogeriatrics, 4*(Suppl 1), 55-69.
2. Schag, C. C., Heinrich, R. L., & Ganz, P. A. (1984). Karnofsky performance status revisited: Reliability, validity, and guidelines. *Journal of Clinical Oncology, 2*(3), 187-193.
3. Nunes, A. F., Bezerra, C. O., Dos Santos Custódio, J., Friedrich, C. F., de Oliveira, I. S., & Lunardi, A. C. (2019). Clinimetric properties of the brief fatigue inventory applied to oncological patients hospitalized for chemotherapy. *Journal of Pain and Symptom Management, 57*(2), 297-303.
4. Ngamkham, S., Vincent, C., Finnegan, L., Holden, J. E., Wang, Z. J., & Wilkie, D. J. (2012). The McGill Pain Questionnaire as a multidimensional measure in people with cancer: An integrative review. *Pain Management Nursing, 13*(1), 27-51.
5. Hearn, J., & Higginson, I. J. (1999). Development and validation of a core outcome measure for palliative care: The palliative care outcome scale. Palliative Care Core Audit Project Advisory Group. *Quality in Health Care, 8*(4), 219-227.
6. Portenoy, R. K., Thaler, H. T., Kornblith, A. B., Lepore, J. M., Friedlander-Klar, H., Kiyasu, E., et al. (1994). The Memorial Symptom Assessment Scale: An instrument for the evaluation of symptom prevalence, characteristics and distress. *European Journal of Cancer, 30A*(9), 1326–1336.

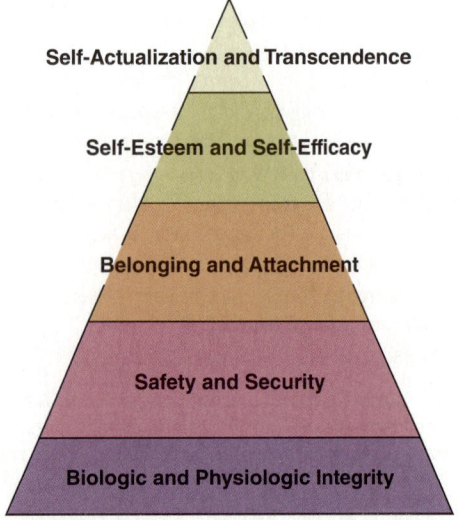

Fig. 27.4 Hierarchy of a dying person's needs. (Modified from Touhy, T. A., & Jett, K. F. [2020]. *Ebersole & Hess' toward healthy aging: Human needs and nursing response* [10th ed.]. St. Louis, MO: Elsevier.)

hierarchy, addressing basic needs first (Zalenski and Raspa, 2006):

- Relief of pain and dyspnea
- Address personal and social fears; these include fear of falling and fear of death
- The need for belonging does not end with terminal illness; the thought of dying alone can induce fear; a life review can be an intimate experience, revealing personal thoughts and feelings
- Likewise, discussing their accomplishments and values with the person can help restore self-esteem, lost due to suffering and disability
- As death approaches and material needs can no longer be met, nonmaterial needs can be satisfied, and "transcendence" can be achieved

Careful assessment of a dying person's needs may indicate individualized strategies for meeting those needs.

Take Actions (Nursing Interventions)

As death nears, physiologic changes occur in cardiac, circulation, and urinary functions, food and fluid intake, the skin, respiratory system, and mental status. Table 27.3 describes these signs of impending death.

Pain and active dying. Pain management is the top priority during the dying process. Pain may have a powerful, negative effect on a patient's quality of life. The pain experience is complex, and its management is often difficult. A stepped-care approach is recommended, with the use of aspirin or acetaminophen for mild pain, a moderate opiate such as codeine or oxycodone for more constant pain, and a strong opiate such as morphine for severe pain, and neurologic procedures for uncontrolled pain (Chapman, 2011) (Fig. 27.5). Pain medication should be given around the clock to promote stable blood levels. Nursing responsibilities include careful pain assessment, education of patients and family caregivers regarding pain medication, and close communication with the prescriber for changes in medication as needed. Attention must be given to a patient's emotional state because psychosocial factors and emotional pain may accentuate physical pain (Wiech and Tracey, 2009). In the nonverbal person, behavior change is a reliable indicator of pain. Assessment tools such as the Pain Assessment in Advanced Dementia Scale are reliable and may be used to aid pain assessment (Agrace, 2021).

Respiratory changes. Changes in breathing are expected as death nears. Patients may experience Kussmaul respirations, which are constant, deep, rapid breaths. These occur as the body attempts to maintain acid-base balance. Cheyne-Stokes respirations are rapid breaths interspersed with periods of apnea. This type of breathing occurs due to a decrease in perfusion of the respiratory center of the brain and indicate death is very close. Terminal secretions develop when the person can no longer swallow their saliva. This occurs as the person becomes less responsive. Side-to-side repositioning is the most effective intervention. Additionally, anticholinergic drugs (i.e., hyoscyamine, atropine drops, and glycopyrrolate) may be useful in reducing saliva production. It is important for nurses to reassure family members that these breathing patterns do not indicate pain and suffering (Agrace, 2021; Hospice Foundation of America, n.d.).

Patients who are dying may also experience dyspnea. When this occurs, discomfort may be alleviated by elevating the head of the bed, directing a fan toward the person's face to reduce

TABLE 27.3 Common Signs of Impending Death

Physiologic Changes	Signs/Symptoms
Cardiac and Circulation Changes	
Decreased blood perfusion	Skin may become mottled and discolored and feel cool to touch
Decreased cerebral perfusion	Decreased level of consciousness; delirium; drowsiness/disorientation
Decrease in cardiac output and intravascular volume	Tachycardia (heart rate > 100), hypotension (low blood pressure)
	Cyanosis (discoloration in skin due to lack of oxygenated blood)
Urinary Function	
Decreased urinary output	Possible urinary incontinence
	Concentrated urine
Food and Fluids	
Decreased interest in food and fluid	Weight loss/dehydration
Swallowing difficulties	Food pocketed in cheeks or mouth/choking with eating/coughing after eating
Skin	
Skin may become mottled or discolored	Patches of purplish or dark pinkish color can be noted on extremities
Respiratory	
Terminal secretions	Noisy respirations caused by accumulation of secretions in upper airway due to decreased consciousness and inability to cough
Dyspnea	Shortness of breath
Notable changes in breathing	Irregular respiratory pattern
General Changes	
Profound weakness and fatigue	Drowsy for extended periods; sleeping more
Decreased alertness	More withdrawn and detached from surroundings; may appear to be in a comatose-like state and may communicate nonverbally (e.g., squeezing hands, purposeful eye movements, wiggle toes)
Near-death awareness	May include symbolic talk, patient speaking and/or seeing persons/loved ones that others cannot see, knowing when death will occur, preparing for travel

From Stanford School of Medicine – Palliative Care (n.d.) "Signs of Impending Death". Retrieved from https://swap.stanford.edu/was/20180315000323/https://palliative.stanford.edu/transition-to-death/signs-of-impending-death/.

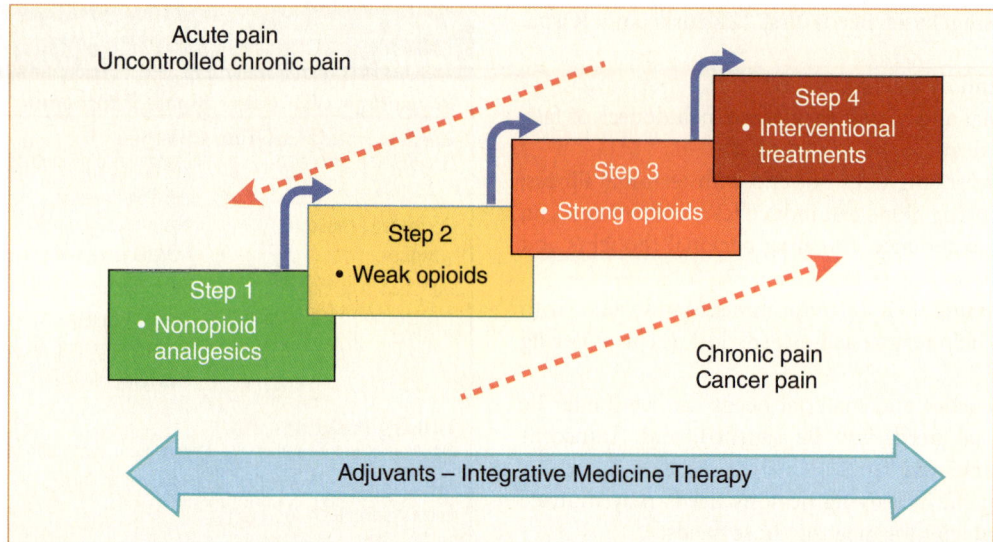

Fig. 27.5 A depiction of the revised World Health Organization's pain relief ladder. In addition to providing a bidirectional approach, the additional "interventional" step 4 includes invasive and minimally invasive treatments. (Redrawn from Mestdagh, F., Steyaert, A., & Lavand'homme, P. [2023]. Cancer pain management: A narrative review of current concepts, strategies, and techniques. *Current Oncology, 30*[7], 6838-6858.)

shortness of breath, and using short-acting opioids (Agrace, 2021; Hospice Foundation of America, n.d.).

Skin changes. Skin changes occur as the body attempts to compensate for decreased cardiac output and a change in peripheral circulation, as the body conserves oxygenated blood for vital organs. As death nears, the hands and feet become cool and pale. It may take on a dusky/grey tone, and skin around the mouth and nose becomes cyanotic (Agrace, 2021). Pressure injuries may develop, particularly if the person is bedbound or has experienced significant weight loss. Open wounds can appear quickly. Nursing care includes pain management, keeping the wounds clean, and preventing infection. Aggressive treatment is not required and may increase pain (Hospice Foundation of America, n.d.). For the bedridden patient who is dying and experiencing altered skin integrity, the benefits of indwelling catheter placement may outweigh the risks of developing an infection.

General changes. As death nears, most persons become less responsive and may develop mental status changes that vary from mild anxiety to delirium. Restlessness in a dying patient may have many causes, including constipation, urinary retention, sepsis, hypoxia, drug toxicity, increased pain, or unresolved psychosocial issues. Restlessness can be resolved if the cause can be identified and effective treatment implemented. Pharmacologic management may be necessary if restlessness continues and is upsetting for the patient and family. "Terminal restlessness" is usually only treated if the behaviors place the person or others at harm. Options include mild tranquilizers called *benzodiazepines* and antipsychotic drugs called *phenothiazines* (Agrace, 2021; Morrow, 2023).

Constipation is common among older adults who require opioids for pain and whose diets and activities are restricted. Adding fiber to a patient's diet or giving bulk-forming laxatives may not be practical if the person cannot maintain sufficient fluid intake and diet. Stool softeners and oral cathartics may be more effective; however, suppositories, enemas, and manual disimpaction may also be necessary, but the benefit versus potential increase in pain must be weighed. Careful assessment and individualized management of constipation are essential.

Food and fluids. Oral nutrition and hydration should be maintained if a patient can swallow safely. Food and fluids should never be pushed. Pushing food and fluids can lead to aspiration pneumonia and gastric discomfort. Dehydration and anorexia are often of greater concern to family members than to the dying patients, who may not be experiencing any resulting discomfort. In many cases, intravenous fluids and feedings are not appropriate (see Nutritional Considerations box). Palliative care providers and nurses know that medically assisted nutrition and hydration rarely benefit patients at the end of life. Adequate hydration may, in fact, increase respiratory secretions. Nasogastric tube feedings, total parenteral nutrition, and intravenous hydration increase infections and may decrease survival time. Additional fluids may also contribute to edema caused by impaired circulation in older adults. The only documented side effect of dehydration is dry mouth, which may be relieved by administering saliva substitutes, ice chips, and glycerin swabs and by promoting good oral care. If adequate oral care is provided, it is believed that patients at the end of life do not suffer from dehydration. Individual assessment and thoughtful decision-making that includes the patient and family regarding hydration and nutrition are important (ANA, 2017; Hospice Foundation of America, n.d.).

CHAPTER 27 Loss and End-of-Life Issues

NEXT-GENERATION NCLEX® EXAMINATION-STYLE CASE STUDY

Scenario: The nurse is caring for a patient admitted to inpatient hospice with end-stage dementia.

Nurses' Notes

0730

- Report received from night shift. The patient had a restless night and received morphine sulfate 20 mg oral solution twice. Last dose at 0630, with moderate relief. No bowel movements for the past 2 days; tube feeding residuals vary from 75 mL to 125 mL every 4 hours. Changed wet incontinence pads twice during the night.
- Hospice comfort pack checked: drugs available include acetaminophen suppository, haloperidol oral solution, atropine solution, lorazepam, morphine sulfate solution, and prochlorperazine and bisacodyl suppositories.
- On assessment this morning, only response to verbal stimuli or touch is groaning; eyes are half open but patient does not follow speaker with eyes; tearing noted; lying on side curled in fetal position; frail; skin of feet and hands has become mottled and cold; drooling – clear and light tan fluid; incontinence pad with scant dark amber urine with strong odor; liquid, light tan stool covers incontinence pad; perineal area with maceration and erythema; breathing is labored and congested with rhonchi throughout; peripheral pulses weak, S_1 S_2 present with faint S_3. Nonpitting edema in bilateral lower extremities. Abdomen with hypoactive bowel sounds throughout – PEG tube in place with serosanguinous drainage at entrance. Area of erythema extending 2.5 cm around entry site.
- Blood pressure 78/42; heart rate 58; respirations 10; temperature 101.8° F (38.8° C); oxygen saturation 88% on 2 L per nasal canula.
- Adult child who is power-of-attorney notified of change in condition. The patient's child states they will notify their siblings, and everyone will come to the hospital as soon as they can. Requested for a priest to come and provide The Last Rights.

For each end-of-life symptom, select the appropriate nursing action to ensure the patient experiences a good death. More than one finding may be selected for each symptom.

Symptom	Nursing Action
Oral secretions	☐ Give atropine sulfate ☐ Position on side ☐ Perform chest physical therapy
Fever	☐ Place cool wash cloth on forehead ☐ Administer acetaminophen 325 mg 2 tabs by mouth ☐ Encourage consumption of clear liquids
Decreased urine output	☐ Begin IV normal saline 125 mL/hr ☐ Replace incontinence pads ☐ Provide gentle perineal care
Loose stool	☐ Administer bisacodyl suppository as ordered ☐ Discontinue PEG feedings ☐ Provide gentle perineal care

🍐 NUTRITIONAL CONSIDERATIONS

Loss of appetite frequently accompanies the dying process. Families usually consider providing food as part of basic human caring and something they can do to prolong the patient's life. For the dying person, however, eating may be an unpleasant and unwanted experience. Artificial feeding with nasogastric or gastrostomy tubes or intravenous nutrition frequently leads to further complications and earlier death. Because eating and food are often closely tied to many fond memories of loved ones, this is a difficult area and potential source of conflict between patients and their caregivers. Patients and families need to know that anorexia is a normal part of dying, and they need to have open discussion on the meaning of food and nutrition. Perhaps other meaningful and symbolic ways of providing sustenance may be achieved without artificial feeding.

Effective communication skills such as maintaining eye contact, sensitive use of touch, and clarifying statements through reflection (i.e., restating the message as it is understood and asking for verification of its meaning) are important.

Another important role of the nurse is to educate and support families and caregivers. Caregivers experience a multitude of issues, including decreased energy levels, health problems, deep grief, and fears about life without their loved ones. Nurses must be sensitive to caregiver needs and provide education, psychologic support, and referrals for additional services.

The role of a social support system is very important during the bereavement process. As a result, it is important that the nurse assess social support networks and help mobilize support for patients and caregivers, if necessary (Ekberg et al, 2021).

As caregivers, nurses are not immune to intense feelings of grief after the death of a person that they have cared for. These feelings may occur whenever close relationships develop between nurses and patients, especially in long-term care and hospice settings. A dying person may have certain characteristics that invoke memories of previous unresolved losses that the nurse has experienced. Such grief needs to be recognized, accepted, and evaluated, just as any other experience of loss and grief needs to be assessed. The first step is for the nurse to recognize unresolved grief. The next step may be to express their thoughts and feelings to a coworker, friend, or family member. If additional help is needed, sources such as employee assistance programs, clergy, or other counselors may be contacted.

HOSPICE

Hospice care was founded on the philosophy of compassionate, humane care for the person who is dying and their families. Although a hospice may be where dying people go, in the United States, the term *hospice* usually refers to a philosophy of care implemented wherever the patient may be dying — at home, the hospital, or a nursing facility. The basic goal of hospice care is palliative care plus support services, helping the dying person live as fully as possible with the highest quality of life on a day-to-day basis. During the dying process and the bereavement period, physical, emotional, social, and spiritual care is provided by an interdisciplinary team consisting of the patients, their families, health-care professionals, and volunteers (American Cancer Society, 2019; Egan City and Labyak, 2010).

PALLIATIVE CARE

The term *palliative care* refers to "an approach that improves the quality of life of patients and their families facing the problems associated with life-threatening illness, through the prevention and relief of suffering using early identification and impeccable assessment and treatment of pain and other problems, physical, psychosocial, and spiritual" (WHO, 2020). Offering palliative care before hospice care yields many benefits. It differs from hospice care in that curative treatment can be obtained through palliative care but not hospice care. This approach has successfully guided the care of dying patients and their families provided by interdisciplinary health-care teams (NIH and NIA, 2021).

For many older adults, home is the preferred place to die. Home care may or may not include hospice or palliative care. Many older persons die at home, cared for only by their family or sometimes visiting nurses or home health aides. In these situations, caregivers' goals are often like hospice goals; however, the dying person and family do not benefit from an interdisciplinary team and an organized approach to follow-up care.

LEGISLATIVE INITIATIVES

Legislative initiatives regarding death and dying include the Patient Self-Determination Act, which became law in 1991; it requires all health-care facilities receiving Medicare and Medicaid reimbursement to recognize advance directives. These instructions for care (living wills and durable powers-of-attorney) guide families and health-care providers should the patient be incapable of decision-making (NIH and NIA, 2022). Yadav et al (2017) reviewed studies from 2011 to 2016 and found no increase in the number of patients with advanced directives; despite efforts and initiatives, only 36.7% of people have completed these documents, including living wills.

Nurses caring for very ill older adults must understand the legal status of advance directives, living wills, and DNR orders.

As natural extensions of a patient's right to self-determination, these preferences should be adhered to by the nurse (House et al, 2022).

EVIDENCE-BASED PRACTICE

Nursing Students' Knowledge and Attitudes About End-Of-Life Care

Background
Nurses play a key role in the multiprofessional palliative care team, and they are expected to take time to care for dying patients at their bedside. Studies vary greatly regarding the level of end-of-life care knowledge and attitudes of nursing students. Disparities also exist in nursing students' knowledge and attitudes about end-of-life care across geographic regions, genders, and academic years. Inadequate knowledge hinders them from delivering high-quality end-of-life care after graduation, and consequently, the increasing needs and demands of patients are not being satisfied.

Sample/Setting
Twenty-six cross-sectional studies of medium or high quality from 13 countries met the eligibility criteria, involving 9749 nursing students.

Method
This review was conducted under the guidance of the Preferred Reporting Items for Systematic Reviews and Meta-Analyses (PRISMA) guidelines. Eligibility criteria included the following:
- Population was nursing students, including interns who had not yet graduated
- Knowledge and attitudes about end-of-life care were evaluated using Palliative Care Quiz for Nursing (PCQN) and Frommelt Attitudes Toward Care of the Dying (FATCOD), respectively
- Study was quantitative, with extractable means and standard deviations
- Study design was observational, including cross-sectional, case-control, and cohort studies; 26 studies ultimately met requirements based on eligibility criteria

Findings
Nursing students demonstrated insufficient knowledge about end-of-life care, with a pooled mean score of 7.50 (95% CI, 6.55–8.45); of these, knowledge about philosophy and principles, psychosocial and spiritual care, and pain and symptom management were all deficient, with pooled mean scores of 1.49 (95% CI, 0.78–2.21), 1.00 (95% CI, 0.35–1.65), and 3.44 (95% CI, 2.25–4.63), respectively. Conversely, nursing students showed positive attitudes toward end-of-life care, with a pooled mean score of 102.97 (95% CI, 99.43–106.51). The subgroup analysis revealed that male nursing students had lower pooled mean scores for end-of-life care knowledge and attitudes.

Implications
The authors found a knowledge deficit among nursing students about end-of-life care, including knowledge about philosophy and principles, psychosocial and spiritual care, and pain and symptom management. There is a mismatch between nursing students' knowledge and attitudes about end-of-life care, they have a positive attitude but lack the necessary knowledge. Male nursing students seem to have a greater deficit of knowledge and a relatively conservative attitude toward end-of-life care. These findings may provide a significant reference for nursing educators to adjust educational strategies promptly.

Data from Wang, W., Wu, C., Bai, D., Chen, H., Cai, M., Gao, J., et al. (2022). A meta-analysis of nursing students' knowledge and attitudes about end-of-life care. *Nurse Education Today*, 119, 105570.

HOME CARE

1. Homebound older adults who have lost a spouse or significant other may manifest grief through physical symptoms.
2. Homebound older adults may develop crises of faith and express anger at God. It is important for the home care nurse to avoid being judgmental and to allow the older adult to verbalize anger and grief.
3. Refer to an advanced practice nurse or other health professional skilled in working with complicated grieving if the homebound older adult experiences dysfunctional grieving.
4. Loss of a spouse or significant other, coupled with living alone, puts homebound older adults at risk for depression.
5. Assess the terminally ill, homebound older adult's feelings toward their own death.
6. Provide family members and caregivers information related to the stages of dying and the physiologic changes that accompany them.
7. Use hospice care to help dying homebound older adults live as fully as possible on a day-to-day basis.
8. If hospice care is not available, home care nurses may support the homebound, terminally ill older adult through the dying process.

SUMMARY

It is important for gerontological nurses to have a thorough understanding of the strategies related to caring for older adults who are grieving or dying. Part of understanding involves examination of the nurse's own value system and prior experience with grief and death. It is hoped that care and support for grieving or dying older persons will improve with increased knowledge and positive attitudes. This improvement should benefit both older adults and nurses, who have much knowledge and wisdom to gain from those who have the most experience in life.

KEY POINTS

- *Grief* is the acute reaction to one's perception of loss, *mourning* is the longer process of resolving acute grief reactions, and *bereavement* is the state of having experienced a significant loss.
- Grief involves many changes over time, is a natural response to all kinds of losses (not just death) and is based on one's unique perception of a loss.
- Worden (2009) views the grief process as active, involving the following four tasks of mourning: (1) accepting the reality of the loss, (2) working through the pain of grief, (3) adjusting to an environment in which the deceased is missing, and (4) emotionally relocating the deceased and moving on with life.
- Human beings respond as whole people, and their grief manifests itself in physical symptoms, psychologic responses, changes in socialization patterns, and spiritual issues concerning life's meaning.
- Nursing care activities that assist in the grieving process include helping the survivor express feelings, providing time to grieve, explaining "normal" grieving behaviors, examining defenses, and coping styles, identifying pathologic conditions, and making appropriate referrals.
- Age-related changes predispose older persons to greater potential problems in areas such as hygiene and skin care, nutrition, elimination, mobility, transfers, rest, sleep, pain, respiratory management, and cognitive and behavioral functioning.
- Nursing strategies for assisting dying older persons include delivering excellent physical care, using good communication skills, conducting a life review, and educating and supporting family caregivers.
- Hospice programs help dying persons live as fully as possible on a day-to-day basis by providing symptom control, addressing the psychologic needs of patients, supporting family caregivers, dealing with environmental problems, and assisting patients with spiritual concerns.

CLINICAL JUDGMENT EXERCISES

1. An 80-year-old is admitted to the hospital with pneumonia and weakness. The patient lives alone; their children are supportive and help around the house, but do not live with the patient. The patient's spouse of 51 years died within the last 6 months. The patient is grieving the loss but is relieved and feels guilty as the spouse was abusive. How should the nurse assist the patient in coping with their loss?

2. A 75-year-old is dying from metastatic prostate cancer with bone involvement. The patient's family has not been very close. They now want to become closer and have as much time with your patient as possible. How should the hospice nurse prepare this family to work through their anticipatory grieving?

REFERENCES

Agency for Healthcare Research and Quality (AHRQ). (2021). *Research protocol: Assessment tools for palliative care.* Rockville, MD: Effective Healthcare Program, AHRQ. Retrieved from https://effectivehealthcare.ahrq.gov/products/palliative-care-tools/research-protocol. Accessed July 31, 2023.

Agrace. (2021). *Clinical practice guidelines. Active dying: Overview.* Agrace.org [website]. Retrieved from https://www.agrace.org/wp-content/uploads/2016/10/Clinical-practice-guidelines-Active-Dying-10-20-2021-FNL.pdf. Accessed July 31, 2023.

American Cancer Society. (2019). *Hospice care: What is hospice care?* Retrieved from https://www.cancer.org/treatment/end-of-life-care/hospice-care/what-is-hospice-care.html. Accessed July 31, 2023.

American Nurses Association (ANA). (2017). *Position statement: Nutrition and hydration at the end of life.* Retrieved from https://www.nursingworld.org/~4ad4a8/globalassets/docs/ana/nutrition-and-hydration-at-end-of-life.pdf. Accessed July 31, 2023.

Anderson, F., Downing, G. M., Hill, J., Casorso, L., & Lerch, N. (1996). Palliative performance scale (PPS): A new tool. *Journal of Palliative Care, 12*(1), 5–11.

Balk, D. E. (2013). Life span issues and loss, grief, and mourning: Adulthood. In D. K. Meagher & D. E. Balk (Eds.), *Handbook of Thanatology* (2nd ed.). Northbrook, IL: Association for Death Education and Counseling.

Bauld, C. M., Letcher, P., & Olsson, C. A. (2021). Supporting the dying and bereaved during COVID-19. *Australian Psychologist, 56*(4), 269–273. doi:10.1080/00050067.2021.1937924.

Bettinger, J. J., Wegrzyn, E., & Fudin, J. (2017). Pain management in the elderly: Focus on safe prescribing. *Practical Pain Management, 17*(3).

Brandt, A. (2021). *Making meaning: A way to heal after trauma and loss.* Psychology Today [website]. Retrieved from https://www.psychologytoday.com/us/blog/mindful-anger/202110/making-meaning-way-heal-after-trauma-and-loss. Accessed July 31, 2023.

Burbank, P. M. (1992). An exploratory study: Assessing the meaning in life among older adult clients. *Journal of Gerontological Nursing, 18*(9), 19–28. doi:10.3928/0098-9134-19920901-06.

Cancer.net Editorial Board. (2022). *Understanding grief and loss.* Cancer.net [website]. Retrieved from https://www.cancer.net/coping-with-cancer/managing-emotions/grief-and-loss/understanding-grief-and-loss. Accessed July 31, 2023.

Carlsson, M., & Gunningberg, L. (2017). Unavoidable pressure ulcers at the end of life and nurse understanding. *British Journal of Nursing, 26*(Suppl. 20), S6–S17. doi:10.12968/bjon.2017.26.Sup20.S6.

Carr, D., Boerner, K., & Moorman, S. (2020). Bereavement in the time of coronavirus: Unprecedented challenges demand novel interventions. *Journal of Aging and Social Policy, 32*(4-5), 425–431. doi:10.1080/08959420.2020.1764320.

Centers for Disease Control and Prevention (CDC), & National Center for Health Statistics. (2021). *National vital statistics system, mortality 1999-2020.* CDC WONDER Online Database. Data are from the Multiple Cause of Death Files, 1999-2020, as compiled from data provided by the 57 vital statistics jurisdictions through the Vital Statistics Cooperative Program. Retrieved from http://wonder.cdc.gov/ucd-icd10.html. Accessed July 31, 2023.

Chapman, S. (2011). Assessment and management of patients with cancer pain. *Cancer Nursing Practice, 10*(10), 28–36. doi:10.7748/cnp2011.12.10.10.28.c8867.

Corless, I. (2010). Bereavement. In B. R. Ferrell & N. Coyle (Eds.), *Textbook of palliative nursing* (3rd ed.). New York: Oxford University Press.

Corr, C. A., & Corr, D. M. (2013). *Death and dying, life and living* (7th ed.). Belmont, CA: Wadsworth.

Damarell, R. A., Morgan, D. D., Tieman, J. J., & Healey, D. (2020). Bolstering general practitioner palliative care: A critical review of support provided by Australian guidelines for life-limiting chronic conditions. *Healthcare, 8*(4), 553. doi:10.3390/healthcare8040553.

Derby, S., O'Mahoney, S., & Tickoo, R. (2010). Elderly patients. In B. R. Ferrell & N. Coyle (Eds.), *Textbook of palliative nursing* (3rd ed.). New York, NY: Oxford University Press.

Doka, K. J. (1993). The spiritual needs of the dying. In K. J. Doka (Ed.), *Death and spirituality.* Amityville, NY: Baywood.

Doka, K. J. (2013). Historical and contemporary perspectives on loss, grief, and mourning. In D. K. Meagher & D. E. Balk (Eds.), *Handbook of thanatology* (2nd ed.). Northbrook, IL: Association for Death Education and Counseling.

Egan City, K. A., & Labyak, M. J. (2010). Hospice palliative care for the 21st century: A model for quality end-of-life care. In B. R. Ferrell & N. Coyle (Eds.), *Textbook of palliative nursing* (3rd ed.). New York: Oxford University Press.

Ekberg, S., Parry, R., Land, V., Ekberg, K., Pino, M., Antaki, C., et al. (2021). Communicating with patients and families about illness progression and end of life: A review of studies using direct observation of clinical practice. *BMC Palliative Care, 20*(1), 186. doi:10.1186/s12904-021-00876-2.

Ernstmeyer, K., & Christman, E. (2021). Chapter 17 Grief and Loss. https://www.ncbi.nlm.nih.gov/books/NBK591827/. Accessed 17 August 2024.

Familydoctor.org Editorial Staff. (2022). *Helping older adults deal with life-changing events.* familydoctor.org [website]. Retrieved from https://familydoctor.org/helping-older-adults-deal-with-life-changing-events/. Accessed July 31, 2023.

Fanjul, L. (2022). *Anticipatory grief: Preparing for a loved one's end of life* [Fact Sheet]. CancerCare [website]. Retrieved from https://www.cancercare.org/publications/385-anticipatory_grief_preparing_for_a_loved_one_s_end_of_life. Accessed July 31, 2023.

Florida Crisis Consortium. (n. d.). *The process of grieving.* New Jersey Department of Human Services [website]. Retrieved from https://www.state.nj.us/humanservices/emergency/FCC_ESF8_ProcessOfGrieving.pdf. Accessed July 31, 2023.

Frazer Consultants. (2018). *Grief theories series: Continuing bonds theory.* Frazer Consultants [blog]. Retrieved from https://web.frazerconsultants.com/grief-theories-series-continuing-bonds-theory/. Accessed August 25, 2024.

Funeral Guide. (2021). *The dual process model.* Funeral Guide [website]. Retrieved from https://www.funeralguide.co.uk/help-resources/bereavement-support/the-grieving-process/the-dual-process-model. Accessed July 31, 2023.

Gire, J. (2014). How Death Imitates Life: Cultural Influences on Conceptions of Death and Dying. *Online Readings in Psychology and Culture, 6*(2). doi:10.9707/2307-0919.1120.

Hairston, S., & Pathak, N. (2019). *How grief shows up in your body.* WebMD [website]. Retrieved from https://www.webmd.com/special-reports/grief-stages/20190711/how-grief-affects-your-body-and-mind. Accessed July 31, 2023.

Hibberd, R. (2013). Meaning reconstruction in bereavement: Sense and significance. *Death Studies, 37*(7), 670–692. doi:10.1080/07481187.2012.692453.

Holland, J. M., Currier, J. M., & Neimeyer, R. A. (2006). Meaning reconstruction in the first two years of bereavement: The role of sense-making and benefit-finding. *Omega: Journal of Death and Dying, 53*(3), 174–191. doi:10.2190/FKM2-YJTY-F9VV-9XWY.

Hospice Foundation of America. (n. d.). *Signs of approaching death.* HospiceFoundation.org [website]. Retrieved from https://hospicefoundation.org/Hospice-Care/Signs-of-Approaching-Death. Accessed July 31, 2023.

House, S. A., Schoo, C., & Ogilvie, W. A. (2022). *Advance directives.* StatPearls [Internet]. Retrieved from https://www.ncbi.nlm.nih.gov/books/NBK459133/. Accessed July 31, 2023.

Hughes, R. G., Bakos, A. D., O'Mara, A., & Kovner, C. T. (2005). Palliative wound care at the end of life. *Home Health Care Management & Practice*, 17(3), 196–202. doi:10.1177/1084822304271815.

Kaiser Family Foundation (KFF). (2023). *Global COVID-19 Tracker.* KFF [website]. Retrieved from https://www.kff.org/coronavirus-covid-19/issue-brief/global-covid-19-tracker/. Accessed July 31, 2023.

Kelly, L. (2021). *16 different types of grief people experience.* Talkspace [website]. Retrieved from https://www.talkspace.com/blog/types-of-grief/. Accessed July 31, 2023.

Klass, D., Silverman, P. R., & Nickman, S. L. (2006). *Continuing bonds: New understandings of grief.* Washington, DC: Taylor & Francis.

Kolcaba, K., & DiMarco, M. A. (2005). Comfort Theory and its application to pediatric nursing. *Pediatric Nursing*, 31(3), 187–194.

Lund, D. A. (1989). Conclusions about bereavement in later life and implications for interventions and future research. In D. A. Lund (Ed.), *Older bereaved spouses: Research with practical applications.* New York: Hemisphere.

Marie Curie. (2022). *Providing spiritual care.* Marie Curie [website]. Retrieved from https://www.mariecurie.org.uk/professionals/palliative-care-knowledge-zone/individual-needs/spiritual-care. Accessed July 31, 2023.

Mendoza, M. A. (2020). *Complicated spiritual grief.* Psychology Today [website]. Retrieved from https://www.psychologytoday.com/us/blog/understanding-grief/202006/complicated-spiritual-grief. Accessed July 31, 2023.

Morrow, A. (2023). *End of life concerns: Recognizing terminal restlessness at the end of life.* Verywellhealth [website]. Retrieved from https://www.verywellhealth.com/terminal-restlessness-1132271. Accessed July 31, 2023.

National Consensus Project for Quality Palliative Care. (2018). *Clinical practice guidelines for quality palliative care* (4th ed.). Richmond, VA: National Coalition for Hospice and Palliative Care.

National Institutes of Health (NIH), & National Institute on Aging (NIA). (2021). *End of life: What are palliative care and hospice care?* Retrieved from https://www.nia.nih.gov/health/what-are-palliative-care-and-hospice-care. Accessed July 31, 2023.

National Institutes of Health (NIH), & National Institute on Aging (NIA). (2022). *Advance care planning: Advance directives for health care.* Retrieved from https://www.nia.nih.gov/health/advance-care-planning-health-care-directives. Accessed July 31, 2023.

Neimeyer, R. A. (2000). Searching for the meaning of meaning: Grief therapy and the process of reconstruction. *Death Studies*, 24(6), 541–558. doi:10.1080/07481180050121480.

Nolan, R., Kirkland, C., & Davis, R. (2021). LGBT* after loss: A mixed-method analysis on the effect of partner bereavement on interpersonal relationships and subsequent partnerships. *Omega (Westport)*, 82(4), 646–667. doi:10.1177/0030222819831524.

NursingAnswers.net. (2018). *Palliative care lecture: Holistic assessment and care.* Retrieved from https://nursinganswers.net/lectures/nursing/palliative-care/3-detailed.php?vref=1. Accessed July 31, 2023.

Patlamazoglou, L., Simmonds, J. G., & Snell, T. L. (2018). Same-sex partner bereavement: Non-HIV-related loss and new research directions. *Omega (Westport)*, 78(2), 178–196. doi:10.1177/0030222817690160.

PDQ Supportive and Palliative Care Editorial Board. (2022). PDQ grief, bereavement, and coping with loss (PDQ®): Health Professional Version. In: *PDQ cancer information summaries* [Internet]. Bethesda, MD: National Cancer Institute. Retrieved from https://www.ncbi.nlm.nih.gov/books/NBK66052/. Accessed July 31, 2023.

PDQ® Supportive and Palliative Care Editorial Board. (2021). *PDQ grief, bereavement, and loss.* Bethesda, MD: National Cancer Institute. Retrieved from https://www.cancer.gov/about-cancer/advanced-cancer/caregivers/planning/bereavement-pdq. Accessed July 31, 2023.

Purrington, J. (2021). Psychological adjustment to spousal bereavement in older adults: A systematic review. *Omega (Westport)*, 88(1), 302228211043702. doi:10.1177/00302228211043702.

Quinn, B. G. (2022). Providing palliative and end of life care for people with advanced disease. *Nursing Standard*, 37(6), 60–65. doi:10.7748/ns.2022.e11780.

ReachOut Australia. (n. d.). *Common reactions to death.* Reachout.com [website]. Retrieved from https://au.reachout.com/articles/common-reactions-to-death. Accessed July 31, 2023.

Şahn, D. S., & Büken, N. Ö. (2020). Death anxiety and concept of good death in the elderly. *Turkish Journal of Geriatrics*, 23(1), 18–26. doi:10.31086/tjgeri.2020.133.

Schladitz, K., Löbner, M., Stein, J., Weyerer, S., Werle, J., Wagner, M., et al. (2021). Grief and loss in old age: Exploration of the association between grief and depression. *Journal of Affective Disorders*, 283, 285–292. doi:10.1016/j.jad.2021.02.008.

Sinha, A., Deshwal, H., & Vashisht, R. (2023). *End-of-life evaluation and management of pain.* StatPearls [Internet]. Retrieved from https://www.ncbi.nlm.nih.gov/books/NBK568753/. Accessed July 31, 2023.

Social Work Portal. (n.d.). The ultimate guide to the biopsychosocial spiritual model of mental health. https://www.socialworkportal.com/biopsychosocial-spiritual-model/#Biopsychosocial-Spiritual-Factors. Accessed 25 August 2024.

Stroebe, M., & Schut, H. (2010). The dual process model of coping with bereavement: A decade on. *Omega (Westport)*, 61(4), 273–289. doi:10.2190/OM.61.4.b.

Sutton, J. (2022). *13 types of grief + how to treat loss in therapy.* PositivePsychology.com [website]. Retrieved from https://positivepsychology.com/grief-types/. Accessed July 31, 2023.

Tinnirello, A., Mazzoleni, S., & Santi, C. (2021). Chronic pain in the elderly: Mechanisms and distinctive features. *Biomolecules*, 11(8), 1256. doi:10.3390/biom11081256.

Touhy, T. A., & Jett, K. F. (Eds.). (2020). *Ebersole & Hess' toward healthy aging: Human needs and nursing response* (10th ed.). St. Louis: Elsevier.

Weitzner, M. A., Moody, L. N., & McMillan, S. C. (1997). Symptom management issues in hospice care. *The American Journal of Hospice & Palliative Care*, 14(4), 190–195. doi:10.1177/104990919701400501.

Wiech, K., & Tracey, I. (2009). The influence of negative emotions on pain: Behavioral effects and neural mechanisms. *NeuroImage*, 47(3), 987–994. doi:10.1016/j.neuroimage.2009.05.059.

Worden, J. W. (2009). *Grief counseling and grief therapy: A handbook for the mental health practitioner* (4th ed.). New York: Springer.

World Health Organization (WHO). (2020). *Palliative care: Key facts.* Retrieved from https://www.who.int/news-room/fact-sheets/detail/palliative-care. Accessed July 31, 2023.

Yadav, K. N., Gabler, N. B., Cooney, E., Kent, S., Kim, J., Herbst, N., et al. (2017). Approximately one in three US adults completes any type of advance directive for end-of-life care. *Health Affairs (Project Hope)*, 36(7), 1244–1251. doi:10.1377/hlthaff.2017.0175.

Zalenski, R. J., & Raspa, R. (2006). Maslow's hierarchy of needs: A framework for achieving human potential in hospice. *Journal of Palliative Medicine*, 9(5), 1120–1127. doi:10.1089/jpm.2006.9.1120.

Appendix A

Resources and Advocacy Groups for Older Adults

AARP
601 E Street NW
Washington, DC 20049
(888) 687-2277
http://www.aarp.org

ADA Information Line
(800) 514-0301 (voice)
(800) 514-0383 TTY
http://www.ada.gov

Administration for Community Living
330 C Street SW
Washington, DC 20201
(202) 401-4634
https://www.acl.gov

Advancing Care Excellence for Seniors
The Watergate
2600 Virginia Avenue, NW | Eighth Floor
Washington, DC 20037
(800) 669-1656
https://www.nln.org/education/teaching-resources/professional-development-programsteaching-resourcesace-all/ace-s

Alzheimer's Association National Office
225 N. Michigan Avenue, Fl. 17
Chicago, IL 60601
(800) 272-3900 (24/7 help line)
https://www.alz.org/

American Academy of Physical Medicine and Rehabilitation
330 N. Wabash Avenue, Suite 2500
Chicago, IL 60611-7617
(847) 737-6000
https://www.aapmr.org/

American Heart Association
National Center
7272 Greenville Ave
Dallas, TX 75231
(800) 242-8721
https://www.heart.org/

American Parkinson Disease Association
135 Parkinson Avenue
Staten Island, NY 10305
(800) 223-2732
https://www.apdaparkinson.org/

American Printing House for the Blind, Inc.
1839 Frankfort Ave.
Louisville, KY 40206-0085
800-223-1839 toll-free
502-895-2405
www.aph.org

Arthritis Foundation
PO Box 7669
Atlanta, GA 30357-0669
(800) 283-7800
https://www.arthritis.org/

Association of Rehabilitation Nurses
8735 W. Higgins Road, Suite 300
Chicago, IL 60631-2738
(800) 229-7530
https://rehabnurse.org/

Caregiver Action Network
1130 Connecticut Ave. NW, Ste. 501
Washington, DC 20036
202-454-3970
info@caregiveraction.org
http://caregiveraction.org

Centers for Disease Control and Prevention
(800) 232-4636
https://www.cdc.gov/chronicdisease/index.htm

Department of Housing and Urban Development
451 Seventh St. SW
Washington, DC 20410
202-708-1112
202-708-1455 TTY
www.hud.gov

APPENDIX A Resources and Advocacy Groups for Older Adults

Eldercare Locator
800-677-1116 toll-free
https://eldercare.acl.gov/Public/Index.aspx

Five-Star Quality Rating System
U.S. Centers for Medicare & Medicaid Services
7500 Security Boulevard
Baltimore, MD 21244
https://www.cms.gov/medicare/provider-enrollment-and-certification/certificationandcomplianc/fsqrs

Hartford Institute for Geriatric Nursing
433 First Avenue, 5th Floor
New York, NY 10010
https://hign.org/

Healthy People 2030
https://health.gov/healthypeople/objectives-and-data/browse-objectives/older-adults

The John A Hartford Foundation
55 East 59th Street, 16th Floor
New York, NY 10022-1713
(212) 832-7788
https://www.johnahartford.org/

Lions Club International Foundation
300 W. Twenty-second St.
Oak Brook, IL 60523
630-571-5466
https://lionsclubs.org

Lighthouse for the Blind, Inc.
359 E. Parkcenter Circle South
San Bernardino, CA 92408
(909) 884-3121
info@ielighthousefortheblind.org
https://ielighthousefortheblind.org

Meals on Wheels America
1550 Crystal Drive, Suite 1004
Arlington, VA 22202
https://www.mealsonwheelsamerica.org/

National Adult Protective Services Association
1612 K St. NW #200
Washington, DC 20006
202-370-6292
www.napsa-now.org

National Association of Area Agencies on Aging (n4a)
1100 New Jersey Ave. SE, Ste. 350
Washington, DC 20003
202-872-0888
202-872-0057 fax
info@n4a.org
www.n4a.org

National Association of Nutrition and Aging Services Programs
1612 K St., NW, Ste. 200
Washington, DC 20006
202-682-6899
202-223-2099 fax
pcarlson@nanasp.org
www.nanasp.org

National Council on Aging
251 18th Street South, Suite 500
Arlington, VA 22202
https://ncoa.org/

National Council on Disability
1331 F Street NW, Suite 850
Washington, DC 20004
(202) 272-2004
(202) 272-2074 TTY
https://www.ncd.gov/

National Hospice and Palliative Care Organization
1731 King St.
Alexandria, VA 22314
703-837-1500
703-837-1233 fax
www.nhpco.org

National Institute on Aging
Building 31, Room 5C27
31 Center Drive, MSC 2292
Bethesda, MD 20892
(800) 222-2225
(800) 222-4225 TTY
https://www.nia.nih.gov/

National Kidney Foundation
30 East 33rd Street
New York, NY 10016
(855) 653-2273
https://www.kidney.org/

National Resource Center on Native American Aging
Center for Rural Health
University of North Dakota
School of Medicine & Health Sciences, Suite E231
1301 North Columbia Road, Stop 9037
Grand Forks, ND 58202-9037
(800) 896-7628 or (701) 777-0676
https://www.nrcnaa.org/

National Stroke Association
9707 E. Easter Lane
Centennial, CO 80112
(800) STROKES
(800) 787-6537

Program of All-Inclusive Care for the Elderly
Centers for Medicare & Medicaid Services
7500 Security Boulevard
Baltimore, MD 21244
https://medicaid.gov/medicaid/long-term-services-supports/
 program-all-inclusive-care-elderly/index.html

Substance Abuse and Mental Health Services Administration
5600 Fishers Lane
Rockville, MD 20857
(877) 726-4727
https://www.samhsa.gov/resources-serving-older-adults
https://www.stroke.org/en/

USAging
100 New Jersey Avenue, SE, Suite 350
Washington, DC 20003
(202) 872-0888
https://www.usaging.org/

US Department of Veterans Affairs
Benefits hotline: (800) 827-1000
https://www.benefits.va.gov/persona/veteran-elderly.asp

INDEX

Note: Page numbers followed by "f" indicate figures, "t" indicate tables, and "b" indicate boxes.

A

AAA. *See* Area Agencies on Aging
AARP. *See* American Association of Retired Persons
Abandonment, 20
Abdomen
   acute, 361
   pain in, 361, 361f
   wall of, age-related changes in, 358t
Absorption, in pharmacokinetics, 212
Abuse
   alcohol, 225–227
      assessment of, 226, 226t
      BMAST for, 224
      CAGE tool for, 224
      evaluation of, 227
      interventions of, 226–227
      prevalence of, 225–226
   defined, 145
   emotional, 20, 145
   financial, 145
   institutional, 20
   physical, 20, 145
   psychologic, 145
   sexual, 20, 145
Access services, for older adults, 514b
Accessory apartment, 516t
Accessory organs, disorders of, 374–381
Accreditation, by TJC, 19
Acebutolol, 294–296t
ACEIs. *See* Angiotensin-converting enzyme inhibitors
Acetaminophen, 174
Acetaminophen/hydrocodone (Vicodin, Norco), 96t
Acetylcholine (ACh), 446t
ACh. *See* Acetylcholine
Acquired gout, 426
Acrochordons, 239, 239f
Actinic keratosis, 244–246, 245f
Action, 83
Activities of daily living (ADLs), 117–118
   instrumental, 118
   Katz Index of, 49, 49f
Activity, 117–121
   activities of daily living (ADLs), 117–118
   Alzheimer disease effect on, 120–121
   dementia and, 120–121
   home care in, 121b
   intolerance of, 540
   lifestyle changes in, 118–120
   loss of partner and, 119–120
   patterns in, assessment of, 88
   physical exercise, 118
   relocation and, 118–119, 119b, 119f
   retirement and, 118
Acupuncture, 225
Acute abdomen, 361
Acute care for elders (ACE) units, 49–51
Acute care setting, 506
   adverse drug reactions in, 507
   assessment of function in, 50b

Acute care setting *(Continued)*
   critical care in, 510–511
   environment, 507–509, 509b
   falls in, 507–508
   hazards of immobility in, 509
   health status and, 9–10
   infection in, 509
   nursing in, 509–511
   older adults' characteristics in, 506–507
   philosophy of care in, 507, 508f
   risk in, 507–509
   safety features of, 509, 509b
   trauma care in, 510–511
Acute grief responses, 573
Acute kidney injury (AKI), 398–399, 399b
Acute respiratory tract infections, coughing and, 330
ADA. *See* Americans with Disabilities Act
Adaptation, with chronic illness, 538
Adenosine receptor antagonist, for Parkinson disease, 465t
Adhesion, in intestine, 370f
ADLs. *See* Activities of daily living
Adoptive cell transfer, 561
Adrenal cortex, 483t
Adrenal medulla, 483t
Adrenopause, 483
Adult. *See* Older adults
Adult day care, 459
Adult day care services, 516–517
Adult protective services, 21
Adult respiratory distress syndrome, 349
Advance Health Directive, 63t
Advance medical directives, 26
Advocacy, need for, 77
Affective assessment, of older adult, 51–54, 51t, 52f, 53f
Affordable Care Act (ACA), 25
Age cohorts
   Great Depression and, 70–71
   World War II, 70–71
Ageism, 11
Age-related changes
   in approaching death, 577–578
   contributing to falling, 126–127
      cardiovascular factors, 126
      hearing as, 126
      musculoskeletal factors as, 126–127
      neurologic factors as, 127
      vision as, 126
   in nature of disease and disability, 38
   in pharmacokinetics, 212t
   in sleep, 109–110, 109b
   in smell, 286
   in taste, 286
Age-related disorders, in history taking, 44t
Age-related macular degeneration (AMD), 276–277
Aggression, nonpharmacological management of, 457t

Aging
   cancer and, 551–553, 552f
   cardiovascular system and, 290–291
   gastrointestinal system and, 357–360, 358–359b, 358t
   hearing and, 281
   immune system and, 183, 183b
   integumentary function and, 237–238, 237b
      in dermal appendages, 237
      in dermatoporosis, 237–238
      in dermis, 237
      in epidermis, 237
      in subcutaneous fat, 237
   musculoskeletal system and, 414–415
   pain and, 164
   in place, 7
   respiratory system and, 325–328, 326t, 327t
   sexuality and, 150–162, 150b
   urinary function and, 388–389, 389f
   vision and, 271f, 272
Aging population, increasing, 60
Agitation, nonpharmacological management of, 457t
AKI. *See* Acute kidney injury
Albumin, 99, 202t, 204
Albuterol (Ventolin, Proventil), 96t
Alcohol
   abuse of, 225–227
      assessment of, 226, 226t
      BMAST for, 224
      CAGE tool for, 224
      evaluation of, 227
      interventions of, 226–227
      prevalence of, 225–226
   sexuality and, 154t
   sleep and, 112
   trends in, 229
   use of, advantages and disadvantages of, 86t
Aldosterone antagonist
   adverse effects of, 294–296t
   for CHD, 311t
Alkaline phosphatase, serum levels of, 202t, 205
Alkylating agents, for cancer, 560t
Allergies, in health history format, 46
Alopecia, 564
Alpha$_1$-blockers, adverse effects of, 294–296t
Alpha$_2$-agonists, adverse effects of, 294–296t
Altered thought processes. *See* Cognitive disorders
Alzheimer disease (AD), 451–453
   activity affected by, 120–121
   clinical manifestations of, 452–453, 452f
   death from, 535t
   diagnostic evaluation of, 453
   genetic factors for, 452
   mild, 453
   moderate, 453
   nonpharmacological management of, 453
   pharmacological management of, 453
   preclinical, 452
   risk factors for, 451–452
   severe, 453

591

INDEX

Amebiasis, 369
American Nurses Association (ANA), 2-3, 19
American Social Security program, 5-6
American Society for Parenteral and Enteral Nutrition (ASPEN), 98
Americans with Disabilities Act (ADA), 543
Amiloride, 294-296t
Amlodipine, 294-296t
Amlodipine (Norvasc), 96t
Ampullary disequilibrium, 285
Amputation, 435-437
    assessment of, 435
    evaluation of, 436-437
    nursing care guidelines for, 435-437
    nursing care plan for, 436-437b
    nursing interventions for, 435-436
    patient problems in, 435
    planning for, 435
    postoperative care in, 435-436
    preoperative care in, 435
    prosthetic fitting and adaptation in, 436
    rehabilitative care in, 436
Amylase, serum levels of, 202t, 203-204
ANA. *See* American Nurses Association
Analgesics
    as first-line approach, 174
    nonopioid, 174
    opioid, 174-176, 220
    for pain, 171
Androgens in Men Study (AIMS), 152
Andropause, 491
Anemia, 127b, 318-320
    assessment of, 319, 320b
    chemotherapy-induced, 562
    diagnosis of, 319
    diagnostic tests, procedures, and treatment of, 319
    evaluation of, 320
    interventions for, 320
    pernicious, 367
    planning for, 319
    prognosis of, 319
Anesthesia, lung function and, 329
Angina, 298
Angiomas, cherry, 238, 238f
Angioplasty, percutaneous transluminal coronary, 300
Angiotensin receptor blockers, 220
Angiotensin-converting enzyme inhibitors (ACEIs), 294-296t, 311t
Anions, 200
Anorexia, 361
    of aging, 95
    in cancer, 564
Anorgasmia, 152
Anterior cerebral artery, 469
Anterior pituitary gland, 483t
Anthropometrics, 99
Antianxiety medications, sexuality and, 154t
Antibiotics
    antitumor, for cancer, 560t
    for COPD, 336
Anticholinergics
    for asthma, 332
    for COPD, 336
    for Parkinson disease, 465t
Anticipatory grief, 575
Anticipatory nausea and vomiting, 562-563

Anticoagulants, 200b, 299-300
Anticonvulsants
    for pain, 176
    sexuality and, 154t
Antidepressants, 218-219
    profiles of, 219t
    sexuality and, 154t
Antiepileptics, 154t
Antihistamines, sexuality and, 154t
Antihypertensives, 154t, 220
Anti-inflammatory agents, for asthma, 331
Antimalarials, 427t
Antimetabolites, for cancer, 560t
Antimicrobials, 220
Antiplatelets, 299-300
Antipsychotics, 154t, 218, 456
    for dementia, 456, 458-459b
Antirheumatics, 427t
Antiseptic solution, 261
Antitumor antibiotics, for cancer, 560t
Anus, age-related changes in, 358t
Anxiety, 473-474
    nonpharmacological management of, 457t
Anxiolytics, 218
Aortic regurgitation, 308b
Aortic stenosis, 307, 308b
Apartment, accessory, 516t
Apathy, nonpharmacological management of, 457t
Apnea, obstructive sleep, 352-353
    assessment of, 353
    diagnosis of, 353
    diagnostic tests and procedures for, 352
    evaluation after, 353
    intervention for, 353, 353f
    planning for, 353
    prognosis of, 353
    treatment of, 352-353
Appendages, dermal, age-related changes in, 237
Arcus senilis, 272
Area Agencies on Aging (AAA), 77, 515
Aromatherapy, 527
Arrhythmia, 127b, 303-305
    assessment of, 304
    diagnosis of, 304
    diagnostic tests and procedures for, 303
    evaluation of, 305
    interventions for, 304-305
    planning for, 304
    prognosis of, 304
    symptoms of, 304
    treatment of, 303-304, 305b
Arterial blood gas testing
    bicarbonate in, 207
    blood pH in, 207, 207t
    carbon dioxide in, 207
    components of, 207-208, 207t
    oxygen saturation in, 208
    partial pressure of oxygen in, 207
Arterial insufficiency, 318t
Arterial ulcers, 248-249, 248t
Arthritis
    gouty, 426-428, 428f
        assessment of, 428
        evaluation of, 428
        nursing care guidelines for, 428
        nursing interventions for, 428
        patient problems in, 428
        planning for, 428

Arthritis *(Continued)*
    osteoarthritis, 420-423, 421f
        assessment of, 421
        benefits of shared yoga intervention for, 421-422b
        evaluation of, 423
        nursing care guidelines for, 421-423
        nursing interventions for, 421-423
        patient problems in, 421
        planning for of, 421
        rheumatoid arthritis *versus,* 425t
    rheumatoid, 186, 424-426, 424f
        assessment of, 425
        deformities of, 425f
        drugs for, 427t
        evaluation of, 426
        nursing care guidelines for, 425-426
        nursing interventions for, 425-426
        osteoarthritis *versus,* 425t
        patient problems in, 425
        planning for, 425
Ascites, 378
Aspartate aminotransferase, 205
ASPEN. *See* American Society for Parenteral and Enteral Nutrition
Aspiration, coughing and, 330
Aspirin, 174, 300, 427t
Assessment, 36-56, 36b. *See also* Cognitive function; Health history
    affective, 51-54, 51t, 52f, 53f
    cognitive, 51-54, 51t, 52f, 53f
    functional status, 48-51, 49f, 50b
    interrelationship between physical and psychosocial aspects of aging in, 37-38, 37t
    laboratory data in, 54
    nature of disease and disability in, 38-42
        age-related changes, 38
        atypical presentation of illness, 38-39, 39b, 39t
        cognitive assessment, 40-42, 40b, 41t
    pain, 169-173, 170t
    prevention and, 85-89
    social, 54, 55f
    special considerations affecting, 37-42
    tailoring, 42, 42b
Assisted living facility, 514, 516t
Assisted suicide, 30-31
Assisted-listening devices, 284b
Association for Advancement of Retired People (AARP), Grief and Loss, 567
Asthma, 330-334
    assessment of, 332, 332f
    classification of, 333t
    diagnosis of, 333, 333t
    evaluation after, 334
    intervention for, 333-334
    planning for, 333
    prognosis of, 331
    treatment of, 331-332
        long-term control medications for, 331
        quick-relief medications for, 331-332
        stepwise approach to, 332
Asymptomatic bacteriuria, 403-404, 404-405b
Ataxia, of aging, vestibular, 285
Atenolol, 294-296t
Atherosclerosis, 298
Atorvastatin (Lipitor), 96t
Atrial fibrillation, 303-304, 306
Atrioventricular (AV) node, 290

Atrophic AMD, 276
Attitude, 43
Auranofin, 427t
Autoimmune diseases, 182
Autoimmune thyroiditis, 497–498
Autoimmunity, 185–186
Autolysis, 259b
Automobile safety, 144–145
Autonomy, 25–30
Awakenings, nocturnal, 109
Azilsartan, 294–296t

B

Baby Boomers, 460
Baby boomers, 71
Bacillus Calmette-Guérin (BCG), 561
Bacteria, in urine, 206–207, 206t, 208b
Bacteriuria, 208b
Balance
    abnormalities of, 128t
    hearing and, 280–286
    Tinetti test of, 128f
Barbiturates, 218
Barium enemas, 84t
Basal cell carcinoma, 246, 246f
Basophils, in hematology test, 197t, 198
Beers Criteria for Potentially Inappropriate Medication Use in Older Adults, 213
Behavior modification
    fall prevention with, 129–130, 130t
    smoking cessation with, 228
Behavioral and psychological symptoms of dementia (BPSD), treatment of, 456, 457t
Behavioral variant frontotemporal dementia, 454
Belching, 362
Benazepril, 294–296t
Benign paroxysmal positional vertigo, 285
Benign prostatic hyperplasia (BPH), 408–410, 409–410b, 409b
    assessment of, 408–409
    drugs for, sexuality and, 154t
    nursing interventions for, 409–410
    patient problems in, 409
    planning for, 409
Benzodiazepines, 218
Bereavement, 572–573
Beta-blockers
    adverse effects of, 294–296t
    for CAD, 299
    for CHD, 311t
    for hypertension, 293
Beta$_2$-agonists, for COPD, 335–336
Betaxolol, 294–296t
Bicarbonate, 207
Biguanides, for type 2 diabetes mellitus, 489t
Bile ducts, 359
Biographic data, in health history format, 44
Biophysical agents, 266
Bisoprolol, 294–296t
Bladder
    age-related changes in, 388–389
    cancer, 408
    diary, 393f
    habits, 392
    retraining, 395
Blepharitis, 273
Bloating, 362

Blood. *See also* Arterial blood gas testing; Fecal occult blood test; Hematology test
    cells
        red, 197t, 198
        white, 197t, 198
    oxygen-carrying capacity of, 327
    pH of, 207, 207t
    therapeutic drug monitoring in, 208
    in urine, 206t, 207
    vessels, age-related changes in, 290–291
Blood chemistry testing
    albumin in, 202t, 204
    alkaline phosphatase in, 202t, 205
    amylase in, 202t, 203–204
    aspartate aminotransferase in, 202t, 205
    brain natriuretic peptide in, 205
    calcium in, 202t, 203
    chloride in, 202t, 203
    cholesterol in, total, 202t, 204
    components of, 200–206, 202t
    creatine kinase in, 202t, 205
    creatinine in, 202t, 204
    electrolytes in, 200–203
    glucose, 202t, 203
    lactate dehydrogenase in, 205
    magnesium in, 202t, 203
    phosphorus in, 202t, 203
    potassium in, 201, 202t
    prealbumin in, 204
    protein in, total, 202t, 204
    PSA in, 206
    sodium in, 201, 202t
    of thyroid function, 205–206
    triglycerides in, 204
    troponin in, 205
    TSH in, 205–206, 205t
    urea nitrogen in, 202t, 204
Blood urea nitrogen (BUN), 202t, 204
BMI. *See* Body mass index
Body mass index (BMI), 297
Bone. *See also* Fractures
    metastases, prostate cancer with, 175b
Bone marrow suppression, 562
    coping with, 562
Borborygmi, 371
Boutonnière deformity, 425f
Bowel
    obstructions, 370f
    training, 364b
BPH. *See* Benign prostatic hyperplasia
Bradyarrhythmias, 306
Brain, 445, 445f
Brain natriuretic peptide, 205
Breast cancer, 554–555
    early detection of, 554
    risk factors for, 554
    screening for, 551b
    sexuality and, 155
    signs and symptoms of, 554
    survival in, 555
    treatment of, 554–555
Breast self-examination, 554
Breathing
    diaphragmatic, 339b, 339f
    mechanics of, 326t
    pattern, 326t
    pursed-lip, 339b, 339f

Breathing *(Continued)*
    retraining, 339
    sleep and, 326t
Brief Michigan Alcoholism Screening Test (BMAST), 224
Bristol stool chart, 362–363, 362f
Brittle bone disease, 428–429
Bronchitis, chronic, coughing and, 330, 334
Bronchodilators, for COPD, 335
Buck extension, 416f
Bullectomy, 336
Bumetanide, 294–296t
BUN. *See* Blood urea nitrogen
Bundle of His, 290
Bunions, 439, 439f
Burn injuries, 138–139. *See also* Fire

C

CABG. *See* Coronary artery bypass graft
Cachexia, 97
    in cancer, 564
CAD. *See* Coronary artery disease
Caffeine
    products with, 394
    sleep and, 111
CAGE tool, 224
Calcium
    dietary sources of, 430t
    serum levels of, 202t, 203
Calcium channel blockers, 215t, 293, 294–296t, 299
Calluses, 438
Calories
    in renal diet, 402b
    for type 2 diabetes mellitus, 491b
CAM. *See* Complementary and alternative medicine
Cancer, 549, 549b. *See also* Basal cell carcinoma; Melanoma; Squamous cell carcinoma
    aging and, 551–553, 552f
    breast, 554–555
        cultural considerations in, 551b
        early detection of, 554
        risk factors for, 554
        signs and symptoms of, 554
        survival in, 555
        treatment of, 554–555
    colorectal, 383–384, 556
        assessment of, 384
        early detection of, 556
        evaluation of, 384
        nursing interventions for, 384
        patient problems with, 384
        planning for, 384
        risk factors of, 556
        screening, 84t
        sexuality and, 155
        signs and symptoms of, 556
        treatment of, 556
    complications with, 561–564, 563b
        alopecia as, 564
        anorexia as, 564
        bone marrow suppression as, 562
        cachexia as, 564
        diarrhea as, 564
        nausea and vomiting, 562–563
    coughing and, 330
    death from, 535t
    depression and, 566

INDEX

Cancer (Continued)
  esophageal, 381–382
    assessment of, 381
    evaluation of, 381–382
    nursing care plan for, 382b
    nursing interventions for, 381
    patient problems with, 381
    planning for, 381
  gastric, 382–383
    assessment of, 383
    evaluation of, 383
    nursing interventions for, 383
    patient problems with, 383
    planning for, 383
  of gastrointestinal system, 381–385
  grief and loss and, 566–567
  home care for, 568b
  immune function and, 185
  incidence of, 549–550, 550t
  lung, 341–342, 553–554
    assessment of, 342
    diagnosis of, 342
    diagnostic tests and procedures for, 341, 341t
    early detection of, 554
    evaluation after, 342
    intervention for, 342
    planning for, 342
    risk factors of, 553
    signs and symptoms of, 553
    treatment for, 341, 554
  oral, 381
  prostate, 410–411, 555–556
    assessment of, 410
    with bone metastases, 175b
    early detection of, 555
    evaluation of, 411
    nursing care plan for, 411b
    nursing interventions for, 410–411
    patient problems with, 410
    planning for, 410
    risk factors for, 555
    screening for, advantages and disadvantages of, 86t
    sexuality and, 155
    signs and symptoms of, 555
    treatment for, 555–556
  quality of life with, 564–566, 565–566b, 565f
  racial and ethnic patterns of, 550–551, 551b
  resources and support with, 567–568
  screening for, 556–557
  social isolation and loneliness, 567
  treatment of, 557–561
    bone marrow/stem transplant as, 561
    chemotherapy for, 559, 560t
    hormone therapy for, 561
    immunotherapy for, 561
    radiation therapy for, 558–559
    surgery for, 558
    targeted therapy for, 559
Candesartan, 294–296t
Candida albicans, 364
Candidiasis, 242–243, 242f
Cane, 420f
Cannabis, 228–229
  assessment of, 228
  evaluation of, 228–229
  interventions of, 228–229
  prevalence of, 228

Capsaicin cream, 427t
Captopril, 294–296t
Carbohydrates, for type 2 diabetes mellitus, 491b
Carbon dioxide, 207
Carbon monoxide, poisoning with, 139–140, 140b
Cardiac arrhythmias, 306
Cardiac glycosides, for CHD, 311t
Cardiac rehabilitation, 301
Cardiogenic pulmonary edema, 349
  diagnostic tests and procedures for, 349
  prognosis of, 349
  treatment of, 349
Cardiopulmonary resuscitation (CPR), 26
Cardiovascular disease (CVD), 291–320, 291b
  anemia, 318–320
    assessment of, 319, 320b
    diagnosis of, 319
    diagnostic tests, procedures, and treatment of, 319
    evaluation of, 320
    interventions for, 320
    planning for, 319
    prognosis of, 319
  arrhythmia, 127b, 303–305
    assessment of, 304
    diagnosis of, 304
    diagnostic tests and procedures for, 303
    evaluation of, 305
    interventions for, 304–305
    planning for, 304
    prognosis of, 304
    symptoms of, 304
    treatment of, 303–304, 305b
  chronic venous insufficiency, 316–318
    assessment of, 318, 318t
    diagnosis of, 318
    diagnostic tests and procedures for, 317
    evaluation of, 318
    interventions for, 318
    planning for, 318
    treatment of, 317–318
  congestive heart failure, 309–314, 310t, 313–314b
    assessment of, 312–314, 313–314b
    case study, 314b
    coughing and, 330
    diagnosis of, 312
    diagnostic tests and procedures for, 310, 310b
    diastolic, 312
    evaluation of, 313–314
    interventions for, 313
    planning for, 312–313
    presentation of, 39t
    prognosis of, 312
    systolic, 311–312
    treatment of, 311–312, 311t
      ACEIs in, 311t
      aldosterone antagonist in, 311t
      beta-blockers in, 311t
      cardiac glycosides in, 311t
      diuretics in, 311t
      sympathomimetics in, 311t
  coronary artery disease, 298–303
    assessment of, 300–303, 301b
    diagnosis of, 300–301
    diagnostic tests and procedures for, 298–299
    evaluation of, 302–303
    in female, 300
    intervention of, 301–302

Cardiovascular disease (Continued)
    nonpharmacologic treatment of, 300
      CABG in, 300
      PTCA in, 300
      stents for, 300
    pharmacologic treatment of, 299–300
      anticoagulants in, 299–300
      antiplatelets in, 299–300
      beta-blockers in, 299
      calcium channel blockers in, 299
      fibrinolytics in, 299–300
      lipid-lowering drugs in, 300
      nitrates in, 299
    planning for, 301
    prognosis of, 300
    symptoms of, 298b
  hypertension, 291–296, 291b
    assessment of, 293
    drug-induced, 292
    evaluation of, 296
    heart disease and, 290
    intervention for, 296
    patient problems of, 293–296
    pharmacologic treatment of, 292–293, 294–296t
      beta-blockers for, 293
      calcium channel blockers for, 293
      diuretics for, 293
    planning for, 296
    primary, 292
    prognosis of, 293
    secondary, 292
  orthostatic hypotension, 305–306
    assessment of, 305–306
    diagnosis of, 306
    evaluation of, 306
    intervention for, 306
    planning for, 306
  peripheral artery disease, 315–317, 316b
    assessment of, 316, 316b
    diagnosis of, 316
    diagnostic tests and procedures for, 315
    evaluation of, 316–317, 317b
    interventions for, 316
    planning for, 316
    prognosis of, 315–316
    surgical procedures for, 315
    treatment of, 315
  risk factors for, 291b, 296–298, 297b
    diabetes mellitus as, 297
    diet as, 296–297
    estrogen as, 298
    hypertension as, 290
    menopause as, 298
    obesity as, 297
    physical activity as, 297
    sedentary lifestyle as, 297
    smoking as, 297
    stress as, 298
  syncope, 306–307
    assessment of, 307
    diagnosis of, 307
    evaluation of, 307
    intervention for, 307
    planning for, 307
  valvular heart disease, 307–309
    assessment of, 308
    diagnosis of, 308

Cardiovascular disease *(Continued)*
    diagnostic tests and procedures for, 307–308
    evaluation of, 309
    interventions for, 308–309
    manifestations of, 308b
    planning for, 308
    prognosis of, 308
    treatment of, 308
Cardiovascular factors, fall related to, 126
Cardiovascular function, 290, 290b. *See also* Cardiovascular system
Cardiovascular system
    age-related changes in, 290–291
    conduction system in, 290
    drugs for, 219–220
    exercise program for, 291
    home care for, 321b
    response to stress and exercise of, 291
    vessels in, 290–291
Care. *See also* Acute care setting; Family; Home care; Palliative care
    community standard of, 19
    continuity of, 511–513, 512b
    critical, 510–511, 511t
    day, 516–517
    intensive, 510
    long-term, 516t, 519–520, 519t, 520b
    settings, 512, 527b
    special, 514
    subacute, 514
    TJC accreditation of, 19
    trauma, 510–511
Care facility, family and, 67–68
Care setting. *see* Acute care setting; Home care; Hospitals; Nursing facilities; Nursing homes
Caregivers
    chronic illness effect on, 541
    family, 61
        education of, 65–66, 65b
        respite programs in, 65–66
        support groups for, 66
    stress, nursing implications of, 541
Caregiving, family, 63–65
Carvedilol, 294–296t
Casts and cast care, 419–420, 420b
Cataracts, 274–276
    nursing care plan for, 274–276, 276b
    surgery, home care after, 275b
Catechol-O-methyltransferase (COMT), for Parkinson disease, 465t
Catheter, indwelling, 404b
Cations, 200
CCRC. *See* Continuing care retirement community
Central nervous system (CNS), 444–447
Cerebral infarction, 469
Cerebrovascular accident (CVA), 469–473, 469f
    assessment for, 472
    clinical manifestations of, 469
    complications of, 469–470
    diagnostic evaluation of, 470
    evaluation for, 473
    intervention for, 472–473
    levels of prevention for, 470t
    management of, 470–472
        long-term, 471–472
        medical and pharmacologic therapy for, 470–471

Cerebrovascular accident *(Continued)*
    patient problems of, 472
    planning for, 472
    risk factors for, 469
Cerebrovascular disease, death from, 535t
Certification, 3, 4b
Cerumen impaction, 281–282
Cervical smear test, 84t
    advantages and disadvantages of, 86t
Charcot joint, 128t
CHD. *See* Coronary heart disease
Chemical restraints, 23–24
Chemotherapy
    for cancer, 560t
    effects of, 190–191b
    myelosuppressive toxicities of, 561–562b
    nutritional consequences of, 563b
    pharmacodynamics of, 559
    pharmacokinetics of, 559
    for prostate cancer, 555
Chemotherapy-induced nausea and vomiting (CINV), 562–563
Cherry angiomas, 238, 238f
Chest pain, assessment of, 301b
Chest physiotherapy (CPT), COPD and, 339
CHF. *See* Congestive heart failure
Chloride, 202t, 203
Chlorothiazide, 294–296t
Chlorthalidone, 294–296t
Cholecystitis, 374–375
    assessment of, 375
    evaluation of, 375
    nursing interventions for, 375
    patient problems with, 375
    planning for, 375
Cholelithiasis, 374–375
    assessment of, 375
    evaluation of, 375
    nursing interventions for, 375
    patient problems with, 375
    planning for, 375
Cholestasis, 380
Cholesterol
    HDL, 202t, 204
    heart disease risk and, 296–297
    LDL, 202t, 204–205
Cholinesterase inhibitors, for dementia, 454
Chronic cancer-related pain (CRP), 166b
Chronic Care Model, 538–539
Chronic conditions, definition of, 507, 535
Chronic disease, health status affected by, 9
Chronic grief, 575
Chronic illness, 534–546
    activity intolerance from, 540
    adaptation with, 538
    adherence in, 537
    case study in, 546b
    deaths from, 535t
    definition of, 546
    experience of, 536
    family and caregivers affected by, 541
    fatigue from, 540
    health within, 536
    immobility from, 540
    life issues with, 545
    pain from, 540
    patient-centered approach in, 537, 537b
    physiologic needs with, 540–541

Chronic illness *(Continued)*
    powerlessness from, 539
    prevalence of, 535–536, 536t
    psychosocial adaptation, nursing interventions to assist, 539–540
    psychosocial needs with, 538
    quality of life and, 538
    sexual activity and, 540–541
    social isolation from, 539
    as stigma, 539
    trajectory framework of, 538
Chronic kidney disease (CKD), 399–403, 399b, 400b
Chronic lower respiratory disease, death from, 535t
Chronic obstructive pulmonary disease (COPD), 334–341
    antibiotics for, 336
    anticholinergics for, 336
    assessment of, 336–341
    $beta_2$-agonists for, 335–336
    breathing retraining for, 339
    bronchodilators for, 335
    chest physiotherapy for, 339
    diagnosis of, 336–337
    diagnostic tests and procedures for, 334–335, 335t
    evaluation after, 341
    exacerbations for, 340–341
    glucocorticosteroids for, 336
    home oxygen therapy for, 340
    intervention for, 337–341
    medications for, 339–340, 340b
    nursing care plan for, 337–338b
    nutrition and, 95, 338–339, 339b
    oxygen therapy for, 336
    planning for, 337
    pulmonary hygiene for, 339, 340b
    pulmonary rehabilitation, 338–340
    self-management in ethno-cultural communities, 330b
    self-monitoring for, 340–341
    signs and symptoms of, 334
    smoking cessation and, 338, 338t
    surgical options for, 336
    treatment for, 335–336
    vaccines for, 336
Chronic postsurgical pain (CPSP), 166b
Chronic posttraumatic pain (CPSP), 166b
Chronic primary headache, 166b
Chronic primary musculoskeletal pain (CPMP), 166b
Chronic primary pain (CPP), 166b
Chronic primary visceral pain (CPVP), 166b
Chronic secondary headache, 166b
Chronic secondary musculoskeletal pain (CMP), 166b
Chronic secondary pain, 166b
Chronic venous insufficiency, 316–318
    assessment of, 318, 318t
    diagnosis of, 318
    diagnostic tests and procedures for, 317
    evaluation of, 318
    interventions for, 318
    planning for, 318
    treatment of, 317–318
Chronic widespread pain (CWP), 166b
Chronicity, 534–541

Cigarettes. See Nicotine; Smoking; Smoking cessation
Circadian rhythm, sleep and, 109
Cirrhosis
　assessment of, 379
　clinical manifestations of, 379f
　evaluation of, 380
　nursing interventions for, 380
　patient problems with, 379
　planning for, 379–380
　secondary to alcohol use disorder, 378–380
CKD. see Chronic kidney disease
Claudication, intermittent, in PAD, 315
Clavicular fracture, 419, 420b, 420f
Clinically Aligned Pain Assessment Tool (CAPA), 173t
Clonidine, 294–296t
Clostridium botulinum, 369
Clostridium difficile, 186, 189b
Codeine, 175
Cognitive assessment, of older adult, 51–54, 51t, 52f, 53f
Cognitive behavioral therapy (CBT), for depression, 449
Cognitive disorders
　associated with altered thought processes, 448–460
　case study on, 466–468b, 478b
　problems and conditions in, 460–475
　resources for, 459–460
　　adult day care, 459
　　community mental health centers, 460
　　family support groups as, 459
　　home health care, 459–460
　　legal services, 460
　　long-term care services, 460
　　psychiatric hospitals, 460
　　respite services, 459
Cognitive function, 444–478
　assessment of
　　depression, 447
　　functional, 448–449
　　evaluation of, 446–447
　　home care and, 472–473b, 515
　　in typical aging, 447, 448t
Cognitive status, in critical care, 511t
Cognitively impaired patients, urinary function in, 396–397
Cognitively intact patients, urinary function in, 395–396
Coital positioning, for older couples, 159f
Colles fractures, 419
Colon, sigmoid, volvulus of, 370f
Colonoscopy, 84t
　advantages and disadvantages of, 86t
Colon polyps, 373–374
　assessment of, 374
　evaluation of, 374
　nursing interventions for, 374
　patient problems with, 374
　planning for, 374
Colorectal cancer, 383–384, 556
　assessment of, 384
　early detection of, 556
　evaluation of, 384
　nursing interventions for, 384
　patient problems with, 384
　planning for, 384

Colorectal cancer *(Continued)*
　risk factors of, 556
　screening, 84t
　sexuality and, 155
　signs and symptoms of, 556
　treatment of, 556
Colorectal screening, 84t
Columbia Suicide Severity Rating Scale (C-SSRS), 460
Comfort theory, 577, 577f
Comminuted fracture, 415f
Common grief, 575
Communication, between patient's directives and family desires, 30
Community-acquired infections, 184
Community-acquired pneumonia, 185, 345
Community-based services, 514
　for older adults, 514b
　profile of, 515–517
Community health centers, 72b
Community standard of care, 19
Community mental health centers, in cognitive disorder, 460
Competency framework, in geriatric nursing education, 13b, 14f
Complementary and alternative medicine (CAM). *See also* Herbal remedies
　for pain, 177
　for sleep, 117, 117b
Complex grief, 575
Complex regional pain syndrome (CRPS), 166b
Complex sleep apnea syndrome (CompSAS), 112
Complicated grief, 575
Conduction system, age-related changes in, 290
Confusion Assessment Method (CAM), 40, 40b, 450
Congestive heart failure (CHF), 309–314, 310t, 313–314b
　assessment of, 312–314, 313–314b
　case study, 314b
　coughing and, 330
　diagnosis of, 312
　diagnostic tests and procedures for, 310, 310b
　diastolic, 312
　evaluation of, 313–314
　interventions for, 313
　planning for, 312–313
　presentation of, 39t
　prognosis of, 312
　systolic, 311–312
　treatment of, 311–312, 311t
　　ACEIs in, 311t
　　aldosterone antagonist in, 311t
　　beta-blockers in, 311t
　　cardiac glycosides in, 311t
　　diuretics in, 311t
　　sympathomimetics in, 311t
Congregate housing, 516t
Constipation, 362–363, 577
　high-fiber foods to relieve, 176b
　from opioids, 176b
　from polypharmacy, 362–363
　as side effect of opioid, 175–176, 176b
Contemplation, 82–83
Continuing care retirement community (CCRC), 516t
Continuity of care, 511–513, 512b, 516t
Continuous ambulator peritoneal dialysis, 401b

Continuous cycle peritoneal dialysis, 401b
Continuum of care, 10–11
Cooling fans, injuries from, 140–141
COPD. *See* Chronic obstructive pulmonary disease
Coping, patterns in, assessment of, 87
Corns, 438, 438f
Coronary artery bypass graft (CABG), 300
Coronary artery disease (CAD), 298–303
　assessment of, 300–303, 301b
　diagnosis of, 300–301
　diagnostic tests and procedures for, 298–299
　evaluation of, 302–303
　in female, 300
　intervention of, 301–302
　nonpharmacologic treatment of, 300
　　CABG in, 300
　　PTCA in, 300
　　stents for, 300
　pharmacologic treatment of, 299–300
　　anticoagulants in, 299–300
　　antiplatelets in, 299–300
　　beta-blockers in, 299
　　calcium channel blockers in, 299
　　fibrinolytics in, 299–300
　　lipid-lowering drugs in, 300
　　nitrates in, 299
　planning for, 301
　prognosis of, 300
　symptoms of, 298b
Coronary heart disease (CHD), 290. see also Coronary artery disease
Corticobasal syndrome, 454
Corticosteroids, for asthma, 332
Cough, 330
Coumadin. see Warfarin
CPR. *See* Cardiopulmonary resuscitation
Cramps, muscle, 440
C-reactive protein, in hematology test, 200
Creatine kinase, serum levels of, 202t, 205
Creatinine, 204
　clearance of, 204
　serum levels of, 202t, 204
Credential, 4b
Crepitus, 420–421
Crime, prevention of, 144
Critical care, 510–511, 511t
Cromolyn, 331
Cues to action, 83
Cultural awareness
　in breast cancer screening, 551b
　cultural assessment and, 42b
　health literacy, 45b
　interviewer and, 42b
　nutritional needs, 47b
　skin assessment in darkly pigmented skin, 238b
Cultural competency, 536–537
Curbs, as risk factor for falling, 129
CVD. *See* Cardiovascular disease
Cyanosis, 336
Cytokines, for cancer, 561

D

DASH diet, 320b
Dating, 151
Day care services, 516–517
Daytime napping, 110
Daytime sleepiness, 109–110

INDEX

D-dimer test, 197t, 200
Death and dying
　age-related changes in, 577–578
　approaching, 577–584
　assessment in, 578–581, 579t, 580f
　case study, 583b
　causes of, leading, 535t
　comfort theory in, 577, 577f
　evidence-based practice, 584b
　general health care needs in, 577
　hospice in, 584
　interventions for, 581–584, 581t, 582f
　legislative initiatives in, 584–585
　nursing care in, 578–584
　nutritional considerations, 583b
　palliative care in, 584
Debridement, 259b
Decisions, practice, 30–32
Deep vein thrombosis (DVT), 317
Degenerative joint disease, 420
Degradation changes, in endocrine system, 484t
Dehydration, 95–97, 200–201
Delirium, 450–451
　characteristics of, 511t
　clinical features of, 449t
　clinical manifestations of, 450
　dementia *versus*, 41t
　management of, 450–451
　　nonpharmacologic interventions for, 450–451
　　pharmacotherapy for, 451
　risk factors for, 450
Delirium tremens, 226b
Dementia, 451–459
　activity and, 120–121
　advanced, feeding tubes in, 365b
　assessment for, 456
　characteristics of, 511t
　clinical features of, 449t
　delirium *versus*, 41t
　frontotemporal, 454
　interventions for, 456–459
　Lewy body, 454
　mixed, 455
　nonpharmacological measures, 456, 458f
　nutrition and, 95
　patient problems of, 456
　person-centered care, 455–456
　planning for, 456
　reversible, 451, 452b
　sexuality and, 155
　sleep and, 112
　vascular, 453
Demerol. *See* Meperidine
Demographic profile
　of drug use, 211
　education in, 8
　employment in, 8
　gender in, 6–7
　geographic distribution in, 7–8
　income in, 8, 8f
　living arrangements in, 7, 7f
　marital status in, 6–7
　of older Americans, 6, 6f
　of older population, 6
　poverty in, 8, 8f
　race and ethnicity in, 7
Dental caries, malnutrition and, 97
Dependence, in family, 67

Depression, 31b, 448–450
　assessment for, 447
　cancer and, 566
　characteristics of, 511t
　clinical manifestations of, 448–449
　diagnosis of, 449
　drugs for, 449–450
　evaluation for, 173
　immune function affected by, 184
　nonpharmacological management of, 457t
　in older adults, 53
　presentation of, 39t
　sleep and, 112
　treatment of, 449–450
Dermatitis, seborrheic, 239, 239f
Dermatoporosis, 237–238, 238f
Dermatoses, inflammatory, 239
Dermis, age-related changes in, 237
Detrusor, abnormal contractions of, caffeine and, 394
Diabetes mellitus
　death from, 535t
　diagnosis and classification of, 203t
　heart disease and, 297
　screening for, 84t
　type 2, 486–496
　　assessment of, 488–490
　　evaluation of, 493–496
　　medical management of, 487–488, 488t, 489t
　　nursing care guidelines for, 488–496, 494b
　　nursing interventions for, 490–493
　　　diet in, 490–491, 491b
　　　education in, 490
　　　emergency identification in, 491, 491t
　　　exercise in, 491–492
　　　insulin and oral hypoglycemic drugs, 490–491
　　　lifestyle changes in, 492
　　　monitoring in, 491
　　　sick day management in, 492, 492b
　　　skin alterations in, 492–493, 492b, 493f
　　　wound infections in, 493
　　pathophysiology of, 486, 487f
　　patient problems in, 490
　　planning for, 490
　　signs and symptoms of, 487
Diabetic foot lesions, 248t, 249–250
Diabetic retinopathy, 277
Diagnostic and Statistical Manual of Mental Disorders, Text Revision (DSM-5-TR)
　definition of, 223
　for substance use disorders, 224
Dialysis, peritoneal, 401b, 403f
Diaphragmatic breathing, 339b, 339f
Diarrhea, 362
　cancer and, 564
Diet
　DASH, 320b
　for diabetes mellitus, 490–491, 491b
　healthy, components of, 100–101, 100f
　heart disease and, 296–297
　history, 98–99, 98b
　monitoring of, advantages and disadvantages of, 86t
　sleep affected by, 111–112
Dietary supplements, 221
Difficulty recalling, in history taking, 44t
Dihydropyridines, adverse effects of, 294–296t

Diltiazem, 294–296t
Disability
　Americans with Disabilities Act (ADA) and, 543
　life issues with, 545
　management of, 545
Disasters, 143
Disbelief, in grief, 573
Discomfort, sleep and, 111
Disease, defined, 546
Disease-modifying antirheumatic drugs (DMARDs), 426
Disenfranchised grief, 574–575
Disequilibrium, 285
Disinhibited behavior, nonpharmacological management of, 457t
Dislocation, 418
Disorder, unusual manifestations of, in history taking, 44t
Distraction, 178
Distribution, in pharmacokinetics, 212
Disturbed sleep, 112
Diuretics
　adverse effects of, 294–296t
　for CHD, 311t
　for hypertension, 293
　sexuality and, 154t
Diverticula, 373
Diverticulitis, 372b, 373
　assessment of, 373
　evaluation of, 373
　nursing interventions for, 373
　obstruction resulting from, 372b
　patient problems with, 373
　planning for, 373
Diverticulosis, 373
　assessment of, 373
　evaluation of, 373
　nursing interventions for, 373
　patient problems with, 373
　planning for, 373
Dizziness, 285
Domestic elder abuse, 20
Domestic violence, 145
Do-not-resuscitate (DNR) order, 26, 63t
Dopamine (DA), 446t
Dopamine agonists, for Parkinson disease, 465t
Dopaminergics, for Parkinson disease, 465t
Dose-response relationship, 553
Doxazosin, 294–296t
Doxepin, in sleep, 116–117
Dressing, wound, types of, 263–266, 264t
Driving, family and, 61–62, 62b
Drug administration, in nursing facilities, 523
Drug-disease interaction, 214, 215t
Drug-disease interactions, 214, 215t
Drug-drug interactions, 214, 214t
Drug-food interactions, 214, 215t
Drug-induced hepatitis, 380–381
Drug-induced hypothyroidism, 497–498
Drug-nutrient interactions, 95, 96t
Drugs, 211, 211b. *see also* Medications
　adherence to, 221–223
　　list for problems, reviewing, 222–223
　　risk factors, 222
　　strategies for, 222
　alcohol and, 225–227
　Beers criteria on, 213

Drugs (Continued)
  for BPH, sexuality and, 154t
  cardiovascular, 219–220
  commonly used, 218–221
  for depression, 449–450
  errors, 216–217
  in health history format, 46
  in home care setting, 223b
  inappropriate, for older patients, 213
  interactions with, 214
    drug-disease, 214, 215t
    drug-drug, 214, 214t
    drug-food, 214, 215t
  over-the-counter, 216t, 221
  for Parkinson disease, 464, 465t
  prescription, 227
  promoting sleep, 116–117, 117b
  quality of life and, 214
  response to, aging and, 211–213
  safe of, 228b
  use of, demographics of, 211
Dry eyes, 272
Dry mouth, 286–287
Dry skin, prevention and treatment of, 241b
Dual-energy x-ray absorptiometry (DXA), in nutritional assessment, 99
Dual-process model, 576f
Duloxetine, 450
Dumping syndrome, 369
Duodenal ulcers, 368–369
Durable power of attorney for health care (DPAHC), 30
Dynamics, in family, 66
Dyspareunia, 153
Dysphagia, 101, 101–103t, 365–366
  assessment of, 365
  diet for, 472
  evaluation of, 366
  nursing interventions for, 365
  patient problems with, 365
  planning for, 365
Dyspnea, 329–330
  in older adults, 577

E

Ear
  age-related changes in, 281
  anatomy of, 280f
  health promotion/illness prevention for, 285b
Ease, 577
ECG. See Electrocardiography
ECHO. See Elder Cottage Housing Opportunity
Edges, as risk factor for falling, 129
Education, 178
  demographic profile in, 8
  for diabetes mellitus, 490
  of family caregivers, 65–66, 65b
  in gerontologic nursing, 11–14
  in nursing, 11–14
  socioeconomic factors, 73–74, 73f, 74b
Ejaculation
  premature, 152
  retarded, 152
Elder abuse, 145
  emotional, 20, 145
  financial, 145
  institutional, 20
  nursing training on, 20

Elder abuse (Continued)
  physical, 20, 145
  protective services and, 20–21, 20t
  psychologic, 145
  sexual, 20, 145
Elder Cottage Housing Opportunity (ECHO), 516t
Elderly-onset rheumatoid arthritis (EORA), 424
Electrocardiography (ECG)
  aging changes reflected by, 290
  for arrhythmia, 303
  for valvular disease, 307–308
Electroconvulsive therapy (ECT), 450
Electrolytes, 200–203
Electronic health records, in assessment of older adult, 44
Elimination, pattern of, 89
Emergency identification, in type 2 diabetes mellitus, 491, 491t
Emotional abuse, 20, 145
Emphysema, 334
Employment, 61
  in demographics, 8
Empowerment, of older adult, support for, 90
Enalapril, 294–296t
Encephalopathy, 379
Endocrine function, 481–502, 502b
Endocrine system, 481–482
  aging changes in, 484t
  case study, 495–496b
  feedback loops in, 484f
  glands, 482f, 483t
  home care, 502b
  pathophysiology of, 484t, 485–501
  physiology of, 481–484, 482f
Endocrinology of aging, 481
End-of-life
  care planning model, 63f
  health care decisions, 62–63, 63f, 63t
  in nursing facility care, 525
Enemas, barium, 84t
Enteral nutrition, 103–104
Enteritis, 369–370. see also Gastritis
Environment, sleep and, 110–111
Environmental influence, 70, 70b
EORA. See Elderly-onset rheumatoid arthritis
Eosinophils, in hematology test, 197t, 198
Epidermis, age-related changes in, 237
Epinephrine (Epi), 446t
Epithelialization, 259b
Eplerenone, 294–296t
Eprosartan, 294–296t
Epworth Sleepiness Scale, 115f
Equipment, in assessment of older adult, 48
Erectile dysfunction (ED), 151, 152, 499–500
Erythrocyte sedimentation rate, in hematology test, 200
Eschar, 259b
Escherichia coli, extended spectrum b-lactamase-positive, 187
Esophageal cancer, 381–382
  assessment of, 381
  evaluation of, 381–382
  nursing care plan for, 382b
  nursing interventions for, 381
  patient problems with, 381
  planning for, 381
Esophageal reconstruction, nutritional consequences of, 563b

Esophagectomy, nutritional consequences of, 563b
Esophagitis, 366
Esophagogastrectomy, nutritional consequences of, 563b
Esophagus, age-related changes in, 358t, 359
Estrogen, heart disease and, 298
Ethambutol, 344t
Ethics
  of assisted suicide, 30–31
  committees, 31–32
  dilemmas in, 30–31
  nurses' code, 30–32
Ethnicity, in demographics, 7
Euthanasia, 30–31
Evidence-based practice, 13b, 14f
  depression, 31b
  for pressure injuries, 254b
  sensory impairments in older adults, 272b
  spousal self-euthanasia, 31b
Excretion, in pharmacokinetics, 213
Exercise(s), 178
  advantages and disadvantages of, 86t
  capacity for, 326t
  for diabetes mellitus, 491–492
  Kegel, 396b
  lung function and, 328
  patterns in, assessment of, 88
  pelvic floor muscle, 395
  programs, 291
  response to, age-related changes in, 291
Expenditure, health care and, 9
Experimentation, law on, 31
Expiratory reserve volume, 327t
Extremity, lower, ulcers of, 248–250, 248t
Exudate, 259b
Eye drops, administering, 275b
Eyes
  aging and, 272b
  anatomy of, 271f
  dry, 272
  health promotion/illness prevention for, 272b
  injuries of, emergency treatment for, 278b

F

Facility. See Hospitals; Nursing facilities; Nursing homes
Falls, 125–137
  in acute care setting, 507–508
  age-related changes contributing to, 126–127
    cardiovascular factors, 126
    hearing as, 126
    musculoskeletal factors as, 126–127
    neurologic factors as, 127
    vision as, 126
  antecedents of, 130–131
  classification of, 130–131, 131b
  consequences of, 131–132
    physical injury as, 131
    psychologic trauma as, 131–132
  definition of, 125–126, 125b
  diary, 136b
  emergency treatment for, 137b, 508b
  evidence-based practice, 140–141b
  extrinsic risk for, 128–129
  factor contributing to, 130t
  fear of, 131–132, 131b
  health history in, 132, 132t, 133f
  intrinsic risk for, 127–128

Falls (Continued)
  meaning of, 126
  nursing management of, 136–137, 137b
  physical examination in, 132
  prevention guidelines, 125b
  prevention program for, 417b
  risk for, 127–130, 127b, 131t, 137b, 415
  serious injury in, 129, 129b
  special testing of, 132–136
  Tinetti test in, 128f
  treatable causes of, 127b
Family
  assessing, 66–67
  caregivers
    education of, 65–66, 65b
    respite programs in, 65–66
    support groups for, 66
  caregiving, 63–65
  chronic illness effect on, 541
  common late-life issues and decisions, 61–65
    care facility, deciding about, 67–68
    changes in living arrangements, 67–68
    driving, 61–62, 62b
    end-of-life health care decisions, 62–63, 63f, 63t
    family caregiving, 63–65
    financial and legal concerns, 62
  function of, 60–61
  influences, 59–69, 60b
  past relationships in, 66
  role of, 60–61
Family history, in health history format, 47
Family profile, in health history format, 44
Fasting plasma glucose, 203
Fat
  subcutaneous, age-related changes in, 237
  for type 2 diabetes mellitus, 491
Fatigue
  chronic illness with, 540
  in rheumatoid arthritis, 426
Fear
  of falls, 131–132, 131b
  in history taking, 44t
Fecal incontinence, 363–364
Fecal occult blood test, 84t
  advantages and disadvantages of, 86t
Federal housing assistance programs, 73b
Feeding tubes, in advanced dementia, 365b
Felodipine, 294–296t
Female sexual dysfunction (FSD), 499–500
Fentanyl, 175–176
Fiber, for type 2 diabetes mellitus, 491b
Fibrinolytics
  for CAD, 299–300
  for stroke, 471b
Financial abuse, 145
Financial concerns, family and, 62
Financial exploitation, 20
Fire
  cigarette smoking and, 138, 138b
  fireplace hazards and, 138
  kitchen hazards and, 139
  safety tips, 139, 139b
  space heaters and, 139
Firearms, 145–146
Flashers, 271
Flatus, 362
Floaters, 272

Floor surfaces, as risk factor for falling, 129
Fluid, in renal diet, 402b
Foam dressings, 264t
Folic acid, in hematology test, 197t, 198–199
Food. See also Nutrition
  drug interactions with, 214, 215t
  handling, 141
  illnesses from, 141
  recall of, 98
Foot
  infection, diabetes mellitus with, 494b
  patient education on, 439
  problems with, 438–439
  ulcers, with diabetes mellitus, 492b
Fosinopril, 294–296t
Foster home care, 516t
Fractures
  clavicular, 419, 420b, 420f
  Colles, 419
  comminuted, 415f
  definition of, 415
  emergency treatment of, 415b
  greenstick, 415f
  hip, 416–419, 416f, 419b
    assessment of, 417
    Buck extension for, 416, 416f
    evaluation after, 418–419
    intervention for, 418f
    Küntscher nail for, 416f
    Neufeld nails and screws for, 416f
    nursing care guidelines for, 417–419
    nursing intervention for, 417–418, 418b
    patient problems in, 417
    planning for, 417
  oblique, 415f
  pathologic, 415f
  spiral, 415f
  stress, 415f
  transverse, 415f
Frailty, with acute myocardial infarction, 291b
Friction, 252, 259b
Friendly visitors, telephone monitoring and, 517
Frontotemporal dementia (FTD), 454
Fullness, 362
Function, enhancement of, 543
Functional decline, in history taking, 44t
Functional incontinence, 391
  diagnosis of, 394
  nursing care plan for, 398b
  planning for, 394
Functional Pain Scale (FPS), 171, 171t
Functional residual capacity (FRC), 327t
Functional status
  assessment of, 48–51, 49f, 50b
  in health status, 9
  home care and, 514–515
Functioning, 60
Furosemide, 294–296t

G

Gabapentin (Neurontin, Neuraptine), 96t
Gait
  abnormalities of, 128t
  in Parkinson disease, 463b
  Tinetti test of, 128f
Gallbladder, age-related changes in, 360
Gallstones, age-related changes in, 359
Gamma-aminobutyric acid (GABA), 446t

Gas exchange, 325
Gas, GI symptoms with, 362
Gastrectomy, nutritional consequences of, 563b
Gastric cancer, 382–383
  assessment of, 383
  evaluation of, 383
  nursing interventions for, 383
  patient problems with, 383
  planning for, 383
Gastric mucosa, degeneration of, 367
Gastric secretions, 359
Gastric ulcers, 368
Gastritis, 367–368
  assessment of, 367
  evaluation of, 368
  nursing interventions for, 368
  patient problems with, 367
  planning for, 367–368
  stress-induced, 367
Gastroesophageal reflux disease (GERD), 366
  assessment of, 366
  cough and, 330
  evaluation of, 367
  nursing interventions for, 367
  patient problems with, 367
  planning for, 367
Gastrointestinal function, 357–386, 357b
Gastrointestinal (GI) system
  age-related changes in, 357–360, 358–359b, 358t
  cancers of, 381–385
  diseases of, 364–374
    prevention of, 360
  home care for, 385b
  symptoms in, 360–364
Gauze, 264t
Gender, demographic profile in, 6–7
Generalist nurse, roles of, 3
Generation X, 71
Genome, 552
Geographic distribution, demographic profile in, 7–8
Geographic location, of residence, 76
GERD. See Gastroesophageal reflux disease
Geriatric Depression Scale (GDS), 449
Geriatric Depression Scale: Short Form, 53, 53f
Geriatrics, definition of, 5
Gerontic nursing, definition of, 5
Gerontologic clinical nurse specialist. See Nurse specialist, gerontologic clinical
Gerontologic nurse. See Nurse, gerontologic
Gerontologic nurse practitioner. See Nurse practitioner, gerontologic
Gerontologic nursing. See also Nursing
  American Nurses Credentialing Center eligibility requirement for, 4b
  competency statements, 11b
  definition of, 5
  educator, core competencies for, 12–13b
  effect of an aging population on, 11–15
  foundations of specialty of, 2–5
  overview of, 1–16, 2b
  professional origins of, 2–3
  roles of, 3–5
  standards of practice of, 3
Gerontology
  baby boomers in, 2
  definition of, 5

INDEX

GI. *See* Gastrointestinal system
GI system. *See* Gastrointestinal (GI) system
Gingivitis, 364–365
    assessment of, 364
    evaluation of, 365
    nursing interventions for, 364–365
    patient problems with, 364
    planning for, 364
Glaucoma, 273–274
    acute angle-closure, 273
    assessment of, 273
    chronic open-angle, 273
    evaluation for, 274
    nursing care guidelines for, 273–274
    nursing intervention for, 274, 274b
    patient problems for, 273–274
    patient with, 274b
    planning for, 274
    screening for, 84t
    secondary, 273
Glucocorticosteroids, for COPD, 336
Glucose, in urine, 206, 206t
a-Glucosidase inhibitors, for type 2 diabetes mellitus, 489t
Glutamate (Glu), 446t
Glycohemoglobin, 203
Glycosylated hemoglobin, 202t
Goiter, 497f
Gout, 199, 426, 428f
Gouty arthritis, 426–428, 428f
    assessment of, 428
    evaluation of, 428
    nursing care guidelines for, 428
    nursing interventions for, 428
    patient problems in, 428
    planning for, 428
Grab bars, as risk factor for falling, 129
Granulation tissue, 259b
Graying of America, 5
Great Depression, 70–71
Greenstick fracture, 415f
Grief, 573–575, 573b, 574f
    cancer and, 566–567
    during COVID-19 pandemic, 575b
    definition of, 572
    physical symptoms of, 573
    psychologic responses in, 573
    social responses on, 573–574
    spiritual aspects of, 574
    types of, 574–575
Guanfacine, 294–296t
Guided reminiscence, 43
Guilt, in grief, 573
Gum disease, periodontal, 357–358

H

Habits, bladder, 392
Habit training, 396
Hallux valgus, 425f, 439, 439f
Haloperidol, 451
Hammer toe, 128t
Hammertoe, 439, 439f
HDL. *See* High-density lipoprotein
Health. *See also* Mental health
    management pattern, assessment of, 87
    optimal, 82
    perception of, 87
Health Belief Model, 83

Health care
    agents, 26–27, 27b
    continuum of, 10–11
    delivery settings, 9, 506, 506b
    expenditure and use of, 9
Health Care Proxy or Medical Power of Attorney, 63t
Health history, 42–48. *See also specific condition*
    electronic health records, 44
    equipment and skills in, 48
    format, 44–47, 45t
        allergies, 46
        drugs, 46
        family history, 47
        family profile, 44
        immunization and health screening status, 46
        living environment profile, 45
        nutrition, 46–47, 47b
        occupational profile, 44–45
        patient profile or biographic data, 44
        present health status, 45, 46t
        previous health status, 47
        recreation or leisure profile, 45
        resources or support systems used, 45
        review of systems, 47
        typical day, description of, 45
    interviewer, 43–44, 43b
    patient, 44, 44t
    physical assessment, 47–48
Health insurance, 74–75, 74f
Health Insurance Portability and Accountability Act of 1996 (HIPAA), 19–20
Health literacy, 45b
Health patterns
    activity or exercise, 88
    cognitive or perceptual, 88
    coping or stress-tolerance, 87
    elimination, 89
    health perception or health management, 87
    nutritional or metabolic, 87
    roles or relationships, 87
    self-perception or self-concept, 87
    sexuality or reproductive, 89
    value or belief, 88, 88b
Health perception, patterns in, assessment of, 87
Health promotion, 544–545, 544f
    advantages and disadvantages of, 86t
    areas of, relevant to older adults, 82b
    assessment and, 85–89
    barriers to, disease prevention, 82
    essentials of, aging adults, 81–82
    evaluation and, 90
    for eyes, 272b
    illness/disability prevention and, 81, 81b
    interventions and, 89–90
    models of, 82–83
    nursing role in, 85–90
    osteoporosis, 432b
    planning and, 89
    for respiratory system, 328b
    terminology in, 82
Health Promotion Model, 83
Health screening status, in health history format, 46
Health status
    acute care setting and, 9–10
    chronic disease in, 9
    continuum of care, 10–11
    functional ability in, 9

Health status *(Continued)*
    health care delivery and, 9
    health care expenditure and, 9
    home care and, 10
    nursing facilities and, 10
    of older adults, 8–11
    self-assessed, 9
    socioeconomic status and, 74–76, 74b, 74f
Healthcare policy, 18–19, 18b, 32b
Hearing, 280–286
    age-related changes in, 281
    falls related to, 126
    problems and conditions in, 281–286
Hearing loss, 283
    assessment of, 283, 283b
    evaluation of, 278, 285
    nursing interventions for, 284–285, 284b, 285b
    patient problems in, 283
    planning for, 284
Heart block, 304
Heart disease. *see also* Coronary heart disease
    causing death, 290
    death from, 535t
    risk factors for, 291b, 296–298, 297b
        diabetes mellitus as, 297
        diet as, 296–297
        estrogen as, 298
        hypertension as, 290
        menopause as, 298
        obesity as, 297
        physical activity as, 297
        sedentary lifestyle as, 297
        smoking as, 297
        stress as, 298
Heart failure, 309–314
    definition of, 310t
    presentation of, 39t
    stages of, 310t
Heat and cold, 177
Heberden nodes, 420–421, 421f
Helicobacter pylori, 368
Heloma durum, 438
Hematocrit, in hematology test, 197t
Hematology test, 197t, 198–200
    C-reactive protein in, 200
    D-dimer test in, 197t, 200
    erythrocyte sedimentation rate in, 200
    folic acid in, 197t, 198–199
    hematocrit in, 197t
    hemoglobin in, 197t
    iron in, 197t, 199
    partial thromboplastin time in, 197t, 200
    platelets in, 197t, 200
    prothrombin time in, 197t, 199–200
    red blood cells in, 197t, 198
    TIBC in, 197t, 199
    uric acid in, 197t, 199
    vitamin B_{12} in, 197t, 199
    white blood cells in, 197t, 198
Hemiparesis, 128t
Hemodialysis, 401b, 403f
Hemoglobin, in hematology test, 197t
Hemorrhoids, 374
    assessment of, 374
    evaluation of, 374
    nursing interventions for, 374
    patient problems with, 374
    planning for, 374

Heparin, 299–300
Hepatitis, 376–378
  assessment of, 378
  drug-induced, 380–381
  evaluation of, 378
  nursing interventions for, 378
  patient problems with, 378
  planning for, 378
  viral, 377t
Hepatitis A virus (HAV), 376, 377t
Hepatitis B virus (HBV), 376, 377t
  vaccination for, 84t
Hepatitis C virus (HCV), 376, 377t
Hepatitis D virus (HDV), 376
Hepatitis E virus (HEV), 377
Hepatitis G virus (HGV), 377
HER2, 552
Herbal remedies, 117b
Hernia
  hiatal, 366, 366f
  strangulated inguinal, 370f
Herpes zoster, 243–245, 243f, 245b
HHA. See Home health aide
Hiatal hernia, 366, 366f
High-density lipoprotein (HDL), 202t, 204
Hip
  fracture, 416–419, 416f, 419b
    assessment of, 417
    Buck extension for, 416, 416f
    evaluation after, 418–419
    intervention for, 418f
    Küntscher nail for, 416f
    Neufeld nails and screws for, 416f
    nursing care guidelines for, 417–419
    nursing intervention for, 417–418, 418b
    patient problems in, 417
    planning for, 417
  surgery, precautions after, 423b
HIPAA. See Health Insurance Portability and Accountability Act of 1996
Hippocampal sclerosis, 455
Histamine blockers, sexuality and, 154t
HIV. See Human immunodeficiency virus
Holistic biopsychosocial spiritual model, 574f
Home
  burn injuries in, 138–139
  carbon monoxide poisoning in, 139–140, 140b
  foodborne illnesses in, 141
  knife injuries in, 139
  medication storage in, 143–144
  portable electric cooling fans at, 140–141
  safety in, 137b, 138–141
  sharing, 516t
Home care, 511–513, 512b, 517–518
  agency, role of, 513
  benefits of, 511–513
  cancer, 568b
  in cognitive disorder, 459–460
  cognitive function and, 452b, 515
  drugs and aging in, 223b
  for end-of-life, 585b
  with facility-based agencies, 518
  factors affecting health care needs of older adults, 514–517
  functional status and, 514–515
  for gastrointestinal system, 385b
  health status and, 10
  HHA's role in, 513–514

Home care (Continued)
  with home health agency, 513, 518
  immune function and, 191b
  indicators for, 512b
  nurse's role in, 513
  OASIS in, 514
  organizations, 517
  pain and, 178b
  plan of treatment in, 513–514
  with proprietary agencies, 518
  safety and, 146b
  sexuality in, 161b
  substance use disorders and, 229b
Home environments, sleep and, 110
Home health agency, 513, 518
Home health aide (HHA), 513–514
Homemaker services, 517
Hormone replacement therapy (HRT), 482–483
Hormone therapy, for prostate cancer, 555
Hormones
  estrogen, 298
  sexuality and, 154t
  thyroid-stimulating, 205–206, 205t
Hospice, 528–530
  location of, 530
  Medicare benefit of, 529
  palliative care and, 528–529
  philosophy of, 528–530
  services, 529
Hospitals. See also Acute care setting
  psychiatric, 460
  risk in, 507–509
  sleep and, 110
  as technologic system, 507
Household chemical emergencies, 140
Housing, 76b, 77. See also Living arrangements
  congregate, 516t
  options for older adults, 515, 516t
  subsidized, 77
Human Genome Project, 552
Human immunodeficiency virus (HIV), 153–155, 186
Hydralazine, 294–296t
Hydration, 582. see also Dehydration
Hydrocephalus, normal pressure, 454–455
Hydrochlorothiazide, 294–296t
Hydrocodone, 175
Hydrocolloid dressing, 264t
Hydrogel, 264t
Hygiene
  oral, 364–365
  pulmonary, 339, 340b
  sleep, 116
Hypercapnia, 329
Hyperglycemia, heart disease from, 297
Hypersecretion, in endocrine system, 484t
Hypertension, 291–296, 291b
  assessment of, 293
  drug-induced, 292
  evaluation of, 296
  heart disease and, 290
  intervention for, 296
  patient problems of, 293–296
  pharmacologic treatment of, 292–293, 294–296t
    beta-blockers for, 293
    calcium channel blockers for, 293
    diuretics for, 293
  planning for, 296

Hypertension (Continued)
  primary, 292
  prognosis of, 293
  secondary, 292
Hypertension retinopathy, 277
Hyperthermia, 141–143
Hyperthyroidism, 205–206, 497
  medical management of, 497
  nursing care guidelines for, 497, 498t
  pathophysiology of, 497, 497f
  presentation of, 39t
  signs and symptoms of, 497
Hypertonic dehydration, 95–96
Hypnosis, 178
Hypnotics, 218
Hypoglycemia, 127b
Hypoglycemic drugs, for diabetes mellitus, 490–491
Hypokalemia, 201b
Hyponatremia, 201
Hyporesponsiveness, in endocrine system, 484t
Hyposecretion, in endocrine system, 484t
Hypotension, 127b. See also Orthostatic hypotension
Hypothalamic-pituitary-adrenal (HPA) axis, 483
Hypothalamus, 108, 483t
Hypothermia, 141–143
Hypothyroidism, 205–206, 497–498
  medical management of, 498
  nursing care guidelines for, 498, 499t
  pathophysiology of, 497–498
  presentation of, 39t
  primary, 497
  secondary, 497
  signs and symptoms of, 498
  tertiary, 497
Hypotonic dehydration, 95–96
Hypoxemia, 329

I

ICU. See Intensive care unit (ICU)
Identification, emergency, in type 2 diabetes mellitus, 491, 491t
Idiosyncratic toxicity, of drugs, 380
Ileocecal intussusception, 370f
Ileus, paralytic, 370
Illness
  atypical presentation of, 38–39, 39b, 39t
  defined, 546
  foodborne, 141
  prevention. see Health promotion
Immobility
  from chronic illness, 540
  hazards from, in acute care setting, 509
  lung function and, 328
Immune system
  age-related changes in, 183, 183b
  cancer and, 185
  chemotherapy effects on, 190–191b
  depression's effect on, 184
  drug effects on, 184
  home care and, 191b
  medications' effect on, 184
  nutritional factors on, 183–184
  psychosocial factors, 184
Immunizations, 46, 83
Immunocompetence, factors affecting, 183–184
Immunologic theory, 182–183

Immunomodulators, for asthma, 331
Immunosuppressives, 427t
Immunotherapy, for cancer, 561
Impact Act of 2014, 543, 544t
Inactivity, physical, heart disease from, 297. *See also* Immobility
Inappropriate/impulsive sexual behavior, nonpharmacological management of, 457t
Income
　demographics of, 8, 8f
　socioeconomic factors and, 71-72, 71f, 72f
Incontinence
　bowel training and, 364b
　fecal, 363-364
　in nursing facilities, 522
Indapamide, 294-296t
Independence, in family, 67
Indwelling catheter, 404b
Infection, 182-192. *see also* Urinary tract infection
　in acute care setting, 509
　assessment of, 187-188, 187b
　chain of, 184-185
　common problems and conditions, 185-186
　control of, in nursing facilities, 524-525
　evaluation of, 189-191
　with *Helicobacter pylori*, 368
　home care for, 191b
　nursing care guidelines for, 187-191
　nursing interventions for, 188-189
　nutritional interventions for, 189
　patient problems in, 188
　planning for, 188
　psychosocial intervention for, 189
　with significant healthcare-associated pathogens, 186-187
Inflammation, common problems and conditions, 185-186
Inflammatory dermatoses, 239
Influenza, 185
　death from, 535t
　vaccination for, 84t
Informed consent, 25
In-home services, for older adults, 514b
Insomnia, 109
Inspiratory reserve volume (IRV), 327t
Institutional abuse, 20
Institutionalization, factors associated with, 519
Instrumental activities of daily living (IADL), 118. *See also* Activities of daily living
Insulin
　deficiency, pathophysiology of, 487f
　for hypoglycemia, 490-491
Insulin glargine injection (Lantus Solostar), 96t
Insurance. *See* Health Insurance Portability and Accountability Act of 1996
Integumentary function, 236, 236b
　age-related changes, 237-238, 237b
　　in dermal appendages, 237
　　in dermatoporosis, 237-238
　　in dermis, 237
　　in epidermis, 237
　　in subcutaneous fat, 237
　common problems, and conditions, 238-246
　　actinic keratosis, 244-246, 245f
　　candidiasis, 242-243, 242f
　　cherry angiomas, 238, 238f
　　herpes zoster, 243-245, 243f, 245b
　　inflammatory dermatoses in, 239

Integumentary function *(Continued)*
　　intertrigo, 239, 239f
　　malignant skin growths in, 246-248
　　pruritus, 241-242
　　psoriasis in, 240-241
　　seborrheic dermatitis, 239, 239f
　　seborrheic keratoses, 238-239, 238f
　　skin tags, 239, 239f
Intensive care unit (ICU), 510
Interaction pattern, grief and, 573
Interface pressure, 259b
Internal carotid, 469
International Dysphagia Diet Standardization Initiative (IDDSI), 101
Interpersonal psychotherapy (IPT), for depression, 449
Interstitial lung disease, coughing and, 330
Intertrigo, 239, 239f
Interventions, prevention and, 89-90
Interviewer, in assessment of older adult, 43-44, 43b
Intestinal obstruction, 370-372, 370f
　assessment of, 371
　complications of, 371
　evaluation of, 372
　nursing interventions for, 372
　patient problems with, 371
　planning for, 371-372
Intestinal resection, nutritional consequences of, 563b
Intestine, adhesion in, 370f
Intimacy
　importance of, 150-152
　older adult needs for, 150
Intraarticular drugs, 427t
Intussusception, from polyp, 370f
Ions, 200
Irbesartan, 294-296t
Iron
　deficiency of, 183-184
　in hematology test, 197t, 199
　TIBC of, 197t, 199
Ischemic heart disease, 298
Ischemic ulcer, 248
Isoniazid, 344t
Isotonic dehydration, 95-96
Isradipine, 294-296t

J

Jaundice, 377-378
Joint
　Charcot, 128t
　replacement of, complications after, 422

K

Katz Index of ADLs, 49, 49f
Kegel exercises, 396b
Keratoses
　actinic, 244-246, 245f
　seborrheic, 238-239, 238f
Ketones, in urine, 206t, 207
Kidney
　age-related changes, 398
　problems and conditions in, 398-411
Kidney injury
　acute, 398-399, 399b
　assessment of, 400, 401b
　chronic, 399-403, 399b, 400b

Kidney injury *(Continued)*
　evaluation of, 403
　management of, 403b
　nursing interventions for, 401-403
　patient problems with, 400-401
　planning for, 401
Kinetic labyrinth, 280
Knee, replacement surgery for, 422
Knife injuries, in home, 139
Küntscher nail, 416f
Kyphosis, 325, 429f

L

Labetalol, 294-296t
Laboratory and diagnostic tests, 195-209, 196b
　arterial blood gas testing
　　bicarbonate in, 207
　　blood pH in, 207, 207t
　　carbon dioxide in, 207
　　components of, 207-208, 207t
　　oxygen saturation in, 208
　　partial pressure of oxygen in, 207
　blood chemistry testing
　　albumin in, 202t, 204
　　alkaline phosphatase in, 202t, 205
　　amylase in, 202t, 203-204
　　aspartate aminotransferase in, 202t, 205
　　brain natriuretic peptide in, 205
　　calcium in, 202t, 203
　　chloride in, 202t, 203
　　cholesterol in, total, 202t, 204
　　components of, 200-206, 202t
　　creatine kinase in, 202t, 205
　　creatinine in, 202t, 204
　　electrolytes in, 200-203
　　glucose, 202t, 203
　　lactate dehydrogenase in, 205
　　magnesium in, 202t, 203
　　phosphorus in, 202t, 203
　　potassium in, 201, 202t
　　prealbumin in, 204
　　protein in, total, 202t, 204
　　PSA in, 206
　　sodium in, 201, 202t
　　of thyroid function, 205-206
　　triglycerides in, 204
　　troponin in, 205
　　TSH in, 205-206, 205t
　　urea nitrogen in, 202t, 204
　hematology test, 197t, 198-200
　　C-reactive protein in, 200
　　D-dimer test in, 197t, 200
　　erythrocyte sedimentation rate in, 200
　　folic acid in, 197t, 198-199
　　hematocrit in, 197t
　　hemoglobin in, 197t
　　iron in, 197t, 199
　　partial thromboplastin time in, 197t, 200
　　platelets in, 197t, 200
　　prothrombin time in, 197t, 199-200
　　red blood cells in, 197t, 198
　　TIBC in, 197t, 199
　　uric acid in, 197t, 199
　　vitamin B_{12} in, 197t, 199
　　white blood cells in, 197t, 198
　sexuality and, 157b
　therapeutic drug monitoring in, 208
　urinalysis, 206-207, 206t

Laboratory data, in assessment of older adult, 54
Laboratory values, in nutritional assessment, 99
Lactate dehydrogenase, 205
Large intestine, age-related changes in, 358t, 359
Law. *See also* Omnibus Budget Reconciliation Act of 1987
    on advance medical directives, 26
    on DNR, 26
    on experimentation and research, 31
    HIPAA as, 19–20
    on living will, 26–27
    for Medicare and Medicaid, 21, 22f
    on organ donation, 31
    overview of relevant, 19–20
    power of attorney, 30
    professional standards and, 18–19
    sources of, 19
    state, 19
Laxatives, for constipation, 363
LDL. *See* Low-density lipoprotein
Legal services, in cognitive disorder, 460
Legal tools, 26–30
Legislation, rehabilitation and, 542–543
Leisure profile, in health history format, 45
Lesbian, gay, bisexual, and transgender older adults (LGBT), 156
Leukocytes, in hematology test, 197t, 198
Leukotriene antagonists, for asthma, 331
Levorphanol (Levo-Dromoran), 176t
Levothyroxine (Levothroid, Synthroid), 96t
Lewy body dementia (DLB), 454
Libido, loss of, 152
Life review, 581
Lifestyle changes
    activity and, 118–120
    for diabetes mellitus, 492
    sleep and, 111
    for urinary incontinence, 394–395, 395b
Lighting
    as risk factor for falling, 129
    sleep and, 110, 114b
Lipitor. *See* Atorvastatin
Lipoprotein. *See* High-density lipoprotein; Low-density lipoprotein
Lisinopril (Prinivil, Zestril), 96t, 294–296t
Liver, age-related changes in, 358t, 360
Liver cancer, 385
Living arrangements, 60
    changes in, 67–68
    demographic profile in, 7, 7f
    in older adults, 7, 7f
Living environment profile, in health history format, 45
Living will, 26–27, 27b, 63t
Location, geographic, of residence, 76
Loneliness, cancer and, 567
Long-acting beta$_2$-agonists (LABAs), for asthma, 331
Long-term care, 516t, 519–520, 519t, 520b
Long-term care facilities, 10. *See also* Nursing facilities; Nursing homes
    activity and, 119b
    sleep and, 110
Lopressor. *See* Metoprolol
Lordosis, 429f
Losartan, 294–296t

Loss, 572, 572b
    cancer and, 566–567
    during COVID-19 pandemic, 575b
    definition of, 572
Low-density lipoprotein (LDL), 202t, 204–205
Lower extremity ulcers, 248–250, 248t
Low-vision aids, 277b
Lung
    capacity of, 327t
    defense mechanisms of, 326t
    function of, 328–329
        anesthesia and, 329
        exercise and, 328
        immobility and, 328
        obesity and, 329
        smoking and, 328–329
        surgery and, 329
    volume of, 327t
Lung cancer, 341–342, 553–554
    assessment of, 342
    diagnosis of, 342
    diagnostic tests and procedures for, 341, 341t
    early detection of, 554
    evaluation after, 342
    intervention for, 342
    planning for, 342
    risk factors of, 553
    signs and symptoms of, 553
    treatment for, 341, 554
Lymphocytes
    in hematology test, 197t, 198
    total count of, 99

M

Macular degeneration
    age-related, 276–277
    dry, 276
    wet, 276
Macular disequilibrium, 285
Magnesium, serum levels of, 202t, 203
Maintenance, 83
Malignant skin growths, 246–248
    analyze cues, and prioritize hypotheses (patient problems) in, 248
    assessment for, 247
    basal cell carcinoma in, 246
    evaluation of, 248
    melanoma in, 246–247
    nursing interventions in, 248
    planning, 248
    squamous cell carcinoma in, 246
Malnutrition, 94–98
    dental caries and, 97
    immune function and, 183
Mammography, 84t
    advantages and disadvantages of, 86t
    in breast tumors, 554
MAOIs. *See* Monoamine oxidase inhibitors
Marijuana, sexuality and, 154t
Marital status, demographic profile in, 6–7
Massage, 177
MAST. *See* Michigan Alcoholism Screening Test
Masturbation, 151
Material exploitation, 20
Meals-on-Wheels, 313, 517
Meaning making, in mourning, 576–577

Medicaid, 75
    laws on, 21, 22f
    rehabilitation reimbursed by, 542
Medical directives, advance, 26
Medicare, 74–76
    hospice benefit by, 529
    laws on, 21, 22f
    Part A, 75, 75t
    Part B, 75, 75t
    Part C, 75, 75t
    Part D, 75–76, 75t
    rehabilitation reimbursed by, 542
    reimbursement by, for secondary prevention, 84t
Medications. *See also* Chemotherapy; Drugs; Polypharmacy
    adjuvant, 176–177
    for asthma, 331
    for CAD, 299–300
    for constipation, 363b
    for hypertension, 292–293, 294–296t
    immune function affected by, 184
    sexuality and, 153
Medigap policy, 75–76
Melanoma, 246–247, 247f
    acral-lentiginous, 247
    lentigo maligna, 247
    nodular, 247
    superficial spreading, 247
Ménière's disease, 285–286
Menopause, 491
    genitourinary syndrome of, 153
    heart disease and, 298
Mental health
    centers, community, 460
    in nursing facilities, 525
    resources, 475–476, 476f
Mental status, assessment, 51t
Meperidine (Demerol), 176t
Mesenteric occlusion, 370f
Metabolic syndrome, 485
    assessment of, 486t
    clinical judgment (nursing process) applied to, 485, 486t
    evaluation of, 486t
    medical management of, 485, 485b
    nursing interventions for, 486t
    pathophysiology of, 485
    patient problems in, 486t
    planning for, 486t
    signs and symptoms of, 485
Metabolism
    patterns in, assessment of, 87
    in pharmacokinetics, 212–213
Metered-dose inhaler, 335–336, 340b
Metformin (Glucophage XL, Gluformin), 96t
Methicillin-resistant *Staphylococcus aureus* (MRSA), 187
Methyldopa, 294–296t
Metolazone, 294–296t
Metoprolol (Lopressor, Toprol-XL), 96t, 294–296t
Michigan Alcoholism Screening Test (MAST), 224
Micronutrient deficiency, 97
Middle cerebral artery, 469
Mid-upper arm muscle circumference (MUAC), 99
Minerals, for type 2 diabetes mellitus, 491b
Minerals, in renal diet, 402b
Mini Nutritional Assessment, 98

INDEX

Mini Nutritional Assessment (MNA), 98
Mini-Cog, 53
Mini-Mental State Examination (MMSE), 447
Minoxidil, 294–296t
Mirtazapine, 116–117, 450
Mitotic inhibitors, for cancer, 560t
Mitral regurgitation, 307, 308b
Mitral stenosis, 307, 308b
Mixed incontinence, 391, 397–398b
MNA-short form (SF), 98
Modified Caregiver Strain Index, 64, 64f
Moexipril, 294–296t
Monoamine oxidase inhibitors (MAOIs), for Parkinson disease, 465t
Monoclonal antibodies, for cancer, 561
Monocytes, in hematology test, 197t
Montreal Cognitive Assessment (MoCA), 51, 52f, 446–447
Motility, decrease in, 357
Mourning, 575–577
    definition of, 572
    meaning making in, 576–577
Muscle
    cramps, 440
    pelvic floor exercises, 395, 396b
    strength of, decline in, 326
Musculoskeletal function, 414, 414b
    age-related changes in, 414–415
    home care for, 440b
    problems with, 414
Musculoskeletal system
    falls related to, 126–127
    problems and conditions of, 415–440, 415f
Music therapy, 178, 527
Myelodysplastic syndrome (MDS), 200
Myelosuppressive toxicities, of chemotherapy, 561–562b
Myocardial infarction
    frailty with, 291b
    intervention for, 302–303b
    presentation of, 39t
MyPlate, 100, 100f

N

Nadolol, 294–296t
Nail disorders, 439
Napping, daytime, 110
National Association for Home Care and Hospice (NAHC), 567
National Guidelines for Nursing Delegation, 14, 15b
National Hospice and Palliative Care Organization (NHPCO), 567
Natural disasters, 143
Nausea, 360
    in cancer, 562–563
    interventions for, 360
Nebulizer, 339–340
Nedocromil, 331
Neglect, 20, 145
Nerve stimulation, peripheral, with TENS, 178
Nervous system, central, 444–447
Neufeld nails and screws, 416f
Neuralgia, postherpetic, 243
Neurologic function, 444–478
Neurologic system, falls related to, 127
Neurons, 445, 446f, 447f

Neuropathic pain, chronic, 166b
Neuropathy, peripheral, 128t
Neurotransmitters, 445, 446t
Neutropenia, chemotherapy-induced, 562
Neutrophils, in hematology test, 197t, 198
Nicardipine, 294–296t
Nicotine, 228
    assessment of, 228
    evaluation of, 228
    interventions of, 228
    prevalence of, 228
Nifedipine, 294–296t
Nisoldipine, 294–296t
Nitrates, for CAD, 299
Nitrites, 207
Nocturia, 388–389
    management of, 395b
Nocturnal awakenings, 109
Nocturnal disruption, nonpharmacological management of, 457t
Noise, sleep and, 110
Noncardiogenic pulmonary edema, 349
    diagnostic tests and procedures for, 349
    prognosis of, 349
    treatment of, 349
Nondihydropyridines, adverse effects of, 294–296t
Nonpharmacological therapies, for sleep, 116
Nonprescription agents, 220–221
Non-rapid eye movement (NREM) sleep, 108, 109t
Nonsteroidal antiinflammatory drugs (NSAIDs), 427t
Norco. See Acetaminophen/hydrocodone
Norepinephrine (NE), 446t
Normal grief, 575
Normal pressure hydrocephalus (NPH), 454–455
Norton Risk Assessment Scale, 253, 253f
Norvasc. See Amlodipine
NSAIDs. See Nonsteroidal antiinflammatory drugs
Nurse, gerontologic
    association of
        ANA, 2–3, 19
        visiting nurses, 518
    certification of, 4b
    characteristics of, 513
    credential for, 4b
    ethical code for, 30–32
    in home care, 513
    role of, 85–90
Nurse practitioner, gerontologic
    certification of, 4b
    in nursing facility, 527–528
    roles of, 4–5
Nurse specialist, gerontologic clinical
    certification of, 4b
    roles of, 3–4
Nursing
    in acute care setting, 509–511
    care delivery systems, 525–526
    department of, 525
    education in, 11–14
    in elder abuse, 20
    gerontologic
        American Nurses Credentialing Center eligibility requirement for, 4b
        competency statements, 11b
        definition of, 5

Nursing (Continued)
    educator, core competencies for, 12–13b
    effect of an aging population on, 11–15
    foundations of specialty of, 2–5
    overview of, 1–16, 2b
    professional origins of, 2–3
    roles of, 3–5
    standards of practice of, 3
    practice of, 14–15
    research, 15
    -specific competency and expertise, 510
    terminology of, 5
Nursing facilities
    admission agreement for, 23
    assisted living in, 516t
    care models in, 519–520
    certification of, 24–25
    clinical aspects of, 520–525
    creativity in, 527
    DNR guidelines in, 26
    end-of-life care in, 525
    enforcement mechanisms for, 25
    future of, 528
    guidelines for DNR policies in, 26
    health status and, 10
    infection control in, 524–525
    innovations in, 527–528
    management of, 525–526
    nurse practitioners in, 527–528
    nursing home as, 10
    quality of care in, 23
    reform, 21–25, 22b, 22t
    resident assessment in, 521, 521f
    resident rights in, 23
    sanctions of, 25
    skilled, 21
    unnecessary drug use in, 23–24
    urinary incontinence in, 24
Nursing-focused assessment, 36
Nursing homes
    falls in, 415
    as nursing facility, 10
Nutrition, 93–105., 94b. See also Malnutrition
    assessment of, 98–99
        anthropometrics in, 99
        diet history in, 98–99, 98b
        laboratory values in, 99
    cancer treatment and, 563b
    COPD and, 338–339, 339b
    dehydration and, 95–97
    drug-nutrient interactions and, 95, 96t
    in dying process, 583b
    dysphagia and, 101, 101–103t
    enteral, 103–104
    evidence-based strategies to improve, 99–104
    in health history format, 46–47, 47b
    healthy diet and, 100–101, 100f
    immune function affected by, 183–184
    micronutrient deficiency and, 97
    in nursing facilities, 522–523
    parenteral, 104, 104b
    patient problems associated with, 99, 100b
    patterns in, assessment of, 87
    risk in older adults, factors influencing, 95
    screening for, 98–99
    service, 517
    specialized, 103–104, 103b

O

OAA. See Older Americans Act
OARS. See Older Adults Resources and Services (OARS) Multidimensional Functional Assessment Questionnaire
OASIS. See Outcome and Assessment Information Set
Obesity
  abdominal, low-calorie sweetener use and, 485b
  heart disease and, 297
Oblique fracture, 415f
OBRA. See Omnibus Budget Reconciliation Act of 1987
Obstructive sleep apnea (OSA), 352–353
  assessment of, 353
  diagnosis of, 353
  diagnostic tests and procedures for, 352
  evaluation after, 353
  intervention for, 353, 353f
  planning for, 353
  prognosis of, 353
  treatment of, 352–353
Occupational profile, in health history format, 44–45
Occupational Safety and Health Administration (OSHA), 524
"Old age," definition of, 5
Older adults
  abuse of, 145
  in acute care setting, 506–507
  assessment of, 36–56, 36b
    cognitive and affective, 51–54, 51t, 52f, 53f
    functional status, 48–51, 49f, 50b
    interrelationship between physical and psychosocial aspects of aging in, 37–38, 37t
    laboratory data in, 54
    nature of disease and disability in, 38–42
      age-related changes, 38
      atypical presentation of illness, 38–39, 39b, 39t
      cognitive assessment, 40–42, 40b, 41t
    social, 54, 55f
    special considerations affecting, 37–42
    tailoring, 42, 42b
  community-based services for, 514b
  demographics of, 5
  evaluating sexual risk in, 156t
  factors influencing nutritional risk in, 95
  health status of, 8–11
  homebound, sleep in, 116
  homeless, 77
  hypothermia and hyperthermia in, 141–143
  living arrangements of, 7, 7f
  needs for sexuality, 150
  neglect of, 145
  pain in. See Pain
  strategies to maintain sexual health in, 160b
Older Adults Resources and Services (OARS) Multidimensional Functional Assessment Questionnaire, 54, 55f
Older Americans Act (OAA), 515–517
Olmesartan, 294–296t
Omeprazole (Prilosec, Zegerid), 96t
Omnibus Budget Reconciliation Act of 1987 (OBRA), 21
  enforcement mechanisms with, 25
  facility survey and certification and, 24–25

Omnibus Budget Reconciliation Act of 1987 (Continued)
  provision of service in, 23–24
  quality of care in, 23
  regulatory "level A" requirements by, 519b
  resident rights in, 23
  restraint in, 23–24
  three major parts of, 22–25
  urinary incontinence in, 24
Oncology Nursing Society, 175–176
Onychauxis, 439
Onychomycosis, 439
Opioid analgesics, 220
Opioids
  to avoid in pain management of older adults, 176t
  sexuality and, 154t
  side effect of, 175–176, 176b
Oral cancer, 381
Oral cavity, age-related changes in, 357–359
Oral glucose tolerance test, 203
Oral health, 97–98
Oral hygiene, 364–365
Oral mucositis, chemotherapy-induced, 563–564
Oral nutrition, in older adults, 582
Organ donation, law on, 31
Orgasm, age-related changes to, 152
Orofacial pain (OFP), 166b
Orthostatic hypotension, 305–306
  assessment of, 305–306
  diagnosis of, 306
  evaluation of, 306
  intervention for, 306
  planning for, 306
OSA. See Obstructive sleep apnea
OSHA. See Occupational Safety and Health Administration
Osteitis deformans. See Paget's disease
Osteoarthritis, 420–423, 421f
  assessment of, 421
  benefits of shared yoga intervention for, 421–422b
  evaluation of, 423
  nursing care guidelines for, 421–423
  nursing interventions for, 421–423
  patient problems in, 421
  planning for of, 421
  rheumatoid arthritis versus, 425t
Osteomyelitis, 434–435
Osteoporosis, 84t, 127b, 130t, 428–433, 429f, 430t
  assessment of, 431
  evaluation of, 432–433
  with fractured thoracic vertebrae, 432–433b
  health promotion/illness prevention for, 432b
  nursing care guidelines for, 431–433
  nursing interventions for, 432
  patient problems in, 431
  planning for, 431–432
  primary, 498–499
    medical management of, 499
    nursing care guidelines for, 499, 500t
    pathophysiology of, 498–499
    signs and symptoms of, 499
  risk factors for development of, 429b
  screening for, 84t
Outcome and Assessment Information Set (OASIS), 514
Ovaries, 483t

Overall Benefit of Analgesic Score (OBAS), 173b
Overflow incontinence, 390–391
  diagnosis of, 394
  planning for, 394
Over-the-counter medications
  safety of, 216t
  use of, 221
Oxycodone, 175
Oxygen
  in blood, 327
  partial pressure of, 207
  saturation, 208
Oxygen therapy
  for COPD, 336
  home, 340
Oxygenation, 325, 326t
Oxyphenbutazone, 427t

P

Pacemaker, for arrhythmia, 305b
PAD. See Peripheral artery disease
Paget's disease, 433–434
Pain, 164–179., 164b. See also Palliative care
  abdominal, 361, 361f
  aging and, 164
  assessment of, 169–173, 170t
    culture and, 169–171, 171b
    functional impairment in, 172–173
    functional scale, 173t
    history in, 171
    pharmacologic treatment for, 173–178, 174f
    physical examination in, 172
    quality of life, 173
    self-treatment for, 171
    tools, 171–173, 172f
  chest, assessment of, 301b
  from chronic illness, 540
  classification of, 166b
  controlling of, by team approach, 168b
  definition of, 165
  depression and, 173
  diary of, 172f
  home care and, 178b
  management of, 177b
    barriers to, 167–168, 168f
    CAM in, 177
    cognitive therapy in, 178
    dementia, 168
    planning for, 178
  neuropathic, 166b
  pathophysiology of, 167
  perception of, 167
  scope of problem of, 165
  sleep and, 111
  unrelieved, consequences of, 165–167
Pain Assessment in Advanced Dementia (PAINAD), 169t
Palliative care, 528–529
  definition of, 584
Palliative Performance Scale (PPSv2), 580, 580t
Pancreas, 483t
  age-related changes in, 358t, 359–360
Pancreatectomy, nutritional consequences of, 563b
Pancreatic cancer, 384–385
  assessment of, 384
  evaluation of, 385
  nursing interventions for, 385

INDEX

Pancreatic cancer (Continued)
  patient problems with, 385
  planning for, 385
Pancreatitis, 375–376
  acute, amylase in, 203–204
  assessment of, 376
  evaluation of, 376
  nursing interventions for, 376
  patient problems with, 376
  planning for, 376
Pannus, 424
Papanicolaou test, 84t
Paralytic ileus, 370
Parathyroid, 483t
Parenteral nutrition, 104, 104b
Parietal pathways, 361
Parkinson disease (PD), 462–468, 463f
  assessment for, 464
  clinical manifestations of, 463
  diagnostic studies in, 464
  drugs for, 464, 465t
  evaluation of, 466–468
  interventions for, 466
  management of, 464
  patient problems of, 464
  planning for, 466
  postural and gait terms for, 463b
  risk factors for, 462–463
  surgical therapy for, 464
Partial thromboplastin time (PTT), in hematology test, 197t, 200
Partner, loss of
  activity and, 119–120
  sleep and, 111
Pathologic fracture, 415f
Patient education, on foot care, 439
Patient, in assessment of older adult, 44, 44t
Patient profile, in health history format, 44
Patient Self-Determination Act (PSDA), 25
Pelvic examination, 84t
Pelvic floor muscle exercises, 395, 396b
Penbutolol, 294–296t
Penicillamine, 427t
Pentazocine, 176t
PEPSI COLA framework, 578–580, 579t
Peptic ulcer disease (PUD), 368–369, 368f
  assessment of, 369
  evaluation of, 369
  nursing interventions for, 369
  patient problems with, 369
  planning for, 369
Perceived barriers, 83
Perceived benefits, 83
Perceived severity, 83
Perceived susceptibility, 83
Percutaneous transluminal coronary angioplasty (PTCA), 300
Perindopril, 294–296t
Periodic limb movement in sleep (PLMS), 113–114
Periodontal gum disease, 357–358
Periodontitis, 364–365
  assessment of, 364
  evaluation of, 365
  nursing interventions for, 364–365
  patient problems with, 364
  planning for, 364
Peripheral arterial occlusive disease (PAOD), 248

Peripheral artery disease (PAD), 315–317, 316b
  assessment of, 316, 316b
  diagnosis of, 316
  diagnostic tests and procedures for, 315
  evaluation of, 316–317, 317b
  interventions for, 316
  planning for, 316
  prognosis of, 315–316
  surgical procedures for, 315
  treatment of, 315
Peripheral nerve stimulation, with TENS, 178
Peripheral vascular disease (PVD), 292
Peritoneal dialysis, 401b
Pernicious anemia, 367
Persistent grief, 575
Personal emergency response systems (PERSs), 517
Person-centered care, 520b
PERSs. See Personal emergency response systems
Pessaries, 395–396, 397f
pH
  arterial, 327
  of blood, 207, 207t
  of urine, 206t, 207
Phantom limb pain, 435
Phantom limb sensation, 435
Pharmacodynamics, 213
  age-related changes in, 213
  in chemotherapy, 559
Pharmacokinetics
  absorption in, 212
  age-related changes in, 212t
  changes, 211–213
  in chemotherapy, 559
  distribution in, 212
  excretion in, 213
  metabolism in, 212–213
Pharmacologic contributors, risk factors in, 214–217
Pharynx, age-related changes in, 357–359
Phenylbutazone, 427t
Phosphatase, alkaline, 202t, 205
Phosphodiesterase 5 (PDE 5) inhibitors, 152
Phosphorus, serum levels of, 202t, 203
Physical abuse, 20, 145
Physical examination, 84t
  after falls, 132
  pain assessment with, 172
  of urinary incontinence, 392
Physical exercise, 118
Physical fitness, enhancement of, 543
Physical restraints, 23–24
Physical therapy, pain management with, 178
Physician Orders for Life-Sustaining Treatment (POLST), 27–30, 28f, 63t
Physician-assisted suicide, 30
Pick's disease, 454
Pindolol, 294–296t
Pineal gland, 483t
Plan, do, check, act cycle, 512b
Planning
  family and, 61
  prevention and, 89
Plasma, 198
Platelets, in hematology test, 197t, 200
PLISSIT model, 156–157
PLMS. See Periodic limb movement in sleep
Pneumococcal infection, vaccination, 84t

Pneumonia, 185, 190b, 344–348
  aspiration, 346
  assessment of, 347
  community-acquired, 345, 345t
  death from, 535t
  diagnosis of, 348
  diagnostic tests and procedures for, 346
  evaluation after, 348
  health care–associated, 345
  hospital-acquired, 345
  intervention for, 348
  nosocomial, 345
  planning for, 348
  presentation of, 39t
  prognosis of, 347
  treatment for, 346–347, 347t
  ventilator-associated, 345
  viral, 345–346
Podagra, 426–428
Polycythemia, 198
Polymyalgia rheumatica (PMR), 437–438
  assessment of, 437
  evaluation of, 438
  nursing care guidelines for, 437–438
  nursing interventions for, 438
  patient problems in, 437–438
  planning for, 438
Polyp(s)
  colon, 373–374
  intussusception from, 370f
Polypharmacy, 84–85, 215–216, 217f
  adverse drug reaction with, 507
  constipation from, 362–363
Porous bone disease, 428–429
Portal hypertension, 378–379
Posterior pituitary, 483t
Postfall syndrome, 306
Postherpetic neuralgia, 243
Potassium
  hypokalemia and, 201b
  in renal diet, 402b
  serum levels of, 201, 202t
Poverty, in demographics, 8, 8f
Power of attorney, 30
Prazosin, 294–296t
Prealbumin, 204
  in nutritional assessment, 99
Precontemplation, 82
Preparation, 83
Presbycusis, 126, 283–285
Presbyopia, 273
Prescription drugs, 227
  assessment of, 227
  evaluation of, 227
  interventions of, 227
  prevalence of, 227
Present health status, in health history format, 45, 46t
Pressure injuries, 250–266
  definitions of terms for, 257, 259b
  epidemiology of, 251
  etiology of, 251–253, 251f, 252f
  evidence-based practice for, 254b
  general care guidelines for, 265t
  home care for, 266b
  management of, 257–266
    biophysical agents in, 266
    debridement for, 261–263

Pressure injuries (Continued)
    nursing care plan for, 265b
    principles of, 257
    physiology of wound healing and, 257
    preventive strategies for, 254–257, 256f, 260b
    risk assessment tools for, 253–254, 253f, 255f
    staging criteria for, 257, 258b, 258f, 259f
Pressure Ulcer Scale for Healing (PUSH) Tool, 262f
Pressure ulcers. See Pressure injuries
Prevention
    assessment and, 85–89
    of disease, 83–85
    evaluation and, 90
    interventions and, 89–90
    Medicare reimbursement for, 84t
    planning and, 89
    primary, 82, 83–85, 84t
    secondary, 82, 84t, 85
    tertiary, 82, 85
Previous health status, in health history format, 47
Primary gout, 426
Primary hypothyroidism, 497
Primary progressive aphasia, 454
Prinivil. See Lisinopril
Problem, magnitude of, 125
Professional standards, 18–19
Progressive relaxation, 177–178
Progressive supranuclear palsy (PSP), 454
Prolonged grief, 575
Prompted voiding, 396–397, 397b
Propranolol, 294–296t
Propulsive gait, in Parkinson disease, 463b
Prostate cancer, 410–411, 555–556
    assessment of, 410
    with bone metastases, 175b
    early detection of, 555
    evaluation of, 411
    nursing care plan for, 411b
    nursing interventions for, 410–411
    patient problems with, 410
    planning for, 410
    risk factors for, 555
    screening for, advantages and disadvantages of, 86t
    sexuality and, 155
    signs and symptoms of, 555
    treatment for, 555–556
Prostate, examination of, 84t
Prostate-specific antigen (PSA), 206
Prosthesis, fitting of, 436
Protamine sulfate, 299–300
Protective services, 20–21
    elder abuse and, 20–21, 20t
Protein
    in blood chemistry testing, 202t, 204
    C-reactive, 200
    HDL, 202t, 204
    LDL, 202t, 204–205
    for type 2 diabetes mellitus, 491b
    in urine, 206, 206t
Proteinuria, 206
Prothrombin time, in hematology test, 197t, 199–200
Proventil. See Albuterol
Pruritus, 241–242, 281
    evaluation after, 242
    nursing interventions in, 241–242
    patient problems in, 241

Pruritus (Continued)
    planning in, 241
    recognize cues (assessment) of, 241
PSDA. See Patient Self-Determination Act
Psoriasis, 240–241
    assessment of, 240
    evaluation in, 241
    nursing interventions for, 240–241
    patient problems in, 240
    planning for, 240
Psychiatric hospitals, in cognitive disorder, 460
Psychologic abuse, 145
Psychologic trauma, falls and, 131–132
Psychotic symptoms, nonpharmacological management of, 457t
PTCA. See Percutaneous transluminal coronary angioplasty
PUD. See Peptic ulcer disease
Pulmonary disease
    obstructive, 330–341
    restrictive, 341–348
Pulmonary edema
    assessment of, 349
    cardiogenic, 349
        diagnostic tests and procedures for, 349
        prognosis of, 349
        treatment of, 349
    diagnosis of, 349–350
    evaluation after, 350
    intervention for, 350
    noncardiogenic
        diagnostic tests and procedures for, 349
        prognosis of, 349
        treatment of, 349
    planning for, 350
Pulmonary emboli, 350–352
    assessment of, 351
    diagnosis of, 351
    diagnostic tests and procedures for, 351
    evaluation after, 352
    intervention for, 351–352
    planning for, 351
    prognosis of, 351
    treatment for, 351
Pulmonary function. see Lung
Pulmonary hygiene, for COPD, 339, 340b
Pulmonary rehabilitation, COPD and, 338–340
Pursed-lip breathing, 339b, 339f
PVD. See Peripheral vascular disease
Pyrazinamide, 344t

Q

Quad cane, 420f
Quality of life
    chronic illness and, 538
    drugs and, 214
    health-related, 537
    in pain assessment, 173
    transitioning from hospital to home, 537b
Quinapril, 294–296t
Quinine sulfate, 440

R

Race, in demographics, 7
Radiation therapy
    for cancer, 558–559
    nutritional consequences of, 563b
Rails, as risk factor for falling, 129

Ramelteon, in sleep, 116–117
Ramipril, 294–296t
Random blood sugar, 203
Rapid eye movement (REM) sleep, 108, 109t
Reactive hyperemia, 259b
Recreation profile, in health history format, 45
Recreational drugs, sexuality and, 154t
Rectum, age-related changes in, 358t
Red blood cells
    in bone marrow suppression, 562
    in hematology test, 197t, 198
Referral pathways, 361
Regret, in grief, 573
Rehabilitation, 541–546
    care environments of, 542, 542f
    fitness enhancement with, 543
    functional assessment in, 543
    functional enhancement with, 543
    in nursing facilities, 523–524
    nursing strategies in, 545–546
    public policy and legislation in, 542–543
    reimbursement issues for, 542
Relaxation, progressive, 177–178
Relief, 577
Religion, grief and, 574
Relocation
    activity and, 118–119, 119b, 119f
    sleep and, 111
REM sleep. See Rapid eye movement (REM) sleep
Reminiscence therapy (RT), for depression, 449
Renal diet, 402b
Repetitive transcranial magnetic stimulation (rTMS), 450
Research
    on gerontologic nursing, 15
    law on, 31
    nursing, 15
    on rights, 31
Reserpine, 294–296t
Resident rights, 520
Residual volume, 327t
Residual volume/total lung capacity (RV/TLC), 327t
Resources
    for cancer, 567–568
    for cognitive disorders, 459–460
    in health history format, 45
Respiratory disorders. see Adult respiratory distress syndrome
Respiratory function, 325–354, 325b
    home care for, 353b
Respiratory rate, 326
Respiratory system. see also Lung
    age-related changes in, 325–328, 326t, 327t
    alterations in, 330
    gas exchange in, 325
    health promotion for, 328b
    symptoms common in older patients, 329–330
Respite care, 517
Respite programs, family caregivers and, 65–66
Respite programs, in cognitive disorder, 459
Rest patterns, 88
Restlessness, in older adults, 582
Restraints, OBRA's requirements for, 23–24
Resuscitation. See Cardiopulmonary resuscitation; Do-not-resuscitate (DNR) order

Retinal disorders, 276–278
  age-related macular degeneration in, 276–277
  assessment of, 277
  diabetic retinopathy in, 277
  evaluation of, 278
  hypertension retinopathy in, 277
  nursing interventions for, 277–278
  patient problems in, 277
  planning for, 277
  retinal detachment in, 277
Retinopathy, diabetic, 277
Retirement
  activity and, 118
  benefits, 71
  communities, 77, 516t
  sleep and, 111
Retropulsion, in Parkinson disease, 463b
Reversible dementia, causes of, 452b
Review of systems, in health history format, 47
Rheumatic fever, causing valvular disease, 307
Rheumatoid arthritis (RA), 186, 424–426, 424f
  assessment of, 425
  deformities of, 425f
  drugs for, 427t
  evaluation of, 426
  nursing care guidelines for, 425–426
  nursing interventions for, 425–426
  osteoarthritis *versus*, 425t
  patient problems in, 425
  planning for, 425
Ribs, age-related changes in, 325
Rifampin, 344t
Rights
  in experimentation and research, 31
  resident
    bill of, 23b
    OBRA's requirements for, 23
  to self-determination, 25
Roles, in family, 66–67
Roommate, sleep and, 111
Rosuvastatin (Crestor), 96t
Russell traction, 416

S

Safety, 124–147, 124b
  automobile, 144–145
  with fire, 139, 139b
  in home, 137b, 138–141
  OSHA on, 524
  of over-the-counter medications, 216t
  seasonal, 141–143
Salicylates, 427t
Salmonella, 369
Salts, 200
Sanctions, 25
Sarcopenia, 97, 97b
SARS. *See* Severe acute respiratory syndrome
Schizophrenia, 474–475
Sclerosis, hippocampal, 455
Scoliosis, 325, 429f
Screening. *See also* Mammography
  alcoholism
    with BMAST, 224
    with MAST, 224
  for cancer, 556–557
    breast, 551b
  colorectal, 84t
  for colorectal cancer, 84t

Screening (Continued)
  for diabetes, 84t
  for glaucoma, 84t
  Medicare reimbursement for, 84t
  nutritional, 98–99
  for osteoporosis, 84t
  for substance use disorder, 224
Seborrheic dermatitis, 239, 239f
Seborrheic keratoses, 238–239, 238f
Secondary hypothyroidism, 497
Sedentary lifestyle, heart disease from, 297
Selective serotonin reuptake inhibitors (SSRIs), 218
Self-determination, 25–30. *See also* Patient Self-Determination Act
Self-efficacy, 83
Self-neglect, 20
Senior. *See* Older adults
Senior centers, multipurpose, 516
Sensory deficits, in history taking, 44t
Sensory function, 270–288, 287b
  hearing and balance, 280–286
  taste and smell, 286–287
  touch, 287
  vision, 270–280
Serotonin (5-HT), 446t
Serum. *See* Blood chemistry testing
Serum sex hormone-binding globulin (SHBG), 152
Severe acute respiratory syndrome (SARS), 346
Sexual abuse, 20, 145
Sexual activity, chronic illness and, 540–541
Sexual behavior, inappropriate/impulsive, nonpharmacological management of, 457t
Sexual dysfunction, 158b, 499–501
  medical management of, 500–501
  nursing care guidelines for, 501, 501t
  pathophysiology of, 500
  signs and symptoms of, 500
Sexual expression, in nursing homes, exploration of knowledge, attitudes, and experiences with, 157b
Sexual function, conditions affecting, 153b
Sexuality, 150–162, 150b
  barriers to, environmental and psychosocial, 155–156
  coital positioning for older couples, 159f
  female, 159b
  genitourinary syndrome of menopause, 153
  in home care, 161b
  illness, surgery, and medication, 153, 154t
  lesbian, gay, bisexual, and transgender older adults, 156
  loss of libido in, 152
  male, 159–160b
  normal changes of aging in, 152–153
  nursing care guidelines for, 156–161
    assessment of, 156–158
    evaluation in, 161
    interventions in, 159–161
    patient problems in, 158
    planning in, 158–159
  nursing management of
    laboratory tests in, 157b
    reluctance to, 152
  older adult needs for, 150
  pathologic conditions affecting, 153–155, 153b
    dementia as, 155
    human immunodeficiency virus as, 153–155

Sexuality (Continued)
    malignancies as, 155
    physiologic changes in, 152–153
    questions on, 156b
Sexually transmitted infections (STIs), 160b
Shear stress, 252f
Shearing, 252, 252f
Shearing force, 259b
Shingles, 243–245
Shock, in grief, 573
Sick days, 492
Sick sinus syndrome, 304
Sighted guide, 279–280, 279b
Sigmoid colon, volvulus of, 370f
Sigmoidoscopy, flexible, 84t
Silent generation, 70–71
Sinoatrial (SA) node, 290
Sinus syndrome, sick, 304
Sinus tract, 259b
Skills, in assessment of older adult, 48
Skin. *See also* Integumentary function
  age-related changes in, 237–238, 237b
  care for, in nursing facility, 521–522
  common problems and conditions of, 238–246
  dry, prevention and treatment of, 241b
  growths of
    benign, 238–239
    malignant, 246–248
    premalignant, 244–246
Skin tags, 239, 239f
SLE. *See* Systemic lupus erythematosus
Sleep, 108–117
  age-related changes in, 109–110, 109b
  biologic brain functions responsible for, 108
  breathing and, 326t
  circadian rhythm and, 109
  disorders and conditions, 112–114
  factors affecting, 110–112
    dementia and disturbed sleep, 112
    depression, 112
    dietary influences, 111–112
    environment, 110–111
    home environments, 110
    lifestyle changes, 111
    pain and discomfort, 111
  further assessment of, 115–116, 115f
  getting good night's, 116–117
    complementary and alternative medicines in, 117, 117b
    drugs used to, 116–117, 117b
    in homebound older adults, 116
    nonpharmacological therapies, 116
    sleep hygiene, 116
  history, components of, 114–115, 114b
  home care in, 121b
  hygiene, 116
  insomnia and, 109
  latency, 109
  patterns, disturbance, 113b
  stages of, 108, 109t
Sleep apnea, 112–113, 113b
Sleep disturbance, nonpharmacological management of, 457t
Sleep restriction therapy, 116
Small intestine, age-related changes in, 358t, 359
Smell, 286–287
  age-related changes in, 286
  problems and conditions of, 286–287

Smoking, 328–329. See also Nicotine
  cigarette, fire risk with, 138, 138b
  heart disease and, 297
Smoking cessation, 83–84, 296, 328–329
  advantages and disadvantages of, 86t
  with behavior modification, 228
  components of, 328–329
  COPD and, 338
  counseling for, 84t
Social isolation
  cancer and, 567
  from chronic illness, 539
Social media, 32, 32b
Social responses, on grief, 573–574
Social Security, 71–72
Social Security Disability Insurance (SSDI), 72
Social-Ecologic Model, motivation with, 89t
Socialization, grief and, 573
Socioeconomic factors, 70–76, 70b
  education, 73–74, 73f, 74b
  generational differences and, 70–71
  health status and, 74–76, 74b, 74f
  income and, 71–72, 71f, 72f
Sodium
  in renal diet, 402b
  serum levels of, 201, 202t
  for type 2 diabetes mellitus, 491b
Somatic pathways, 361
Somatopause, 495–496
Somatotropin, 483–484
Special care units, 514
SPICES acronym, in assessment of older adult, 48
Spinal cord, 445–446
Spinal stenosis, 423–424, 423f
Spiral fracture, 415f
Spirituality, grief and, 574
Spironolactone, 294–296t
Spousal self-euthanasia, 31b
Squamous cell carcinoma, 246, 247f
SSRIs. See Selective serotonin reuptake inhibitors
Standard of care, 19
Staphylococcus aureus, 187, 369
Stasis ulcers, 249
Statins, sexuality and, 154t
Stenosis, spinal, 423–424, 423f
Stents, for CAD, 300
Steps, as risk factor for falling, 128–129, 129f
Steroids, 427t
Stimulus control therapy, 116
Stomach, age-related changes in, 358t, 359
Stomatitis, 190–191b
Strangulated inguinal hernia, 370f
Stress
  heart disease and, 298
  managing, 65b
  response to, age-related changes in, 291
  tolerance to, patterns, 87
Stress fracture, 415f
Stress incontinence, 389–390
  diagnosis of, 392
  planning for, 394
Stroke, 469
  levels of prevention for, 470t
Stump shrinker, 436
Subacute care, 514
Subclinical hyperthyroidism, 497

Subcutaneous fat, age-related changes in, 237
Subjective Global Assessment (SGA), 98
Subsidized housing, 77
Substance Abuse and Mental Health Services Administration (SAMHSA), 460
Substance use disorders (SUD), 155, 223–224. See also Alcohol; Nicotine
  assessment of, 224–225
    screening tools for, 224–225
  definitions and common usage of, 223
  difficulty in identification of, 223
  evaluation for, 225
  history of, 224
  home care and, 229b
  intervention for, 225
  nursing caveats, 225
  nursing interventions of, 225
  patient problems of, 225
  physiologic changes with, 223–224
  psychological changes with, 224, 224f
  sociologic changes with, 224
  trends in, 229
Suicide, 30–31, 460–462
  assessment for, 460, 461f
  assisted, 30–31
  evaluation for, 462
  with firearms, 145
  interventions for, 462
  patient problems of, 460
  planning for, 460–462
  risk factors for, 460, 461b
Sulfonylureas, for type 2 diabetes mellitus, 489t
"Sundowning," nonpharmacological management of, 457t
Supplemental Nutrition Assistance Program (SNAP), 72b
Supplemental Security Income (SSI), 72
Supplements, dietary, 221
Support
  for cancer, 567–568
  groups
    for family caregivers, 66
    family, in cognitive disorder, 459
  systems, in health history format, 45
Surgery
  for breast cancer, 552, 554–555
  for cancer, 558
  for cataracts, 275b
  hip, 422, 423b
  for knee replacement, 422
  lung function and, 329
  nutritional consequences of, 563b
  for Parkinson disease, 464
Survivor benefits, 72
Suvorexant, in sleep, 116–117
Swan-neck deformity, 425f
Sympathomimetics, for CHD, 311t
Symptoms, underreporting of, in history taking, 44t
Syncope, with cardiac causes, 306–307
  assessment of, 307
  diagnosis of, 307
  evaluation of, 307
  intervention for, 307
  planning for, 307
Systemic lupus erythematosus (SLE), 186

T

Targeted therapy, for cancer, 559
Taste, 286–287
  age-related changes in, 286
  buds, age-related changes in, 358
  problems and conditions of, 286–287
Tazarotene, 240
Teeth, loss of, 357–358
Telephone monitoring, 517
Telmisartan, 294–296t
Temperature, sleep and, 110–111
Terazosin, 294–296t
Tertiary hypothyroidism, 497
Testes, 483t
The Cancer Genome Atlas (TCGA) project, 552–553
The Joint Commission (TJC), 19
Therapeutic drug monitoring, 208
Thiazolidinediones (TZDs), for type 2 diabetes mellitus, 489t
Thought process. See Cognitive function
Thrombocytopenia, chemotherapy-induced, 562
Thromboplastin time, partial, in hematology test, 197t, 200
Thrush, 364
Thymus, 483t
Thyroid, 483t. See also Hyperthyroidism
  feedback loops in, 484f
  functional testing of, 205–206, 205t
Thyroid storm, 497
Thyroid-stimulating hormone (TSH), 205–206, 205t
Thyrotoxic crisis, 497
Thyroxine, 205–206, 205t
Tidal volume, 327t
Timolol, 294–296t
Tinetti Balance and Gait Evaluation, 128f
Tinnitus, 282–283
  assessment of, 282, 282b
  evaluation of, 283
  nursing interventions for, 282–283
  patient problems in, 282
  planning for, 282
Tissue tolerance, 259b
Tobacco use. See also Nicotine; Smoking
  disorder, 228
  sexuality and, 154t
Toenail, problems of, 439
Toileting, scheduled, 396
Tophaceous gout, 428f
Tophi, 426
Topoisomerase inhibitors, for cancer, 560t
Toprol-XL. See Metoprolol
Torsemide, 294–296t
Total iron binding capacity (TIBC), in hematology test, 197t, 199
Total lung capacity, 327t
Total patient care, 526
Touch, 287
  importance of, 151
Touch therapy, 527
Trabeculectomy, 274
Trace element deficiency, 183–184
Trajectory framework, 538
Trandolapril, 294–296t
Transcendence, 577
Transferrin, in nutritional assessment, 99
Transparent film dressing, 264t
Transportation, 77, 78f, 517

Transtheoretical Model, 82–83
Transverse fracture, 415f
Trauma
    care, 510–511
    psychologic, fall resulting in, 131–132
Trazodone, 116–117
Triamterene, 294–296t
Triceps skinfold (TSF), 99
Trichinosis, 369
Triglycerides, serum levels of, 204
Triiodothyronine, 205–206, 205t
Troponin, serum levels of, 205
TSH. See Thyroid-stimulating hormone
Tuberculosis, 342–344
    assessment of, 343
    diagnosis of, 343
    diagnostic tests and procedures for, 343
    evaluation for, 344
    intervention for, 344, 344t
    planning for, 344
    prognosis of, 343
    treatment for, 343
Tumor initiation, 551–552
Tumor necrosis factor (TNF) inhibitors, 426
Tumor progression, 552
Tumor promotion, 551–552
Typical day, description of, in health history format, 45

U

UI. See Urinary incontinence
Ulcers. See also Pressure injuries
    arterial, 248–249, 248t
    duodenal, 368–369
    gastric, 368
    lower extremity, 248–250, 248t
    peptic, 368–369, 368f
    stress, 367
    venous, 248t, 249
Ulnar drift, 425f
Undermining, 259b
Unintentional injuries, death from, 535t
United States Preventive Services Task Force (USPSTF), 84t
Urea nitrogen, blood test of, 202t, 204
Urge incontinence, 389
    diagnosis of, 392
    planning for, 394
Uric acid, in hematology test, 197t, 199
Urinalysis, 206–207, 206t
Urinary function, 388–412, 388b
    case study, 405–407b
    health promotion/illness prevention in, 411b
    home care in, 411b
    problems and conditions in, 389–391
Urinary incontinence (UI), 388
    assessment of, 391–392
        bladder habits, 392, 393f
        environmental, 391–392
        functional, 391
        history in, 391
        physical examination, 392
        psychosocial, 392
    cognitively impaired patients and, 396–397
    diagnosis of, 391, 392–394
    established, 389–391
        functional incontinence as, 391
        mixed incontinence as, 391

Urinary incontinence (Continued)
        overflow incontinence as, 390–391
        stress incontinence as, 389–390
        urge incontinence as, 389
    evaluation of, 397–398, 397–398b, 398b
    nursing facility requirements regarding, OBRA's, 24
    nursing interventions for, 394–397
        bladder retraining as, 395
        habit training as, 396
        lifestyle modifications as, 394–395, 395b
        pelvic floor muscle exercises as, 395, 396b, 397b
        prompted voiding as, 396–397, 397b
        scheduled toileting as, 396
    planning for, 394
    prevalence of, 389
    transient, 389
        causes of, 390t
Urinary tract, age-related changes in, 388–389, 389f
Urinary tract infection (UTI), 127b, 403–407
    assessment of, 404
    evaluation of, 404–407
    nursing interventions for, 404
    patient problems with, 404
    planning for, 404
    presentation of, 39t
Urine
    bacteria in, 206–207, 206t, 208b
    blood in, 206t, 207
    glucose in, 206, 206t
    ketones in, 206t, 207
    leukocytes in, 206t, 207
    pH of, 206t, 207
    protein in, 206, 206t
UTI. See Urinary tract infection

V

Vaccinations, 83
Vaccine therapy, for prostate cancer, 555–556
Valsartan, 294–296t
Values, health patterns of, 88, 88b
Valvular heart disease (VHD), 307–309
    assessment of, 308
    diagnosis of, 308
    diagnostic tests and procedures for, 307–308
    evaluation of, 309
    interventions for, 308–309
    manifestations of, 308b
    planning for, 308
    prognosis of, 308
    treatment of, 308
Vancomycin-resistant *Enterococcus* (VRE), 186–187
Varicose veins, 316–317
Vascular dementia (VaD), 453
Vasodilators, direct, adverse effects of, 294–296t
Vasovagal syncope, 306
Venous insufficiency, 318t
Venous ulcers, 248t, 249, 316–317
Ventilation, 325, 326t
Ventolin. See Albuterol
Ventricular tachycardia, 306
Verapamil, 294–296t
Vertebrae, age-related changes in, 325
Vertebral artery, 469
Vertigo, 285
Vestibule, 280
VHD. See Valvular heart disease
Vicodin. See Acetaminophen/hydrocodone

Visceral pain pathways, 361
Vision, 270–280
    age-related changes in, 271f, 272
    common complaints in, 272
        dry eyes in, 272
        floaters and flashers in, 272
    common problems and conditions with, 272–280
    effects of sensory impairments, in older adults, 272b
    falls related to, 126
Visiting nurse association (VNA), 518
Visual impairment, 278–280
    assessment of, 278
    evaluation of, 280
    nursing interventions for, 279–280, 279b
    patient problems in, 279
    planning in, 279
Visualization, 177
Vital capacity, 327t
Vitamin B_{12}
    deficiency of, 367
    in hematology test, 197t, 199
Vitamin K, 299–300
    as anticoagulant, 200b
Vitamins
    in renal diet, 402b
    for type 2 diabetes mellitus, 491b
Voiding, prompted, 396–397, 397b
Volvulus, of sigmoid colon, 370f
Vomiting, 360
    in cancer, 562–563
    interventions for, 360
    stimuli involved in, 360f
Vulnerable populations, inappropriate drugs in, 215b

W

Walkers, 418f
    as assistive devices, 420f
    use of, 418b
Wandering, nonpharmacological management of, 457t
Warfarin, 299–300
White blood cells
    in bone marrow suppression, 562
    in hematology test, 197t, 198
Widowhood, 573
Wills, living, 26–27, 27b
Women
    postmenopausal, 152–153
    sexuality of, 159b
World War II, 70–71
Wound
    care principles for, 263–266
    dressing types for, 263–266, 264t
    healing, physiology of, 257

X

Xerosis, prevention and treatment of, 241b
Xerostomia, 97, 286–287

Z

Zestril. See Lisinopril
Zinc, 184
Zoonoses, 184